Small Animal Cardiovascular Medicine

About the Authors

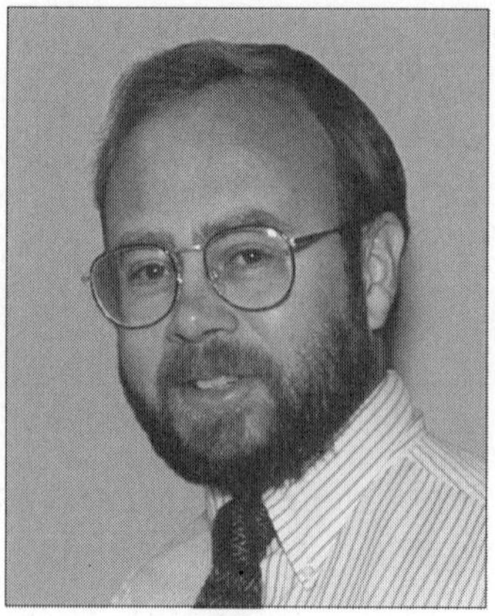

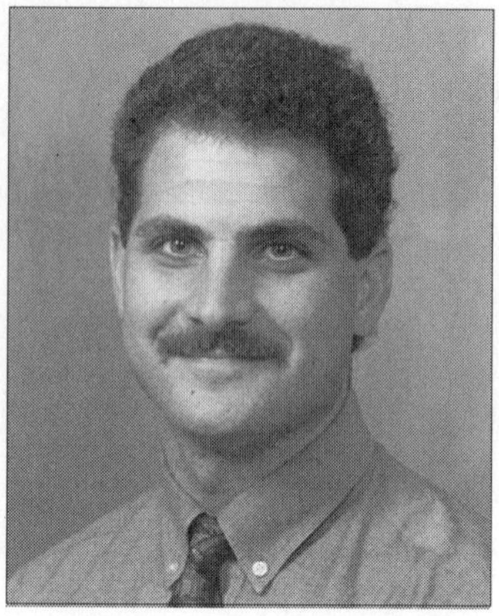

Mark D. Kittleson, DVM, PhD, Diplomate ACVIM (Cardiology), Professor, Department of Medicine and Epidemiology, Associate Director, Veterinary Medical Teaching Hospital, School of Veterinary Medicine, University of California, Davis. Dr. Kittleson is a graduate of the University of Minnesota. He completed his residency training in internal medicine at Kansas State University and received his PhD in Veterinary Cardiovascular Physiology and Pharmacology from the Ohio State University under the mentorship of Dr. Robert Hamlin. He served as a faculty member at Michigan State University for 4 years, and for the past 14 years has been a faculty member at University of California, Davis. Dr. Kittleson is an active and well-recognized veterinary clinical cardiovascular researcher, teacher, and clinician. His areas of particular expertise and interest include feline dilated and hypertrophic cardiomyopathies, canine myxomatous atrioventricular valve degeneration, heart failure, and heart failure therapy. He received the Ralston Purina Small Animal Research Award for his work related to feline dilated cardiomyopathy and taurine deficiency in 1989. Dr. Kittleson has served as the President of the Specialty of Cardiology in the American College of Veterinary Internal Medicine (ACVIM) and as Associate Editor of Cardiology for the Journal of Veterinary Internal Medicine. He is currently a member of the Board of Regents of the ACVIM, serving in an ascending position that culminates as Chairperson of the Board.

Richard D. Kienle, DVM, Diplomate ACVIM (Cardiology), Mission Valley Veterinary Cardiology, Gilroy, California. Dr. Kienle is a graduate of Texas A&M University and completed his residency training in Cardiology at the University of California, Davis. Dr. Kienle served as a postdoctoral fellow under the leadership of Dr. Mark Kittleson and served as a clinical instructor and lecturer at the University of California, Davis, for 2 years. Dr. Kienle is an active and recognized clinician and is continuing to develop a solid reputation as a consultant in the human medical and biotech industries. In 1996, Dr. Kienle founded Mission Valley Veterinary Cardiology, a consultation service providing clinical support in cardiology for veterinarians practicing in the south Bay Area, California, and consultation services for medical device and pharmaceutical manufacturers in Silicon Valley. Dr. Kienle's areas of particular expertise and interest include noninvasive imaging, congenital heart disease, interventional therapy, and arrhythmias.

Small Animal Cardiovascular Medicine

MARK D. KITTLESON, DVM, PhD

Department of Medicine and Epidemiology
Veterinary Medical Teaching Hospital
School of Veterinary Medicine
University of California, Davis
Davis, California

RICHARD D. KIENLE, DVM

Mission Valley Veterinary Cardiology
Gilroy, California

With 834 illustrations

Mosby

St. Louis Baltimore Boston Carlsbad Chicago Minneapolis New York Philadelphia Portland
London Milan Sydney Tokyo Toronto

Mosby
Dedicated to Publishing Excellence

A Times Mirror Company

Publisher: John A. Schrefer
Executive Editor: Linda Duncan
Senior Developmental Editor: Teri Merchant
Project Manager: Mark Spann
Production Editor: Beth Hayes
Book Design Manager: Judi Lang
Manufacturing Supervisor: Karen Boehme

Cover Photos: Clockwise from upper left: Foxglove plant *Digitalis purpurea;* two-dimensional and color flow Doppler echocardiogram from a dog with severe mitral regurgitation; American cocker spaniel with cyanosis resulting from tetralogy of Fallot; pathology specimen (heart) from a dog with dilated cardiomyopathy.

Printed in the United States of America
Composition by Graphic World, Inc.
Lithography/color plate lithography by Graphic World, Inc.
Color plate printing by Coral Graphic Services

Mosby, Inc.
11830 Westline Industrial Drive
St. Louis, MO 63146

Library of Congress Cataloging in Publication Data

Kittleson, Mark D.
Small animal cardiovascular medicine / Mark D. Kittleson, Richard D. Kienle.
p. cm.
Includes bibliographical references and index.
ISBN 0-8151-5140-3
1. Dogs—Diseases. 2. Cats—Diseases. 3. Veterinary cardiology.
I. Kienle, Richard D. II. Title.
SF992.C37K58 1998 97-49052
636.089'61—DC21 CIP

98 00 01 02 / 9 8 7 6 5 4 3 2 1

Preface

"The heart of animals is the foundation of their life, the sovereign of everything within them, the sun of their microcosm."

William Harvey
De Motu Cordis et Sanguinis, 1628

This textbook is primarily the result of a collaboration between the two authors. As opposed to a textbook that has multiple authors, we believe this collaboration has given this book a more cohesive approach to small animal cardiovascular medicine. It is a much more labor-intensive process than a multiauthor text, but we hope our readers find it worth the effort. *"An inveterate and incurable itch for writing besets many, and grows old in their sick hearts"* (Juvenal).

Readers of veterinary cardiology texts fall into six categories: veterinary students, practicing veterinarians, postgraduate clinical veterinarians (interns and residents), veterinary specialists other than veterinary cardiologists, veterinary cardiology residents, and veterinary cardiologists. We have not attempted to satisfy all of the needs of veterinary cardiologists. We have, however, tried to write a text that can be used by students, interns, residents, practicing veterinarians, and other specialists. Chapters 1, 2, and 9 are basic chapters that are primarily aimed at students. However, all of the material is relevant, and an attempt has been made to build on this basic material in later chapters. No textbook can be all-inclusive. Because of this, each chapter has a select list of references. We have not attempted to provide an exhaustive list of references, although the reference list for some chapters is extensive. Rather we have attempted to provide references that we feel are particularly useful or that document key points or facts within a given chapter.

Cardiology is a specialty and a discipline that relies heavily on physiologic and pharmacologic principles. Because of this, we have included sections on these disciplines that we believe are clinically relevant to the practice of clinical cardiology. Basic principles of pathophysiology have been built into each chapter. Although these basic principles are not required to make a diagnosis or to treat a disease, we feel that they are essential for any individual that wants to understand a disease process or concept. We feel that if a clinician understands the pathophysiology of a disease or disease process, he or she does a much better job of identifying clinical abnormalities and of determining the significance of these abnormalities. Understanding the pathophysiology also gives a clinician insight into how a disease might be treated in a particular patient and especially how to modify therapy in the patient that does not respond in the expected way. The same also can be said for our approach to pharmacology and drug therapy. Cardiology is a discipline that depends heavily on logic. As with everything, some memorization of facts is required. However, once the basic facts of a particular area are learned, we feel that most principles of cardiovascular medicine can be approached by thinking about logical consequences of a perturbation in the cardiovascular system. Because of this belief, we have attempted to present our material in a manner that is conducive to logical thinking. We have attempted to stay away from presenting facts without logical reasoning for these facts or presenting principles without providing explanations for these principles. This may make this textbook less useful for the person that wants to quickly find out only the facts about a particular disease (e.g., how to diagnose the disease quickly and what dose of a drug to administer). This text is designed to be read by the clinician who wants to know the pathophysiology of a disease, wants to know why a disease behaves as it does, and wants to know why a particular disease is treated as it is. However, we have tried to provide a complete index and relevant tables so that information can be found quickly if needed.

> *"Insofar as the concatenation of their perceptions is due to the principle of memory alone, men act like the lower animals, resembling empirical physicians whose methods are those of mere practice without theory. Indeed, in three-fourths of our actions we are nothing but empirics. For instance, when we expect that there will be daylight to-morrow, we do so empirically, because it has always happened until now. It is only the astronomer who thinks it on rational grounds."*
>
> Leibniz, *Monadology*

This text contains a large number of figures devoted to echocardiography. We fully realize that not everyone has access to this technology. For those individuals who do not have access to echocardiography, the figures are presented as teaching examples. Echocardiography is an excellent teaching tool. Two-dimensional echocardiography provides a picture of the abnormal anatomy present in a particular disease. Color flow Doppler allows one to visualize the disturbed blood flow that creates a heart murmur and creates an anatomic change. So rather than just talking about a lesion such as mitral regurgitation, one can actually see the leak with color flow Doppler, see the diseased valves, and visualize and measure the changes that have occurred in the affected chambers with two-dimensional echocardiography. This provides an intuitive insight into the disease process that cannot be gained by trying to visualize what is happening by reading a description. Spectral Doppler is excellent for teaching pathophysiologic principles, especially related to pressure gradients and measuring pressures in the heart noninvasively. For the individual who is starting to use echocardiography or has the ability to do echocardiography but doesn't use it enough because of lack of understanding, we hope that the presentations in this text will teach the value of the technology and provide examples that are clinically relevant. For the individual who is already using echocardiography, we hope that we have provided a set of examples to compare with the images acquired. Almost all of the echocardiographic images were acquired using an Acuson 128XP/10 ultrasound machine.

Veterinary cardiology is a small specialty. Unlike human cardiology, there are a limited number of people involved in veterinary cardiovascular research. Consequently, the foundation of veterinary cardiology is not always solidly based on well-studied principles. Instead, much of veterinary cardiology is based on the clinical experience of experts, basic research, and extrapolations from human cardiology. Because of this, the specialty has tended to breed two types of individuals—those that tend to believe everything espoused in human cardiology and those that are skeptical of all we do. *It was, of course, a grand and impressive thing to do, to mistrust the obvious, and to pin one's faith in things which could not be seen!* (Galen). We believe both extremes are dangerous and have tried to stay on the middle ground in this book. Many areas of cardiology are controversial. We have tried to present this type of material in a balanced manner but are ourselves biased by our reading and clinical experiences.

We would like to acknowledge the contributions of several people to this book. This book would never have come to fruition without the patient guidance of Linda Duncan and Beth Hayes at Mosby. Mentors, including Drs. Stan Harris, Bob Hamlin, and George Eyster, have made major contributions to our knowledge and abilities. *"I say with Didacus Stella, a dwarf standing on the shoulders of a giant may see farther than a giant himself"* (Robert Burton). Many of the pictures for this book were acquired by former residents while under our supervision. These individuals also contributed to research projects and journal club presentations that helped formulate some of the knowledge that went into this book. In chronologic order they are: Drs. Grant Knowlen, Bari Olivier, Jerry Woodfield, Paul Pion, Laura DeLellis, Carroll Loyer, Bill Brown, Lori Siemens, Mark Rishniw, Mark Oyama, and Brad Gavaghan. This is an incredible group of colleagues and friends. Thank you all. Dr. Matt Mellema edited a large number of chapters in this book. We thank him for his effort and his many suggestions. We would also like to acknowledge the clinical support of Dr. Bill Thomas and the technical support of Lynne Johnson, Colette Williams, Jan Lansing, Kathi Greene, and Dr. Kathleen Backus. And we are extremely thankful for the continual support of each of our wives, our children, and our parents.

"Ah, nothing is too late, till the tired heart shall cease to palpitate" (Longfellow).

Mark D. Kittleson
Richard D. Kienle

Contents

Small Animal Cardiovascular Medicine

CHAPTER 1

Cardiac Embryology and Anatomy

A developmental analysis of various cardiac anomalies can be gained by correlating embryonic cardiac morphology and development with the anatomic features of malformed hearts. A thorough anatomic knowledge of the normal heart and pathologic conditions, both during development and in the adult, is necessary for the competent evaluation of the cardiovascular system. Detailed accounts of the normal development of the cardiovascular system and cardiac morphogenesis are beyond the scope of this text and are provided elsewhere.[1-3]

Cardiac Embryology

HEART TUBE FORMATION

The heart takes origin as paired endocardial heart tubes that arise from splanchnic mesoderm (cardiogenic cords) just ventral to the pericardial coeloms on either side of the embryo.[4] As the lateral folds develop, the heart tubes gradually fuse (from cranial to caudal) to form a single tube consisting of mesoderm, endoderm, and extracellular material (cardiac jelly). The surrounding mesenchyme thickens to form the myoepicardial mantle. At this stage, the endocardial heart tube is separated from the myoepicardial mantle by the cardiac jelly. The inner endocardial tube is destined to become the endocardium, and the myoepicardial mantle is destined to become the myocardium and epicardium.[4,5] The cardiac jelly is later incorporated into both the myocardium and endocardial cushion tissue.

As the embryo continues to develop, the single tube elongates and forms alternate dilations and constrictions that delineate the tube into primitive chambers. From cranial to caudal these chambers are the truncus arteriosus, the bulbus cordis, the primitive ventricle, and the sinus venosus (Figure 1-1). The truncus arteriosus bulges cranially and forms the aortic sac (which is fixed by the brachial arches). The sinus venosus lies outside the pericardial cavity and is fixed in position by the septum transversum (the primitive diaphragm).

CARDIAC LOOP FORMATION

The bulboventricular portion of the heart tube grows rapidly, and, because the two ends are fixed, is forced to bend to adapt to the available pericardial space. Normally, the bend is cranial and to the right, forming the bulboventricular sulcus and bulboventricular fold (see Figure 1-1). Torsion during the bend forces the tube to twist. This twist is at least in part responsible for the position of the truncus and conus swellings. The atrioventricular junction is forced laterally to the left, as is the primitive ventricle. At this stage, the right side of the pericardial cavity is occupied by the bulbus cordis. Also during this stage, the small right atrium and the primitive left atrium dilate and fuse to form a single atrium and single sinus venosus with right and left horns. This growth and dilation occur mainly in a dorsocranial direction, so that the atrium lies more cranially and dorsal to the bulbous cordis and ventricle. A distinct atrioventricular canal (between the single atrium and the primitive ventricle) and a primary interventricular foramen (between the primitive ventricle and the bulbus cordis) are now apparent because the junctions of the primitive chambers remain relatively narrow.[6]

In the later stages of cardiac loop formation, two diverticula appear along the ventral border of the endocardial tube on either side of the primary interventricular foramen, first at the expense of the cardiac jelly and later of the myoepicardial mantle.[4] These diverticula expand the capacity of these chambers and give them a trabeculated appearance. Although at this stage the primitive heart is still a single tube, the outward appearance strongly suggests its future four-chambered anatomy (see Figure 1-1). The primitive ventricle will become the adult left ventricle, and the trabeculated portion of the proximal bulbus cordis will become the adult right ventricle.[6] The middle third of the bulbus cordis, now called the *conus cordis,* will form the outflow portions of both ventricles, and the terminal third of the bulbus cordis (truncus arteriosus) will develop the proximal parts of the ascending aorta and main pulmonary artery.[5,6]

FORMATION OF THE CARDIAC SEPTA

The partitioning of the heart into four chambers, four valves, and two great arteries involves the formation of seven individual septa.[6] Of these, three are formed passively (septum secundum, the muscular portion of the ventricular septum, and the aorticopulmonary septum); three are formed actively (the atrioventricular canal septum, the spiral septum, and the truncal septum); and one starts passively but is completed by active septation (the septum primum).

Sinus venosus. The right horn of the sinus venosus enlarges, and the left horn decreases in size and importance. This is primarily a result of shunting of blood into the right vitelline, umbilical, and anterior cardinal veins.[5] The right horn of the sinus venosus becomes completely incorporated into the expanding right atrium to form its dorsal wall. In the mature animal this region, the sinus venarum, has a smooth internal surface. The left horn of the sinus venosus does not incorporate into the left atrium. Instead it reduces in size and becomes the coronary sinus.[6]

Atrial septation. The atrial division occurs because of development of two separate septa: the septum primum and the septum secundum (Figure 1-2). The septum primum is produced by an indentation in the roof of the common atrium made by the truncus arteriosus. As it extends ventrally toward the atrioventricular canal, it forms the ostium, or foramen, primum. Fusion of the septum primum with the endocardial cushion tissue at the atrioventricular canal closes the ostium primum. Before closure of the ostium

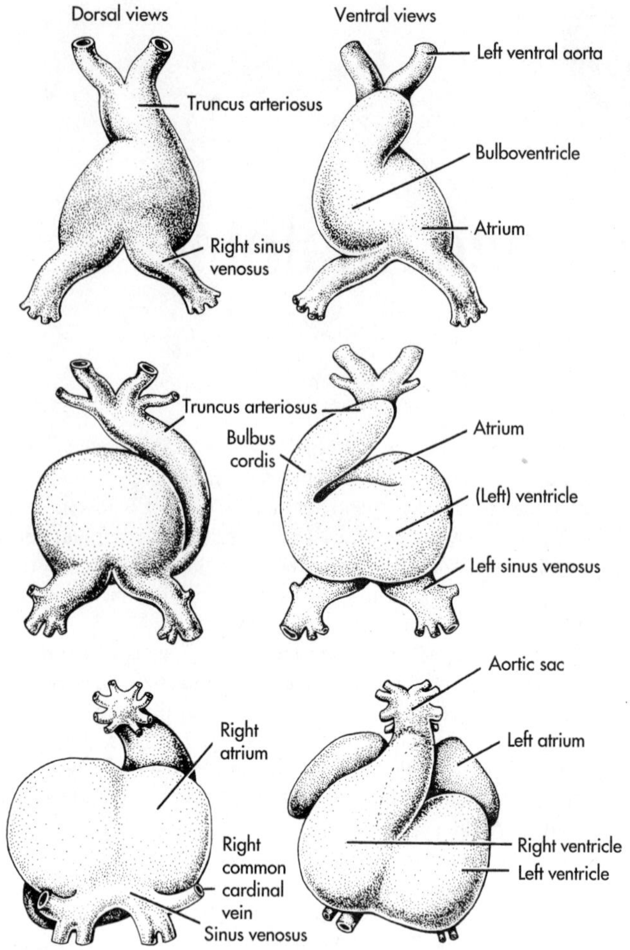

FIGURE 1-1 Dorsal *(left)* and ventral *(right)* external views of cardiac loop formation. Embryonic stages from top to bottom are the neurula, 15-somite, and 4-mm stages. (From Noden DM, DeLahunta A: *The embryology of domestic animals: developmental mechanisms and malformations,* Baltimore, 1985, Williams & Wilkins.)

primum, perforations occur in the cranial portion of the septum primum. These perforations coalesce to form the ostium, or foramen, secundum, maintaining communication between right and left atria. As the growth of the atria proceeds, a second septum, the septum secundum, forms to the right of the septum primum from the cranial margin of the atrium. One portion of the septum secundum extends caudally along the dorsal wall, and the other portion extends caudally along the atrioventricular cushions. An opening remains in the septum secundum, the foramen ovale, which is covered by the septum primum. Eventually the septum primum and septum secundum fuse to form the intraatrial septum; however, anatomic closure of the foramen ovale does not occur until after birth.

Atrioventricular canal. The mesoderm in the atrioventricular (AV) canal proliferates, producing bulges on the dorsal and ventral walls of the AV canal. These bulges, called *AV endocardial cushions,* are initially filled with cardiac jelly but are later invaded by mesenchymal cells. The AV endocardial cushions actively grow. This is most pronounced on the two regions located in the median plane. These regions eventually fuse, forming a single endocardial cushion and dividing the AV canal into right and left AV orifices (see Figure 1-2).

Truncus arteriosus and conus cordis. Paired endocardial cushions (ridges) also develop within the bulbus cordis and truncus arteriosus. The truncal cushions form first and expand into the lumen of the truncus from the right and left sides. They eventually fuse to form the truncal septum, which has a slight spiral, rotating progressively clockwise distally.[5] The bulbar cushions arise from the right dorsal and left ventral margins of the heart wall and are continuous with the truncal ridges. The spiral orientation of the bulbar cushions produces the spiral septum when they ultimately fuse with each other and with the truncal septum. Simultaneously, invagination of the dorsal wall of the distal truncus arteriosus (the aortic sac) forms a short thick aorticopulmonary septum, the leading edge of which fuses the distal face of the truncal septum.[6] This now continuous septum divides the bulbus cordis and truncus arteriosus into the aorta and main pulmonary artery. Because of the spiral orientation of the spiral and truncal septa, the pulmonary artery twists around the ascending aorta.

Ventricular septation. Growth of the primitive ventricle during cardiac loop development results in a shift of the single AV canal to the center of the heart. Once the AV and bulbar cushions form and fuse, only closure of the primary interventricular foramen remains to complete ventricular septation. The growth and expansion of the interventricular septum occurs passively as a result of caudal expansion of the ventricle combined with elongation along the midline. Enlargement of the ventricles is accomplished by centrifugal growth of the myocardium followed by increasing diverticulation and formation of the trabeculae that started during cardiac loop development. The medial walls of the growing ventricles appose and fuse, forming most of the muscular interventricular septum. Separation begins from the apex by an extension of the trabeculation process and growth of the interventricular septum toward the AV canal (see Figure 1-2). Completion of ventricular septation results from fusion of three tissues: the right bulbar ridge, the left bulbar ridge, and the fused endocardial cushions with the interventricular septum.[4,5] The primary interventricular foramen never closes, and, in the developed heart, gives rise to the aortic vestibule (the connection of the left ventricle to the aorta).[6] Once complete, the left AV canal and aorta are in communication with the left ventricle, and the pulmonary trunk and the right AV canal are fused with the right ventricle.

Formation of the valves. The AV valves form from a combination of growth of AV endocardial cushion tissue (the septal leaflets of the mitral and tricuspid valve) and from diverticulation and undermining of the ventricular wall (Fig. 1-2).[5] The primordia of semilunar valves are small tubercles of subendocardial tissue that form on each of the truncal ridges. Small tubercles also form on the walls opposite the fused truncal swellings. The semilunar cusps and sinuses of Valsalva are formed by a process of excavation of these swellings in a proximal direction.[6]

FORMATION OF THE MAJOR BLOOD VESSELS

The early embryonic arterial system consists of paired ventral aortae that are continuous with the heart tube caudally, six pairs of aortic arches, and paired dorsal aortae. Paired vitelline arteries and paired umbilical arteries connect the dorsal aortae with the yolk sac and allantois, respectively. Three main venous systems can be distinguished in the embryo: (1) the vitelline venous system, which carries blood from the yolk sac to the sinus venosus, (2) the umbilical venous system, which collects oxygenated blood from the chorion (placenta) and carries it to the sinus venosus, and (3) the cardinal venous system, which returns blood from the body of the embryo to the right and left sinus horns.[4]

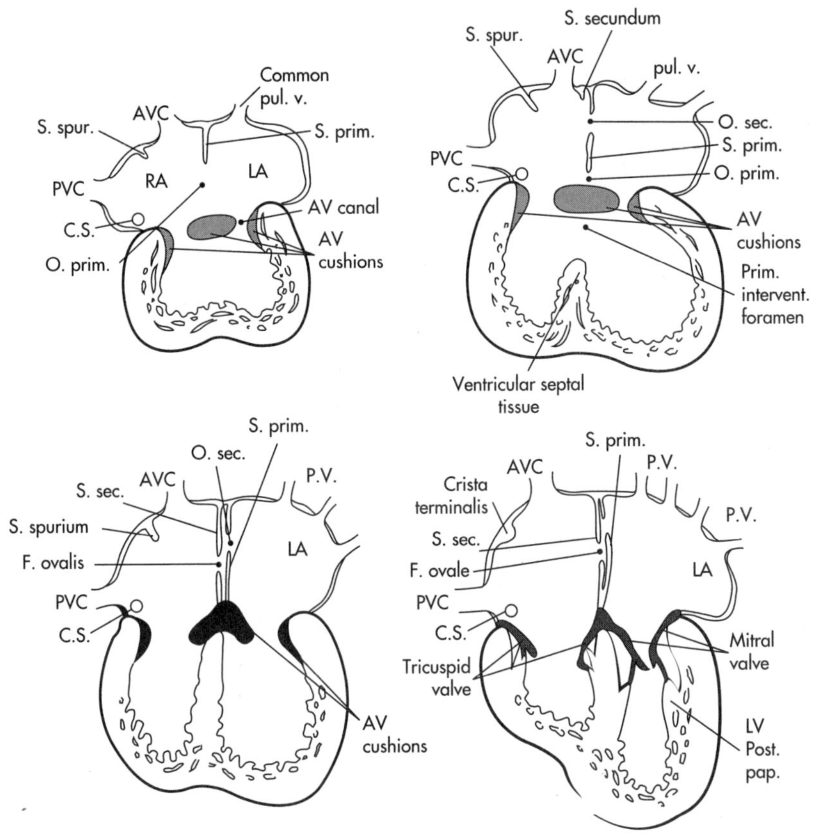

FIGURE 1-2 Diagrammatic representation of septal development. **A** through **D**, Drawings illustrate the development of the atrial and ventricular septa and the formation of the atrioventricular valve from endocardial cushion tissue. *AVC,* anterior vena cava; *cs,* coronary sinus; F. *ovalis,* fossa ovalis; F. *ovale,* foramen ovale; *LA,* left atrium; *O. sec,* ostium secundum; *O. prim,* ostium primum; *PV,* pulmonary veins; *PVC,* posterior vena cava; *RA,* right atrium; *S. sec,* septum secundum; *S. prim,* septum primum; *S. spur,* septum spurium. (From Bishop SP: Developmental anatomy of the heart and great vessels. In Fox PR, ed: *Canine and feline cardiology,* New York, 1988, Churchill Livingstone.)

The aortic arch system. The cranial portions of the dorsal aortae become the first pair of aortic arches as the paired heart tubes fuse and realign. Although a total of six pairs of aortic arches develop, they are not all present at the same time.[7] Several pairs of intersegmental arteries also develop along the dorsal aortae.[4,7] These aortic arches and intersegmental arteries are greatly modified during development to form the major components of the fully developed arterial system (Color Plate 1; Table 1-1).

Major systemic veins. The maturation of the embryonic venous system is a complex process and discussion will only involve a brief account of how the major systemic veins are formed. Development of the caudal vena cava results from a series of changes related to shifting venous flow from the left to the right side of the body.[4] The caudal vena cava is composed of four main segments: (1) a hepatic segment derived from part of the right vitelline vein and hepatic sinusoids, (2) a prerenal segment derived from the right subcardinal vein, (3) a renal segment derived from the subsupracardinal anastomosis, and (4) a postrenal segment derived from the right supracardinal vein.[6] The cranial vena cava eventually forms from the right anterior cardinal vein and the right common cardinal vein. The left anterior cardinal vein becomes the left brachiocephalic vein, and the renal veins develop from remnants of the subcardinal veins and the right subsupracardinal anastomosis. The supracardinal veins ultimately form the azygos and hemiazygos veins.

Pulmonary veins. The primitive pulmonary vein develops as an outgrowth of the dorsal left atrial wall, just to the left of the septum primum. It gains connections with the splanchnic plexus of veins in the region of the lung buds. As the atrium expands, the primitive pulmonary vein and its four main branches are gradually incorporated into the left atrium to form the larger, smooth part of the adult dorsal left atrial wall.[6]

TABLE 1-1

Embryonic origin of the major arteries

Embryologic structure	*Adult structure*
Truncus arteriosus	Proximal ascending aorta and main pulmonary artery
Aortic sac (distal truncus)	Distal ascending aorta, brachiocephalic artery, and aortic arch
First aortic arches	Regress; some parts maxillary arteries
Second aortic arches	Regress
Third aortic arches	Common carotid arteries and proximal internal carotid arteries
Fourth aortic arches	Right, proximal right subclavian; left, aortic arch
Fifth aortic arches	Regress
Sixth aortic arches	Right, proximal right pulmonary artery Left, proximal left pulmonary artery and ductus arteriosus
Right dorsal aorta	Right subclavian artery
Left dorsal aorta	Distal aortic arch
Seventh intersegmental	Right subclavian artery Left subclavian artery

From Moore KL. In Moore KL, editor: *The developing human,* Philadelphia, 1982, WB Saunders; Netter FH. In Yonkman FF, Netter FH, editors: *The Ciba collection of medical illustrators,* vol 5, Rochester, NY, 1974.

FETAL AND TRANSITIONAL CIRCULATION

Circulation in the primitive heart

Muscular contractions begin during early cardiac loop development.[8] Because the muscular layers of the primitive atrium and ventricle are continuous, contractions proceed as a wave of peristalsis along the heart tube, beginning in the sinus venosus and continuing through the truncus arteriosus. Initially, flow is bidirectional, with an "ebb-and-flow" motion, but by the end of the fourth week of gestation, coordinated contractions allow unidirectional flow. Venous flow entering the sinus venosus through the sinoatrial orifice is controlled by the sinoatrial valve and a structure in the dorsal wall of the right atrium, the septum spurium. Venous flow enters the ventricle through the singular atrioventricular canal. Blood is pumped from the ventricle into the bulbus cordis, truncus arteriosus, and aortic arches and dorsal aortae, eventually reaching the umbilical and vitelline arteries.

Fetal circulation. In the fetus, pulmonary alveoli are filled with amniotic fluid, and respiratory exchange of oxygen and carbon dioxide is carried out by the maternal lungs. Metabolism in the fetus depends critically on the umbilical artery and veins and requires little blood flow to the fetal lungs. Consequently, the fetal circulation is set up as a double circuit with parallel flow and crossover proximal and distal to the ventricles. Although the fetal circulation is designed to serve prenatal needs, it also permits rapid modifications at birth that help to establish a postnatal circulatory pattern (Color Plate 2).

The umbilical veins carry well-oxygenated blood (85% of hemoglobin is saturated with oxygen) from the placental chorionic villi to the caudal vena cava. Only about 50% of this blood passes through the hepatic sinusoids. The remainder by-passes the hepatic circulation through the ductus venosus directly into the caudal vena cava. A sphincter (either anatomic or physiologic) regulates flow through the ductus venosus, allowing more blood to be shunted to the portal vein when contracted. The blood entering the right atrium from the caudal vena cava is composed of flow from the ductus venosus, hepatic vein, and caudal body venous drainage. It is primarily diverted by the crista dividens, a small ridge in the medial right atrial wall, across the foramen ovale into the left atrium, left ventricle, and aorta. This allows the heart, head, and neck structures to receive well-oxygenated blood (65% hemoglobin saturation after mixing). A small amount of blood from the caudal vena cava is diverted, again by the crista dividens, to remain in the right atrium and is mixed with cranial vena caval flow.

Poorly oxygenated blood (50% hemoglobin saturation) in the right atrium, containing mostly cranial vena caval blood, passes to the right ventricle and pulmonary artery. Because pulmonary vascular resistance is high, only 5% to 10% of right ventricular output passes through the pulmonary circulation. The remainder is diverted through the ductus arteriosus into the aorta, distal to the head and neck branches. Between 40% and 50% of aortic flow enters the umbilical arteries and returns to the chorionic villi of the placenta. The remainder circulates through the caudal portion of the embryo. Thus two parallel circuits are present that serve to deliver highly oxygenated blood to the brain and heart and less oxygenated blood to the placenta (Color Plate 2).

Circulatory changes at birth. At birth and during the subsequent neonatal period, changes occur in the circulatory system that result in two separate circuits connected in series (see Chapter 2). Almost immediately, when the placenta ceases to function, the three shunts that permit most of the blood to bypass the hepatic and pulmonary circulations also cease to function. First, the sphincter in the ductus venosus constricts tightly so that all the blood reaching the liver must pass through the hepatic sinusoids. The exact mechanism responsible for closure of the ductus venosus is not well understood but is in part influenced by the reduction in caudal vena caval and right atrial pressure that occurs with removal of the placental circulation.[4,9]

Aeration of the lungs is associated with a precipitous fall in pulmonary vascular resistance and an increase in pulmonary blood flow. These changes are mitigated by the sudden suspension in air of the pulmonary vessels previously supported by fluid media. This reduced extravascular pressure allows collapsed vessels to open and already open vessels to dilate. However, the fall in pulmonary vascular resistance is probably more importantly related to vasodilation associated with the sudden increase in oxygen tension.[9] As a result, pulmonary pressure falls dramatically, pulmonary blood flow increases, and left atrial pressure rises slightly as a result of greater venous return. Removal of the placental circulation also causes an increase in systemic vascular resistance and a reduction in caudal vena caval and right atrial pressures. These changes have two important effects on the fetal pattern of circulation. First, the foramen ovale functionally closes because of the increase in left atrial pressure combined with a fall in right atrial pressure as the valve of the foramen ovale (septum primum) is pressed against the septum secundum. Also, flow across the ductus arteriosus ceases because of the relative changes in systemic and pulmonary vascular resistance. The musculature in the ductus arteriosus is also sensitive to the changes in oxygen tension and contracts when exposed to the increased oxygen content of the aortic blood.[4,9] This constriction of the ductus is also mediated by local prostaglandins and bradykinin.[9] The ductus arteriosus is completely or partially open in most puppies that are 4 days of age. By 6 to 8 days of age, the ductus arteriosus is either functionally or anatomically closed in most puppies.[10]

The change from fetal to adult circulation is not sudden. The ductus venosus, ductus arteriosus, and foramen ovale remain potential channels for blood flow after birth. Initially, the closure of these shunts is only functional. Anatomic closure occurs later in the neonatal period, resulting primarily from the proliferation of endothelial and fibrous tissues.[4] Also, the right ventricle and the muscular portion of the pulmonary arteries are thicker than adult arteries because of the high resistance of the right circuit in the fetus. In the weeks following birth, progressive atrophy of the pulmonary arterial smooth muscle occurs and the left ventricle grows progressively.[4,11]

During the embryonic and fetal growth periods, increases in heart mass are predominantly by cell multiplication (hyperplasia). Cellular hyperplasia continues into the early neonatal period but is eventually replaced by cellular hypertrophy.[11] In the dog, this switch occurs at approximately 2 weeks of age.[11] After that, virtually all increases in cardiac mass are accomplished by hypertrophy.

Gross Cardiac Anatomy

Dog and cat hearts are similar in structure and orientation. Consequently, they are treated as one in this discussion, with clinically significant differences highlighted. The dog is used as the model in the illustrations.

ORIENTATION OF THE HEART WITHIN THE THORACIC CAVITY

The heart lies nestled within the thoracic cavity, extending from about the third to the sixth intercostal space. The heart is contained within the mediastinum, the central space between the pleural cavities and the partition that separates the left and right pleural spaces. The lung almost surrounds the heart laterally, cranially, dorsally, and caudally. The ventral portion of the heart lies on the floor of the thoracic cavity, touching the tissue surrounding the sternebrae. The cranial portion of the heart touches the cranial mediastinum, and the dorsal portion of the heart touches the medial mediastinum.[12] The trachea and mainstem bronchi and the esophagus, along with lymph nodes and vascular structures such as the aortic arch and the proximal portion of the descending aorta, lie within the medial mediastinum on top of the heart (Color Plates 3 and 4). Caudally, the heart, primarily the left ventricle, is in contact with the diaphragm. The heart is conical, with the pointed, or apical, portion lying ventral and somewhat caudal. The base of the heart is the dorsal part of the heart. The heart in most dogs and cats lies at an angle within the chest, with the apex lying more caudally than the base. In deep-chested dogs, however, the heart is more upright and the apex may lie immediately ventral to the base.

The canine heart lies such that the left heart (the left ventricle and left atrium) lies caudally and a bit to the left, and the right heart (the right atrium and right ventricle) lies cranial to the left heart and to the right (Color Plates 3 and 4). The atria are dorsal to the ventricles. The body of the left atrium is situated dorsally to the left ventricle. The left auricle extends cranially and to the left from the body of the left atrium to lie on the left lateral aspect of the heart. The body of the right atrium is dorsal to the right ventricle. The right auricle extends cranially to lie along the cranial border of the heart (Color Plate 4).

THE PERICARDIUM

The four chambers of the heart are encased within a fibrous sac, the pericardium (Color Plate 5). The pericardium is divided into the fibrous and the serous pericardia. The fibrous pericardium is the strong outer covering. It attaches to the adventitia of the large vessels entering and leaving the heart at its base (Color Plate 6). At the apex, the fibrous pericardium extends to the diaphragm to form the phrenopericardial ligament. Externally, a thin layer of mediastinal pleura covers the pericardium that attaches to the sternal area. These two attachments hold the pericardium, and so the heart, in a semifixed position within the thorax. The serous pericardium lines the fibrous pericardium and overlies the heart, where it is called the *epicardium.* The serous pericardium is composed of a thin layer of mesothelial cells overlying a lamina propria containing elastic fibers. The portion that lines the fibrous pericardium is called the *parietal layer* of the serous pericardium. Where it overlies the heart, it is called the *visceral layer* of the serous pericardium. These two layers are normally in contact with each other and are moistened by a small amount of fluid secreted by the cells in the serous pericardium. This fluid lubricates the area, allowing the heart to move easily within the pericardial space as it contracts and relaxes. The visceral and parietal layers of the serous pericardium meet above the base of the heart to form an uneven line around the base (the pericardial reflection).

The right and left phrenic nerves course from cranial to caudal across the surface of the pericardium on their respective sides of the heart, beneath the pulmonic valve and left atrium on the left side and beneath the right auricle on the right side (Color Plate 5). The ventral vagal trunk courses parallel more dorsally near the aorta on the left side.

CARDIAC SIZE

The heart of a normal adult dog is approximately 0.7% to 0.8% of body weight (8 g/kg). This, however, varies considerably and has been reported to range from 0.45% to 1.1%.[13] Several variables affect this ratio. Females have smaller hearts than males. Small dogs have higher ratios than large dogs. Certainly an obese, sedentary dog is expected to have a smaller ratio than an athletic dog. As might be expected, the ratio is more uniform in cats. Cats have smaller hearts than dogs, with hearts that are approximately 0.33% of body weight.[14] In one study the percent of body weight ranged from 0.28% to 0.38% in adult cats.

Young animals have different heart weight to body weight ratios than adult animals. In one study, hearts from puppies that were 6 to 11 days old were 0.47% of body weight; whereas in adults the ratio increased to 0.7%.[14] In the same study, hearts from 65-day-old kittens were 0.63% of body weight, and adult hearts were 0.33% of body weight. This study examined seven species. The dog was the only one in which the heart weight to body weight ratio increased with age. In another study, the heart weight to body weight ratio was not different between puppies and adult dogs.[10]

The left ventricle weighs more than the right ventricle in the adult animal. If the right ventricular free wall is excised from the heart and the left ventricle is kept intact (with the interventricular septum considered part of the left ventricle), the left ventricle weighs approximately 3 times the right ventricle in the dog.[14] In the cat this ratio is closer to 3.5. In the neonatal animal, however, this ratio is closer to 1 in dogs and 1.7 in cats. In puppies, a clear line of cleavage can be seen in the interventricular septum, so that the right and left ventricles can be separated. When this is done, the right ventricle weighs more than the left ventricle at birth.[15] Within 3 days, however, the two ventricles weigh the same. This is not due to right ventricular atrophy but to the left ventricle growing more rapidly than the right ventricle. The relative right ventricular hypertrophy at birth is present because the right ventricle must generate the same pressure as the left ventricle in fetal life.

In dogs the left ventricular wall thickness and chamber diameter increase with age, with adults having diameters and wall thicknesses 4 times that of puppies.[10] The ratio of the chamber diameter to the wall thickness does not change. This is expected, because the primary stimulus for growth is wall stress (see Chapter 2). However, heart weight increases 10 to 16 times as fast as wall thickness in growing dogs, because myocytes lengthen more rapidly than they thicken.[10]

THE CARDIAC SURFACE AND MAJOR BLOOD VESSELS

The chambers of the heart are separated on the surface by grooves, or sulci. The coronary groove separates the atria from the ventricles. This groove contains the left circumflex and right coronary arteries and coronary veins, as well as fat. The coronary groove encircles the heart except cranially where the coronary vessels lie beneath the right ventricular outflow tract (Color Plates 7 and 8). The interventricular grooves descend from the coronary groove along the cranial and caudal aspects of the interventricular septum. Consequently, they divide the left ventricle from the right ventricle (Color Plates 7 and 8). They are less indented than the coronary groove and contain less fat. The cranial groove contains the left anterior (cranial) descending coronary artery and vein. It descends along the left border of the right ventricular outflow tract, originating just below the left auricle. The caudal groove contains the caudal branch of the left circumflex coronary artery and vein. Other branches of the coronary vessels descend along the surface of the ventricles in other areas.

When a heart is removed, one can orient oneself quickly to the surface anatomy by grasping the right auricle in one's left fingers and the left auricle in one's right fingers and holding the heart aloft. The right ventricular outflow tract lies between the two auricles, is cranial, and ascends from right to left to the main pulmonary artery (Color Plate 8). Once this orientation is obtained, identifying the remaining structures on the surface of the heart is usually easy. The bodies of the two atria lie caudal to the auricles. Each ventricle lies ventrally to its respective atrium. The body of the right ventricle is on the right side of the heart, but the outflow tract ascends cranially and to the left to join the main pulmonary artery. The main pulmonary artery is short, giving rise to the left and right caudal lobar branches immediately cranial to the body of the left atrium (Color Plate 9). The aorta emerges cranially from the base of the heart, caudal to the right ventricular outflow tract, and to the right of the pulmonary artery. It immediately curves to first ascend toward the spine and then descend beneath the spine. This produces an aortic arch. The brachiocephalic trunk and the left subclavian artery arise from the aorta on the transverse portion of the aorta. These vessels provide blood flow to the head, the front limbs, and the ventral thorax (Color Plates 3, 8, and 9). The ligamentum arteriosum angles forward from the proximal descending aorta to the branching of the main pulmonary artery and the left pulmonary artery branch (Color Plate 8). The cranial vena cava enters the right atrium cranially and dorsally (Color Plates 4, 9, and 10). The caudal vena cava enters the right atrium from its very caudal aspect, lower than the cranial vena cava. The azygos vein enters the base of the cranial vena cava, descending from beneath the thoracic spine (Color Plates 4, 9, and 10). The pulmonary veins enter the dorsal part of the left atrium from the respective lung lobes (Color Plates 7 and 9). The vein from the right cranial and middle lung lobes enters the left atrium immediately dorsal to the interatrial septum.

THE FIBROUS SKELETON

The fibrous skeleton, or base, forms a scaffold that anchors the four cardiac valves (Figures 1-3 and 1-4). It is a fibrous and cartilaginous structure that separates the atria from the ventricles. It forms two fibrous rings that form the annuli (encircling fibrous bases) of each atrioventricular orifice and fibrous cuffs that surround each arterial orifice. This fibrous skeleton also electrically isolates the atria from the ventricles. Only the atrioventricular node, encased in the fibrous base, and the bundle of His, that penetrates it, allow electrical signals to traverse this base. The central fibrous body is a triangular, dense fibrous connection between the region of the noncoronary cusp of the aortic valve, the septal leaflet of the tricuspid valve, the septal leaflet of the mitral valve, and the base of the interatrial septum. The membranous portion of the interventricular septum connects to the central fibrous body. The bundle of His penetrates through this region. The left fibrous trigone connects the caudal aortic wall to the annulus of the mitral valve in the region of the septal leaflet of the mitral valve. The conus ligament connects the aortic and pulmonic valves. Fibrous cords extend from the right and left trigones to encircle the mitral and tricuspid valves to form the valve annuli.

THE VENA CAVAE, AZYGOS VEIN, AND THORACIC DUCT

The cranial vena cava receives blood from the head, neck, chest wall, and thoracic limbs. It courses dorsally to the right auricle, entering the right atrium dorsal to the crista terminalis (Color Plates 9 through 11). The axillary veins from the thoracic limbs join with the external and internal jugular veins from the head to form the right and left brachiocephalic veins. These join to form the cranial vena cava. The costocervical and internal thoracic veins join the cranial vena cava distal to this site. The azygos vein lies along the psoas muscles, primarily under the thoracic vertebrae. Its origin is in the region of the third lumbar vertebra. It courses forward from there, collecting venous blood from the lumbar, subcostal, dorsal intercostal, esophageal, and bronchoesophageal veins. It enters the cranial vena cava near where the vena cava enters the right atrium. The thoracic duct empties lymph into the region where the left external jugular vein joins the axillary vein and cranial vena cava in about one half of dogs. In the others the duct branches, emptying into various veins, including the azygos vein. The thoracic duct drains all of the lymph from the body, except for lymph from the right thoracic limb and the right side of the head and neck. The right lymphatic duct drains these. The thoracic duct originates in the cranial sublumbar region or between the crura of the diaphragm as a continuation of the cisterna chyli. It courses cranially in the thorax along the right dorsal border of the aorta and the ventral border of the azygos vein.

The caudal vena cava begins as the convergence of the common iliac veins ventral to the seventh lumbar vertebra. In the abdomen it ascends retroperitoneally beneath the vertebrae, between the right and left psoas muscles, and to the right of the aorta. During its course, the deep circumflex iliac, renal, testicular or ovarian, phrenicoabdominal, and hepatic veins join it. At the liver, the caudal vena cava dives ventrally and to the right to pass through the caudate lobe of the liver and through the right crus of the diaphragm. The thoracic portion of the cranial vena cava is short. It passes from the diaphragm to enter the caudal border of the right atrium in a groove within the

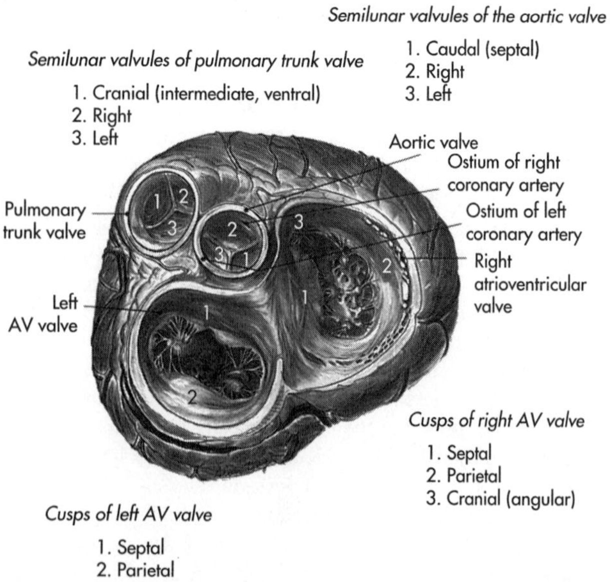

FIGURE 1-3 Fibrous skeleton, valve, and cusps of the heart shown in early ventricular diastole. The atria, auricles, and great vessels have been removed, and the heart is viewed from above. The atrioventricular valves are open as the ventricles fill, and the semilunar valves are closed. (From Anderson WD, Anderson BG: *Atlas of canine anatomy,* Philadelphia, 1994, Lea & Febiger.)

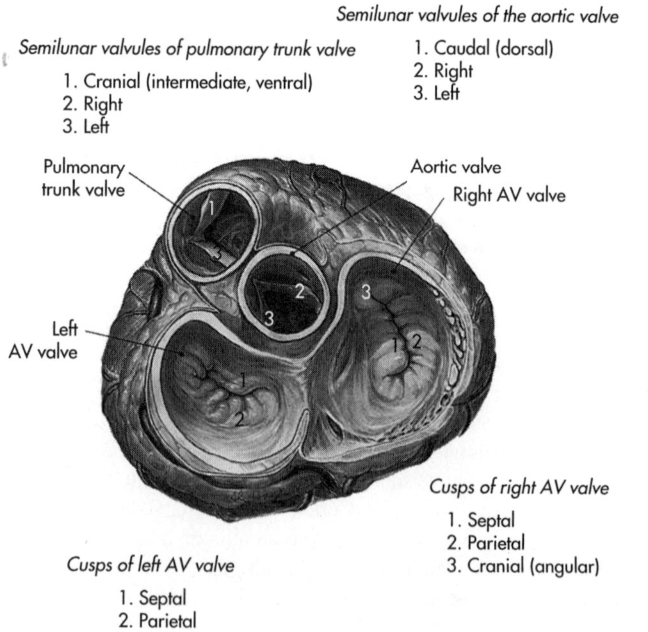

FIGURE 1-4 Same as Figure 1-3 during ventricular systole. The atrioventricular valves are closed, and the semilunar valves are open as the ventricles eject blood into the aorta and pulmonary artery. (From Anderson WD, Anderson BG: *Atlas of canine anatomy,* Philadelphia, 1994, Lea & Febiger.)

intermediate lung lobe. The right phrenic nerve lies in close association with it.

THE RIGHT ATRIUM

The right atrium lies above the right ventricle. It acts as a receiving and holding chamber for deoxygenated systemic venous blood during ventricular systole and as a conduit for blood flow and a pumping chamber in ventricular diastole (Color Plate 11). It is divided into the body of the right atrium and the right auricle. The right auricle is a blind pouch that lies cranial to the body of the right atrium. Whereas the inner body is smooth, the auricle and lateral wall of the right atrium are heavily trabeculated, containing a network of muscular bands, the pectinate muscles, that form hills and furrows on the inner surface (Color Plate 12). These muscles radiate from the crista terminalis, a ridge of tissue that originates near the lateral opening of the cranial vena cava. It separates the body of the right atrium from the medial wall of the right auricle. A ridge of tissue lies in the middle of the body of the right atrium, arising from the intervenous tubercle, a part of the interatrial septum. Caudal to this ridge is the fossa ovalis, the region where the foramen ovale is located in fetal life and in which an ostium secundum atrial septal defect would lie (Color Plate 11).

The right atrium fills with blood returning from the systemic venous system. This blood enters the right atrium via the cranial and caudal vena cavae and the coronary sinus (Color Plate 10). Coronary blood flow enters the great cardiac vein that enters the right atrium via an ostium in the floor of the right atrium, the coronary sinus. The coronary sinus lies slightly caudal and to the left of the septal leaflet of the tricuspid valve (Color Plate 12).

THE TRICUSPID VALVE

The tricuspid valve, or right atrioventricular valve, is a one-way valve that lies within the atrioventricular orifice between the right atrium and right ventricle (Color Plates 12, 13, and 14). It opens passively and maximally during each diastole when the right ventricle relaxes, as blood flows from the right atrium into the right ventricle. It opens to a similar extent again when the right atrium contracts (see Figure 1-3). During ventricular systole, the valve closes, preventing backflow of blood from the ventricle into the atrium (see Figure 1-4). The valve apparatus is composed of two leaflets, an annulus, chordae tendineae, and papillary muscles. The leaflets are anchored to the annulus. The fibrous skeleton of the heart reinforces the annulus for most of the circumference, except along the upper portion of the interventricular septum.

In humans the tricuspid valve has three leaflets. In dogs and cats, only two leaflets are present, the septal and the mural, or parietal, leaflets (see Figures 1-3 and 1-4). The septal leaflet is much smaller than the mural leaflet (Color Plates 12, 13, and 14). It lies medially, above the interventricular septum. It is semicircular in shape. The larger mural leaflet is more mobile than the septal leaflet. It extends from the region of the crista supraventricularis cranially to the most caudal aspect of the right ventricle. Indentations along its free edge give it a scalloped appearance. The junctions between the two leaflets are the cranial and caudal commissures. The atrial surface of the leaflets is smooth and glistening. On the ventricular surface, the valve is divided into a rough zone and a clear zone. The rough zone is irregular and coarse. It is along the edge of the leaflets where the chordae tendineae attach. The clear zone is smooth and translucent. It extends from the rough zone to the base of the leaflets.

The leaflets are anchored by chordae tendineae, papillary muscles, and papillae, which prevent the leaflets from prolapsing back into the right atrium in systole. The chordae tendineae are tough fibrous cords that are extensions of the fibrous layer of the leaflets. They attach the underside of the leaflets, to the papillary muscles and papillae. A variable amount of branching occurs with primary and secondary chordae attaching to the ventricular surface of the leaflets. The right ventricle has a variable number of papillary muscles, all of which attach to the mural leaflet. Most commonly there are three large papillary muscles and a small papillary muscle of the conus (Color Plate 13). The large papillary muscles originate from the apical third of the interventricular septum. The papillary muscle of the conus is the most cranial papillary muscle. It also arises from the interventricular septum along the dorsal region of the crista supraventricularis. The septal leaflet has shorter chordae tendineae that attach to small muscular ridges, or papillae, that lie more dorsal than the papillary muscles along the interventricular septum (Color Plates 12, 13, and 14).

THE RIGHT VENTRICLE

The right ventricle actively pumps blood through the low-resistance pulmonary circuit. It is an angular structure that wraps partially around the left ventricle. Because it pumps through a lower resistance than the left ventricle, its myocardium must generate less force. Consequently, its walls are thinner and have less mass than those of the left ventricle in the adult animal.

The right ventricle is divided into two regions, the caudal body, or inflow, region immediately beneath the tricuspid valve orifice and the outflow tract, or infundibulum, that ascends cranially and to the left (Color Plates 13 and 14). The right ventricle can be mimicked by wrapping the left hand around a ball, with the thumb fully extended. When this is done, the body of the hand is the body of the right ventricle and the thumb is the outflow tract extending upward and to the left. Blood flows through the tricuspid valve in diastole and into the body. In systole some of this blood and the blood in the outflow tract are ejected into the pulmonary circulation through the pulmonic valve. The body of the right ventricle contains the papillary muscles. Dorsal to the papillary muscles, along the interventricular septum, the body is smooth (Color Plate 14). The interventricular septum is heavily trabeculated ventral to the papillary muscles (apically), as is the free wall that encompasses the body. The outflow tract is smooth, both along the septum and along the free wall. The body and the outflow tract are separated from each other by an indistinct ridge of tissue, the crista supraventricularis, located along the interventricular septum. The papillary muscle of the conus originates from this crest (Color Plate 13).

The moderator band is a thin muscular strand that runs from the interventricular septum to the free wall of the right ventricle. It carries the right bundle branch to the free wall. The moderator band most commonly originates near the base of the largest papillary muscle. One anastomosing strand or a loose plexus of anastomosing strands may exist.

THE PULMONIC VALVE

The pulmonic valve lies cranial, to the left and dorsal to the tricuspid valve (Color Plate 15). The annuli of these two valves are separate. The pulmonic valve consists of an annulus and three cusps. The cusps are thin, semitransparent structures anchored to the annulus at their base. The cusps are shaped like three symmetric triangles that meet in the middle to close the orifice in diastole (see Figure 1-3). In systole they are forced dorsally to lie against the wall of the main pulmonary artery (see Figure 1-4). Position names them as *cranial, right,* and *left* cusps. The right and left cusps are partially contiguous with the left and right aortic valve cusps. When closed, the lines of cusp apposition (the linea alba) form small linear ridges that radiate from the center to the annulus, resembling a "peace sign" or the Mercedes Benz logo, depending on the orientation.

THE PULMONARY ARTERIES

The pulmonary arteries carry deoxygenated blood from the right ventricle to the lungs. The main pulmonary artery arises from the pulmonic valve to arch dorsally and caudally to the left of the aortic root and dorsal to the left auricle. Caudal to the aortic root and immediately before it reaches the body of the left atrium, the pulmonary artery splits into left and right branches (Color Plate 9). The ligamentum arteriosum joins the proximal portion of the left branch of the pulmonary artery (Color Plate 8). The right caudal lobar branch runs caudal to the root of the aorta and across the top of the right atrium to emerge lateral to the right bronchus. The left caudal branch courses across the top of the left auricle to emerge lateral to the left bronchus.

THE PULMONARY VEINS

The pulmonary veins return oxygenated blood from the pulmonary capillaries in the lungs to the left atrium. These veins enter the left atrium from its dorsal aspect (Color Plate 9). Six veins are present, three from the right lung and three from the left lung. It is common for two veins to merge into one vein before entering the left atrium. Consequently, four to six pulmonary vein ostia are present in the roof of the left atrium in dogs. Cats generally have four openings.

THE LEFT ATRIUM

The left atrium fills with oxygenated blood from the pulmonary veins. It is divided into the body of the left atrium and the auricle. The smooth and glistening body of the left atrium lies immediately dorsal to the left ventricle (Color Plate 16). It is on the dorsocaudal aspect of the heart and lies immediately beneath the carina of the trachea and the mainstem bronchi. It is also directly caudal to the branching of the main pulmonary artery into its caudal lobar branches (Color Plate 9). The left auricle extends cranially from the body of the left atrium to lie immediately beneath the main pulmonary artery (Color Plate 8). It lies flush with the left ventricular free wall below it. The left auricle is heavily trabeculated. In contrast to the right atrium, the pectinate muscles of the left atrium are confined to the auricle and no distinct muscle ridge separates the trabeculated appendage from the smooth endocardial surface of the atrial free wall.

The interatrial septum separates the right and left atria. This septum starts cranially just caudal to the aorta and runs caudally and to the left between the two atria.

THE MITRAL VALVE

The mitral valve (left atrioventricular valve) is a one-way valve that lies within the atrioventricular orifice between the left atrium and left ventricle. The valve apparatus consists of two leaflets, a valve annulus, chordae tendineae, and papillary muscles. The two leaflets are the septal, or anterior, and the mural (posterior or parietal) leaflets (see Figures 1-3 and 1-4). The surface area of the two leaflets exceeds that of the atrioventricular orifice. During early diastole the two leaflets open wide so that the septal leaflet lies close to and parallel with the interventricular septum. The mural leaflet lies close to and parallel with the free wall (see Figure 1-3). As opposed to the tricuspid valve, the septal leaflet is the larger leaflet, being 2 to 3 times the size of the mural leaflet (Color Plate 16). The base of the septal leaflet is continuous with the root of the aorta (see Figures 1-3, 1-4, and Color Plate 17). Like the tricuspid valve, the atrial surface of the leaflets is smooth. Rough and clear zones can be identified on the ventricular surface. Two commissures are present where the valves meet. Besides the two large leaflets, smaller commissural cusps may also be present. Ventral to each commissure is a papillary muscle. These papillary muscles are larger than the papillary muscles in the right ventricle and have been termed the *dorsal* and *ventral* papillary muscles. We would prefer other terminology, because this orientation is probably not true in deep-chested dogs in which the heart is upright. The ventral papillary muscle is cranial to the dorsal papillary muscle. Consequently, cranial and caudal papillary muscles would be appropriate. The cranial papillary muscle lies more toward the left auricle, and the caudal papillary muscle lies more toward the caudal aspect of the body of the left atrium. Consequently, the cranial papillary muscle has been termed the *subauricular* papillary muscle and the caudal termed the *subatrial* papillary muscle.[16] Both papillary muscles start within a few millimeters of the apex as what appear to be deep-rooted structures that extend upward to form a thick, tapering trunk (Color Plate 16). Stout chordae tendineae emerge from the papillary muscles at their tips to fix to the underside of the mitral valve leaflets. Each leaflet receives chordae from each papillary muscle. The chordae start at the papillary muscle as single strands that branch, usually only into secondary, but sometimes into tertiary, chordae tendineae.

THE LEFT VENTRICLE

The left ventricle is the largest structure in the heart. It pumps blood through the high-resistance systemic circulation. The myocardium of the left ventricle is approximately 3 times the thickness of the right ventricle (Color Plates 17 and 18). It occupies the left and caudal regions of the heart. The left ventricle's shape is conical, with the tip at the apex (Color Plate 17). When it is open, the septal leaflet of the mitral valve physiologically divides the left ventricle into an inflow and an outflow region (Color Plate 17). The inflow region extends from the mitral valve annulus to the apex. It includes the papillary muscles. The outflow tract begins at the apex and extends to the aortic valve, which lies at the base of the heart, cranial to the septal leaflet of the mitral valve. It is bounded medially by the interventricular septum but has no anatomic lateral border in systole.

The left ventricle also has trabeculations (trabeculae carnae), but they are not nearly as deep as those in the right ventricle (Color Plate 16). Usually no bands cross the ventricular cavity, but in some hearts single or, rarely, multiple cords may traverse the ventricular cavity (Color Plate 17). These cords are sometimes referred to as *false tendons.* A fine network of short muscular strands passes from the interventricular septum to the cranial papillary muscle. They probably carry terminal branches of the left bundle branch.

The membranous septum lies beneath the junction of the left and the caudal noncoronary aortic cusps at the crest of the interventricular septum. It blends with the muscle of the interventricular septum and with the tissue of the caudal noncoronary cusp.

The left bundle branch cannot be seen in a gross specimen. However, it can be visualized by placing an iodine-containing solution on the interventricular septum. It then can be seen starting at the base beneath the membranous septum as a discrete band and branching as it descends to become a fan-shaped structure along the septum.

THE AORTIC VALVE

The aortic valve apparatus is formed by the fibrous annulus, the root of the aorta, and three aortic valve cusps (Color Plate 17). The cusps are similar in shape to the pulmonic valve cusps but are slightly thicker. The root of the aorta bulges slightly behind each valve cusp beyond the annulus to form the sinuses of Valsalva. The ostia of the right and left coronary arteries lie within two of these sinuses. The sinuses prevent the coronary ostia from being closed over by the open aortic valve cusps in systole. The coronary cusps are named for their position and the position of the coronary ostia (see Figures 1-3 and 1-4). The cusp associated with the ostium of the right coronary artery is called the *right cusp* of the aortic valve, and the cusp associated with the left coronary artery is called the *left cusp.* The

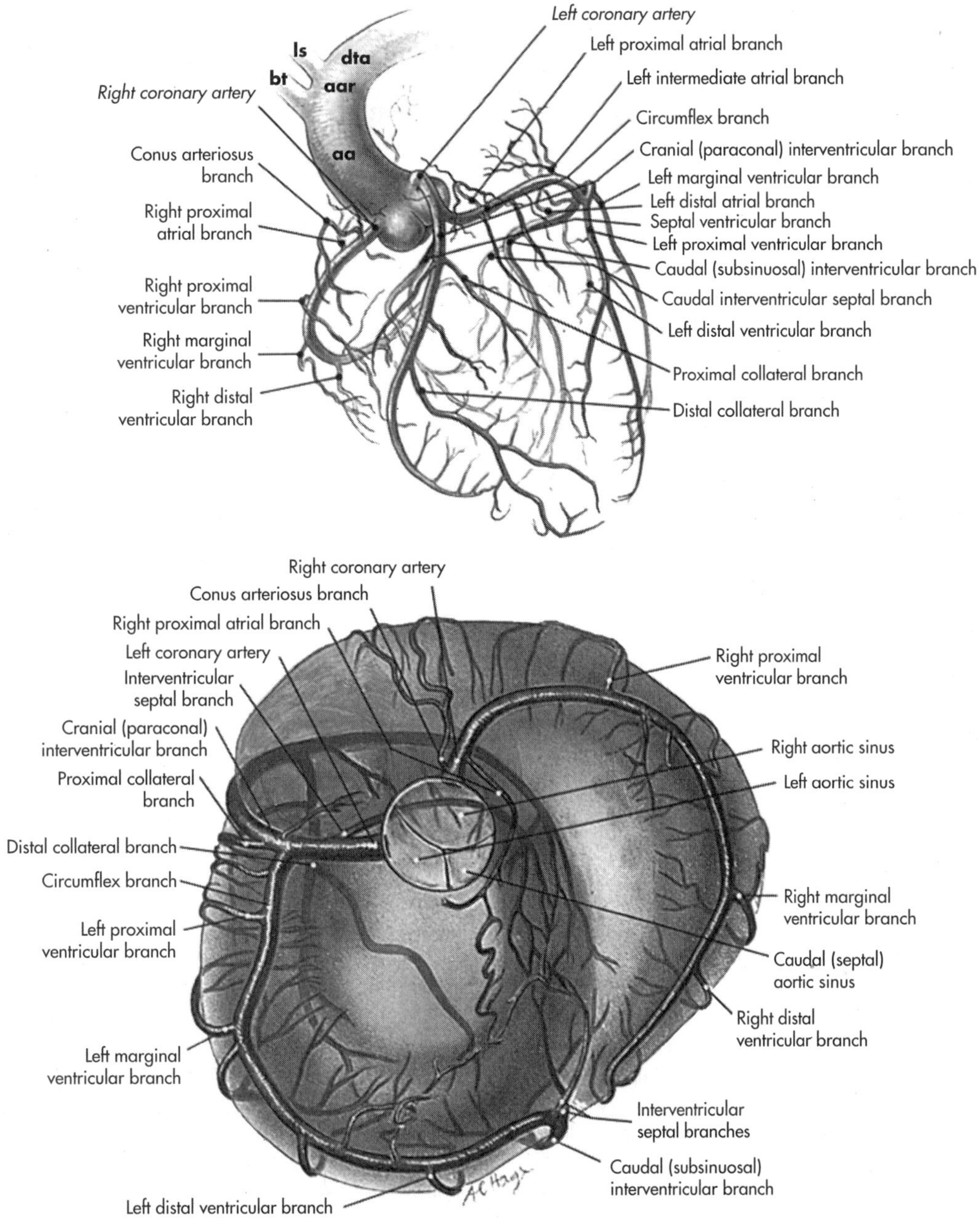

FIGURE 1-5 Coronary vasculature viewed laterally *(top)* and from above *(bottom)* after removal of the atria. The right and left coronary arteries originate from ostia behind the aortic valve cusps. The left coronary artery branches into the cranial paraconal interventricular (left anterior descending) coronary artery and left circumflex coronary artery. An interventricular septal branch also originates near this branch point. The left circumflex coronary artery terminates as the caudal interventricular branch, descending between the left and right ventricles. *aa,* Ascending aorta; *aar,* aortic arch; *dta,* descending thoracic aorta; *bt,* brachiocephalic trunk; *ls,* left subclavian artery. (From Anderson WD, Anderson BG: *Atlas of canine anatomy,* Philadelphia, 1994, Lea & Febiger.)

cusp that is not associated with a coronary artery is called the *noncoronary,* or *caudal, cusp* of the aortic valve. In the middle of the free edge of each valve cusp is a small nodule. The free edges where each cusp contacts the adjacent cusp are called the *lunulae.*

The commissure between the left and right cusps of the aortic valve is closest to the pulmonic valve, and so the linea alba points outward toward the pulmonic valve (see Figures 1-3 and 1-4). The linea alba between the left and noncoronary cusps points toward the left atrium. The linea alba between the noncoronary and the right coronary cusps points at the tricuspid valve. The lineae alba are visualized on an echocardiogram, and their orientation is important for determining the echocardiographic anatomy of the root of the aorta. In their usual orientation on an echocardiogram, they resemble the Mercedes Benz logo.

THE AORTA

The aorta consists of three segments, the ascending aorta, transverse arch, and descending aorta (Color Plate 19). The ascending aorta is short and arises from the cranial aspect of the heart, immediately behind the right auricle and the tissue at the junction of the right ventricle outflow tract and the pulmonic valve (Color Plate 19). The ascending aorta is oriented in the same way as the left ventricle, angling dorsally and cranially as it emerges from the left ventricle. This segment enlarges as a poststenotic dilation with subaortic stenosis. Once the aorta is above the plane of the main pulmonary artery, it curves backward as the transverse segment, which is also short. The brachiocephalic trunk and the right subclavian artery emerge from the transverse aorta in both dogs and cats. Once the aorta has turned completely, it is the descending aorta. The descending aorta is divided into thoracic and abdominal portions. The ligamentum arteriosum lies on the left lateral/ventral portion of the proximal descending aorta, coursing ventrally and slightly cranially to the junction of the main and left pulmonary arteries (Color Plate 8). The descending aorta courses within the dorsal mediastinum beneath the spine. It starts to the left of the vertebral column but gradually moves to the right, so that it is on the midline by the time it crosses through the diaphragm. As it descends, it sends arterial branches to the vertebrae and spine (see Figure 1-1). In the abdomen, the aorta lies within the retroperitoneum. Major arterial branches come off the aorta to supply the liver, gastrointestinal tract, kidneys, and genital organs as the aorta traverses the abdomen. The aorta terminates beneath the sixth or seventh lumbar vertebrae to branch into the two external iliac and the common iliac arteries. This is termed the aortic trifurcation and is the common site for thromboemboli to lodge in cats. The common iliac artery divides into the two internal iliac and the middle sacral arteries. The external iliac arteries descend to become the femoral arteries, the arteries commonly palpated during the physical examination.

THE CORONARY ARTERIES

The two major coronary arteries, the right and left main coronary arteries, arise from the root of the aorta (Figure 1-5). The ostium of the left main coronary artery is within the left sinus of the aortic root (Color Plate 19). The left main artery is short, being only about 5 mm long in a medium-size dog. It emerges from the aorta beneath the pulmonary trunk and branches beneath the left auricle into the left circumflex and left anterior descending (cranial [paraconal] interventricular) coronary arteries. In some dogs, an interventricular septal branch (the septal perforator) originates as a separate branch from the left main coronary artery. In most others it originates from the left anterior descending coronary artery. The left circumflex coronary artery first can be visualized in the coronary groove immediately caudal to the left auricle. It continues to encircle the heart between the left atrium and the left ventricle. It terminates by diving ventrally at the caudal aspect of the heart as the caudal interventricular branch. The left circumflex coronary artery has branches that supply most of the left atrium and the caudolateral left ventricular free wall. The major ventricular branches can be seen as they descend from the atrioventricular groove along the lateral wall. The left anterior descending coronary artery can first be visualized emerging from beneath the tip of the left auricle, descending to the apex. It also gives off branches that fan out as they descend toward the apex. The left anterior descending coronary artery often curves around immediately cranial to the apex and may anastomose with the caudal interventricular branch. The left anterior descending coronary artery supplies the craniolateral free wall of the left ventricle and part of the cranial interventricular septum and right ventricular outflow tract. The septal branch enters the interventricular septum and runs apically, giving off branches along its course.

The smaller right coronary artery originates from the right coronary ostium. It mimics the course of the left circumflex coronary artery, lying in the right atrioventricular groove. Its course first can be visualized as it emerges beneath the caudal aspect of the right auricle. The right coronary artery supplies about two thirds of the right ventricular free wall with blood. It also supplies the right atrium and portions of the proximal aorta and pulmonary artery. A larger atrial branch supplies the sinoatrial node.

THE CORONARY VEINS

The great cardiac vein initially ascends from the apex of the heart along with the left anterior descending coronary artery and then circles the heart in the atrioventricular groove, along with the left circumflex coronary artery. It empties into the caudal aspect of the body of the right atrium. The dilated terminal opening of the great cardiac vein where it empties into the right atrium is the coronary sinus (Color Plate 12). The coronary sinus can be catheterized. When a catheter is manipulated into the coronary sinus, it can be seen to wrap around the backside of the heart on fluoroscopy. The dorsal or caudal vein of the left ventricle and the oblique vein of the left atrium enter the terminal portion of the great cardiac vein before it enters the right atrium. The oblique vein of the left atrium is a vestige of the embryonic left cardinal vein, as is the coronary sinus, which can remain patent to form a persistent cranial vena cava. Several other smaller cardiac veins exist as paired structures that lie on either side of the arteries.

REFERENCES

1. Los JA: Embryology. In Watson H, ed: *Pediatric cardiology,* London, 1968, Lloyd Luke Ltd.
2. Anderson RH, Ashley GT: Anatomic development of the cardiovascular system. In Davies J, Dobbing J, eds: *Scientific foundations of pediatrics,* London, 1974, Heinemann.
3. Icardo JM: The growing heart: an anatomical perspective. In Zak R, ed: *Growth of the heart in health and disease,* New York, 1984, Raven.
4. Moore KL: *The developing human,* Philadelphia, 1982, WB Saunders.
5. Noden DM, DeLahunta A: Cardiovascular system. II. Heart. In Noden DM, DeLahunta A, eds: *The embryology of domestic animals: developmental mechanisms and malformations,* Baltimore, 1985, Williams & Wilkins.
6. Netter FH: Embryology. In Yonkman FF, Netter FH, eds: *The Ciba collection of medical illustrations: the heart,* vol 5, Rochester, NY, 1974, Case-Hoyt Corp.
7. Noden DM, DeLahunta A: Cardiovascular system. I. Blood and arteries. In Noden DM, DeLahunta A, eds: *The embryology of domestic animals: developmental mechanisms and malformations.* Baltimore, 1985, Williams & Wilkins.
8. Manasek FJ: Embryonic development of the heart. I. A light and electron microscopic study of myocardial development in the chick embryo, *J Morphol* 25:329, 1968.
9. Friedman WF: Congenital heart disease in infancy and childhood. In Braunwald E, ed: *Heart disease: a textbook of cardiovascular medicine,* ed 4, Philadelphia, 1992, WB Saunders.
10. House EW, Ederstrom HE: Anatomical changes with age in the heart and ductus arteriosus in the dog after birth, *Anat Rec* 160:289, 1968.
11. Bishop SP: Developmental anatomy of the heart and great vessels. In Fox PR, ed: *Canine and feline cardiology,* New York, 1988, Churchill Livingstone.
12. Rogers KS, Walker MA: Disorders of the mediastinum, *Compend Contin Educ Pract Vet* 19:69, 1997.
13. Northrup DW, Van Liere EJ, Stickney JC: The effect of age, sex, and body size on the heart weight: body weight ratio in the dog, *Anat Rec* 128:411, 1957.
14. Lee JC, Taylor FN, Downing SE: A comparison of ventricular weights and geometry in newborn, young, and adult mammals, *J Appl Physiol* 38:147, 1975.
15. Kirk GR, Smith DM, Hutcheson DP, et al: Postnatal growth of the dog heart, *J Anat* 119:461, 1975.
16. Anderson WD, Anderson BG: *Atlas of canine anatomy,* Philadelphia, 1994, Lea & Febiger.

CHAPTER 2

Normal Clinical Cardiovascular Physiology

The Cardiovascular System

An enormous amount of literature exists describing normal cardiovascular physiology. The purpose of this chapter is to provide a foundation of the principles that govern cardiovascular performance necessary to engage in clinical practice. More complete and detailed discussions of cardiovascular physiology are found elsewhere.[1-3] The electrical activity of the heart is explained in the chapter on electrocardiography.

The normal cardiovascular system is set up as a circuit (circulatory system). A blood cell can be tracked from one point in the system back to the same point (i.e., it moves in a circle) (Color Plate 20). Two circulations, the systemic circulation and the pulmonary circulation, are joined in series to form the global circulation. Appropriate valves within the normal circulation ensure one-way flow of blood. Oxygenated blood flows from the pulmonary capillaries into the pulmonary veins that drain into the left heart (the left atrium and left ventricle). The left ventricle fills with oxygenated blood when it relaxes (diastole) and pumps the oxygenated blood into the systemic circulation when it contracts (systole) (Figure 2-1). The systemic circulation consists of the aorta, systemic arteries, systemic arterioles, systemic capillaries, and systemic venules and veins. Elastic recoil of large arteries continues to propel blood forward when the heart relaxes (diastole), which makes the circulation more efficient (Color Plate 21).[1] The systemic circulation is a high-pressure system with a mean blood pressure in the large systemic arteries of approximately 100 mm Hg (Figure 2-2). This high pressure is required to maintain blood flow to organs that lie above the heart (i.e., to overcome gravitational forces) and to force blood flow through vascular beds that have high resistance to blood flow (e.g., heart, kidneys, brain). Circulations to various body organs are arranged in parallel. The systemic arterioles provide the greatest resistance to blood flow. This occurs because the arterioles (30 μm) are much smaller in diameter than small arteries (4 mm). Consequently, mean pressure decreases from 100 mm Hg to 20 mm Hg across the systemic arteriolar bed. Arterioles contain smooth muscle that contracts and relaxes to change the resistance to blood flow. Capillaries are 0.5 μm in diameter and made up of only endothelium. Within capillary beds, oxygen diffuses from the blood across this endothelial layer to the mitochondria within the cells and carbon dioxide diffuses into the capillary blood. Deoxygenated blood flows into systemic venules to systemic veins and ultimately to the vena cavae. The vena cavae drain into the right heart (the right atrium and right ventricle). The right ventricle fills and pumps blood into the pulmonary artery and the pulmonary circulation (Figure 2-3). The lung capillary bed has a low resistance to flow. Consequently, the pressure within the pulmonary circulation is much lower than in the systemic circulation, with a mean blood pressure in the pulmonary artery of approximately 15 mm Hg. Oxygen diffuses from the alveoli within the lungs to the capillary blood, and carbon dioxide diffuses into the alveoli to be expelled during exhalation. Average blood flow (mL/min) is the same in the pulmonary circulation and the systemic circulation in the normal animal. Blood volumes (mL) in each circulation, however, are vastly different.

The number and cross-sectional area of vessels increases dramatically from the aorta to the capillaries. In a 20-kg dog, there are about 100,000 arteries, 3 million arterioles, and 3 billion capillaries.[1] The cross-sectional area of the aorta is 3 cm^2; the systemic arteries, 40 cm^2; the systemic arterioles, 55 cm^2; and the capillaries, 1300 cm^2. Because of this change in cross-sectional area, blood flow velocity in the arteries is approximately 10% of aortic flow velocity and in the capillaries is less than 1% of aortic flow velocity. Normal aortic flow velocity is approximately 1 m/sec.

The systemic circulation contains about 80%, the pulmonary circulation about 15%, and the heart about 5% of the total blood volume.[1] The aorta, systemic arteries, and systemic arterioles contain approximately 10% of the total blood volume, and the systemic capillaries contain about 5%. The systemic veins contain the vast majority of the blood volume (65%). Consequently, venoconstriction and venodilation can shift large quantities of blood into or out of other parts of the circulation.

The mammalian cardiovascular system has three basic, yet essential, functions: (1) maintenance of normal hydrostatic pressure in the arteries, (2) maintenance of normal blood flow to tissues, and (3) maintenance of normal hydrostatic pressure in the capillaries and veins. If normal values for these variables are present at rest and during exercise, the cardiovascular system is usually defined as functioning normally. The normally high hydrostatic pressure in the systemic arteries is required to ensure normal flow through the organ vascular beds that have a high innate resistance to blood flow (e.g., brain, kidney, heart) and to maintain flow to organs above the heart (e.g., brain). For example, systemic arterial blood pressure is approximately twice as high in giraffes as in other mammals to maintain normal brain blood flow despite the exaggerated height of the brain above the heart in this species.[2] A normal blood flow is required to: (1) deliver oxygen and other nutrient transport to the tissues (2) remove metabolic waste (e.g., carbon dioxide) from the tissues, and (3) transport messages (hormonal) from one part of the body to the other. Normal venous and capillary pressures are needed to prevent edema formation. In addition, the physical components of the cardiovascular system possess important endocrine, autocrine, and apocrine functions.

The overall performance of the heart rests on a delicate and balanced interplay between the inotropic state of the heart (contrac-

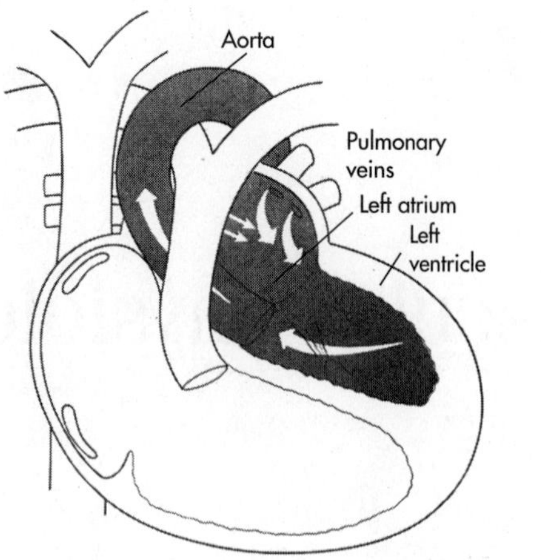

FIGURE 2-1 During systole, the left ventricle contracts and pushes blood into the aorta and through the systemic circulation. The left atrium continues to fill during ventricular systole. (Redrawn From Phillips RE, Feeney MK: *Cardiac rhythms: a systematic approach to interpretation,* ed 3, Philadelphia, 1990, WB Saunders.)

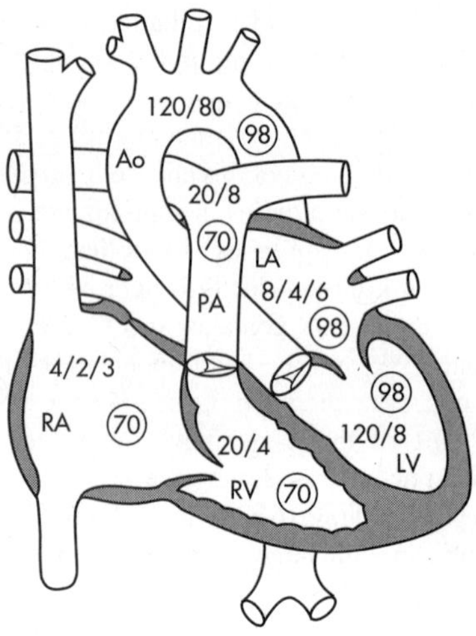

FIGURE 2-2 Normal pressures (systolic/diastolic/mean) and oxygen saturations (in circles) in the chambers of the heart, systemic circulation, and pulmonary circulation. *RA,* right atrium; *RV,* right ventricle; *PA,* pulmonary artery; *LA,* left atrium; *LV,* left ventricle; *Ao,* aorta.

tility), forces opposing the pumping action of the heart (afterload), and forces acting to fill the heart during its quiescent phase (preload). Cardiac performance is influenced by several factors, including heart rate, ventriculoatrial coupling, ventricular synchrony, and pericardial properties, and may be further modified by neural control, drugs, hormones, and metabolic products. In cardiovascular disease, hypertrophy is a major influence on ventricular performance.

The Cardiac Cycle

The heart contracts and relaxes in a cyclical fashion (Figure 2-4) in response to electrical depolarization of cells and calcium movements within the cell. The period of ventricular contraction is termed *systole,* and the period of relaxation is called *diastole.* Systole and diastole are further divided into phases of cardiac activity. Although atria also have periods of systole and diastole, this discussion focuses on ventricular contraction and relaxation. The left ventricle is used as the example in this discussion. The right ventricular cardiac cycle is similar.

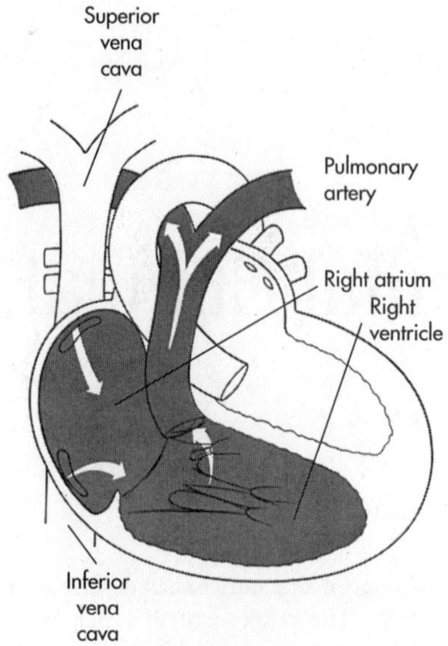

FIGURE 2-3 In systole the right ventricle pumps blood into the pulmonary artery and through the pulmonary circulation. The right atrium fills as blood returns from the systemic veins into the cranial (superior) and caudal (inferior) vena cavae. (Redrawn from Phillips RE, Feeney MK: *Cardiac rhythms: a systematic approach to interpretation,* ed 3, Philadelphia, 1990, WB Saunders.)

SYSTOLE

The end of diastole and the beginning of systole coincide. During diastole the left ventricle fills to maximum volume (Figure 2-5). The volume in the left ventricle at this stage is the end-diastolic volume (EDV). Electrical systole precedes mechanical systole and is recorded as the onset of the QRS complex on the electrocardiogram. At the onset of ventricular mechanical systole, the myocardium tenses and pressure begins to rise within the ventricular chamber. When the ventricle tenses, blood moves toward the path of least resistance—toward the mitral valve orifice. This drags the mitral valve leaflets upward and forces the mitral valve closed as left ventricular pressure exceeds left atrial pressure (Figure 2-6). The first heart sound occurs at this point. For a short time (30 to 50 msec) after mitral closure, both the mitral and aortic valves are closed. Because blood is an incompressible fluid, the blood volume within the chamber cannot change during this phase. Consequently, this initial phase of systole is called *isovolumic* or *isovolumetric* systole or contraction. It is characterized by a rapid increase in intraventricular pressure. The velocity of the pressure rise (dP/dt) during isovolumic systole is a sensitive but nonspecific measure of myocardial contractile function. Isovolumic systole lasts until the aortic valve is forced open. The aortic valve opens when the ventricle is able to generate enough force to overcome forces opposing its contraction. This occurs when or slightly before pressure in the left ventricle exceeds aortic pressure. The opening of the aortic valve heralds the onset of ventricular ejection. Ejection lasts until the end of systole, when the aortic valve closes. At this stage the ventricle achieves the smallest possible volume for that systolic interval. This volume is the end-systolic volume (ESV). The EDV minus the ESV is the total stroke volume (TSV) of the ventricle, the amount of blood ejected

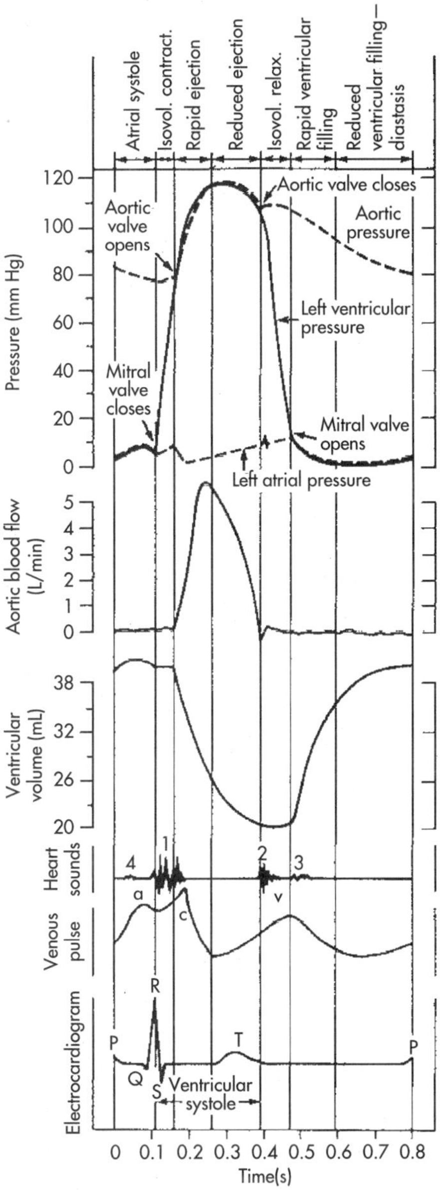

FIGURE 2-4 Schematic drawings of left heart pressures, aortic flow, left ventricular volume, heart sounds, venous pressure, and electrocardiogram on the same time scale. Events within the cardiac cycle are labeled. (From Berne RM, Levy MN: *Cardiovascular physiology,* ed 7, St Louis, 1992, Mosby.)

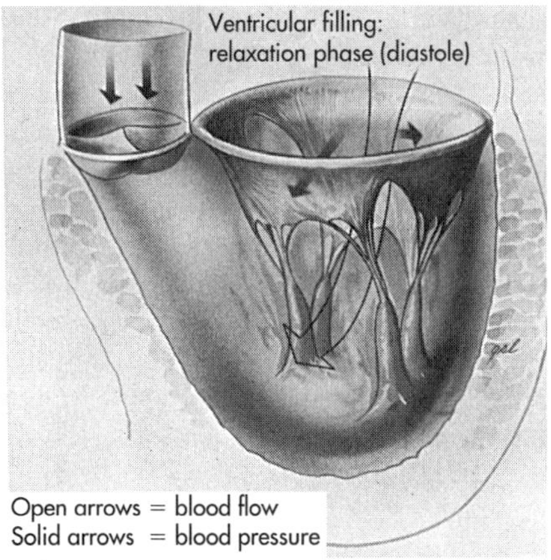

FIGURE 2-5 During ventricular diastole, blood flows from the left atrium into the left ventricle through the open mitral valve when the left ventricular diastolic pressure equalizes with the left atrial pressure. The aortic valve is closed when aortic pressure exceeds left ventricular diastolic pressure. (From Phillips RE, Feeney MK: *Cardiac rhythms: a systematic approach to interpretation,* ed 3, Philadelphia, 1990, WB Saunders.)

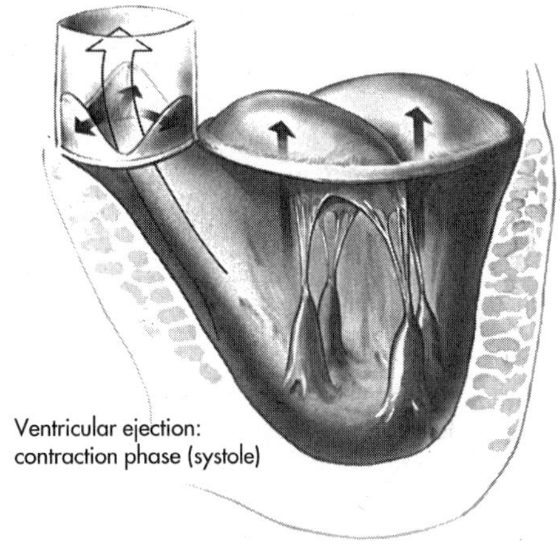

FIGURE 2-6 During ventricular systole, the mitral valve closes when left ventricular pressure exceeds left atrial pressure, and the aortic valve opens and blood flows into the aorta when left ventricular systolic pressure equalizes with aortic pressure. Arrows are as in Figure 2-5. (From Phillips RE, Feeney MK: *Cardiac rhythms: a systematic approach to interpretation,* ed 3, Philadelphia, 1990, WB Saunders.)

during systole. Aortic valve closure is generally considered the end of systole and the onset of diastole. However, actual sarcomere (contractile element) relaxation probably occurs slightly before this event. The end of systole occurs immediately after the T wave on the electrocardiogram. The second heart sound coincides with aortic valve closure.

DIASTOLE

Once the aortic valve closes, both valves are closed again for a short period. Again, volume cannot change, so this period of early diastolic relaxation is called *isovolumic* or *isovolumetric* relaxation. It is characterized by a rapid decrease in intraventricular pressure. Its rate of fall is primarily determined by the rapidity of calcium movement off the contractile proteins. When ventricular force decreases to the point that blood is no longer forced against the mitral valve leaflets, the leaflets open. This allows blood to rush from the atrium to the ventricle at the time that left ventricular and left atrial pressures equalize. This heralds the start of the rapid ventricular filling phase of diastole. Rapid ventricular filling occurs during early diastole as atrial blood 'dumps' into the ventricle. In a dog or a cat with a slow heart rate, this phase can best be appreciated by examining an M-mode echocardiogram of the mitral valve. Rapid ventricular filling occurs during the time that the mitral valve opens wide in early diastole. Filling peaks at the E point on the mitral valve M-mode recording and then decreases rapidly. A third heart sound (gallop sound) may be heard in a patient with cardiac disease at or near the peak of rapid ventricular filling. Immediately following rapid ventricular filling is slow ventricular filling. This phase does not occur in a patient with a fast heart rate when diastole is shortened. On an M-mode echocardiogram, the mitral valve leaflets drift partially closed as blood flow through the mitral valve orifice slows. Atrial systole occurs next and follows the P wave on the electrocardiogram. Atrial systole forces more blood into the ventricle, contributing about 20% of the filling volume in a normal animal. In a patient with a slow heart rate, the mitral valve has time to drift partially closed and atrial systole reopens the valve. This is observed on an M-mode echocardiogram as the A point. In patients with a fast heart rate, rapid ventricular filling and atrial systole occur very close together, resulting in the mitral valve opening only once during diastole. In a canine or feline patient with cardiac disease, atrial systole may create a low-frequency sound, the fourth heart sound (gallop sound).

Myocardial Metabolism

Myocardial metabolism is similar to metabolism in all other parts of the body. This section focuses on the unique aspects of myocardial metabolism. The reader is referred to other sources for a more complete discussion of general metabolism.[3]

Metabolism, more specifically catabolism, is the process of breaking larger molecules down into smaller molecules. Catabolism of glycogen to pyruvate and fatty acids to acetyl-CoA provide the basic substrates for producing high-energy phosphate bonds to produce the large amount of mechanical work performed by the heart. Fatty acids are the major source of energy in the heart. The central role of ATP as an energy source for contraction and the limited energy reserves in the heart require a high rate of ATP production. As much as 5% of the total ATP and creatine phosphate are consumed with each beat, and the glycogen and triglyceride stores in the heart are able to support cardiac function for no more than 6 to 12 minutes if they are not replaced.[4] These processes require a continuous supply of oxygen, because anaerobic glycolysis can supply no more than 5% to 7% of normal energy requirements through the metabolism of pyruvate to lactate. Myocardial oxygen consumption is primarily determined by a basal requirement, myocardial contractility, systolic wall stress, and heart rate. It correlates on a per beat basis to the area within a pressure or wall stress–volume loop.[5] Basal oxygen consumption in a noncontracting heart is only about 20% of that of the contracting organ.[6]

Metabolism can be organized into three steps: (1) cellular acquisition of substrate, (2) the use of substrates to produce ATP, and (3) processes that govern the use of ATP. Catabolic pathways allow for the processing of each of the major energy substrates to produce ATP. Flux through these pathways is governed by availability of the substrate and by enzymatic activities.

CARBOHYDRATE METABOLISM

Carbohydrate metabolism in cardiac muscle is no different from that in other tissues and involves five main processes.[7] (1) *Glucose* is carried across the cell membrane by facilitated diffusion, the rate of which is increased by insulin, anoxia, and increased cardiac work. (2) *Glycogen synthesis* occurs when excess glucose in the cytoplasm is converted to glycogen, a large insoluble carbohydrate polymer. Cardiac glycogen quantities are constant but in a constant state of turnover. Glycogen stores increase during fasting and decrease in the fed state, probably in response to blood fatty acid concentration. (3) *Glycogenolysis* occurs when glycogen is broken down by the concerted action of two enzymes to yield glucose. The breakdown is stimulated by cyclic AMP or by a decrease in intracellular high-energy phosphate concentration. (4) *Glycolysis* occurs when glucose is degraded to pyruvate within the cytoplasm. This series of ten reactions is the centerpiece of CH_20 metabolism. The process yields two pyruvate molecules and a net production of two ATP. NADH is also produced. The ATP production occurs whether or not oxygen is present. Pyruvate is converted to lactate when oxygen is not present. When oxygen is present, pyruvate is converted to acetyl CoA that enters the citric acid (Krebs) cycle. (5) *Pyruvate metabolism* occurs when pyruvate is metabolized within the mitochondria aerobically to acetyl-CoA, anaerobically to lactate, or anaerobically to alanine. Acetyl-CoA then enters the Krebs cycle.

Carbohydrate metabolism is controlled by changes in workload, substrate availability, and hormonal status. Under resting conditions, except after a carbohydrate meal, both glycogenolysis and glycolysis are inhibited and cardiac muscle preferentially uses fatty acids as energy substrates.

LIPID METABOLISM

In the resting postabsorptive state, the principle energy source for the heart is free fatty acid (FA). Long-chain FAs are transported in the bloodstream bound to albumin. FA uptake by the cell is passive. Uptake is controlled by the circulating FA concentration and the circulating molar ratio of FA to its carrier albumin.

Intracellular FAs are stored by an FA–binding protein and are converted to FA-acyl-CoA by thiokinase that requires ATP, reduced CoA, and Mg. FA-acyl-CoA is either converted to triglycerides or combined with carnitine by carnitine acyl transferase I to produce acyl carnitine. This is transported across the outer mitochondrial membrane.[7] Acyl carnitine is transported across the inner mitochondrial membrane by carnitine translocase. Once in the mitochondria, acyl carnitine is converted back to acyl-CoA by carnitine acyl transferase II. Acyl-CoA is then converted to acetyl-CoA by beta oxidation, also producing some ATP. The acetyl-CoA is metabolized in the Krebs cycle to produce ATP.

Ketone bodies (acetoacetate and β-hydroxybutyrate) may also be metabolized by the heart to produce ATP. Generally, they are not an important source of energy but may be used during starvation or diabetic ketoacidosis.

FINAL COMMON PATHWAYS

Most energy production in the myocardium is ultimately funneled through two common pathways (under aerobic conditions): the Krebs cycle and oxidative phosphorylation. The Krebs cycle is the final pathway for oxidation of acetyl-CoA produced from pyruvate, from beta oxidation of FAs, and from acetoacetate. This is a series of reactions that results in the oxidation of acetyl-CoA to carbon dioxide and water within the mitochondrial matrix. These reactions produce a small number of ATP molecules. More importantly they are responsible for producing the majority of the reducing equivalents (NADH and $FADH_2$) for the respiratory (electron transport) chain. The respiratory chain is the site of the oxidative phosphorylation of ADP to ATP. It consists of a sequence of hydrogen and electron carriers on the inner mitochondrial membrane.[7] Hydrogen is removed from NADH by NADH dehydrogenase (a flavoprotein). NADH dehydrogenase is oxidized by ubiquinone (coenzyme Q), and the electron from hydrogen is transferred to the first portion of the electron transport chain. The proton is donated from the mitochondrial membrane to the surrounding medium. The electron carriers are iron-containing hemoproteins or cytochromes, which transfer electrons by alternating between reduced and oxidized states (ferric and ferrous forms). Cytochrome oxidase within the chain reduces oxygen, and the proton generated by the oxidation of ubiquinone combines with the reduced hydrogen to form water. During electron transfer along the respiratory chain, three ADP molecules are phosphorylated to form ATP. The exact mechanism by which ADP phosphorylation is coupled to the respiratory chain is unknown. This process releases a great deal of energy, most of which is conserved through the coupled production of ATP. The net result is that one molecule of glucose yields 38 molecules of ATP during aerobic metabolism. Total oxidation of glucose to CO_2 and water yields 686,000 cal/mole. Only 56,000 cal/mole are produced with anaerobic metabolism. Once ATP is formed, it is immediately converted to phosphocreatine by creatine kinase in the mitochondria.[7] Phosphocreatine can then be transferred throughout the cytosol to sites of usage, where another creatine kinase converts it back to ATP.

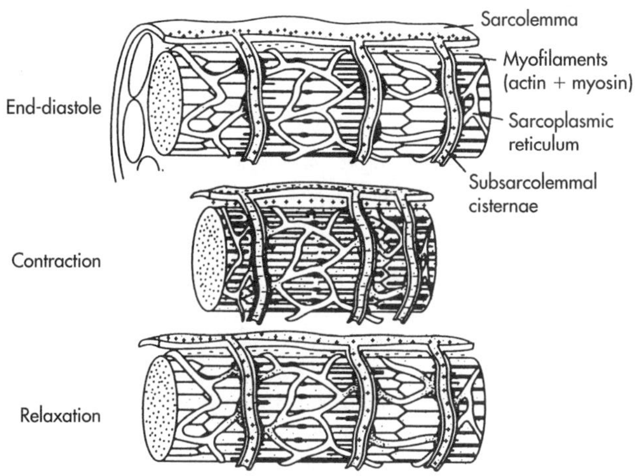

FIGURE 2-7 Schematic drawing of the myofibrils within a myocyte contracting and relaxing. The changes in membrane electrical charge *(+/–)* and calcium ion concentration *(dots)* are indicated. (From Giuliani EM, Gersh BJ, McGoon MD et al, eds: *Mayo clinic practice of cardiology,* St Louis, 1996, Mosby.)

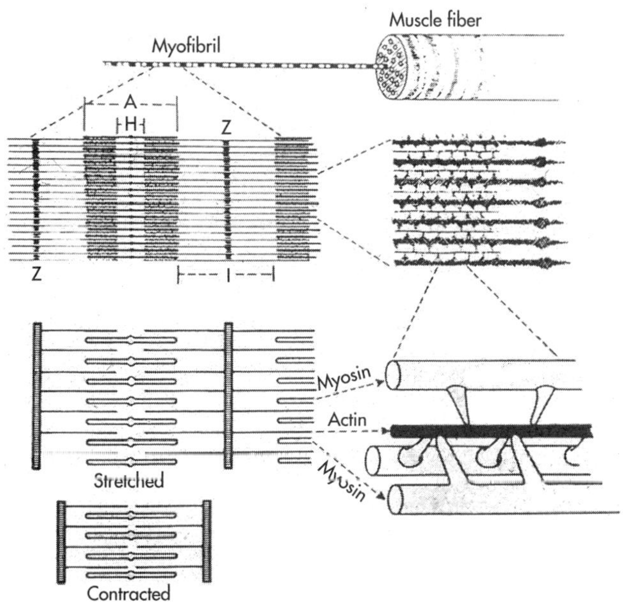

FIGURE 2-8 Schematic diagram of the ultrastructure of myofibrils and sarcomeres (myofilaments). The sarcomere is depicted in a relaxed (stretched) and contracted state. It is made up of actin and myosin, which overlap and interact to form the A, H and I bands and Z lines. (From Myerson RM, Pastor BH: *Congestive heart failure,* St Louis, 1967, Mosby.)

Ultrastructure of Cardiac Muscle

The cardiac muscle is composed of myocytes and a connective tissue matrix. Each myocyte has a sarcolemma (cell membrane) and consists of numerous myofibrils (contractile elements, or sarcomeres, connected in series) that are incompletely separated by clefts of cytoplasm containing mitochondria and membranous T tubules (Figure 2-7). The myofibrils constitute about 50% of the myocyte mass. There are also centrally located nuclei (usually two/cell), a complex sarcoplasmic reticulum, and numerous mitochondria (located in close apposition to myofibrils and just under the sarcolemma). Cardiac myocytes are arranged as a syncytium, with the cells connected through intercalated discs. The heart is divided by a fibrous ring into a ventricular syncytium and an atrial syncytium.

Myofibrils are composed of longitudinally repeating sarcomeres, the fundamental contractile unit of striated muscle (Figure 2-8). A sarcomere is delineated at each end by a Z line. The thin actin filaments project from the Z lines toward the center. The larger, thick myosin filaments, which project from the center of the sarcomere (M line), array themselves longitudinally with the actin filaments. Resting sarcomere length ranges from 1.6 to 2.2 μm, depending in part on the resting tension exerted on the muscle.

Cardiac muscle is striated muscle. The striations are due to the overlap of contractile filaments (actin and myosin) in the sarcomere (Figure 2-9). The region of overlap, the darker area, is the A band. A lighter area, the I band, is the region where only thin filaments (actin) are present. The H band, also lighter, is the region where only thick filaments (myosin) are present. The thin filaments overlap and interdigitate in a tetragonal array at the Z line, held together by cross

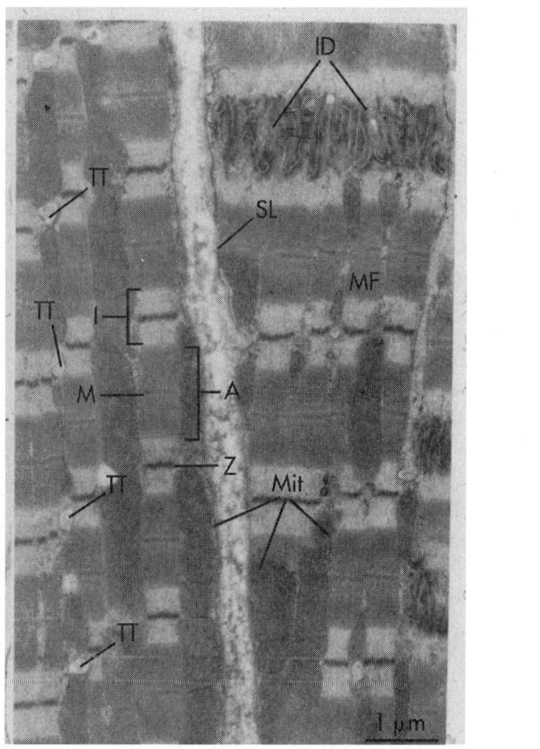

FIGURE 2-9 Medium-magnification photomicrograph of myofibrils within monkey ventricular myocytes. The A and I bands and Z lines are labeled as in Figure 2-8. T tubules *(TT)* are situated near the Z bands of adjoining sarcomeres. The interwoven nature of an intercalated disc *(ID)* can be seen. Mitochondria *(Mit)* and the sarcolemma *(SL)* are labeled. (From Berne RM, Levy MN: *Cardiovascular physiology,* ed 7, St Louis, 1992, Mosby.)

connecting Z filaments. The thin filaments, in turn, form a hexagonal array around each thick filament, each being equidistant from three myosin filaments. Other filaments containing titan and nebulin appear to link thick filaments and Z bands in skeletal muscle and resist movements of thick filaments away from the center of the sarcomere and limit sarcomere distension.

Contractile Proteins and Sarcomere Contraction

THICK FILAMENTS

Thick filaments are composed of myosin molecules arranged in parallel. Each myosin molecule consists of a tail that confers stability and two globular heads that hydrolyze ATP and interact with actin (Color Plate 22). Myosin is composed of heavy chains and light chains. The heavy chains coil around each other to form an α-helical tail that divides to form two globular heads. Two light chains bind to the head at the region where the head joins the tail. Each globular head has a site for ATP binding and hydrolysis and a separate site for actin binding.

Myosin molecules aggregate in a particular pattern to form thick filaments that are 1.6 μm in length. Each filament contains 300 to 400 myosin heads. The heads project laterally and are directed toward the ends of the filament (six heads in each 43 nM). The middle portion of the filament is smooth where the tails of the myosin molecules are closely packed together.

Myosin can be separated into three isoenzyme components—V_1, V_2, and V_3—that have different heavy chain composition. Two chemically distinct heavy chains exist: α and β. V_1 and V_3 are composed of two α-chains and two β-chains, respectively, and V_2 is a heterodimer ($\alpha\beta$). V_1 myosin ATPase activity in the head region is high, and intrinsic muscle contraction speed is fast; whereas V_3 ATPase activity is lower and speed is slower. Abnormal conditions such as hypertrophy and thyroid imbalances alter the levels of myosin isoenzymes. Normal human and canine adult myocardium contains primarily the V_3 isoenzyme.

Myosin-binding protein C is a protein associated with the rod portion of myosin. It wraps around myosin transversely as 10-nM wide proteins at 43-nM intervals. The protein appears to bridge the gap between myosin and actin. Its physiologic action may be to help prevent interaction of myosin and actin at low calcium concentration.[8]

THIN FILAMENTS

Each thin filament contains three major proteins: (1) two strands of fibrous actin; (2) tropomyosin, which stretches along each strand of actin; and (3) a large globular protein, troponin. The actin filament is a double α-helix of two strands of F-actin. Each F-actin is composed of multiple globular units (G-actin monomers). G-actin monomers spontaneously assemble into F-actin at physiologic concentrations of ATP and Mg^{++}. Actin interacts with the globular heads of myosin to form cross-bridges during contraction. Actin is about 1 μm in length and projects inward from the Z lines that anchor the actin filaments.

Troponin and tropomyosin are regulatory proteins. Tropomyosin is a rod-shaped, fibrous molecule formed as a double-stranded α-helical polypeptide chain. In diastole, tropomyosin filaments lie just outside each of the two major grooves formed by the twisted actin filaments. Troponin is a globular protein that contains three functionally distinctive peptides, TnI, TnC, and TnT. Troponin is located at intervals of 365 nM along the actin filament. Troponin C binds calcium and causes a conformational change in tropomyosin; troponin I inhibits the magnesium-stimulated actomyosin ATPase; troponin T attaches troponin to tropomyosin.

MECHANICS OF SARCOMERE CONTRACTION

In the resting state, tropomyosin blocks the myosin binding sites on the actin filament. The binding of calcium to troponin C displaces troponin I, causing a conformational change in tropomyosin. This exposes actin to the binding sites on the globular myosin heads. Without ATP, actin and myosin bind avidly to each other (affinity of myosin for actin = 10^7 M^{-1}). This occurs during severe hypoxia, ischemia, or death and results in rigor. In the presence of ATP, the affinity is much less (10^4 M^{-1}). ATP is cleaved by the myosin ATPase when actin and myosin are allowed to interact. When P_i is liberated, the affinity of myosin for actin increases to 10^6 M^{-1}, meaning that myosin and actin bind together at this step. It is assumed that the energy derived from the hydrolysis of ATP at this step is used for force generation and movement of the myosin molecules. It is also assumed that the myosin molecule moves like a ratchet with the hinge points on myosin flexing during binding and stretching again when detached to find another binding site. Detachment occurs when the ADP and P_i are released and a new ATP is bound to the myosin head to cause actin and myosin to dissociate. If high enough concentrations of calcium are present, the cycle repeats, with the myosin continuing to ratchet and the sarcomere continuing to shorten. The motion produced by one cycle is very small and must be repetitive to cause significant shortening. If calcium concentration falls, the calcium displaces off troponin and tropomyosin again blocks the active sites on the actin filament and the muscle relaxes. The force of isometric contraction and the rate of sarcomere shortening during isotonic contraction are related to the number of cross-bridges and therefore the calcium concentration.

EXCITATION-CONTRACTION COUPLING

Calcium channels in the cell membrane. A complete understanding of excitation-contraction (E-C) coupling has not yet been achieved. Overall, however, the processes are reasonably well understood.[9] The process involves both calcium fluxes across the cell membrane and calcium fluxes within the cell (Figure 2-10). Normally, extracellular calcium concentration is in the millimolar range, and cytosolic concentration is about 10,000 times lower. Consequently, a large chemical gradient for calcium entry into the cell exists. Calcium can only move into the cell through channels. These channels are closed during diastole. E-C coupling starts with L-type calcium channels opening. L (long-lasting)-type calcium channels act as calcium conduits across the cell membrane. They are inactivated, or "blocked," by dihydropyridine compounds, such as nifedipine, as well as phenylalkylamines, such as verapamil, and benzothiazepines, such as diltiazem. The cardiac cell membrane also contains a few T-type calcium channels that probably do not contribute to E-C coupling. The structure of L-type calcium channels is complex. They contain five protein subunits. The α_1 subunit is the active unit in that it forms the pore through which calcium enters the cell. It contains four repeated units of homology, and each repeat contains five hydrophobic helices and one positively charged hydrophilic helix. The positively charged helix is thought to sense a change in voltage during depolarization. L-type calcium channels in the cell membrane open during phase 2 of the action potential, when the membrane channel is no longer negative. This voltage-related event allows a small amount of calcium to cross from the extracellular space into a localized region of the cell. This amount of calcium is not enough to cause muscle contraction. Instead, it is thought that the calcium that crosses during this phase stimulates intracellular structures to release more calcium. The primary

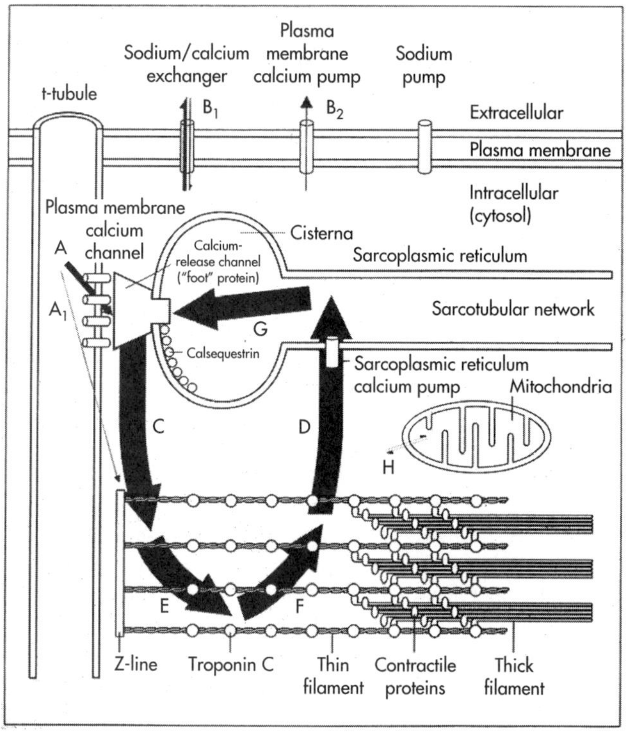

FIGURE 2-10 Schematic drawing of the sarcolemma (plasma membrane), sarcoplasmic reticulum (SR), and sarcomeric proteins (actin, myosin, troponin C) and the contraction-activating calcium movement within the cell. Calcium enters the myocyte, primarily from T tubules, when voltage-regulated L-type (plasma membrane) calcium channels open during phase 2 of the action potential. The SR releases calcium in response, increasing intracellular calcium concentration. Calcium ions bind to troponin C, creating a conformational change in the tropomyosin, allowing actin and myosin to interact and contract. In diastole, the SR calcium pump pumps calcium ions into the SR, decreasing intracellular calcium concentration to a diastolic level. Calcium no longer binds to troponin, and tropomyosin conforms to prevent actin and myosin from interacting. Relaxation of the myofilament occurs. Excess calcium that entered the cell to trigger the SR calcium release is extruded from the cell by the Na-Ca exchanger. (From Braunwald E: *Atlas of heart diseases: heart failure—cardiac function and dysfunction,* St Louis, 1995, Mosby.)

structure that binds and releases this additional calcium is the sarcoplasmic reticulum.

The sarcoplasmic reticulum. The sarcoplasmic reticulum (SR) in mammalian myocardium is a membrane-limited structure that forms a network within the cell that surrounds the myofibrils, running longitudinally to the myofibrils (see Figure 2-7). The inside of the SR does not directly communicate with the extracellular space or the cytoplasm. The function of the SR is to actively pump calcium into its lumen, to store calcium in diastole, and to release calcium in systole. The SR's membrane has two proteins to accomplish these tasks, a Ca-ATPase pump and a calcium release channel.[10] The Ca-ATPase protein is a single-chain polypeptide with high-affinity calcium-binding sites and both high- and low-affinity ATP-binding sites. The Ca-ATPase pump is activated by high intracellular calcium concentration and actively pumps calcium into the SR in diastole. This rapidly decreases the intracellular calcium concentration to approximately 10^{-7} M. Proteins within the SR, primarily calsequestrin, bind calcium once it is pumped into the lumen. Calsequestrin has a strong negative charge. Binding affinity is low and binding capacity is high, allowing for rapid movement of large amounts of calcium in and out of the SR. Calcium release channels lie within the SR membrane to act as a conduit for calcium release from the SR. Their structure differs considerably from L-type calcium channels. They are stimulated by calcium that enters through the L-type calcium channels to rapidly release calcium in systole to increase intracellular calcium concentration to approximately 10^{-5} M (100-fold change from diastole to systole). Because ryanodine interacts with the calcium-release channel, this channel is also known as the ryanodine receptor. The SR has close associations with the transverse tubular system (T system). T tubules are continuous with the cell membrane and so communicate with the extracellular space. The T tubule system runs perpendicular to the long axis of the myocardial cell. The T tubules and the SR come into close contact at the Z line, where they form "triads." Triads consist of a T tubule with terminal sections of the SR on either side. These terminal portions of SR are called *junctional* SR. The junctional SR membrane and the T-tubular membrane are separated by a 12-nM gap. This gap is bridged by so-called foot proteins that have been identified as calcium-release channels. About seven calcium-release channels are present for every L-type calcium channel in the T tubule along this junction. Because of the close association between these two structures at this point, it is believed that calcium entering through the L-type calcium channels in the T-tubules at the Z lines stimulates calcium release from the SR through the calcium-release channels in the junctional SR.

Once calcium is released by the SR, intracellular calcium concentration increases rapidly. At this higher calcium concentration, calcium binds to troponin C. Calcium binding to this site results in a conformational change in the troponin-tropomyosin complex. This results in tropomyosin no longer inhibiting actin from interacting with myosin, as follows. At low calcium concentration, TnI binds tightly to actin and interacts closely with TnT and tropomyosin. When calcium interacts with TnC, TnC binds tightly to TnI. This weakens the TnI-actin interaction and changes the TnT-TnI-actin interaction in such a way that the actin myofilaments move deeper into the groove of the thin filament, exposing actin to the actin-binding sites on the globular head of myosin.[11] When this occurs in the presence of ATP, sarcomere contraction occurs. Repolarization results in the calcium channels on the cell membrane and T tubules and the calcium-release channels on the SR closing. The SR then actively pumps calcium back into its space, resulting in myocardial relaxation.

Sodium-Calcium exchange. Calcium that enters the cell through the L-type calcium channels during systole must exit the cell during diastole to maintain homeostasis. The sodium-calcium exchange system in the cell membrane is the primary mechanism for the cell to extrude calcium in diastole.[12] This system is located primarily in the T tubules and exchanges three sodium ions for one calcium ion moving in the opposite direction. It can move calcium in either direction. However, because intracellular sodium concentration is kept low by the Na^+, K^+-ATPase pumps, calcium is primarily moved out of the cell. About 20% of the calcium released by the SR is moved out of the cell with each beat. Because of the large quantities of calcium extruded via this mechanism over time, small changes in the function of this system can be very important to regulating calcium movement within the cell and so to contractile performance. The cardiac sodium/calcium exchanger is activated by intracellular calcium concentration and by intracellular ATP and inactivated by intracellular sodium. The sodium-calcium exchange mechanism is very sensitive to intracellular sodium concentration. The effect of intracellular sodium on blocking calcium efflux is a square function and its effect on contractility is proportional to the sixth or seventh power. Digitalis glycosides take advantage of this mechanism. By poisoning Na, K-ATPase pumps, intracellular sodium concentration increases, which inactivates the pump, decreasing calcium efflux, and increasing contractility (Figure 2-11).

CELLULAR REGULATION OF MYOCARDIAL FORCE GENERATION

The number of active cross-bridges (actin-myosin interaction sites) determines the force of contraction that occurs. In a normal heart, enough calcium is released from the SR to bring the myofilaments to 10% to 25% of full activation.[11] This means there is the ability to recruit more cross-bridges and so alter force generation.

One means of recruiting more cross-bridges is to increase the amount of calcium released from the SR in systole. Increased calcium release translates into a higher intracellular concentration of calcium, resulting in more troponin-calcium interaction. The greater this interaction, the more cross-bridges that will form. The amount of calcium that enters through the L-type calcium channels is one regulatory mechanism for determining the amount of calcium released by the SR.[13] L-type calcium channels are regulated by several factors. Cyclic AMP-mediated protein kinase phosphorylation of modulating regions of the calcium channel protein results in a channel becoming functional.[14] Consequently, it is thought that channels that are not phosphorylated do not function as well. Catecholamines are the primary activators of cyclic AMP in clinical situations. A calmodulin-mediated protein kinase also phosphorylates the L-type calcium channel but at another site.

Calmodulin is a high-affinity calcium-binding protein that belongs to the same family as troponin C.[15] It responds to transient increases in cytosolic free calcium concentration that result from cell activation by extracellular signals such as hormones, neurotransmitters, and membrane depolarization. Calmodulin has many functions, one of which is to activate cyclic nucleotide phosphodiesterase. Cyclic GMP has an opposite effect to cyclic AMP on the L-type calcium channel, presumably through phosphorylation of yet another regulatory protein. Acidosis also affects slow calcium channels. Function is depressed or blocked at pHs between 6.1 and 6.8. Fast sodium channels are not blocked at this pH, resulting in electromechanical dissociation.

Calcium release also varies with the amount of calcium stored within the SR in diastole (i.e., increased calcium uptake and storage in diastole results in more calcium for release in systole). Calcium storage is primarily controlled by the calcium ATPase pump that actively pumps calcium into the SR during diastole.[10] Catecholamines (e.g., epinephrine, norepinephrine) are primary regulators of calcium movement into the SR. They primarily act to alter this movement and so myocardial contractility by stimulating β-adrenergic receptors. β-Adrenergic receptors are protein structures that lie within the sarcolemma. The receptor protein spans the cell membrane 7 times and has a long intracytoplasmic portion between spanning segments 5 and 6.[16] The receptor is coupled to GTP-binding (G) proteins in the cell membrane.[17] The two GTP-binding proteins are G_s and G_i. The intrinsic GTPase activities of these two G proteins are activated by stimulatory and inhibitory hormones. β-Adrenergic receptors stimulate G_s, which activates adenyl cyclase activity in the cell membrane, which acts on ATP to form cyclic AMP. Cyclic AMP goes on to stimulate cAMP-dependent protein kinase within the cell. The calcium ATPase pump activity is closely regulated by phospholamban, another SR membrane protein. There appears to be a protein-protein interaction between the calcium ATPase pump and phospholamban. Catecholamine-induced increases in intracellular cyclic AMP result in stimulation of cAMP-dependent protein kinase that phosphorylates a serine residue on phospholamban. Phosphorylation at this site results in enhanced calcium ATPase pump activity. Phospholamban may act as an inhibitor of the calcium ATPase pump in its dephosphorylated state such that phosphorylation results in a release of the inhibition. Calmodulin stimulates activation of another protein kinase that interacts at a separate but specific site on phospholamban that produces similar responses. Stimulation of the calcium ATPase pump results initially in faster relaxation as the calcium is removed from the cytoplasm and troponin more rapidly. This is quickly followed by an increase in contractility as the increased stored calcium is released during systole to increase intracellular calcium concentration and interact with more troponin molecules.

Many myofilament proteins are substrates for different protein kinases and phosphatases that phosphorylate and dephosphorylate these various proteins. Phosphorylation of these proteins alters their properties such that the force-generating properties of the sarcomere are altered. Phosphorylation is controlled by several factors, including β-receptor stimulation. On the thin filament the three components of troponin can be phosphorylated and dephosphorylated.[11] Phosphorylation of TnI by cAMP-dependent protein kinase reduces the affinity of TnC for calcium. This may serve as a negative feedback mechanism and may also enhance relaxation by increasing the rate of calcium dissociation from troponin in diastole. Myosin-binding protein C and light chains are substrates on the thick filaments. The effect of phosphorylation of myosin-binding protein C is unknown at this time. Light chains are phosphorylated by

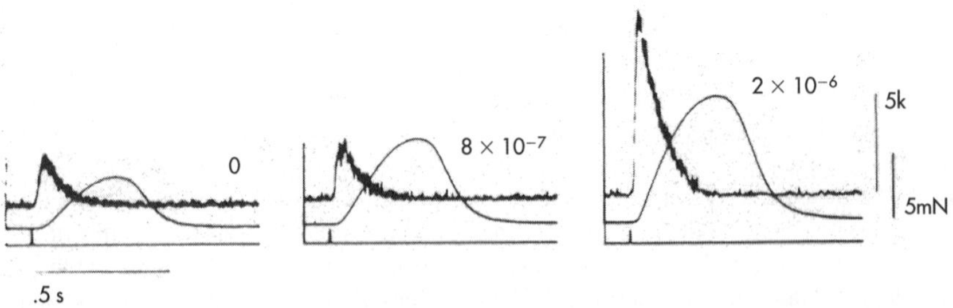

FIGURE 2-11 Simultaneous recordings of intracellular calcium concentration and myocardial isometric tension development before (0) and after (8×10^{-7} and 2×10^{-6}) addition of acetylstrophanthidin, a digitalis glycoside. Intracellular calcium concentration has been measured using the bioluminescent dye, aequorin. Note the delay in tension development after the increase in intracellular calcium concentration and the marked delay in relaxation following the decrease in calcium concentration. The increase in intracellular calcium concentration results in an increase in tension development. (From Giuliani EM, Gersh BJ, McGoon MD et al, eds: *Mayo clinic practice of cardiology,* St Louis, 1996, Mosby.)

calmodulin-dependent kinase, myosin light-chain kinase, and protein kinase C. Phosphorylation of this protein may enhance force generation at low calcium concentration.[18]

Starling's law of the heart states that stroke volume increases as end-diastolic pressure and volume increase in the intact heart. This is a reflection of the fact that isometric tension increases in isolated muscle as end-diastolic length is increased. At the sarcomere level, force of sarcomere contraction increases when sarcomere length is increased, such that the sarcomere contracts down to the same end-systolic length as control. Normal sarcomere length is approximately 2 μm at an end-diastolic pressure of 10 mm Hg. The sarcomere contracts down to an end-systolic length of 1.5 μm.[19] Maximum sarcomere stretch is to 2.2 μm. If contracting against the same force with no change in the calcium milieu surrounding the sarcomere, a sarcomere stretched to this extent would also contract down to 1.5 μm. The molecular basis for Starling's law is now becoming clear. There is convincing evidence that the affinity of the myofilaments, most likely TnC, for calcium increases as sarcomere length increases.[20] This results in more calcium being bound to troponin for any given intracellular calcium concentration, which frees more cross-bridges for interaction. The exact mechanism by which sarcomere length changes affect the sensitivity of TnC for calcium is unknown.

Calcium movement within the myocyte is not the only determinant of myocyte and sarcomere performance. ATP availability clearly is important, and ATP deficiency results in impaired performance. Isoforms of the contractile proteins also regulate cardiac activity. Myosin isoforms exist that change speed of contraction, as explained above. Troponin T isoforms also exist. Change from one troponin isoform to another results in changes in myofibrillar ATPase activity, sensitivity of myofilaments to calcium, and sarcomere length dependence of myofilament sensitivity to calcium.[21]

Systolic Function of the Heart

THE NORMAL CONTRACTION

The heart's ability to pump an adequate amount of blood to peripheral tissues (an adequate forward cardiac output [stroke volume × heart rate]) is determined by at least six factors: the usual four factors taught in cardiovascular physiology that deal with the normal heart—preload, afterload, contractility, and heart rate—and two additional factors that must be considered when cardiovascular disease is present—cardiac hypertrophy and leaks in the cardiovascular system.[22] These factors, their interrelationships, and their effect on cardiac output are depicted in Figure 2-12. Note that preload, afterload, and contractility determine systolic wall motion. This is the amount of wall motion or contraction seen on an echocardiogram. It is measured by calculating the shortening fraction. When examining how these factors change in cardiovascular disease, we will concentrate on how they change the end-diastolic volume (EDV) of the ventricle, the end-systolic volume (ESV) of the ventricle, the wall thickness, and the ability of the ventricle to eject blood into the aorta. Ventricular synchrony, the coordination and pattern of ventricular activation and contraction is another determinant. It, however, will not be dealt with in this discussion.

EDV is the maximum volume the ventricle achieves at the very end of diastole, and ESV is the minimum volume the ventricle achieves at the end of ejection. EDV is determined by the size of the

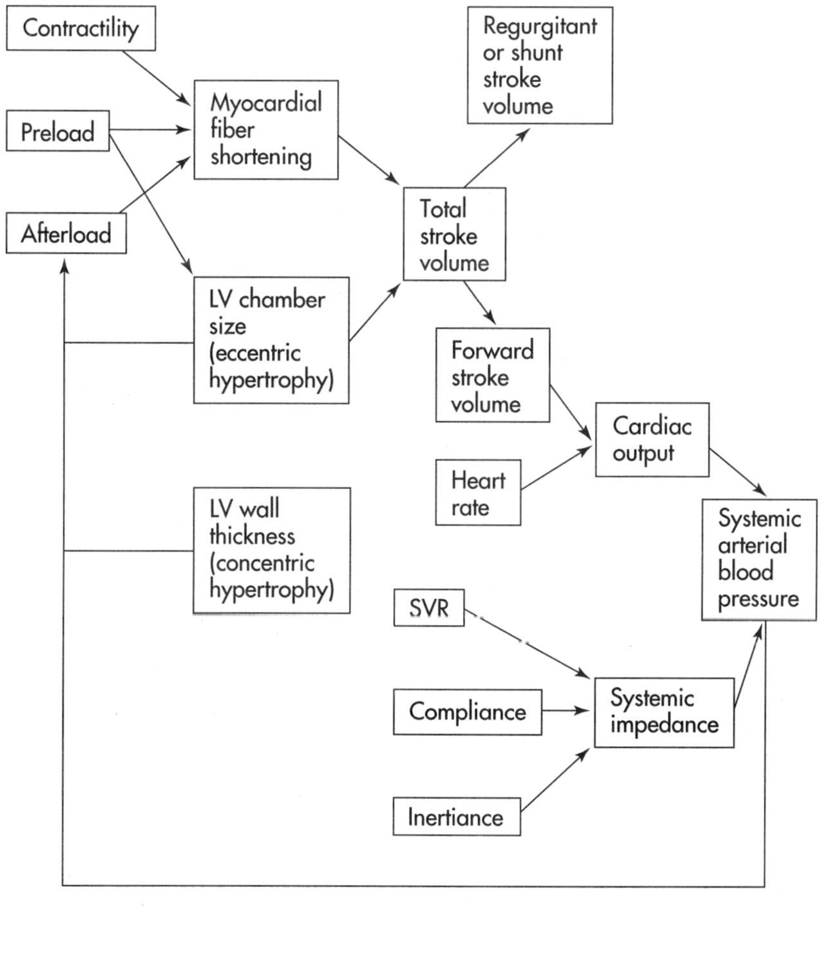

FIGURE 2-12 Diagram of the factors involved in systolic function of the heart, the factors that determine cardiac output, and the factors involved in determining systemic arterial blood pressure and their interrelationships. *SVR*, Systemic vascular resistance; *LV*, left ventricle.

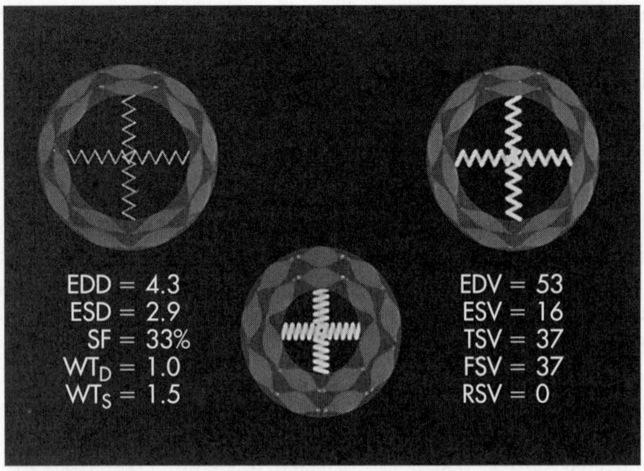

FIGURE 2-13 Cross-sections of a normal left ventricle at end-diastole *(upper left),* just before the aortic valve opening *(upper right),* and at end-systole *(lower center)* from a 28-kg (1 m^2 body surface area) dog. The muscles in the wall of the ventricle represent contractile elements (sarcomeres). The springs in the chamber represent intraventricular pressure. The thicker the spring, the greater the pressure. *EDD,* end-diastolic diameter (cm/m^2); *ESD.* end-systolic diameter (cm/m^2); *SF,* shortening fraction (%); WT_D, wall thickness in diastole (cm/m^2); WT_S, wall thickness at end-systole (cm/m^2); *EDV,* end-diastolic volume (mL/m^2); *ESV,* end-systolic volume (mL/m^2); *TSV,* total stroke volume (mL/m^2); *FSV,* forward stroke volume (mL/m^2); *RSV,* regurgitant stroke volume (mL/m^2).

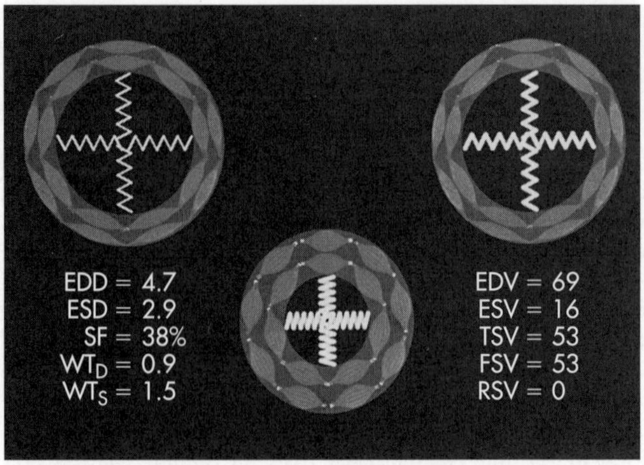

FIGURE 2-14 Cross-sections of a normal left ventricle with maximum preload. Note the increased spring thickness compared with Figure 2-13 in the left ventricular cross-section at the upper left, representing increased end-diastolic pressure. End-diastolic diameter and volume are increased. These changes produce increases in shortening fraction and stroke volume. Abbreviations as in Figure 2-13.

patient, preload (the force stretching the myocardium at the end of diastole), the diastolic properties of the heart (relaxation and compliance), and the amount of eccentric hypertrophy (how much the heart has been stimulated to grow following chronic stretch).[19] The size of the patient is factored out in this discussion by indexing (dividing) volumes and flows to (by) body surface area. ESV is determined mostly by contractility (the inherent ability of the heart to contract with a certain velocity, force, and extent of contraction independent of any forces) and afterload (the force opposing contraction throughout systole).[19] ESV also may become larger as the chamber grows larger through eccentric hypertrophy. EDV minus ESV equals the total stroke volume (TSV) of the ventricle. This TSV may be totally ejected into the aorta if no leaks are present or may be ejected into the aorta and some other structure if a leak is present (e.g., into the left atrium in mitral regurgitation or pulmonary circulation in a ventricular septal defect). Forward stroke volume (amount of blood ejected into the aorta during systole) can be increased by a decrease in afterload or an increase in myocardial contractility, preload, or chamber size brought about by hypertrophy, or the presence of a leak.

Figure 2-13 depicts cross-sections of a left ventricle from a normal animal that has 1 m^2 of body surface area (weighs 25 to 30 kg). The diameter of the left ventricle at the end of diastole in a normal dog of this size is 4.3 cm.[23] For the rest of this discussion volumes are presented based on cubing a diameter and then dividing by 1.5. This formula is based on studies in the literature on dog ventricles and determining left ventricular mass and volume.[24,25] This method probably is not totally accurate but provides an approximation and is presented for illustration purposes only. The approximate chamber volume at the end of diastole in this dog is 53 mL/m^2.

In a normal dog the wall thickness is 1 cm/m^2.[23] End-diastolic pressure in the upper left of Figure 2-13 is depicted as a flimsy spring in the center of the chamber, pushing out against the myocardium. The muscles that encircle the left ventricular cavity represent the sarcomeres (contractile units) of the myocardium. Each muscle represents thousands of sarcomeres. The upper right of Figure 2-13 has the same measurements as before but depicts the ventricle at the instant before the aortic valve opens. The spring in the middle now depicts a systolic pressure in the ventricle. The spring is thicker than it was in diastole, because peak systolic pressure (120 to 160 mm Hg) is much higher than diastolic pressure (0 to 10 mm Hg). The lower center cross-section in Figure 2-13 is the ventricle at the end of systole, when maximum contraction has taken place. The ventricle has contracted as far as it can in the time allotted. The chamber diameter at the end of systole is now 2.9 cm/m^2, and the ESV is 16 mL/m^2. The wall has thickened to 1.5 cm/m^2. The volume of the wall is 114 mL. To obtain an estimate of the wall mass or the weight of the heart, the wall volume is taken times 1.05 g/mL, the density of the myocardium. Consequently, the left ventricular mass is approximately 120 g. Subtracting ESV from EDV gives the total amount of blood the chamber has ejected during systole (TSV). The percentage change in diameter from diastole to systole or the shortening fraction (end-diastolic diameter – end-systolic diameter/end-diastolic diameter) is 33%. This figure provides a number that describes the amount of wall motion (contraction) that is seen on an echocardiogram. The percentage of blood ejected during systole or the ejection fraction (EDV – ESV/EDV) is 69%. The percent change in wall thickness from diastole to systole or the thickening fraction (end-diastolic wall thickness – end-systolic wall thickness/end-diastolic wall thickness) is 50%.

PRELOAD

Preload is the first determinant of systolic wall motion (contraction). It is the force that determines the amount of stretch placed on a myocardial sarcomere (the contractile elements in the myocardial cell) at the end of diastole.[19] This increase in diastolic force stretches the sarcomeres and increases EDV. The sarcomeres respond to the increased stretch by contracting more forcefully to expel the increased quantity of blood taken in during diastole. In Figure 2-14 end-diastolic pressure has been increased by infusing a crystalloid solution intravenously to increase venous return to the heart. The increase in end-diastolic pressure is depicted as a thicker spring within the left ventricular cavity, which is pushing out against the myocardium.

Starling's law of the heart states that increased sarcomere stretch (acute increase in EDV) results in a more forceful contraction to expel the increased volume, and decreased stretch results in the opposite.[22,26,27] This gives the heart the ability to regulate stroke volume on a beat-to-beat basis and allows the body to acutely increase cardiac output by increasing venous return to the heart.[28] For example, during inspiration intrapleural pressure decreases, which increases venous return to the right heart and pools blood in the pulmonary vasculature, resulting in a decrease in venous return to the left heart. On expiration, intrapleural pressure increases, forcing more blood back into the left heart and decreasing venous return to the right heart. Because of Starling's law, left ventricular stroke volume decreases with inspiration and increases with expiration without any change in myocardial contractility; the opposite occurs in the right heart. This allows stroke volume to change on a beat-to-beat basis and keeps right ventricular and left ventricular stroke volumes equal over time.[22] The increase in force of contraction associated with an increase in end-diastolic sarcomere length apparently is due to increased affinity of the myofilament (troponin C) for calcium during systole.[20,29,30]

What is the force that determines this degree of sarcomere stretch? If all of the sarcomeres were aligned so that they pointed toward the center of the chamber, this force would simply be the pressure in the left ventricular cavity at the end of diastole (the force provided by the coiled spring). However, they are aligned circumferentially around the chamber. Therefore one must calculate the tension or stress stretching the sarcomeres apart.[31,32]

Diastolic wall stress (σ) is determined by the pressure in the ventricular chamber at end-diastole (P_{ed}), the radius of the chamber at end-diastole (r_{ed}), and the wall thickness at end-diastole (h_{ed}) and is approximated by the formula: $\sigma = (P_{ed} \times r_{ed})/2h_{ed}$.[33] This is Laplace's law. It calculates the force producing the stretch and is explained more fully in the section on afterload. The amount of sarcomere stretch is also determined by the compliance of that chamber, the orientation of the sarcomere to the forces acting upon it, and the number of sarcomeres in series within the cell. Figure 2-14 provides literature values for the maximum increase in EDV achieved with an increase in preload in dogs.[34] As can be seen, the spring at the end of diastole is thicker (end-diastolic pressure is increased) and stroke volume has increased 16 mL/m^2, or 43%, above baseline, because EDV has increased and ESV has remained the same. This is the maximum change that can be achieved by an increase in preload. This is a small change compared with changes that can be affected in EDV by a change in the amount of eccentric hypertrophy. Even though the left ventricular wall is thinner at the end of diastole, left ventricular weight is normal (120 g).

AFTERLOAD

Afterload is the force that opposes muscle shortening (impedes contraction) and is the second determinant of wall motion (shortening fraction). Systolic wall stress is the force that most accurately predicts myocardial shortening and so is the best estimate of afterload.[35] If the myocardium was arranged as a linear strip of muscle with a weight attached to one end and the other end fixed, afterload would be the mass of the weight that the muscle had to lift during contraction. In the heart, the weight, or force, that the muscle has to overcome to shorten and eject blood is approximated by calculating systolic *(s)* wall stress: $\sigma_s = (P_s \times r_s)/2h_s$. Based on this formula, afterload is increased whenever intraventricular pressure is increased, chamber volume (radius) is increased, or ventricular wall thickness is decreased during systole. The force producing contraction and the force opposing contraction are equal and opposite. Consequently, another way to think about afterload is as the force

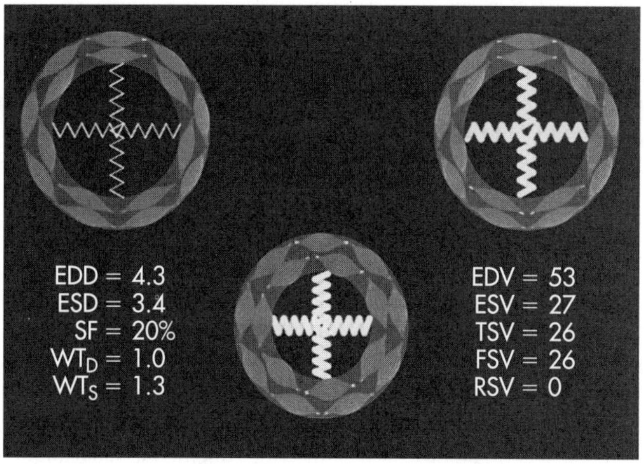

FIGURE 2-15 Cross-sections of a normal left ventricle in which systolic pressure has been increased by infusing a vasopressor to increase afterload. Note the increased spring thickness in the upper right and lower center cross-sections, representing increased systolic pressure. The increase in afterload results in increases in end-systolic diameter and end-systolic volume. Abbreviations as in Figure 2-13.

required to achieve a certain intraventricular pressure during systole. During systole in Figure 2-13, intraventricular pressure increases to 140 mm Hg. A certain myocardial force is needed to generate this intraventricular force. Intraventricular pressure has been increased in Figure 2-15. This could represent a situation in which a drug or hormone, such as angiotensin II, has been administered to constrict systemic arterioles or acute aortic stenosis has been produced. Systolic intraventricular pressure is now much greater than it was previously (e.g., 210 mm Hg vs. 140 mm Hg). Intraventricular pressure is represented by a spring. The spring in systole is thicker than in Figure 2-13, and consequently it takes a greater force to compress it than the normal spring. The myocardium must generate a larger force to generate this intraventricular pressure. This is relatively easy to understand on an intuitive basis. An increase in the chamber radius can also increase systolic wall stress (afterload). This is intuitively more difficult to understand. One must remember physical principles. An experiment that can be performed while sitting in a chair demonstrates this. Place the palms of the hands together in front of the chest. Then generate a force in the biceps (this represents the force generated in the myocardium) by pushing the hands together. This produces a resultant pressure between the palms (which represents systolic intraventricular pressure). Take note of the force generated by the biceps at this time. Maintain the same pressure between the palms and move the hands away from the chest. Feel the greater force in the biceps required to maintain the same pressure between the palms. If the heart muscle could feel the same thing, the same feeling would be generated when the intraventricular pressure remained constant but the chamber radius increased. In this situation, a greater force is required to generate a "normal" systolic intraventricular pressure. The corollary to this is that a greater force impedes ventricular contraction when the chamber radius is increased and systolic intraventricular pressure is "normal."

Afterload is highly dependent on systolic intraventricular pressure. The pressure that a ventricle generates during systole is usually the same as the systolic systemic arterial blood pressure (unless aortic stenosis is present) and is determined by aortic input impedance, stroke volume, and velocity of flow into the aorta. Impedance is the force opposing forward flow in a system in which pulsed or cyclic flow is present (e.g., cardiovascular system).[36] Resistance is the similar opposing force in a system in which the flow is constant rather than cyclic. It is calculated by dividing average pressure by average flow (cardiac output). The radius of the systemic arterioles is the primary determinant of resistance and impedance. Consequently, both can be manipulated with vasodilators and vasoconstrictors. Impedance is also influenced by the stiffness of the aorta and several other factors. Heart failure stimulates the constriction of systemic arterioles and stiffening of the aorta by increasing sympathetic tone and increasing the circulating concentration of angiotensin II.

An increase in systolic wall stress results in increased end-systolic diameter and volume if contractility remains the same. The increased force against which the ventricle contracts impedes contraction, resulting in increased end-systolic values. A corollary is lifting a weight with your biceps muscle. If you are lifting a 25-lb weight, you may be able to lift that weight 2 feet in one second with maximum effort. If you then tried to lift a 50-lb weight, you would find that you would only be able to lift it 1 foot in the same amount of time with the same effort. In Figure 2-15, end-systolic diameter has increased from 2.9 to 3.2 cm, resulting in a decrease in shortening fraction (the amount of contraction). ESV has increased, resulting in a decrease in stroke volume.

MYOCARDIAL CONTRACTILITY

The third determinant of systolic wall motion (contraction) is myocardial contractility. Contraction and myocardial contractility are different. Contractility is an inherent myocardial cellular property. It can be changed by intracellular and extracellular influences. Contractility, preload, and afterload influence the force and velocity with which and the extent to which the sarcomere contracts. Consequently, they change the amount of wall motion or contraction. Contractility is myocardial performance (force, velocity, and extent of contraction) independent of preload and afterload.[22] The primary determinants of contractility are discussed above. They include, but are not limited to, increased amount and rate of calcium release by the sarcoplasmic reticulum, phosphorylation of proteins within the cell, and cellular ATP production.

The effects of administering a positive inotropic agent (an agent to increase contractility) are depicted in Figure 2-16. Note that ESD and ESV have decreased, whereas the spring thickness has remained normal. This means the ventricle can contract farther than it did in Figure 2-13, against the same afterload. The administration of a positive inotropic agent (e.g., dobutamine) has increased contractility, which has increased the strength of the contraction. There are no known drugs that increase skeletal muscle contractility. Spinach is the only make-believe agent able to do this. A corollary to giving a positive inotropic drug to increase myocardial contractility is Popeye lifting weights before and after eating spinach. If he can lift a 25-lb weight 2 feet in 1 second before eating spinach, he may be able to lift it 3 feet after eating spinach. Kryptonite is a make-believe example of a skeletal muscle negative inotropic agent for Superman.

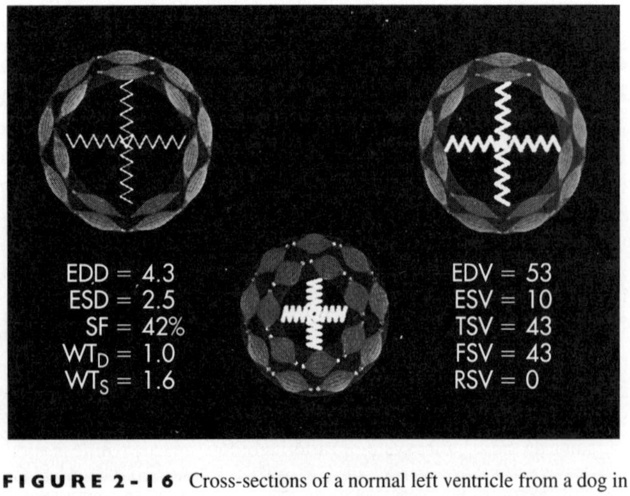

FIGURE 2-16 Cross-sections of a normal left ventricle from a dog in which contractility has been increased by infusing a β-adrenergic receptor agonist. End-systolic diameter and volume are decreased from Figure 2-13. Shortening fraction and stroke volume are also increased. Abbreviations as in Figure 2-13.

Myocardial contractility is highly dependent on intracellular calcium fluxes, as explained above. Increasing the amount of calcium released from the sarcoplasmic reticulum and increasing the rate at which it is released are two means of increasing contractility. The rate of tension rise (dP/dt) probably reflects the rate at which Ca^{++} is bound to troponin. Maximal velocity at which the heart muscle contracts is probably determined by the rate of actin-myosin interaction and the type of myosin ATPase.

Preload (the amount of sarcomere stretch) also changes force development characteristics of the myocardium, probably through changes in intracellular Ca^{++} kinetics. Apparently when muscle length increases, troponin increases its sensitivity for Ca^{++}. This, however, is not considered a change in contractility because it does not affect a change in ESV.

The contractile properties of a myocardial cell have several other determinants, some of which we are probably unaware. The ability of the cell to produce energy for contraction plays a role in determining contractility. Decreases in intracellular ATP concentration have been demonstrated in myocardium from patients with myocardial failure (decreased myocardial contractility) and could be contributing to the alteration in contractility. Changes in the type of myosin in the sarcomere have been demonstrated in certain diseases in some species. In other species it appears that calcium movement in the cell changes in response to types of hemodynamic stress.[4] This results in the speed of contraction changing but does not necessarily affect the extent to which the myocardium contracts.[37] This is similar to the situation in skeletal muscle, where there are "slow twitch" and "fast twitch" types of fibers. In the myocardium, certain abnormalities would benefit from a change in the contractile speed of the sarcomere, and clinically we certainly see differences in contractile velocity in different diseases. In our clinical experience, in mitral regurgitation an increased velocity of contraction should be beneficial and appears to occur.[38] Think what would happen if contraction was very slow so that pressure built up slowly in mitral regurgitation. If the contraction was made slow enough, all of the blood would leak into the left atrium before the aortic valve ever opened. Rapid ejection allows the left ventricle to eject blood more efficiently in this disease. In aortic stenosis, slow ejection should be beneficial and more efficient.[38] Slower contraction allows for a lesser increase in left ventricular pressure during systole and requires less oxygen consumption. In dogs, the activity of the myosin ATPase decreases in association with aortic stenosis, which should result in a slower contraction.[39] Therefore one can theorize that myocardial fibers might change to more fast twitch fibers in diseases such as mitral regurgitation (volume overloads) and to more slow twitch fibers in diseases such as aortic stenosis (pressure overloads).

HEART RATE

The rate of diastolic depolarization and the threshold potential in the sinus node normally control the heart rate. The rate of diastolic depolarization is altered by a variety of influences, such as temperature, metabolic rate, sympathetic tone, and parasympathetic tone.[19] Diverse influences, such as fever, thyrotoxicosis, excitement, and exercise, cause an increase in heart rate. Each situation that results in heart rate elevation does so because the body is demanding an

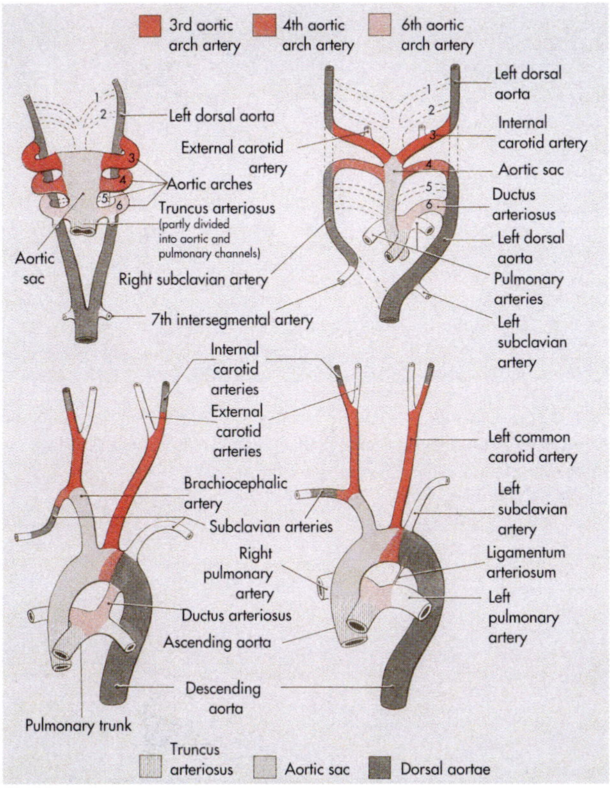

COLOR PLATE 1 Schematic drawings illustrating the transformation of the truncus arteriosus, aortic sac, aortic arches, and dorsal aorta into the adult arterial pattern. **A,** Six weeks. **B,** Seven weeks. **C,** Eight weeks. **D,** Neonatal. (From Moore KL: *The developing human,* Philadelphia, 1982, WB Saunders.)

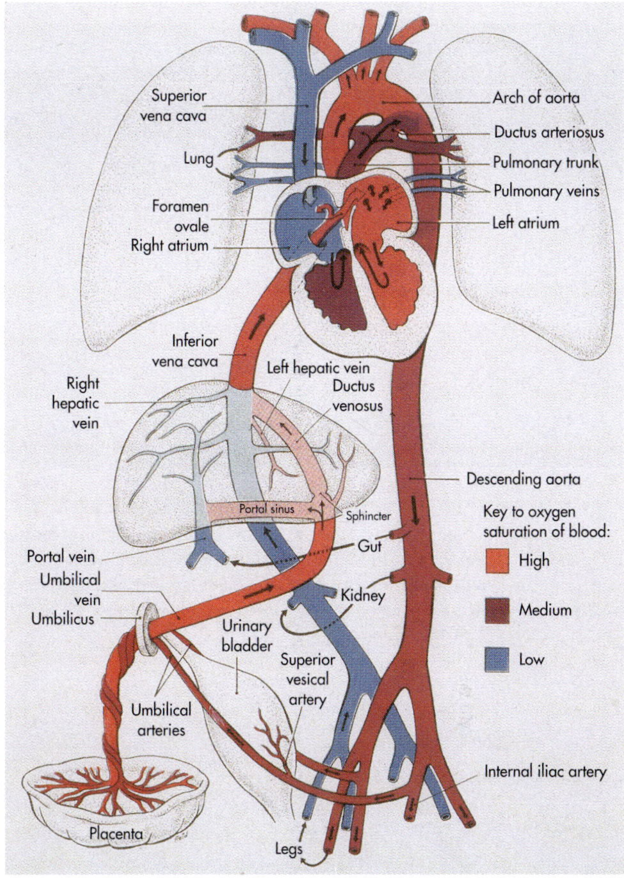

COLOR PLATE 2 Schematic drawings illustrating the transformation of the truncus arteriosus, aortic sac, aortic arches, and dorsal aorta into the adult arterial pattern. **A,** Six weeks. **B,** Seven weeks. **C,** Eight weeks. **D,** Neonatal. (From Moore KL: *The developing human,* Philadelphia, 1982, WB Saunders.)

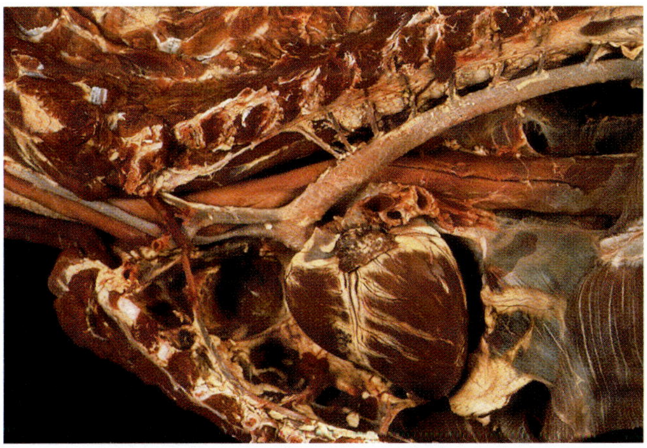

COLOR PLATE 3 Dog chest. The left chest wall, lung, and pericardium have been removed. Most of the cardiac surface is occupied by the left ventricle. It lies caudally, next to the diaphragm, and is separated from the right ventricle by the cranial interventricular groove. The left auricle lies on the dorsal aspect of this groove. The aorta emerges from the heart to curve caudally and descend beneath the spine, to the left of the esophagus. The brachiocephalic trunk and left subclavian artery course cranially from the aorta to give rise to the carotid arteries, arteries of the forelimbs, and internal thoracic arteries (coursing along the sternum). (Courtesy Dr. Carroll Loyer.)

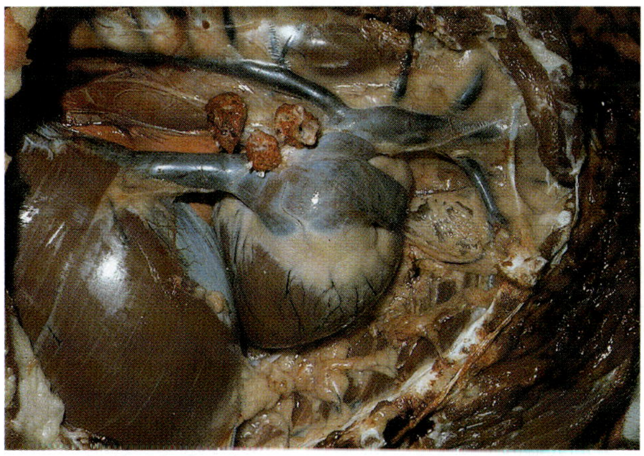

COLOR PLATE 4 Similar view to Color Plate 3 but from the right side. The ventral portion of the heart is the right ventricle. The dorsal portion is the right atrium. The right auricle wraps around the front of the heart. The cranial vena cava is short, starting as a confluence of veins in the cranial chest and ending where it empties into the right atrium. The azygos vein emerges from beneath the spine to drain into the cranial vena cava. The caudal vena cava emerges from the diaphragm to course forward into the caudal aspect of the right atrium. (Courtesy Dr. Bari Olivier.)

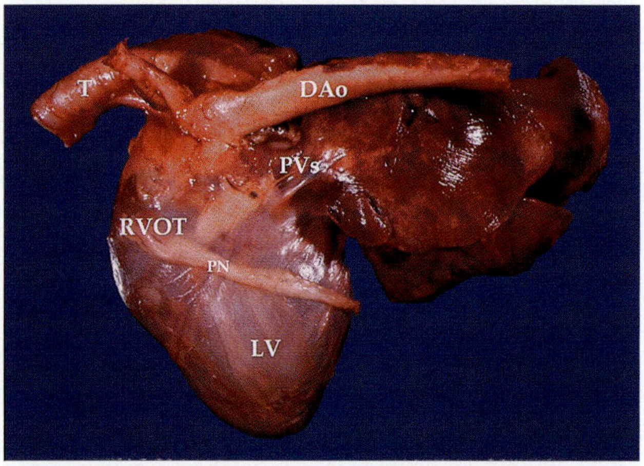

COLOR PLATE 5 The heart and lungs have been removed from the thoracic space, and the left lung reflected dorsally. The orientation is similar to Color Plate 3, but the heart is confined within the pericardial sac. The left phrenic nerve *(PN)* crosses the pericardium in its course to the diaphragm. *DAo,* descending aorta; *T,* trachea; *RVOT,* right ventricular outflow tract; *PVs,* pulmonary veins; *LV,* left ventricle.

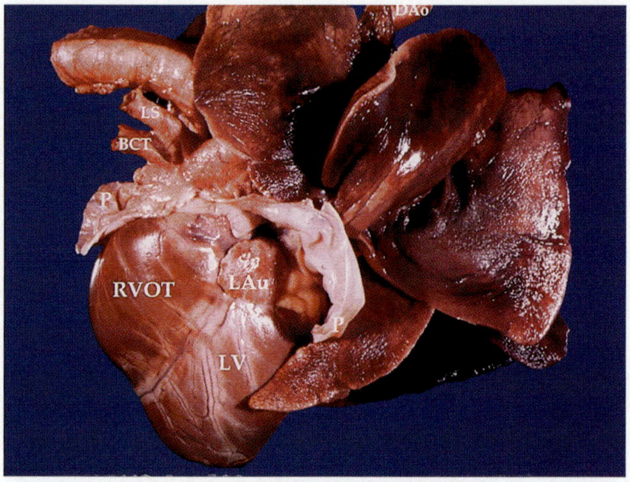

COLOR PLATE 6 Similar view to Color Plate 5, but the pericardium *(P)* has been incised and reflected dorsally and caudally. Structures are same as in Color Plate 3. Abbreviations are same as Color Plate 5, plus *LAu,* Left auricle; *BCT,* brachiocephalic trunk; *LS,* left subclavian artery.

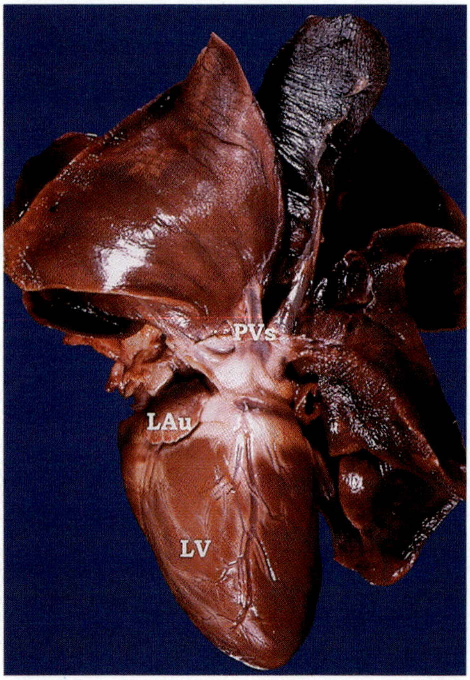

COLOR PLATE 7 With the lungs reflected dorsally, the heart has been rotated slightly so more of the caudal heart is visible. Fat in the atrioventricular groove can be readily seen between the left atrium and left ventricle *(LV).* The pulmonary veins *(PVs)* lie between the lung lobes and left atrium. The left auricle *(LAu)* lies immediately above the cranial interventricular groove. The large coronary artery descends from the left circumflex coronary artery along the lateral left ventricular free wall.

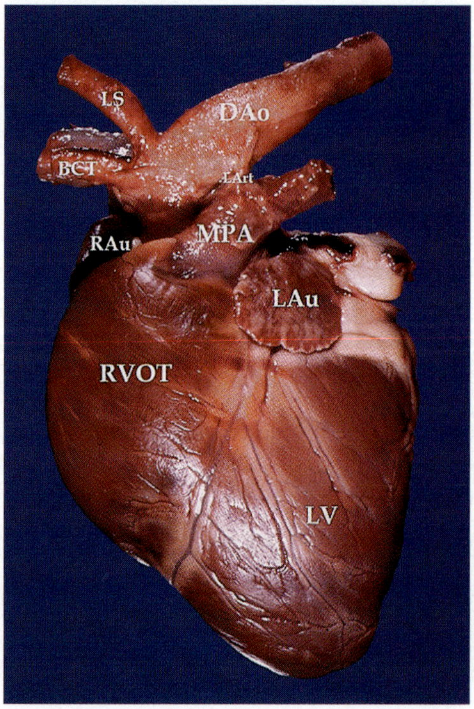

COLOR PLATE 8 Lungs have been removed to reveal the major cardiac structures that can be visualized from the left side. The right ventricular outflow tract *(RVOT)* ascends from the body of the right ventricle across the cranial aspect of the heart to give rise to the main pulmonary artery *(MPA).* The left auricle *(LAu)* is on the left lateral surface. The right auricle *(RAu)* wraps around cranially. The ligamentum arteriosum descends from the proximal descending aorta *(DAo)* to the origin of the left pulmonary artery branch. *LV,* Left ventricle, *BCT,* brachiocephalic trunk.

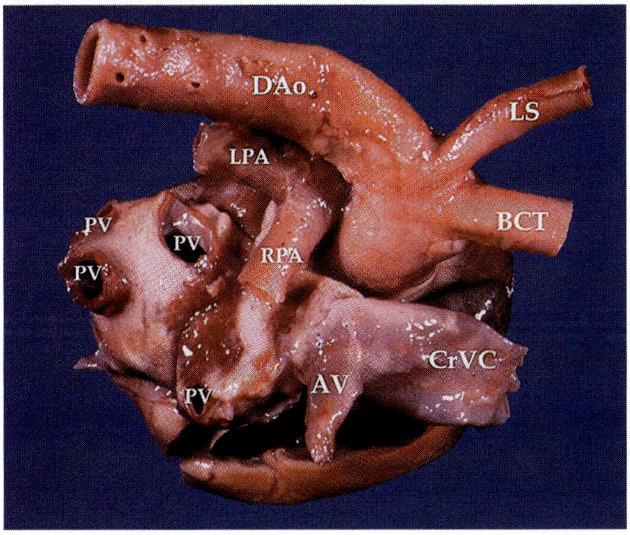

COLOR PLATE 9 Base of the heart viewed from above. The aorta emerges from the cranial aspect of the left ventricle to form the aortic arch and then descend beneath the spine. The brachiocephalic trunk *(BCT)* and left subclavian *(LS)* artery originate from the aortic arch. The main pulmonary artery divides into the right and left pulmonary arteries (*RPA* and *LPA*) immediately caudal to the aorta. Four ostia for the pulmonary veins *(PV)* can be seen in the roof of the body of the left atrium. The cranial vena cava *(CrVC)* lies to the right of the aorta. The azygos vein *(AV)* enters the cranial vena cava at its junction with the right atrium. *DAo,* Decending aorta.

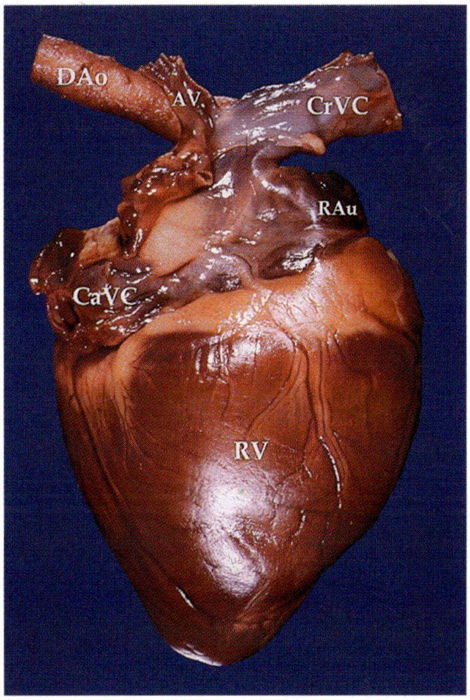

COLOR PLATE 10 Heart viewed from the right. Similar to Color Plate 4. The caudal interventricular coronary artery descends along the caudal aspect of the heart between the right ventricle *(RV)* and left ventricle. The cranial vena cava *(CrVC)* can be seen as it enters the body of the right atrium from its dorsal aspect. The caudal vena cava *(CaVC)* enters the caudal aspect of the right atrium much lower. *RAu,* Right auricle; *DAo,* descending aorta.

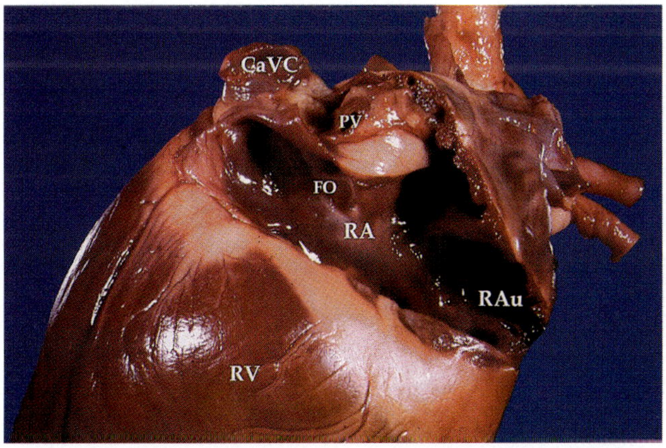

COLOR PLATE 11 Opened right atrium. The lateral wall has been reflected dorsally and placed on top of the roof of the right atrium. One of the right pulmonary veins *(PV)* can still be seen from this view. The caudal vena cava *(CaVC)* is intact on the caudal aspect of the heart. The label for the right atrium *(RA)* is placed on the intervenous tubercle on the interatrial septum. Behind this is the fossa ovalis *(FO)*. The crista terminalis can be seen as another ridge of tissue passing from the interatrial septum to the lateral wall of the right atrium cranial to the intervenous tubercle, between the right atrium and right auricle *(RAu)*. *RV,* Right ventricle.

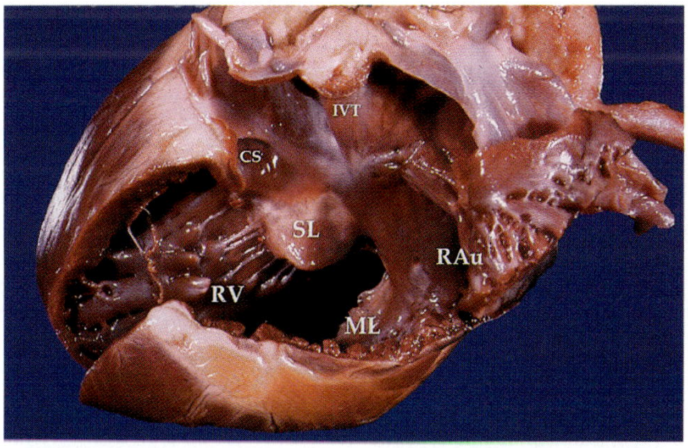

COLOR PLATE 12 Right atrium, tricuspid valve, and right ventricle *(RV)* viewed from above. The crista terminalis is in better view than in Color Plate 11. The heavy trabeculations of the lateral wall of the right atrium can be clearly visualized. The coronary sinus *(CS)* lies on the floor of the right atrium, just caudal to the septal leaflet *(SL)* of the tricuspid valve. The chordae tendineae of the septal leaflet can be seen to attach to the papillae along the interventricular septum. A small portion of the mural leaflet *(ML)* of the tricuspid valve can be seen. Its chordal attachments have been severed. *RAu,* Right auricle; *IVT,* intervenous tubercle.

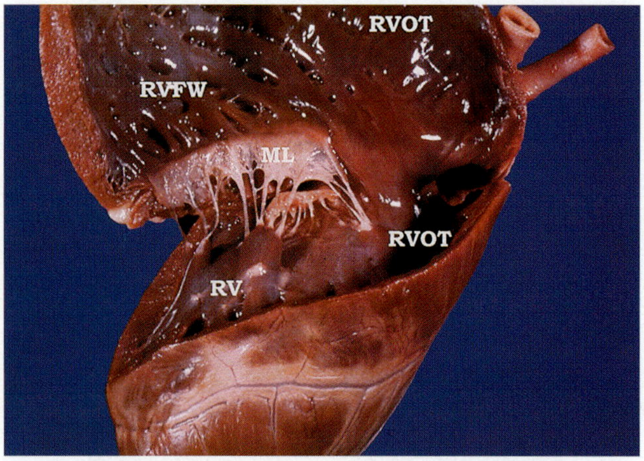

COLOR PLATE 13 Right ventricular chamber viewed with the right ventricular free wall *(RVFW)* displaced dorsally. The deep trabeculations in the part of the RVFW that encircles the body of the right ventricle can be seen. The large mural leaflet *(ML)* of the tricuspid valve is attached by chordae tendineae to the papillary muscles that originate from the apical region of the right ventricle. A smaller papillary muscle (papillary muscle of conus) originates from the crista supraventricularis immediately left of the RVOT label. The smooth right ventricular outflow tract *(RVOT)* ascends to the pulmonic valve. *RV,* Right ventricle.

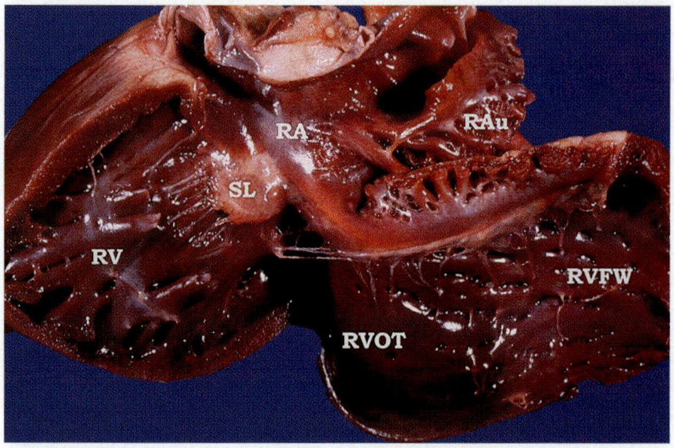

COLOR PLATE 14 The right ventricular free wall *(RVFW)* has been displaced cranially. The heavy trabeculations of the right atrial free wall and right auricle *(RAu)* can be seen. The right ventricle *(RV)* label is placed on the interventricular septum. The dorsal portion of the interventricular septum between the septal leaflet of the tricuspid valve and the papillary muscles is smooth and called the *inlet septum.* The apical portion, below the papillary muscles, is heavily trabeculated and is called the *trabecular septum.* The right ventricular free wall *(RVFW)* overlying the body is also heavily trabeculated. The right ventricular outflow tract *(RVOT)* has no trabeculations. *SL,* Septal leaflet of tricuspid valve; *RA,* right atrium.

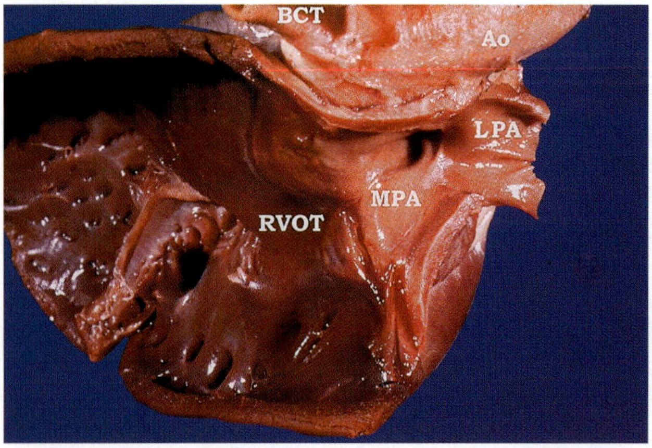

COLOR PLATE 15 The pulmonic valve lies between the right ventricular outflow tract *(RVOT)* and main pulmonary artery *(MPA).* Its cusps are translucent and therefore difficult to see. One has been cut, and other two are cup-shaped, lying against the wall of the proximal MPA. The commissure of these two cusps lies immediately to the left of the MPA label. *RPA,* Right pulmonary artery; *BCT,* brachiocephalic trunk; *Ao,* aorta.

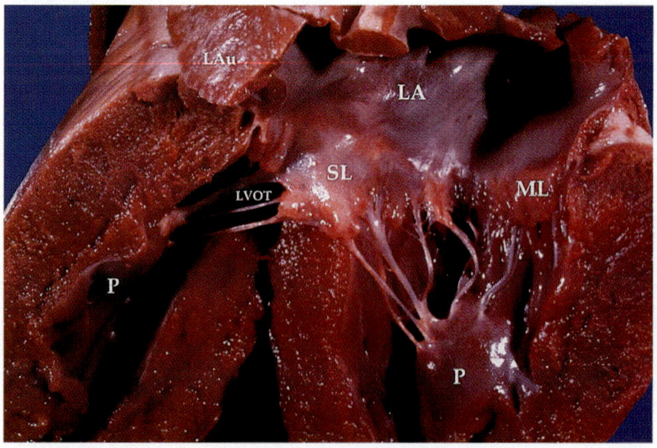

COLOR PLATE 16 The left ventricle and left atrium have been cut open longitudinally to show the thicker left ventricular myocardium, papillary muscles *(P),* larger septal leaflet *(SL),* and smaller mural leaflet *(ML)* of the mitral valve, left atrium *(LA),* and left auricle *(LAu).* The chordae tendineae from the caudal papillary muscle can be seen extending to both mitral valve leaflets. The left ventricular myocardium has contracted after death (similar to rigor mortis) and so is thicker than in diastole in a living dog. *LVOT,* left ventricular outflow tract.

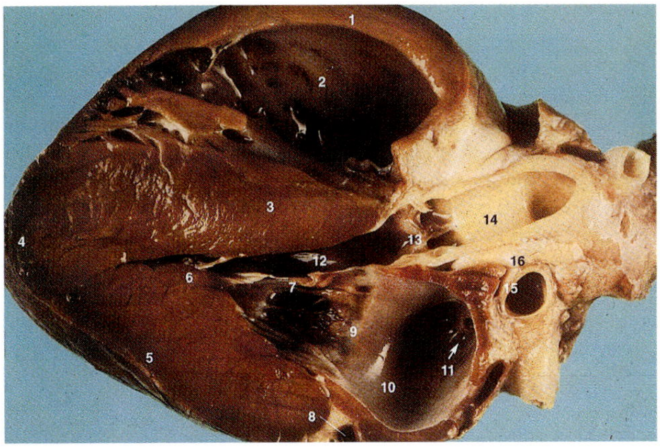

COLOR PLATE 17 The heart has been cut longitudinally to reveal the left ventricle, right ventricle, left atrium, and proximal aorta. This view is similar to the longitudinal view seen with a two-dimensional echocardiogram. The chordae tendineae of the caudal papillary muscle can be seen attached to the septal leaflet of the mitral valve, which is open. The inflow portion of the left ventricle lies ventral *(left of picture)* to the open mitral valve. The outflow tract lies between open the septal leaflet and interventricular septum, beneath the aortic valve. The base of the septal leaflet of the mitral valve is in continuity with the root of the aorta. The two cusps of the aortic valve are visible and look like two cups lying at the junction of the left ventricle and aorta. *1,* Right ventricular free wall; *2,* right ventricular cavity; *3,* interventricular septum; *4,* apex of the heart; *5,* left ventricular free wall; *6,* papillary muscle; *7,* chordae tendineae; *8,* left circumflex coronary artery; *9,* mitral valve; *10,* left atrium; *11,* left auricle; *12,* left ventricular outflow tract; *13,* aortic valve; *14,* aorta; *15,* right main branch of the pulmonary artery; *16,* base of the heart. (From Boyd JS: *A color atlas of clinical anatomy of the dog and cat,* St Louis, 1995, Mosby.)

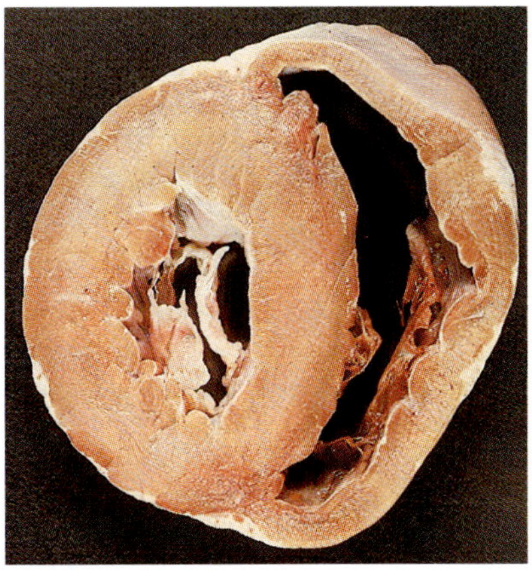

COLOR PLATE 18 The heart has been cut in cross-section at the level of the ventricles, immediately below the atrioventricular (AV) valves and immediately above the AV valves. The heart has then been turned over so the AV valve leaflets are viewed from underneath. The left ventricle is to the left of the figure, and the right ventricle is to the right. The left ventricular myocardium is thicker than the right ventricular myocardium. The left ventricle is circular; the right ventricle wraps around the left ventricle. The right ventricular outflow tract is to the top of the figure.

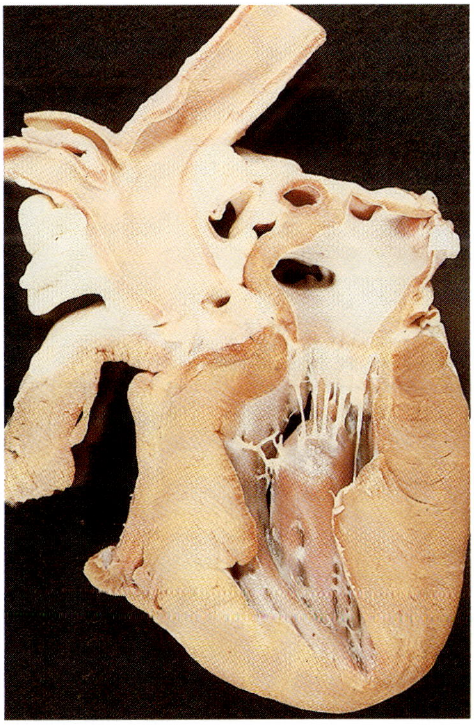

COLOR PLATE 19 Longitudinal section of heart. Ascending, transverse, and proximal descending aorta; brachiocephalic trunk; and left subclavian artery can be seen. The ostium of the left coronary artery can be seen behind the left coronary cusp of the aortic valve.

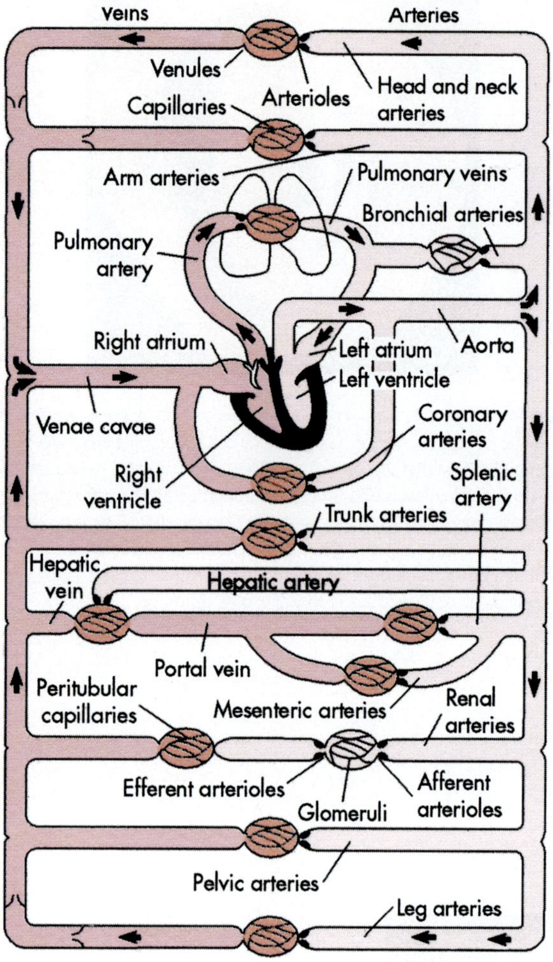

COLOR PLATE 20 Schematic diagram of the circulatory system. The pulmonary circulation consists of the pulmonary artery, pulmonary microvasculature, and pulmonary veins; the remainder is the systemic circulation. The oxygenated blood is light pink, and the deoxygenated blood is dark pink. The arterioles are drawn as crescent-shaped thickenings before the capillary beds. The capillary beds are thin lines within cells (brown areas of increased width between arteries and veins). (From Berne RM, Levy MN: *Cardiovascular physiology,* St Louis, 1992, Mosby.)

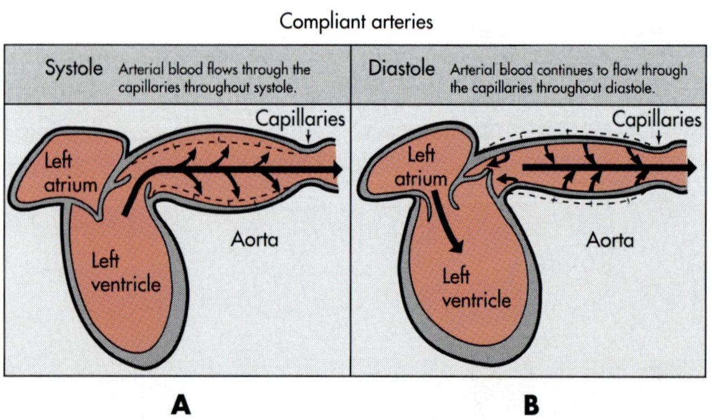

COLOR PLATE 21 **A,** Schematic drawing of the left heart and aorta during systole. The aorta distends in systole as blood is pumped into it. Impedance to blood flow is less than if the aorta was rigid. **B,** Left heart and aorta during diastole. During diastole, the elastic recoil of the aorta continues to propel the blood forward. (From Berne RM, Levy MN: *Cardiovascular physiology,* St Louis, 1992, Mosby.)

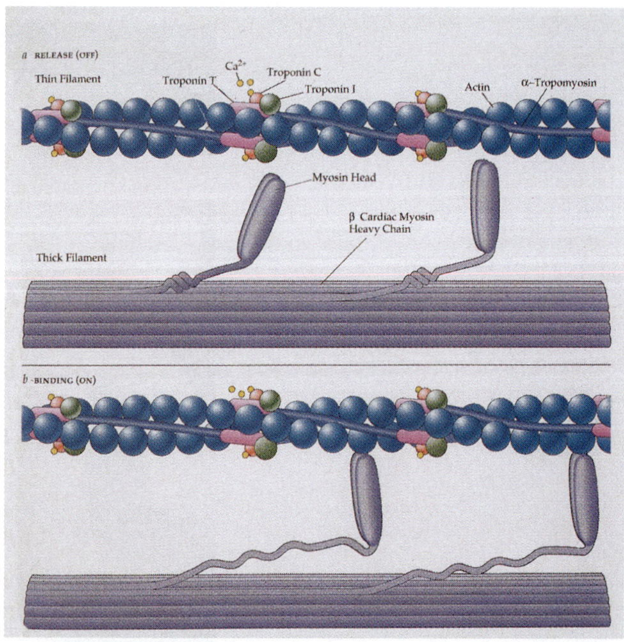

COLOR PLATE 22 **A,** Drawing of the contractile proteins during relaxation. During relaxation, the intracellular calcium concentration is low and tropomyosin inhibits actin from interacting with myosin. **B,** During systole, the cytoplasmic calcium concentration is high, binding to troponin C and resulting in a conformational change in tropomyosin. When tropomyosin moves, actin and myosin can interact in presence of ATP, which causes the contractile element (sarcomere) to contract. (From Seidman CE, Seidman JG: Gene mutations that cause familial hypertrophic cardiomyopathy. In Haber E, ed: *Molecular cardiovascular medicine,* New York, 1995, Scientific American.)

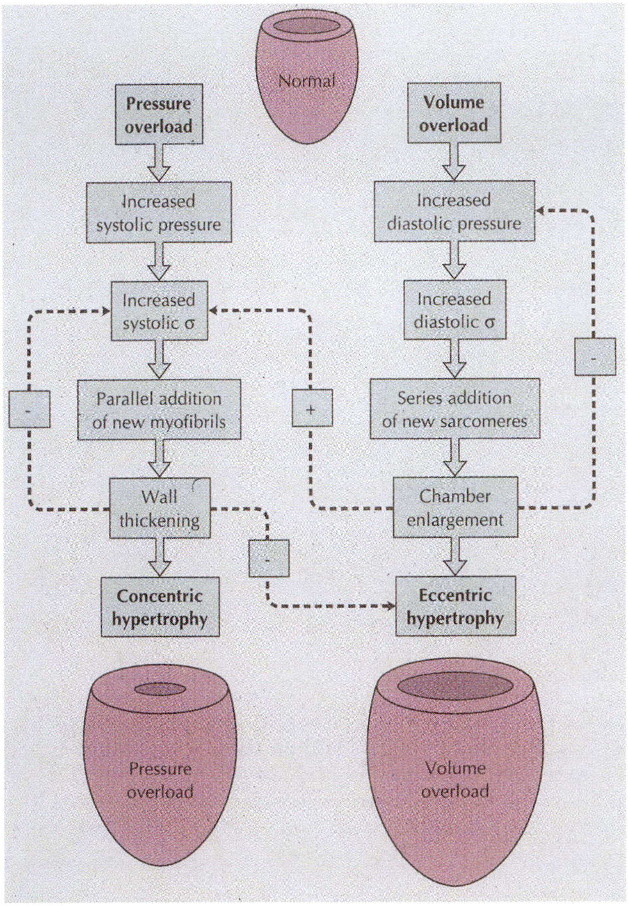

COLOR PLATE 23 Schematic drawings of a normal left ventricle, a left ventricle with volume overload (eccentric) hypertrophy, and a left ventricle with pressure overload (concentric) hypertrophy. δ, Wall stress.

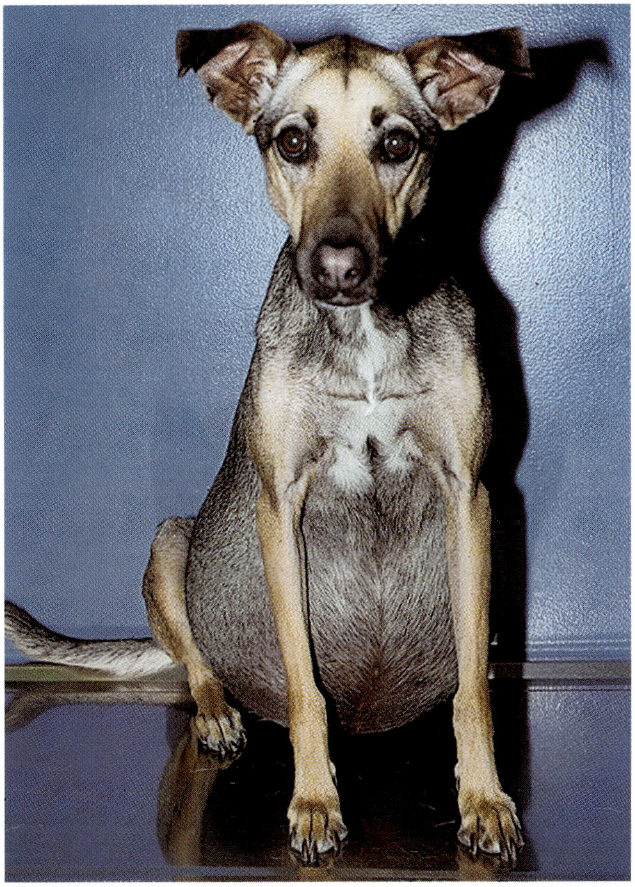

COLOR PLATE 24 Severe ascites in a dog with severe pulmonic stenosis and severe tricuspid regurgitation. The abdomen is markedly distended.

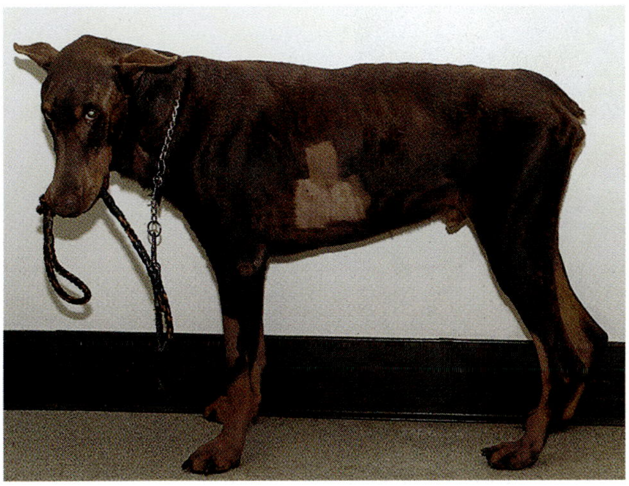

COLOR PLATE 25 Weight loss in Doberman pinscher with dilated cardiomyopathy (cardiac cachexia). The primary problem was accumulation of pleural effusion that required draining once a week.

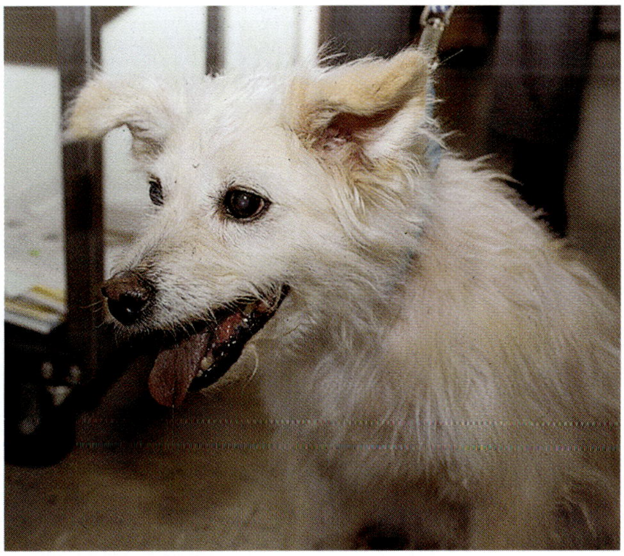

COLOR PLATE 26 Central cyanosis in a dog with severe mitral regurgitation and pulmonary edema leading to hypoxemia. The dog's pulmonary capillary wedge pressure was 35 mm Hg, and his arterial oxygen tension was 43 mm Hg.

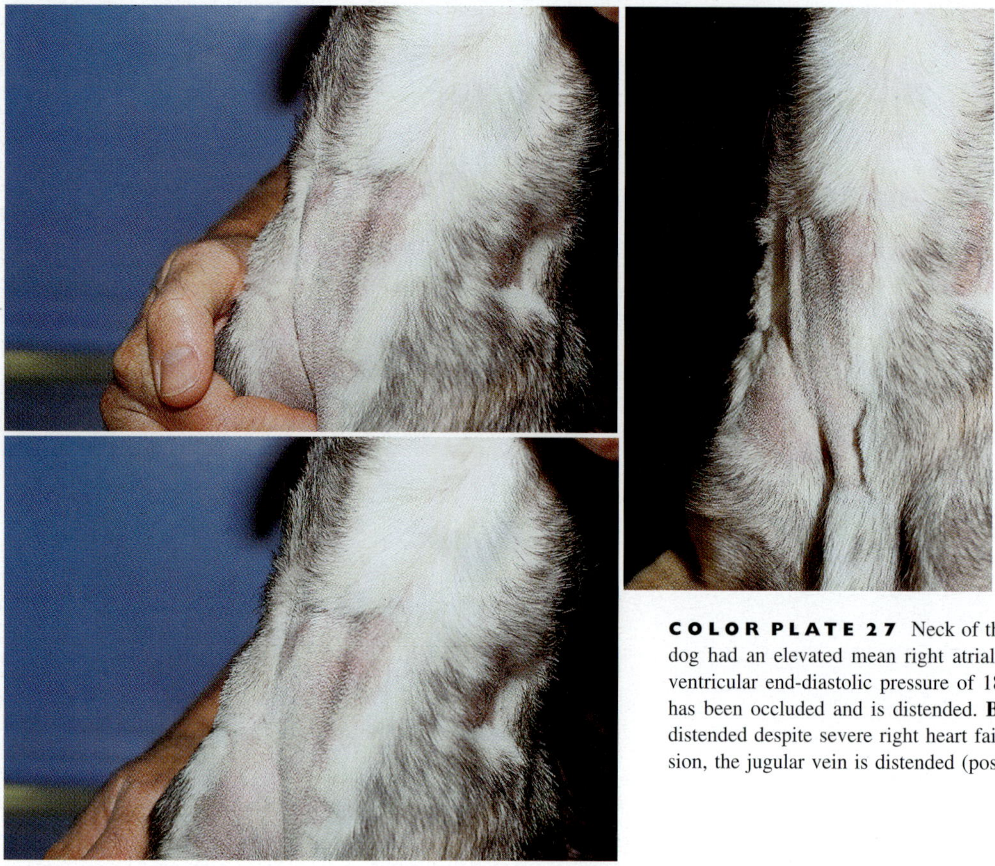

COLOR PLATE 27 Neck of the dog shown in Color Plate 24. This dog had an elevated mean right atrial pressure of 13 mm Hg and a right ventricular end-diastolic pressure of 18 mm Hg. **A,** The right jugular vein has been occluded and is distended. **B,** Without occlusion, the vein is not distended despite severe right heart failure. **C,** During abdominal compression, the jugular vein is distended (positive hepatojugular reflux test).

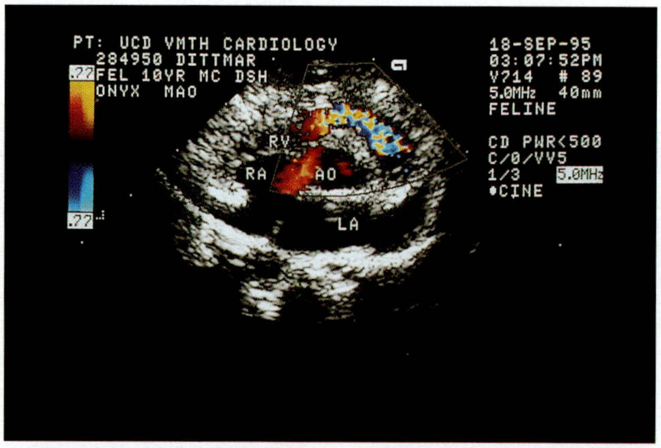

COLOR PLATE 28 Recording of color flow Doppler from a cat with a heart murmur but no evidence of cardiac disease. The region of turbulence in the right ventricular outflow tract presumably created the murmur in this cat. The peak flow velocity was 2.3 m/sec. *RV,* Right ventricle; *RA,* right atrium; *AO,* aorta; *LA,* left atrium.

increased cardiac output, usually because it needs a greater supply of oxygen. The increase in heart rate is generally beneficial to the rest of the body but may be detrimental to the heart. For example, tachydysrhythmia may be detrimental because of inadequate ventricular filling time or because it produces myocardial failure when the ventricular rate achieves 210 to 260 beats/min for prolonged periods in the dog.[40]

HYPERTROPHY

In chronic heart disease the aforementioned factors are not the only factors that determine the ability of the left ventricle to pump blood. Hypertrophy is an extremely important factor in chronic heart disease and so warrants detailed consideration. Hypertrophy is an increase in the weight of an organ as a result of increase in cell size with no change in cell number. It is similar to the physiologic property of growth, although growth may also occur via hyperplasia (increase in cell number). The increase in cell size in myocardium is caused by sarcomere hyperplasia (increased numbers of contractile elements). The method by which the cell increases sarcomere numbers is thought to involve the intercalated discs that proliferate and lay down new sarcomeres.[41] Hypertrophy occurs in response to increased systolic pressure (a pressure overload) or in response to increased diastolic pressure and volume (a volume overload) (Color Plate 23). The two forms of hypertrophy are eccentric, or volume overload, hypertrophy and concentric, or pressure overload, hypertrophy.[31,42]

Concentric hypertrophy. Concentric hypertrophy is the form of hypertrophy that clinicians are used to thinking about. It is characterized by a thick wall and a normal chamber size.[43] Concentric hypertrophy occurs in response to an increase in systolic intraventricular pressure (a pressure overload) and systolic wall stress such as occurs with aortic stenosis and systemic hypertension. Concentric hypertrophy is usually produced to normalize afterload when afterload is increased by an increase in systolic intraventricular pressure.[41,44]

If one were to create aortic stenosis experimentally, the heart would start with normal EDV, normal ESV, and normal wall thickness. The stenosis would increase systolic intraventricular pressure as depicted in Figure 2-15. This would result in an increase in systolic wall stress ($[P \times r]/2h$) or afterload. This increased force would push out against the walls of the left ventricle, making it more difficult for them to contract inward. Therefore the walls could not contract as far inward, and ESV would increase. This would result in a decrease in stroke volume. To compensate for this, the heart increases its wall thickness and in so doing decreases systolic wall stress or afterload (note that the increase in pressure in the numerator is compensated for by the increase in wall thickness in the denominator). By doing this over time it allows the ESV to come back to normal with no change in contractility, as seen in Figure 2-17.

The major stimulus for hypertrophy appears to be an increase in wall tension or stress (systolic or diastolic) that triggers the sarcomeres to replicate within the cells.[45,46] It has been noted that sodium influx into the cell increases in response to an increased load in isolated myocardial cells, and that myocardial protein synthesis varies directly with sodium influx.[47] Consequently, deformation-dependent sodium influx may be one of the signals that transduces change in load (force) into increased actin and myosin synthesis and so myocardial hypertrophy. In the study that identified sodium influx as a signal for cell growth, ouabain, a digitalis glycoside, inhibited protein synthesis.[45] Besides mechanical factors, neurohumoral factors such as α_1-adrenoreceptor stimulation, angiotensin II, endothelin, and myotrophin, a newly described factor produced in the myocardium, appear to induce myocardial hypertrophy.[48-51] Mechanical and humoral factors may interact to produce hypertrophy. Recent studies have demonstrated that mechanical stretching of myocytes results in autocrine secretion of angiotensin II.[52] This local production of angiotensin II then stimulates the type 1 angiotensin receptor. This receptor is coupled to a G protein (G_q) that ultimately stimulates $p12^{ras}$ through phosphorylation of tyrosine in intermediary proteins by a tyrosine kinase.[53] Ras proteins are protooncogenes that stimulate cell growth. Angiotensin II also stimulates other protooncogenes. Its effects not only occur through activation of protein kinases but also through activation of phospholipase C activity.[54] In addition, angiotensin II induces phosphorylation of insulin receptor substrate, a substrate for growth hormone.[54]

In concentric hypertrophy, sarcomeres would be expected to replicate in parallel (side by side), resulting in wider cells and a thicker wall. Myocardial fiber diameter is increased in human patients with aortic stenosis.[55] The percentage of the cell occupied by sarcomeres is increased when myocardial cells grow larger.[56] In other words what appears to be cellular hypertrophy is in reality sarcomere hyperplasia. There is, however, evidence to suggest that some cellular hyperplasia may also occur in concentric hypertrophy.[57,58]

In dogs, concentric hypertrophy is a very efficient means of compensating for even severe pressure overloads. Most dogs with severe subaortic stenosis have normal EDVs and ESVs. Myocardial failure (decreased myocardial contractility) secondary to subaortic stenosis is rare in dogs. We have seen only a small number of dogs with significant myocardial failure and heart failure secondary to subaortic stenosis. In one study of dogs with experimentally produced severe aortic stenosis (peak systolic intraventricular pressure = 254 ± 14 mm Hg, wall thickness = 18.4 ± 1.2 mm), left ventricular function was normal at rest. In humans, indexes of left ventricular function may be decreased in patients with aortic stenosis. However, one study has suggested that this may be due to inadequate concentric hypertrophy and a resultant inappropriately high systolic wall stress rather than myocardial failure.[59] In dogs with moderate (81% increase in left ventricular mass) experimentally produced aortic stenosis, myocardial oxygenation was normal, which may help explain why myocardial failure is so uncommon in this disease.[60] However, the thickened walls that are seen secondary to congenital pressure overloads in dogs and cats may be more due to myocyte hyperplasia than to hypertrophy in certain situations. During fetal life, myocytes have the ability to replicate (hyperplasia). Lesions such as pulmonic stenosis are present in the fetal heart and so may

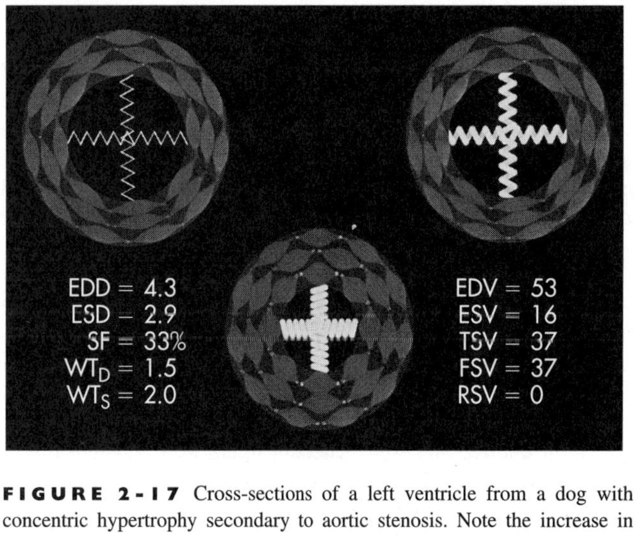

FIGURE 2-17 Cross-sections of a left ventricle from a dog with concentric hypertrophy secondary to aortic stenosis. Note the increase in spring thickness in systole, the increased wall thickness as result of addition of another row of contractile elements, and the normal hemodynamic variables. Abbreviations as in Figure 2-13.

stimulate myocyte replication. A lesion like subaortic stenosis that develops after birth would more likely stimulate sarcomere hyperplasia and hypertrophy.

Eccentric hypertrophy. Eccentric hypertrophy is quite different from concentric hypertrophy. Eccentric hypertrophy occurs whenever it is advantageous for the heart to increase its EDV (volume overload) and is commonly inappropriately referred to as *dilation.* It is characterized by an increase in left ventricular chamber volume or diameter with a relatively normal wall thickness (Color Plate 23).[43] Obviously, the weight of such a left ventricle is greater than normal. An increase in weight could occur because of either cellular hypertrophy or cellular hyperplasia with or without increases in interstitial cellular components. In eccentric hypertrophy it appears that most of the increase is due to cellular hypertrophy caused by replication of sarcomeres in series (end-to-end).[42] This results in cells that are longer than normal. Increases in interstitial components, including increased fibrosis, also may occur.[42]

An increase in EDV is advantageous in many forms of heart disease because in a larger heart more blood is ejected for any given amount of contraction or percent of myocardial fiber shortening (e.g., shortening fraction). A 5-kg dog and a 30-kg dog have the same shortening fraction, but the larger dog has a much larger stroke volume because of its larger heart (i.e., its larger EDV). Eccentric hypertrophy occurs in many diseases, from dilated cardiomyopathy to mitral regurgitation. It occurs in diseases in which leaks are present, such as mitral regurgitation and patent ductus arteriosus, so that the TSV of the left ventricle can increase to compensate for the leak (increased EDV coupled with normal wall motion leads to an increase in TSV). In dilated cardiomyopathy eccentric hypertrophy occurs so that stroke volume can remain normal when myocardial fiber shortening (shortening fraction) decreases. Eccentric hypertrophy, put simply, is the process of the heart growing larger in a structurally similar way to the way it would grow in a maturing dog or cat. The major differences are that the wall tends to not thicken as much and capillary density does not increase proportionately.[42] It is very similar to the type of growth stimulated in the heart by strenuous running exercise.[42] In clinical practice it is not unusual to see a 10-kg dog with heart disease with a left ventricular chamber the same size as that of a normal 25-kg dog.

Eccentric hypertrophy (commonly called *dilation*) is the result of a process that usually starts with a decrease in forward cardiac output (blood flow into the aorta) that occurs either in response to a decrease in myocardial contractility or the presence of a leak.[43] The body, especially the kidneys, senses the decrease in blood flow and the net result is that the kidneys are forced to retain more sodium and water.[19] The sodium and water retention causes an increase in blood volume and an increase in venous return to the heart. This increase in venous return increases preload (end-diastolic wall stress) and consequently places chronic stretch on the myocardium. It is thought that the myocardium senses and responds to this increased chronic stretch. It is also thought that sarcomere replication occurs in series (end-to-end) in response.[43] This results in longer cells and a larger ventricular chamber. Again the heart grows larger through sarcomere hyperplasia. The same factors mentioned previously that are responsible for concentric hypertrophy are also probably responsible for eccentric hypertrophy. A heart with eccentric hypertrophy is commonly called a *dilated* heart, and it is true that the chamber is dilated. The term *dilated,* however, generally refers to a structure that is passively distended with a substance, such as a balloon filled with air. In this situation the mass of the balloon does not change and consequently the wall thins as distension occurs. This is usually not the situation that occurs in chronic left ventricular disease. The ventricle does not passively distend very well. It is a stiff structure that is more like a basketball than a balloon. It can be distended to take advantage of Starling's law, but this sort of distension only increases EDV by 30% to 40%, as illustrated previously. The EDV can be increased by more than 200% in chronic diseases via eccentric hypertrophy. Simply stated, a left ventricle generally cannot become extremely enlarged through simple distension (this is not always true in human medicine, in which infarcted myocardium can distend tremendously). Eccentric hypertrophy is a better means of compensating for chronic ventricular disease than is a simple increase in preload affecting Starling's law. Stating that a ventricle is "dilated" should be avoided, because it depicts the wrong process of cardiac enlargement. Also, stating that "increased preload" is the mechanism of compensation in volume overload should be avoided, because eccentric hypertrophy is the variable that is greatly affecting left ventricular function. Any heart that has an end-diastolic pressure greater than 20 mm Hg is stretched to its maximum (sarcomere length = 2.2 to 2.28 μm) and so has no preload reserve.[61,62] Consequently, one cannot realistically increase preload further in such a heart.[19]

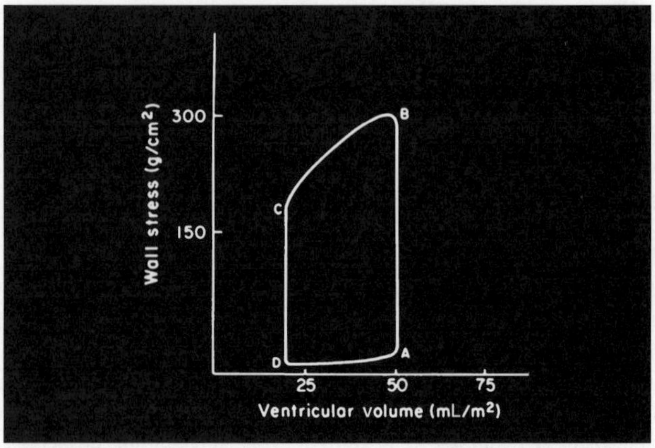

FIGURE 2-18 Wall stress–volume loop from a normal 28-kg dog. Various stages of the cardiac cycle are labeled. *A,* End-diastole and closure of the mitral valve. *B,* Onset of ejection and aortic valve opening. *C,* End-systole and aortic valve closure. *D,* Onset of ventricular filling and mitral valve opening. *A* – *D* = Stroke volume.

WALL-STRESS VOLUME LOOPS

One of the best means of depicting systolic left ventricular function, especially in the face of left ventricular disease, and to determine left ventricular contractility is to plot left ventricular wall stress vs. left ventricular volume.[63,64] An illustration of a perceived normal left ventricular wall stress–volume loop is depicted in Figure 2-18. In this type of analysis, end-diastolic wall stress is preload. Afterload is the wall stress throughout systole and so is constantly changing. End-systolic wall stress is most commonly used to depict afterload.[65]

The ESV in the lower center part of Figure 2-16 is determined by contractility and afterload.[66] To separate contractility from afterload, one can alter afterload, as in Figure 2-19.[67] In this figure, a vasopressor has been infused to increase systolic intraventricular pressure and so increase afterload (systolic wall stress). Refer to Figure 2-15 to see the net result of this type of perturbation. One should readily appreciate that as systolic wall stress is increased, ESV increases. This is logical. As the force opposing contraction increases, the myocardium is unable to shorten and move as well as

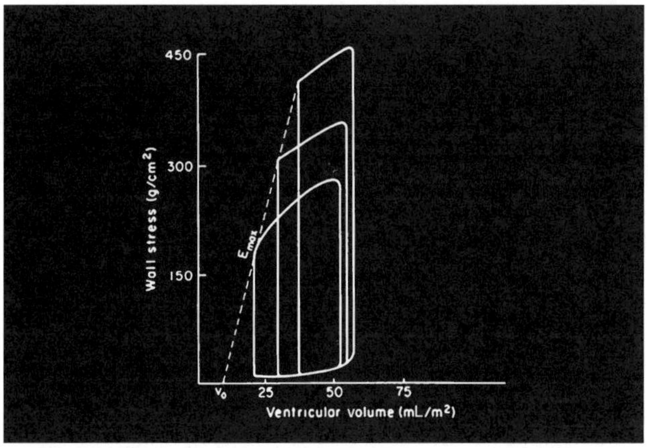

FIGURE 2-19 Wall stress–volume loops from a normal left ventricle from a 28-kg dog. A vasopressor has been infused to increase systolic intraventricular pressure. Consequently, systolic wall stress has been increased, resulting in two new wall stress–volume loops with larger end-systolic volumes. A line connecting the end-systolic wall stress–volume points has been drawn. This line has slope that represents the maximal elastance of muscle *(Emax)* and an *x*-axis intercept that represents the theoretic end-systolic volume that would be attained if afterload was zero *(V_0)*.

long as contractility does not change. It is the same as a person lifting weights. The heavier the weight, the shorter the distance it can be lifted in a given period for a given amount of muscular effort. If one draws a line connecting several end-systolic wall stress–volume points, one can define contractility.[68] The slope of this line is labeled E_{max} and the *x*-axis intercept is labeled V_0. E_{max} represents the maximal elastance of the ventricle, and V_0 is the theoretic volume the chamber could empty to if afterload were zero. This line shows what the ESV will be for any given afterload at the contractility defined by this line. When contractility decreases, the slope of the line flattens and V_0 shifts to the right. When contractility is increased, the slope becomes steeper and V_0 shifts to the left.[68] In other words, when contractility decreases, the ESV is greater for any given systolic wall stress (afterload), because the myocardium is weaker and cannot contract down to a normal ESV. When contractility increases, the opposite occurs.

Blood Flow

VASCULAR SMOOTH MUSCLE

Vascular smooth muscle is similar to the smooth muscle of the GI tract and other organs. The contractile apparatus is not arranged in sarcomeres, but myosin and actin are present. Cross-sections of vascular smooth muscles shows that about 15 actin filaments are disposed around each myosin filament in a rosette pattern. The chemical characteristics of smooth muscle filaments are similar but not exactly the same as in striated muscle. Actin filaments are attached to structures called dense bodies, some of which are in turn attached to the cell membrane and others are held in place by a scaffold of structural protein cross-attachments from one dense body to another. Despite the relative paucity of thick filaments there is still sufficient cross-bridge formation, and studies have shown that smooth muscle can generate the same strength per unit cross-sectional area as striated muscle. The actions of calcium movements are "slow" in smooth muscle cells, and hence the duration of contraction is seconds rather than tens of milliseconds, as in striated muscle.

Receptors

Vascular smooth muscle cells possess numerous receptors. Those of the autonomic nervous system are most important, but receptors for histamine, serotonin, ATP, and other vasoactive substances are also present in many vessels.

α-Adrenergic receptors. Subtypes 1 and 2 of α-adrenergic receptors are both found. Agonist binding leads to smooth muscle contraction. Presynaptic α_2-receptors inhibit the release of norepinephrine from the nerve ending and serve as a feedback loop that modulates extraneural concentration of the transmitter.

β-Adrenergic receptors. β-adrenergic receptors, found in most vessels, inhibit contraction and thus relax smooth muscle. All subtypes (β_1, β_2, and β_3) exist, with β_2 more prominent. Both α- and β-adrenergic receptors exist in the same vessels and share the same transmitter (norepinephrine). The net effect on the action of the smooth muscle depends on the affinity and numbers of the two classes of receptors. The alpha effect usually, but not always, predominates.

Muscarinic receptors. Cholinergic receptors of the muscarinic type are found in many vessels. They are found on both endothelial and smooth muscle cells. Binding of acetylcholine to smooth muscle causes contraction.

Factors other than receptors also affect smooth vascular tone in systemic arterioles and precapillary sphincters. Shear stress on the endothelium releases nitric oxide (NO), resulting in smooth muscle relaxation. Local metabolites (e.g., K^+, ATP, adenosine, oxygen) control the contraction of precapillary sphincters.

STEADY FLOW AND VASCULAR RESISTANCE

Because of the mechanical nature of the heart and blood vessels, physical principles can be applied to analyze cardiovascular function. Hemodynamics involve principles that relate the physical movement of blood and the strength of contraction to the physical properties of the structures involved. Most methods employ classic laws of force and motion expressed in forms appropriate to the unusual nature of the system.

Steady flow denotes the absence of pulsations and a continuous stream moving at a constant velocity. Although the cardiovascular system is pulsatile, some concepts of steady flow apply.

Viscosity. Because fluids (blood) have no fixed shape they tend to move in laminae, or layers, of different velocities. The differences in velocity arise, in part, as a result of frictional drag imposed by the walls of the vessels and the individual properties of the fluid (viscosity). Fluids in which the viscosity is not directly influenced by the absolute velocity are said to be *Newtonian* fluids. Blood is not entirely a Newtonian fluid.[69] Its apparent viscosity increases with increasing cellular content and rises at low shear rates. The viscosity of blood is a relevant factor in the relationship between pressure, flow, and the dimensions of the container. However, across the range of normal hematocrits and blood flows, the viscosity of canine blood is relatively constant (approximately 0.03 to 0.04 poise at 37° C).[70]

Poiseuille's law and vascular resistance. Resistance to flow provided by blood vessels (vascular resistance) is a primary determinant of blood pressure in the vascular system. Because pressure is a primary determinant of afterload (systolic wall stress), resistance is an important determinant of afterload. Relative resistance between the systemic and pulmonary circulations are important determinants of shunt flow in congenital cardiac abnormalities such as PDA and ventricular septal defect.

Poiseuille's law states that the ratio of driving pressure to blood flow is a function of the physical properties of the system (resistance). The motion of blood through a tube depends not only on the force applied (pressure) but also the length and radius of the tube and blood viscosity (which determine resistance). In a sense, the system opposes the flow (Q) to an extent determined by its dimensions. The mathematical relation is:

$$Q = \frac{\pi r^4 (P_1 - P_2)}{8\eta L}$$

where r = radius of the vessel; P_1 and P_2 = pressures on either end of the vessel; η = viscosity of blood; and L = length of the vessel. Poiseuille's Law has been firmly established for the special conditions of steady laminar flow in cylindrical tubes. Even under pulsatile conditions, Poiseuille's law approximates the relationships between mean pressure and flow averaged over an integral number of cardiac cycles.

Resistance, flow, and pressure in a steady-flow system are related as follows:

$$Q = \frac{(P_1 - P_2)}{R}$$

where R = resistance, P_x = pressure downstream and upstream, and Q = flow. This equation resembles Ohm's law of electrical resistance, which relates the ratio of voltage to electrical current (current = voltage/resistance). Obviously, none of these conditions are satisfied perfectly by mammalian circulatory systems, yet the true relationships depart only moderately from Poiseuille's law.

Combining the equations for Poiseuille's law and resistance we get the following relationship:

$$R = \frac{8\eta L}{\pi r^4}$$

From this relationship it can be readily appreciated that the radius of the resistance vessels is the major variable that determines vascular resistance. For this relationship to be valid, flow must be laminar and the following conditions must be met: (1) the conduit must be cylindrical, (2) flow must be steady (not pulsatile), and (3) the viscosity must be Newtonian.

Resistance in a vascular bed in various animals is inversely proportional to body size, a relationship that arises from the architecture of the circulation and the effects of parallel, in contrast with series, connections of resistances. Vascular resistance can be indexed to body size by multiplying resistance times body surface area (Table 2-1).

If three tubes are connected in sequence, total resistance is a combination of the individual resistances (as in electrical circuits):

$$\text{Series: } R_T = R_1 + R_2 + R_3$$

TABLE 2-1

Typical vascular resistances at rest (dyne sec/cm^5 or dyne sec/cm^5 m^2)

Vascular bed	*Dog (20 kg; 0.75 m²)*	*Man (70 kg; 1.75 m²)*	*Resistance index (1 m²)*
Pulmonary	400	175	300
Systemic	3000	1300	2250
Splanchnic	11,700	5100	8800
Renal (both)	14,600	6300	11,000
Cerebral	23,400	10,100	17,500

When the resistances are connected in parallel, a reciprocal relationship applies:

$$\text{Parallel: } \frac{1}{R_T} = \frac{1}{R_1} + \frac{1}{R_2} + \frac{1}{R_3}$$

To illustrate what type of difference this creates, pretend that the average resistance index of all of the vessels other than the splanchnic, renal, and cerebral vessels was 300 dyne sec/cm^5 m^2, as in the example in Table 2-1. If the vascular beds from all of these areas were connected in series, the resistance index to flow would be 39,550 dyne sec/cm^5 m^2. Because they are connected in parallel, the resistance index is 1416 dyne sec/cm^5 m^2.

All mammals basically have the same number of large vessels; they differ, however, in the periphery, where the number of small vessels with parallel connections increases with increasing size of the animal (hence, the lower resistance). The increased number of vessels carries a proportionate increase in flow such that pressure stays the same despite body size. The resistance in the mammalian circulation is concentrated in the microcirculation (arterioles).

The units for vascular resistance may be expressed as dyne sec/cm^5 (absolute resistance units) or as mm Hg/L/min (Wood's units or hybrid resistance units). One absolute resistance unit equals 80 times one hybrid unit. Resistance is calculated in clinical medicine using Ohm's law (above) by measuring flow and pressure.

PULSATILE FLOW AND VASCULAR IMPEDANCE

In a pulsatile system, resistance is no longer the only factor that helps determine flow. Resistance is still the primary factor, however. In addition to resistance, compliance, inertance, and reflectance factor into making up a variable called *impedance.* Impedance is one of the factors that determines the force a ventricle must generate to eject blood.

Compliance. Compliance is primarily determined by the compliance or stiffness of the aorta (Color Plate 21). If 30 mL of blood is ejected into a very stiff aorta and systolic pressure increases to 200 mm Hg, administering a drug that relaxes the smooth muscle in the aorta will decrease systolic pressure to, for example, 150 mm Hg. The more compliant aorta will accommodate more blood and the ventricle will eject against a lesser pressure. Consequently, stroke volume will increase.

Compliance describes the elastic behavior of a hollow vessel or chamber. It refers to changes in capacity (volume) in relation to changes in transmural pressure and is expressed as:

$$C = \frac{\Delta V}{\Delta P}$$

Compliance and stiffness are related in a reciprocal way; a vessel that is stiff is incompliant. Distensibility and compliance are synonymous. Compliance becomes very important in pulsatile flow systems. Aortic compliance is a major determinant of flow and the relationship between pressure and flow.

The compliance of vessels is determined by the elasticity of the constituents that make up their walls. Although elastic fibers and smooth muscle are quite elastic, the collagen network of the adventitia and collagen fibers in the media are not. The mechanical behavior of the vessel is also influenced by the way these elements are interconnected. In simple elastic substances, stress (force) and strain (distension or stretch) are directly proportional. This is not so with blood vessels, mainly because of the heterogeneous makeup of the vascular wall, but also in part because of the relative stiffness of collagen.

Blood vessels become stiffer (increased elastic modulus) as they are distended, much like a ventricle. Vessels are readily distended when the radius is relatively small; a small increase in stress is accompanied by a large increase in the radius (strain). At large radii the vessel is stiff; small increments in stress produce only small increments in the radius. The steepness of the right-hand portion of a vessel stress-strain relationship develops as the stiff collagen network bears more and more of the stress.

Smooth muscle contraction reduces the radius at any given pressure and shifts the stress-strain curve upward and to the left. Muscle contraction combined with an increase in transmural pressure may leave the radius unchanged. Smooth muscle contraction in the aorta produces clinically significant changes in aortic compliance.

Inertance. Inertance is the force required to start a column of blood moving (inertia). It is reasonable to suspect that inertance changes when body position changes. For example, it is much easier to start blood moving in a person that is lying down vs. one that is standing. It is more difficult to start moving that column of blood in a person that is standing on his head.

Reflectance. Reflectance refers to the fact that pressure and flow waveforms reflect back, primarily from branching sites within the vasculature, adding to the force against which a ventricle must eject. The reflected waves originate mainly from sites where small peripheral arteries divide, resulting in abrupt changes in the vessel diameter. They also originate from the aorta as it progressively changes diameter. When waves reflect, the wave observed at any point in the vascular system is a sum of a forward-moving and a retrograde wave. Waves may be in phase at some points, creating larger waves, but may be as much as 180 degrees out of phase at other points, resulting in wave diminution.

PULSATILE HEMODYNAMICS

Pulsatile hemodynamics are concerned with sinusoidal waves of pressure and flow oscillating around some positive average value. The waves that occur in the circulation are not sinusoidal. However, pressure and flow waveforms can be broken down into sinusoids at their harmonic constituents using Fourier analysis. Each harmonic waveform has a certain amplitude and frequency. For example, if the heart rate is 120 beats/min in a dog, its pressure waveform in the aorta will have a basic sine wave frequency of 2 Hz (2 cycles/sec). This sine wave would have a similar amplitude to the amplitude of the pressure waveform. However, it would look nothing like the original waveform. If a smaller waveform at 4 Hz was added to the basic waveform, the resultant waveform would start to look a little more like the original waveform but still would look very different. As one continued to add in faster and smaller sinusoidal waveforms (harmonics), the resultant waveform would look more and more like the original pressure waveform. Ultimately, one would have a family of waveforms, each described by its frequency and amplitude, that would constitute the original waveform.

In contrast to resistance, which is mean pressure divided by mean flow, impedance is the ratio of sinusoidal components of pressure and flow at each harmonic frequency. Impedance, similar to resistance, expresses a determinant of the force against which the ventricle must eject and determines the amount of work the ventricle must produce for a given pulsatile flow. Vascular impedance in any part of the circulation can be calculated by frequency analysis of pressure and flow pulsations that are simultaneously recorded. The impedance amplitude at any given harmonic frequency is the ratio of the pressure to flow amplitudes, and the phase difference between the pressure and flow sinusoids is the impedance phase angle. The ratio of mean arterial pressure and mean flow is impedance at a frequency of zero and is the same thing as input resistance. Resistance is the same as in a steady-flow system and so is determined primarily by the cross-sectional area of the systemic arteriolar vascular bed on the systemic side. Resistance is considerably higher than the impedance to pulsatile waves (i.e., the ratio of pressure to flow at the different harmonics is less than mean pressure divided by mean flow). The impedance observed in any artery is the input impedance of the vascular bed it supplies. Aortic input impedance defines the impedance that must be overcome by the ventricle to eject blood into the aorta. In the aorta, pressure may precede flow or flow may precede pressure (good evidence that it is not pressure that pushes blood flow through the vasculature but rather the force of ventricular contraction). The relationship between pressure and flow is a phase angle. Negative phase angles indicate that flow leads pressure, and positive phase angles indicate that pressure precedes flow.

Pressure waves travel primarily in an antegrade fashion through the vasculature. However, some portions of these waves are reflected back in the system to combine with waveforms traveling forward. This results in an increase in impedance, primarily at low frequencies. Reflections do not affect mean pressure and flow or resistance and have very little effect on the ratio between pressure and flow at higher frequencies. Vasoconstriction increases reflections, thus increasing low-frequency impedance oscillations. Vasodilation has the opposite effect. The ratio of pressure to flow at higher frequencies is primarily determined by vessel properties, specifically the compliance of the aorta. An average of the pressure-flow ratio at higher frequencies is often called the *characteristic impedance* (Z_o).

LAMINAR FLOW VS. TURBULENT FLOW

Laminar flow means all fluid layers move in a longitudinal direction without eddies of radial deviation (Figure 2-20). In a straight tube this consists of a set of concentric, cylindrical shells. The most rapid motion occurs centrally, and velocity progressively decreases toward the wall of the tube, forming a parabolic velocity profile (Newtonian or parabolic flow).

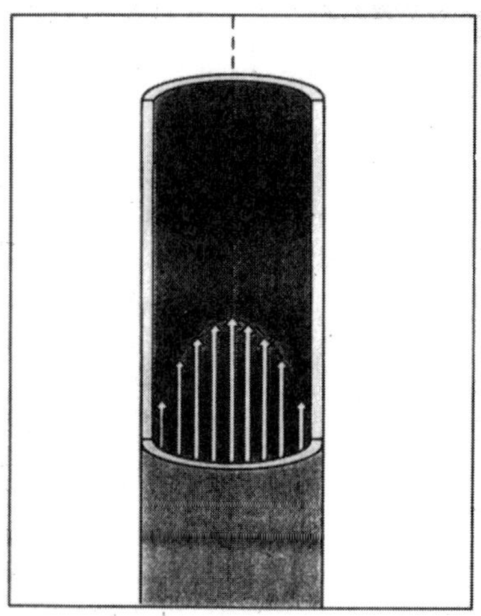

FIGURE 2-20 Schematic drawing of laminar blood flow. Flow velocity is similar across the vessel, with the flow velocity in the center marginally greater than along the sides. Flow is streamlined, with no radial or circumferential motion. (From Berne RM, Levy MN: *Cardiovascular Physiology,* ed 9, St. Louis, 1996, Mosby.)

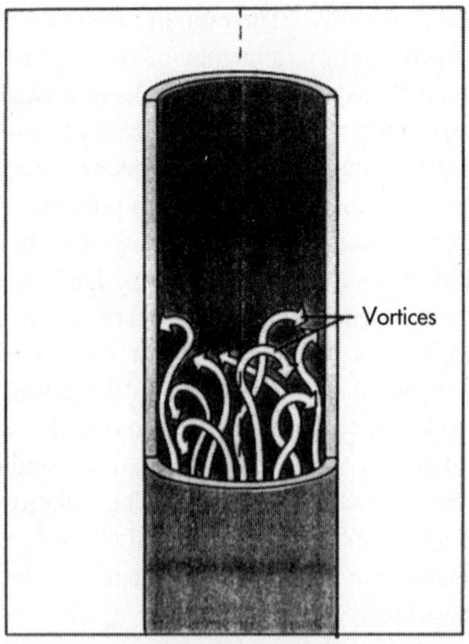

FIGURE 2-21 Schematic drawing of turbulent blood flow. High-velocity blood flow is disturbed, with the blood cells moving axially, radially, and circumferentially. Vortices (whirlpools) may develop. (From Berne RM, Levy MN: *Cardiovascular Physiology,* ed 9, St. Louis, 1996, Mosby.)

Laminar flow can be disturbed under certain conditions, producing eddies and vortices (i.e., turbulence) (Figure 2-21). Sharp bends or obstructions are most common, but other conditions also produce turbulence. The significance of turbulence is that it dissipates energy, and Poiseuille's Law no longer applies, because the pressure drop is much greater than the equation would predict.

The critical factors leading to turbulent blood flow have been mathematically described as Reynolds number:

$$N_R = \frac{2r\bar{v}\rho}{\eta}$$

where r = radius, v = velocity, ρ = fluid density, and η = viscosity. The higher the number, the greater the likelihood of turbulence. The critical number, based on empiric observations, is 2300. Reynolds number rarely achieves the turbulence-producing levels in the normal cardiovascular system, and flow is generally laminar. Reynolds number in the human aorta and pulmonary artery is about 1600.

As can be deduced from the formula, Reynolds number, and so the possibility for turbulence, increases as blood flow velocity increases, blood viscosity decreases, or the area into which blood is flowing increases (abruptly). For example, turbulence can easily be produced in water by increasing velocity. A finger over the end of a garden hose to increase resistance will increase velocity of flow from the end of the hose. Turbulence can be seen and heard such as molasses, as the water squirts out the end of the hose. Water is a very-low-viscosity fluid. With a very viscous fluid, such as molasses, flowing through the same hose to achieve the same velocity, it would be more difficult to produce turbulence even if the same velocity was achieved.

HYDRAULIC ENERGY

Hydraulic energy is important to the understanding of flow and pressure. It is especially important for understanding the relationship between pressure gradient and change in velocity, a concept that is used frequently when interpreting Doppler ultrasound.

Poiseuille's law defines a fall in hydraulic energy along a tube under certain conditions of steady flow. The heart supplies the energy, and the motion of blood through the vessels dissipates the energy. In addition, the inertia of blood must be overcome, and the heart must work against gravitational influences. The Poiseuille equation only includes one of the three types of energy associated with blood flow (pressure energy). Energy is the product of force and distance (dyne cm). Hemodynamics deal with pressure, kinetic, and gravitational energy.

Poiseuille ignored kinetic and gravitational influences because he used low velocities in horizontal tubes. Similar situations exist in vivo, and, largely, pressure energy is much larger than the other two. When the kinetic and gravitational influences are absent, pressure falls linearly along the length of the tube. If the cross-sectional area changes abruptly, however, kinetic energy can be converted to pressure, or vice versa, a phenomenon described by Bernoulli.

Bernoulli's principle states that if flow is maintained across a change in cross-sectional area, the change in pressure is equal and opposite to the change in kinetic energy (ignoring gravitational forces). By simplifying the equation, for clinical application, the change in pressure is related to the change in velocity:

$$P_2 - P_1 = 4(V_2 - V_1)^2$$

Lateral and end pressures are another situation in which kinetic energy must be taken into account. Needles or catheters placed into a stream of blood to bring the blood that impinges on them to almost zero velocity, so that its kinetic energy is converted to local pressure. This phenomenon has no effect on laterally placed openings (lateral pressure), but when an end-hole catheter is used (end pressure) the pressure detected is higher by an amount equivalent of the kinetic energy. The effect is reversed if the opening faces downstream. Normally, the difference is less than 1 mm Hg, but may increase to more than 10 mm Hg in high-velocity jets.

PULSE PRESSURE

Arterial pulse pressure (systolic – diastolic pressure) is the force felt by one's fingers when palpating a pulse. It is related to the stroke volume, the velocity of ejection, and the elastic modulus of the vessel. The stiffer the vessel, the larger the pulse pressure for a given stroke volume. In addition, the larger the stroke volume or the more rapidly it is ejected, the greater the pulse pressure.

These simple rules are all that is necessary to explain physiologic changes in pulsatile blood pressure in most conditions. The principle is straightforward: resistance and mean flow themselves do not affect systolic and diastolic pressure, but the mean pressure they determine carries those oscillations up or down with it.

Neurohumoral Control of the Circulation

Although the completely denervated heart in a cardiac transplant patient performs well, the normal individual has numerous mechanisms for controlling the cardiovascular system. These include central nervous system control, hormonal control, and local control. These mechanisms alter vascular tone, myocardial contractility, heart rate, and blood volume to ensure adequate blood pressure and blood flow to all organs at a normal venous pressure. Control of pressure, blood volume, and flow are considered separately.

NEUROHUMORAL CONTROL OF SYSTEMIC BLOOD PRESSURE AND FLOW

Nervous control. As explained previously, systemic blood pressure is primarily determined by systemic vascular resistance, cardiac output, and blood volume. The central nervous system has numerous inputs from the cardiovascular system to sense changes in function and numerous outputs to the cardiovascular system to alter function (Figure 2-22). Afferent connections come from the aortic barorecep-

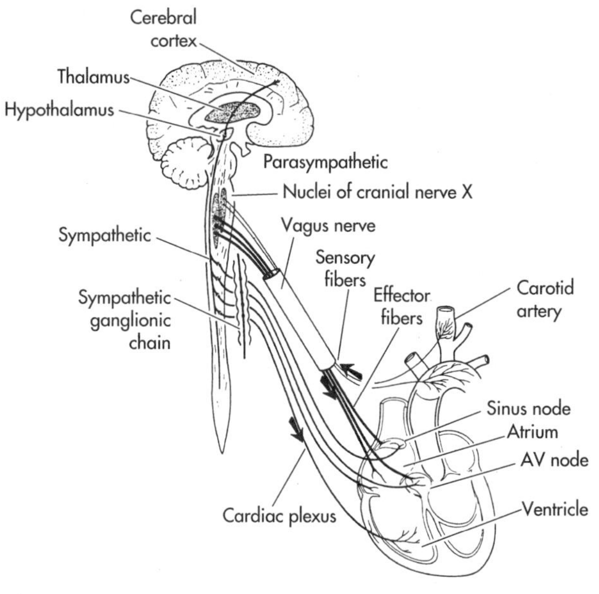

FIGURE 2-22 Drawing of the autonomic nervous system. (Modified from Phillips RE, Feeney MK: *Cardiac rhythms: a systematic approach to interpretation,* ed 3, Philadelphia, 1990, WB Saunders.)

tors and chemoreceptors, the carotid sinuses and bodies, and the cardiopulmonary receptors.[3] The baroreceptors in the aortic arch and the carotid sinuses sense change in pressure within the systemic arterial system. The glossopharyngeal nerve carries afferent nerve traffic to the medulla from the carotid sinuses, and the vagus nerve carries the same nerve traffic from the aortic baroreceptors. When these regions sense a decrease in blood pressure, the sympathetic nervous system is activated and the parasympathetic nervous system is suppressed. The net result is an increase in heart rate, myocardial contractility, and systemic arteriolar constriction that bring blood pressure back to normal. Sympathetic stimulation of venous receptors produces venoconstriction and increases venous return to the heart. Increased sympathetic nerve traffic to the kidneys increases renin release and, ultimately, increased sodium retention. The opposite occurs when the mechanoreceptors in these regions sense an increase in blood pressure.

Changes in blood pressure result in profound changes in the efferent neural system, or autonomic nervous system. The autonomic nervous system is divided into two major divisions: the sympathetic, or thoracolumbar, division and the parasympathetic, or craniosacral, division.[3] Cells of the sympathetic division originate in the lateral horn of spinal grey matter from the eighth cervical segment to the third lumbar segment. Their myelinated axons exit the spinal cord via the ventral roots and pass to numerous sympathetic ganglia that lie as a chain along either side of the vertebral column. Excision of the stellate and upper four cervical ganglia disables most postganglionic innervation to the heart and major blood vessels. In the cat, most of the synapses that eventually reach the heart are in the stellate ganglia, whereas in the dog they are in the middle, or caudal, cervical ganglia.[71] Acetylcholine acts as the neurotransmitter between preganglionic and postganglionic fibers in the ganglia. Unmyelinated postganglionic fibers leave the ganglia to join peripheral nerves that innervate vascular smooth muscle and the heart. The heart is served by the superior, middle, and inferior cardiac nerves. Sympathetic activation results in stimulation of adrenergic receptors on the heart and blood vessels, primarily by norepinephrine. Epinephrine is also released, but the majority of this catecholamine is supplied by the adrenal medulla. Norepinephrine stimulates both α- and β-adrenergic receptors. In most regions of the body, α_1- adrenergic receptors predominate on vascular smooth muscle. α_1-Adrenergic receptor stimulation results in smooth muscle contraction (vasoconstriction). Vascular smooth muscle also contains β_2-adrenergic receptors, which produce vasodilation if the α- adrenergic receptors are blocked. In the myocardium, β_1-adrenergic receptors predominate. Stimulation results in increases in contractility and heart rate. β_2-Adrenergic receptors also are present but to a lesser extent in ventricular myocardium. β_2-Adrenergic receptors appear to be more prevalent in the sinus node and produce more chronotropic than inotropic affects when administered parenterally, whereas β_1-adrenergic receptors produce more of an inotropic effect.[72] Recently, β_3-adrenoreceptors have been identified in myocardium.[73] β_3-Adrenoreceptors have little in common with other β receptors. They share only about 40% to 50% of the amino acid sequence of other β receptors, and they are activated by agonists that have little effect on the other types of β receptors. In the myocardium they produce a decrease in myocardial contractility.

α_1-Adrenergic receptors, like β-adrenoreceptors, are coupled to G proteins in cardiac cell membranes. Instead of stimulating cyclic AMP production in the myocardium, however, receptor stimulation results in production of phospholipase C, which results in the formation of 1,4,5-triphosphate (IP_3) and diacylglycerol (DAG). IP_3 mobilizes intracellular calcium, and DAG stimulates protein kinase C to phosphorylate intracellular proteins and enhance calcium fluxes.[16] α_1-Adrenergic receptor stimulation may also stimulate phosphodiesterases, enzymes that break down cyclic AMP. α_2-Adrenergic receptors are situated on adrenergic nerve terminals, where they inhibit the release of norepinephrine.

Cells that provide central parasympathetic efferent activity to the body originate in the midbrain and medulla and in the midsacral spinal segments. Medullary centers, particularly the dorsal motor nucleus of the vagus, control the cardiovascular system via efferent nerve fibers that leave the brainstem via the vagus nerve. Preganglionic fibers are myelinated and synapse with unmyelinated postganglionic fibers in parasympathetic ganglia that lie within or close to organs. Ganglionic cells reside within the walls of the heart. Parasympathetic fiber input to the atria is much greater than to the ventricles. Acetylcholine is released from terminal nerve fibers to stimulate muscarinic receptors. Muscarinic receptors are coupled to G_i, the inhibitory G protein.[16] This decreases cyclic AMP production within the myocardial cell. Muscarinic receptors also stimulate phospholipase C production with the same effects as with α_1-adrenergic receptor stimulation. Muscarinic receptors may also increase cyclic GMP production within the cell, which may counter the effects of cyclic AMP. Within the sinus node, muscarinic receptors act on the inward-rectifying potassium channel to decrease the rate of depolarization. In normal subjects, this vagal influence outweighs sympathetic input influence to control the heart rate. At the vascular level, muscarinic stimulation results in vasodilation. This acts through bradykinin in some vascular beds.[3]

Humoral control. Hormones also act to produce vasoconstriction and maintain blood pressure. Angiotensin II, vasopressin (antidiuretic hormone), and endothelin are potent vasoconstrictive agents present in low concentrations in the normal individual. When blood flow is decreased, such as in hypovolemia and heart failure, these agents are present in higher concentrations to counter the effect of low blood flow on systemic pressure.[74] They increase systemic vascular resistance by stimulating smooth muscle contraction in systemic arterioles and so help bring blood pressure back to normal.

Angiotensin II is an octapeptide formed when the angiotensin-converting enzyme cleaves two amino acids from the decapeptide angiotensin I. The process is started by another enzyme, renin, cleaving 10 amino acids from the polypeptide angiotensinogen to form angiotensin I. Renin is released to help maintain blood pressure in response to increased sympathetic discharge to the juxtaglomerular apparatus and to activation of baroreceptors in the renal vascular bed. Angiotensin II binds to two types of receptors, AT1 and AT2.[75] AT1 receptors are GTP-binding membrane proteins with seven transmembrane-spanning domains, much like β-receptors. AT2 receptors are similar in structure, but the cellular signaling mechanism has not been worked out. Angiotensin receptors are present in both the heart and vascular smooth muscle. In the heart, the AT2:AT1 receptor ratio is 2:1.[76] In the systemic vasculature, the AT1 receptor predominates. In the vasculature, angiotensin II directly produces smooth muscle contraction. In addition, it enhances the activity of the sympathetic nervous system by blocking reuptake of norepinephrine and facilitating norepinephrine release. Angiotensin II has a positive inotropic effect by stimulating AT1 receptors in the myocardium. It also is a mitogen, stimulating myocardial growth via hypertrophy.

Arginine vasopressin (antidiuretic hormone) is a pituitary hormone that also stimulates two types of receptors, V_1 and V_2. Stimulation of V_1 receptors results in vasoconstriction, and stimulation of V_2 receptors results in renal water retention.[77] Consequently, vasopressin helps maintain blood pressure via vasoconstriction, although probably to a lesser degree than angiotensin II.

The endothelins (ETs) are potent vasoconstrictors released by endothelial cells throughout the body. Three types of endothelins have been identified: ET-1, ET-2, and ET-3.[78] ET-1 is a 21-amino acid peptide that is produced by the vascular endothelium. Endothelins bind to two types of endothelin receptors, type A (ET_A) and type B (ET_B). The ET_A receptor has a greater affinity for ET-1 than for ET-3, whereas the ET_B receptor has similar affinities for all ET isoforms. ET-1 is a potent vasoconstrictor. Norepinephrine and angiotensin II enhance the release of endothelins. The circulating concentration of ET-1 is increased in human patients and experimental dogs with heart failure, presumably to help maintain blood pressure.[79] The endothelins also increase contractility and heart rate and stimulate hypertrophy. They are degraded by endothelin-converting enzyme.

NEUROHUMORAL CONTROL OF BLOOD VOLUME

Blood volume is an important determinant of blood pressure and venous return to the heart. Venous return is an important determinant of cardiac size and cardiac output. Consequently, regulation of blood volume is important in regulation of arterial blood pressure and blood flow. It is also an important determinant of venous and capillary pressures, as evidenced by patients with heart failure. In severe heart failure, blood volume is increased by 25% to 30% above normal. This increase in blood volume results in increased diastolic intraventricular pressures, which result in increased venous and capillary pressures behind the affected ventricle.

Neural control of blood volume starts with mechanoreceptors found in the walls of the atria and ventricles and at junctions of the vena cavae and pulmonary veins with the atria. They are found within the subendocardium and along the coronary vessels in the subepicardium. They sense change in volume within the chambers. Afferent nerves from these sensors course to the medulla in the sympathetic and parasympathetic trunks and are important in regulating systemic resistance, heart rate, and blood volume. Unmyelinated vagal afferents originate from the atria and ventricles, where they sense changes in chamber volume and force of contraction. An increase in either of these results in sympathetic nervous system inhibition and enhanced parasympathetic activity. Increased stretch of these receptors activates the sympathetic nervous system to eject the increased volume that they sense.

Water and sodium intake and output primarily determine blood volume. The kidney is the dominant organ in blood volume control because of its ability to alter water and sodium output. However, hormonal effects on thirst and sodium appetite are also major contributors to volume control. The baroreceptors in the atria directly alter vasopressin (antidiuretic hormone) secretion.[3] Antidiuretic hormone (ADH) secretion is suppressed by atrial stretch and enhanced by decreased atrial volume. Osmoreceptors also regulate ADH secretion, but the volume receptors in the body produce a stronger effect on ADH release. ADH secretion results in retention of water in the collecting system of the kidney. It also stimulates thirst. Atrial stretch also results in the release of atrial natriuretic factor (ANF) from storage granules in the atria, causing diuresis.

Sodium excretion is primarily controlled by the kidneys. Regulation of renal sodium excretion is controlled by numerous factors, but the renin-angiotensin-aldosterone system is one of the major factors in this control (Figure 2-23). Renin is an enzyme that is secreted from the granular cells of the juxtaglomerular apparatus. Renin secretion is controlled by several variables, including (1) the amount of baroreceptor stimulation in the afferent arterioles, (2) the composition of tubular fluid that reaches the macula densa, (3) the amount of sympathetic stimulation by the renal sympathetic nerves, and (4) prostaglandins. Decreased blood volume or decreased cardiac output results in decreased renal blood flow and so afferent arteriolar pressure, increased sympathetic nervous stimulation, and decreased sodium flux by the macula densa, culminating in increased renin release. This ultimately results in angiotensin II stimulating aldosterone release by the adrenal cortex (zona glomerulosa). Aldosterone is a steroid hormone that has primary effects on the distal tubule/collecting ducts. It stimulates sodium reabsorption and secretion of K^+ and H^+ and binds to intracellular receptors in the nucleus to stimulate expression of several genes. New proteins are produced that modulate the activity of ion transport in the membranes of the epithelial cells. Aldosterone's primary effect is to stimulate sodium uptake into the vascular space. Water follows sodium, resulting in increased plasma volume. Angiotensin II also stimulates thirst and, possibly, salt appetite.

Angiotensin II also has an indirect effect on renal sodium retention and blood volume. When cardiac output decreases, renal blood flow decreases. This decrease is probably disproportionately high compared with other organs because of afferent (the arteriole entering the glomerulus) renal arteriolar constriction, which occurs secondary to sympathetic stimulation.[80] A decrease in renal blood flow results in a decrease in glomerular filtration rate and an increase in blood urea nitrogen and serum creatinine concentration. To increase filtration back to or toward normal, the efferent arteriole leaving the glomerulus constricts secondary to angiotensin II stimulation.[81,82] The afferent arteriole, although constricted, is constricted less than the efferent arteriole. The net effect is an increase in the pressure above normal within the glomerular capillaries, which increases the percentage of filtrate squeezed from the blood (the filtration fraction increases). This increase maintains a normal glomerular filtration rate, whereas total renal blood flow is reduced. The increase in filtration fraction that occurs when renal blood flow is reduced results in the blood within the efferent arteriole and peritubular capillaries being relatively dehydrated, or hyperosmolar, compared with normal.[83] The plasma protein concentration (oncotic pressure) within these vessels is increased, and the hydrostatic pressure is decreased.[84] Therefore as blood traverses the peritubular capillaries a greater percentage of sodium and water are

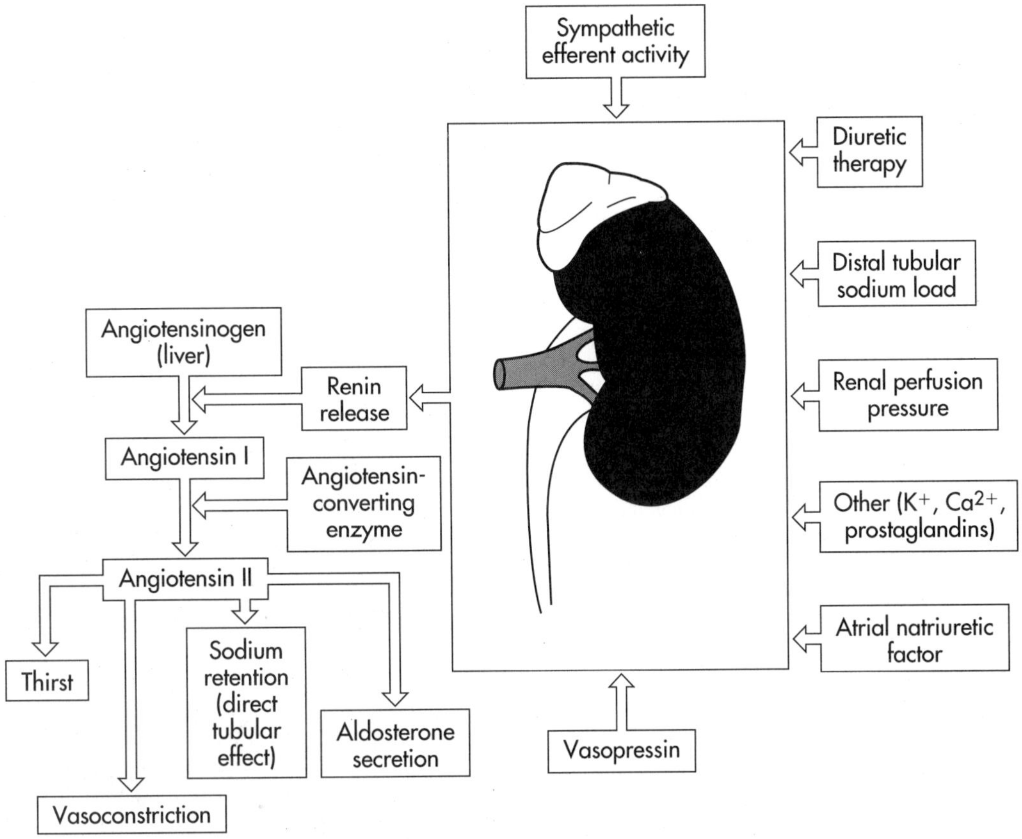

FIGURE 2-23 Schematic drawing of the renin-angiotensin-aldosterone system, hormonal effects, and variables that influence renin release.

resorbed back into the vascular space from the proximal tubules. This also helps increase blood volume.

In addition to these mechanisms, sodium excretion is also controlled by changes in glomerular filtration rate (GFR) and a "third factor" effect.[3] Changes in GFR produce only minor changes and are not discussed. When GFR and aldosterone secretion are controlled experimentally, sodium excretion is still regulated. Consequently, a third factor or more factors must be involved. Despite intense scrutiny, this third factor has not been identified. Most likely this factor is really a combination of factors. These include the effects of the sympathetic nervous system, angiotensin II, and ANF factor on sodium excretion. Sympathetic stimulation of the kidneys directly results in sodium reabsorption in the proximal tubule, as well as stimulating renin secretion. Angiotensin II also directly stimulates proximal tubular sodium reabsorption. ANF inhibits sodium reabsorption in the collecting ducts.

ANF is an important hormone in blood volume regulation. It is a 28-amino acid peptide that is synthesized primarily in the right atrial and left atrial myocytes.[85] The hormone is released into the bloodstream following atrial stretch and tachycardia. The primary target organ is the kidney. ANF binds to renal receptors in the nephron. At the glomerular level, it increases GFR by dilating the afferent arteriole, constricting the efferent arteriole, and increasing glomerular permeability by relaxing mesangial cells.[86] This results in increased sodium filtration into the proximal tubule. It also directly depresses sodium reabsorption in the medullary collecting ducts. Along with these primary effects, ANF has several other effects. These include antagonism of renin and aldosterone synthesis, antagonism of angiotensin II–mediated vasoconstriction, thirst and sodium hunger, inhibition of aldosterone secretion, inhibition of ADH secretion, inhibition of the sympathetic nervous system, and vasodilatory effects. Despite all these actions, the increased plasma concentration of this hormone identified in patients with congestive heart failure fails to overcome the effects of the other hormones and factors that promote sodium retention. We interpret this to mean that ANF is a weak hormone compared with angiotensin II, aldosterone, and the catecholamines.

NEUROHUMORAL CONTROL OF BLOOD FLOW

Pressure and volume sensors (mechanoreceptors) in the cardiovascular system are well studied and understood. Flow receptors are poorly understood. There are three variables within the cardiovascular system that are tightly controlled. They are systemic arterial blood pressure, venous and capillary pressures through regulation of blood volume, and venous oxygen tension. Venous oxygen tension is a measure of the adequacy of blood flow to tissue. It is determined by the ratio of oxygen delivery to oxygen consumption. The ratio of oxygen delivery to oxygen consumption is kept tightly controlled such that mixed venous oxygen tension in the pulmonary artery is close to 40 mm Hg in a normal resting animal. This variable is constant across mammalian species.[87] It therefore makes sense that this variable must have some means of control rather than this being the fortuitous end result of all other control mechanisms. Oxygen is critical for the maintenance of life forms on earth. It is required for aerobic metabolism. Despite this, very little is known about how organisms are capable of sensing oxygen availability in tissues.[88] Chemoreceptors exist within the carotid bodies and aortic arch to sense changes in arterial oxygen tension and so regulate respiration. Similar oxygen-sensitive ion channels (receptors) are present in many regions of the body.[88] These ion channels are open and allow potassium current to flow when oxygen is present. Hypoxemia closes them. These channels are present in pulmonary myocytes, where they mediate hypoxemia-induced pulmonary vasoconstriction.[88] The oxygen sensor on these ion channels may be a heme-linked protein, like the protein that is sensitive to hypoxemia in the kidneys that results in erythropoietin production.[89] Such chemoreceptors have not been identified in systemic vasculature, but it is tempting to predict their existence based on teleologic reasoning. In this reasoning, oxygen sensors would lie at the end of capillary beds, where oxygen tension is lowest. They would then modulate vasomotion to increase or decrease flow through a particular vascular bed. Oxygen sensors would also be placed in the pulmonary veins or other large systemic veins to modulate gross cardiovascular function by modulating the autonomic nervous system and blood volume control. There certainly is evidence for oxygen sensors in the microvasculature that modulate small systemic vessel tone. For example, in cat skeletal muscle, decreasing the oxygen saturation of the air surrounding the muscle results in vasodilation, especially of the small arterioles.[90] Coronary autoregulation of blood flow is coupled very closely to myocardial oxygen consumption. One modeling study has concluded that tissue oxygen tension controls coronary blood flow.[91] In another study coronary sinus oxygen tension correlated with coronary vascular resistance.[92] To our knowledge, no one has examined structures that carry systemic venous blood for evidence of oxygen sensors.

The kidneys are also thought to control blood flow via the ability of the macula densa to sense changes in sodium flux. Decreased renal blood flow results in decreased sodium presentation to the macula densa with resultant renin secretion. Renin secretion ultimately results in aldosterone production, sodium and water retention, increased blood volume, increased venous return to the heart, and increased cardiac output (blood flow).

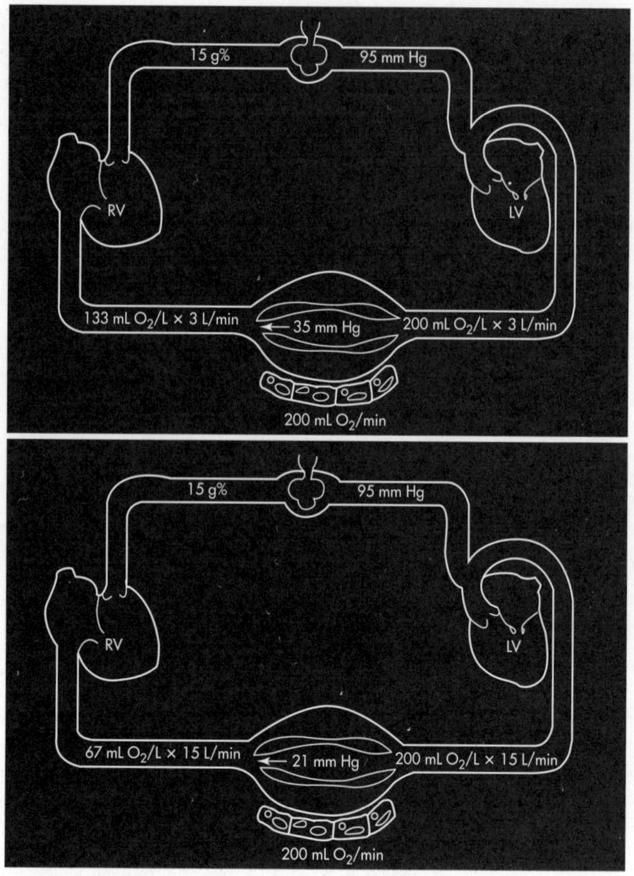

FIGURE 2-24 Schematic diagrams of the circulation, depicting the balance between hemoglobin concentration (g%), arterial oxygen tension (mm Hg), arterial oxygen content (mL O_2/L), cardiac output (L/min), oxygen delivery (cardiac output × arterial oxygen content), tissue oxygen consumption (mL O_2/min), and resultant end-capillary or venous oxygen tension (mm Hg). **A,** Values in this diagram are normal for a 25-kg dog (1 m^2 body surface area) and result in a normal venous oxygen tension of 35 mm Hg. **B,** Low cardiac output (1.5 L/min in this example) results in decreased tissue oxygen delivery and decreased venous oxygen tension.

Oxygen Delivery, Oxygen Consumption, and Venous Oxygen Tension

Venous oxygen tension is an important, but often ignored, variable in cardiovascular physiology and medicine. As stated previously, it is a measure of the adequacy of tissue oxygen delivery and can be predicted by examining the ratio of oxygen delivery to oxygen consumption. Oxygen delivery is the number of milliliters of oxygen delivered to the body. It is calculated by multiplying cardiac output (or index to obtain oxygen delivery index) by systemic arterial oxygen content. Arterial oxygen content is determined by multiplying hemoglobin concentration times oxygen saturation of hemoglobin times the number of milliliters of oxygen that each gram of hemoglobin can carry (1.34 mL). Oxygen saturation is determined by oxygen tension and the shape of the oxyhemoglobin dissociation curve. Oxygen saturation can be directly measured or calculated by knowing oxygen tension and examining a nomogram relating oxygen tension, blood pH, and blood temperature to hemoglobin saturation. Oxygen consumption can be directly measured by collecting expired gas and determining the difference between inspired and expired oxygen content. It can also be determined by calculating the amount of oxygen being carried away from the tissues in venous blood (the opposite of oxygen delivery) and subtracting that from oxygen delivery. A ratio of oxygen delivery to oxygen consumption at rest is usually about 4 and results in a venous oxygen tension of 40 mm Hg (Figure 2-24). A ratio of 1 would give a venous oxygen tension of zero, which is physiologically impossible. A ratio of 1.5 is severely decreased and results in anaerobiosis.

In almost all situations, the body attempts to deliver an adequate supply of oxygen to tissues that need it. As oxygen consumption increases and decreases in a particular organ, blood flow increases and decreases in concert. At the capillary level, oxygen delivery to the mitochondria depends on the pressure difference (gradient) between capillary blood and mitochondria and the diffusion distance.[87] The diffusion distance is usually constant. Mitochondrial oxygen tension (Po_2) is constant at about 1 mm Hg. Consequently, the pressure difference, or driving pressure, is primarily determined by the capillary oxygen tension. Capillary oxygen tension at the arterial end of the capillary bed is the same as arterial blood. It gradually decreases across the capillary bed as oxygen is forced out of the capillaries to the mitochondria. It reaches its lowest value at the end of the capillary bed, where the capillaries join the venous circulation. As one might deduce, end-capillary oxygen tension and venous oxygen tension are equal. The cells at the end of the capillary bed are most susceptible to hypoxia, because oxygen tension is lowest at this point. Consequently, it makes sense that the cardiovascular system would try to maintain this value at a level that ensures adequate oxygen supply to these cells. We know that when end-capillary (venous) oxygen tension decreases to below approximately 24 mm Hg in working skeletal muscle that oxygen delivery to the mitochondria becomes inadequate and anaerobic metabolism must be used. This is manifested as an increase in blood lactate concentration. Consequently, the cardiovascular system must try to keep venous oxygen tension greater than 24 mm Hg in all vascular beds. The value for venous oxygen tension varies from organ to organ. Myocardium is constantly working and so has a high resting oxygen consumption. As a result, the oxygen tension in coronary sinus blood is lower than anywhere else in the body, usually in the 25- to 30-mm Hg range. All other venous circulations have oxygen tensions greater than 30 mm Hg. Kidneys have much more blood flow than is required to maintain metabolism, because they are filtering blood. Consequently, renal venous oxygen tension is higher than other vascular beds. Blood sampled from the pulmonary artery is termed *mixed venous blood* because it is a mixture of venous blood from all vascular beds. In normal resting animals, mixed venous oxygen tension is almost always greater than 30 mm Hg. The ability of the cardiovascular system to deliver adequate oxygen can be overwhelmed. The best example of this is exercise. With exercise, oxygen consumption in skeletal muscle increases dramatically. Even though the cardiovascular system responds dramatically to this demand for increased oxygen delivery, its response is usually submaximal and with severe exercise is inadequate. At moderate exercise levels, oxygen tension from venous blood that is draining working skeletal muscle is decreased, usually into the 25- to 30-mm Hg range (similar to venous blood draining cardiac muscle). With severe exercise, oxygen tension can decrease to very low levels, often less than 15 mm Hg. This results in inadequate delivery of oxygen to skeletal muscle, lactic acidosis, and muscle fatigue.

Normal Pressures, Volumes, and Flow

Pressure, flow, and volume change throughout the cardiac cycle. A general knowledge of normal pressures, flows, and volumes within the cardiovascular system is necessary to understand many of the changes that occur during the cardiac cycle and in disease.

GREAT VESSEL AND SYSTOLIC VENTRICULAR PRESSURES

Systolic pressure in the cardiovascular system is generated by the contraction of a ventricle that ejects blood against an impedance to blood flow.[19] The resistance to blood flow results in blood being ejected into a circulation at a rate faster than its runoff into capillary beds. Left ventricular peak systolic pressure in a normal animal is approximately 5 to 6 times that of right ventricular peak systolic pressure. This occurs because the impedance (i.e., resistance plus other factors explained above) to blood flow through the systemic circulation is approximately 5 to 6 times that through the pulmonary circulation. Normal peak systolic pressure in the left ventricle is in the 90- to 150-mm Hg range. In the right ventricle, peak systolic pressure is in the 15- to 30-mm Hg range. The systemic circulation has several vascular beds that have very high innate resistances, including the heart and kidneys. The kidneys need a high resistance so that high glomerular capillary pressures can be generated to filter metabolic waste products from the blood in an efficient manner. The heart has high resistance to blood flow during systole when the myocardium contracts around the blood vessels. Because it is critical to produce blood flow through such organs, pressure in the systemic circuit must be high. Conversely, the lungs do not have nor do they need a high resistance. Consequently, resistance is low and pressure is low. Resistance to blood flow through the lungs is similar to resistance to blood flow through many other tissues in the systemic circuit.

Peak systolic pressures in the aorta and main pulmonary artery are very similar to peak systolic pressures in the respective ventricle. It is commonly believed that pressure in the left ventricle must be greater than pressure in the aorta to produce blood flow. This comes from the mistaken belief that pressure 'pushes' blood flow through the circulation. In reality, the ventricles push blood flow through the circulation, and pressure is a product of the flow that is produced and the resistance to that flow. It is a resultant force that opposes motion. Flow and flow velocity are related to pressure differences across structures and vascular beds, but pressure is not the force that produces flow in the proximal aorta. This becomes clear when one realizes that flow can precede pressure in the aorta and that if left ventricular pressure exceeds aortic pressure, it does so for only a short period in the early part of ejection.[93]

Diastolic pressure in the great arteries is generally measured at the end of diastole, when these pressures are lowest. Normal diastolic pressure in the aorta is in the 60- to 100-mm Hg range and in the pulmonary artery is in the 5- to 15-mm Hg range.

On the systemic side, the strength of a pulse that is palpated is an estimation of the pulse pressure. Normal pulse pressure is in the 40- to 80-mm Hg range. A pulse pressure of 40 mm Hg, for example, would be generated by a systolic pressure of 140 mm Hg and a diastolic pressure of 100 mm Hg. The same pulse pressure would be generated with a systolic pressure of 100 mm Hg and a diastolic pressure of 60 mm Hg. The pulse pressure changes as it moves from the aorta to the distal arteries. Systolic blood pressure increases, and the upstroke of the pressure waveform becomes steeper. The dicrotic notch also disappears. The dicrotic notch is a rapid decrease and then increase in aortic pressure that occurs when the aortic valve closes and the cardiohemic system oscillates.

The average, or mean, blood pressure can be estimated by dividing the pulse pressure by 3 and adding this to diastolic pressure. It can also be measured by electrically damping the pressure waveform so that very little oscillation occurs. Normal mean aortic pressure is in the 70- to 100-mm Hg range. Mean pulmonary artery pressure is in the 10- to 20-mm Hg range.

VENTRICULAR DIASTOLIC AND ATRIAL PRESSURES

Ventricular diastolic pressure usually is measured at the end of diastole and is low compared with systolic pressure. This pressure is primarily determined by the blood volume in the chamber and the compliance of the chamber. Because the left ventricle is a thicker and therefore stiffer structure than the right ventricle, left ventricular diastolic pressure is usually higher than right ventricular diastolic pressure. Normal left ventricular diastolic pressure is in the 4- to 12-mm Hg range, and normal right ventricular diastolic pressure is in the 0- to 5-mm Hg range.

During diastole the mitral and tricuspid valves are open, so there is very little resistance to flow. Consequently, atrial pressures and ventricular pressures are very similar. Normal mean left atrial pressure is in the 4- to 12-mm Hg range, and normal right atrial pressure is in the 0- to 5-mm Hg range. Atrial pressures also oscillate or pulsate as volume within the chamber changes over time, atrial muscle contracts and relaxes over time, and atrial compliance changes with disease. The resultant waveforms are described in Chapter 3.

VASCULAR FLOW

Cardiac output is the amount of flow through the cardiovascular system per minute. Cardiac output divided by heart rate equals average stroke volume. Stroke volume is the amount of blood ejected from a ventricle with each beat. Cardiac output and stroke volume are commonly divided by body surface area to produce an index that is the same for animals of different size. For example, a 10-kg dog has about 0.5 m^2 of body surface area and may have a stroke volume of 15 mL. A 25-kg dog has a body surface area of approximately 1 m^2 and may have a stroke volume of 30 mL. Each dog would have a stroke volume index of 30 mL/m^2. The normal cardiac index for our laboratory in conscious but resting dogs is 3.9 +/– 0.4 L/min/m^2, measured by thermodilution. This means that cardiac index varies

TABLE 2-2

Normal hemodynamic variables in dogs ($n = 12$)

Hemodynamic variable	*Mean*	*SD*
PaO_2 (mm Hg) (temperature corrected)	111	6
Arterial O_2 saturation (%)	95.5	1.1
Arterial (HGB) (g/dL)	15.1	1.5
Arterial O_2 content (mL O_2/L)	188	18
O_2 Delivery index (mL O_2/min/m^2)	730	77
Femoral vein PO_2 (mm Hg)	41	2
Venous O_2 saturation (%)	66	3
Venous O_2 content (mL O_2/L)	133	16
Venous O_2 effluent index (mL O_2/min/m^2)	517	66
O_2 Consumption index (mL O_2/min/m^2)	212	29
Atrioventricular O_2 difference (mL O_2/L)	55	8
O_2 Extraction (%)	29	4

SD, Standard deviation.

between approximately 3.1 and 4.7 L/min/m^2 in normal resting dogs in our laboratory. The normal stroke volume index (stroke volume/body surface area) in dogs in our laboratory averages 41 mL/m^2. Normal range is between approximately 30 and 50 mL/m^2. Other normal hemodynamic variables for our laboratory are listed in Table 2-2.

REFERENCES

1. Berne RM, Levy NL: *Cardiovascular physiology,* ed 7, St Louis, 1992, Mosby.
2. Van Citters RL, Kemper WS, Franklin DL: Blood flow and pressure in the giraffe carotid artery, *Comp Biochem Physiol* 24:1035, 1968.
3. West JB, ed: *Best and Taylor's physiological basis of medical practice,* ed 12, Baltimore, 1990, Williams & Wilkins.
4. Morgan HE, Neely JR: Metabolic regulation and myocardial function. In Hurst JW, Schlant RC, eds: *The heart,* ed 7, New York, 1990, McGraw-Hill.
5. Monroe RG, French GN: Left ventricular pressure-volume relationships and myocardial oxygen consumption in the isolated heart, *Circ Res* 9:362, 1961.
6. Braunwald E: Control of myocardial oxygen consumption: physiologic and clinical considerations, *Am J Cardiol* 27:416, 1971.
7. Opie LH: Substrate and energy metabolism of the heart. In Sperelakis N, ed: *Physiology and pathophysiology of the heart,* ed 3, Boston, 1995, Kluwer.
8. Hofmann PA, Hartzell HC, Moss RL: Alterations in Ca^{++} sensitive tension due to partial extraction of C-protein from rat skinned cardiac myocytes and rabbit skeletal muscle fibers, *J Gen Physiol* 97:1141, 1991.
9. Katz AM: Calcium channel diversity in the cardiovascular system, *J Am Coll Cardiol* 28:522, 1996.
10. Tada M, Kadoma M: Uptake of calcium by sarcoplasmic reticulum and its regulation and functional consequences. In Sperelakis N, ed: *Physiology and pathophysiology of the heart,* ed 3, Boston, 1995, Kluwer.
11. Solaro RJ: Control mechanisms regulating contractile activity of cardiac myofilaments. In Sperelakis N, ed: *Physiology and pathophysiology of the heart,* ed 3, Boston, 1995, Kluwer.
12. Reeves JP: Cardiac sodium-calcium exchange system. In Sperelakis N, ed: *Physiology and pathophysiology of the heart,* ed 3, Boston, 1995, Kluwer.
13. Shuba LM, McDonald TF: Excitation-contraction coupling: relationship of calcium currents to contraction. In Sperelakis N, ed: *Physiology and pathophysiology of the heart,* ed 3, Boston, 1995, Kluwer.
14. Sperelakis N, Josephson I: Slow action potential and properties of the myocardial slow Ca channels. In Sperelakis N, ed: *Physiology and pathophysiology of the heart,* ed 3, Boston, 1995, Kluwer.
15. Kargacin GJ, Walsh MP: Contractile proteins of smooth muscle. In Sperelakis N, ed: *Physiology and pathophysiology of the heart,* ed 3, Boston, 1995, Kluwer.
16. Wisler PL, Green FJ, Watanabe AM: Cardiovascular adrenergic and muscarinic cholinergic receptors. In Chatterjee K, Cheitlin MD, Karliner J et al, eds: *Cardiology: an illustrated text/reference,* Philadelphia, 1991, JB Lippincott.
17. Feder D, Im MJ, Pfeuffer T et al: The hormonal regulation of adenylate cyclase, *Biochem Soc Symp* 52:145, 1986.
18. Crow MT, Kushmerick MJ: Myosin light chain phosphorylation is associated with a decrease in the energy cost for contraction in fast twitch mouse muscle, *J Biol Chem* 257:2121, 1982.
19. Schlant RC, Sonnenblick EH: Normal physiology of the cardiovascular system. In Hurst JW, Schlant RC, eds: *The heart,* ed 7, New York, 1990, McGraw-Hill.
20. Allen DG, Kentish JC: The cellular basis of the length-tension relation in cardiac muscle, *J Mol Cell Cardiol* 17:821, 1985.
21. Saba Z, Nassar R, Ungerleider RM et al: Cardiac troponin T isoform expression correlates with pathophysiological descriptors in patients who underwent corrective surgery for congenital heart disease, *Circulation* 94:472, 1996.
22. Braunwald E, Sonnenblick EH, Ross JJ: Contraction of the normal heart. In Braunwald E, ed: *Heart disease: a textbook of cardiovascular medicine,* Philadelphia, 1980, WB Saunders.
23. Boon J, Wingfield WE, Miller CW: Echocardiographic indices in the normal dog, *Vet Radiol* 24:214, 1993.
24. Wyatt HL, Heng MK, Meerbaum S et al: Cross-sectional echocardiography. I. Analysis of mathematic models for quantifying mass of the left ventricle in dogs, *Circulation* 60:1104, 1979.
25. Wyatt HL, Heng MK, Meerbaum S et al: Cross-sectional echocardiography. II. Analysis of mathematic models for quantifying volume of the formalin-fixed left ventricle, *Circulation* 61:1119, 1980.
26. Jacob R, Dierberger B, Gulch RW et al: Geometric and muscle physiological factors of the Frank-Starling mechanisms, *Basic Res Cardiol* 88:86, 1993.
27. ter Keurs HE, de Tombe PP, Backx PH et al: Rheology of myocardium: the relation between force, velocity, sarcomere length and activation in rat cardiac muscle, *Biorheology* 28:161, 1991.
28. Jacob R, Dierberger B, Kissling G: Functional significance of the Frank-Starling mechanism under physiological and pathophysiological conditions, *Eur Heart J* 3(suppl E):7, 1992.
29. Lakatta EG: Starling's law of the heart is explained by an intimate interaction of muscle length and myofilament calcium activation, *J Am Coll Cardiol* 10:1157, 1987.
30. Babu A, Sonnenblick E, Gulati J: Molecular basis for the influence of muscle length on myocardial performance, *Science* 240:74, 1988.
31. Spotnitz HM, Sonnenblick EH: Structural conditions in the hypertrophied and failing heart, *Am J Cardiol* 32:398, 1993.
32. Stillwell GK: The law of Laplace: some clinical applications, *Mayo Clin Proc* 48:863, 1973.
33. Yin FC: Ventricular wall stress, *Circ Res* 49:829, 1981.
34. Mahler F, Ross JJ, O'Rourke RA et al: Effects of changes in preload, afterload and inotropic state on ejection and isovolumic phase measures of contractility in the conscious dog, *Am J Cardiol* 35:626, 1995.
35. Covell JW, Pouleur H, Ross JJ: Left ventricular wall stress and aortic input impedance, *Fed Proc* 39:202, 1980.
36. Westerhof N, Elzinga G, Sipkema P et al: Quantitative analysis of arterial system and heart by means of pressure flow relations. In Hwan NHC, Norman NA, eds: *Cardiovascular flow dynamics and measurements.* Baltimore, 1977, University Park.
37. Effron MB, Bhatnagar GM, Spurgeon HA et al: Changes in myosin isoenzymes, ATPase activity, and contraction duration in rat cardiac muscle with aging can be modulated by thyroxine, *Circ Res* 60:238, 1987.
38. Alpert NR, Mulieri LA, Litten RZ: Functional significance of altered myosin adenosine triphosphatase activity in enlarged hearts, *Am J Cardiol* 44:946, 1979.
39. Wikman-Coffelt J, Walsh R, Fenner C et al: Effects of severe hemodynamic pressure overload on the properties of canine left ventricular myosin: mechanism by which myosin ATPase activity is lowered during chronic increased hemodynamic stress, *J Mol Cell Cardiol* 8:263, 1976.

40. Wilson JR, Douglas P, Hickey WF et al: Experimental congestive heart failure produced by rapid ventricular pacing in the dog: cardiac effects, *Circulation* 75:857, 1987.
41. Dhalla NS, Heyliger CE, Beamish RE et al: Pathophysiological aspects of myocardial hypertrophy, *Can J Cardiol* 3:183, 1987.
42. Anversa P, Ricci R, Olivetti G: Quantitative structural analysis of the myocardium during physiologic growth and induced cardiac hypertrophy: a review, *J Am Coll Cardiol* 7:1140, 1986.
43. Grossman W, Jones D, McLaurin LP. Wall stress and patterns of hypertrophy in the human left ventricle, *J Clin Invest* 56:56, 1975.
44. Fanburg BL: Experimental cardiac hypertrophy, *N Engl J Med* 282:723, 1970.
45. Morgan HE, Gordon EE, Kira Y et al: Biochemical mechanisms of cardiac hypertrophy, *Annu Rev Physiol* 49:533, 1987.
46. Cooper G4: Cardiocyte adaptation to chronically altered load, *Annu Rev Physiol* 49:501, 1987.
47. Kent RL, Hoober JK, Cooper IV: Load responsiveness of protein synthesis in adult mammalian myocardium: role of cardiac deformation linked to sodium influx, *Circ Res* 64:74, 1989.
48. Tamai J, Hori M, Kagiya T et al: Role of alpha 1-adrenoceptor activity in progression of cardiac hypertrophy in guinea pig hearts with pressure overload, *Cardiovasc Res* 23:315, 1989.
49. Katz AM: Angiotensin II: hemodynamic regulator or growth factor? *J Mol Cell Cardiol* 22:739, 1990 (editorial).
50. Sen S, Kundu G, Mekhail N et al: Myotrophin: purification of a novel peptide from spontaneously hypertensive rat heart that influences myocardial growth, *J Biol Chem* 265:16635, 1990.
51. Honda M, Morioka S, Yamada S et al: Study of cardiac hypertrophy: humoral factors that stimulate protein metabolism of cultured rat heart cells, *Jpn Circ J* 53:795, 1989.
52. Sadoshima J, Xu Y, Slayter HS et al: Autocrine release of angiotensin II mediates stretch-induced hypertrophy of cardiac myocytes in vitro, *Cell* 75:977, 1973.
53. Sadoshima J, Izumo S: The heterotrimeric G q protein-coupled angiotensin II receptor activates p21 ras via the tyrosine kinase-Shc-Grb2-Sos pathway in cardiac myocytes, *EMBO J* 15:775, 1996.
54. Saad MJ, Velloso LA, Carvalho CR: Angiotensin II induces tyrosine phosphorylation of insulin receptor substrate 1 and its association with phosphatidylinositol 3-kinase in rat heart, *Biochem J* 310:741, 1995.
55. Krayenbuehl HP, Hess OM, Schneider J et al: Physiologic or pathologic hypertrophy, *Eur Heart J* 4(suppl A):29, 1983.
56. Page E, McCallister LP: Quantitative electron microscopic description of heart muscle cells: application to normal, hypertrophied and thyroxin-stimulated hearts, *Am J Cardiol* 31:172, 1973.
57. Ferrans VJ, Rodriguez ER: Evidence of myocyte hyperplasia in hypertrophic cardiomyopathy and other disorders with myocardial hypertrophy. *Z Kardiol* 76(suppl3):20, 1987.
58. Olivetti G, Ricci R, Anversa P: Hyperplasia of myocyte nuclei in long-term cardiac hypertrophy in rats, *J Clin Invest* 80:1818, 1987.
59. Gunther S, Grossman W: Determinants of ventricular function in pressure-overload hypertrophy in man, *Circulation* 59:679, 1979.
60. Scholz PM, Grover GJ, Mackenzie JW et al: Regional oxygen supply and consumption balance in experimental left ventricular hypertrophy, *Basic Res Cardiol* 85:575, 1990.
61. Yoran C, Covell JW, Ross JJ: Structural basis for the ascending limb of left ventricular function, *Circ Res* 32:297, 1973.
62. Komamura K, Shannon RP, Ihara T et al: Exhaustion of Frank-Starling mechanism in conscious dogs with heart failure, *Am J Physiol* 265: H1119, 1993.
63. Pouleur H, Rousseau MF, van Eyll C et al: Assessment of left ventricular contractility from late systolic stress-volume relations, *Circulation* 65:1204, 1982.
64. Mirsky I, Aoyagi T, Crocker VM et al: Preload dependence of fiber shortening rate in conscious dogs with left ventricular hypertrophy, *J Am Coll Cardiol* 15:890, 1990.
65. Reichek N, Wilson J, St John Sutton M et al: Noninvasive determination of left ventricular end-systolic stress: validation of the method and initial application, *Circulation* 65:99, 1982.
66. Maughan WL, Sunagawa K: Factors affecting the end-systolic pressure-volume relationship, *Fed Proc* 43:2408, 1984.
67. Little WC, Freeman GL, O'Rourke RA: Simultaneous determination of left ventricular end-systolic pressure-volume and pressure-dimension relationships in closed-chest dogs, *Circulation* 71:1301, 1985.
68. Sagawa K, Suga H, Shoukas AA et al: End-systolic pressure/volume ratio: a new index of contractility, *Am J Cardiol* 40:748, 1977.
69. Singh M, Balakrishnan S: Viscosity of oscillating non-Newtonian fluids: an empirical approach as applied to blood, *Biorheology* 11:351, 1994.
70. Oka S: Pressure development in a non-Newtonian flow through a tapered tube, *Biorheology* 10:207, 1973.
71. Levy MN, Martin PJ: Autonomic neural control of cardiac function. In Sperelakis N, ed: *Physiology and pathophysiology of the heart,* ed 3, Boston, 1995, Kluwer.
72. Lindemann JP, Watanabe AM: Mechanisms of adrenergic and cholinergic regulation of myocardial contractility. In Sperelakis N, ed: *Physiology and pathophysiology of the heart,* ed 3, Boston, 1995, Kluwer.
73. Gauthier C, Tavernier G, Charpentier F et al: Functional $beta_3$-adrenoreceptors in the human heart, *J Clin Invest* 98:556, 1996.
74. Cavero PG, Miller WL, Heublein DM et al: Endothelin in experimental congestive heart failure in the anesthetized dog, *Am J Physiol* 259:F312, 1990.
75. Timmermans PB, Wong PC, Chiu AT et al: Angiotensin II receptors and angiotensin II receptor antagonists, *Pharmacol Rev* 45:205, 1993.
76. Regitz-Zagrosek V, Friedel N, Heymann A et al: Regulation, chamber localization, and subtype distribution of angiotensin II receptors in human hearts, *Circulation* 91:1461, 1995.
77. Naitoh M, Suzuki H, Murakami M et al: Effects of oral AVP receptor antagonists OPC-21268 and OPC-31260 on congestive heart failure in conscious dogs, *Am J Physiol* 267:H2245, 1994.
78. Yanagisawa M, Masaki T: Molecular biology and biochemistry of the endothelins, *Trends Pharmacol Sci* 10:374, 1989.
79. Shimoyama H, Sabbah HN, Borzak S et al: Short-term hemodynamic effects of endothelin receptor blockade in dogs with chronic heart failure, *Circulation* 94:779, 1996.
80. Mason DT, Tonken MJ: *Management of fluid and electrolyte disturbances in congestive heart failure,* New York, 1975, Science and Medicine.
81. Ichikawa I, Kon V, Pfeffer MA et al: Role of angiotensin II in the altered renal function of heart failure, *Kidney Int Suppl* 20:S213, 1987.
82. Packer M, Lee WH, Kessler PD: Preservation of glomerular filtration rate in human heart failure by activation of the renin-angiotensin system, *Circulation* 74:766, 1986.
83. Cannon PJ: The kidney in heart failure, *N Engl J Med* 296:26, 1977.
84. Liu FY, Cogan MG: Role of angiotensin II in glomerulotubular balance, *Am J Physiol* 259:F72, 1990.
85. Ries PA, Jergens AE: Atrial natriuretic factor: an introduction, *Compend Cont Educ Pract Vet* 17:1029, 1995.
86. Cogan MG: Renal effects of atrial natriuretic factor, *Annu Rev Physiol* 52:699, 1990.
87. Clemmer TP: Oxygen transport, *Int Anesthesiol Clin* 19:21, 1981.
88. Lopez-Barneo J: Oxygen-sensitive ion channels: how ubiquitous are they? *Trends Neurosci* 17:133, 1994.
89. Galson DL, Blanchard KL, Fandrey J et al: Cis elements that regulate the erythropoietin gene, *Ann N Y Acad Sci* 718:21, 1994.
90. Sullivan SM, Johnson PC: Effect of oxygen on blood flow autoregulation in cat sartorius muscle, *Am J Physiol* 241:H807, 1981.
91. Spaan JA, Dankelman J: Theoretical analysis of coronary blood flow and tissue oxygen pressure-control, *Adv Exp Med Biol* 346:189, 1993.
92. Kang YH, Mallet RT, Bunger R: Coronary autoregulation and purine release in normoxic heart at various cytoplasmic phosphorylation potentials: disparate effects of adenosine, *Pflugers Arch* 421:188, 1992.
93. Spencer MP, Greiss FC: Dynamics of ventricular ejection, *Circ Res* 10:274, 1962.

CHAPTER 3

Signalment, History, and Physical Examination

Signalment

Signalment is the age, breed, and sex of a patient. All are important variables to know when attempting to determine a diagnosis, a prognosis, and a therapeutic plan for a particular patient.

Age determination often provides useful information. Congenital heart defects, although not confined to young dogs, are most commonly identified in dogs and cats younger than age 3 and frequently younger than age 6 months. We more commonly identify acquired diseases, such as myxomatous degeneration of the atrioventricular valves and hyperthyroidism, in middle-age to older animals. Exceptions to the rule occur here as in every other phase of clinical medicine, however, so one must always be careful. We sometimes diagnose patent ductus arteriosus in geriatric animals, and myxomatous atrioventricular valve degeneration is known to produce heart murmurs in Cavalier King Charles spaniels as early as age 2.

Determining the breed of an animal is particularly important in veterinary cardiovascular medicine. Most of the dogs examined in clinical veterinary medicine with heart disease are purebred dogs. A listing of the common cardiovascular diseases seen in particular dog and cat breeds is presented in Table 3-1. One must be aware that exceptions to rules exist and only use the breed of animal as a general guide. Assuming that every Doberman pinscher with heart failure has dilated cardiomyopathy is common. Myxomatous mitral valve disease leading to severe mitral regurgitation, however, can occur in this breed and may have different therapy and prognosis. A left basilar heart murmur in a boxer most likely is due to subaortic stenosis, but other congenital abnormalities exist in this breed, including pulmonic stenosis.

Noting the sex of an animal is less important than noting age and breed. Some diseases do have sex predilections, but clinically significant sex-linked abnormalities are uncommon.

History

Taking the history should start by determining the client's primary complaint. Often the client has been rehearsing his or her story to tell to the veterinarian about the problems that the patient is having. Letting the client speak first allows him or her to tell the story without bias by the veterinarian. Following this, the veterinarian should question the client about specific aspects of the story. The veterinarian should then take a detailed history of any past medical or surgical problems and current medications being administered. The veterinarian should also ask questions about any other common problems observed in a particular species.

Frequently, in patients with cardiac disease there is no history of a clinical problem. The first clue that an animal has heart disease often is the auscultation of a heart murmur. Common owner complaints for an animal with cardiac disease include difficulty breathing (dyspnea), breathing too rapidly (tachypnea), coughing, abdominal swelling (ascites), fainting (syncope), turning blue (cyanosis), not eating well or not eating at all (anorexia), losing weight, or inability to exercise normally (exercise intolerance). Rarely, clients complain that the pet is coughing up blood (hemoptysis), has turned yellow (jaundice), or has swollen legs or swelling on the ventral abdomen (peripheral or ventral edema).

RESPIRATORY ABNORMALITIES

Dyspnea can take many forms in cardiac disease. In the animal that exercises, it may only occur during or after exercise (exertional dyspnea). Because dyspnea is a normal result of strenuous exercise, the veterinarian must try to determine if the client's complaint is the result of an abnormality or a variation on normality. For example, a client may complain that a dog is having difficulty breathing during exercise. On further questioning, the veterinarian may determine that this occurs only on hot summer days in a dog that only exercises once a week. This may be normal for this dog. Many pets do not exercise to any significant degree. Consequently, more commonly, owners do not note dyspnea until it is evident at rest. Dyspnea is more difficult to detect in animals than in humans, because animals cannot complain that they are having difficulty breathing. Instead, the owner must observe the forceful nature of the breathing pattern. Consequently, animals are commonly presented with severe dyspnea, because the owner has been unable to see the milder dyspnea that preceded the severe form. Dyspnea in humans commonly occurs because pulmonary edema makes the lung stiffer or pleural effusion decreases lung capacity, resulting in a greater effort required to ventilate. This probably also is true in dogs and cats. Dyspnea is also due to the inability to oxygenate properly, primarily because of poor diffusion capacity caused by pulmonary edema. When dogs or cats present with severe dyspnea as a result of pulmonary edema or pleural effusion, they generally have a marked inspiratory effort and may have an expiratory effort to their breathing pattern. Other dogs may be primarily hyperpneic, with rapid, deep respirations. These dogs usually still look distressed because of their inability to oxygenate. Presumably they feel anxious because of their inability to ventilate properly (air hunger). Occasionally, dogs develop dyspnea

TABLE 3-1

Breed and sex predilections for cardiac abnormalities

Abnormality	*Sex predisposition*	*Breed predisposition*
Patent ductus arteriosus	Female	Miniature and toy poodles, German shepherd, Amerian cocker spaniel, collie, Pomeranian, Shetland sheepdog
Subaortic stenosis	None	Newfoundland, golden retriever, English bulldog, boxer, German shepherd, German short-haired pointer
Pulmonic stenosis	None	English bulldog, fox terrier, miniature schnauzer, Chihuahua, beagle, Samoyed, boxer, bull mastiff, American cocker spaniel, West Highland white terrier, Boykin spaniel
Tetralogy of Fallot	None	Keeshond
Atrial septal defect	None	Boxer, Samoyed
Ventricular septal defect	None	English springer spaniel
Mitral valve dysplasia	None	English bulldog, great Dane, keeshond
Tricuspid valve dysplasia	None	Labrador retriever
Persistent right aortic arch	None	German shepherd, Irish setter
Aortic and carotid body tumors	None	Boston terrier, boxer
Dilated cardiomyopathy	Male	Doberman pinscher, boxer, great Dane, Saint Bernard, Newfoundland, Irish wolfhound, American cocker spaniel
Hypertrophic cardiomyopathy	Male (?)	Maine coon cat, Persian cat, American shorthair cat, Norwegian forest cat
Sick sinus syndrome	Female	Miniature schnauzer
Myxomatous atrioventricular valve degeneration	Male (?)	Small-breed dogs

or coughing when lying down or asleep. When this occurs at night, it is called *paroxysmal nocturnal dyspnea* or *coughing.* This is a common feature of heart failure in humans. This finding has been extrapolated to the veterinary literature as a common finding in dogs with heart failure. In our experience, this finding can occur but is not a common owner complaint. Orthopnea is breathing difficulty when lying down. Many dogs with severe dyspnea refuse to lie down because they become more distressed in this position. Instead they sit or stand, although they become so tired at times it appears that they are trying to fall asleep in these positions. These dogs commonly become more distressed when they are forced to lie down for radiographic or echocardiographic procedures. Forcing such an animal to lie down can precipitate an agonal event. Some animals show no dyspnea when upright but develop dyspnea when forced to lie on their side (trepopnea).

Coughing is a common sign of heart failure in dogs. It is less common in cats. Unfortunately, small dogs prone to developing heart failure secondary to mitral regurgitation as a result of myxomatous mitral valve degeneration also commonly have concomitant respiratory disease. Consequently, it is difficult to determine if the cough is due to respiratory or cardiac disease. These dogs commonly have a left apical systolic heart murmur and evidence of respiratory disease on their thoracic radiographs. Radiographic findings commonly include evidence of collapsing trachea, collapsing mainstem bronchi, or chronic lower airway disease, along with left atrial enlargement and interstitial densities in the caudodorsal lung fields. These densities are due to either pulmonary edema or an expiratory film in an old, obese dog. Often there is no definitive way to determine if the cough in such an animal is due to respiratory disease or to heart failure. We can make a few generalizations. It is more common for dogs with loud, "honking" types of cough to have respiratory disease. However, dogs with pulmonary edema can have the exact same type of cough. Dogs with softer coughs more commonly have pulmonary edema. This type of cough is more common in large dogs with pulmonary edema as a result of dilated cardiomyopathy that are not prone to developing concomitant respiratory disease. Auscultatory evidence of loud snaps, crackles, and wheezes in the lung fields is more common in dogs with respiratory disease than in dogs with pulmonary edema, although severe pulmonary edema can cause abnormal lung sounds. Pulmonary edema is most commonly associated with either radiographic or echocardiographic evidence of severe left atrial enlargement. Pulmonary edema can be present in the presence of mild-to-moderate left atrial enlargement but only in acute mitral regurgitation, which occurs most commonly secondary to a ruptured chorda tendineae. When differentiation is impossible, furosemide (usually 2 mg/kg q8 to 12h to a virgin patient or an increase in the dose in a patient already receiving furosemide) can be administered to evaluate the dog's response. Unfortunately, furosemide can act as a bronchodilator. Consequently, a positive response (reduction in the cough) cannot always be interpreted as evidence of pulmonary edema.

Cats may cough more with heart failure than suspected. Differentiating coughing from vomiting in cats is difficult for owners (and many veterinarians). Consequently, whenever an owner presents a cat and complains of the animal vomiting, coughing should be ruled out. The trachea should be compressed vigorously in these animals in the presence of the owner (one should be able to make a normal cat cough at least once), and both the client and the veterinarian should assess the response. An animal coughing at home usually has a protracted bout of coughing following tracheal compression. Normal animals usually will cough and/or gag once or twice and then stop.

A clinician also should be able to elicit a cough in a normal dog by vigorously compressing and manipulating the trachea. A normal dog should cough once or twice after this and then stop. Dogs presented for coughing commonly cough with lesser degrees of tracheal manipulation and have more prolonged bouts of coughing after manipulation. This response is commonly misinterpreted as the patient having "tracheitis" or "tracheobronchitis." This type of coughing, however, does not localize the cough to the trachea. Once the cough reflex in such an animal is initiated, cough receptors all along the respiratory tract can be stimulated to continue the coughing. Veterinarians treat many animals with lower airway disease, lung disease, and heart failure inappropriately with antibiotics because the animals cough with trachea manipulation and so are assumed to have "tracheobronchitis." Tracheobronchitis is usually an infectious process in dogs. If there is no history of recent exposure to other dogs, the clinician should be wary of making the diagnosis of tracheobronchitis.

Almost all patients that are dyspneic are also tachypneic. Tachypnea usually precedes clinical evidence of dyspnea. Tachypnea is a more subtle clinical sign, however, so owners commonly miss this sign. Once an animal has been diagnosed with pulmonary edema or pleural effusion, owners can be instructed to count their pet's respiratory rate at rest or while asleep. This is to detect recurrence or disappearance of tachypnea associated with pulmonary edema or pleural effusion. A normal dog's respiratory rate should be less than 30 breaths/min when at rest. A respiratory rate exceeding 50 breaths/min at rest is clear evidence that respiratory function is abnormal, and the veterinarian should be contacted.

ASCITES

Abdominal swelling can be due to gas, tissue, or fluid distension. Fluid distension may be due to a transudate (ascites) or an exudate. Right heart failure commonly produces ascites in dogs (Color Plate 24). Ascites secondary to heart failure is less common in cats. Right heart failure as a result of tricuspid valve dysplasia is the most common cardiac reason for ascites in cats. Ascites secondary to right heart failure generally accumulates slowly, although owners commonly think of it as an acute event because they do not notice the increase in abdominal size until it is severe. Chronic pericardial tamponade can result in subacute (days) accumulation of peritoneal fluid. Moderate accumulations of fluid in the peritoneal space usually can be balloted. Mild accumulations are impossible to ballot. Large accumulations may tense the abdominal wall so that a fluid wave cannot be produced. Large accumulations place pressure on the diaphragm, which impedes breathing. Consequently, dogs with severe ascites may be dyspneic or tachypneic.

SYNCOPE

Syncope (fainting) is defined as an episodic and transient loss of consciousness and postural tone.[1] It most commonly occurs because of a brief cessation of blood flow to the brain as a result of either a bradyarrhythmia or short period of asystole or a burst of nonsustained and severe tachycardia. However, syncope, episodic collapse, and episodic weakness can occur secondary to many abnormalities (see Chapter 28). Although syncope can occur in patients with heart failure, it is not a sign of heart failure. When an owner presents an animal because it appears to be fainting or having episodes of weakness, collapse, or seizure activity, the clinician must obtain an accurate history. Generally these "events" or "episodes" are most commonly cardiogenic or neurogenic. Distinguishing between seizures and episodic collapse or syncope can be very difficult, especially if the owner cannot provide a detailed and accurate history of at least one witnessed event (see Chapter 28).

WEIGHT LOSS

Weight loss and failure to grow properly can be indications of cardiac disease. The cardiovascular system should be examined carefully in a puppy or kitten that is failing to thrive. Many animals, however, with even severe congenital heart disease grow normally. Consequently, a normal growth pattern should not be used to rule out severe cardiac disease in a young animal. Weight loss can occur in animals with acquired cardiac disease leading to heart failure (cardiac cachexia) (Color Plate 25).

WEAKNESS

Generalized weakness can occur secondary to cardiac disease. Dogs and cats with advanced heart failure can be weak. This is due to poor perfusion resulting in decreased oxygen delivery to skeletal muscles or to generalized muscle wasting or both. Dogs with severe tachycardia (a heart rate usually greater than 300 beats/min) or severe bradycardia (a heart rate usually less than 30 beats/min) have a severely decreased cardiac output and so poor tissue perfusion and weakness. The decrease in cardiac output occurs with the tachycardia because of inadequate ventricular filling time and with the bradycardia because of the slow heart rate.

EXERCISE INTOLERANCE

Exercise intolerance is an occasional complaint by an owner of an animal with cardiac disease. It is not a more common complaint, because many animals do not exercise vigorously. It is more common in dogs with subaortic stenosis than in other cardiac disease. Owners of dogs with pulmonic stenosis often describe an increase in activity following successful balloon valvuloplasty. Consequently, it appears these dog owners often may not recognize exercise intolerance or decreased activity resulting from cardiac disease. Exercise intolerance as a result of cardiac disease also can be an early indication of heart failure. Whatever the cause, exercise intolerance is due to inadequate oxygen delivery to exercising muscle. This occurs because of inadequate blood flow, decreased arterial oxygen tension, or decreased hemoglobin concentration. In patients with heart disease, the decreased blood flow occurs most commonly because of poor pumping performance by the left ventricle. A decrease in arterial oxygen tension is usually secondary to pulmonary edema or pleural effusion.

CYANOSIS

Cyanosis is commonly both a historical finding and a physical sign. It is a blue to blue-gray discoloration of the mucous membranes, usually resulting from an increased quantity of reduced (deoxygenated) hemoglobin (Color Plate 26). Rarely, it is due to abnormal hemoglobin pigments in the blood (e.g., congenital methemoglobinemia). Cyanosis can be central or peripheral in origin. Peripheral cyanosis is due to the stasis of blood in capillary beds resulting in increased extraction of oxygen in the capillary beds. This is most commonly due to low cardiac output with peripheral vasoconstriction. The decrease in cardiac output must be severe for peripheral cyanosis to become evident. To demonstrate this, one can take a rubber band and place it around a finger to completely occlude blood flow and note that it takes almost 1 minute of no flow to produce obvious cyanosis in the finger.

Central cyanosis primarily is due to decreased arterial oxygen tension and saturation resulting in an increased concentration of systemic arterial deoxygenated hemoglobin. Cyanosis occurs in humans when more than 4 g/dL of deoxygenated hemoglobin is present in circulation. This occurs when arterial hemoglobin saturation decreases below 85%. This degree of subtle change is rarely noted in dogs or cats. Usually arterial saturation is less than 70% and arterial oxygen tension is less than 40 mm Hg before cyanosis is noted in animals. Consequently, cyanosis is an extremely insensitive means of detecting hypoxemia in dogs and cats. In Caucasian humans, cyanosis can be detected as a bluish color to the normally white or light pink skin. In dogs and cats, the darker pink color of the mucous membranes competes with the blue color of deoxygenated blood, making it more difficult to detect. Lighting conditions also affect ability to detect cyanosis.

In cardiovascular medicine, cyanosis is most common in patients with arterial hypoxemia as a result of right-to-left shunts such as tetralogy of Fallot. Dogs that are cyanotic at rest with this disorder routinely have arterial oxygen tensions between 30 and 35 mm Hg, oxygen saturations less than 65%, and greater than 6 g/dL of deoxygenated hemoglobin. Amazingly, cyanosis in humans can be visualized when the amount of blood shunting right to left exceeds the left ventricular output by only 25%.[1] This amount is probably greater in dogs. Patients with right-to-left shunts with hypoxemia usually also have polycythemia. The increased red cell mass results in a greater quantity of reduced hemoglobin and so contributes to the cyanosis. Cyanosis is commonly exacerbated with exercise. During exercise, peripheral vascular resistance decreases and pulmonary vascular resistance remains fixed in patients with right-to-left shunts. Consequently, the percentage of venous blood shunted into the systemic circulation during exercise increases.

Physical Examination

A careful physical examination should be performed on any patient suspected of having cardiac disease. Most animals with severe cardiac disease have some physical abnormality identified. The ability of the clinician to identify mild-to-moderate cardiac disease depends primarily on the type of disease present. For example, dogs with mitral regurgitation have a heart murmur that is present from very early disease until death. Consequently, detection of a heart murmur is a very sensitive diagnostic test for mitral regurgitation. On the other hand, dogs with dilated cardiomyopathy have no abnormalities on physical examination until the late stages of the disease are present. Other, more sensitive diagnostic tests, such as echocardiography, must be used to detect diseases such as dilated cardiomyopathy before end-stage disease. Although the physical examination is a valuable diagnostic tool, it is fallible, and the clinician must know its limitations and disadvantages in different diseases, just as for any other diagnostic test.

The patient with suspected cardiac disease should first undergo general inspection and observation, in which general condition and attitude are noted. Conformation and mobility should be assessed and an accurate weight obtained. A general physical examination should be performed to identify abnormalities of other organ systems.

HEAD AND NECK

Examination of the head and neck should include examining the color of the mucous membranes. Normal mucous membrane color is light to dark pink. Cyanosis may be observed as a blue to bluish-gray mucous membrane color. This may be more evident in tongue color than in the color of the gums. Dark red to muddy red mucous membrane color may be observed in animals with polycythemia, whereas pale mucous membrane color may suggest anemia or decreased perfusion. Rarely, icterus is present in a patient with cardiac disease.

Measurement of capillary refill time should be done on every patient. Measurement of capillary refill time consists of applying digital pressure to oral mucous membranes that are visibly pink to blanch the color, releasing the pressure and then measuring the time it takes for the color to return. The clinician should attempt to standardize this examination, by examining capillary refill time of buccal mucous membranes or of the mucous membranes of the gums. Capillary refill time varies with the amount of pressure applied and the site used for measurement. Consequently, it varies among clinicians. If moderate pressure is applied to the buccal mucous membranes, capillary refill time is generally from 1 to 2 seconds. The same amount of pressure applied to the mucous membranes of the gums results in a capillary refill time that is usually less than 1 second in the normal animal. Capillary refill time is an insensitive means of evaluating tissue blood flow. Many dogs with heart failure and a low cardiac output still have a normal capillary refill time.

The jugular veins should be examined carefully in any case of suspected cardiac disease (Color Plate 27). Neck hair may require clipping or wetting for identification of the jugular veins in dogs and cats with thick or long neck hair. A jugular vein should be initially identified with the animal in a sitting or standing position with the head moderately extended. In a normal animal the vein should be distended by placing enough pressure at the thoracic inlet to occlude jugular vein flow, resulting in jugular vein distension. Thoracic inlet pressure should then be released and the vein observed to determine the rate of vein collapse. In an animal with cardiac disease, the vein may be distended or pulsating, in which case it should be observed without occlusion. Distended jugular veins indicate increased systemic venous pressure or occlusion of the venous system between the jugular veins and the right heart. An increase in systemic venous pressure is most commonly secondary to an increase in right ventricular diastolic pressure. Because the tricuspid valve is open in diastole and because the tricuspid valve annulus provides very little resistance, right ventricular diastolic pressure and right atrial pressures are approximately equal. No valves are present between the right atrium and the systemic veins. Consequently, whatever pressure is present in the right atrium is also present in the systemic veins that are at the same height as the right atrium. The pressure in the veins is like pressure in any other semistatic system. That is, the pressure is greatest at the lowest levels and decreases further up the neck. For example, if the pressure in the right atrium is 5 cm of water (about 3 mm Hg), the pressure will be zero 5 cm above the right atrium. In addition the column of blood will rise 5 cm above the right atrium. Because of this, as right atrial pressure increases, the jugular veins become distended farther and farther up the neck. For the same reason, the amount of jugular vein distension should vary with animal size. The fact that cats do not normally have jugular vein distension must mean that their normal right atrial pressure is less than 2 to 3 cm of water, whereas in most dogs, up to 7 to 8 cm of water is considered normal. Jugular vein distension is not 100% sensitive for congestive right heart failure (elevated right ventricular diastolic and right atrial pressures). In our estimation, approximately 70% of dogs with right heart failure have jugular vein distension. A more sensitive noninvasive means of identifying increased systemic venous pressure is to examine hepatic vein size via ultrasound examination. One must be careful interpreting jugular vein distension in cats. We have noted instances in which jugular veins have been distended when the cat was in sternal recumbency but not distended when sitting or standing. These cats have not had right heart failure but have had left heart failure and a positive hepatojugular reflux test, as described below.

Jugular vein pulsation may also be observed in patients with cardiac disease. A normal venous waveform is presented in Figure 3-1. Jugular vein pulsation may be due to exaggerated *a* waves, cannon *a* waves, or prominent *v* waves. The *a* wave of any venous or atrial pressure wave recording occurs during atrial systole. An increase in atrial systolic pressure may occur secondary to decreased right ventricular compliance. A decrease in right ventricular compliance may occur with right ventricular hypertrophy, restrictive right ventricular disease, constrictive pericarditis, and so on. The deceased right ventricular compliance must be severe to result in jugular vein

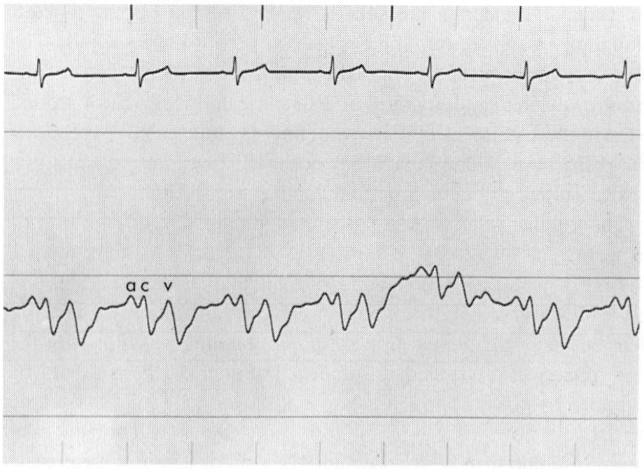

FIGURE 3-1 Right atrial pressure tracing from an anesthetized dog with pulmonic stenosis. Scale is from 0 to 20 mm Hg. Mean pressure is slightly increased at 6 to 7 mm Hg. The first four beats are inscribed during an expiratory pause. The fifth beat occurs during positive pressure ventilation. The *a* wave occurs coincident with the *P* wave on the electrocardiogram. This is followed by the *c* wave that occurs during isovolumic contraction coincident with the QRS complex. Following the *c* wave, the pressure wave decreases, forming the negative *x* wave. The *x* descent occurs as the tricuspid valve is displaced apically during ejection. This is followed by the positive *v* wave, which is produced by atrial filling while the tricuspid valve is closed. Following the *v* wave is the negative *y* wave. The *y* descent occurs when the tricuspid valve opens and blood from the right atrium rushes into the right ventricle. The *y* ascent occurs as the right atrium and ventricle continue to fill with blood.

pulsation, and a severe decrease in right ventricular compliance generally results in an overall increase in right ventricular diastolic pressure, with resultant jugular vein distension. Cannon *a* waves may occur with atrioventricular dissociation when the atria contract against a closed tricuspid valve, as in third-degree atrioventricular block. Prominent *v* waves occur secondary to tricuspid regurgitation. The *v* wave occurs during ventricular systole and is increased when the atrial volume is increased by the regurgitation of blood into the right atrium.

Patients with overt right heart failure may have obviously distended jugular veins. More subtle heart failure may be detected by performing the hepatojugular or abdominojugular reflux test. This test is performed by applying sustained pressure to the abdomen with one or both hands. This technique is generally accepted as a test for detecting right heart failure. In humans, however, it has been recently demonstrated that a positive test most closely correlates with increased pulmonary capillary wedge pressure (left heart failure).[2] It also correlates with right atrial pressure, however. Most likely this test is an indication of increased blood volume in the peripheral venous system and so can be positive with either left or right heart failure.

EXTREMITIES

The femoral pulse should be evaluated carefully in every patient. This should be done with the patient standing. The clinician may stand behind the animal and palpate both femoral arteries at once. The femoral arteries should be palpated high on the limb, so that the artery is palpated within or just below the femoral triangle, where the least amount of fat and muscle overlie the artery. The index or middle finger or both should be placed over the artery lightly to start. In most dogs, the artery itself can be palpated. Digital pressure should then be applied with sufficient strength to occlude arterial flow, so that no pulsation directly beneath the fingers is identified. Digital pressure should then be gradually decreased until the maximum pulsation is felt. The maximum pulsation occurs when digital pressure is equal to mean arterial blood pressure. A digital pressure more or less than this will result in feeling a "weaker" than real pulse pressure. Reporting a weak pulse in an animal with a normal pulse pressure because of improper technique is a common mistake.

The pulse pressure (the pressure felt on digital palpation of the pulse) is systolic systemic blood pressure minus diastolic systemic blood pressure. A normal blood pressure of 120 mm Hg systolic and 80 mm Hg diastolic results in a pulse pressure of 40 mm Hg. A patient with a systolic blood pressure of 200 mm Hg and a diastolic blood pressure of 160 mm Hg also will have a pulse pressure of 40 mm Hg. Consequently, absolute blood pressure cannot be determined by digital palpation of pulse pressure.

Pulse pressure can be decreased or increased or have an altered configuration. A decrease in pulse pressure can occur if stroke volume is decreased, as in patients with heart failure or hypovolemia, or if peripheral vascular resistance is decreased or arterial compliance increased. In most patients with a decreased stroke volume, arterial resistance increases and arterial compliance decreases to keep systemic blood pressure within the normal range. These changes may also keep pulse pressure normal. In humans, pulse pressure correlates well with cardiac output in patients with heart failure.[3] In our experience, canine patients with decreased stroke volumes commonly have normal pulses until the stroke volume becomes markedly reduced. Therefore examining pulse pressure is an insensitive means of identifying decreased stroke volume in a patient with chronic cardiac disease. Patients with severely decreased stroke volumes or very acute decreases in stroke volume are more likely to have weak pulses.

An increase in pulse pressure can occur because of an increase in systolic blood pressure, a decrease in diastolic blood pressure, or both. In cardiovascular disease, an increase in systolic blood pressure usually is caused by an increase in stroke volume. A decrease in diastolic blood pressure usually is due to runoff of blood into some other portion of the cardiovascular system during diastole. These abnormalities commonly occur in concert. For example, in aortic regurgitation the left ventricle increases the stroke volume pumped into the aorta to compensate for the amount of blood volume lost through the regurgitation. Consequently, the systolic blood pressure in severe aortic regurgitation is commonly increased. During diastole, blood flows back into the left ventricle, as well as the systemic vasculature, resulting in the diastolic blood pressure decreasing to a lower than normal level. Consequently, dogs with aortic regurgitation commonly have an increase in pulse pressure, called a *bounding pulse.* Bounding pulses can also be felt in patients with a patent ductus arteriosus, arteriovenous fistula, severe bradycardia, thyrotoxicosis, fever, and anemia. The pressure may rise and then fall sharply in these patients as blood flows through the shunt or regurgitant lesion, resulting in a pulse described as a "waterhammer" pulse.

Alteration in pulse conformation also may occur. Dogs with severe subaortic stenosis may have a weak pulse or may have a pulse pressure that increases more slowly and peaks later during systole (pulsus parvus et tardus). This occurs because the velocity of shortening may be reduced, and the ejection time may be longer in severe subaortic stenosis. Some dogs with subaortic stenosis, however, have pulses that are indistinguishable from normal. Conversely, dogs with mitral regurgitation commonly have a brisk pulse that rises more rapidly in systole and lasts a shorter time. This occurs

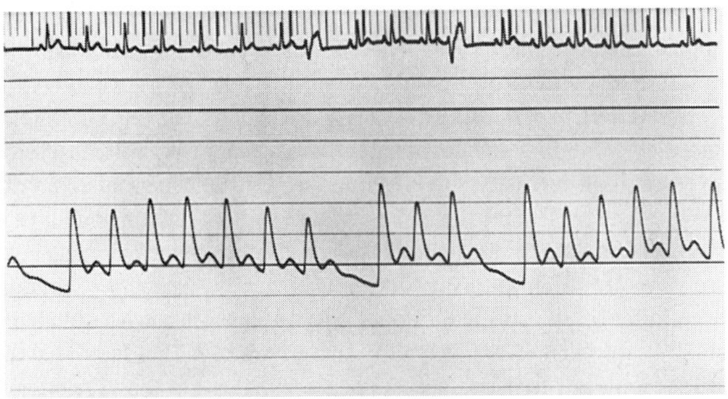

FIGURE 3-2 Simultaneous recordings of an ECG and systemic arterial blood pressure in an anesthetized dog with premature ventricular contractions. Scale is from 0 *(baseline)* to 200 mm Hg *(top line)*. There is about a 200-msec delay between QRS complexes and pressure tracings. Heavy time lines along the top represent 1 second. Systolic pressure varies but is approximately 120 mm Hg, and diastolic pressure is approximately 80 mm Hg, giving a pulse pressure of 40 mm Hg. The first seven beats are sinus beats. The eighth beat is a premature ventricular contraction. No pressure pulse is generated by depolarization. Pulse pressure is increased on the following beat, because diastolic pressure has time to decrease to a lower level and systolic pressure is increased by increased force of contraction of the beat following the premature beat (postextrasystolic potentiation). The same thing occurs three beats later.

because the left ventricle ejects blood at a higher velocity and the ejection time is shorter in mitral regurgitation.

Other pulse abnormalities include pulsus paradoxus, pulse deficits, and pulsus alternans. Pulsus paradoxus is an increase in pulse pressure on expiration and a decrease on inspiration. This occurs normally but is exaggerated in pericardial tamponade. Pulse deficits occur with cardiac tachyarrhythmias in which beats occur so rapidly that the ventricle does not have time to fill enough to result in ejection of blood (Figure 3-2). Examples include fast atrial fibrillation and ventricular premature beats. Pulsus alternans is alternating strong and weak pulses and is a rare finding unless one calls the pulse associated with ventricular bigeminy pulsus alternans. The correct term for this abnormality is *pulsus bigeminus.* Pulse pressure alternates erratically in patients with atrial fibrillation. Pulse deficits are also present.

The extremities also should be examined for the presence of edema. Peripheral, subcutaneous edema is not a common finding in dogs and cats with cardiovascular disease. It may occasionally be seen in dogs or cats with right heart failure. The extremities are usually colder than the trunk in dogs and cats with severely low cardiac output caused by heart failure. This may also be true of the ears. The caudal extremities are cold in cats and dogs with a saddle thromboembolus.

THORAX

The thorax should be palpated and any abnormalities in thorax shape noted. The precordial impulse should be palpated. Normally the heart is felt best in the region of the left apex, that is, on the left side of the chest in the region of the fourth to fifth intercostal spaces at the costochondral junction. Palpation of the precordial impulse rarely gives valuable information unless a cardiac thrill (palpable heart murmur) is felt. Feeling a strong apex beat is commonly but wrongly equated with a "strongly" contracting heart. When one feels the apex beat of the heart, one is *not* feeling the heart strike the chest wall. Instead, one is feeling the myocardium generate tension through the chest wall (much the same as feeling the biceps muscle tense during contraction). The wall tension can be recorded and is called an *apexcardiogram.*[4] Wall tension is calculated by multiplying the left ventricular chamber pressure times the left ventricular chamber radius (see Chapter 2). In dilated cardiomyopathy, the systolic pressure in the left ventricle is usually normal to mildly decreased and the chamber radius is increased. Consequently, a dog with dilated cardiomyopathy, a condition defined by a decrease in myocardial contractility and contraction, often has a stronger apex beat than a dog with a normal heart.

Palpation of the precordial impulse may reveal a cardiac thrill. A thrill is the ability to feel the vibrations created by turbulence within the heart through the chest wall. The location of this thrill is always the region where a heart murmur is heard best.

Auscultation. Auscultation is the act of listening for sounds within the body. Cardiac auscultation is usually the act of listening to heart sounds and murmurs through a stethoscope. Abnormal cardiac sounds are commonly generated in cardiac disease. Consequently, cardiac auscultation is the most valuable physical examination procedure for suspected cardiac disease.

Auscultation of the lungs also should be performed in every patient. Respiratory auscultation is more commonly abnormal in patients with primary respiratory disease. It also may be abnormal in patients with secondary respiratory abnormalities such as pulmonary edema and pleural effusion. However, auscultation of the lungs is not a sensitive means of detecting pulmonary edema or pleural effusion in dogs and cats. Many patients have pulmonary edema without any auscultatory abnormalities other than increased bronchovesicular sounds as a result of hyperpnea (moving more air through their airways). Therefore one should never rely on detecting abnormal lung sounds to identify pulmonary edema in dogs and cats. In human medicine, abnormal lung sounds are commonly identified in patients with pulmonary edema. The sounds associated with pulmonary edema are described as fine crackles that occur at the end of a forced inspiration.[5,6] When physicians listen to patients, they ask them to breathe deeply to accentuate sounds. Consequently, they can hear fine crackles at the end of a deep inspiration. Veterinarians cannot ask their patients to breathe deeply and so the ability to hear these sounds in our patients is markedly reduced. Patients with severe pulmonary edema resulting in free fluid in the airways are more likely to have audible crackles.

Stethoscopes. Veterinarians should choose a suitable stethoscope and then become used to its characteristics by using it frequently. A suitable stethoscope should fit the ears snugly and comfortably and should have a diaphragm and a bell. Veterinarians routinely auscult various sizes of animals, from cats to large dogs. The same size stethoscope is not appropriate for all animals. If one uses an adult stethoscope on a cat, a murmur cannot be localized accurately. Conversely, if one uses a pediatric stethoscope on a large dog, it often will distort the sounds and decrease the sound intensity. Consequently, a veterinarian should purchase a stethoscope on which the heads can be easily switched (e.g., a Sprague-Rapaport type) or purchase two stethoscopes, one adult size and one pediatric size.

Auscultatory sounds range in frequency and intensity. To optimize the intensity of sounds of different frequency, using both the diaphragm and the bell is often necessary. Routine use of both modes when listening to canine patients is preferred. The diaphragm is used to filter out low-frequency sounds (less than 300 Hz) so that higher-frequency sounds are accentuated. To do this, the diaphragm must be intact and rigid. The frequency of the heart sounds ausculted with a diaphragm can be changed by pressing more firmly or lightly during the examination. When listening with the diaphragm, the head of the stethoscope usually should be pressed firmly against the chest. The bell is used to listen to low-frequency sounds. To do this, the bell is placed gently against the chest. If the bell is placed firmly against the chest, the skin is tensed between the edges of the bell, making a diaphragm. The bell is used to listen to low-frequency sounds, such as third and fourth heart sounds in dogs. Third and fourth heart sounds in cats are commonly higher-frequency sounds than they are in dogs and are usually readily ausculted with a diaphragm. Third and fourth heart sounds are generated by the heart vibrating. The smaller heart of cats vibrates at a higher frequency than that of dogs and humans. Consequently, the rule of using the bell to listen to gallop sounds often is not true for cats.

Technique. Whenever an animal is ausculted, it should be in a standing or sitting position. Listening to recumbent animals is fraught with error. Recumbency results in the heart lying against the chest wall. This predisposes to the formation of rubbing sounds that can be mistaken for heart murmurs. The position of the heart may also change, resulting in incorrect localization of heart sounds.

When ausculting an animal, a routine should be used to decrease the chance of missing important information. Initial palpation should identify the left apex beat. The stethoscope should be placed over this region first. This is the so-called mitral region and is the region where the murmur of mitral regurgitation is heard best. Generally the first heart sound is also loudest at this point. The stethoscope should be "inched" from the left apex to the left base. The left base is approximately two rib spaces forward from the apex and dorsal, about ¼ of the chest height up from the left apex. While the stethoscope is being moved cranially and dorsally, the examiner should listen carefully at each point, concentrating on each heart sound and each phase of the cardiac cycle. The left heart base is the region where the heart can be heard well, the first heart sound is softer than at the apex, and the second heart sound is prominent. Murmurs of aortic and pulmonic stenosis are commonly heard well in this region. Textbooks commonly divide this region into aortic and pulmonic regions, as if the murmurs of aortic and pulmonic stenosis can be distinguished by the exact region of their intensity at the left heart base. This may be feasible in a very large dog but is totally impractical in a small dog or cat and should not be attempted. Instead, describing the murmur as loudest at the left heart base is sufficient. While on the left side of the chest, one should take time, especially in puppies, to slide the stethoscope head forward into the left axillary region to listen carefully for the murmur of a patent ductus arteriosus. Next, the right apex beat should be palpated, and the stethoscope head moved to this region. This is the so-called tricuspid region, where the murmur of tricuspid regurgitation is heard best. One may also choose to listen to the right heart base, a region where the murmur of tricuspid regurgitation and the murmur of subaortic stenosis may be heard best on occasion. Besides ausculting these regions, whenever an auscultatory abnormality is encountered, one should "inch" the head of the stethoscope over all regions of the heart to identify the region where the abnormality is heard best or to identify new abnormalities. In so doing, the entire region of the chest where heart sounds can be heard should be ausculted.

Unfortunately a textbook cannot demonstrate heart murmurs and abnormal heart sounds. Even recorded heart sounds and murmurs only provide a starting point for becoming proficient at identifying abnormal cardiac sounds. The only true methods of becoming proficient at auscultation are listening to many animals' heart sounds by oneself or listening with a mentor, switching the stethoscope between mentor and student or using a double-headed stethoscope. Once an abnormal sound is heard, it is never forgotten. An analogy can be made between listening to the distinctive sounds of a tuba versus the sounds of a flute. Once heard, they are never forgotten and never confused. Likewise, the harsh, blowing systolic murmur of mitral regurgitation, once heard, will never be confused with the soft, blowing diastolic murmur of aortic regurgitation; nor will the high-frequency snap of a systolic click be confused with the low-frequency thud of a gallop sound in a dog.

Transient heart sounds. Four heart sounds can be potentially ausculted. The first and second heart sounds are normally ausculted and are high-intensity, high-frequency transients associated with valve closures. The third and fourth heart sounds (gallop sounds) are not heard in normal dogs and only rarely heard in normal cats. They are low- to high-intensity and low- to high-frequency sounds, depending on the species. In dogs they are usually of low intensity and low frequency. In cats, gallop sounds are often loud and may be louder than the first and second heart sounds, and they are higher frequency than in dogs. Size is a primary determinant of frequency. This can be readily appreciated by comparing the pitch of a large bell (e.g., the Liberty Bell) with that of a small bell.

The first heart sound occurs at the onset of systole and is associated with the closure of the atrioventricular (mitral and tricuspid) valves (Figure 3-3). This coincides with the QRS complex on the electrocardiogram. The exact source of the first and second heart sounds remains controversial. The most popular explanation is to say that the rapid deceleration of blood causes the first heart sound, setting the entire cardiohemic system into vibration. The intensity of the first heart sound is dependent on several variables, including (1) the velocity of valve closure, (2) ventricular contractility, (3) the integrity of the valve, (4) the mobility of the valve, (5) the transmission characteristics of the thoracic cavity, and (6) the physical characteristics of the vibrating structures.

The velocity of valve closure is related to the time that the valve has to accelerate and to acceleration. The position of the valve at the onset of ventricular systole determines the time that the valve has to accelerate. If the valve is wide open, it attains maximum velocity by the time it coapts and the loudest sound is produced. If it is almost closed, however, it will not have time to achieve the same velocity and the sound will be softer. Ventricular contractility determines acceleration of the valve to closure. Contractility is related to ventricular dP/dt, a factor known to change the intensity of the first heart sound. Exercise and catecholamine infusion both increase the intensity of the first heart sound by increasing contractility. Varying

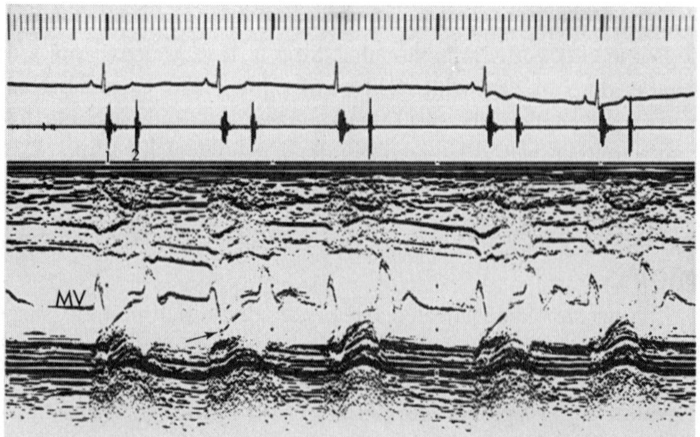

FIGURE 3-3 Simultaneous recordings of an ECG *(top)*, a phonocardiogram *(between ECG and echocardiogram)*, and an M-mode echocardiogram from a normal dog. The first heart sound (1) coincides with the end of the QRS complex and closure of the mitral valve (MV) leaflets on the echocardiogram *(arrow)*. The second heart sound (2) occurs at the end of the T wave.

the P-R interval changes the opening of the mitral valve leaflets at the onset of systole. Consequently, it changes the first heart sound intensity. In mitral regurgitation, the mitral valve leaflets open wide in diastole and is one reason the first heart sound is increased in mitral regurgitation.

The second heart sound is associated with closure of the semilunar valves (aortic and pulmonic). It occurs at the end of ventricular ejection (at the end of systole), after the T wave on the electrocardiogram (see Figure 3-3). The second heart sound has two components, one associated with the closure of the aortic valve and one with closure of the pulmonic valve. Normally these two components occur simultaneously in dogs and cats or so close together that the human ear cannot distinguish the separation between the two. The normal human ear requires approximately a 30- to 50-msec separation between two sounds to detect both sounds. The intensity of these two components is dependent on the force closing the valves and other determinants of transmitting sound to the body surface. Consequently, pulmonary and systemic hypertension increase the intensity of the second heart sound. This change, however, is subtle. So much variation is present between animals that it is difficult to detect a change in second heart sound intensity unless a patient is followed over time.

On occasion the second heart sound may become split. This occurrence is much less frequent as an audible event in veterinary medicine than in human medicine, probably because of patient size differences and faster heart rates. The most common situation in which we have detected a split second heart sound is in dogs with right-to-left shunting patent ductus arteriosus, although it can be appreciated in other patients with severe pulmonary hypertension. In a right-to-left shunting patent ductus arteriosus, there is no heart murmur to mask the split sound. Pulmonary hypertension is severe in this disease. This increases right ventricular afterload and prolongs right ventricular ejection time, whereas left ventricular ejection time remains normal to decreased. The result is that the pulmonic valve closes later than the aortic valve. Heartworm disease is commonly listed in the veterinary literature as a frequent cause of a split second heart sound. However, a split second heart sound is only identified in dogs with severe pulmonary hypertension, and, in most heartworm

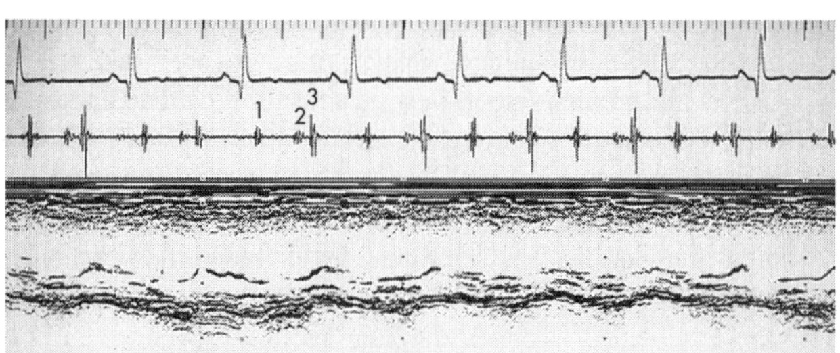

FIGURE 3-4 Simultaneous recordings of an ECG, a phonocardiogram, and an M-mode echocardiogram from a dog with dilated cardiomyopathy. There is slight time delay between the ECG and the phonocardiogram. A third heart sound *(3)* is present and occurs coincident with maximal opening of mitral valve *(E point)* in early diastole. *1*, First heart sound; *2*, second heart sound.

cases, pulmonary hypertension is mild to moderate. Consequently, identification of a split second heart sound in heartworm disease depends on the number of severe cases identified. Theoretically, bundle branch blocks, premature ventricular contractions, and pacing should result in split second heart sounds, but clinically this split is often too subtle to detect except via phonocardiography. These abnormalities can also result in a split first heart sound.

The third heart sound is not audible in normal dogs and almost never audible in normal cats. When audible, it is called a *gallop sound* or *rhythm* or an *audible third heart sound.* It may also be called a *protodiastolic gallop sound.* The third heart sound is a sound that occurs at the peak of rapid ventricular filling or shortly after that. It coincides with the initial maximal opening of the mitral valve on an echocardiogram (Figure 3-4). It is generated by the ventricular walls vibrating, primarily the left ventricular walls.[7,8] Ventricular walls can vibrate in diastole with enough intensity to produce an audible sound for two reasons. First, they vibrate when they are stiffer than normal, such that during rapid ventricular filling the left ventricle reaches the end of its distensibility very quickly, resulting in the walls vibrating. The closing of a door is an example of this. A normal heart may be compared to a door with a lot of weather stripping. Rapid ventricular filling may be compared to closing that door forcefully. Because of the weather stripping (cushioning), very little sound is generated. If the cushioning is removed (the structure made stiffer), a louder sound is generated when the door is forcefully closed. Hypertrophic cardiomyopathy makes the left ventricle stiffer than normal, which can result in an audible third heart sound. Second, the walls can vibrate when a large volume of blood dumps into a normal left ventricle in early diastole, such that the ventricle again reaches the end of its distensibility rapidly and then shudders. This may be compared to slamming the door. With severe mitral regurgitation, a large volume of blood is pumped into the left atrium in systole and then "dumps" rapidly and forcefully into the left ventricle during rapid ventricular filling. In this situation the third heart sound may become loud enough to be mistaken for the second heart sound at the end of a pansystolic heart murmur. Occasionally a third heart sound can be loud enough to be felt by placing fingers lightly over the left apex beat. Third heart sounds are heard best with the bell of the stethoscope in dogs and are readily audible with the diaphragm in cats. The smaller cat heart apparently and sensically vibrates at a higher frequency.

The fourth heart sound is a low-frequency sound generated during atrial systole (late ventricular diastole). It is also caused by ventricular wall vibration. This occurs because the atria are trying to force blood into an already overdistended ventricle or because the atria are forcing blood into a stiff ventricle. Atrial contraction must be present for production of an audible fourth heart sound. Consequently, the fourth heart sound cannot be present in patients with atrial fibrillation. Fourth heart sounds are most commonly heard in feline patients with cardiomyopathies and in canine patients with third-degree atrioventricular block. In the latter, soft fourth heart sounds sometimes may be heard in the background of normal heart sounds (Figure 3-5).

When the heart rate is greater than 160 to 180 beats/min rapid ventricular filling and atrial systole occur very close together, making it impossible to tell if the gallop sound is an audible third or fourth heart sound or both. In this situation, the audible sound is called a *summation gallop sound.* This occurs most frequently in cats.

Ejection sounds are generated by the semilunar valves or within the great vessels during early systole. They have similar frequencies with the first heart sound and so may be confused with the first heart sound. They occur most commonly in dogs with valvular pulmonic

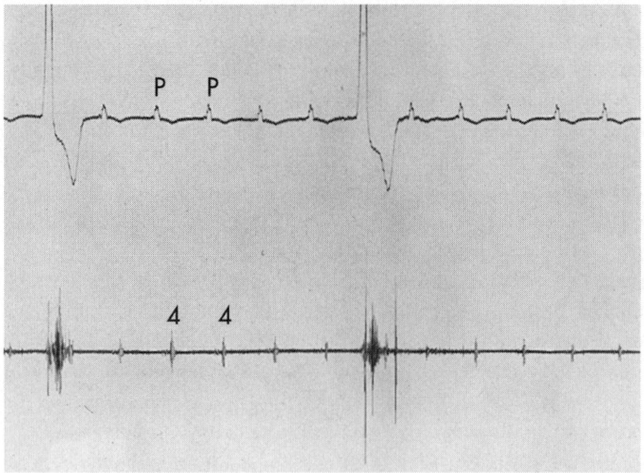

FIGURE 3-5 Recording of an ECG and a phonocardiogram from a dog with third-degree atrioventricular block. Low-intensity fourth heart *(4)* sounds are recorded that coincide with each P wave.

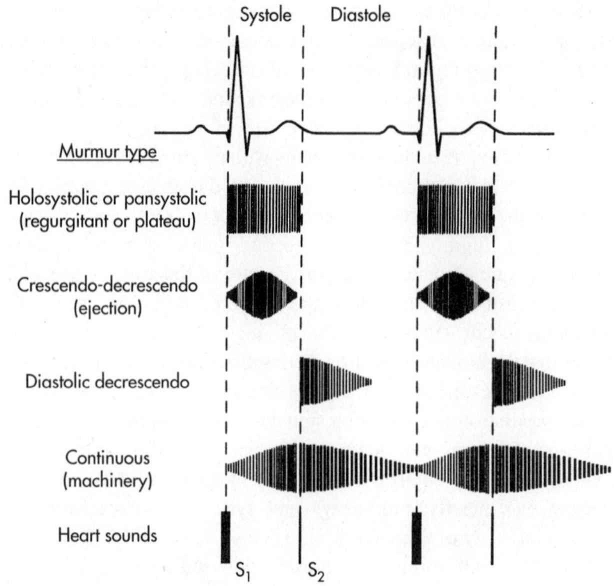

FIGURE 3-6 Schematic drawing of the shapes of various types of heart murmurs most commonly ausculted in dogs and cats.

stenosis and are probably due to immobile leaflets snapping open in early systole.

The other heart sound commonly identified in dogs is a systolic click. Systolic clicks are high-frequency sounds that occur in systole, creating three audible heart sounds. Systolic clicks are commonly mistaken for gallop sounds (third and fourth heart sounds). They occur almost exclusively in dogs with early mitral valve disease. In humans, systolic clicks are heard in patients with mitral valve prolapse. The sound is generated by the valve as it buckles into the left atrium. A similar mechanism is probably responsible for the generation of this sound in dogs.

Heart murmurs. A heart murmur is defined as a prolonged series of auditory vibrations emanating from the heart or blood vessels. The sounds produced can be characterized by their location, intensity (loudness), frequency (pitch), timing, quality, and configuration (Figure 3-6). Murmurs are generated by two basic mechanisms. The most common is turbulence of blood flow. The less common cause is vibration of a cardiac structure, usually part of a valve leaflet or chordal structure. The former creates a harsh or blowing sound. The latter creates a murmur with a single frequency. This usually is described as a musical murmur, although the single frequency may be honking or grunting in character and not musical to most people's ears.

Blood flow turbulence can be created by high-velocity flow, flow from a narrow region into a larger area, or low blood viscosity. The relationship of these variables is defined by the Reynolds number, a number generated by the formula:

$$\text{Reynolds number} = \frac{\text{(Area) (Velocity) (Density)}}{\text{Viscosity}}$$

Most murmurs are heard in animals with cardiac disease. By examining this equation, the clinician can appreciate that not all heart murmurs are due to cardiovascular disease. Blood flow can become turbulent in some normal animals or become turbulent for reasons other than cardiac disease. Puppies tend to have larger stroke volumes for the size of their great vessels than adult dogs. When excited in an examination room, their stroke volume may increase even further, creating an "innocent" heart murmur that disappears as the dog matures. The classic example of increased flow creating a murmur is that of an atrial septal defect. The flow through a large atrial septal defect does not create a murmur. The flow into the right ventricle in diastole in this situation forces the right ventricle to expel a much greater quantity of blood, however. The increased flow results in an increased blood flow velocity through the region of the pulmonic valve. This can create turbulence and a soft left basilar heart murmur. Anemia is a classic example of a means of creating a nonpathologic or physiologic heart murmur. Anemia decreases blood viscosity. Producing turbulence in a more viscous medium is more difficult (e.g., in molasses) than in a less viscous medium. As packed cell volume decreases, blood becomes more like water, making it easier for turbulence to develop. Stroke volume also increases in anemic patients to compensate for the loss of oxygen-carrying units (red blood cells). The combination of the decreased viscosity and the increased stroke volume (increased velocity) can produce a heart murmur. Some normal cats have heart murmurs. We have noted that some of these cats have turbulent blood flow in the region of the right ventricular outflow tract (Color Plate 28).[9] Although blood flow velocity is increased and blood flow is turbulent as a result, there is no evidence that there is structural disease in these cats.

Common causes of pathologic heart murmurs are listed in Box 3-1. Almost all turbulent blood flow as a result of cardiac disease is due to high-velocity flow through a narrow orifice. The peak velocity can be measured using spectral Doppler echocardiography and can be displayed graphically with color flow Doppler. When the Reynolds' number reaches a critical level, blood flow becomes turbulent. Turbulent blood flow is characterized by red cells traveling at multiple velocities, as opposed to laminar flow, in which all of the red cells in a certain area travel at the same velocity. Laminar vs. turbulent blood flow is demonstrated in rivers that have rapids. Laminar flow is the part of the river where the flow rate is slow, with all of the water in one region traveling at the same velocity. Increased velocity occurs when the river narrows, and turbulent flow occurs when the velocity reaches a critical velocity. Turbulent flow creates sound, and turbulent flow in river rapids demonstrates this fact. Use of a garden hose also demonstrates this fact. When the orifice at the end of a hose is partially occluded, flow velocity of the water stream increases and, with further occlusion, becomes turbulent. At this time, sound is generated in the same manner that sound is generated in the cardiovascular system.

The force generated by turbulent blood flow, and so the intensity of the murmur at its origin, is determined by blood flow velocity (cm/sec) and the rate of flow (cm^3/sec or g/sec) (velocity × flow = force [dynes or g cm/sec^2]). The intensity of the heart murmur at the surface, however, is determined by many variables, including the intensity of the heart murmur at its origin, the direction of the turbulent jet in relation to the region ausculted, the character of the tissues between the turbulent jet and the area being ausculted, and the frequency of the murmur.

Although the intensity of a heart murmur is not directly correlated with the severity of a lesion, in certain cardiac diseases, such as mitral regurgitation, at least a rough correlation exists.[10] Consequently, describing the intensity of a murmur in an individual patient is useful. However, in certain cardiac diseases, such as ventricular septal defect, small defects can result in very loud heart murmurs, whereas in other diseases, such as atrial septal defect, a very large defect may be associated with no heart murmur.

Murmurs are most commonly graded on a 1 to 6 scale, with a grade 1 murmur the softest and a grade 6 the loudest. A grade 1 murmur is very soft and is heard only in a quiet room and after close concentration and adjustment of the stethoscope. A grade 2 murmur is faint but can be easily heard. A grade 3 murmur is moderately loud. A grade 4 murmur is loud. A grade 5 murmur is very loud and can be heard with just the edge of the stethoscope placed on the chest. This intensity of murmur also has a palpable thrill. A grade 6 murmur has a thrill and can be heard with the stethoscope just removed from contact with the chest.

Location is an important clue to the origin of a heart murmur. The murmurs that occur secondary to aortic and pulmonic stenosis, for example, are most commonly heard best at the left heart base. The murmur of mitral regurgitation is usually heard best at the left apex. The murmur caused by patent ductus arteriosus is best heard on the cranial left thorax, in the left axillary region. The clinician should note the location where the heart murmur is heard best (the point of maximal intensity, or PMI) and where else the murmur can be heard on the chest wall or elsewhere. The location to where the murmur radiates may also give important clues about the source of the murmur. For example, the murmur secondary to subaortic stenosis may also be heard on the ventral neck (because of turbulence in the carotid arteries) and at the right heart base.

Murmurs are described relative to their timing in the cardiac cycle. Systolic murmurs may start immediately after the first heart sound and last until the second heart sound (holosystolic murmur), may start immediately after the first heart sound and last through the second heart sound (pansystolic), or, more rarely, last only a portion of systole. A pansystolic murmur lasts through the second heart sound because the left ventricular systolic pressure is greater than left atrial pressure for a short time after aortic valve closure. Diastolic murmurs most commonly start immediately after the second heart sound and last through the first portion or most of diastole. Continuous murmurs last throughout systole and diastole. Their intensity usually peaks at the time of the second heart sound (Figure 3-7).

The configuration of a heart murmur varies with the type of lesion present. Determining the shape of a murmur via auscultation may be difficult because of tachycardia in many animals. Classically, however, regurgitant lesions (e.g., mitral and tricuspid regurgitation) create murmurs that have the same intensity throughout the time that the murmur is generated (plateau murmur) (Figure 3-8). Blood flow velocity increases in direct correlation to the increase in pressure, and regurgitant flow begins as soon as the ventricle starts to generate pressure. Because the rapid upstroke of the left ventricular pressure trace only takes a few milliseconds, the murmur attains its maximal intensity very quickly. Conversely, during ventricular relaxation, the left ventricular pressure trace decreases very rapidly, such that the murmur intensity decreases rapidly. Stenotic lesions (e.g., aortic and pulmonic stenoses) create murmurs that may build in intensity in systole and then taper in intensity (crescendo-decrescendo, or ejection quality, murmur) (Figure 3-9). These murmurs do not begin until ejection begins. This is shortly after the onset of systole that theoretically should occur a short time after the first heart sound. The time is so short, however, that one does not generally appreciate this. The increase in systolic pressure after semilunar valve opening is

BOX 3-1

Principal causes of pathologic heart murmurs in dogs and cats

I. SYSTOLIC MURMURS
  A. Plateau murmurs
    1. Atrioventricular valve regurgitation
    2. Left-to-right shunting ventricular septal defect
  B. Ejection murmurs
    1. Aortic
      a. Obstructive (fixed or dynamic stenosis)
      b. Increased flow (aortic regurgitation, hyperthyroidism)
    2. Pulmonic
      a. Obstructive (fixed stenosis)
      b. Increased flow (left-to-right shunt at cardiac level)

II. DIASTOLIC MURMURS
  A. Early diastolic murmurs (high or mixed frequency)
    1. Aortic regurgitation (bacterial endocarditis; with ventricular septal defect)
    2. Pulmonary regurgitation (rarely audible)
  B. Middiastolic murmurs (low frequency)
    1. Mitral stenosis (rare)
    2. Functional atrioventricular valve stenosis (ventricular septal defect, atrial septal defect; rarely audible)

III. CONTINUOUS MURMURS
  A. Patent ductus arteriosus (95% of cases)
  B. Ruptured aneurysm of a sinus of Valsalva (rare)
  C. Aorticopulmonary window (rare)

IV. TO-AND-FRO MURMURS
  A. Ventricular septal defect with aortic regurgitation (most common)
  B. Aortic stenosis and significant aortic regurgitation (uncommon)
  C. Pulmonic stenosis and significant pulmonic regurgitation (rare)

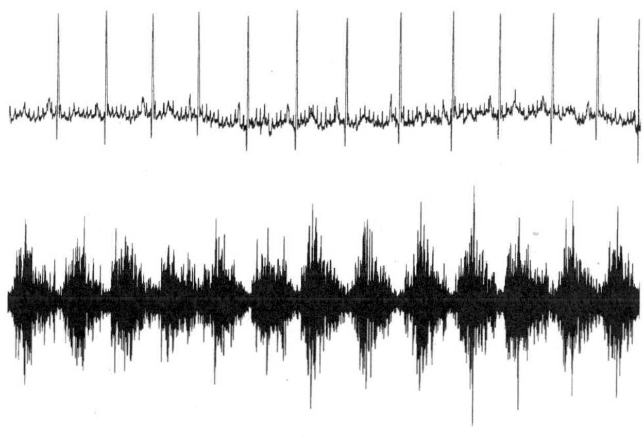

FIGURE 3-7 Recordings of an ECG and a phonocardiogram from a dog with a continuous heart murmur resulting from a patent ductus arteriosus. A baseline artifact is present on the ECG. The murmur lasts throughout systole and diastole and peaks in intensity at the end of systole.

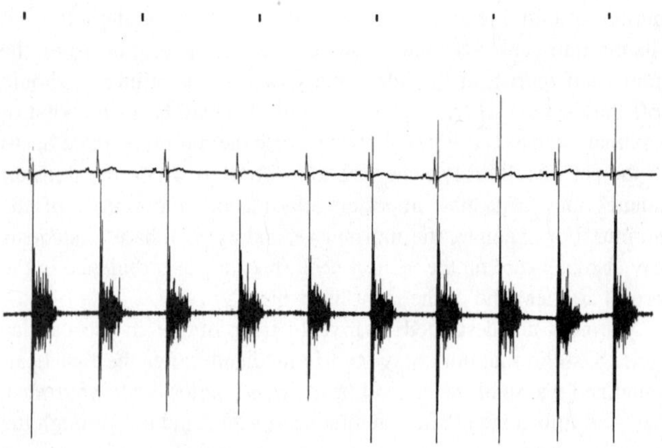

FIGURE 3-8 Simultaneous recordings of a phonocardiogram and an ECG from a dog with a grade 4/6 pansystolic heart murmur resulting from severe mitral regurgitation. The first heart sound is very loud. The murmur's configuration is plateau to slightly decrescendo. The second heart sound cannot be readily identified.

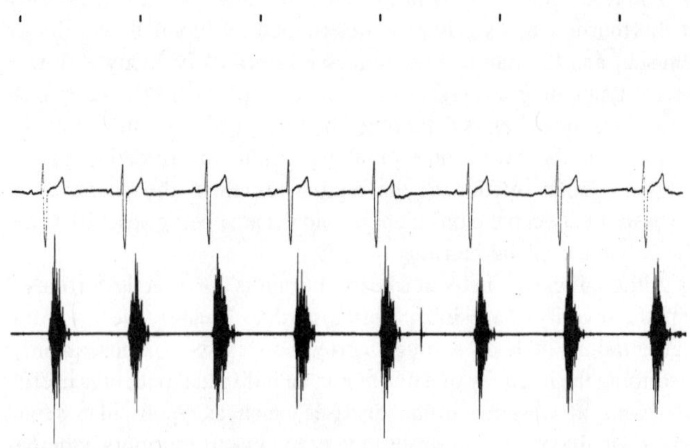

FIGURE 3-9 Recordings of an ECG and a phonocardiogram from a young dog with severe pulmonic stenosis. The murmur begins immediately in systole, increases in intensity to peak in midsystole, and then decreases in intensity (crescendo-decrescendo murmur). The second heart sound can be visualized and is soft.

more gradual than during isovolumic systole, so the murmur should increase in intensity more gradually. This slower increase in intensity is often subtle and may not be appreciated. During the latter part of systole, ejection slows. Consequently, pressure and flow velocity slow, resulting in a diminution in murmur intensity. This decrease is often also subtle and may be appreciated on a phonocardiogram but less well appreciated on auscultation. Examination of the increase and decrease in velocity of blood flow through a stenotic lesion with spectral (continuous wave) Doppler allows appreciation of the speed at which these velocities increase and decrease and why the murmurs are not always as classically described in humans. A continuous heart murmur clearly increases and decreases in intensity over time. The murmur is generally loudest at the end of ejection and decreases in intensity through diastole. The murmur may cease in late diastole, especially in dogs with slow heart rates. The murmur then increases in intensity again at the onset of ejection. Diastolic heart murmurs usually have a decrescendo configuration, decreasing in intensity through diastole (see Figure 3-6).

The character of a heart murmur should be noted. Most systolic heart murmurs have multiple frequencies present and are described as *harsh*. This can be demonstrated by placing the back of the tongue close to the roof of the mouth and blowing out forcefully. The murmur of aortic insufficiency is usually softer and with fewer frequencies and is described as *blowing*. This can be demonstrated by blowing air with moderate force through lips parted about 2 cm. The murmur created by a patent ductus arteriosus can be described as sounding like wind blowing through a tunnel.

The frequency of most heart murmurs is mixed and in the midrange. Occasionally heart murmurs will be a single frequency, creating pure tones. These may be high-frequency musical tones or lower-frequency "honks" or "grunts." Musical murmurs are most commonly identified in dogs with mitral regurgitation and thought to be the result of a portion of the mitral valve apparatus vibrating at a certain frequency as blood rushes past the affected structure. Musical murmurs are often loud but are most commonly identified in animals with mild disease.

REFERENCES

1. Braunwald E: Examination of the patient. In Braunwald E, ed: *Heart disease: a textbook of cardiovascular medicine,* ed 4, Philadelphia, 1992, WB Saunders.
2. Ewy GA: The abdominojugular test: technique and hemodynamic correlates *Ann Intern Med* 109:456, 1988 (erratum 109[12]:997, 1988).
3. Stevenson LW, Perloff JK: The limited reliability of physical signs for estimating hemodynamics in chronic heart failure, *JAMA* 261:884, 1989.
4. Denys BG, Aubert AE, Denef B et al: Relationship between apex-cardiogram, left ventricular pressure and wall stress, *J Biomed Eng* 4:9, 1982.
5. Kotlikoff MI, Gillespie JR: Lung sounds in veterinary medicine. II. Deriving clinical information from lung sounds, *Compend Cont Educ* 6:462, 1996.
6. Forgacs P: Lung sounds, *Chest* 63:1, 1969.
7. Ozawa Y, Smith D, Craige E: Origin of the third heart sound. I. Studies in dogs, *Circulation* 67:393, 1983.
8. Glower DD, Murrah RL, Olsen CO et al: Mechanical correlates of the third heart sound, *J Am Coll Cardiol* 19:450, 1992 (see comments).
9. Rishniw M, Thomas WP, Kienle RD: Dynamic right mid-ventricular obstruction in 50 cats, *J Vet Intern Med* 10:159, 1996 (abstract).
10. Haggstrom J, Kvart C, Hansson K: Heart sounds and murmurs: changes related to severity of chronic valvular disease in the Cavalier King Charles spaniel, *J Vet Intern Med* 9:75, 1995.

CHAPTER 4

Radiography of the Cardiovascular System

This chapter is presented from a cardiologist's, not from a radiologist's, viewpoint. Consequently, we are not presenting material on thoracic radiograph technique. Numerous veterinary radiology textbooks provide this type of information. Normal thoracic radiographic anatomy is presented in Figures 4-1 and 4-2.

Thoracic radiographs provide a wealth of knowledge about many patients with cardiovascular disease. Detecting cardiac enlargement makes the diagnosis of significant cardiac disease much more likely. Identifying specific chamber or great vessel enlargement often provides clues as to the nature of a cardiac disease (Table 4-1). Identifying pulmonary edema or pleural effusion is a direct means of diagnosing heart failure in patients that have cardiac disease. Determining the size of the pulmonary vessels may provide clues regarding pulmonary vascular flows and pressures. The severity of the changes detected on thoracic radiographs often correlates with the severity of the disease and so with the prognosis. Thoracic radiographs are very useful for evaluating the effectiveness of heart failure therapy.

Although thoracic radiographs are useful, thoracic radiography is not an ideal tool for evaluating patients with cardiovascular disease. It is an inaccurate tool for determining overall cardiac size and for determining the size of the ventricles and the right atrium. Echocardiography has supplanted thoracic radiography for determining the size of these chambers in most situations. Thoracic radiography does not definitively distinguish cardiogenic pulmonary edema from other pulmonary disease. Identifying a radiographic pattern consistent with pulmonary edema can only accomplish this in association with severe left heart disease. The same can be said for pleural effusion.

Thoracic radiology was the first means of objectively identifying changes in cardiac size and shape with any degree of accuracy. Because it was the first modality, it is still sacrosanct to many clinicians. Few instances exist in which a thoracic radiograph is not indicated in a patient with heart disease. However, these instances do exist. Just because the technology is available does not mean that a thoracic radiograph is required in every patient with cardiovascular disease. For example, a dog with mild subaortic stenosis would be expected to have a heart murmur and Doppler evidence of the stenosis but would not be expected to have any radiographic changes of clinical significance. Neither is it necessary to evaluate the thoracic radiographs before performing other examinations, such as echocardiography. Although it may be a good exercise to read the radiographs in a blinded fashion, performing diagnostic tests in the order in which they were invented is not necessary.

Before 1980, the diagnosis of cardiac disease relied on physical examination, an electrocardiogram, and thoracic radiographs. One study suggests that the diagnosis of congenital heart disease could be made based primarily on thoracic radiographs and the electrocardiogram in about 25% of cases, primarily based on physical examination in 15% of cases, required invasive diagnostic tests (cardiac catheterization/angiocardiography, surgery) in 30% of cases, and was not made until necropsy in about 30%.[1] These numbers have changed drastically since the arrival of medical ultrasound. Today it is very unusual that a congenital cardiac abnormality is not diagnosed before necropsy. Careful echocardiographic evaluation results in a definitive diagnosis in more than 90% of cases. Thoracic radiographs commonly contribute to the diagnosis but still provide definitive evidence of the specific congenital or acquired cardiac abnormality in less than 50% of cases. However, this is very lesion specific. For example, it is common to identify a main pulmonary artery bulge on a dorsoventral thoracic radiograph in a dog with severe pulmonic stenosis. It is less common to identify the proximal aortic bulge on the lateral radiograph of a dog with subaortic stenosis.

Radiographic Interpretation: Philosophy

Thoracic radiography is one of the most important diagnostic tests used in small animal cardiovascular medicine. It is also the most difficult to interpret. Thoracic radiography is used primarily in cardiovascular medicine to identify generalized cardiac enlargement, specific cardiac chamber or great vessel enlargement, pulmonary parenchymal and vascular abnormalities that occur secondary to cardiovascular disease, and pleural effusion. Thoracic radiography often enables the clinician to assess the severity of many cardiac diseases. The ability to identify and assess cardiac abnormalities varies with the abnormality, the patient, and the clinician. For decades, thoracic radiographs were the primary means of assessing cardiac size in veterinary medicine. Because no other method for making this determination existed, most veterinarians became very adept at assessing changes on thoracic radiographs. However, because there was no other readily available method for comparison, veterinarians could not determine the accuracy of their assessments. Because there was no means of questioning an interpretation of a thoracic radiograph, belief in interpretations was predicated on the clinical skills, experience, and confidence of the interpreter. However, even the most skilled interpreters had no means of determining if their assessments were accurate. With the advent of cardiac ultrasound, a means for determining accuracy became available. Our impression from comparing thoracic radiographs and cardiac ultrasound examinations for the past 12 years is that determining overall cardiac size and cardiac chamber size from a chest radiograph in a

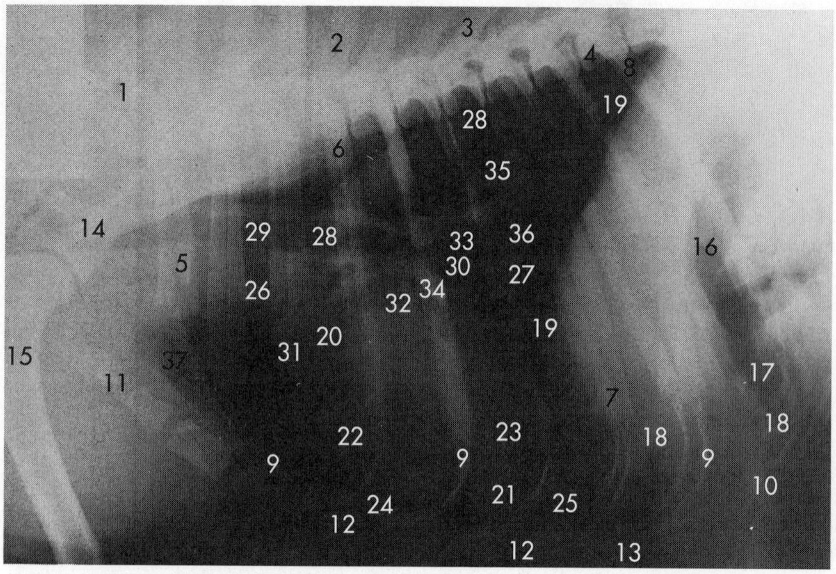

FIGURE 4-1 Normal lateral thoracic radiographic anatomy of the dog. *1,* First thoracic vertebra; *2,* fourth thoracic vertebra; *3,* seventh thoracic vertebra; *4,* tenth thoracic vertebra; *5,* first rib; *6,* fourth rib; *7,* seventh rib; *8,* tenth rib; *9,* costal cartilage; *10,* costal arch; *11,* manubrium sterni; *12,* sternebrae; *13,* xiphoid process; *14,* scapula; *15,* humerus; *16,* stomach; *17,* small intestine; *18,* caudal edge of liver; *19,* diaphragm; *20,* base of the heart at the region of the right atrium; *21, a*pex of the heart; *22,* cranial border of the heart (right heart); *23,* caudal region of the heart (left heart); *24,* ventral border of the heart; *25,* sternopericardiac ligament; *26,* cranial mediastinum; *27,* caudal vena cava; *28,* proximal descending aorta underlying the trachea; *29,* trachea; *30,* bronchus to right caudal lung lobe; *31,* bronchus to cranial lung lobe; *32,* bronchus to middle lung lobe; *33,* bronchus to left caudal lung lobe; *34,* bronchus to accessory lung lobe of right lung; *35,* confluence of pulmonary arteries and veins and bronchi from the caudal lung lobes; *36,* lung; *37,* pleural cupula. (From Boyd JS: *A color atlas of clinical anatomy of the dog & cat,* St Louis, 1995, Mosby.)

TABLE 4-1

Radiographic changes commonly observed with various moderate to severe cardiac diseases

Abnormality	*LV*	*LA*	*Ao*	*RV*	*RA*	*MPA*	*Pulmonary*	*Other*
Patent ductus arteriosus	+[a]	+	+[b]	0	0	+/0	+/0 artery +/0 vein	Left heart failure
Aortic stenosis	+[c]	0	+[d]	0	0	0	0 artery 0 vein	
Pulmonic stenosis	0	0	0	+[e]	0	+	0 artery 0 vein	
Ventricular septal defect	+	+	0	+/0	0	0	+/0 artery +/0 vein	Left heart failure
Atrial septal defect	0	0	0	+	+	0	+/0 artery +/0 vein	
Tetralogy of Fallot	0	0	0	+/0	0	+/–	0/– artery 0/– vein	
Mitral regurgitation	+	+[f]	0	0	0	0	0 artery +/0 vein	Left heart failure
Tricuspid regurgitation	0/–	0	0	+	+	0	0 artery 0 vein	Right heart failure
Dilated CM	+	+	0	+/0	+/0	0	0 artery +/0 vein	Left heart failure Right heart failure
Hypertrophic CM	+/0	+	0	0	0	0	0 artery +/0 vein	Left heart failure
Unclassified CM	+/0	+	0	0	+/0	0	0 artery +/0 vein	Left heart failure Right heart failure
Heartworm disease	0	0	0	+/0	+/0	+/0	+ artery 0 vein	Right heart failure Pulmonary infiltrates

CM, Cardiomyopathy.
[a] Cardiac silhouette commonly appears longer than normal because of left ventricular enlargement.
[b] A bulge in the descending aorta is commonly seen on the dorsoventral radiograph.
[c] The left ventricle may or may not appear enlarged and commonly does not appear to be as enlarged as in a volume overload.
[d] The ascending aorta is enlarged.
[e] The right ventricle may or may not appear enlarged and is usually not as prominent as in right ventricular volume overload.
[f] The left atrium is usually more prominent than the other cardiac chambers in this disease.

dog is fraught with error. At our institution, it is common for radiologists now to examine the cardiac silhouette on a chest radiograph and then hold off final judgment until they see the echocardiographic report because they have been wrong so often in the past. Consequently, echocardiography has supplanted the chest radiograph for determining overall cardiac size and specific chamber enlargement in most situations because it is a much more accurate tool. The one exception to this rule is determination of left atrial size; in this case the thoracic radiograph is usually as good or sometimes better at detecting enlargement.

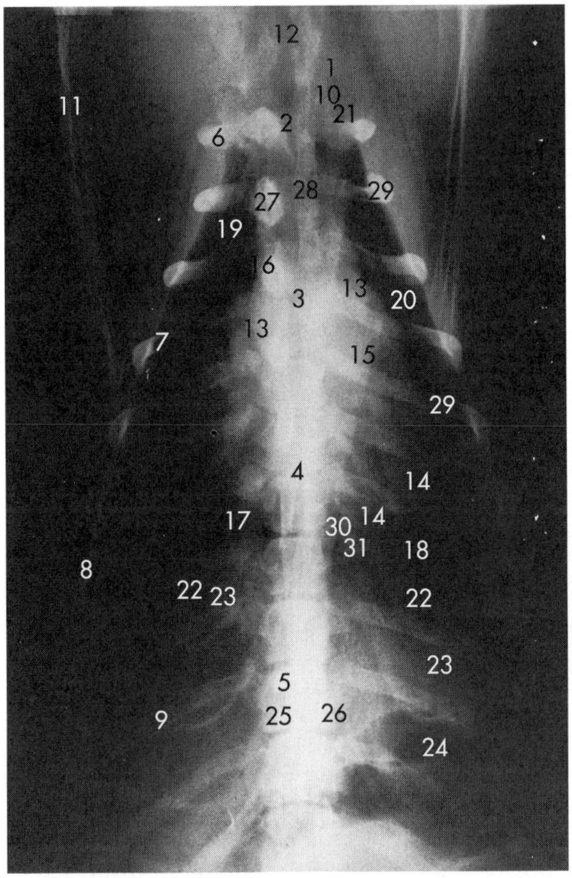

FIGURE 4-2 Normal ventrodorsal thoracic radiographic anatomy of the dog. *1,* Seventh cervical vertebra; *2,* first thoracic vertebra; *3,* fourth thoracic vertebra; *4,* seventh thoracic vertebra; *5,* tenth thoracic vertebra; *6,* first rib; *7,* fourth rib; *8,* seventh rib; *9,* tenth rib; *10,* sternebra; *11,* scapula; *12,* trachea; *13,* base of the heart (the *13* on the right of the figure is in the region of the main pulmonary artery, and the *13* on the left is in a region where the right auricle and right ventricular outflow tract overlie each other); *14,* apex of the heart; *15,* descending aorta; *16,* cranial mediastinum; *17,* caudal vena cava; *18,* sternopericardiac ligament; *19,* right cranial lung lobe; *20,* left lung; *21,* pleural cupula; *22,* diaphragm; *23,* liver; *24,* stomach; *25,* cranial articular process of vertebra; *26,* caudal articular process of vertebra; *27,* spinous process; *28,* costal fovea; *29,* body of rib; *30,* head of rib; *31,* costal cartilage. (From Boyd JS: *A color atlas of clinical anatomy of the dog & cat,* St Louis, 1995, Mosby.)

Interpreting the Size of the Cardiac Silhouette

Determining overall cardiac size and specific chamber size on thoracic radiographs is an art. This means that experience improves the ability of the examiner to determine these variables accurately. However, even experienced examiners, in our experience, make many mistakes, especially when interpreting overall cardiac size and the size of the ventricles. Why is cardiac size so difficult to determine on thoracic radiographs? There are several reasons. First, when looking at the cardiac silhouette one must remember that this is in effect a shadow of the heart. To see how difficult it is to determine the size and shape of a complex structure by looking at a shadow, take a heart and section it so that you can see the four chambers. Then take the specimen outside to a sunny area and project the shadow of the heart onto a smooth surface. Obviously this does give an idea of the size and shape of the entire heart. However, the information gained is possibly 20% of that gleaned from looking at the organ itself. Although someone may be able to identify a best friend by looking at the shadow of a profile, identifying a casual acquaintance in this manner would be much more difficult. The chest radiograph is an examination of shadows. Consequently, identifying familiar changes is often easy, but when the changes are unfamiliar, confidence is lost and mistakes are made. Postmortem examination of the heart is akin to looking directly at a face. Echocardiography is more like looking at a face than it is looking at a shadow in profile.

Second, cardiac size is usually evaluated subjectively. This means that when one looks at a thoracic radiograph, one subjectively determines if the size of the heart is normal or altered. To make this determination one compares the size of the heart to the size of the thoracic space. Many examiners fail to consider this simple fact. This is a major mistake, especially when evaluating canine patients. Because the size of the cardiac silhouette is subjectively compared with the size of the thoracic space, increases and decreases in thoracic cavity size and confirmation make the cardiac silhouette appear larger or smaller. Dogs come in many shapes and sizes. Cardiac size and dog size are generally linearly correlated. Dog shape, however, is a variable that changes from dog to dog and that markedly alters the impression of cardiac size. Dogs can be divided into those that are shallow -, normal -, or deep-chested when examined from the lateral aspect and narrow -, normal -, or barrel-chested when examined from a dorsoventral approach. The cardiac silhouette always appears larger than expected in dogs with shallow or narrow thoracic cavities and smaller than expected in dogs with deep or barrel-shaped thoracic cavities.

Thoracic radiographs from a normal young Labrador retriever are presented in Figure 4-3. This type of dog has a "normal" chest confirmation (i.e., not shallow, deep, narrow, or barrel in shape). This is the type of dog classically shown to veterinary students and veterinary practitioners in continuing education courses. Unfortunately, this type of dog is probably the minority of dogs examined. Figure 4-4 shows thoracic radiographs from a normal older basset hound—the other end of the spectrum. This type of dog has both a narrow and a shallow chest confirmation. The resultant decrease in chest size makes the heart appear larger than normal, on both the lateral and dorsoventral views. Luckily, this is not a popular breed and so we are not forced to determine cardiac size on too many of these dogs. The thoracic radiographs in Figure 4-5 are from a normal young Boston terrier. This dog has a shallow chest on its lateral radiograph and a normal- to barrel-shaped chest on its dorsoventral radiograph. Because of the dog's shallow chest, the cardiac silhouette looks large on the lateral radiograph. Note, however, that it looks normal on the dorsoventral view. This type of chest confirmation is common. We see it in Lhasa apsos, dachshunds, Shi-Tzus, and many others. Another example is presented in Figure 4-6. Determining cardiac size from a lateral chest radiograph is difficult. This chest conformation makes it even more difficult. Our recommendation is to concentrate on the dorsoventral view in this type of dog. The thoracic radiographs in Figure 4-7 are from a normal young whippet. This type of dog has a narrow chest on the dorsoventral view and a normal chest on the lateral view. Consequently, the dog appears to have cardiomegaly on the dorsoventral view. The thoracic radiographs in Figure 4-8 are from a normal, young Irish setter. This is a deep-chested dog. The large and deep chest on the lateral view makes the heart look small. Because the chest is deep, the heart lies in the chest cavity in a more upright position. This results in a smaller and

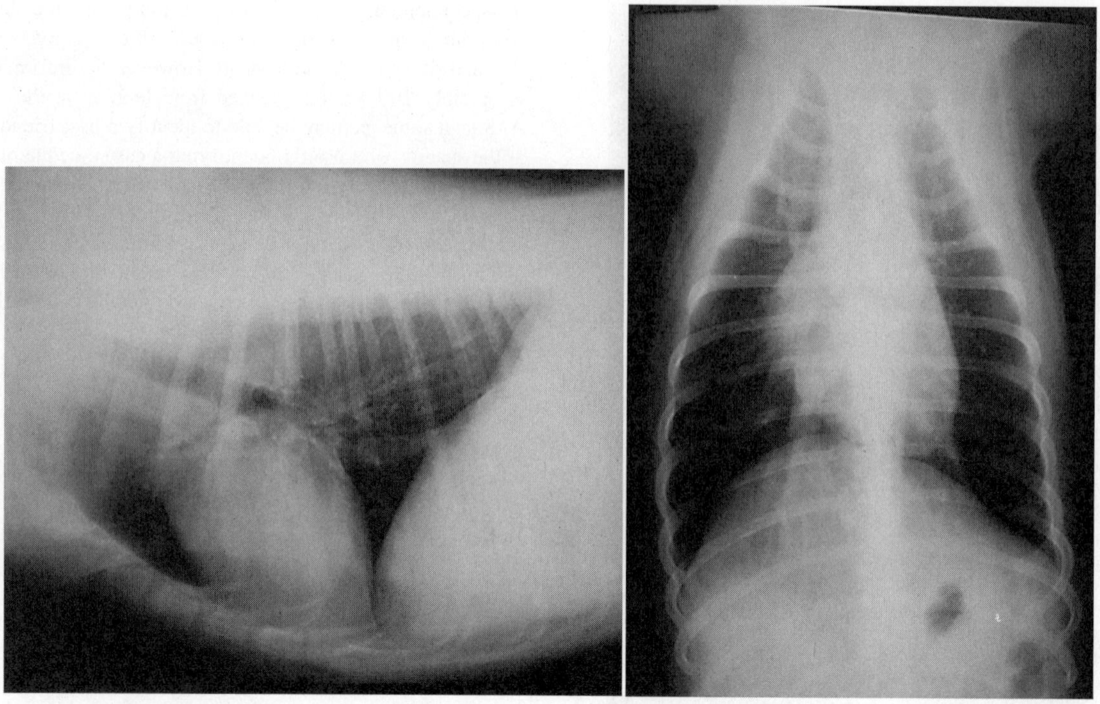

FIGURE 4-3 Thoracic radiographs from a normal 1-year-old Labrador retriever. This breed has a normal chest configuration.

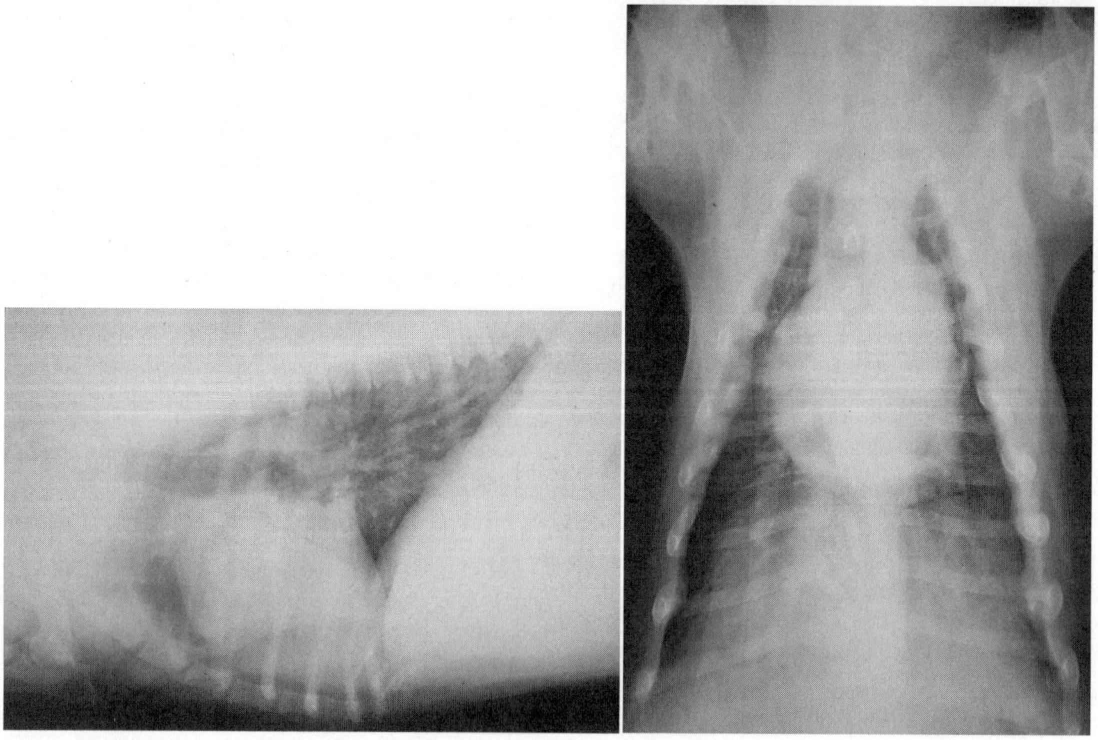

FIGURE 4-4 Thoracic radiographs from an 8-year-old basset hound. The thorax is shallow on the lateral view and narrow on the dorsoventral view. Consequently, the cardiac silhouette appears to be large on both views. Cardiac ultrasound was normal.

rounder cardiac silhouette on the dorsoventral view, and, consequently, the heart also looks small in this view.

Besides chest confirmation, the position of the diaphragm also affects the size of the thoracic cavity and, consequently, the interpretation of the cardiac silhouette size. The phase of respiration is a major factor that determines the position of the diaphragm (Figure 4-9). In human medicine, thoracic radiographs are always taken on maximum inspiration. We only rarely achieve this in veterinary medicine because we cannot tell our patients to "take a deep breath and hold it." All of us have been taught to take thoracic

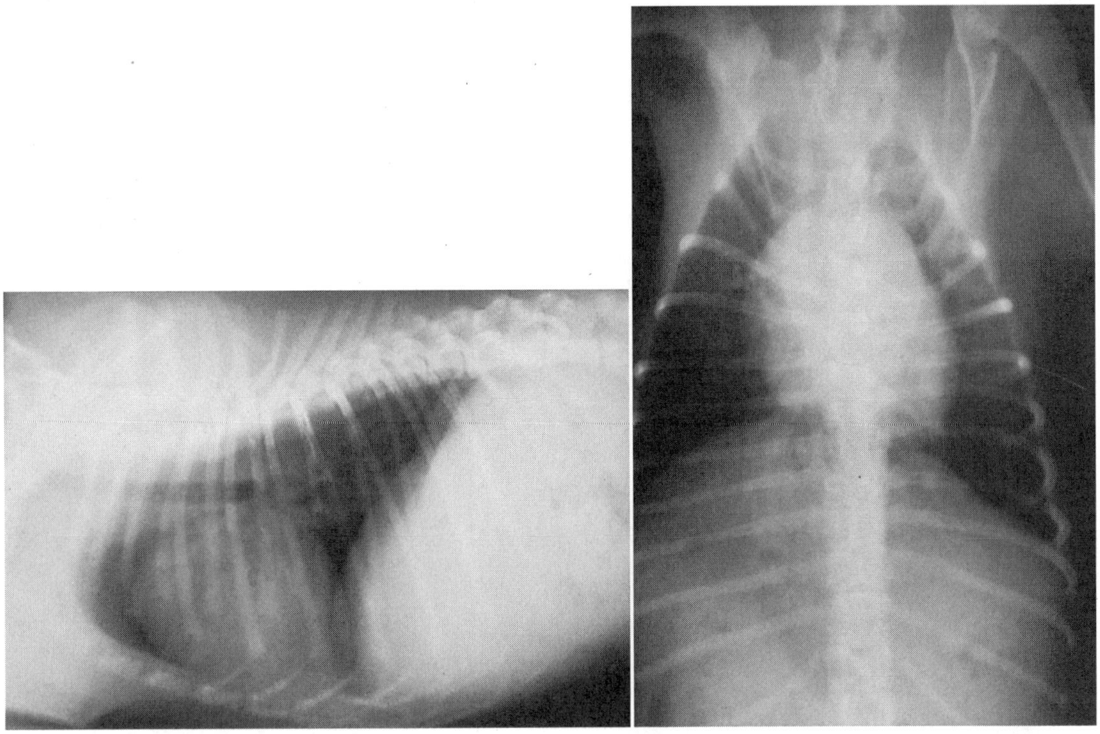

FIGURE 4-5 Thoracic radiographs from a normal 5-month-old Boston terrier. The thorax is shallow on the lateral view and wide (barrel-chested) on the dorsoventral view. Because of this, the cardiac silhouette appears to be large on the lateral view and normal to small on the dorsoventral view.

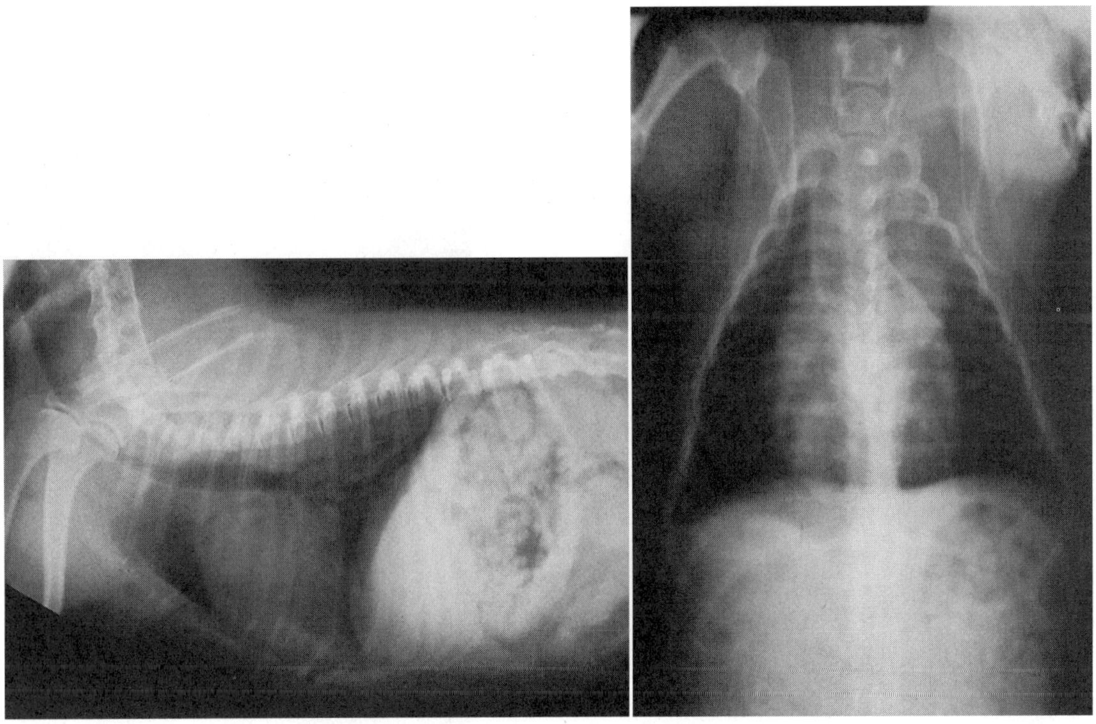

FIGURE 4-6 Thoracic radiographs from a normal 7-year-old Yorkshire terrier. The thorax is similarly shaped to that of the dog in Figure 4-3 on the lateral view but is normal on the dorsoventral view. This chest configuration is common in small-breed dogs, including dachshunds, Lhasa apsos, and Maltese.

radiographs on dogs and cats during inspiration. This is an admirable goal in theory, but in reality the difference in lung volume between end-expiration and end-inspiration in a eupneic animal is very small. Consequently, taking a thoracic radiograph during inspiration, although still best, is a poor substitute for the situation achieved in humans. Therefore we often are forced to read thoracic radiographs that look little different from end-expiratory films. Obesity complicates this situation in many dogs. Abdominal fat accumulation

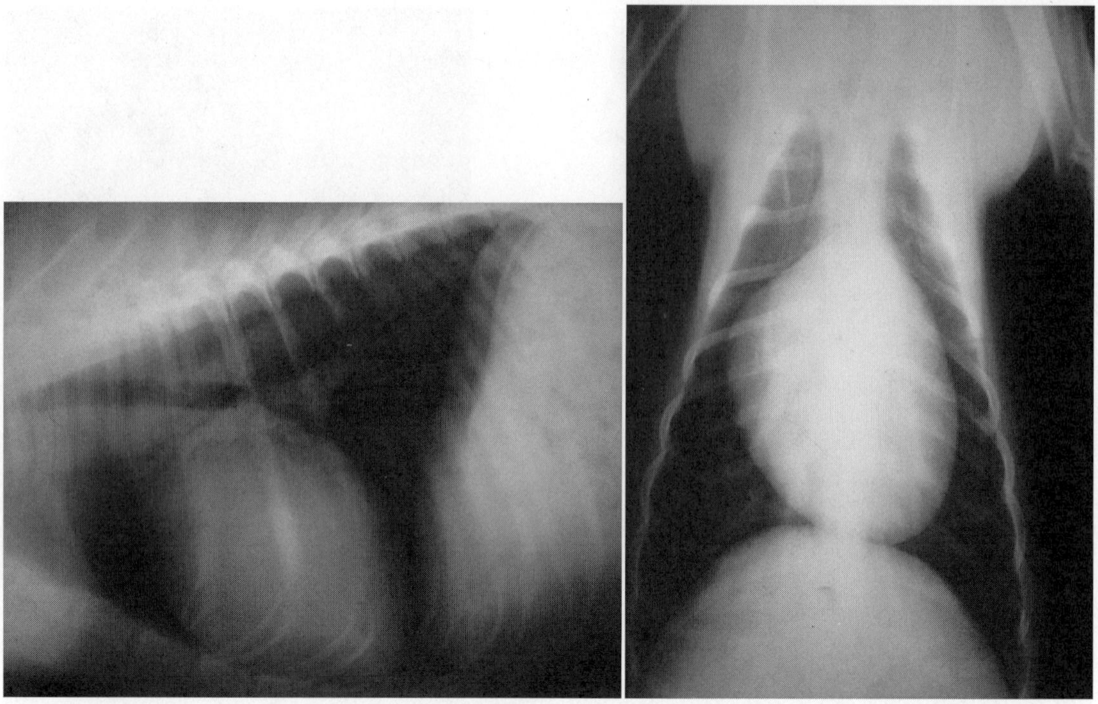

FIGURE 4-7 Thoracic radiographs from a normal 4-year-old whippet. The dog's chest configuration is normal on the lateral view and narrow on the dorsoventral view. Consequently, the cardiac silhouette looks large on the dorsoventral view.

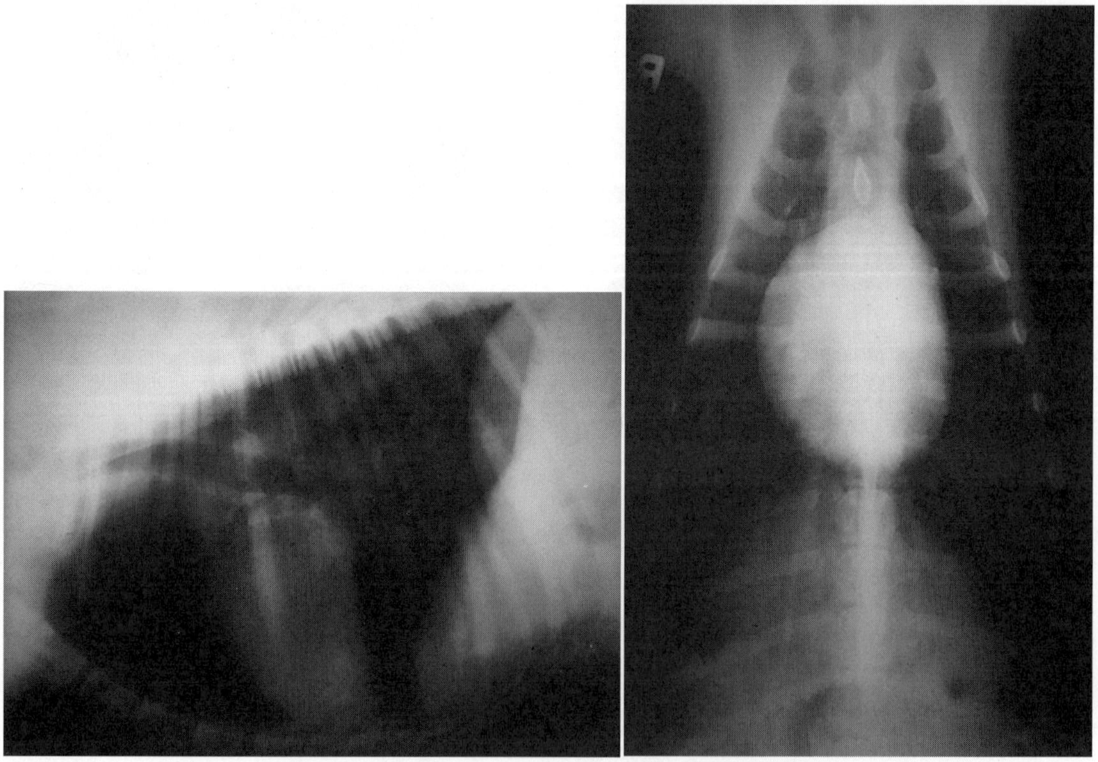

FIGURE 4-8 Thoracic radiographs from a normal 8-year-old Irish setter. In this deep-chested breed, the heart appears small on the lateral view because of the thoracic size. The heart is more upright in the chest because of the configuration. Consequently, on the dorsoventral view the heart is rounder and appears smaller than normal.

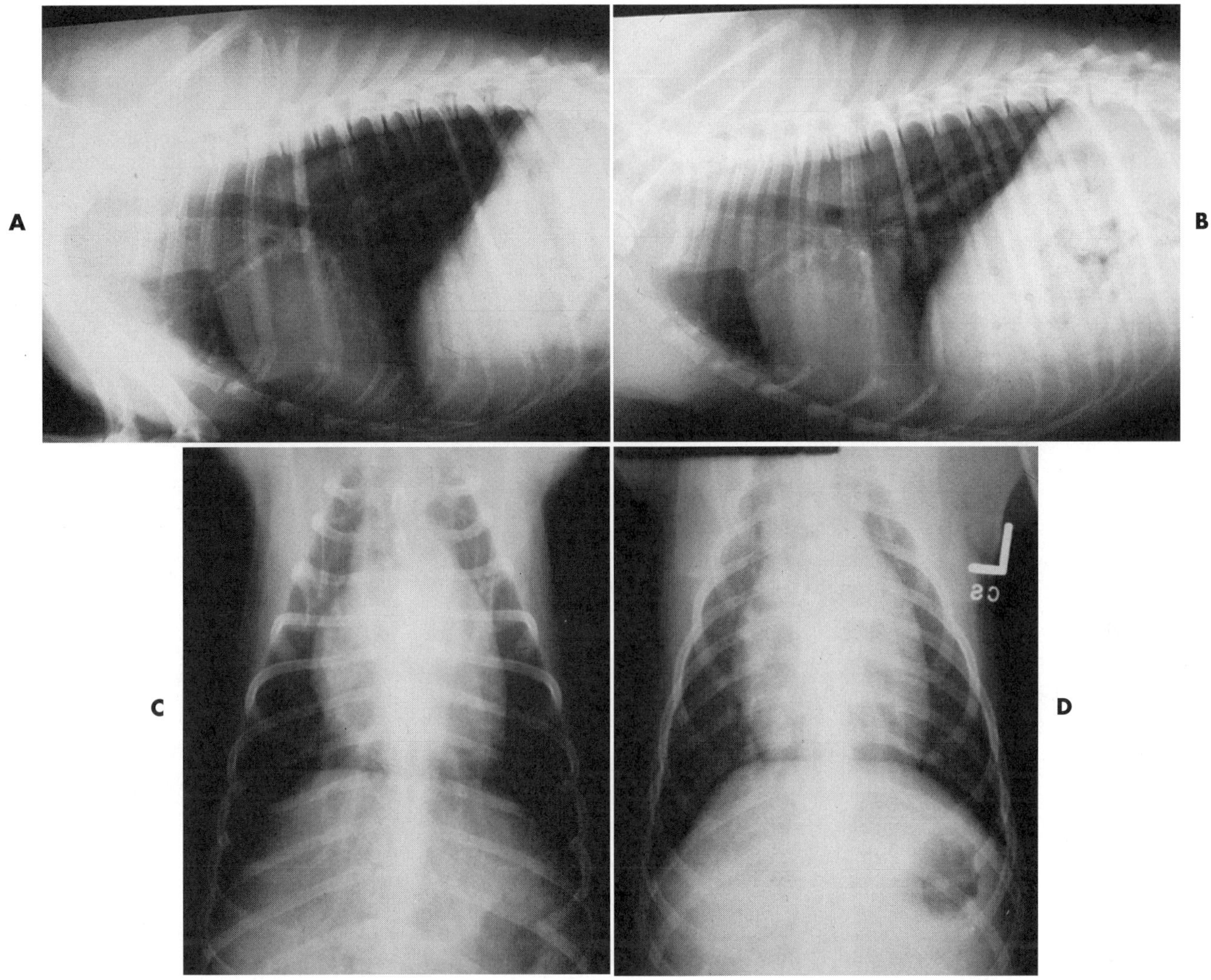

FIGURE 4-9 Two sets of thoracic radiographs from a dog taken during inspiration (**A** and **C**) and expiration (**B** and **D**). On the lateral views (**A** and **B**), the diaphragm becomes more curvilinear on inspiration and the caudodorsal lung fields are larger. On the dorsoventral views (**C** and **D**), the diaphragm is primarily between the ninth and tenth ribs on expiration and between the tenth and eleventh ribs on inspiration. The apex of the cardiac silhouette is pushed to the left on expiration, and the entire cardiac silhouette appears larger.

commonly displaces the diaphragm forward, decreasing the size of the thoracic cavity and making the cardiac silhouette look larger. In addition, obese dogs also may have accumulation of fat in their thoracic cavity, especially in the pericardial space. The two sets of radiographs in Figure 4-10 are taken from an American cocker spaniel at ages 7 months and 2 years. This dog was presented because of a heart murmur. The only abnormality identified was one thickened pulmonary valve leaflet that produced no stenosis. We interpreted the cardiac silhouette as normal. When the dog returned, the heart was still normal on ultrasound examination. The cardiac silhouette on this dog appeared to be larger on thoracic radiographs. This apparent increase in size is due to a decrease in the size of the thoracic cavity and an accumulation of intrapericardial fat. The intrapericardial fat can be best appreciated on the lateral view. On the dorsoventral view, most of the fat appears to have accumulated in the region where the right atrium is commonly identified. This is a common finding and is commonly mistaken for right heart enlargement. The last radiograph in Figure 4-10 is a dorsoventral view that is slightly oblique. This maneuver rotates the area of fat accumulation area so that it is now even more prominent. This makes the interpretation of right atrial enlargement even more enticing.

Besides the differences in thoracic cavity size and shape, the heart itself changes somewhat in size and configuration in normal dogs and cats between systole and diastole and between inspiration and expiration. These changes are relatively small, however, and can generally be ignored.[2] The position of the heart in the thoracic cavity changes the configuration of the silhouette. The confirmation of the thoracic cavity primarily determines the position. As mentioned previously, the heart is in an upright position in deep-chested dogs. This makes it look small and round on the dosoventral view. Conversely, in shallow-chested dogs, the heart is obliquely positioned in the chest. This produces an oblong shape on the dorsoventral view.

In summary, the many variables that change thoracic cavity size

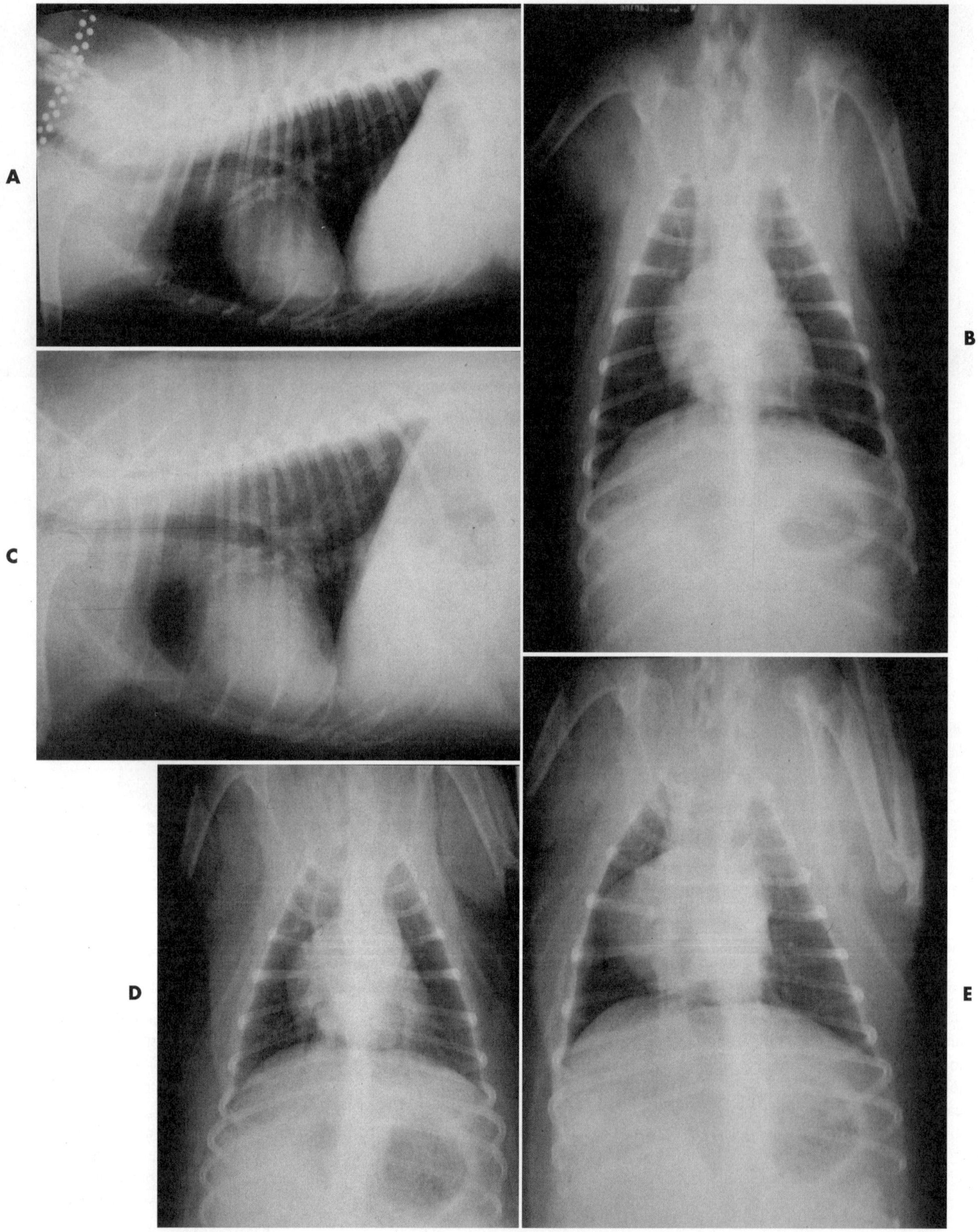

FIGURE 4-10 Two sets of radiographs from a normal American cocker spaniel taken at less than 1 year of age (**A** and **B**) and again 2 years later (**C** through **E**). The dog became obese over time. Intrapericardial fat can be visualized on the lateral view (**C**) as a less dense silhouette cranial to the cardiac silhouette. On the dorsoventral views (**D** and **E**), abdominal fat has pushed the diaphragm cranially, reducing the size of the thoracic cavity and making the cardiac silhouette appear larger. It has also accumulated in the region of the right atrium, making this area appear larger in **D.** In **E,** the radiograph has been taken from a slightly oblique angle. This makes the right atrial region appear even larger.

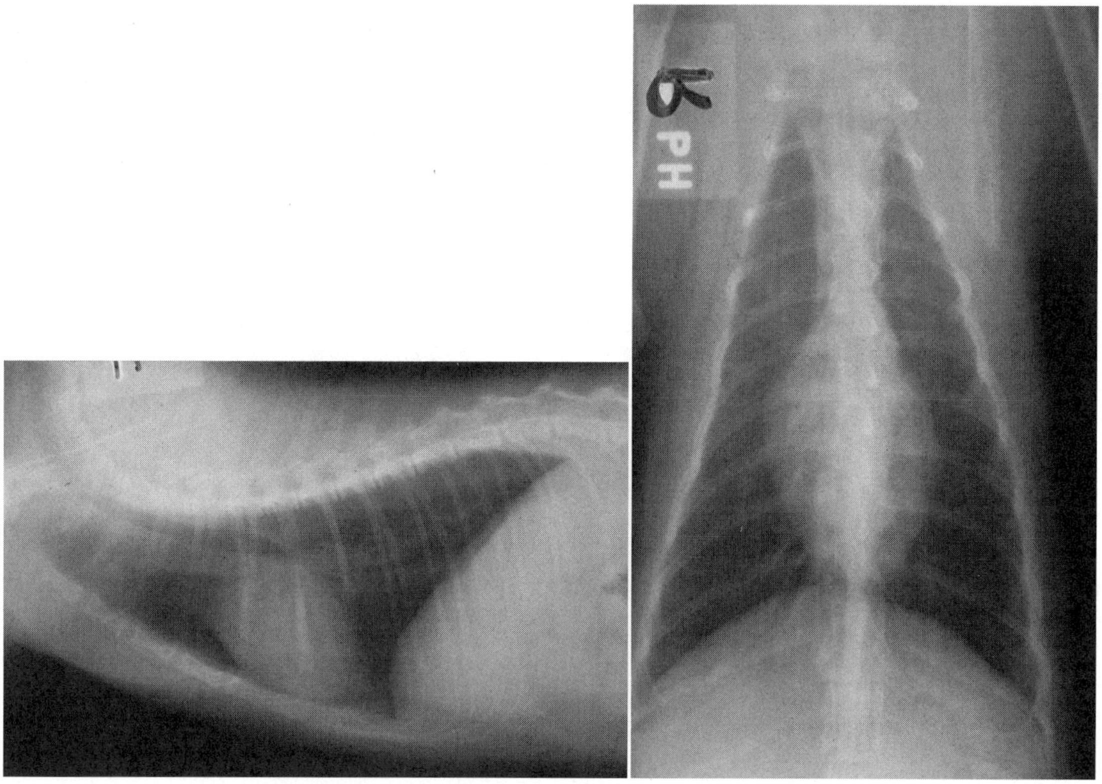

FIGURE 4-11 Thoracic radiographs of a normal young cat.

and configuration make it difficult to interpret the size of the cardiac silhouette in a normal dog. Consequently, distinguishing normal from abnormal in a patient can be difficult. Many veterinarians overinterpret thoracic radiographs and believe that cardiomegaly is present when it is not. As stated previously by Suter and Gomez,[3] "The differences among normal hearts of varying canine breeds or the differences between hearts radiographed at inspiration or expiration are often greater than the differences among normal and diseased hearts." This portion of the chapter demonstrates some of the variability seen in normal canine thoracic radiographs, to make veterinarians that interpret thoracic radiographs more cautious in their interpretation. Unfortunately, space does not permit examples of normal from all breeds or chest confirmations.

Chest confirmation and cardiac position are more uniform in cats (Figure 4-11). However, obesity and phase of respiration do alter the appearance of cardiac size. In some cats the relationship between the heart and the thoracic cavity changes with age.[4] In about 40% of cats older than 10 years the cardiac silhouette assumes a more horizontal alignment in the thoracic cavity, with more sternal contact (Figure 4-12). This is not due to a change in cardiac size, because measurements of cardiac size in old normal cats are no different from young normal cats.[4] Consequently, this change is likely the result of an age-related change in chest conformation. Old cats also sometimes have an aortic bulge that is readily discerned on a dorsoventral radiograph. In one study, this abnormality occurred in 28% of the old cats examined and in none of the younger cats (cats younger than 7 years).[4] The reason for this change is unknown. It does not appear to be due to systemic hypertension or hyperthyroidism, because no evidence of the cardiac changes that commonly occur secondary to these diseases was found in the above study. This abnormality occurs at the junction of the aortic arch and descending aorta, which is known as the aortic isthmus. This is the area where the aorta becomes fixed to the thorax by pleural reflections, intercostal arteries, and the left subclavian artery. In humans, the aorta tends to lengthen and widen with age.[5] It is possible that these changes also occur in cats and result in this aortic bulge.

CARDIAC MENSURATION

If subjectively evaluating cardiac size is difficult, then it might stand to reason that identifying a means of measuring the size of the cardiac silhouette might improve our ability to detect cardiac enlargement. Although individuals have tried this approach over the years, no method has proven accurate or reliable. Recently, Buchanan and Bücheler[6] studied normal dogs using a standardized measurement system, with the thoracic vertebral bodies as the unit of measure. A good correlation exists between heart weight and body length of normal dogs.[7] Consequently, one might assume that cardiac size and vertebral body lengths might correlate. The above study found good correlation between heart size and the length of thoracic vertebrae. To measure the heart, they drew a line on a lateral view, from the bottom of the left mainstem bronchus to the apex of the heart and used calipers to determine the length of the heart. Once the caliper distance had been determined, they repositioned the calipers over the thoracic vertebrae, with the starting point at the cranial edge of the fourth thoracic vertebra. They then measured the distance in vertebrae *(v)*. A line perpendicular to the original line was drawn where the heart was widest and that distance measured in vertebrae. The sum of the two measurements was determined to be between 8.5 and 10.6 *v* (9.7 ± 0.5 *v*) in 100 normal dogs of varying chest confirmations. The chest configuration had no influence on the measurement. A similar scheme was used on ventrodorsal and dorsoventral radiographs. Here they measured the heart in its longest

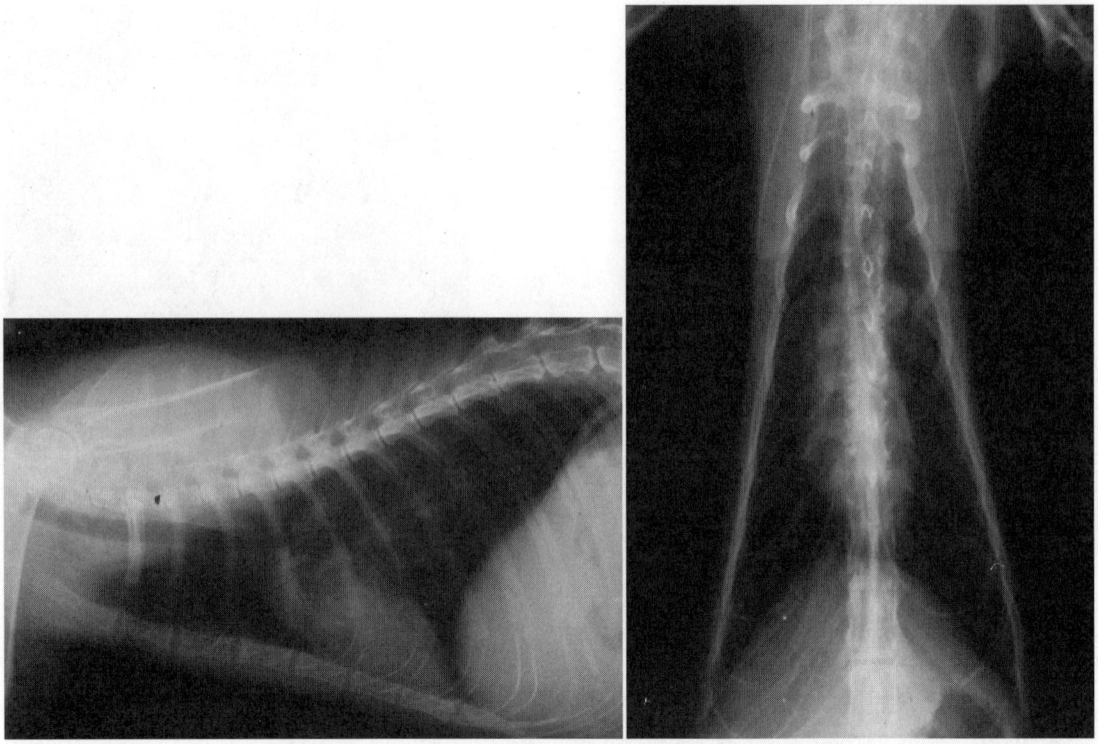

FIGURE 4-12 Thoracic radiographs from an 11-year-old cat. There is a prominent bulge in the proximal descending aorta on the dorsoventral view. On the lateral view, the heart appears to lie in a more horizontal position than in Figure 4-11. These are normal findings in an old cat.

dimension and its widest dimension and found it to be 10.2 *v,* on average. This measurement was slightly more variable than the measurement from the lateral view. Although intriguing, this study so far only has determined normal values for dogs. This system has not been tested to determine what happens in cardiac disease and how much overlap there is between dogs with cardiac disease (mild to severe) and normal dogs.

Normal Radiographic Cardiovascular Anatomy

The heart on a thoracic radiograph is an opaque silhouette. Blood, myocardium, pericardium, pericardial fluid, valves, coronary arteries and veins, and fat are included in this silhouette. Because these have similar attenuation characteristics, little to no contrast exists between them. Consequently, they cannot be distinguished from each other. Only the borders of the heart and overlying structures, such as the aorta, can be clearly identified. Deviations in the cardiac border suggest enlargement of particular cardiac structures.

In the dorsoventral view, the right side of the animal is placed on the viewbox to the left of the examiner, and the left side of the animal is placed to the right, with the cranial end of the radiograph pointed up. The lung outlines the normal cardiac silhouette on the right and left sides (see Figure 4-2). The cardiac silhouette appears like a lopsided egg or a reverse *D.*[8] It is rounded cranially and on the right side. The apex lies to the left of the vertebrae and sternebrae and is a rounded point at the most caudal aspect of the rounded right heart border. The left heart border is straighter than the right side. The cardiac silhouette on the dorsoventral view can be labeled like a clock face in this view (Figure 4-13).[9] At the 11-o'clock to 1-o'clock position, the cardiac silhouette blends with the cranial mediastinum. A portion of the ascending and transverse aorta and the initial portion of the descending aorta (the aortic arch) are the primary cardiac structures that diverge from the cardiac silhouette within this region (Figures 4-2 and 4-14). The aortic arch is difficult to distinguish from other structures in a normal animal, however, because it is surrounded by other mediastinal structures and obscured by the vertebrae and sternebrae. The main pulmonary artery is situated at the 1-o'clock to 2-o'clock position (Figure 4-15). When the pulmonary artery is of normal size it does not protrude beyond the cardiac silhouette and is normally not identified. The left auricle protrudes from the cardiac silhouette at the 2-o'clock to 3-o'clock position when it is enlarged. The left auricle enlarges in concert with the body of the left atrium in almost all situations. When normal, the auricle merges with the lateral border of the left ventricle and cannot be identified. When the left auricle and atrium are enlarged similarly to the left ventricle, the left auricular border and the left ventricular border merge so that one cannot see the enlarged left auricle. The lateral border of the left ventricle lies between 2 o'clock to 3 o'clock and 5 o'clock (the cardiac apex) (Figure 4-14). The body of the left atrium does not contribute to the formation of the cardiac silhouette on the dorsoventral view. It lies within the silhouette, dorsal to the left ventricle, and between the mainstem bronchi (Figure 4-16). The lateral border of the right ventricle extends from approximately 6 o'clock to about 12 o'clock. The body of the right ventricle encompasses the 6-o'clock to 9-o'clock position, and the right ventricular outflow tract is responsible for the rest (see Figure 4-15). The lateral border of the body of the right atrium and right auricle lie between 9 o'clock and 11 o'clock. They cannot be identified as separate structures from the right ventricular outflow tract in the normal animal.

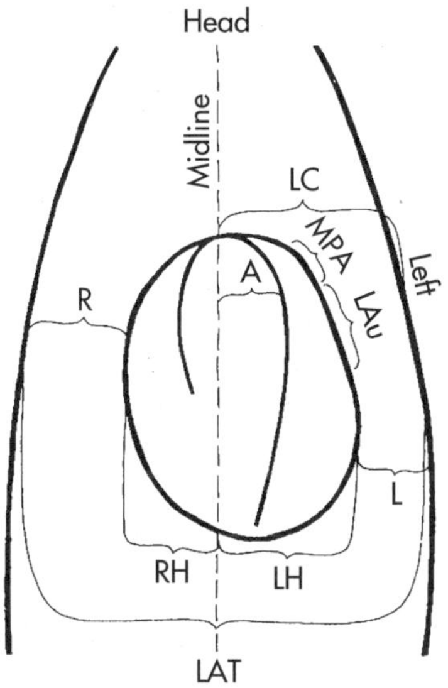

FIGURE 4-13 The position of the cardiac chambers and the great vessels on a dorsoventral view. In a clock-face analogy, the arch of the aorta *(A)* is at the 12-o'clock position and the main pulmonary artery *(MPA)* is at the 1-o'clock to 2-o'clock position. Continuing around the clock face, the left auricle *(LAu)* appears at the 2-o'clock to 3-o'clock position when it is enlarged and the left ventricle is at the 3-o'clock to 6-o'clock position. The right ventricle encompasses the 6-o'clock to 12-o'clock position. The right atrium is in the 9-o'clock to 12-o'clock position.

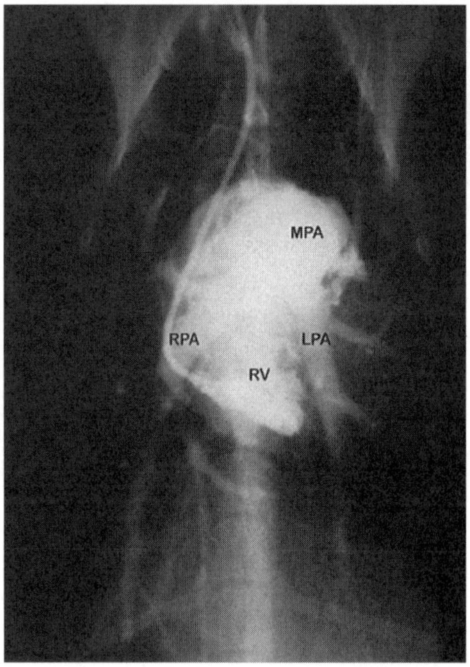

FIGURE 4-15 A dorsoventral radiograph taken after injecting a contrast agent into the caudal portion of the body of the right ventricle *(RV)*. The main pulmonary artery *(MPA)* and pulmonary artery branches are also outlined. The left caudal lobar pulmonary artery *(LPA)* and the right caudal lobar pulmonary artery *(RPA)* are labeled.

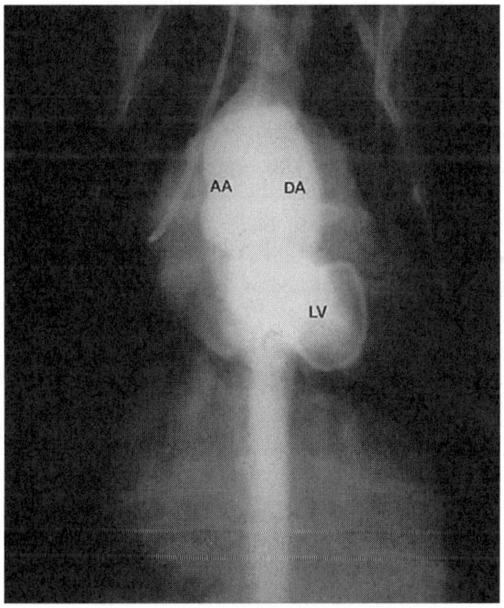

FIGURE 4-14 An angiocardiogram of the left ventricle and aorta from a normal dog. A catheter has been placed via the carotid artery into the left ventricle. The apex of the left ventricle *(LV)* is outlined in this dorsoventral view. The root of the aorta lies immediately to the right of the spine. The ascending aorta *(AA)* is to the right of the spine. The aortic arch is immediately beneath the spine and immediately cranial to the heart. The descending aorta *(DA)* is to the left of the spine.

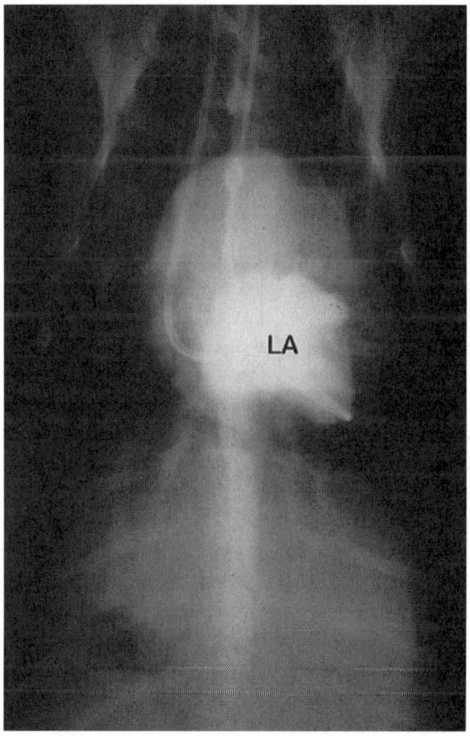

FIGURE 4-16 An angiocardiogram of the left atrium *(LA)* from a normal dog on a dorsoventral radiograph. The catheter was passed retrograde across the mitral valve.

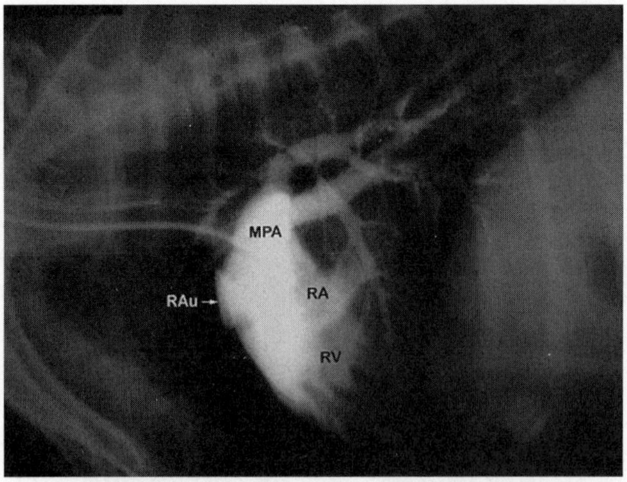

FIGURE 4-17 An angiocardiogram of the right heart and pulmonary vasculature from a normal dog. The contrast agent was injected into the right atrium. The right auricle *(RAu)* can be seen as a small pouch cranial to the heart. The body of the right atrium *(RA)* and the right ventricular outflow tract and main pulmonary artery *(MPA)* overlie one another. There is a small amount of contrast material in the proximal caudal vena cava. The body of the right ventricle *(RV)* is heavily trabeculated.

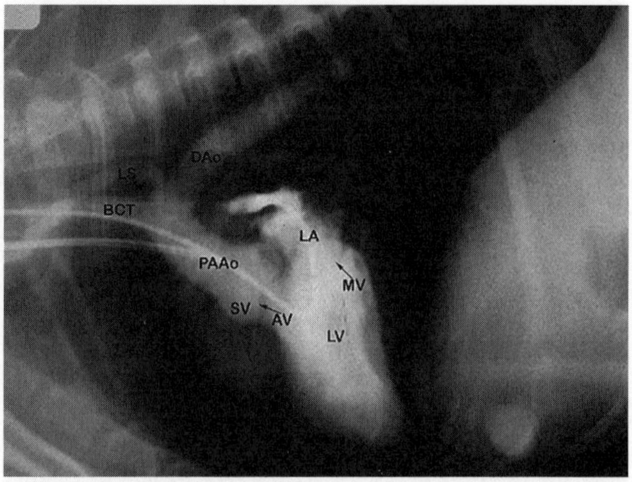

FIGURE 4-18 An angiocardiogram of the left heart taken from a lateral view following injection of contrast material into a pulmonary vein. The catheter has been passed retrograde across the mitral valve. The left atrium *(LA)*, left ventricle *(LV)*, and aorta are outlined. One sinus of Valsalva *(SV)* is labeled as are the proximal ascending aorta *(PAAo)*, descending aorta *(DAo)*, brachiocephalic trunk *(BCT)*, and left subclavian artery *(LS)*. The mitral valve *(MV)* leaflets and aortic valve *(AV)* cusps produce thin lucent lines between the left atrium and left ventricle and the left ventricle and aorta respectively.

Several vascular structures are identified on a normal dorsoventral thoracic radiograph. The caudal vena cava crosses from the diaphragm to the right atrium immediately to the right (of the animal) of the confluence of the sternebrae and vertebrae. It is best visualized in the short space between the diaphragm and the heart but can be followed for a short distance within the diaphragm and the cardiac silhouette (see Figure 4-2). The caudal and cranial pulmonary lobar vessels can be identified. The caudal lobar vessels lie on either side of the caudal lobar bronchi, with the arteries lying lateral and the veins lying medial to the bronchi (Figure 4-15). Usually, the arteries are better visualized than the veins. The right caudal lobar vein often is obscured by the caudal vena cava. The left caudal pulmonary vein is visualized for only a short distance in the left, caudal portion of the chest cavity before it courses centrally and is obscured by vertebrae and sternebrae. The left and right caudal lobar pulmonary arteries usually can be readily identified as they course from cranial to caudal across the cardiac silhouette and as they emerge from the cardiac silhouette into the lung fields. In some dogs, the caudal lobar vessels can be well visualized as they course across the silhouette of the diaphragm. The cranial lobar vessels emerge cranially from the cardiac silhouette, again on either side of the cranial lobar bronchi. The combination of the artery, bronchus, and vein on either side of the chest look like the arms of a ballerina extended overhead. The descending aorta emerges from behind the shadow of the vertebrae and sternebrae to descend the length of the thorax to the left (of the animal) of this shadow (see Figures 4-2 and 4-14).

On the lateral view, the radiograph is positioned on the viewbox, with the vertebrae on top and the head pointed toward the left of the examiner. The shape of the cardiac silhouette is determined by the configuration of the chest. In deep-chested dogs it is almost that of an upside down pyramid, with only the apex resting on the sternum. As the chest becomes more shallow, the apex is shifted caudally and a greater portion of the right ventricle contacts the sternum. In cats, the cardiac silhouette position is similar to that of a normal- to shallow-chested dog. On the lateral view, the dorsal border (the base) of the heart lies directly beneath the trachea, carina, and mainstem bronchi. The base of the heart is primarily formed by the two atria and the vessels entering and leaving the heart. The right atrium lies cranial and the left atrium lies caudal, beneath and caudal to the carina (Figures 4-17 and 4-18). The aorta emerges from the cranial, basilar region of the cardiac silhouette to course dorsally and then caudally beneath the vertebral column. It usually can be visualized (see Figures 4-1 and 4-18). The main pulmonary artery emerges from the cardiac silhouette slightly caudal to the aorta and is generally obscured by the aorta and other basilar structures. The main pulmonary artery branches in the region of the carina, and the caudal lobar branches course caudally from that point slightly beneath the aorta (Figures 4-19 and 4-20). The pulmonary veins course back to the left atrium in this same region. One cannot usually distinguish between the arteries and the veins at this site. The caudal vena cava emerges from the cardiac silhouette in the region of the caudal portion of the left atrial shadow and courses caudally to the diaphragm (see Figure 4-1). The cranial border of the cardiac silhouette is primarily composed of the right ventricular outflow tract and the cranial boundary of the body of the right ventricle (Figure 4-20). The right atrium is located dorsally but rarely protrudes cranially far enough to alter this border. The right auricle, however, does contribute to the cranial border. The ascending aorta and proximal main pulmonary artery are located dorsally but do not normally contribute to the cranial border of the cardiac silhouette. The caudal border of the cardiac silhouette is formed by the left heart. The left atrium is dorsal, lying immediately cranial and dorsal to the silhouette of the caudal vena cava (see Figure 4-18). The caudal border of the left ventricle lies ventrally from this region to the apex (see Figure 4-18). The body of the right ventricle does not contribute to the shape of the caudal cardiac silhouette but does overlie a large portion of the left ventricle in this view (Figure 4-21). The cranial lobar bronchi originate from the region of the carina and course cranial, across the cardiac silhouette and into the lung fields. The cranial lobar pulmonary arteries and veins course with the respective bronchi. The arteries are located dorsally to the bronchi, and the veins are located ventrally to the bronchi (see Figure 4-20). The

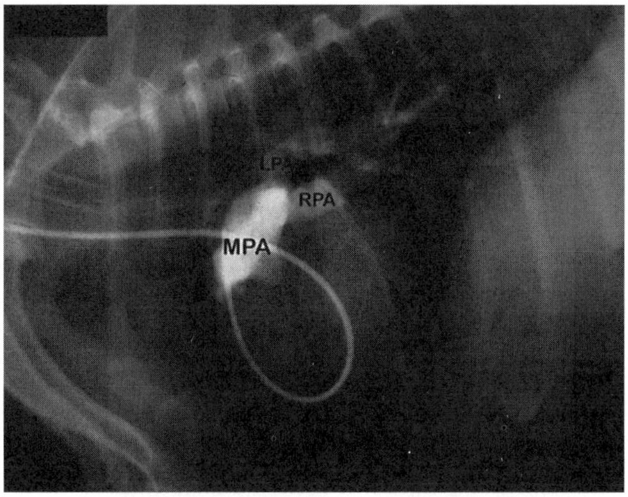

FIGURE 4-19 A radiograph taken following injection of a contrast agent into the main pulmonary artery *(MPA).* The contrast material is prevented from entering into the right ventricle by the pulmonic valve. Consequently, the region of contrast enhancement starts at the pulmonic valve, followed by the main pulmonary artery and the pulmonary artery branches (*LPA* and *RPA*).

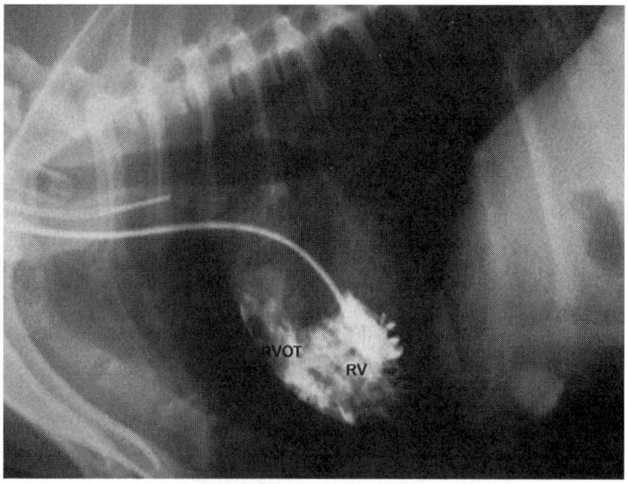

FIGURE 4-21 The contrast material in this angiocardiogram is entirely within the right ventricle. The trabeculated body of the right ventricle *(RV)* is the primary structure outlined. The contrast agent, however, does extend faintly up the right ventricular outflow tract *(RVOT)* to the pulmonic valve region.

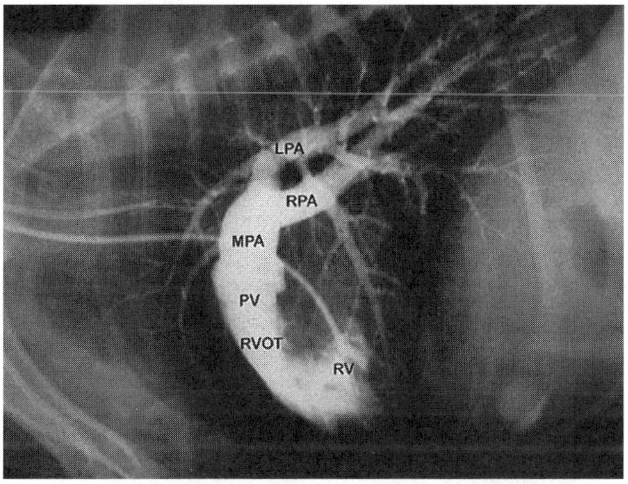

FIGURE 4-20 Contrast material has been injected into the right ventricle. A portion of the trabeculated right ventricular body *(RV)* can be seen. However, the smooth right ventricular outflow tract *(RVOT)* is more clearly visible. The main pulmonary artery *(MPA)* and pulmonary artery branches (*LPA* and *RPA*) are seen as in Figure 4-19.

cranial vena cava is imbedded in the cranial mediastinum and cannot be visualized. At the junction of the craniodorsal cardiac silhouette and the mediastinum is a slight depression commonly called the cranial waist. The caudal waist occurs at the junction of the left atrium and left ventricle.

Generalized Cardiomegaly

The entire cardiac silhouette may appear enlarged in many diseases. True generalized cardiomegaly (all four chambers enlarged) occurs most commonly with acquired cardiovascular disease. Dilated cardiomyopathy or mitral and tricuspid regurgitation are the most common causes (Figure 4-22). Pericardial effusion and peritoneopericardial diaphragmatic hernia can also produce the appearance of generalized cardiomegaly. Chronic severe anemia is an uncommon cause of generalized cardiomegaly. This occurs when the heart enlarges to pump more blood to compensate for the anemia (Figure 4-23). When isolated severe right or left heart enlargement occurs, the cardiac silhouette can appear to be generally enlarged. This is more common with left heart enlargement than right heart enlargement. Consequently, both the left and the right heart can appear to be enlarged in a dog with an abnormality such as a patent ductus arteriosus, in which left heart enlargement only is present (Figure 4-24).

Because so much variation is present between normal animals, it is impossible to detect mild, generalized cardiomegaly unless previous radiographs from the same animal, taken before the onset of disease, are accessible and the radiographic techniques at both times are identical. Moderate and severe generalized cardiomegaly are usually diagnosed subjectively by identifying a larger-than-normal cardiac silhouette. To make this subjective determination, the reviewer must know the appearance of a normal cardiac silhouette. As mentioned previously, one must remember that the size of the cardiac silhouette is being compared with the size of the thoracic space. Consequently, the size of the thoracic space must be evaluated first, and a mental adjustment made when examining radiographs from dogs that have smaller- or larger-than-normal chest cavities. A common mistake is to interpret a normal cardiac silhouette as too large because the chest cavity is smaller than realized.

In the lateral view, generalized cardiomegaly appears as a widening and lengthening of the cardiac silhouette. Normally, the cardiac silhouette is approximately 2.5 to 3 intercostal spaces in width in dogs, although it can approach 3.5 intercostal spaces in dogs with shallow chests.[10] As the silhouette widens, this number increases. Variability from breed to breed makes this difficult to evaluate, however. As the heart increases in size in dorsoventral length, the trachea is displaced dorsally. In a dog with a normal chest configuration and no cardiovascular disease, the angle between the trachea and spine is approximately 30 degrees.[10] However, in normal dogs with shallow chests, this angle is markedly decreased, and in dogs with deep chests, this angle may increase. Consequently, a decrease in this angle is a reliable sign of cardiac

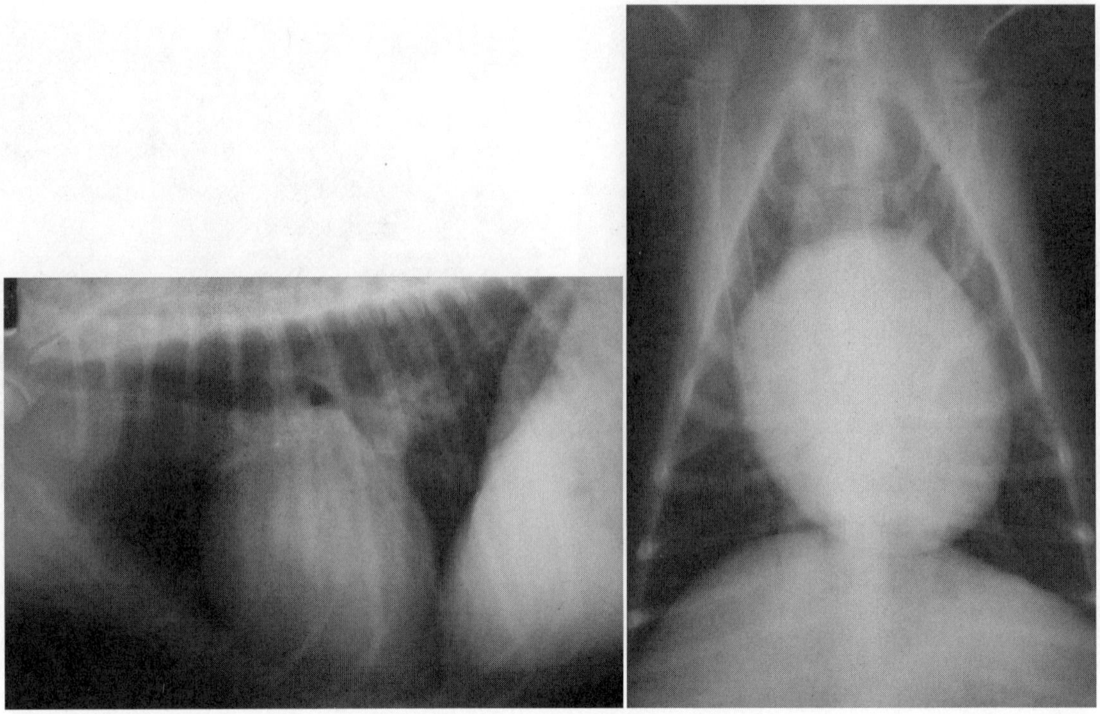

FIGURE 4-22 Generalized cardiomegaly in an American cocker spaniel with dilated cardiomyopathy. On the echocardiogram, all four chambers were enlarged. However, the left heart was larger than the right heart.

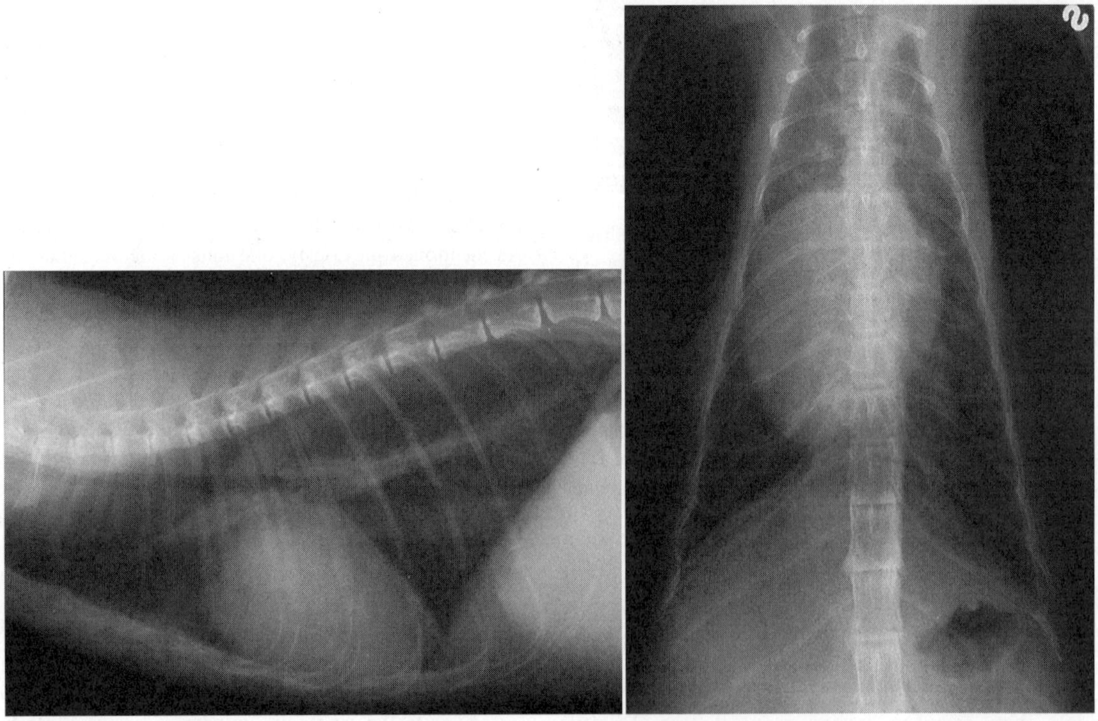

FIGURE 4-23 Generalized cardiomegaly in a 15-month-old Maine coon cat with severe anemia (PCV = 10%). The cardiac apex on the dorsoventral view is shifted to the right.

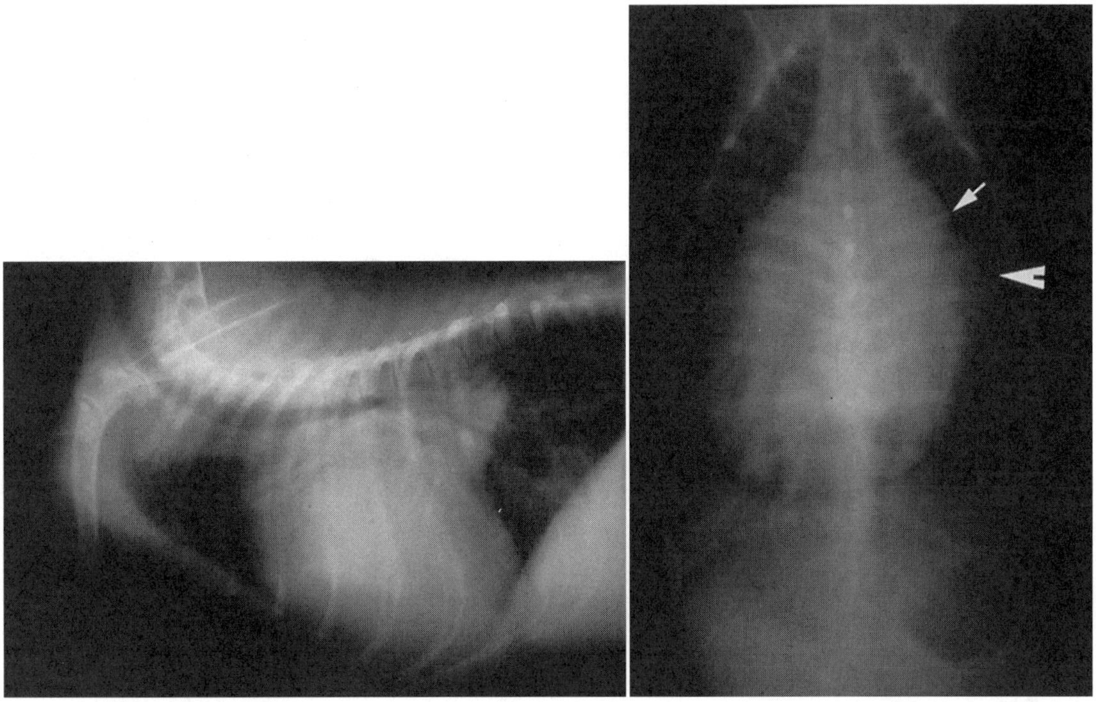

FIGURE 4-24 Radiographs taken from a 5-year-old Maltese with a patent ductus arteriosus. The overall cardiac silhouette appears to be large. The left atrium is clearly enlarged on the lateral view, and a left auricular bulge can be seen on the dorsoventral view *(arrowhead).* The apex of the heart is shifted to the right on the dorsoventral view. This dog was initially interpreted as having right heart enlargement in addition to left heart enlargement. The echocardiogram showed that the dog had only left heart enlargement. A descending aortic bulge (ductal aneurysm) is present *(arrow).*

enlargement in dogs with normal or deep chests. In dogs with shallow chests, however, evaluating this angle is generally futile. In cats, the width of the heart at its widest point on the lateral radiograph is approximately the same as the distance from the cranial border of the fifth rib to the caudal border of the seventh rib.[11] The ratio of the cardiac width to this intercostal distance increases to an average of 1.35 in cats with cardiac enlargement. However, no data have been generated on the sensitivity and specificity of this ratio for detecting cardiac enlargement, and no comparisons have been made with echocardiography. In the ventrodorsal view in cats, the maximum longitudinal length of the heart is approximately the same length as the distance from the cranial edge of the sixth rib to the caudal edge of the tenth rib, measured just distally to the articulation of the ribs with the vertebrae. This ratio increases to an average of 1.3 in cats with cardiomegaly. The ratio of the maximum transverse width of the heart to the width of the thorax at the same level is 0.65 on average for normal cats and increases to 0.85 in cats with cardiomegaly. The same caveats apply to these measures as for the lateral view.

In the dorsoventral view, generalized cardiomegaly results in the cardiac silhouette increasing in diameter and length in dogs (see Figure 4-22). Most commonly, the increase in diameter is more apparent. Any increase in length is generally in the caudal portion of the silhouette. The increase in size usually results in the heart appearing rounder than normal. In a dog with a normal dorsoventral chest configuration, the cardiac silhouette usually encompasses less than two thirds of the diameter of the thoracic space.[12]

Interpreting the Size of Specific Cardiac Chambers

Cardiac enlargement confined to one or two chambers is more common than generalized cardiomegaly, especially in congenital heart disease. However, even with acquired disease, such as mitral regurgitation, the left heart is often much more enlarged than the right heart. Consequently, except for the diseases mentioned in the previous section, one should be looking for specific chamber enlargement. As stated previously, however, specific ventricular chamber enlargement is commonly mistaken for generalized cardiomegaly.

Clinicians are commonly interested in determining cardiac chamber enlargement. Cardiac chambers enlarge in response to cardiovascular disease, and the severity of enlargement often correlates with the severity of the disease. The ability to detect chamber enlargement depends mostly on the specific chamber involved, the type of enlargement, and the chest configuration.

LEFT ATRIAL ENLARGEMENT

Left atrial enlargement is generally easy to detect in both dogs and cats when it is moderate to severe. In dogs, left atrial or auricular enlargement is readily appreciated on lateral and dorsoventral views. In cats, the left atrium is situated more cranially than in dogs, making it difficult to identify on the lateral view. Left atrial pressure and volume overloads create an increase in atrial chamber size, so there is only one type of enlargement that can be present.

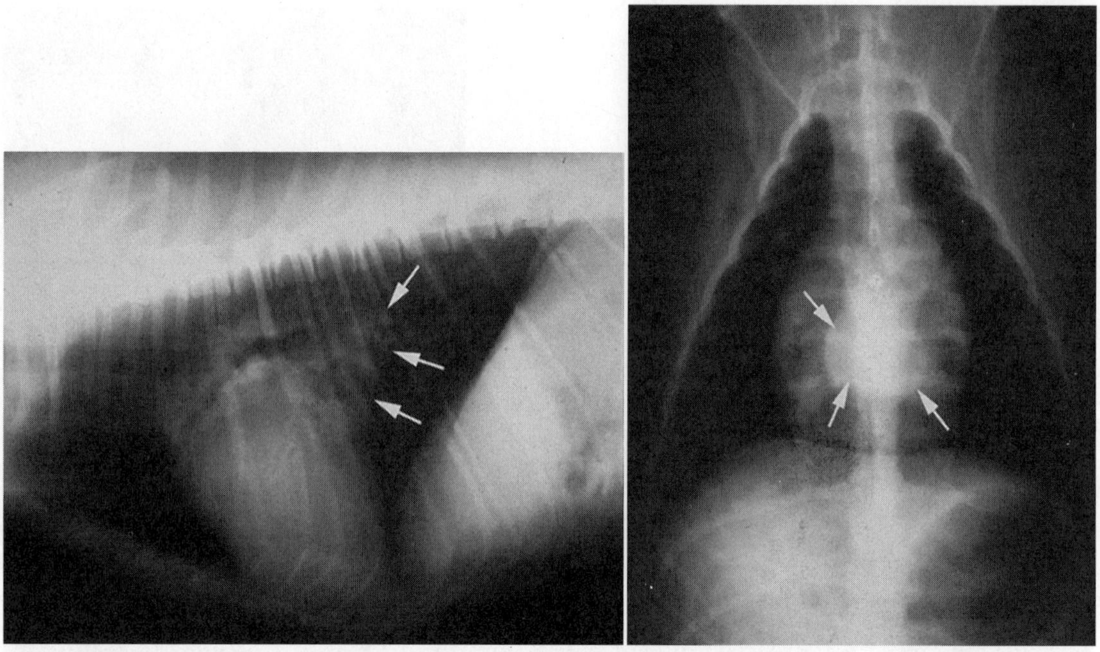

FIGURE 4-25 Isolated left atrial enlargement *(arrows)* in a miniature poodle with mitral regurgitation. The body of the left atrium can be clearly visualized on the lateral view, caudal and ventral to the carina. On the dorsoventral view, the body of the left atrium is seen as a structure denser than the rest of the cardiac silhouette, lying caudally, between the mainstem bronchi.

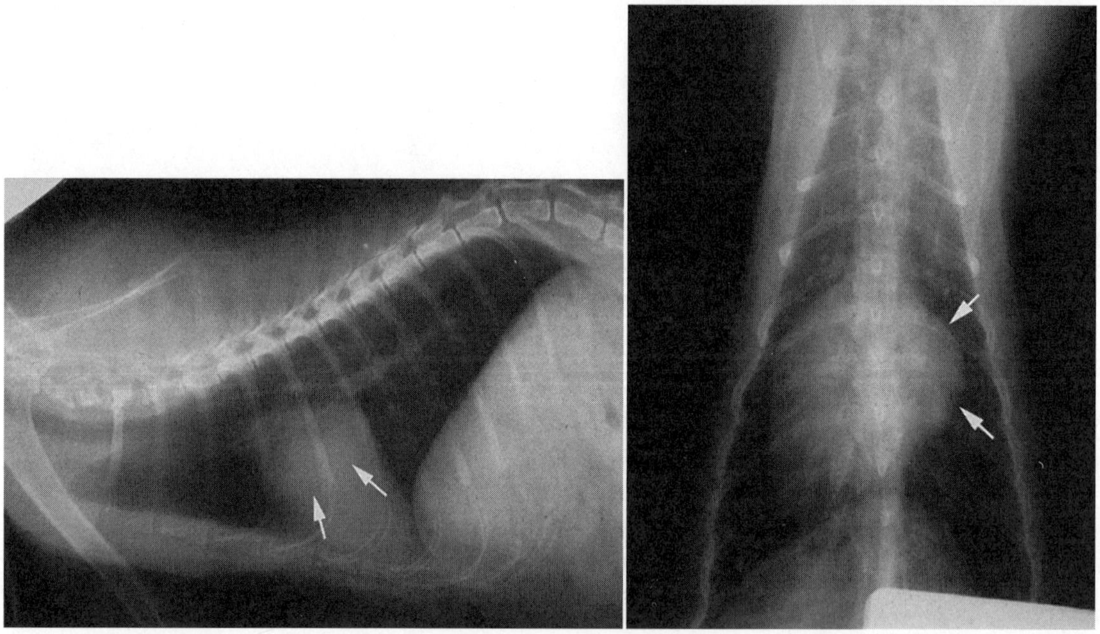

FIGURE 4-26 Left atrial enlargement in a cat with hypertrophic cardiomyopathy. The auricular appendage bulge *(arrows)* on the dorsoventral view occurs in the same place as in a dog. The left atrium can be visualized on the lateral view as a denser region at the base of the heart (arrows are on the ventral border). Compared with dogs, the left atrium lies farther forward and usually cannot be identified in this view. Although the right atrium appears enlarged in this cat, it was not enlarged on an echocardiogram.

Left atrial enlargement is most pronounced in dogs with congenital or acquired mitral regurgitation and in cats with cardiomyopathy of any type (Figures 4-25 and 4-26). On the dorsoventral radiograph, moderate-to-severe left atrial enlargement is most commonly appreciated as an increase in the size of the left auricle. This appears as a bulge in the 2-o'clock to 3-o'clock position in both cats and dogs. This bulge is most prominent when the left auricle and left atrium are increased to a size greater than the left ventricle. This commonly occurs with mitral regurgitation and feline cardiomyopathy. When the left ventricle and left atrium are increased

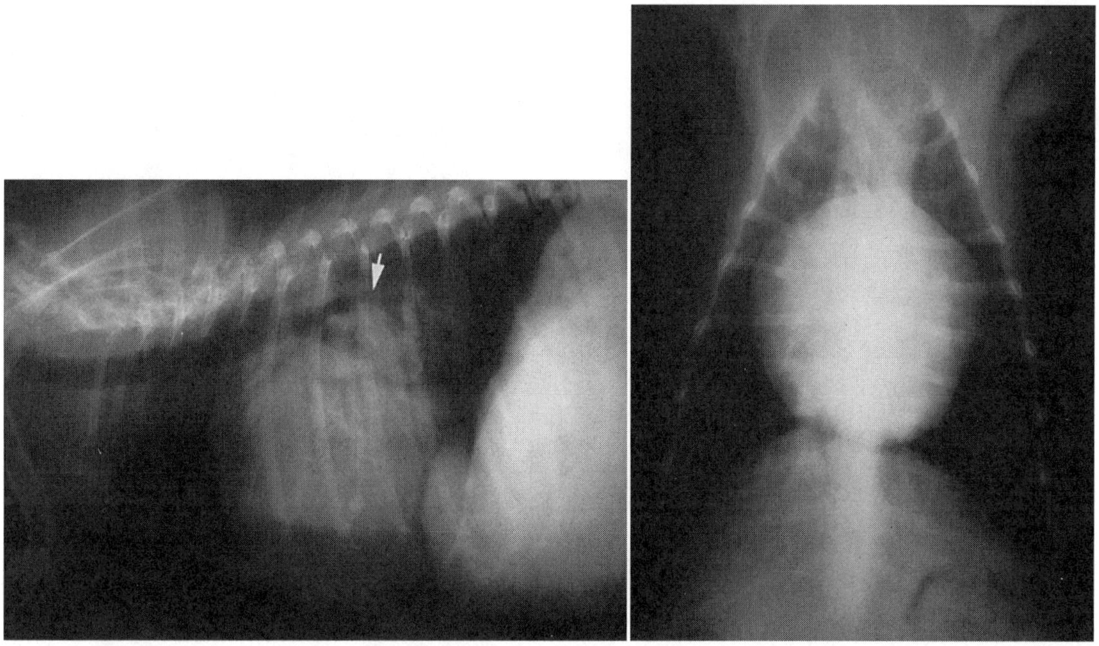

FIGURE 4-27 Severe left atrial and left ventricular enlargement in a dog with severe mitral regurgitation. On the lateral view, the enlarged left atrium has elevated the left mainstem bronchus *(arrow)* above the right mainstem bronchus. The caudal border of the heart is straighter than normal. The cardiac silhouette is enlarged. On the dorsoventral view, there is a prominent left auricular bulge at the 2-o'clock to 3-o'clock position. Although the left ventricle was severely enlarged in this dog, its appearance is not as remarkable.

to a similar degree, the lateral border of the left ventricle and the left auricle may meld together, obliterating the appearance of a bulge in the left auricular area. The body of the left atrium lies between the two caudal mainstem bronchi. The increase in left atrial size may increase the angle between these bronchi, especially by shifting the left mainstem bronchus cranially, giving the mainstem bronchi the appearance of a bowlegged cowboy. In severe left atrial enlargement, the massive amount of blood in the left atrium results in the left atrium becoming denser than the rest of the cardiac silhouette (see Figure 4-25). The left atrium then appears as a round, radiodense region between the two mainstem bronchi. This appearance is most commonly identified in dogs with severe mitral regurgitation.

Enlargement of the left atrium usually is easily identified on the lateral radiograph in dogs. The left atrium is situated more cranially in cats, and left atrial enlargement is commonly not appreciated in this view (see Figure 4-26). In dogs with left atrial enlargement, the enlarged atrium elevates the distal end of the trachea and the left mainstem bronchus (Figure 4-27). The degree of elevation depends on the degree of left atrial enlargement. The combination of the elevation in the trachea and the increase in atrial height results in an increase in the distance between the carina and the caudal waist. In normal dogs, the two caudal mainstem bronchi lie parallel with each other. Commonly, the enlarged left atrium elevates the left caudal mainstem bronchus more than the right mainstem bronchus, resulting in a distinct separation (see Figure 4-27). Severe left atrial enlargement combined with bronchomalacia in small geriatric dogs can result in compression of the left mainstem bronchus between the left atrium and the muscles beneath the spine.

LEFT VENTRICULAR ENLARGEMENT

The ability to detect left ventricular enlargement depends on the type of hypertrophy that is present. Severe left ventricular concentric hypertrophy secondary to a pressure overload results in approximately a 50% increase in wall thickness. In a large dog this means that the two walls of the left ventricle (the free wall and the interventricular septum) increase from 10 mm to 15 mm. This increases the size of the left ventricular shadow by 1 cm (Figure 4-28). In comparison, the left ventricular cavity can increase from 45 mm to 65 mm in diameter (an increase of 2 cm) in the same size dog with a severe volume overload (see Figure 4-27). Consequently, a severe volume overload is generally easier to detect than is a severe pressure overload. Moderate left ventricular enlargement is often difficult to detect. Severe left ventricular enlargement may be difficult to distinguish from biventricular enlargement. Left atrial enlargement often accompanies a left ventricular volume overload and commonly is present in hypertrophic cardiomyopathy.

On the dorsoventral view, moderate-to-severe left ventricular enlargement can appear either as a cardiac silhouette that is longer than normal, more rounded than normal, or both.[12] Dogs with patent ductus arteriosus commonly have a cardiac silhouette that appears longer than normal (Figure 4-29). In dogs with mitral regurgitation, the left heart border usually becomes more convex and may advance toward the left chest wall, decreasing the space between the chest wall and the cardiac silhouette. The apex of the left ventricle may be rotated more to the left but on occasion will be pushed to the right. All these changes are variable and appear differently in dogs with different chest configurations, making it difficult at times to identify left ventricular enlargement accurately in a given patient.

On the lateral view, the caudal cardiac border may become more rounded or straighter than normal (see Figure 4-27). It often extends farther caudally, although this is often difficult to appreciate unless one has a previous radiograph for comparison and the phase of respiration is the same on both radiographs. The caudal waist may become obliterated. The trachea is elevated, but the same caveats with respect to the chest configuration are applicable.

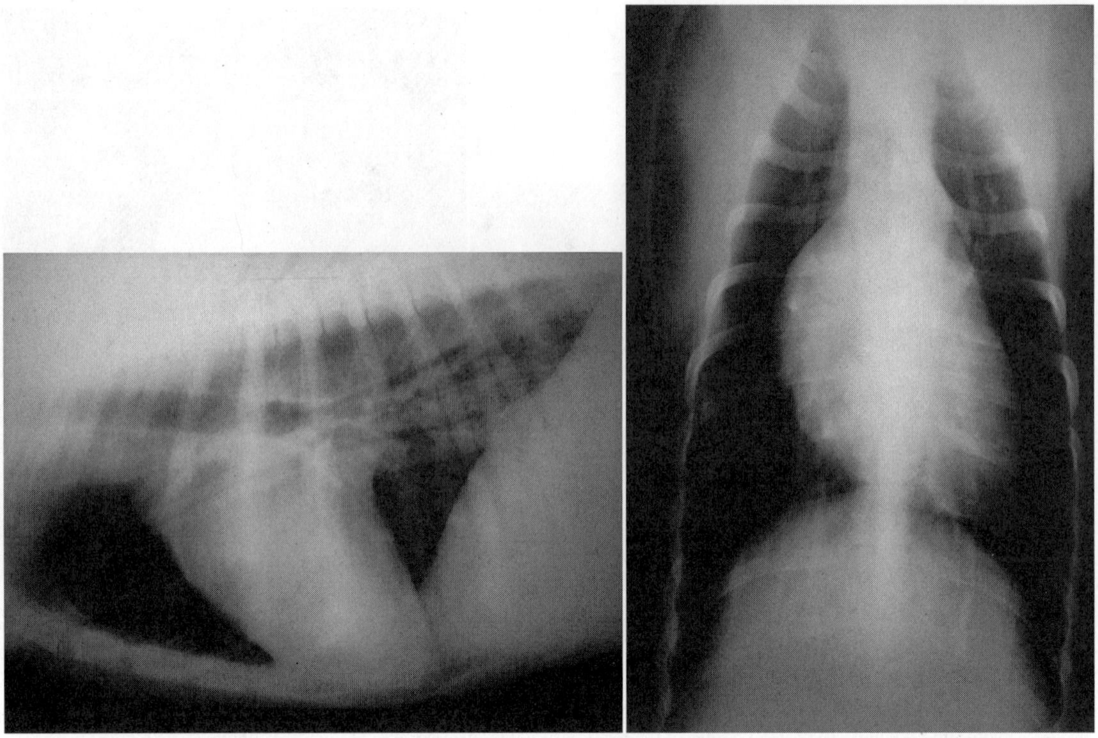

FIGURE 4-28 Thoracic radiographs from a dog with severe subaortic stenosis. Although the left ventricular walls are severely thickened in this dog, the left ventricle does not appear to be severely enlarged. On the lateral view, there is a prominent bulge that obliterates the cranial waist, making the base of the heart appear larger. The bulge is the poststenotic dilation of the ascending aorta. The poststenotic dilation is obscured from view on the dorsoventral radiograph by the vertebrae and sternebrae.

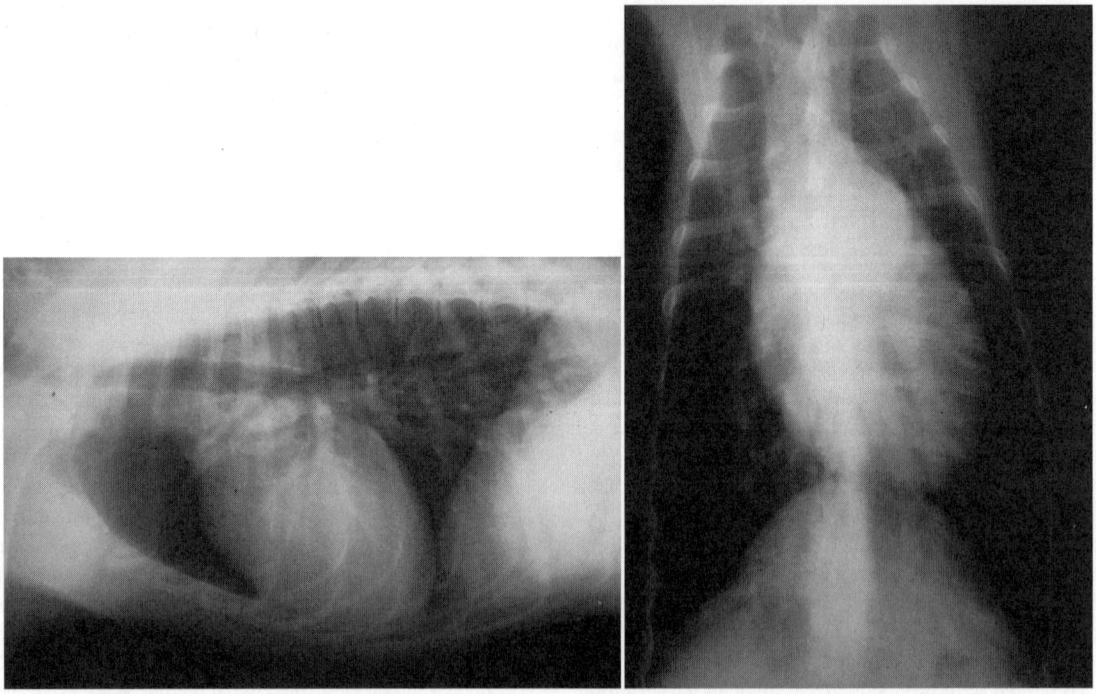

FIGURE 4-29 Thoracic radiographs from a dog with a large patent ductus arteriosus. An echocardiogram from this dog showed moderate-to-severe left ventricular and left atrial volume overloads, with both chambers being similarly increased in size. The primary abnormality seen on the radiographs is an increase in the length of the cardiac silhouette on the dorsoventral view and the bulge on the descending aorta (ductal aneurysm). Because the left ventricle and left atrium are similarly enlarged, a prominent left auricular bulge is not seen.

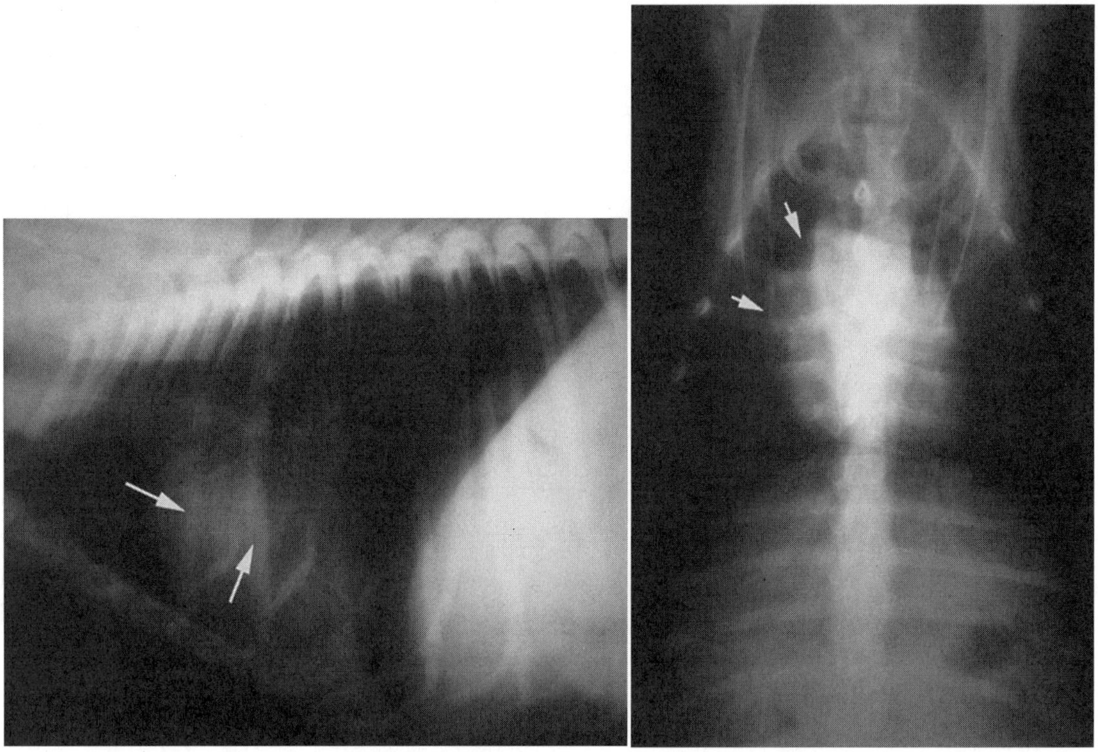

FIGURE 4-30 Thoracic radiographs from a dog with tricuspid regurgitation and moderate right atrial enlargement. On the lateral view, the right auricle is seen as a faint structure bulging cranially from the cardiac silhouette. The body of the right atrium extends caudally from there and is visualized as a structure that is denser than the rest of the cardiac silhouette *(arrows)*. On the dorsoventral view, the right atrium is seen bulging slightly at the 9-o'clock to 12-o'clock position *(arrows)*.

RIGHT ATRIAL ENLARGEMENT

Right atrial enlargement is often difficult to assess unless it is severe. On the lateral view, isolated, moderate-to-severe right atrial enlargement appears as a bulge in the craniodorsal portion of the cardiac silhouette (Figure 4-30). When it is accompanied by right ventricular enlargement, the increase in right atrial size often is not appreciated. The cranial waist may be obliterated by either right atrial or right ventricular outflow tract enlargement. Right atrial enlargement may also displace the part of the trachea that lies cranial to the carina dorsally.

On the dorsoventral view, moderate-to-severe right atrial enlargement can cause a bulge in the cardiac silhouette from 8 o'clock to 12 o'clock (see Figure 4-30). Right ventricular enlargement can also cause an increase in the size of the cardiac silhouette in this region.

RIGHT VENTRICULAR ENLARGEMENT

Right ventricular enlargement must be moderate to severe to be identified consistently in dogs and cats. When accompanied by left ventricular enlargement, the task of identifying the enlargement accurately is compromised.

On a dorsoventral view, right ventricular enlargement increases the size of the cardiac silhouette on the right side of the chest.[12] Classically, the cardiac border looks more convex, and the distance between the chest wall and the right cardiac border decreases (Figure 4-31). A small notch just to the right of the cardiac apex occasionally is identified in dogs with right ventricular enlargement. Also on occasion, the apex may be pushed leftward, making it appear as if there is left ventricular enlargement. The cranial border of the heart may also be increased because of enlargement of the right ventricular outflow tract.

On a lateral radiograph, the cranial portion of the cardiac silhouette is increased in size. This can be determined subjectively, or a measurement of this increase can be attempted by drawing a line from the carina to the cardiac apex and measuring the distance from this line to the cranial border of the heart. This distance is 2 to 2.5 times the distance from the carina-apex line to the caudal border of the heart in a normal dog. It is increased in dogs with right ventricular enlargement. Right ventricular enlargement may displace the portion of the trachea that lies over the cranial heart dorsally. Enlargement of the right ventricle may also displace the apex of the heart dorsally off the sternum, especially in shallow-chested dogs (see Figure 4-31). This latter finding is often not identified (i.e., it is not a sensitive diagnostic test). However, when identified it almost always indicates that the right ventricle is enlarged (i.e., it is a specific test). Right ventricular enlargement may increase the contact of the heart with the sternum. However, increased sternal contact is also observed in dogs with shallow chests and, on occasion, in dogs with left ventricular enlargement. Consequently, this finding is not a specific finding for right ventricular enlargement.

MAIN PULMONARY ARTERY ENLARGEMENT

The main pulmonary artery is most commonly enlarged in dogs with pulmonic stenosis and pulmonary hypertension. Absence of this type of enlargement does not rule out either diagnosis, because the

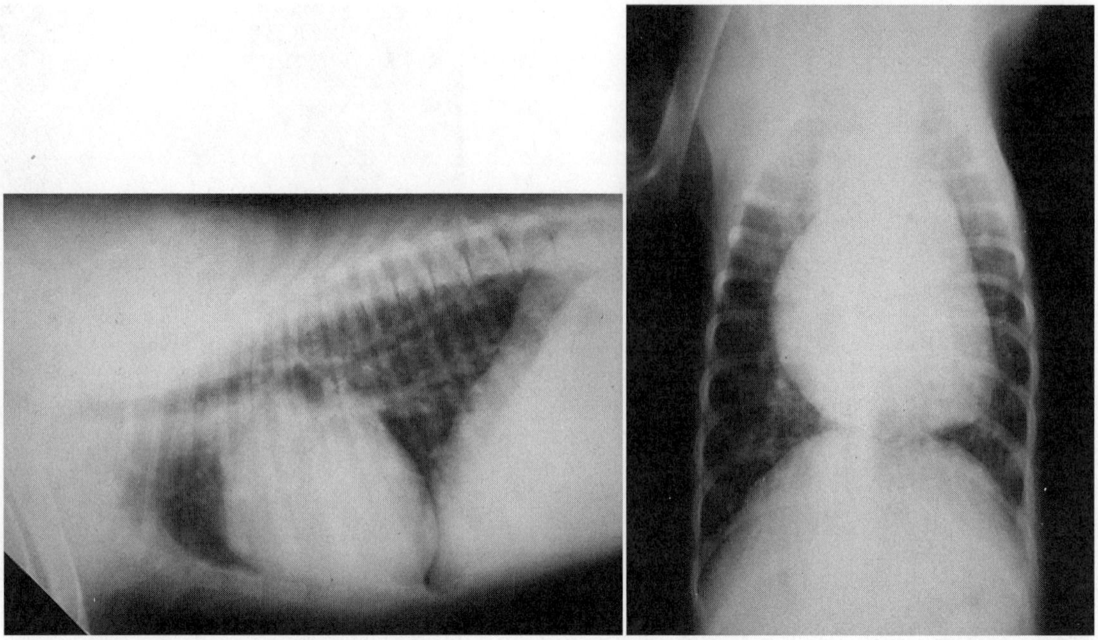

FIGURE 4-31 Right ventricular and atrial enlargement in a dog with severe lung disease leading to pulmonary hypertension (cor pulmonale). On the dorsoventral view, the right side of the cardiac silhouette is enlarged, giving the silhouette the appearance of a larger than normal reverse *D*. The apex of the cardiac silhouette has been pushed to the left by the right heart enlargement. On the lateral view, the cardiac silhouette is enlarged and the cardiac apex is shifted dorsally off of the sternum by the right ventricular enlargement.

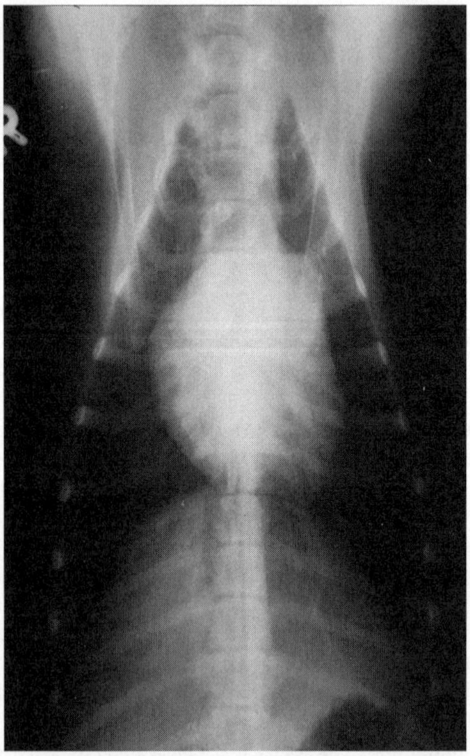

FIGURE 4-32 A dorsoventral radiograph from a dog with pulmonic stenosis. The right heart was enlarged (thickened) on the echocardiogram but does not appear enlarged on the radiograph. There is a bulge at the 1-o'clock position, where the left scapula crosses the cardiac silhouette. The bulge is the main pulmonary artery, which is enlarged because of post-stenotic dilation. The lateral radiograph (not shown) was normal.

enlargement may be mild or obscured by other structures. The main pulmonary artery may be increased in size in some dogs with a severe volume overload of the pulmonary vasculature, as in dogs with patent ductus arteriosus. In pulmonic stenosis, only the proximal portion of the main pulmonary artery is enlarged distal to the stenotic region (poststenotic dilation). In pulmonary hypertension, the pulmonary artery branches also may be enlarged. Main pulmonary artery enlargement is not readily detectable in cats and only becomes detectable when severe enlargement is present.

Enlargement of the main pulmonary artery is most readily identified as a bulge at the 2-o'clock to 3-o'clock position on the dorsoventral view (Figure 4-32). This enlargement must be distinguished from a left auricular bulge and a descending aortic bulge. Main pulmonary artery enlargement is generally not identified on a lateral view, although, rarely, the distended main pulmonary artery may be identified as it crosses the radiolucent trachea in dogs with pulmonic stenosis. Main pulmonary artery enlargement may enlarge the cranial border on the cardiac silhouette on the lateral view in heartworm disease, but in cases of pulmonic stenosis this is rare.

Rarely, the main pulmonary artery segment may be smaller than normal. This occurs most commonly in tetralogy of Fallot.

ENLARGED PULMONARY ARTERY BRANCHES

The pulmonary artery branches should be evaluated for size and character in all dogs and cats evaluated radiographically. Enlargement of the pulmonary arteries can occur with increased pulmonary artery pressure (pulmonary hypertension), with increased pulmonary artery flow (overcirculation), or with pulmonary artery disease, as in dirofilariasis. In animals with overcirculation as a result of a left-to-right shunt, the pulmonary veins should be equally enlarged, although they may not be as readily visible (see Figure 4-29). Overcirculation does not usually result in an increase in the size of the main pulmonary artery to the extent that a bulge is produced on the cardiac silhouette. A decrease in pulmonary artery size can be seen in some patients with pulmonary hypertension, especially those with pulmonary hypertension secondary to pulmonary thromboembolism or severe vasoconstriction.

The caudal lobar branches are usually readily identified on a dorsoventral view, initially as they course across the cardiac silhouette, lateral to the caudal lobar bronchi, and then as they pass through the lung fields and cross the diaphragm. The size of these vessels is usually evaluated subjectively, based on experience. One rule of thumb is that the caudal lobar branches at the level of the seventh rib should be approximately the same width as the width of that rib. Although this may be a valid means of evaluating the size of the vessel at that particular point, patients with pulmonary arteries that are larger or smaller than normal proximal or distal to this point are not detected by this method.

The cranial lobar pulmonary arteries can be seen on a dorsoventral view but are best visualized on the lateral view. In this view, the arteries cross the craniodorsal portion of the cardiac silhouette to emerge in the cranial lung fields. The two arteries are situated dorsally to the cranial lobar bronchi. Depending on the view, the cranial lobar arteries, veins, and bronchi visualized in the cranial lung fields may be clearly separate or may overlie each other, making it difficult to distinguish the two arteries, the two veins, or the arteries from the veins. Normally, the cranial lobar arteries at the level of the fourth intercostal space are approximately 0.75 times the diameter of the proximal third of the fourth rib.[13] When these arteries are enlarged, they are generally 1.2 times the diameter of this rib or greater. The cranial lobar vessels are less frequently involved than the caudal lobar arteries in dogs with heartworm disease. Consequently, one must evaluate the caudal lobar branches in these dogs. In our experience, evaluation of the caudal lobar branches is generally more rewarding for evaluating pulmonary artery size in other conditions also.

ENLARGED PULMONARY VEINS

Pulmonary veins become enlarged either because of high pulmonary vein pressure or increased flow. Pulmonary venous hypertension is almost always secondary to increased left ventricular diastolic and/or left atrial pressures (i.e., left heart failure). In this situation, the veins should be larger than the arteries. Left-to-right shunts result in increased pulmonary blood flow, and pulmonary veins are distended with the increased flow in concert with the pulmonary arteries.

In left heart failure, the pulmonary veins are primarily distended centrally where they join the left atrium. The peripheral veins are less distended or not distended. The central portion of the pulmonary veins may appear larger and denser than the central pulmonary arteries, and the central portions may be triangularly shaped.[10] The distended perihilar veins, along with pulmonary edema, result in increased perihilar density, characteristic of left heart failure. Enlarged pulmonary veins are almost always accompanied by left atrial enlargement, except when acute left heart failure develops. Often, pulmonary venous distension in left heart failure is difficult to appreciate because of the location of the distension. It is often an impression, rather than something one can quantify or defend with confidence. In large left-to-right shunts (e.g., patent ductus arteriosus) the veins may be distended centrally as well as distally (see Figure 4-29).

SEGMENTAL ENLARGEMENT OF THE AORTA

The aorta most commonly enlarges in two regions: the ascending aorta and the proximal descending aorta. The ascending aorta is most commonly enlarged because of poststenotic dilation secondary to subaortic stenosis. Annuloaortic ectasia rarely will cause this type of enlargement. Patent ductus arteriosus commonly results in an aneurysmal dilation at its origin from the proximal descending aorta.

Ascending aortic enlargement is most readily identified on a lateral radiographic view. In this view, the aortic enlargement ("bulge") is observed as an enlargement of the cranial/dorsal region of the cardiac silhouette that obliterates the cranial waist (see Figure 4-28). This region is obscured by the overlying sternebrae and vertebrae on a dorsoventral view. Nevertheless, aortic enlargement can be identified in this region in some dogs, especially if the enlargement is severe.

Aneurysmal enlargement of the proximal descending aorta can only be identified on a dorsoventral view. It is identified as a bulge directed toward the left side of the thorax at the same level as the main pulmonary artery (see Figures 4-24 and 4-29). A bulge in this region is pathognomonic for a dog that has the gene for patent ductus arteriosus and is most commonly identified in a dog with a left-to-right shunting patent ductus arteriosus. Identifying this bulge, however, does not necessarily mean that the dog has a ductus arteriosus that is patent. It can be seen in dogs in which the pulmonary artery end of the ductus arteriosus has successfully closed but the aortic end has not. These dogs have a so-called ductal aneurysm. Dogs with a right-to-left shunting patent ductus arteriosus also often have this radiographic finding.

ENLARGED CAUDAL VENA CAVA

Right heart failure may lead to a demonstrable increase in the size of the caudal vena cava on the dorsoventral and the lateral views. Caudal vena caval size changes with the phase of respiration. Assessment of caudal vena caval enlargement is usually based on subjectively evaluating its size in comparison with normal. In our experience, only severe enlargement associated with severe right heart failure is detectable with any reasonable degree of certainty (Figure 4-33). A recent study has suggested that the caudal vena cava can be measured and compared with vertebral body length.[6] Using this method, maximum caudal vena caval width is almost always less than the length of either the fifth or sixth thoracic vertebrae in normal dogs. It remains to be determined if this method of determining caudal vena caval size is accurate for detecting mild-to-severe enlargement.

Heart Failure

One primary reason for obtaining thoracic radiographs is to detect evidence of heart failure. Although the echocardiogram is much better at detecting and quantitating cardiac enlargement, it cannot, by itself, provide a definitive diagnosis of heart failure. Radiographs often can provide this information.

Radiographic evidence of heart failure is dependent on the identification of pulmonary edema or pleural effusion. Cardiogenic pulmonary edema is always secondary to left heart disease and usually is associated with left atrial enlargement, which is usually severe. Identifying pulmonary edema on a thoracic radiograph does not provide a definitive diagnosis of left heart failure, because pulmonary edema may be caused by other abnormalities. Consequently, one must identify pulmonary edema in association with severe left heart disease to make the diagnosis of left heart failure. This information may be present on the thoracic radiograph as severe left heart enlargement, or an echocardiogram may be required to identify the severe left heart disease.

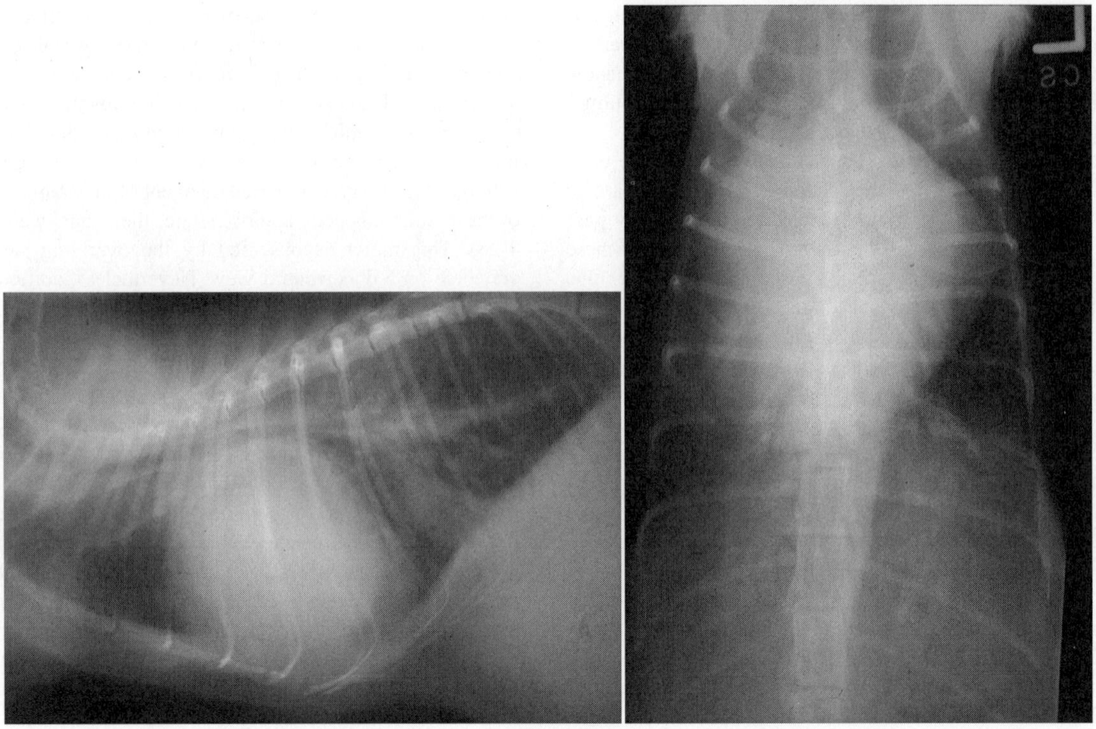

FIGURE 4-33 Thoracic radiographs from a cat with severe mitral and tricuspid valve dysplasias. All four chambers are enlarged, with the right and left atria larger than the ventricles. The cat is in left heart failure, as evidenced by interstitial pulmonary edema in the caudodorsal lung fields. The caudal vena cava is very large because of right heart failure. The left auricle is very prominent on the dorsoventral view.

To identify a pleural effusion as cardiogenic, it is necessary to identify severe heart disease in association with finding pleural effusion. Although a pleural effusion can be readily identified using ultrasound, it is often better quantified by examining a thoracic radiograph. Cardiogenic pleural effusions in dogs are most commonly secondary to a combination of left and right heart failure. Cardiogenic pleural effusions used to be very common in cats with left and right heart failure secondary to dilated cardiomyopathy. Diseases that create both left and right heart failure are less common in cats, because dilated cardiomyopathy has been controlled in the cat population. Right heart failure is a rare cause of pleural effusion in cats. Left heart failure, usually secondary to hypertrophic cardiomyopathy, is more common. Because pleural effusion on a thoracic radiograph usually obscures the cardiac silhouette, identification of the presence of underlying cardiac disease usually requires an ultrasound examination.

Mild pulmonary edema is identified in dogs as a poorly defined increase in the interstitial density of the caudal and dorsal lung fields. This increased density is commonly more dense immediately caudal and dorsal to the left atrium (perihilar) on the lateral radiographic view. The increased density partially obscures the pulmonary vessels. The increased perihilar density may be due to pulmonary edema and enlarged pulmonary veins. Moderate pulmonary edema appears as a more dense veil of interstitial markings. Mild-to-moderate pulmonary edema is usually located centrally. Consequently, it is often not visualized well on a dorsoventral radiograph. Severe pulmonary edema is diagnosed when the fluid invades alveolar spaces, resulting in the lungs having the same or a similar density to soft tissue. This marked increase in density obscures pulmonary vessels. Edema fluid does not encroach on the bronchi unless the edema is very severe. Consequently, the bronchi are visualized within the soft tissue density of the edema-filled lungs (so-called air bronchograms).

In cats, pulmonary edema may appear as it does in dogs or the edema may appear as patchy or unevenly distributed infiltrates in the lungs (Figures 4-33 and 4-34). It may also concentrate in the lung fields immediately caudal to the heart. This pattern must be distinguished from other infiltrative pulmonary diseases.

Pleural effusion is readily identified on thoracic radiographs. Mild pleural effusion most commonly is identified on the lateral radiograph as a line of the effusion that obscures the ventral cardiac silhouette and diaphragmatic shadow (see Figure 4-34).[10] It may also be identified as an increase in the space between the lung and spine immediately above the distal caudal and dorsal lung fields. The quadratus lumborum muscle also lies in this region and can be confused with pleural effusion, especially in cats. Mild pleural effusion may obscure the cardiac silhouette on the dorsoventral view and fluid can be visualized between lung lobes (so-called pleural fissure lines). Obtaining a ventrodorsal view may be helpful. Positioning the animal on its back may allow the fluid to accumulate centrally along the spine, allowing visualization of the cardiac silhouette. With moderate effusions, most of the cardiac silhouette and diaphragmatic shadow are obliterated on the lateral view with the lung lobes displaced dorsally. The edges of the lung lobes are rounded. On the dorsoventral view, the cardiac silhouette cannot be discerned. Pleural fissure lines may be visible and the mediastinum may be wide. With a severe effusion, the lung lobes are compressed dorsally on the lateral view and have a leaflike appearance. All other

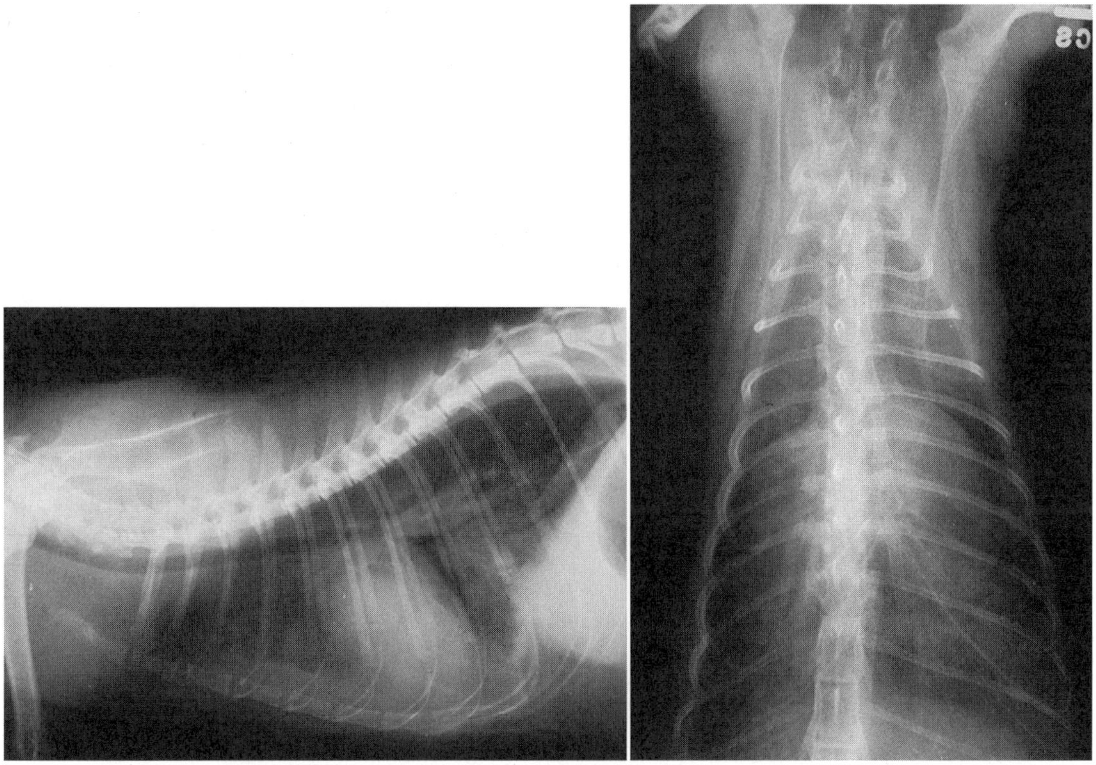

FIGURE 4-34 Thoracic radiographs from a cat with hypertrophic cardiomyopathy and left heart failure. There is pulmonary edema concentrated primarily behind the heart on the lateral view. Pleural effusion is also present. It obscures the cardiac silhouette on the dorsoventral view and is located primarily ventral to the cranial lung lobes and dorsal to the caudal lung lobes on the lateral radiograph.

intrathoracic structures are obscured. On the dorsoventral view, the lung lobes are separated from the chest wall and their borders appear rounded.

Microcardia

Radiographs can also be used to detect a heart that is smaller than normal (microcardia). Microcardia can be seen in patients that are severely dehydrated or that have hypoadrenocorticism (Addison's disease; Figure 4-35). Rarely, microcardia is a congenital abnormality.

Angiocardiography

Injecting radiopaque dye into cardiac chambers or blood vessels allows visualization of the lumenae of these structures radiographically. This is demonstrated in Figures 4-14 through 4-21. Angiocardiography also allows identification of communications between structures and visualization of stenotic regions and valvular regurgitation. Angiocardiography, in conjunction with measuring intracardiac pressures (i.e., cardiac catheterization), used to be a common means of definitively diagnosing many types of cardiovascular abnormalities. Since the advent of cardiac ultrasound, our use of cardiac catheterization has dwindled to the point that our residents get little experience at performing these techniques.

Angiocardiography is an invasive technique performed most commonly in anesthetized patients. Cardiac catheters are introduced into a peripheral vessel, either via surgical exposure or percutaneous puncture of the vessel, as described in Chapter 7. The catheter is then guided into the appropriate vessel or chamber while the clinician observes its progress using fluoroscopy. An iodinated contrast agent is then injected through the catheter to outline the structure of interest.

Several commercial iodinated contrast agents are marketed. The most widely used ionic contrast agents (Renograffin, E. R. Squibb & Sons, Inc., New Brunswick, N.J.; Hypaque, Sanofi Winthrop Pharmaceuticals, New York, N.Y.; and Angiovist, Berlex Laboratories, Wayne, N.J.) are mixtures of meglumine and sodium salts of diatrizoic acid. The sodium concentration is similar to that of blood, and the iodine concentration is between 320 and 370 mg/mL. Their osmolality is approximately 6 times that of blood. The high osmolality results in hemodynamic alterations when the agents are injected. Alterations include an increase in intracardiac diastolic pressures. The increase in diastolic pressures may be harmful to patients with severe cardiac disease and heart failure. Low osmolality contrast agents such as iohexol (Omnipaque, Sinofi Winthrop Pharmaceuticals, New York, N.Y.), iopamidol (Isovue, E. R. Squibb & Sons, Inc., New Brunswick, N.J.), metrizamide (Amipaque, Sinofi Winthrop Pharmaceuticals, New York, N.Y.), and ioversol (Optiray, Mallinckrodt, Inc., St. Louis, Mo.) have been developed for these types of patients. These agents are water-soluble in a noncharged form and so have no associated cation. Their osmolality is approximately 3 times that of blood.

Contrast agents are most commonly injected into cardiac chambers or great vessels in dogs and cats. Selective catheterization

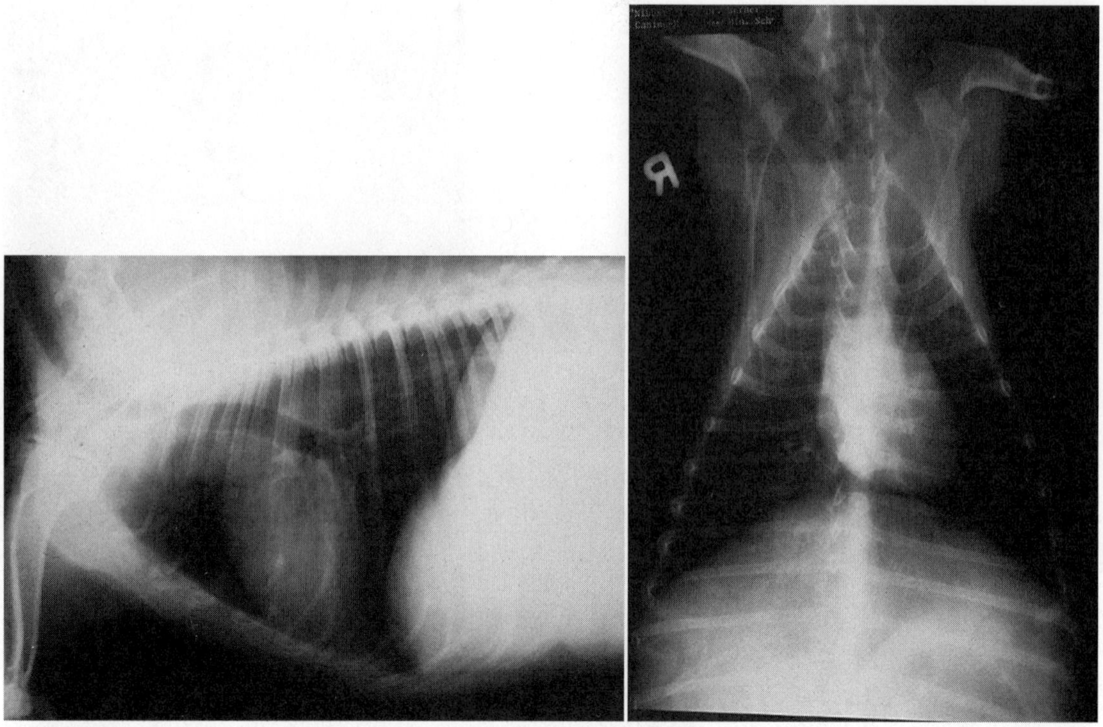

FIGURE 4-35 Microcardia in a severely dehydrated terrier.

of smaller vessels, such as coronary vessels is done less commonly. Injection into a cardiac chamber is accomplished through a cardiac catheter. Examples of commonly used catheters include the pigtail, NIH, and Lehman ventriculographic catheters. These catheters have only side holes. A catheter with just an end hole is unsatisfactory for angiocardiography because it recoils during delivery of the contrast agent and can penetrate the endocardium, resulting in delivery of contrast material into the myocardium ("myocardial staining") or, rarely, myocardial perforation. Ventriculography requires rapid delivery of an adequate quantity of contrast agent. We usually use 0.5 to 1 mL/kg of an ionic contrast agent. In a small dog, this dose can be delivered within 1 to 2 seconds through a hand injection, using the smallest appropriate syringe. For larger dogs, a pressure or flow injector is preferred, because it is impossible to deliver the quantity of contrast agent needed in the time allotted. The automated injector that we use is made by Cordis and allows selection of a volume of delivery, the pressure at which it is injected, and the flow rate, given the characteristics of the catheter used. One must be careful, especially with power injectors, not to inject air. This is especially true on the left side of the heart where one bubble can occlude a coronary artery and result in acute myocardial infarction and sudden death. Small bubbles cause no problems with right-sided injections. However, large quantities of air can replace ventricular blood volume, resulting in clinically significant hemodynamic consequences. Catheters should be flushed frequently to prevent thrombus formation and subsequent thromboembolism. Before a power injection is made, a smaller test injection should be performed to confirm proper catheter position.

Angiography is also performed in veterinary medicine. Contrast agents are most commonly injected into the root of the aorta to diagnose and assess the severity of aortic regurgitation, into the aortic arch to detect a patent ductus arteriosus, into the main pulmonary artery or pulmonary artery branches to detect pulmonary thromboemboli, and into the distal aorta to diagnose systemic thromboembolism. Injections are usually made by hand at a dose of 0.25 to 0.5 mL/kg of an ionic contrast agent. Complications are rare except when pulmonary angiography is attempted in patients with severe pulmonary hypertension. One of our colleagues has witnessed sudden death in two such patients. This complication is also recognized in human patients with primary pulmonary hypertension and, probably, pulmonary hypertension resulting from other causes.[14] In humans, serious complications have most often been associated with large or large cumulative doses of an ionic contrast agent into the main pulmonary artery of patients with pulmonary artery pressures that approach systemic arterial pressure. Consequently, smaller injections and nonionic contrast agents should probably be employed in patients with severe pulmonary hypertension. When looking for pulmonary thromboembolism, a better technique may be to use a double lumen catheter with a latex balloon at its tip, such as a Swan-Ganz catheter or a Berman angiographic catheter. These catheters are advanced into a pulmonary artery branch of interest and inflated. A smaller amount of contrast agent is then injected by hand into the distal lumen of the catheter. The small volume of contrast delivered by hand completely opacifies the regional pulmonary vasculature without producing any hemodynamic consequence.

Adverse reactions to contrast agents are rare. In human medicine they are estimated to occur at a rate of less than 0.05%. We have never witnessed a serious systemic adverse effect from a contrast agent in a clinical patient. However, that does not mean that complications cannot occur, and minor complications are common. Anaphylaxis can occur, usually after the second exposure to an agent. It is rare for dogs or cats to undergo cardiac catheterization more than once, making this complication extremely rare. Renal failure can occur, especially after large amounts of contrast material are administered within a short period. Contrast agents can depress left ventricular function. It is common for blood pressure to decrease modestly and heart rate to increase for a short time after the injection. Depression of contractility is especially evident when contrast agents are administered into a coronary artery. We generally dilute an ionic contrast agent 1:1 with saline before a coronary artery injection to prevent serious problems. Ionic contrast agents are hyperosmolar and so increase intravascular volume. This is of no consequence in a patient with a normal pulmonary capillary pressure. However, in a patient in left heart failure, injections of contrast agents can increase pulmonary capillary pressure further. This can result in exacerbation of pulmonary edema or even intractable pulmonary edema and death. Ventricular premature beats are common during ventriculography and usually are due to mechanical irritation of the endocardium by the catheter or the jet of contrast agent. They usually stop after the injection or after repositioning or removal of the catheter. Serious ventricular arrhythmias or arrhythmias that persist following catheter removal may be treated with intravenous lidocaine.

REFERENCES

1. Mulvihill JJ, Priester WA: Congenital heart disease in dogs: epidemiologic similarities to man, *Teratology* 7:73, 1993.
2. Rankin JS, McHale PA, Arentzen CE et al: The three-dimensional dynamic geometry of the left ventricle in the conscious dog, *Circ Res* 39:304, 1976.
3. Suter PF, Gomez JA: *Diseases of the thorax: radiographic diagnosis,* Davis, Calif, 1981, Venture.
4. Moon ML, Keene BW, Lessard P et al: Age related changes in the feline cardiac silhouette, *Vet Radiol Ultrasound* 34:315, 1993.
5. Eagle KA, De Sanctis RW: Diseases of the aorta. In Braunwald E, ed: *Heart disease: a textbook of cardiovascular medicine,* ed 4, Philadelphia, 1992, WB Saunders.
6. Buchanan JW, Bücheler J: Vertebral scale system to measure canine heart size in radiographs, *J Am Vet Med Assoc* 206:194, 1995.
7. Stunzl H, Teuscher E, Bolliger O: Systematische Untersuchungen am Herzen von Haustieren. I. Mitteilung: Untersuschung am Herzen der Katze, *Zentralbl Veterinarmed* 6:101, 1959.
8. Wyburn RS, Lawson DD: Simple radiography as an aid to the diagnosis of heart disease in the dog, *J Small Anim Pract* 8:163, 1967.
9. Buchanan JW: Radiology of the heart: seminar synopsis, 39th Annual Meeting, American Animal Hospital Association, Las Vegas, *Am Anim Hosp Assoc,* 1972, p 78.
10. Suter PF, Lord PF: *Thoracic radiography: thoracic diseases of the dog and cat,* Peter F. Suter, 1984.
11. van den Broek AHM, Darke PG: Cardiac measurements on thoracic radiographs of cats, *J Small Anim Pract* 28:125, 1987.
12. Hamlin RL: Analysis of the cardiac silhouette in dorsoventral radiographs from dogs with heart disease, *J Am Vet Med Assoc* 153:1446, 1968.
13. Thrall DF, Losonsky JM: A method for evaluating canine pulmonary circulatory dynamics from survey radiographs, *J Am Anim Hosp Assoc* 12:457, 1976.
14. Marsh JD, Glynn M, Torman HA: Pulmonary angiography: application in a new spectrum of patients, *Am J Med* 75:763, 1983.

CHAPTER 5

Electrocardiography: Basic Concepts, Diagnosis of Chamber Enlargement, and Intraventricular Conduction Disturbances

The electrocardiogram (ECG) is a recording of the heart's electrical activity from the surface of the body. It is used primarily as a clinical tool to identify and characterize cardiac arrhythmias and conduction disturbances. The ECG is also used as an adjunctive device to help identify cardiac chamber enlargement. It can also be used as an indicator of certain electrolyte disturbances, particularly hyperkalemia.

The ECG is a surface recording of the changing potentials of the electrical field imparted by the heart's electrical activity over time during the different phases of the cardiac cycle. It is not a direct recording of the heart's electrical activity and provides only a rough approximation of the actual voltages generated by the heart. When an electrode catheter is placed inside the heart and touches the myocardium, electrical potentials measured in volts are recorded. The surface ECG records these potentials in millivolts. If the body were homogeneous like a container of water (a homogeneous volume conductor), the heart's electrical potentials would be conducted to the surface in a direct relationship to the voltage source (the heart). The body is not homogeneous and so this relationship does not exist. This limitation decreases the ability of the surface ECG to accurately determine true voltage changes that occur in association with changes in chamber size. This limits the ability of the ECG to detect chamber enlargement. It does not limit the ability of the ECGs to detect arrhythmias, however, and electrocardiography remains the gold standard in veterinary medicine for diagnosing cardiac arrhythmias.

The electrocardiograph, invented in the late 1800s, is the instrument used to record the surface electrocardiogram. It consists of a conducting unit suspended between the magnetic poles of an electromagnet, an amplifier, electrodes attached to the patient, cables that attach the electrodes to the amplifier, and a recording device. The electrodes pick up the electric potentials on the surface of the body. The electrical potentials pass through the cables to the amplifier. Once the potentials are amplified, they pass through the conducting unit attached directly to a stylus. When a positive potential flows through the conducting unit, a magnetic field is set up that opposes the permanent magnetic field such that the stylus is deflected in one direction. When a negative potential flows through the conducting unit, the stylus is deflected in the opposite direction. The deflection height is directly related to the amount of current, or voltage. In many clinical electrocardiograph machines, the stylus is heated and paper passes underneath the stylus to record its deflections. The recording surface of this paper consists of a thin layer of carbon coated with wax. The heated stylus melts the wax, revealing the carbon underneath. Other recording methods, including light and direct-writing units, are also used.

Electrocardiographic Theory

To understand the genesis of the ECG, one must understand the physical and electrophysiologic events responsible for the transmembrane action potential and the spread of activation in the heart, the equivalent dipole and volume conductor theories, and the lead system.

TRANSMEMBRANE ACTION POTENTIAL

The heart is an electrically charged organ. At rest, most cells in the heart maintain an electrical gradient across the cell membrane. During depolarization, this gradient changes such that polarity is lost or reverses. When one cell is depolarized, it stimulates the cells next to it to depolarize. Depolarization spreads as a wave, from cell to cell through the myocardium. This depolarization wave is detected by an ECG. The electrical activity of the heart is responsible for coordinating the sequence of cardiac activation and contraction.

At rest, cardiac cells maintain an electrical gradient across the cell membrane such that the inside of the cell is negative with respect to the outside of the cell. The inside and outside of a cell are separated by the cell membrane, or sarcolemma. The sarcolemma consists of a phospholipid bilayer with associated membrane proteins. The phospholipids are arranged so that the hydrophobic fatty acyl chains are in the membrane core, and the polar head groups lie at the inner and outer surfaces of the membrane. The bipoles are hydrophobic and very resistant to ion movement. Proteins imbedded in this phospholipid bilayer serve as receptors, ion channels, and pumps. Ion channels are proteins that contain water and span the membrane. The water allows hydrated ions to cross the membrane. Channels are selective to specific ions (e.g., sodium, potassium, or calcium). Channels have gating mechanisms so that they may be open or closed. Transmembrane voltage commonly alters the degree to which the channel is open. Voltage-dependent channel opening is created by rearrangement of charged channel proteins during voltage changes. Channels for different ions act differently. For example, once open, sodium channels remain open for only about 1 ms, whereas calcium channels are open for more than 50 ms.

The resting membrane potential is large in cardiac cells, ranging from –40 mV to –90 mV, with the inside of the cell negative compared with extracellular fluid. The resting ion gradients are also large. Extracellular sodium concentration is 150 mM/L, and intracellular sodium concentration is 25 mM/L. Extracellular potassium concentration is 4 mM/L, and intracellular potassium concentration is 150 mM/L. The concentration gradients are maintained by several factors. The cell membrane is relatively impermeable to sodium ions when the cell is polarized at rest. It is relatively permeable to potassium. Fixed negative charges inside the cell, presumably proteins and polypeptides too large to diffuse out of the cell, attract potassium ions and impair their outward movement. The Na^+-K^+ ATPase pump is activated once depolarization occurs. It lies within the cell membrane and extrudes three sodium ions and pumps in two potassium ions for each molecule of ATP hydrolyzed. The activity of this pump is electrogenic (i.e., more positive charge is pumped out than in). The resting membrane potential is primarily determined by the concentration gradient of potassium ions. The cell membrane is relatively permeable to potassium ions and impermeable to sodium ions, with the potassium ions being held within the cell by the fixed negative charges. The cell acts like a potassium electrode, with potassium leaving the cell along its concentration gradient, leaving the inside of the cell negative with respect to the outside of the cell. If potassium conductance of the cell membrane decreases so potassium cannot freely move out of the cell, the resting membrane potential decreases as the cell membrane starts to act more like a sodium electrode.

The resting membrane potential for Purkinje cells and myocardial cells is –80 to –90 mV. When diastolic depolarization reaches a threshold potential (voltage) in Purkinje cells or when a myocardial cell is depolarized by the cell next to it, fast sodium channels open in the cell membrane, allowing sodium to rush into the cell. Simultaneously, potassium conductance across the cell membrane decreases dramatically as the cell depolarizes. The positively charged sodium ions rushing into the cell depolarize the cell membrane (phase 0 of the action potential) (Figure 5-1). Membrane potential becomes

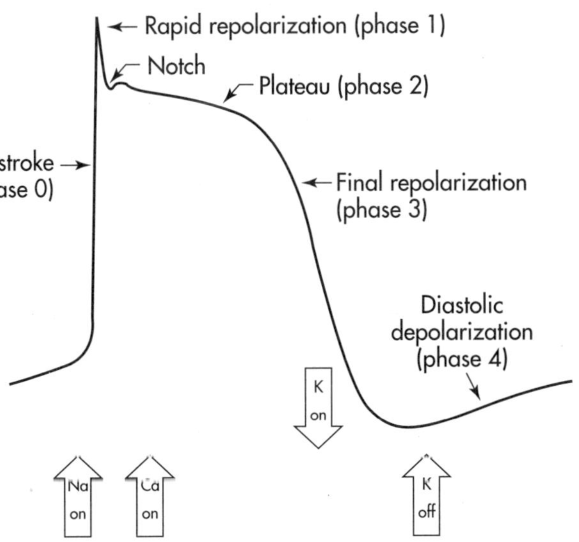

FIGURE 5-1 Schematic drawing of an action potential from a Purkinje fiber. Downward arrows depict movement of ions out of the cell; upright arrows depict movement into the cell. Diastolic depolarization occurs making this an automatic cell. (Redrawn from Cooksey JD, Dunn M, Massie E: *Clinical vectorcardiography and electrocardiography,* Chicago, 1977, Mosby.)

slightly positive during early depolarization but then rapidly repolarizes to a near neutral potential (phase 1) as sodium channels inactivate and a potassium current (I_{to}) turns on briefly. The cell then maintains this neutral potential (phase 2) for 150 to 250 ms (similar time to the Q-T interval) in dogs, depending on the heart rate. During this phase, slow calcium channels in the cell membrane open, allowing calcium to enter the cell and initiate contraction (excitation-contraction coupling; see Chapter 2). The cell membrane becomes relatively impermeable to potassium ions during phase 2 because the resistance to potassium ion transfer increases when the voltage of the cell increases. Conductance to sodium is low during this phase because the sodium channels are closed. At the end of phase 2, the inward slow calcium channels turn off and an outward potassium current (I_K) turns on. As the positively charged potassium ions leave the cell, the membrane potential decreases back to the resting potential. During diastole, another potassium current (I_{K1}) is active and is responsible for maintaining the stable resting potential in atrial, His-Purkinje, and ventricular cells.

CARDIAC PACEMAKERS

Cardiac cells can be divided into automatic and nonautomatic cells (Figure 5-2). Automatic cells (cells said to possess the property of automaticity) can depolarize on their own during phase 4 of the action potential. Automatic cells in the heart include sinus node P cells, AV node N cells, and Purkinje cells. Normal atrial and ventricular myocytes do not spontaneously depolarize (phase 4 is flat).

The sinus node and AV node cells have low resting membrane potentials of –40 to –70 mV. This is thought to be due to the lack of inward potassium channels in these tissues.[1] The resting potential during diastole (phase 4) in these cells is not stable. Instead, membrane potential gradually becomes more positive during diastole. In the sinus node, the cell membrane spontaneously depolarizes, primarily because of the influx of calcium through slow calcium channels and a decrease in the efflux of potassium through I_K. In Purkinje cells, diastolic depolarization occurs primarily because an inward current, I_f, becomes activated. The channel responsible for this current is nonspecific for monovalent cations. The I_f current in Purkinje cells is increased by catecholamines, resulting in an increase in the rate of spontaneous depolarization in phase 4 and so an increase in the rate of depolarization. Cholinergic stimulation has the opposite effect.

When the membrane potential reaches a critical potential, called the *threshold potential,* voltage-gated cell membrane L-type calcium channels in the sinus node open. This allows positively charged ions to enter the cell, which results in cell depolarization (phase 0). The slower calcium current produces a slower upstroke velocity of the action potential in nodal cells. The inside of the cell now becomes positive with respect to the outside of the cell (and the outside negative with respect to the inside of the cell). Depolarization of these cells is slower and the action potential shorter than for myocardial cells (see Figure 5-2). The rate of phase 4 depolarization can be altered. Rate alteration is primarily governed by the sympathetic and parasympathetic nervous systems. Acetylcholine hyperpolarizes the cell and decreases the slope of depolarization. These combine to increase the time that it takes for the cell to reach threshold potential and so decrease the rate of depolarization. This effect is explained by an increase in membrane potassium conductance through the delayed rectifier potassium channel.[1] Presumably, catecholamines have the opposite effect.

The rate of depolarization is different for different types of cells. Sinus node cells depolarize at a rate faster (60 to 180 beats/min in a dog) than AV nodal cells (40 to 60 beats/min in a dog) or Purkinje cells (20 to 40 beats/min in a dog). Consequently, the sinus node normally depolarizes before the other automatic cells have the opportunity to depolarize. Because of this, it normally controls the rate of the heart.

THE SPECIALIZED CONDUCTION SYSTEM

The primary active components of the heart are the myocardium and the specialized conduction system. The specialized conduction system starts at the sinus node and terminates at the Purkinje network in the ventricles (Figure 5-3). The specialized conduction system has two basic functions. First, cells in specific regions of the system are automatic and so can initiate cardiac depolarization. Second, the rest of the system is responsible for conducting the cardiac electrical impulse throughout the heart in a coordinated fashion.

The sinus node. The sinus node is a collection of specialized cells that lie at the junction of the right atrium and the cranial vena cava (Figures 5-3 and 5-4). Cells in the sinus node include nodal, or P cells, transitional cells, and atrial muscle cells closely packed within a fibrous tissue matrix. The P cells are the source of impulse formation. These cells depolarize at a rate faster than any other collection of automatic cells in the heart and so normally control the pacing function of the heart. The transitional cells, or T cells, are responsible for conducting the electrical impulse from the P cells to the internodal tracts and atrial muscle.

The sinus node is richly innervated with sympathetic and parasympathetic fibers. It contains an equivalent concentration of norepinephrine to the rest of the right atrium but has a much higher concentration of acetylcholine. This is physical evidence that cholinergic tone, which slows sinus rate discharge, is high at rest; whereas sympathetic tone, which increases sinus node rate, is lower at rest. The fact that cholinergic tone predominates at rest can be easily demonstrated by administering an anticholinergic agent, such as atropine, and observing the heart rate increase by 50% to 100% and then administering a β-adrenergic blocking agent, such as propranolol, and observing only a minor decrease in the heart rate in a normal dog. The autonomic nervous system not only controls the sinus node rate but also the site within the sinus node that depolarizes first. Normally, depolarization originates in the middle or cranial

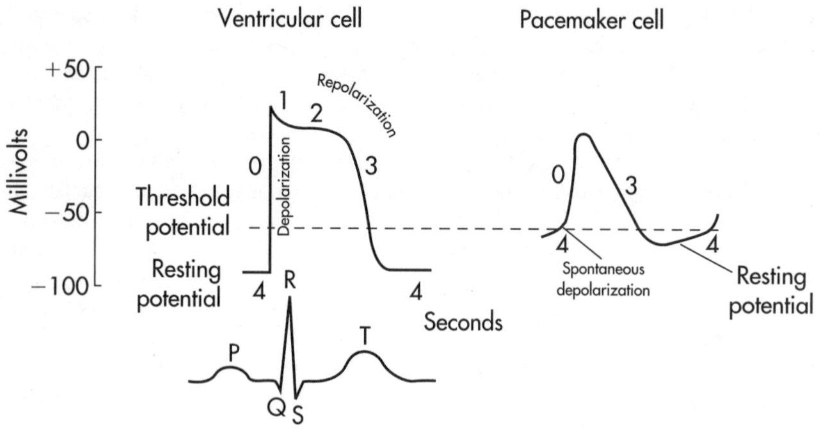

FIGURE 5-2 Schematic action potentials from a ventricular myocyte and a sinus node P cell. The ventricular cell has no spontaneous diastolic depolarization, whereas the pacemaker cell does. The upstroke velocity of phase 0 in the ventricular cell is fast because of fast sodium channel activity, whereas the upstroke velocity of the pacemaker cell is slow because it depolarizes via slow calcium channels. (From Tilley LP: *Essentials of canine and feline electrocardiography,* ed 3, Philadelphia, 1992, Lea & Febiger.)

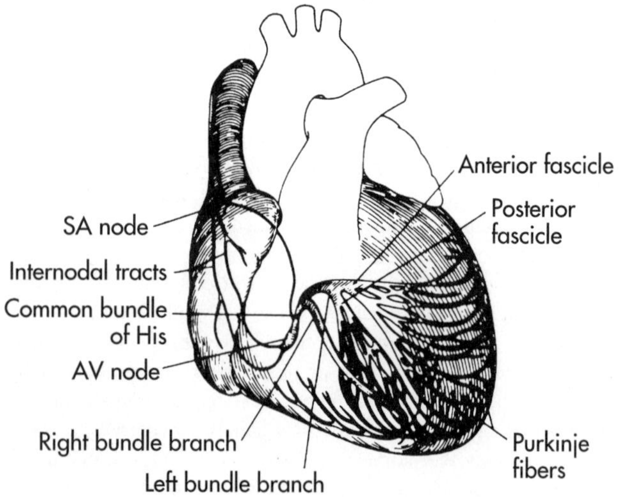

FIGURE 5-3 Drawing of the conduction system. The SA node lies at the junction of the cranial vena cava and the right atrium. The internodal tracts course across the atria to join the atrioventricular (AV) node. The left bundle branch starts as a discrete stalk and then fans out across the left side of the interventricular septum. There is no distinct anatomic division of the left bundle branch into anterior and posterior fascicles. (From Tilley LP: *Essentials of canine and feline electrocardiography,* ed 3, Philadelphia, 1992, Lea & Febiger.)

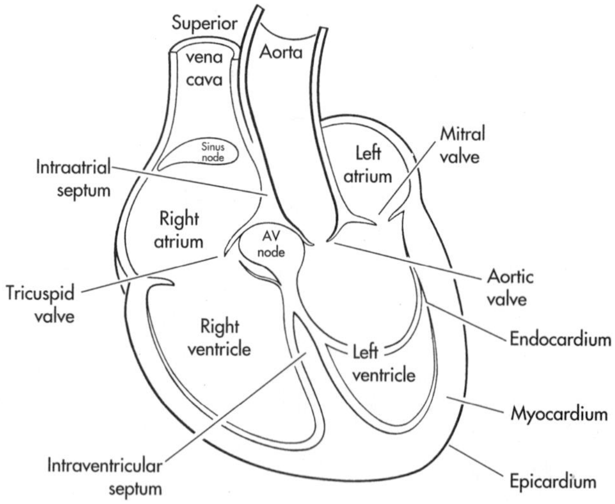

FIGURE 5-4 Schematic representation of the heart and conduction system minus the internodal tracts. There is an exaggerated division in the left bundle branch. (Redrawn from Phillips RE, Feeney MK: *Cardiac rhythms: a systematic approach to interpretation,* ed 3, Philadelphia, 1990, WB Saunders.)

regions of the node, and the cranial internodal pathway is activated first.[2] Vagal stimulation of the sinus node results in the initial site of activation switching to the caudal region of the sinus node, activating the middle and caudal internodal tracts first. Vagal stimulation at times can result in suppression of sinus node activity to the point that the site of pacing moves out of the sinus node to automatic tissue in the region of the coronary sinus. These shifts in the site of pacing (wandering pacemaker) result in changes in the P wave configuration on the ECG during changes in vagal tone. Vagal efferents to the heart converge in ganglions in a fat pad that lies at the junction of the cranial vena cava and the aorta.[3] The vagal efferents that traverse to the sinus node course through another fat pad that lies close to the pulmonary veins returning from the right lung lobes.

The internodal tracts. Internodal tracts connect the sinus node with the AV node (see Figure 5-3). The existence of these tracts or bundles is controversial in humans, although they have been clearly identified in dogs.[4,5] The cranial, or anterior, internodal pathway begins at the sinus node and curves cranially along the cranial vena cava to enter Bachmann's bundle, a large muscle band that preferentially conducts the cardiac impulse from the right atrium to the left atrium. From here the cranial internodal pathway descends along the interatrial septum to the AV node. The middle internodal tract descends along the interatrial septum just cranial to the region of the fossa ovalis. The caudal, or posterior, internodal tract travels along the crista terminalis and descends along the interatrial septum caudal to the coronary sinus to the AV node. The internodal tracts conduct the cardiac electrical impulses quickly from the sinus node to the atrioventricular junctional tissue. Not only do these tracts conduct more rapidly than does atrial muscle, they are also more resistant to the effects of hyperkalemia. In severe hyperkalemia the resting membrane potential of atrial muscle decreases, ultimately resulting in the muscle failing to depolarize and conduct. The internodal pathways continue to conduct the cardiac electrical impulse from the sinus node to the atrioventricular junction, allowing the sinus node to maintain its cardiac pacing function (sinoventricular conduction).[6]

The atrioventricular node. The atrioventricular (AV) junction of the heart has been recently reexamined and redefined in dogs.[5] In this region, the caudal and middle internodal tracts converge to form the proximal AV bundle. The cranial internodal tract joins the distal portion of the proximal AV bundle that then forms the AV node. The AV junctional region is a collection of fibers that are 1 to 2 mm in diameter in the dog. It begins in the floor of the right atrium, a few millimeters cranioventral to the opening of the coronary sinus and craniodorsal to the septal leaflet of the tricuspid valve (see Figure 5-3). From here it courses forward and downward through the fibrous base of the heart. The AV node itself is encased within the central fibrous body. This prevents any atrial fibers from joining it. The AV node connects with the bundle of His, or distal AV bundle, which starts within the central fibrous body and then penetrates it to form the bundle branches. The AV node is generally considered the region of slowest conduction in the specialized conduction system. However, recent evidence shows that conduction through the proximal AV bundle is much slower than through the AV node, accounting for 67% of the delay between the sinus node and the bundle of His.[6] Maximum upstroke velocity (V_{max}) of an action potential correlates well with conduction velocity. One study has shown that V_{max} in proximal AV bundle tissue is 2.5 V/sec, whereas in the AV node it is 7.0 V/sec.[7] V_{max} in the bundle of His is much greater (33 V/sec). Phase 0 of depolarization is much flatter in these cell types than in myocardium (1 to 10 V/s vs. 200 to 800 V/s) (see Figure 5-2). Depolarization velocity determines conduction velocity. As such, conduction velocity in myocardium is faster than in automatic tissue like the AV node (0.5 to 1 m/sec for myocardium vs. 0.01 to 0.1 m/sec for the proximal AV bundle).

When the AV junctional area is experimentally transected in isolated dog hearts between the proximal AV bundle and the AV node, the AV node continues to depolarize at a rate of 36 beats/min.[6] If transection occurs between the AV node and the bundle of His, the Purkinje fibers depolarize at a rate of 24 beats/min. Depolarization rates in live dogs are probably faster, corresponding to the rates of 40 to 60 beats/min for the AV node and 20 to 40 beats/min for Purkinje tissue observed clinically in patients with escape rhythms.

Like the sinus node, the AV junction is richly innervated with cholinergic and adrenergic fibers. Both right and left sympathetic and parasympathetic nerves innervate the AV junction, but the left nerves predominate. After leaving the ganglia in the fat pad at the cranial vena cava–aortic junction, vagal efferents pass through another fat pad that lies between the caudal vena cava and the left atrium.[3]

The bundle branches. The bundle of His divides into two bundle branches immediately beneath the membranous septum. The bundle branches conduct the electrical impulse about 3 times as fast as myocardium (2 to 4 m/sec). They are responsible for rapidly conducting the impulse coming from the bundle of His to the Purkinje fibers. The right bundle branch descends as an unbranched extension of the bundle of His beneath the endocardium on the right side of the interventricular septum (see Figures 5-3 and 5-4). Toward the apex it courses from the interventricular septum to the right ventricular free wall in the moderator band. The left bundle branch descends beneath the endocardium on the left side of the interventricular septum. It branches immediately and spreads out like a fan over the interventricular septum (see Figure 5-3). The left bundle is commonly divided into anterior and posterior fascicles for electrocardiographic purposes (see Figure 5-4). However, no electrophysiologic correlate or anatomic correlate for this division exists.

The Purkinje fibers. The terminal Purkinje fibers connect with the ends of the bundle branches to form an interweaving network of fibers in the subendocardium of both ventricles. In dogs and cats, the Purkinje fibers penetrate about one third of the way into the myocardium, just as they do in humans.[8] The Purkinje fibers are also responsible for rapid (conduction velocity = 2 to 4 m/sec) and orderly distribution of the electrical impulse to both ventricles.

CARDIAC DEPOLARIZATION

Once P cells in the sinus node depolarize, they depolarize cells next to them. A wave of depolarization is set up that travels across the atrial myocardium as depolarization of one cell forces the cells next to it to depolarize, which in turn depolarize more cells (Figure 5-5). The wave of depolarization that starts at the sinus node spreads like a ripple in a pond across the atria and produces atrial contraction. This wave spreads from right to left and from cranial to caudal. The depolarization wave ultimately reaches the AV node. However, the AV node starts to depolarize long before the wave of atrial muscle activation reaches it because of the internodal tracts that connect the sinus node with the AV node.

When the cardiac electrical impulse enters the AV junction, it slows dramatically. This allows for a delay between atrial contraction and ventricular contraction. When the impulse emerges from the AV node into the bundle of His, it speeds dramatically to reach the bundle branches and Purkinje network. The length of the action potential gradually increases as a function of the length from the AV node to reach a maximum near the Purkinje fiber–ventricular muscle junctions. Action potential duration and refractoriness then shorten. This prevents the electrical impulse from reentering the conduction system and producing an arrhythmia. The cardiac impulse then depolarizes the ventricular myocardium, spreading from cell to cell,

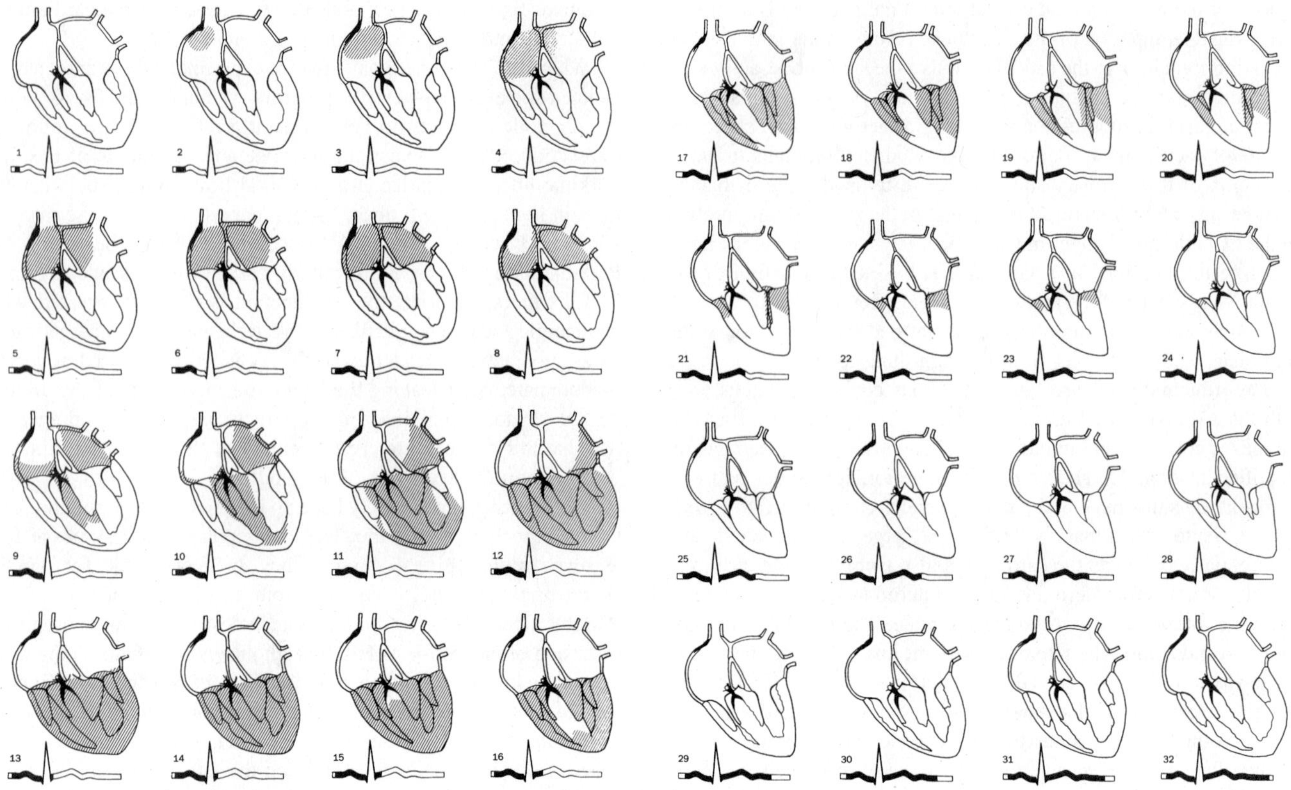

FIGURE 5-5 Schematic drawings of depolarization and repolarization of the heart and their influence on the ECG. Depolarization is depicted as hatch marks. Repolarization is depicted as the hatch marks turning white again. Depolarization of the conduction system is not visualized. (From Hurst JW: *Ventricular electrocardiography,* New York, 1991, Gower Medical.)

from endocardium to epicardium, and from right to left. Figure 5-6 depicts that actual sequence of ventricular activation in dogs. Initial (0 to 3 ms) activation starts toward the apex of the heart, along the left side of the interventricular septum (the right part of the left ventricle) and in the subendocardium of the right ventricle. At this time the waves are traveling primarily left to right and caudal to cranial. Next (5 to 8 ms) the wave spreads circumferentially, encompassing the subendocardiums of both ventricles. The waves are spreading equally in all directions, although there may be a general movement from apex to base. About 10 to 12 ms after ventricular activation starts, the right ventricle, except the basilar region, is completely depolarized. After that, the left ventricle continues to depolarize, with the primary wavefront traveling right to left and cranial to caudal.

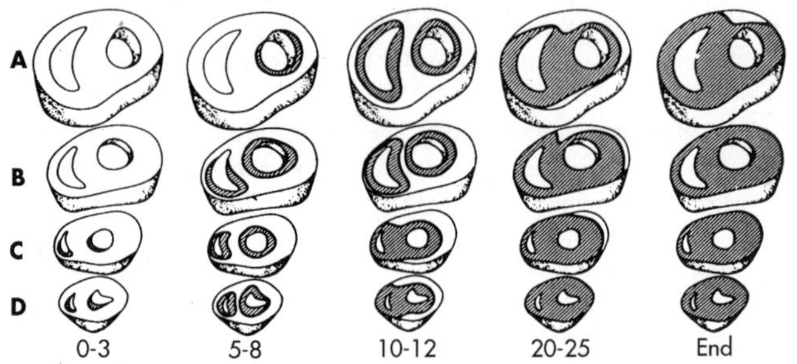

FIGURE 5-6 Map of the sequence of activation of the ventricles in the dog. The ventricles are cut into four cross-sections from base **(A)** to apex **(D).** Five periods are represented starting 0 to 3 ms after activation until the end of activation. The right ventricular cavity is crescent-shaped and to the left, and the left ventricular cavity is round and to the right. Cross-hatched areas represent depolarization. (From Cooksey JD, Dunn M, Massie E: *Clinical vectorcardiography and electrocardiography,* Chicago, 1977, Mosby.)

EQUIVALENT DIPOLE THEORY

A dipole is a positive and negative charge separated by a small distance that generates an electrical force (Figure 5-7). If one dipole is submersed in a conducting medium, such as water, the dipole generates an electric field throughout the conducting medium. A wavefront consists of numerous dipoles. In a homogeneous volume conductor, such as a container of water, the electric field generated by this wavefront is symmetrically distributed. The lines of the electrical field are symmetric in relation to a line that is perpendicular to the dipole and transects it at its midpoint. This theoretic electrical potential can be measured with a galvanometer (e.g., an electrocardiograph) by placing recording electrodes on either side of the medium (i.e., a lead) containing the dipole. This was first performed by Augustus Waller in 1877. The magnitude of the potential measured depends on the strength of the source, how close the electrodes are to the dipole, and the angle of a line drawn from the electrode to the midpoint of the dipole. The relationship is expressed as: $V = m \cos\theta/r^2$, where V = voltage, m = strength of the source, $\cos\theta$ = the cosine of the angle between the wavefront and the lead, and r = the distance the electrodes are from the dipole. Figure 5-7 depicts a line of dipoles (a wavefront) created by depolarizing myocardium. When myocardium is not depolarizing, the inside of the cell is negative with respect to the outside of the cell. Consequently, the outside of the cell must be positive with respect to the inside of the cell. When the cell depolarizes, the charges reverse such that the outside of the cell is negative with respect to the inside

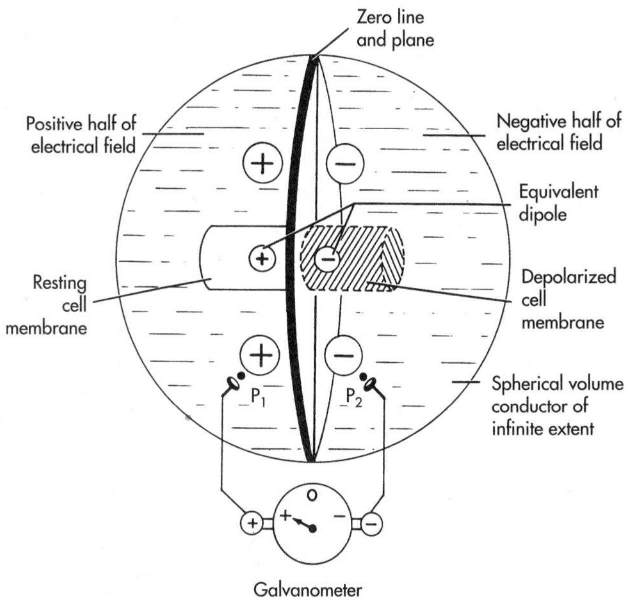

FIGURE 5-7 Schematic representation of equivalent dipoles along the surface of a wavefront. Two electrodes (+ and –) have been placed on either side of the wavefront and attached to a galvanometer to form a lead and record the electric field. The wavefront is spreading from left to right, toward the positive pole, resulting in a positive deflection on the galvanometer. (From Cooksey JD, Dunn M, Massie E: *Clinical vectorcardiography and electrocardiography,* Chicago, 1977, Mosby.)

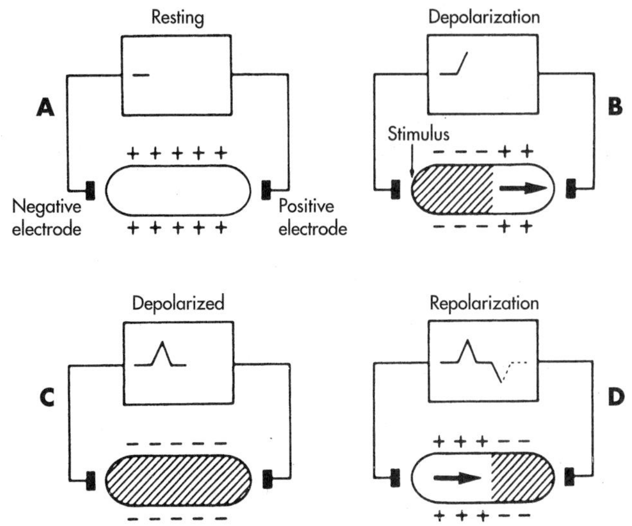

FIGURE 5-8 Similar drawing to Figure 5-7, in which a positive and a negative electrode have been placed on either side of a strip of myocardium. The left end is activated and the wave of depolarization spreads from left to right, toward the positive electrode. This produces a positive (upright by convention) deflection on the recording paper of the electrocardiograph. When fully depolarized the deflection returns to baseline. Repolarization results in the opposite. (From Tilley LP: Essentials of Canine and Feline Electrocardiography, ed 3, Philadelphia, 1992, Lea & Febiger.)

of the cell. The electrocardiograph "sees" a depolarization wavefront as a wavefront with positive charges along the leading edge (cells not yet depolarized) and negative charges along the trailing (depolarized) edge. Consequently, if a positive electrode is placed such that the wavefront travels toward it, it will detect it as a positive potential. Conversely, if the electrodes are reversed, it will detect positive charges coming toward the negative electrode and will record a negative potential.

We can take this one step further by examining a larger strip of myocardium in a water bath (Figure 5-8). Again we can place two electrodes (one positive, one negative) on either side of the myocardium to form a lead. When the myocardium is not depolarizing, the outside of the myocardium is positive with respect to the intracellular milieu. At rest, all of the dipoles cancel each other out, so no net activity is recorded by the ECG. One end of the muscle strip can then be depolarized, stimulating a wave of depolarization to travel from that end to the other. The wavefront has positive charges in front and negative charges behind. Each positive and negative charge is a dipole, each creating a small electrical field. All of the small electrical fields at the wavefront add up to a larger electrical field. To the positive electrode that the wave is traveling toward, this appears as a positively charged wavefront coming at the electrode. Conversely, it also appears as a positive wavefront traveling away from the opposite negative electrode. During depolarization, a positive (upright by convention) deflection is inscribed by the galvanometer or ECG connected to the positive electrode. When depolarization is complete, the ECG recording returns to the baseline. Repolarization occurs as a wavefront traveling in the same direction. However, now the wavefront has negative charges in the leading edge and positive charges along the trailing edge. Consequently, a negative deflection is inscribed.

Let us now alter the three variables that determine the size of the voltage deflection recorded on the ECG. We know that the voltage inscribed will depend on the size of the depolarization wavefront (the voltage source), the distance of the lead from the source *(r),* and the orientation of the lead to the wavefront of dipoles (cosθ). We want to measure the size of the depolarization wavefront because the size of this wavefront should vary with the size of the source (the heart). We also want to measure the direction that the wavefront is traveling because this will change as the heart enlarges or conduction in the heart changes. Moving the electrodes closer to or farther away from the heart increases or decreases the size of the voltage deflection. We factor this out in clinical medicine by always placing the electrodes at fixed anatomic sites (i.e., at the elbows and stifles).

Changing the orientation of the lead (the two electrodes) with the wavefront changes the size of the deflection, as seen in Figure 5-9. This is critically important. This physical fact allows one to determine the direction a wavefront is traveling by using more than one set of electrodes (leads) to examine the wavefront. If the wavefront is traveling parallel with a lead, the largest deflection occurs. If the wavefront is traveling perpendicular to a lead, no deflection occurs. If the lead is somewhere between parallel and perpendicular, a defection somewhere between smallest and largest occurs. By using more than one lead, with each lead oriented in a different direction, one can examine the heights of the deflections in each lead and determine the direction of the wavefront.

In the heart, more than one wavefront may be present or the wavefront may not travel in one simple direction. The other important fact to remember is that the ECG only "sees" the average wavefront. Consequently, if one wavefront is traveling toward the positive pole and another is traveling away from it simultaneously, the smaller electrical field will be subtracted from the other to give an average electrical force. Consequently, although a wavefront is made up of numerous dipoles, the wavefront itself is seen as one large dipole. Each dipole can be represented by a vector (an arrow that represents the direction and magnitude of a dipole). All dipoles have the same magnitude. However if numerous dipoles are present, they will add together to form a larger resultant dipole. As such, a wavefront can be depicted as one vector that represents thousands of smaller vectors by adding and subtracting all the small vectors together.

Now we know that we can record electrical potentials from a strip of myocardium in a beaker of water. In real life, the strip of myocardium is the heart and the beaker of water is the body. The sequence of cardiac activation is more complex than the sequence of activation of a strip of myocardium. Although we pretend that it is, the body is not a homogeneous volume conductor like a beaker of water (Figure 5-10). Still, the same principles apply such that sense can be made of the waveforms derived. We also pretend that the strength of the dipoles along the wavefront of depolarization is uniform. It is not.[9] Myocardial cells are longer than they are wide, and each cell can depolarize contiguous cells. The connections between cells are predominantly at the ends of the cell, and the longitudinal depolarization of myocardium travels 3 times as fast as transverse depolarization. Consequently, the wavefront is not uniform but is strongest parallel to the long axes of the cells.

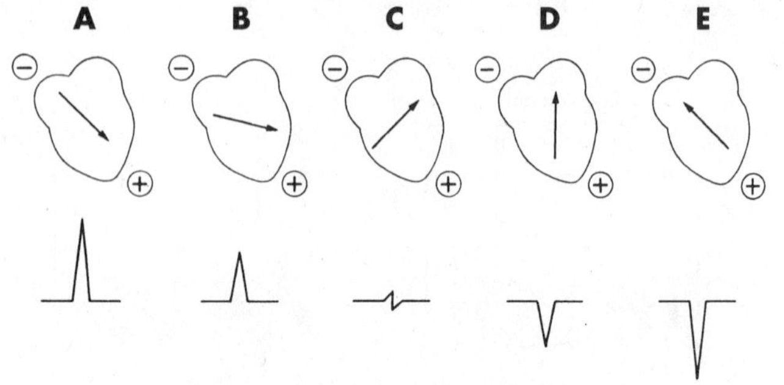

FIGURE 5-9 One of the important things to remember about electrocardiography is that when a wavefront spreads directly toward an electrode, in parallel with a lead, the largest possible deflection will occur. When a wavefront spreads perpendicular to a lead, the smallest or no deflection occurs. In this schematic drawing, average wavefronts of depolarization are represented by a vector. The effect of changing the orientation of the wavefront to the lead depicted (lead II) is shown. (From Tilley LP: *Essentials of canine and feline electrocardiography,* ed 3, Philadelphia, 1992, Lea & Febiger.)

THE LEAD SYSTEM

One goal of recording an ECG is to determine the magnitude of the wavefront and the direction it is traveling. The best way to do this is to use multiple leads to obtain multiple orientations to the average wavefront and to keep these leads a constant distance from the heart. As described in the information presented above, a lead placed parallel with the direction a particular wavefront is moving will get the largest deflection on the ECG, and a lead placed perpendicular to the wavefront that gets a small deflection or no deflection at all. If a wavefront is traveling toward a positive electrode, a positive deflection will be recorded, and if it is traveling toward a negative electrode, a negative deflection will be recorded. All that is necessary now to determine the direction a wavefront is traveling is to either take a lead and move it around to identify the largest deflection or place several different leads and identify the lead with the largest deflection. In clinical medicine the latter is done. When the largest deflection is identified, the height of the complex can be measured to make a rough determination of the average size of the wavefront and so obtain an approximation of the size of a chamber.

Willem Einthoven, a Dutch physiologist, devised the first electrocardiograph in 1902 and the first fixed lead system used to record clinical ECGs.[10] The lead system consisted of three bipolar (one positive and one negative pole or electrode) leads formed by placing three electrodes on three limbs, one on the right front leg, one on the left front leg, and one on the left rear leg (Figure 5-11).

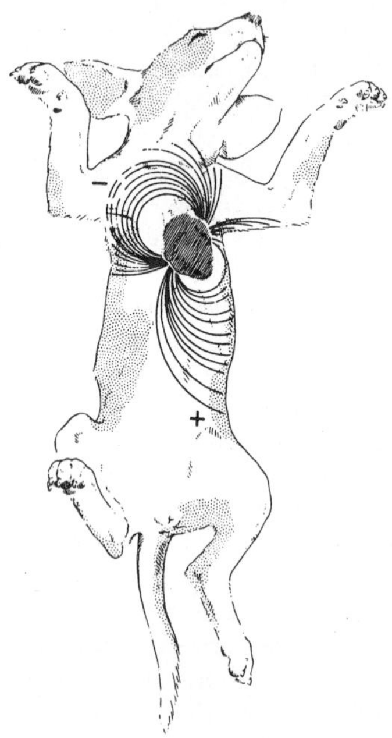

FIGURE 5-10 Electrocardiographic theory depends on the body acting as a homogeneous volume conductor, much like a water bath. Because of its shape and the differing tissues contained in the body it cannot act as such a conductor. However, for clinical work, this variation from perfect theory is probably not significant. This schematic drawing depicts the electrical wavefront spreading throughout the body to the periphery. Electrical potentials are recorded in volts in the heart. By the time they reach the electrodes attached to the body they are recorded in millivolts. (From Edwards NJ: *Bolton's handbook of canine and feline electrocardiography,* ed 2, Philadelphia, 1987, WB Saunders.)

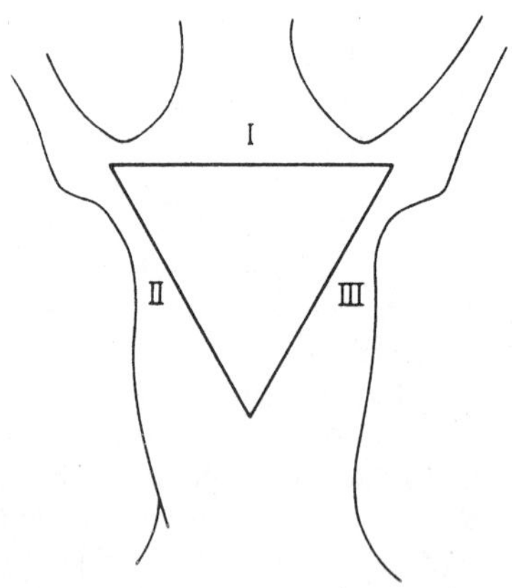

FIGURE 5-11 Einthoven's triangle is made up of three leads (I, II, III) to form an equilateral triangle about the heart. (From Tilley LP: *Essentials of canine and feline electrocardiography,* ed 3, Philadelphia, 1992, Lea & Febiger.)

These leads all lay within one plane (the frontal plane) and formed a triangle (Einthoven's triangle; Figures 5-11 and 5-12). He labeled them leads *I, II,* and *III.* Because the depolarization waves normally spread from right to left and from cranial to caudal in the heart, Einthoven placed the positive electrodes of these leads on the left side of the body and the caudal body so that positive deflections were recorded on the ECG. Einthoven labeled the lead that has a positive electrode on the left front leg and a negative electrode on the right front leg, lead I (Figure 5-13). Lead II had its positive electrode on the left caudal leg and the negative electrode on the right front leg. Lead III also had its positive electrode on the left caudal leg with its negative electrode on the left front leg. Although devised theoretically to be an equilateral triangle about the heart, placing the electrodes on the limbs negated this effect. However, for clinical determinations this lead system is adequate.

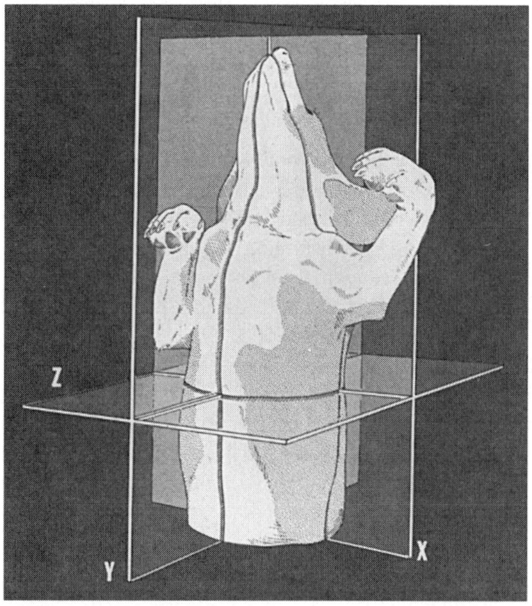

FIGURE 5-12 The three planes of the body: *X* (frontal), *Y* (sagittal), and *Z* (transverse). The limb leads (I to aV_F) lie within the frontal plane, which can be imperfectly defined by leads I and aV_F. The sagittal plane can be approximated by leads aV_F and V_{10}. The transverse plane can be approximated by leads I and V_{10}. (From Edwards NJ: *Bolton's handbook of canine and feline electrocardiography,* ed 2, Philadelphia, 1987, WB Saunders.)

Unipolar leads are used in addition to bipolar leads. They use the same electrodes as leads I, II, and III. These leads use one electrode as the positive electrode and the average of the other two electrodes to form a neutral reference point, rather than having a negative electrode (Figure 5-14). Unipolar leads record one half the voltage of a bipolar lead. To make the deflections produced by these leads comparable to the other three leads, the ECG machine amplifies the deflections of the unipolar leads, effectively doubling their height. Consequently, these leads are called *augmented* leads. This is denoted by placing an *a* in front of the rest of their designations (aV_R, aV_L, and aV_F). Lead aV_L has a positive electrode on the left front leg (the same as lead I) but uses a summation of the forces across lead II as its reference. Lead aV_R is opposite, with the positive electrode on the right front leg and lead III as the reference. Lead aV_F's positive pole is on the left caudal leg and lead I serves as the neutral reference. Because the positive poles of leads aV_R and aV_L are cranial to the heart, their complexes are primarily negative in a normal animal, with aV_R being more negative than aV_L. The complexes in lead aV_F, which is midway between leads II and III, are normally positive.

According to Einthoven's hypothesis, the limb leads reflect activity of all parts of the heart. Unipolar leads attached to the chest were devised later in electrocardiographic history to measure electrical events limited to specific regions of the heart. It was argued that if one could devise an indifferent electrode paired with an exploring electrode, one could place the exploring electrode over different regions of the heart to record activity from a specific region. To create an indifferent electrode, the right front leg, the left front leg, and the left rear leg were electrically connected through resistors to a common junction in the electrocardiograph, named the *central terminal.* This terminal theoretically produces a net voltage of zero. The theory that one could "sample" electrical activity locally was later shown to be inaccurate. Rather, this type of lead acts as if the indifferent electrode is at the anatomic center of the heart and the exploring electrode is a positive electrode at some distance to the heart, albeit a shorter distance than with limb leads. Consequently, the principle value of these leads is that they sample the electrical field in directions (i.e., in a different plane) not covered by the limb leads. A positive exploring electrode placed on the chest coupled with the indifferent electrode is termed a *V (voltage) lead.* To record these leads, the exploring electrode is physically moved from position to position on the chest or multiple exploring electrodes are used. In

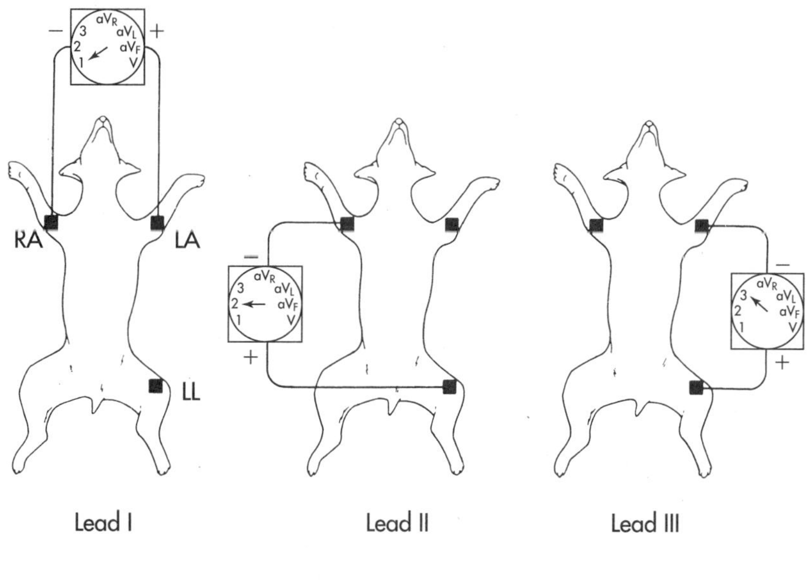

FIGURE 5-13 The three bipolar limb leads and the placement of their electrodes. (From Tilley LP: *Essentials of canine and feline electrocardiography,* ed 3, Philadelphia, 1992, Lea & Febiger.)

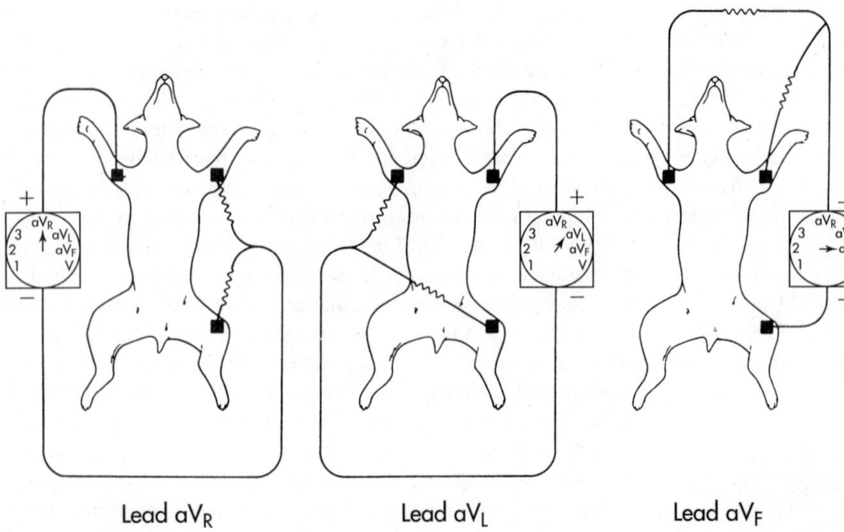

FIGURE 5-14 The three unipolar limb leads and their electrodes. The ECG machine doubles the height of the recordings from these leads to make their height similar to the bipolar leads. (From Tilley LP: *Essentials of canine and feline electrocardiography,* ed 3, Philadelphia, 1992, Lea & Febiger.)

humans, six standard positions are used. The exploring electrode for V_1 is placed in the fourth intercostal space, just to the right of the sternum. The exploring electrode for V_6 is placed in the fourth intercostal space at the midaxillary line. The other chest leads (V_2 to V_5) are spaced equidistant between these two points. In dogs, the use of exploring V leads was described in 1949 by Lannek[11] and was modified by Detweiler and Patterson[12] in 1965. In dogs, the fifth and sixth intercostal spaces are used. Consequently, new terminology was coined for dogs. In dogs and cats, four common positions are used:

CV_{5RL}—Fifth right intercostal space near the edge of the sternum
CV_{6LL}—Sixth left intercostal space near the edge of the sternum
CV_{6LU}—Sixth intercostal space at the costochondral junction
V_{10}—Over the dorsal spinous process of the seventh thoracic vertebra

Chest leads are of limited value in dogs and cats. We rarely use V_{10} or CV_{5RL} clinically because little additional clinical information is gained using these leads (although V_{10} can theoretically be used to determine electrical axes in the transverse and sagittal planes). As outlined below, the left chest leads are more sensitive at detecting right ventricular enlargement than the other leads. At times, P waves can be identified more easily in the left chest leads than other leads. These are the primary reasons for using the chest (V) leads in dogs and cats. In humans they are primarily used to identify the location of myocardial infarction following coronary artery occlusion.

Genesis of the Electrocardiogram

RELATIONSHIP OF DEPOLARIZATION TO ECG DEFLECTIONS

Let us examine the genesis of the ECG using leads I, II, and III. When the sinus node depolarizes, no wavefront of dipoles exists. Consequently, no deflection is recorded on the ECG (see Figure 5-5). Immediately after sinus node depolarization, the atria depolarize from muscle cell to muscle cell. The wavefront starts at the junction of the right atrium and cranial vena cava and spreads from right to left and from cranial to caudal (Figure 5-15). This produces a small upright deflection on the ECG in leads I, II, III, and aV_F and a negative deflection in leads aV_R and aV_L, called the *P wave.* Because the wavefront (the average vector) is spreading directly toward the positive pole of lead II, the largest P wave is recorded in lead II. Because it is mostly perpendicular to lead aV_L (the lead perpendicular to lead II), the P wave in this lead is the smallest. As depolarization is traveling across the atrial myocardium, it spreads rapidly through the internodal tracts to the AV node. Consequently, the AV node starts to depolarize before the P wave is completely inscribed.

Next the cardiac impulse conducts slowly through the AV node, and then rapidly through the bundle of His, bundle branches, and Purkinje network. No deflection is recorded again during this phase, because there is no depolarization wave. Instead, the impulse conducts primarily intracellularly in a linear fashion. Consequently, the ECG returns to the baseline for a short time (30 to 100 ms) after the P wave is inscribed.

When the cardiac impulse reaches ventricular myocardium, wavefronts of depolarization are again created, conducting relatively slowly from muscle cell to muscle cell. As shown previously, depolarization through the ventricles is more complex than through the atria (see Figure 5-6). Spread of initial activity in the septum is from left to right and in the right ventricular wall from endocardium to epicardium (left to right). This results in an average wavefront (the sum of the two wavefronts) that travels toward the right ventricle (Figure 5-16). Because the right side of the heart is positioned cranially and to the right in the chest, the average wavefront travels toward the negative poles and away from the positive poles of leads I, II, III, and aV_F. This produces a negative deflection on the ECG in these leads called the *Q wave.* A Q wave is defined as the first negative deflection of the QRS complex on an ECG. In lead aV_R a positive deflection is produced. Although it is a recording of the same electrical event, in lead aV_R this is called an *R wave,* because the first positive deflection is always called an R wave. Next, a radiation of both wavefronts proceeds circumferentially, spreading outward from the endocardium to the outer surfaces of each ventricle. Because both wavefronts are spreading evenly in all directions, the electrical forces that they produce cancel each other out. Consequently, the ECG returns to baseline 5 to 8 ms after initiation of ventricular depolarization. By 10 to 12 ms after initiation of depolarization, all of the apical right ventricle and interventricular septum are depolarized. The left ventricle and base of the heart depolarize next, with the average wavefront traveling toward the left, caudally and dorsally. The wavefront traveling dorsally is perpendicular to the frontal plane and so does not register a deflection of any magnitude.

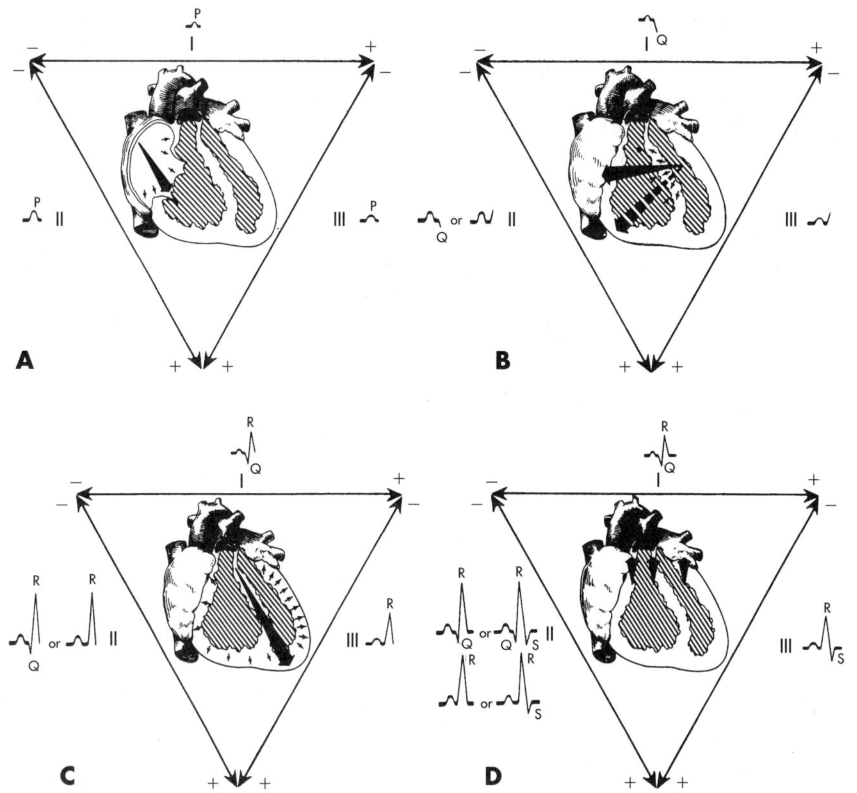

FIGURE 5-15 Schematic representations of the generation of waveforms on the ECG from wavefronts within the heart. **A,** Atrial depolarization results in an average wavefront *(large arrow)* spreading caudally and to the left, parallel with lead II. This produces the P wave. Lead II has the largest P wave. **B,** Early activation of the interventricular septum and right ventricular subendocardium results in the wavefront of ventricular depolarization spreading initially from left to right. This inscribes a negative deflection in lead I (Q wave). At the same time it can spread either slightly caudal to cranial or slightly cranial to caudal. This produces either a Q wave or the beginning of the R wave in lead II. An R wave is depicted in lead III. **C.** Next the rest of the ventricular myocardium is activated. Because the left ventricle is much larger than the right ventricle, it has a larger wavefront, which predominates, drawing the average vector caudally and to the left. This results in an R wave in all the bipolar leads. The R wave in lead II is the largest because it is oriented parallel with the average wavefront. **D,** The last portions of the ventricles activated are the basilar portions. This may produce a terminal negative deflection (S wave) in some leads. (From Edwards NJ: *Bolton's handbook of canine and feline electrocardiography,* ed 2, Philadelphia, 1987, WB Saunders.)

The average wavefront travels toward the positive electrodes in leads I, II, III, and aV_F, producing a positive deflection on the ECG (the R wave). Because the left ventricle is positioned in the thorax more caudally than it is to the left and more leftward than rightward, lead II in a normal dog has the largest R wave. In a heart that lies somewhat horizontally in the chest, the depolarization of the base of the heart at the end of ventricular depolarization may produce a second negative deflection called the *S wave*. This wave is either not present or very small in normal dogs. Once the entire heart is depolarized, the ECG deflection returns to the baseline. Following depolarization, the ventricles repolarize and produce the T wave on the ECG (see below).

Using all six limb leads and knowing where the positive and negative electrodes are positioned allows one to examine the wavefronts of depolarization and determine in which direction the average wavefront is traveling at any point in time (Figure 5-17). By identifying the largest deflection and knowing in which lead it is produced and the orientation of that lead, one can identify the average direction of the average wavefront. This is the same way the direction of a wavefront in a strip of muscle was determined in the beaker experiment. For example, if the R wave in lead I is taller than the R waves in all other leads, the ventricular wave of depolarization must be traveling from right to left and more directly toward the positive pole of lead I than any other lead. If, on the other hand, the largest deflection on the ECG is a terminal negative deflection (an S wave) in lead aV_F, the ventricular wavefront must be traveling toward the negative pole of lead aV_F (from caudal to cranial), toward the head. Because the largest chamber is depolarized last and the right ventricle is situated cranially within the thorax, this must mean that the right ventricle is larger than the left ventricle. Determining the average direction of the ventricular wave of depolarization is called determining the *mean electrical axis.*

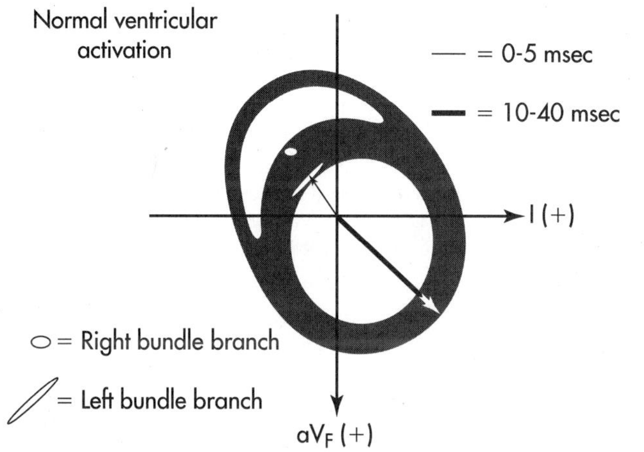

FIGURE 5-16 The dog ventricles depicted in the manner that the ECG "sees" them in the frontal plane in cross-section. Early ventricular activation is cranial and to the right. Most of the QRS complex is generated by the average wavefront *(heavy arrow)* spreading toward the left and caudally.

SIZES OF COMPLEXES: DOGS VS. CATS

Complexes in cats are smaller than in dogs. This is primarily because a dog heart is larger with respect to body size than a cat heart. Average heart weight to body weight ratio in dogs is approximately 0.8%. In cats this number is closer to 0.5%. This makes sense because cats have evolved to be sedentary creatures, whereas dogs have evolved to work.

NAMING THE QRS COMPLEX

The QRS complex represents electrical depolarization of the ventricles. The QRS complexes in all leads are named by a convention that can be confusing. An R wave is defined as the first positive deflection associated with ventricular activation (Figure 5-18). A Q wave is defined as the first negative deflection preceding the R wave. The S wave is defined as the first negative deflection after the R wave. Because the positive electrodes of some leads are attached caudally and to the left of the heart and some are attached cranially and to the right of the heart, the orientations of the QRS complexes are very different, although they represent the same electrical events. For example, leads II and aV_R are close to being opposite to each other. If a Q wave is observed in lead II, a comparable waveform is generated in lead aV_R but is a positive deflection and so termed an R wave. The Q wave in lead II and the R wave in lead aV_R represent the same electrical event. Nevertheless, because the QRS complex is named by convention, these two waveforms are named differently.

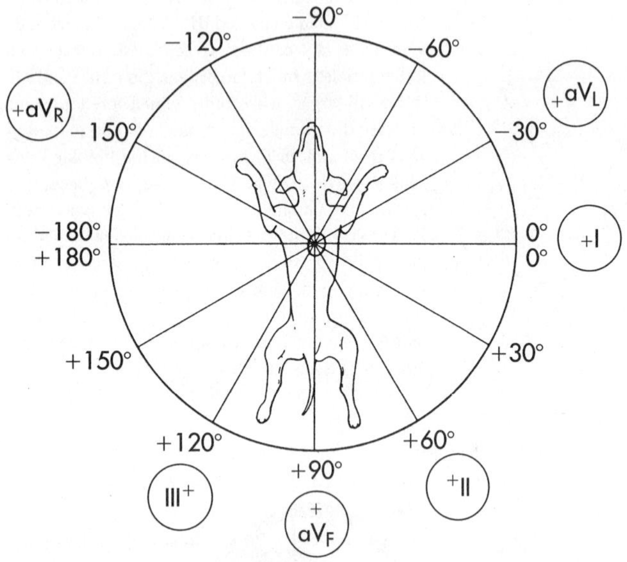

FIGURE 5-17 The hexaxial lead system formed by the six limb leads. This system is used to determine the average atrial and ventricular wavefront directions. (From Tilley LP: *Essentials of canine and feline electrocardiography,* ed 3, Philadelphia, 1992, Lea & Febiger.)

THE T WAVE

The T wave is generated during ventricular repolarization. Phase 3 of the action potential is related to the T wave in the same general way that phase 0 is related to the QRS complex. However, repolarization is an independent and complicated process that does not occur as a propagated wave during normal repolarization.[13] If it occurred as a propagated wave, it would inscribe a complex similar to the QRS complex. Instead the T wave is a much broader wave. In general, in the dog the epicardium repolarizes first and the endocardium last, and the apex repolarizes later than the base.[14] However, multiple areas of potential difference are oriented in many directions, resulting in frequently changing relationships as repolarization is completed in dogs.[15] Consequently, the T wave and its orientation to the QRS complex can change. As opposed to humans, the orientation of the T wave relative to the QRS complex is variable in dogs. In the standard limb leads, the T wave is upright approximately 50% of the time and is negative the other 50% of the time in any given lead.[16]

Recording and Calibrating the ECG

Numerous electrocardiograph machines are available for use. Some use a heated stylus and waxed recording paper, and others record on light-sensitive paper or record the waveforms digitally on a computer and print the waveforms on paper. Electrocardiographic machines commonly employ filters to decrease the baseline artifact. The filter must not limit any high-frequency deflections on the ECG, because this can decrease the size of the QRS complex. Usually, a 50-Hz filter can be used in dogs. Cats have high-frequency components to their ECG QRS complexes that are up to 150 Hz. Consequently, machines that filter anything less than 150 Hz artifactually decrease R and S wave amplitudes.[17] One must be especially careful with computer-generated ECGs and transtelephonic ECGs. If sampling rates are not

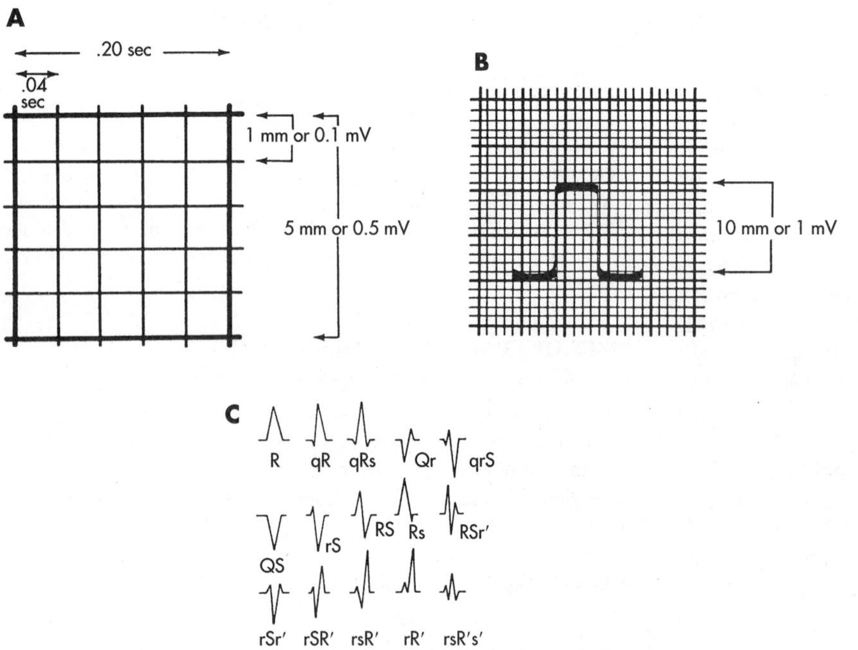

FIGURE 5-18 **A,** A close-up picture of the graph paper used to record electrocardiograms. The paper is divided into 1-mm sections horizontally and vertically. Larger divisions are created by placing heavy lines every 5 mm. The paper speed is 25 mm/sec. Consequently, each millimeter represents 1/25th (0.04) second, and each 5 mm represents 0.2 seconds. The voltage calibration is 1 cm = 1 mV. Consequently, each mm represents 0.1 mV. **B,** A calibration signal produced by generating a 1-mV signal within the machine. The 1-mV signal produces a square wave signal that is 1 cm (10 mm) in height. **C,** The manner in which QRS complexes are labeled. The first positive deflection is always called an R wave. The first negative deflection preceding the R wave is a Q Wave, and the first following it an S wave. The tallest wave is denoted by placing it in capital letters. A completely negative wave is called a QS wave. Second R waves and S waves are denoted as R′ and S′. (From Cooksey JD, Dunn M, Massie E: *Clinical vectorcardiography and electrocardiography,* Chicago, 1977, Mosby.)

fast enough, this acts as a filter that cuts off higher-frequency portions of the complexes.

When recording an ECG, grounding is very important. If the apparatus is not properly grounded, electrical interference, in the form of 60-Hz (cycle) oscillations, will interfere with the recording (Figure 5-19). The source of 60-Hz interference is the alternating current (AC) in the wires that supply electricity to the ECG machine and other devices in a room. A separate electrode is provided to ground the dog to the ECG. In some it comes as a completely separate wire. In others it is incorporated in one of the other wires. Proper grounding also requires proper contact of the electrodes with skin. This is usually accomplished by "wetting" the skin with alcohol or ECG paste to improve electrical contact. One of the most common errors that results in improper grounding and 60-Hz interference is placing too much wetting material on a limb. This results in an electrical bridge between that limb and the one lying under it or between a limb and the table.

To record an ECG, the patient should be placed on its right side, usually on a plastic or rubber mat. The limbs should be perpendicular with the body and slightly separate. The electrodes are commonly attached to the skin with alligator clips, although electrode patches, subcutaneous wires, or metal plates held in place by rubber straps can be used. The electrodes are color-coded. The black electrode is placed on the left front leg at the elbow. The white electrode is placed opposite on the right elbow. The red electrode is attached to the left stifle and the green electrode (ground) is attached to the right stifle (snow [white electrode] and grass [green electrode] are always on the ground [closest to the table]). The sizes of the deflections recorded on the ECG are dependent on the distance between the electrodes of a lead and the heart according to the explanations provided above. Size is a square function so that small changes in distance can make large changes in the amplitude of deflections. Consequently, care should be taken to place the electrodes at the elbows and stifles and care should be taken to orient the limbs perpendicular to the body. The skin can be wetted before or after the electrodes are placed. Care should be taken not to place too much solution or paste during the wetting process.

Electrocardiograms are usually recorded on calibrated paper. The paper is divided by horizontal and vertical lines that occur every 1 mm (see Figure 5-18). This produces small squares that are 1 mm by 1 mm. Every fifth line is heavier on most paper. This produces squares that are 5 mm by 5 mm.

Once the animal holder and patient are comfortable and the electrodes are in place, the ECG machine should be calibrated. On most ECG machines, a 1-mV signal can be sent through the device for calibration by pressing a button or the calibration signal is sent automatically. Usually the ECG machine is calibrated so that this 1-mV signal produces a 1-cm (10 mm) vertical deflection on the paper (so-called standard sensitivity) (see Figure 5-18). By calibrating in this manner, the height of the wave deflections can be measured in mV. When the machine is calibrated such that a 1-mV signal produces a 1-cm deflection, every 1-mm deflection represents 0.1 mV. With most machines, this calibration can be altered to make the complexes larger or smaller. When the calibration is set such that a 1-mV signal produces a 2-cm deflection (so-called double-sensitivity), all of the complexes will be twice as tall as with the previous calibration. This calibration setting is used commonly to record ECGs from cats, because cat ECG complexes are small. Of course, doubling the sensitivity also doubles the size of any artifacts. The calibration can usually also be set so that a 1-mV calibration signal produces a 0.5-cm deflection (so-called half-sensitivity). This calibration setting is commonly used in dogs that have very large QRS complexes because of left ventricular enlargement or because they originate from ectopic sites (e.g., premature ventricular depolarizations).

Following the calibration procedure, the paper speed must be chosen. An ECG can be recorded at any paper speed. However, most clinical ECG machines record at 25 mm/sec and 50 mm/sec. When recorded at 25 mm/sec, 25 of the 1-mm or five of the 5-mm lines pass beneath the stylus each second. Each mm represents $\frac{1}{25}$ of a second, or 0.04 seconds (40 ms), and every 5 mm represents $\frac{1}{5}$ of a second, or 0.2 seconds (see Figure 18). Consequently, five heavy lines represent 1 second. At 50 mm/sec, every mm represents $\frac{1}{50}$ of a second, or 0.02 seconds (20 ms), and every 5 mm represents $\frac{1}{10}$ of a second (Figure 5-20). Ten heavy lines constitute 1 second. Usually, all leads should be recorded first at a paper speed of 50 mm/sec. More accurate measures of intervals, segments, and durations can be made at the faster paper speed. Each lead should be marked on the paper at the time of recording. This can be done

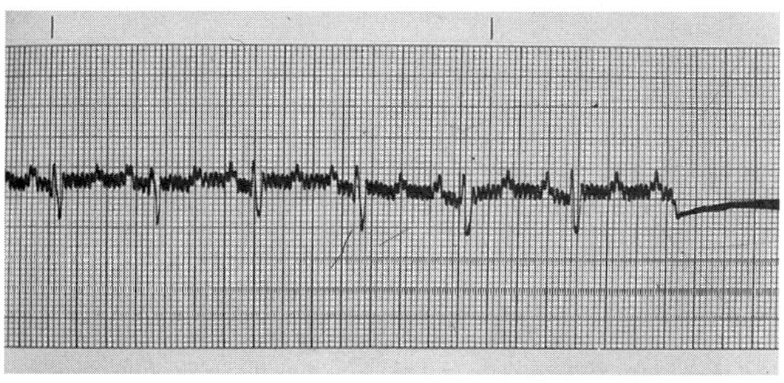

FIGURE 5-19 Example of 60-cycle (Herz) interference from improper grounding. The paper speed is 50 mm/sec. There are six oscillations every 0.1 seconds.

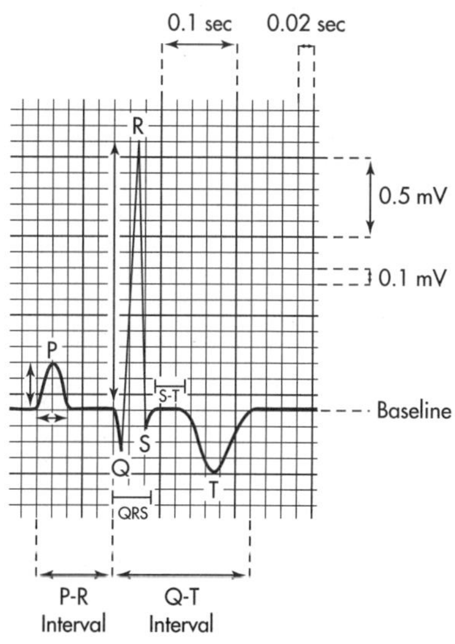

FIGURE 5-20 A normal P-QRS-T complex on electrocardiograph paper. The paper speed is 50 mm/sec, and the calibration is 1 cm = 1 mV. Measurements of P wave height and duration, P-R interval duration, QRS complex height and duration, Q-T interval duration, and ST segment placement are depicted. (From Tilley LP: *Essentials of canine and feline electrocardiography,* ed 3, Philadelphia, 1992, Lea & Febiger.)

manually but usually the machine automatically marks each lead. The lead that produces the largest deflections (usually lead II) should then be chosen and recorded at 25 mm/sec to analyze the cardiac rhythm.

Following recording, the ECG should be analyzed and stored properly. ECGs can be stored by folding them and placing them in holders. Alternatively, they can be cut into sections and placed on storage paper, or larger sheets can be fan-folded and placed in holders or the medical record.

Measuring the ECG

A normal P-QRS-T complex is depicted in Figure 5-20. The ECG should be analyzed in a standard fashion. Haphazard analysis may result in items being missed.

THE NORMAL CANINE AND FELINE ECG

Normal canine and feline ECGs are depicted in Figures 5-21 and 5-22. In each species the P waves are positive (upright) in leads I, II, III, and aV_F. The P wave is always negative in lead aV_R. In each species a Q wave is usually present in leads II, III, and aV_F. A Q wave may also be present in lead I. Leads I, II, III, and aV_F have large R waves, with lead II usually having the largest R wave. These leads, except for lead I, may also have a small S wave but frequently one is not present. Leads aV_R and aV_L have negative deflections that are usually S waves. This wave is usually largest in lead aV_R.

MEASURING THE HEART RATE

Measuring the heart rate gives clues to the cardiac rhythm and usually should be determined first. Initially, an average heart rate should be calculated. One must realize first that the longer the time over which the heart rate is counted, the more accurate the count will be. If counted for 1 minute, the count is accurate to within 1 beat/min. If it is counted for 6 seconds, it is accurate to within 10 beats/min. Consequently, one should attempt to count as long an interval as possible, but usually 6 seconds will suffice. Counting the heart rate on a portion of the ECG recorded at 25 mm/sec is easier and uses less paper. To determine the number of complexes in 6 seconds, identify a segment of the ECG that is 150 mm in length (25 mm/sec × 6 seconds = 150 mm) and count the number of complexes within this span. Six seconds is $\frac{1}{10}$ of a minute, so the number of complexes counted is multiplied by 10 to give the number of complexes in 1 minute. Electrocardiographic paper usually has "hatch" marks along the top or the bottom of the paper, which occur either every 50 mm or 75 mm to aid in identifying a specific length.

The heart rate can also be determined for each beat (the so-called instantaneous heart rate). The ECG is most commonly used to determine heart rhythm. Arrhythmias commonly produce irregularities in the heart rate (varying intervals between complexes). Consequently, the heart rate varies from beat to beat. Determining the rate at which an ectopic focus is firing or the rate at which an escape rhythm is depolarizing at any point is often useful. For example, normally the sinus node acts as the pacemaker of the heart, and normally myocardium cannot depolarize spontaneously. However, damaged myocardium can depolarize spontaneously. It can do this for periods and then stop. If a region of ventricular myocardium was damaged and started to depolarize spontaneously and it did so at a rate faster than the sinus node, it would take over the cardiac rhythm. The faster a ventricular ectopic focus such as this fires, the more malignant the arrhythmia is likely to be. To determine how fast it is firing, the distance between the last sinus complex and the first ventricular premature complex is measured. If 1 second is present between these complexes, there is one complex each second, and the rate at which the ventricular site is firing is 60 beats/min. If 0.5 seconds are between them, that would mean that two complexes are present every second (1/0.5), so the rate would be 120 beats/min. If

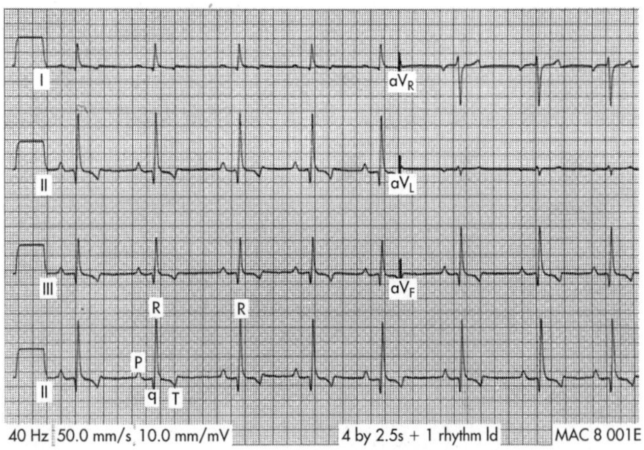

FIGURE 5-21 The six limb leads recorded from a normal 23-kg adult mixed-breed dog. A longer recording of lead II is at the bottom for determining average heart rate and analyzing the cardiac rhythm. Three leads are recorded simultaneously by this machine. The filter has been set at 40 Hz to decrease baseline artifact. This did not alter the height of any complex in this dog. The R wave in lead II is the largest and is positive. Consequently, the mean electrical axis is approximately 60 degrees. Leads I, II, III, and aV_F have a Q wave and an R wave. No S waves are present. Lead aV_R has a small R wave followed by a deep S wave. The P waves in leads aV_R and aV_L are negative. The QRS complex in lead aV_L is isoelectric (the R wave minus the S wave equals zero). The T wave in this dog is opposite in polarity to the R wave. The heart rate is 117 beats/min. There is a mild sinus arrhythmia.

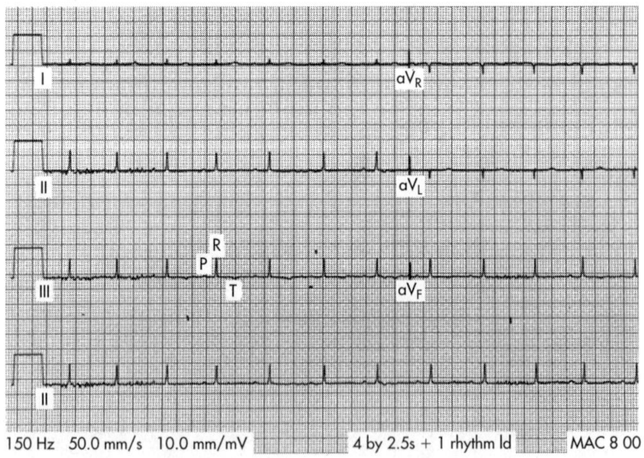

FIGURE 5-22 The six limb leads from a normal adult domestic shorthaired cat. The filter was set at 150 Hz because lower settings decreased the height of the complexes. Consequently, there is more baseline artifact than in the dog. The most artifact occurs before the third complex and is due to shivering. The complexes are much smaller than in the dog. The P waves in all leads are very small and cannot be seen whenever there is the slightest baseline artifact. The R waves in leads II, III, and aV_F are positive and are similar in size. The QRS complex in lead I is the smallest. Therefore the mean electrical axis is likely somewhere between 60 and 120 degrees and probably closer to 90 degrees. Lead I has a small Q wave and a small R wave. Leads II, III, and aV_F only have R waves that are less than 1 mV. The heart rate is 167 beats/min. The rhythm is a sinus rhythm.

there is 0.2 seconds between them, it would mean that there are five beats/sec and so 300 beats/min. The formula for determining this "instantaneous" heart rate is: rate = 60 (sec/min) ÷ R-R interval (sec/beat), where R-R is the distance between two QRS complexes measured in seconds.

MEASURING INTERVALS, HEIGHTS, AND DURATIONS OF THE P-QRS-T COMPLEX

After determining the heart rate, several electrocardiographic complex height and interval measurements are taken (see Figure 5-20). Lead II is always used to measure heights and intervals. Normal values for intervals between complexes, durations of P-QRS-T complexes, and heights of these complexes are listed in Table 5-1. Whenever possible, calipers should be used to make ECG measurements. Whenever measuring intervals, heights, and durations, one must be careful not to include the width of the line in the measurement. Line width can often be 1 mm, which, if included in a measurement, can produce significant error.

The P wave. The P wave begins with the first upward deflection from the baseline and ends with the return to the baseline. The duration of the P wave should be measured from the beginning to the end of the P wave. So as not to include the width of the line in the measurement, one point of the calipers should be placed to the right side of the line where the P wave starts and then opened so that the other point rests on the right side of the line at the end of the P wave. Alternatively, both points can be placed on the left side of the line. Once the calipers have been opened the appropriate distance, the calipers should be lifted and placed on another portion of the paper to measure the distance that the calipers are opened in millimeters. The number of millimeters should then be translated into seconds. The paper speed must be known to determine duration of any complex or interval. Next the P wave height should be measured. This should be from the top of the baseline to the top of the P wave in lead II. The calibration must be known to determine the height in mV. For example, if the calibration is 1 cm = 1 mV and the P wave is 3 mm (0.3 cm) in height, it has deflected 0.3 mV.

The P-R interval. The P-R interval is measured from the first upward deflection of the P wave to the first deflection of the QRS complex. As such, the proper name for this interval should be the P-Q interval. However, P-R interval is ingrained in the medical literature and cannot be changed. One must remember that the P-R interval ends at the onset of the QRS complex.

The P-R interval is primarily a measure of the time it takes for the cardiac impulse to traverse the AV node. The AV node begins to depolarize long before the P wave ends, and so P wave duration has little effect on the P-R interval. Conduction through the internodal paths, the bundle of His, the bundle branches, and the Purkinje network are also represented in the P-R interval but normally represent only a short portion. Abnormalities of P-R duration primarily occur when an AV node abnormality exists. For example, the P-R interval is shortened when the AV node is bypassed, and it is prolonged when the AV node is diseased, and conduction through it is prolonged. However, prolongation of conduction in the bundle of His and both bundle branches can also prolong the P-R interval.

The QRS complex. The onset of the QRS complex is the first deflection of the QRS complex from the baseline, whether negative or positive. The end of the QRS complex can be difficult to ascertain at times. Usually the QRS complex ends when it returns to the baseline. Sometimes, however, it ends above or below the baseline at the so-called J point. When this occurs, the QRS complex ends when the line changes from a thin line to a thick line again. Whenever a QRS complex is inscribed, the line on the paper becomes thinner than the baseline, because the velocity of the tracing increases during ventricular depolarization. One can take advantage of this fact to delineate the end of the QRS complex.

The QRS complex interval or duration is measured in mm from the onset of the QRS complex to the end and recorded in seconds. The height of the R wave is measured in mm from the baseline to the top of the R wave in lead II and recorded in mV.

The ST segment. The ST segment should first be inspected visually to determine if it is at the same level as the rest of the baseline (see Figure 5-20). The ST segment can be elevated or depressed from the baseline. This occurs whenever regional myocardial hypoxia is present. Regional hypoxia is a common finding in human medicine because of coronary artery disease producing regional ischemia and infarction. Regional hypoxia can occur in dogs and cats, but global hypoxia is more common and does not result in any ST segment change.

The Q-T interval. The Q-T interval is measured from the beginning of the QRS complex to the end of the T wave. It represents total electrical systole. The QT interval is markedly affected by heart rate. As the heart rate increases, the QT interval shortens and as heart rate slows, the QT interval lengthens. No set formula for determining a normal QT interval at a particular heart rate has been devised for dogs or cats. This makes it difficult to interpret a particular QT interval in a particular setting.

The T wave. The T wave direction, amplitude, and duration depend on many variables, making changes difficult to interpret. Any changes that are noted are generally nonspecific. Consequently, T wave abnormalities commonly are not recognized and when they are present have little significant clinical meaning. The exception is in hyperkalemia, in which T wave abnormalities can be quite evident. A tall and spiked T wave may be present when the serum potassium concentration is moderately elevated. This disappears when the concentration is markedly elevated. Consequently, many hyperkalemic animals do not have T wave changes.

TABLE 5-1

Normal values for heart rate, intervals between complexes, durations of P-QRS-T complexes, and heights of complexes

	Dog	*Cat*
Heart rate (beats/min): resting-excited	Giant breeds: 60-140 Adult dogs: 70-160 Toy breeds: 80-180 Puppies: Up-220	100 (asleep)-240 (excited)
P wave (upper limit)	Width: 0.04 sec Height: 0.4 mV	Width: 0.04 sec Height: 0.2 mV
P-R interval	0.06-0.13 sec	0.05-0.09 sec
QRS complex (upper limit)	Width: 0.06 sec Height: 3.0 mV	Width: 0.04 sec Height: 0.9 mV
Q-T interval	0.15-0.25 sec depending on heart rate	0.07-0.20 sec depending on heart rate
S-T segment	No more than 0.2-mV elevation or depression	No depression or elevation
T wave	Positive, negative, or biphasic	Positive, negative, or biphasic
Mean electrical axis	+40°-+100°	0°-+160°

THE MEAN ELECTRICAL AXIS

The mean electrical axis (MEA) refers to the average (mean) direction (axis) that a wavefront of dipoles (electrical wavefront) is moving in the heart. The MEA can be applied to atrial depolarization

(P wave), ventricular depolarization (QRS complex), or ventricular repolarization (T wave) but is almost always determined only for ventricular depolarization. As outlined above, the depolarization of the ventricles is more complex than atrial depolarization. Even so, the larger ventricle has a larger wavefront of depolarization or a ventricle without intact conduction will draw the wavefront toward it. Consequently, it is this wavefront that predominates when all of the wavefronts are averaged (which is what an ECG does). The net result is that the direction of the QRS complex deflection (positive or negative) in any particular lead reflects which chamber is larger or which chamber is missing its normal conduction through a bundle branch.

By convention, the frontal plane is treated as if it were a circle with 360 degrees (see Figure 5-17). Also by convention, the left front leg (the positive pole of lead I) is labeled 0 degrees, and the right front leg (the negative pole of lead I) is labeled 180 degrees. The positive pole of lead aV_F is labeled 90 degrees. The negative pole of lead aV_F can be labeled either 270 degrees or –90 degrees. The normal MEA in the dog is 40 degrees to 100 degrees (Figure 5-23). In the cat it is 0 degrees to 160 degrees (Figure 5-24).

The MEA can be calculated several different ways. Based on the previous explanations of how the ECG is generated, the easiest method to determine MEA is to identify the lead with the largest net QRS complex deflection, either positive or negative. To obtain the net deflection, the QRS complex deflections must be algebraically added. For example, if the Q wave in a particular lead is 0.2 mV and the R wave is 2.5 mV, because the Q wave is negative and the R wave is positive, the sum is 2.3 mV (2.5 + –0.2 mV). Normally lead II has the tallest deflection—an R wave (a positive wave). This means that the largest wavefront in the ventricles is traveling more directly toward the positive pole of lead II than any other lead, and the MEA is approximately 60 degrees. This makes sense because the left ventricle is situated within the thorax to the left and caudally (a little more caudal than to the left), and so the wavefront of depolarization of the left ventricle is directly in line with lead II (see Figure 5-16). One can quickly deduce what the other leads should look like in this situation (see Figure 5-21). Lead aV_L should have the smallest QRS complex because it must be the lead that is most perpendicular to the wavefront because it is perpendicular to lead II. Lead aV_R should have a relatively large deflection and should have the largest negative deflection because it is the lead with a positive pole that is most opposite to lead II. Leads I, III, and aV_F should all have positive QRS complexes that are smaller than lead II, and the R wave in lead aV_F should be taller than the R wave in lead III. If, on the other hand, lead I has the largest QRS complex and most of the QRS complex size because of a very deep S wave, one immediately knows that the MEA is 180 degrees and that the largest wavefront is traveling to the right. This means that either the right ventricle is larger than the left ventricle or the right bundle branch is no longer functioning.

As stated at the beginning of this section, there are other means to determine MEA. None are more accurate. Because of the inherent errors in an ECG (the body is not a homogeneous volume conductor, the lead system is not a perfect equilateral triangle, etc.), it is of no value to try to determine the MEA down to the nearest degree. Instead, calculation to within 30 degrees should be sufficient. With that in mind, another method to determine MEA is to find the lead that is most isoelectric (has the smallest QRS complex) and then identify the lead perpendicular to this lead. The direction of the electrical wavefront with respect to the perpendicular lead is then determined and the MEA estimated. This is opposite to the method presented above. One other method is to examine leads I and aV_F, two leads that are perpendicular to each other. The quadrant in which the MEA lies can then be quickly determined. The quadrants are 0 to 90 degrees (quadrant 1), 90 to 180 degrees (quadrant 2), 180 to 270 degrees (quadrant 3), and 270 to 360 degrees (quadrant 4). If the QRS complex in lead 1 is positive, then the MEA has to be in either quadrants 1 or 4. If aV_F is also positive, the MEA must be in quadrant 1. If the QRS complex in lead I is negative, the MEA must be in quadrants 2 or 3. If lead aV_F is negative, the MEA must be in quadrant 3. This is the least accurate method. However, the MEA in most normal dogs is in quadrant 1 (normal MEA in the dog is 40 to 110 degrees). As long as the MEA is in quadrant 1 and the QRS

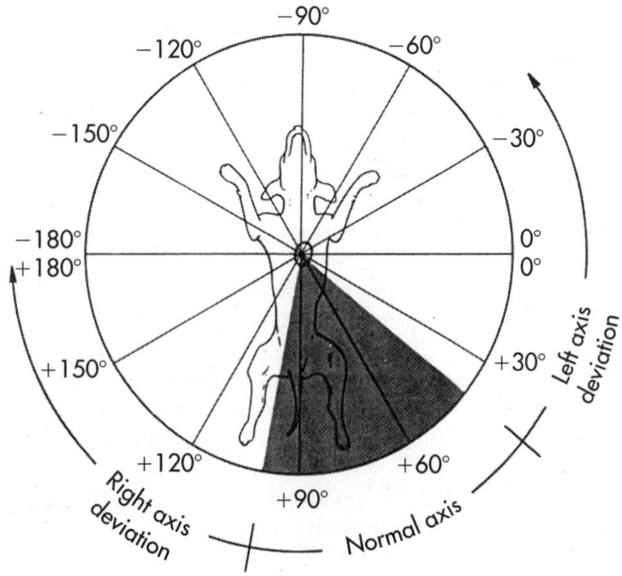

FIGURE 5-23 The hexaxial lead system with the normal mean electrical axis *(shaded area)* and right and left axis deviations for dogs portrayed. (From Tilley LP: *Essentials of canine and feline electrocardiography,* ed 3, Philadelphia, 1992, Lea & Febiger.)

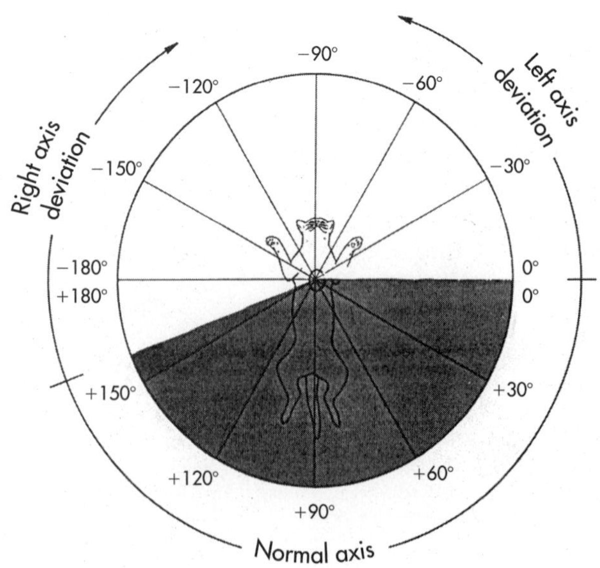

FIGURE 5-24 The same as in Figure 5-23, but for cats. (From Tilley LP: *Essentials of canine and feline electrocardiography,* ed 3, Philadelphia, 1992, Lea & Febiger.)

complex in lead aV_F is taller than or as tall as the one in lead I, the MEA must be normal. In cats the normal MEA is approximately 0 to 160 degrees, so as long as the MEA is in quadrants I or 2 the MEA is usually normal.

Lastly, one can plot out the MEA using leads 1 and aV_F (any two leads can be used, but two leads that are perpendicular to each other makes it easier). First, the algebraic sum of the QRS complex is determined in mV. For example, if the Q wave in lead I is –0.3 mV deep and the R wave is +1.3 mV tall, the algebraic sum is +1.0 mV. Similarly, for lead aV_F, if the Q wave is –0.2 mV and the R wave is +2.2 mV, the algebraic sum is +2.0 mV. This is plotted on graph paper, and in this situation the MEA is 67 degrees. As mentioned previously, this does not mean that the MEA is exactly 67 degrees. Instead, the MEA is probably somewhere between 50 and 80 degrees.

In a heart with normal conduction, the relative sizes of the ventricles determine which ventricle predominates. Consequently, the mean electrical axis is used to determine which chamber (the right ventricle or the left ventricle) is larger. Normally the left ventricle is much larger (3 times the mass) than the right ventricle. Consequently, the ECG primarily "sees" a wavefront of depolarization traveling caudally and to the left. This results in large R waves in leads I, II, III, and aV_F. With severe right heart enlargement, the right ventricular mass can exceed the left ventricular mass. Now the opposite occurs. The right ventricle predominates (has a larger wavefront), and so the ECG "sees" the average of the wavefronts of depolarization traveling cranially and to the right. This results in deep S waves being present in leads I, II, III, and aV_F. This shifts the MEA to the right and cranially.

Ventricular chamber enlargement is not the only variable that can change the MEA. It is also highly dependent on the route of conduction through the ventricles. This is most commonly changed by bundle branch blocks. The bundle branches are responsible for rapidly transmitting the cardiac electrical impulse to the Purkinje network and ventricular myocardium. Conduction velocity in the bundle branches is about 3 times as fast as it is in myocardium. If a bundle branch does not function, instead of the electrical impulse reaching a particular ventricle rapidly via the bundle branch, it must spread through the ventricle from muscle cell to muscle cell, very slowly. This prolongs the QRS complex duration. It may also alter the MEA. For example, if the right bundle branch is diseased and so no longer conducts (a right bundle branch block), the left ventricle still depolarizes normally via the left bundle branch. In this situation, the left ventricle depolarizes normally but the right ventricle depolarizes much more slowly. During the first 3 to 50 ms, instead of the right ventricle depolarizing rapidly and so losing its influence after the first 10 ms or so, the right ventricular depolarization wave continues to influence the average depolarization wave. Consequently, the first part of the QRS complex is canceled into a very small deflection because of these nearly equal depolarization waves traveling in opposite directions. Once the left ventricle is depolarized, the right ventricle continues to depolarize. Because no depolarization wavefront counteracts the right ventricular wavefront, the ECG now only "sees" a wavefront traveling cranially and to the right. This produces deep S waves in leads I, II, III, and aV_F.

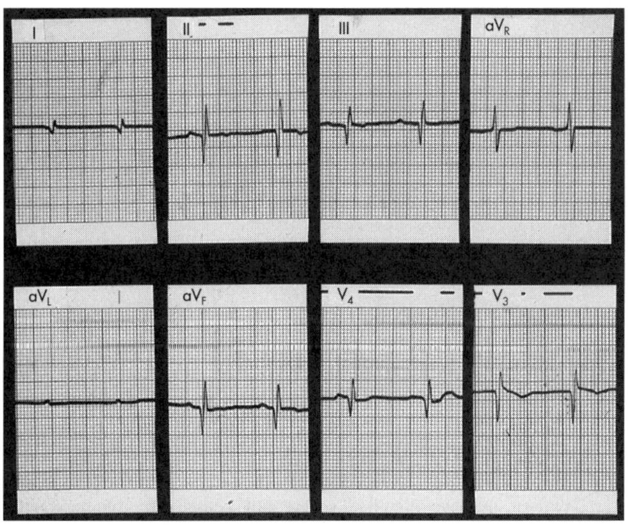

FIGURE 5-25 ECG from a normal 6-year-old Doberman pinscher. All leads are equally positive and negative (isoelectric). This probably is due to a heart that lies vertically within the thoracic cavity.

Occasionally, a dog or cat will have an ECG in which all of the leads have equal positive and negative QRS complex deflections (Figure 5-25). The mean electrical axis is impossible to calculate in this situation. This occurs most commonly in normal, deep-chested dogs.

Chamber Enlargement

Although the ECG is still used to aid in the diagnosis of cardiac chamber enlargement, this method often is insensitive at detecting chamber enlargement (there are many false negative findings). False positive findings are less common. When used for detecting chamber enlargement, the ECG should always be used in conjunction with thoracic radiography and preferably with echocardiography.

RIGHT ATRIAL ENLARGEMENT

Right atrial enlargement is characterized by a tall, peaked P wave, most commonly identified in leads II, III, and aV_F (Figure 5-26). In dogs this means that the P wave in lead II is >0.4 mV and in the cat is >0.2 mV. This increased amplitude results from an increase in the size of the electrical wavefront traveling toward the aforementioned leads. Increased P wave height is commonly termed *P pulmonale* because in human medicine right atrial enlargement is most commonly observed in patients with pulmonary hypertension secondary to chronic lung disease or left heart failure. Although right atrial enlargement is sometimes observed in dogs with only lung disease, it is rarely observed secondary to left heart failure and is more common in dogs with isolated or concomitant tricuspid regurgitation. Consequently, this term is confusing and somewhat inappropriate in veterinary medicine.

Increase in P wave height is a reasonably specific indicator of right atrial enlargement. In other words, whenever a tall, spiked P wave is observed on an ECG from a dog or cat, right atrial enlargement is usually present. Increased P wave height, however, is not a very sensitive indicator of right atrial enlargement. No studies have yet been completed to determine sensitivity. The authors estimate that less than 50% of cases with right atrial enlargement will have the characteristic ECG change.

LEFT ATRIAL ENLARGEMENT

The ECG findings characteristic of left atrial enlargement are a wide P wave and, sometimes, a notched P wave (Figure 5-27). The upper limit for normal P wave duration in the dog and the cat is 0.04 seconds. A wider-than-normal P wave indicates that conduction time through the atria is prolonged. Whereas this could occur with an increase in atrial size, an increase in right atrial size should be able to do this, as well as an increase in left atrial size. The fact that it usually does not suggests that the increase in size may not be the only abnormality that causes the ECG findings. It has been suggested that when the left atrium enlarges, conduction from the right atrium to the left atrium is prolonged or disrupted, resulting in P wave prolongation. A paper from a study in humans with left atrial enlargement secondary to mitral valve disease found no correlation between echocardiographically measured left atrial size and P wave duration.[18] Instead, they found reasonable correlation between percent fibrosis and P wave duration. This suggests that an intramyocardial conduction delay is the cause of the prolonged P wave. A wide, notched P wave is often termed *P mitrale* because mitral valve disease commonly produces an enlarged left atrium and, consequently, the typical ECG changes.

As with the ECG criteria for right atrial enlargement, criteria for left atrial enlargement are very insensitive but reasonably specific. The ECG may be especially insensitive in cats.[19]

LEFT VENTRICULAR HYPERTROPHY

Left ventricular hypertrophy (LVH) increases the size of the electrical wavefront traveling through the left ventricle (Figure 5-28). This results in an increase in the size of the R wave deflection in leads that are parallel with this wavefront, primarily leads II and aV_F in both dogs and cats (Figures 5-29 and 5-30). It can also prolong the QRS complex. Whether this is due to an increase in left ventricular mass or to prolonged conduction secondary to conduction system disease that occurs in response to left ventricular disease is unknown.

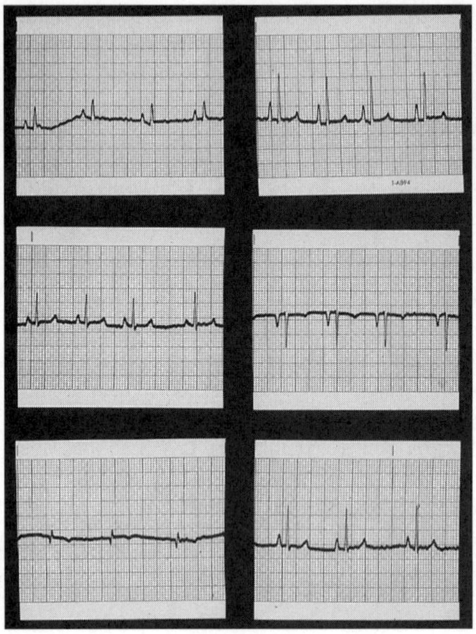

FIGURE 5-26 ECG tracings from all six limb leads from an 8-year-old Yorkshire terrier with chronic respiratory disease. The right heart was enlarged on the thoracic radiographs and the echocardiogram. On the ECG, the P waves are taller than normal in lead II (0.5 mV). This suggests right atrial enlargement. (Paper speed = 25 mm/sec; 1 cm = 1 mV.)

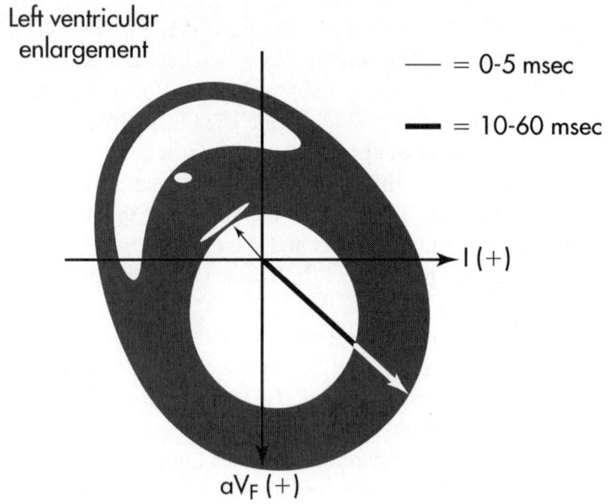

FIGURE 5-28 Schematic drawing depicting the effect of left ventricular hypertrophy on the ECG. The hypertrophy has resulted in a larger wavefront (depicted as a longer arrow) that results in a larger deflection on the ECG *(taller R wave in lead II).* The time for depolarization is also prolonged from 40 to 60 ms and is depicted as a slightly thicker arrow.

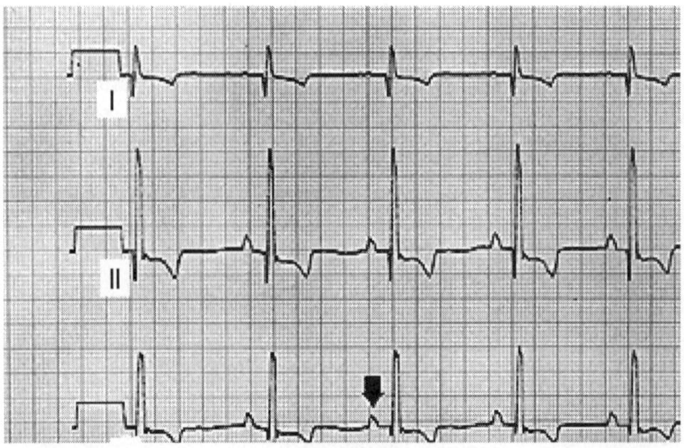

FIGURE 5-27 Lead II ECG tracing recorded from a 6-year-old boxer with dilated cardiomyopathy. The left ventricle and left atrium were severely enlarged on the echocardiogram. On the ECG, the P waves are too wide (0.05 seconds) and some are notched *(arrow).* The R wave height in lead II is too tall (4.2 mV), meaning there is evidence of left ventricular enlargement. ECG is recorded at half sensitivity (Paper speed = 50 mm/sec; 5 mm = 1 mV.)

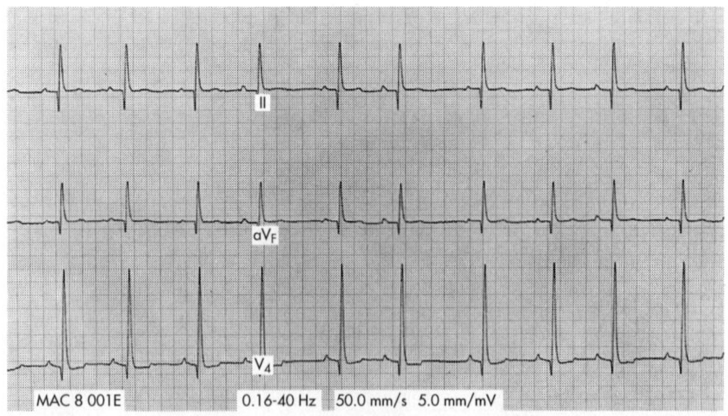

FIGURE 5-29 ECG tracings from two limb leads (leads II and aV_F) from a 1-year-old longhaired Chihuahua weighing 2.5-kg and with a patent ductus arteriosus. The dog had severe left ventricular volume overload hypertrophy on the echocardiogram. The R waves in leads II and CV_6LU (V_4) are too tall (3.5 mV and 7.4 mV respectively). This is consistent with left ventricular hypertrophy. Note that the ECG is recorded at half sensitivity. (Paper speed = 50 mm/sec; 5 mm = 1 mV.)

It should be noted that although a prolongation in QRS complex duration in a dog with a normal mean electrical axis is considered evidence of LVH, in man it is not. Instead, it is considered evidence of left conduction system disease. However, it has been shown in sled dogs that QRS complex duration does prolong with training as left ventricular mass increases.[20]

Although the original report on detection of left ventricular hypertrophy in dogs suggested that the ECG can distinguish between pressure and volume overload hypertrophy, the consensus by veterinary cardiologists today is that it cannot.[21] The original report suggested that an R wave height in lead aV_F more than 3 mV was consistent with volume overload hypertrophy and a left axis deviation (MEA between 30 degrees and −90 degrees) was consistent with pressure overload hypertrophy. The increase in R wave height has withstood the test of time, although lead II is usually used instead of aV_F. The left axis deviation has not. Most recently, a Chinese author, with Dr. David Knight at the University of Pennsylvania, examined 30 dogs with subaortic stenosis and 24 dogs with patent ductus arteriosus and compared them with 30 normal dogs.[22] All of the abnormal dogs had moderate-to-severe LVH. The dogs' ECGs were examined for changes in amplitude and duration of the QRS complex, deviations in the ST segment, abnormal wave deflections, and deviations of the mean electrical axis in the frontal plane. The six most discriminating ECG criteria for detecting left ventricular enlargement used in combination were:

QRS duration greater than 0.06 sec
R wave height in lead II or aV_F greater than 3 mV
R wave height in lead CV_{6LL} greater than 3 mV
R wave height in lead CV_{6LU} greater than 3 mV
R wave height of leads I and aV_F combined greater than 4 mV
R wave height in lead I > 1.5 mV

Fifty-nine percent of the dogs had two or more of the above criteria present, whereas only 7% of the normal dogs had two or more criteria. Of the individual criteria, an R wave height greater than 2.5 mV in leads II, III, or aV_F was detected in 50% of dogs, whereas only 10% of normal dogs had this abnormality. Similarly, 52% of the dogs with LVH had a QRS complex duration greater than 0.06 seconds, and only 7% of the normal dogs had this abnormality. An R wave height greater than 3 mV in leads II or aV_F was less sensitive (33%) at detecting LVH. A left-axis deviation was present in only 10% of the dogs. Dogs with other diseases that cause LVH may differ from the dogs chosen for this study. In our experience, dogs with a patent ductus arteriosus usually have ECG evidence of LVH, whereas in dogs with subaortic stenosis or mitral regurgitation the ECG is less sensitive at detecting LVH. Regardless, the presence of two or more of the above criteria or $R_{II, III, \text{ or } aV_F}$ height greater than 2.5 mV or R_{II} duration greater than 0.06 seconds appear to be the most accurate means of detecting LVH in dogs. It must be noted, however, that these criteria are still insensitive (many dogs have LVH and a normal ECG).

No comparable studies have been performed in cats. Generally, however, an R wave in lead II taller than 1 mV and a QRS complex duration greater than 0.04 seconds are considered evidence of LVH. In one study, only 39% of cats with LVH secondary to dilated or hypertrophic cardiomyopathy had ECG evidence of LVH, whereas some cats with hyperthyroidism had ECG criteria for the presence of LVH but none was present on an echocardiogram.[19]

Nonspecific changes in the ST segment and the T wave can also occur in association with LVH. Because these changes can occur with other abnormalities, they should not be used as any definitive evidence of LVH. They probably are not direct evidence of LVH but instead are evidence of abnormalities in the myocardium that occur secondary to LVH.

RIGHT VENTRICULAR HYPERTROPHY

The classic study of ECG criteria for detecting RVH in dogs ($n = 70$) was published in 1971.[23] The findings from this study are still valid today. The only problem with this study is that the degree of RVH was not categorized. However, it appears that most dogs in this study had moderate-to-severe RVH. All of the dogs with heartworm disease ($n = 26$) had a systolic right ventricular pressure greater than 50 mm Hg. Almost all of the other dogs had pulmonic stenosis, alone or combined with another congenital cardiac defect. The ECG manifestations of right ventricular hypertrophy (RVH) are usually a mirror image of LVH. Instead of observing tall R waves in leads I, II, III, and aV_F (terminal forces directed to the left and caudally), deep S waves are observed in these leads (terminal forces directed cranially and to the right; Figure 5-31). This occurs as right ventricular mass

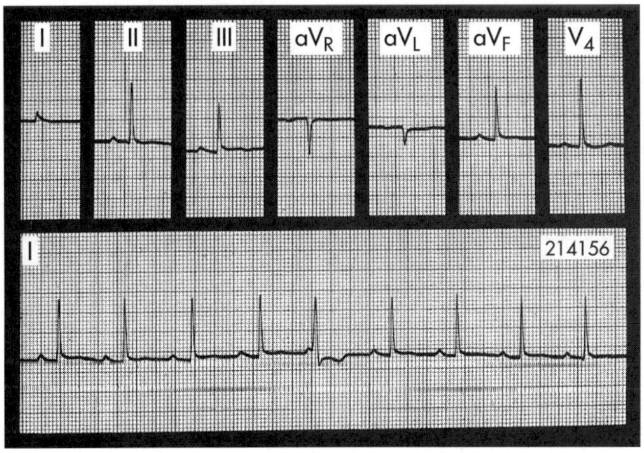

FIGURE 5-30 ECG tracings from all six limb leads and a chest lead from a 12-year-old cat with dilated cardiomyopathy. The R wave height is increased above normal in lead II (1.5 mV), which is consistent with left ventricular hypertrophy. There is a supraventricular premature depolarization (fifth beat) on the rhythm strip at the bottom.

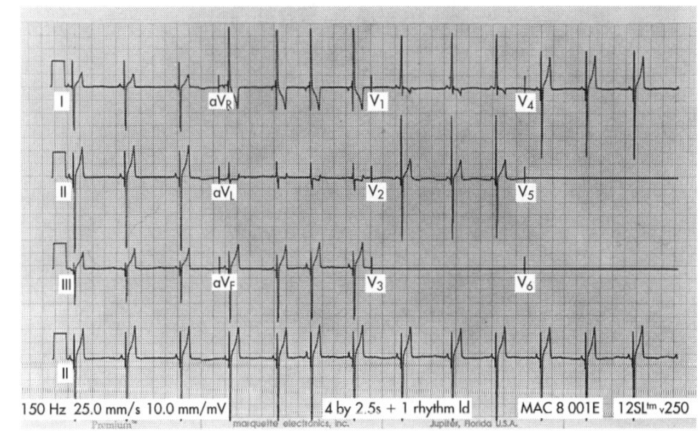

FIGURE 5-31 ECG tracings from all six limb leads and three chest leads (CV_6LU [V_4], CV_6LL [V_2], and CV_5RL [V_1]) from a 10-month-old Tibetan terrier with severe pulmonic stenosis. There are deep S waves in leads I, II, III, and aV_F. The mean electrical axis is oriented cranially and to the right (right axis deviation) because of the deep S waves. There are also deep S waves in the left chest leads. These features are consistent with right ventricular hypertrophy. (Paper speed = 25 mm/sec; 1 cm = 1 mV.)

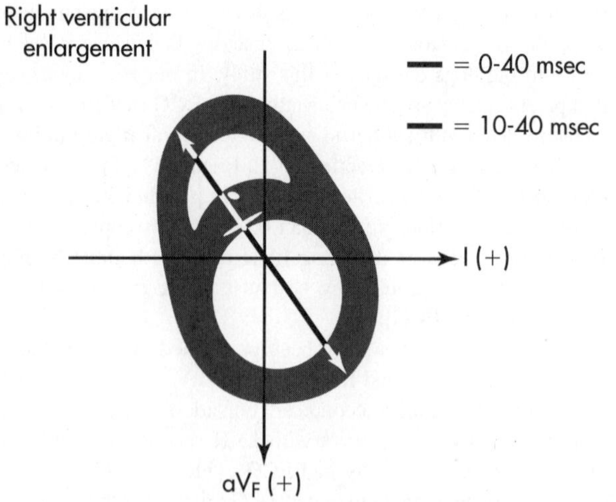

FIGURE 5-32 A drawing of right ventricular hypertrophy and its effect on the ECG. Severe right ventricular hypertrophy has resulted in the wavefront of depolarization spreading toward the right ventricle becoming larger than the one spreading toward the left ventricle. Consequently, the rightward vector predominates resulting in the mean electrical axis shifting cranially and to the right.

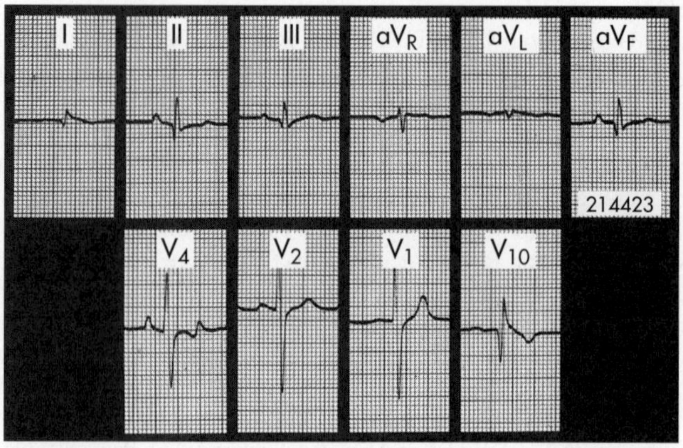

FIGURE 5-33 ECG tracings from all six limb leads and four chest leads (CV_6LU, CV_6LL, CV_5RL, and V_{10}) from a 10-year-old Australian shepherd with pulmonary hypertension. The QRS complexes in the limb leads are normal. However, there are deep S waves present in the left chest leads which is consistent with right ventricular hypertrophy. (Paper speed = 50 mm/sec; 1 cm = 1 mV.)

exceeds left ventricular mass, resulting in the dominant terminal wave of depolarization being directed toward the right ventricle (Figure 5-32). The deep S waves result in the mean electrical axis shifting to the right and cranially (right axis deviation). This is logical because this is where the right ventricle is situated within the thorax. The vast majority of dogs with severe RVH have a mean electrical axis between +90 degrees and –45 degrees in the frontal plane.[23] This usually is due to the presence of an S wave in lead I that is greater than 0.05 mV. Most dogs also have an S wave in the left chest leads greater than 0.8 mV. Some dogs with RVH will only have deep S waves present in the left chest leads (Figure 5-33). Right axis deviation of the mean electrical axis and deep S waves in the left chest leads are the most sensitive means of detecting RVH in dogs.[23] The presence of S waves (greater than 0.35 mV) in leads II and aV_F was less sensitive in the original study, identifying only about 50% of dogs with severe RVH.[23] All these criteria are quite specific (very few false positive findings). Only 0 to 7% of normal dogs have these ECG criteria of RVH. The QRS complex duration is usually normal. However, in some dogs with RVH, the right bundle branch becomes electrically disrupted, resulting in a wide QRS complex and right axis deviation, typical of a right bundle branch block. Whenever this pattern is identified, the presence of right heart enlargement must be confirmed by other means, because some normal dogs can also have a right bundle branch block. Uncommonly, dogs with RVH have deep Q waves present in leads I, II, III, and aV_F, producing a right axis deviation, albeit in the initial rather than the terminal forces. This pattern can also be seen in normal narrow-chested dogs and in golden retrievers with Duchenne's muscular dystrophy.[24]

The ECG is very insensitive at detecting mild-to-moderate RVH. In one study of heartworm dogs with mild, moderate, and severe RVH secondary to heartworm disease assessed radiographically, approximately 25% of dogs with mild or moderate RVH had ECG evidence of RVH.[25] In comparison, 84% of dogs with severe radiographic RVH had ECG evidence of RVH. Again, in this study, both the presence of a deep S wave in one of the left chest leads and a mean electrical axis in the frontal plane greater than 103 degrees as a result of the presence of an S wave in lead I identified approximately 80% of the dogs with severe RVH. Deep S waves in leads II and aV_F only identified about 40% of these dogs.

Similar changes occur in cats with RVH. Deep S waves in leads I, II, III, and aV_F occur most frequently along with a right axis deviation. Deep S waves can also be identified in the left chest leads.

Conduction Disturbances

BUNDLE BRANCH BLOCKS

The left and right bundle branches originate from the bundle of His (see Figure 5-3). Their function is to spread the cardiac electrical impulse rapidly to the Purkinje fibers in both ventricles and to coordinate the depolarization of the ventricles. The bundle branches, like the rest of the conduction system, cannot be seen on gross examination. The right bundle branch descends as a discrete band of tissue along the right side of the interventricular septum, near the crista supraventricularis, toward the apex of the right ventricle. Here it crosses to the right ventricular free wall in a thin, branched muscular strand called the moderator band, or trabecula septomarginalis. The moderator band crosses the lumen of the right ventricle, starting usually near the base of the largest papillary muscle. Here it branches repeatedly. Instead of the usual single strand, the moderator band can be two or more loose anastomosing strands that form a loose plexus (false tendons). The left bundle branch descends toward the apex of the left ventricle on the left side of the interventricular septum. Instead of a discrete band like the right bundle branch, the left bundle branch starts as a wide band that branches and fans out as it descends.

Ventricular depolarization is abnormal in bundle branch blocks. Normally the cardiac electrical impulse proceeds from the AV node through the bundle of His and then rapidly down both left and right bundle branches to the Purkinje fibers. The bundle branches function to spread the cardiac electrical impulse to both ventricles rapidly. If a bundle branch cannot conduct to a particular ventricle, conduction to that ventricle still occurs. However, it must travel from muscle cell to muscle cell. This is a much slower process. Consequently, if a bundle branch is unable to conduct the cardiac electrical impulse,

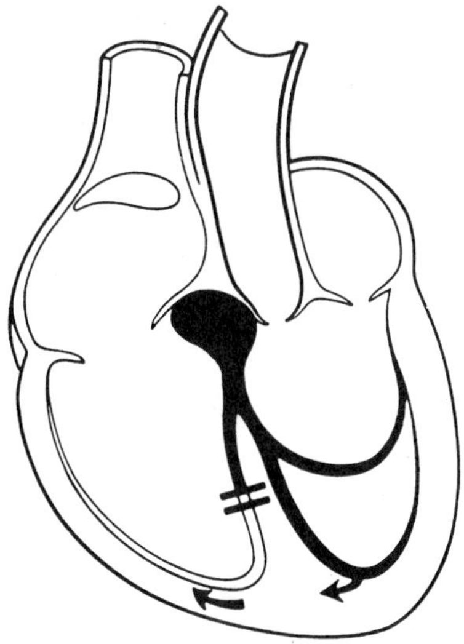

FIGURE 5-34 Schematic drawing of the heart and conduction system showing a complete right bundle branch block. (From Phillips RE and Feeney MK: *Cardiac rhythms: a systematic approach to interpretation,* ed 3, Philadelphia, 1990, WB Saunders.)

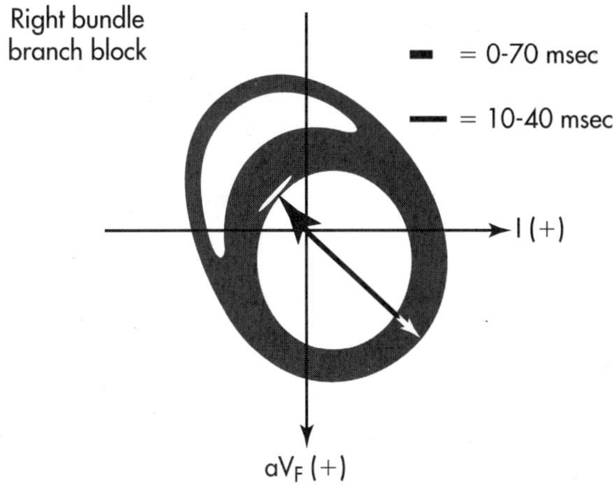

FIGURE 5-35 Drawing of the effect of a right bundle branch block on conduction to the right ventricle. Because of the slow conduction to the right ventricle, the terminal (last) portion of the QRS complex is shifted to the right, producing deep S waves in leads I, II, III, and aV$_F$.

conduction to the unaffected ventricle is normal and conduction to the ventricle served by the abnormal bundle branch is delayed. Complete block of both the right and left bundle branches produces complete (third degree) atrioventricular block.

Bundle branch blocks are usually persistent. However, they can also be intermittent, (i.e., the QRS morphology is normal at times and abnormal at other times).[26] Intermittent bundle branch blocks are most commonly rate-related, that is, they occur at certain heart rates but not at others. Bundle branch blocks can occur when the heart rate increases or decreases to a certain level, but most commonly they emerge at faster heart rates. In this situation, at least some cells in a bundle branch must have a prolonged refractory period.[27] When the heart rate increases to a certain rate, the cardiac electrical impulse finds the bundle branch refractory to stimulation and so conduction, and when it slows the cells have time to repolarize fully, allowing conduction to occur at slower heart rates. For example, if the heart rate is 120 beats/min, the time between each depolarization is 0.5 seconds. If the absolute refractory period of the cells in the left bundle branch is prolonged to 0.51 seconds, every time the electrical impulse reaches the left bundle branch, conduction will not occur. If however, the heart rate slows to 100 beats/min, the time between depolarizations is 0.6 seconds. At this rate, the cells in the left bundle branch have time to repolarize fully before the next electrical impulse stimulates them. Consequently, they are no longer refractory and conduct each impulse.

Right bundle branch block. Right bundle branch block (RBBB) can be complete or incomplete; it occurs because of conduction system disease or secondary to right ventricular enlargement. Rarely, a dog can have a congenital right bundle branch block. The cause of most conduction system disease in dogs and cats is unknown. At the time of diagnosis, all that can be seen histologically are degenerative changes. Disruption by any means of the portion of the bundle branch that courses beneath the endocardium of the interventricular septum results in a marked delay in conduction to the right ventricle (complete RBBB) (Figure 5-34). This results in the right ventricle continuing to be depolarized (instead of the right ventricle being completely depolarized within the first 10 to 20 ms, as normally ocurs) while the normal left ventricle is being depolarized during the

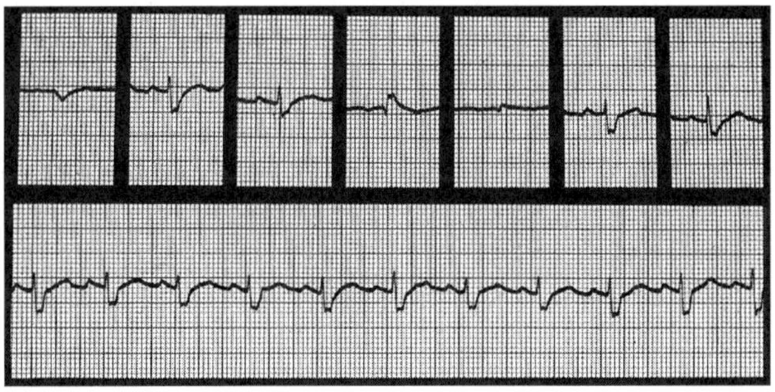

FIGURE 5-36 ECG tracings from the six limb leads from a 14-year-old cat with no cardiac disease. The mean electrical axis is shifted cranially and to the right because of deep S waves in leads I, II, III, and aV$_F$. The S wave is also wide, resulting in the QRS complex duration being greater than normal (0.06 seconds). The diagnosis is right bundle branch block. (Paper speed = 50 mm/sec; 1 cm = 1 mV.)

40 to 50 ms of normal depolarization (Figure 5-35). This decreases the size of the R wave in leads I, II, III, and aV$_F$ (the right ventricular depolarization wave partially cancels the left ventricular depolarization wave), often making it very small. Following complete depolarization of the left ventricle, the right ventricle continues to depolarize, resulting in a late wave of depolarization that travels cranially and to the right. This produces large and wide S waves in leads I, II, III, and aV$_F$. Because conduction time is so prolonged, the QRS complex is wider than normal (greater than 0.06 seconds in the dog and greater than 0.04 seconds in the cat) (Figure 5-36). An incomplete RBBB can occur with disruption of the moderator band. This also prolongs conduction time through the right ventricle but not to the same degree. This results in the R wave becoming smaller (but often not to a noticeable degree) and the appearance of S waves in leads I, II, III, and aV$_F$, without a noticeable increase in QRS complex duration.[28] This pattern mimics that of right ventricular hypertrophy. Theoretically, an increase in right ventricular chamber size can stretch and potentially disrupt moderator band conduction. Conse-

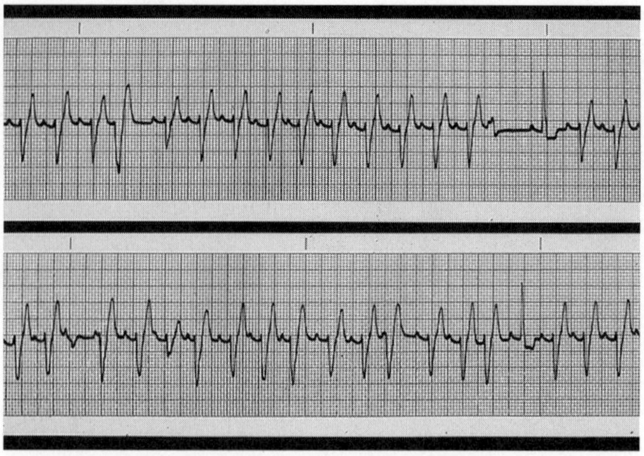

FIGURE 5-37 ECG tracing recorded from a dog with adriamycin cardiotoxicity. The basic rhythm is sinus rhythm with a heart rate of 140 beats/min. There is a right bundle branch block most of the time, as evidenced by the deep S waves and the prolonged QRS complex duration (at least 0.1 seconds). After the fourteenth beat in the first tracing there is an episode of type II second degree atrioventricular block (AV). This gives the right bundle branch time to fully repolarize so that on the next beat it can conduct down both bundle branches, resulting in a normal-appearing QRS complex. This is a rate-dependent bundle branch block. The sinus rate also slows to 130 beats/min at the time of the second-degree AV block, suggesting that increased vagal tone created the AV block. The fourth complex in the top tracing is a premature beat. Ventricular conduction following this premature beat is slightly altered. It is impossible to tell if this is a supraventricular or ventricular premature beat, although it is followed by a compensatory pause suggesting that it may be ventricular in origin. On the third complex of the second tracing, the sinus node abruptly increases its rate to 160 beats/min. This produces more bizarre conduction through the ventricles, as evidenced by the very small and negative QRS complex. The rate stays elevated for the next several beats, with varying conduction patterns. The thirteenth and sixteenth complexes in the second tracing are premature beats. Again, it is impossible to tell if they are supraventricular or ventricular. They are not followed by a compensatory pause, which suggests that they are supraventricular. Notice that their appearance is identical to the fourth complex in the first tracing. Normal conduction occurs after the premature beat. Most likely the right bundle branch was still refractory when the premature beat was generated and so not depolarized by the premature beat, giving it time to fully repolarize before the next sinus beat occurred. For an explanation of premature beats, see Chapter 27. (Paper speed = 25 mm/sec; 1 cm = 1 mV.)

quently, the changes observed with a right ventricular volume overload could be a result of either the increase in right heart mass or to disruption of moderator band function. The pattern of an incomplete RBBB has also been noted in beagles that were from an F_1 generation of beagles with pulmonic stenosis and beagles with a ventricular septal defect. These dogs had right ventricular basilar and conal region thicknesses that were approximately twice normal. This again demonstrates that anatomic abnormalities of the right ventricle must be ruled out whenever an incomplete RBBB pattern is identified.

Right bundle branch block by itself does not cause clinical sequelae. Dogs can have a congenital RBBB, be normal clinically, and live a normal life span.[26] The only hemodynamic abnormality produced by an RBBB is delayed activation of the right ventricle and a prolonged right ventricular ejection time (the time it takes to eject blood in systole). This results in delayed closure of the tricuspid and pulmonic valves and can result in split heart sounds, most commonly a split second heart sound.[26]

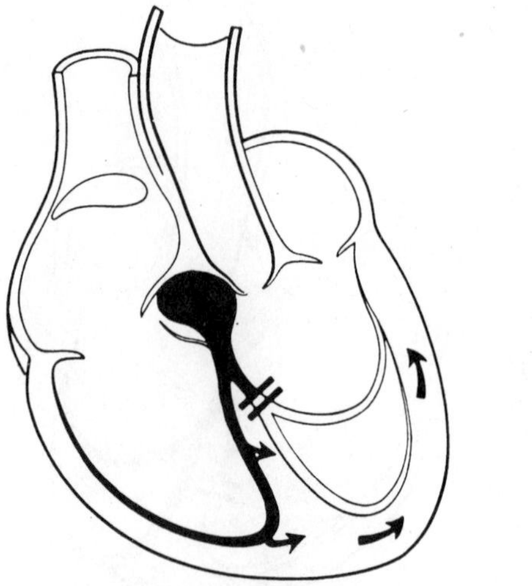

FIGURE 5-38 Drawing similar to Figure 5-33 depicting complete left bundle branch block. (From Phillips RE, Feeney MK: *Cardiac rhythms: a systematic approach to interpretation,* ed 3, Philadelphia, 1990, WB Saunders.)

A rate-dependent RBBB is presented in Figure 5-37. This is from a dog with adriamycin toxicity. The major rhythm is sinus rhythm. A premature ventricular depolarization occurs after the third sinus beat. After the fourteenth QRS complex, a P wave is not followed by a QRS complex (second-degree atrioventricular block). The sinus rate also slows at this time. This gives time for the right bundle branch to repolarize fully and allows it to conduct normally for one beat. After that the sinus rate increases again with no block, resulting in resumption of the RBBB. Note that the fifth QRS complex occurs after a shorter pause and is somewhat shorter than the other QRS complexes. This may reflect a slight improvement in conduction. The dog also has a first degree atrioventricular block (see Chapter 27).

Left bundle branch block. The left bundle branch is a fan-shaped network of interwoven fibers. Complete disruption of the left bundle branch results in delayed depolarization of the left ventricle (Figure 5-38). Because the left ventricle cannot be normally depolarized from the left bundle branch, depolarization must proceed down the right bundle branch and across the interventricular septum to the left ventricle. In this situation the initial depolarization of the ventricles is relatively normal and may produce a small Q wave. After this, the left ventricular depolarization wave predominates like it normally does (Figure 5-39). Consequently, the orientations of the QRS complexes on the ECG are normal (there is no change in the mean electrical axis). Because of the delayed left ventricular activation, one major change noted in the QRS complex is an increase in its duration (it is wider than normal). The other major change that commonly occurs is an increase in the R wave height in the lead most parallel with the left ventricular depolarization wave (usually lead II). The configuration of a QRS complex in a patient with left bundle branch block (LBBB) mimics that of a QRS complex generated by a premature ventricular depolarization that originates from the right ventricle. Besides abnormal ventricular depolarization, ventricular repolarization is also abnormal in LBBB. The T wave in LBBB is always large and opposite in polarity to the QRS complex (Figure 5-40).

LBBB occurs secondary to degenerative conduction system disease, left ventricular myocardial disease, or diseases that produce severe left ventricular hypertrophy. Because the left bundle branch branches early and widely throughout the left ventricle, LBBB

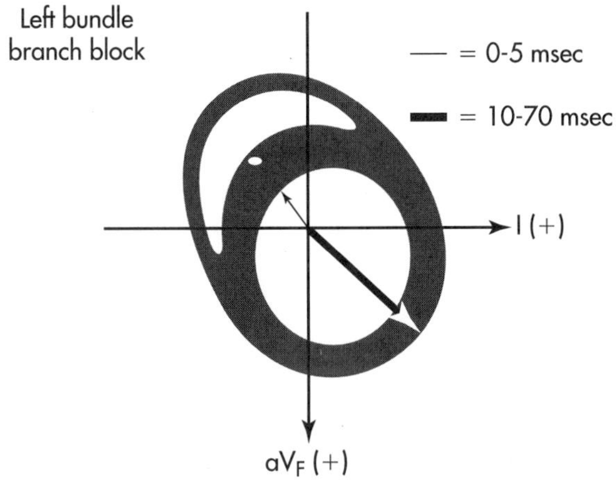

FIGURE 5-39 Drawing of the effect of left bundle branch block on conduction. The size of the wavefront spreading toward the left ventricle is normal, but the duration is longer than normal *(wider arrow),* lasting 70 ms. This results in a wider-than-normal QRS complex with a normal mean electrical axis.

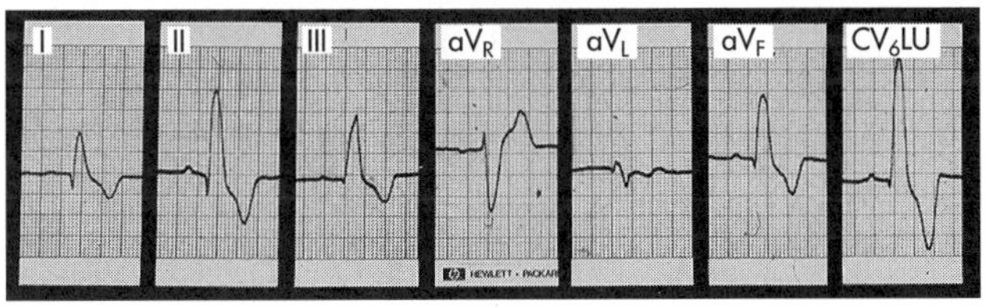

FIGURE 5-40 ECG tracings from the six limb leads from a 7-year-old boxer with dilated cardiomyopathy. The mean electrical axis is normal, but the QRS complex duration is greater than normal (0.1 seconds). The diagnosis is left bundle branch block. (Paper speed = 50 mm/sec; 1 cm = 1 mV.)

usually indicates widespread disease. LBBB almost never occurs by itself as a benign abnormality.

Left axis deviation. A left axis shift or deviation (LAD) is a shift of the mean electrical axis cranially and to the left without an increase in QRS complex duration. The exact boundaries of a left axis shift are uncertain in dogs and cats. It certainly is less than +40 degrees in the dog and less than 0 degrees in the cat, but exactly where this definition ends is unknown. Most likely, anything greater than –60 degrees is a LAD, but this cannot be stated with certainty. Likewise it cannot be stated with certainty that a mean electrical axis between –90 degrees and –60 degrees is either a left or right axis shift.

A left axis shift without an increase in QRS complex duration is commonly called a *left anterior fascicular block* or a *left anterior hemiblock.* These terms originate from a desire by physicians to divide the left bundle branch into two minor branches, or fascicles. This is anatomically incorrect, because no such fascicles exist in humans, dogs, or cats. It also may be electrocardiographically incorrect in the dog. Even if one arbitrarily divides the left bundle branch into anterior and posterior sections and then physically disrupts the anterior portion of the left bundle branch, a LAD is not

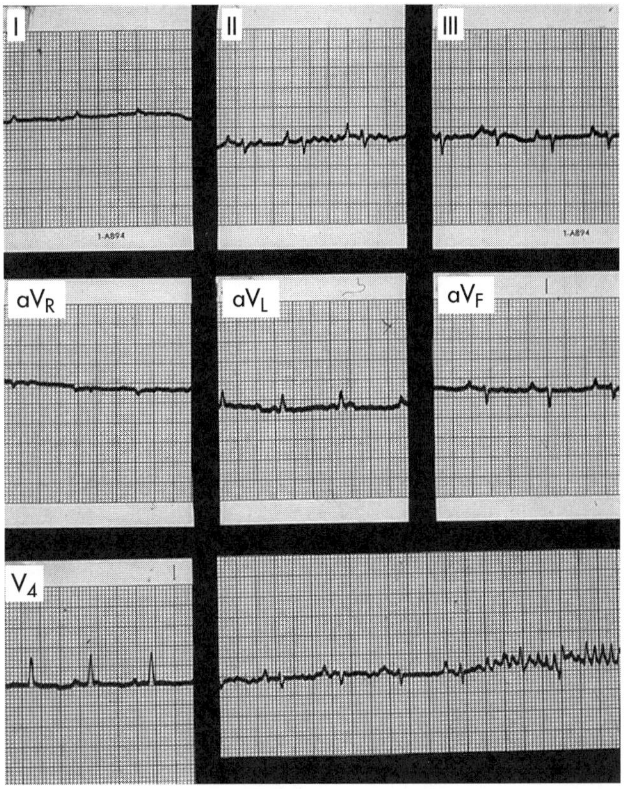

FIGURE 5-41 ECG tracings from the six limb leads from a 1-year-old cat with hypertrophic cardiomyopathy. The mean electrical axis is shifted cranially and to the left (left axis deviation). There is tremor artifact in lead II and severe tremor artifact at the end of the unlabeled lead. (Paper speed = 50 mm/second; 1 cm = 1 mV.)

produced in dogs. Rather, one produces only minor changes in the MEA (going from +70 degrees to +50 degrees in one study).[29] In baboons, similar lesions cause severe LAD. Following physical disruption of all but the very posterior portion of the left bundle branch, the most identified in dogs is the development of small S waves in leads II, III, and aV_F, with no S wave in lead I (Figure 5-41).[30] These small changes do not shift the entire axis. However, the terminal portion of QRS complexes in this situation, in which the terminal portion of the QRS complex is still positive in lead I and is negative in lead aV_F, is directed cranially and to the left (LAD). So, it is theoretically possible that a LAD of the terminal QRS complex is compatible with failure of the anterior portion of the left bundle branch to conduct in dogs.

Left axis deviations are observed in dogs and cats. From the above discussion we clearly do not know what causes LAD in dogs. We do know, however, that this pattern is most commonly identified in cats with hypertrophic cardiomyopathy and that it can also be seen in association with other left ventricular diseases and with hyperkalemia in cats and dogs. Most likely this pattern is caused by myocardial hypertrophy, diffuse disease of the left bundle branch, or both. Because disruption of the cranial portion of the left bundle branch does not cause LAD in dogs, we prefer the term *left axis deviation,* rather than left anterior fascicular block, to describe this electrocardiographic finding.

Right axis deviation. Right axis deviation is deviation of the mean electrical axis to the right and cranially. The exact boundaries are, again, uncertain. In dogs, a mean electrical axis between +110 degrees and –90 degrees is the probable range. In cats that range is probably between +160 degrees and −90 degrees. Right axis deviations are usually associated with right ventricular hypertrophy or RBBB (complete or incomplete). It has been proposed that a left posterior fascicular block can produce a right axis deviation. Experimentally, however, disruption of the caudal portion of the left bundle branch has not changed the mean electrical axis nor has it changed the terminal forces in dogs.[31,32] It has also been suggested that a left anterior fascicular block with a RBBB results in the mean electrical axis moving from a right axis deviation to a marked LAD based on criteria used in humans. However, experimentally, disruption of the cranial portion of the left bundle branch in a dog that already has a RBBB results in a very minor change in the already rightward oriented mean electrical axis.[33]

Artifacts

Numerous artifacts can occur on an ECG. Artifact as a result of 60-cycle (Hz) interference was presented earlier. Tremor or trembling artifact is another common artifact on ECGs from dogs and cats (Figure 5-41). Panting can make the baseline undulate at the frequency of the respiratory rate, and in cat's purring may create characteristic baseline undilates. Switching leads while still recording produces a period during which the baseline is flat. This can mimic sinus arrest. Brief deflections, often created by someone touching an electrode or a patient jerking a limb, can mimic premature ventricular contractions. Artifacts usually can be distinguished from premature ventricular contractions by the fact that they do not have a large, bizarre T wave following them.

REFERENCES

1. Irisawa H, Noma A, Matsuda HL: Electrogenesis of the pacemaker potentials as revealed by atrioventricular nodal experiments. In Sperelakis N, ed: *Physiology and pathophysiology of the heart,* ed 3, Boston, 1995, Kluwer.
2. Goldberg JM: Intra-SA-nodal pacemaker shifts induced by autonomic nerve stimulation in the dog, *Am J Physiol* 229:1116, 1975.
3. Chiou CW, Eble JN, Zipes DP: Efferent vagal innervation of the canine atria and sinus and atrioventricular nodes: the third fat pad, *Circulation* 95:2573, 1997.
4. Josephson ME: *Clinical cardiac electrophysiology: techniques and interpretation,* ed 2, Malvern, Pa, 1993, Lea & Febiger.
5. Racker DK: Atrioventricular node and input pathways: a correlated gross anatomical and histological study of the canine atrioventricular junctional region, *Anat Rec* 224:336, 1989.
6. Racker DK: Sinoventricular transmission in 10 mM K+ by canine atrioventricular nodal inputs: superior atrionodal bundle and proximal atrioventricular bundle, *Circulation* 83:1738, 1991.
7. Tse WW: Transmembrane potentials of canine AV junctional tissues, *Am Heart J* 111:1100, 1986.
8. Hamlin RL, Smith CR: Categorization of common domestic mammals based upon their ventricular activation process, *Ann N Y Acad Sci* 127:195, 1965.
9. Scher AM: Studies of the electrical activity of the ventricles and the origin of the QRS complex, *Acta Cardiol* 50:429, 1995.
10. Fye WB: A history of the origin, evolution, and impact of electrocardiography, *Am J Cardiol* 73:937, 1994 [erratum, 76(8):641, 1995].
11. Lannek N: A clinical and experimental study on the electrocardiogram in dogs, thesis, Stockholm University, Stockholm, 1949.
12. Detweiler DK, Patterson DF: The prevalence and types of cardiovascular disease in dogs, *Ann N Y Acad Sci* 127:481, 1965.
13. Fruehan CT, Baule G, Burgess MJ et al: Differences in the heart as a generator of the QRS and ST-T deflections, *Am Heart J* 77:842, 1969.
14. Kootsey JM, Johnson EA: The origin of the T-wave, *CRC Crit Rev Bioeng* 4:233, 1980.
15. Burgess MJ, Green LS, Millar K et al: The sequence of normal ventricular recovery, *Am Heart J* 84:660, 1972.
16. Hill JD: The electrocardiogram in dogs with standardized body and limb positions, *J Electrocardiol* 1:175, 1968.
17. Schrope DP, Fox PR, Hahn AW et al: Effects of electrocardiograph frequency filters on P-QRS-T amplitudes of the feline electrocardiogram, *Am J Vet Res* 56:1534, 1995.
18. Scott CC, Leier CV, Kilman JW et al: The effect of left atrial histology and dimension on P wave morphology, *J Electrocardiol* 16:363, 1983.
19. Moise NS, Dietze AE, Mezza LE et al: Echocardiography, electrocardiography, and radiography of cats with dilatation cardiomyopathy, hypertrophic cardiomyopathy, and hyperthyroidism, *Am J Vet Res* 47:1476, 1986.
20. Constable PD, Hinchcliff KW, Olson J et al: Athletic heart syndrome in dogs competing in a long-distance sled race, *J Appl Physiol* 76:433, 1994.
21. Hamlin RL: Electrocardiographic detection of ventricular enlargement in the dog, *J Am Vet Med Assoc* 153:1461, 1968.
22. Chen K: Reevaluation and revision of electrocardiographic criteria for the diagnosis of left ventricular hypertrophy in dogs, *J Chinese Vet Soc* 14:359, 1988.
23. Hill JD: Electrocardiographic diagnosis of right ventricular enlargement in dogs, *J Electrocardiol* 4:347, 1971.
24. Moise NS, Valentine BA, Brown CA et al: Duchenne's cardiomyopathy in a canine model: electrocardiographic and echocardiographic studies, *J Am Coll Cardiol* 17:812, 1991.
25. Calvert CA, Losonsky JM, Brown J et al: Comparisons of radiographic and electrocardiographic abnormalities in canine heartworm disease, *Vet Radiol* 27:2, 1986.
26. Bolton GR, Ettinger SJ: Right bundle branch block in the dog, *J Am Vet Med Assoc* 160:1104, 1972.
27. Elizari MV, Lazzari JO, Rosenbaum MB: Phase-3 and phase-4 intermittent left bundle branch block occurring spontaneously in a dog, *Eur J Cardiol* 1:95, 1973.
28. Moore EN, Hoffman BF, Patterson DF et al: Electrocardiographic changes due to delayed activation of the wall of the right ventricle, *Am Heart J* 68:347, 1964.
29. Pruitt RD, Watt TB, Murao S: Left axis deviation: its relation to experimentally induced lesions of the anterior left bundle branch system in canine and primate hearts, *Ann N Y Acad Sci* 127:204, 1965.
30. Gallagher JJ, Ticzon AR, Wallace AG et al: Activation studies following experimental hemiblock in the dog, *Circ Res* 35:752, 1974.
31. Watt TB, Pruitt RD: Left posterior fascicular block in canine and primate hearts: an electrocardiographic study, *Circulation* 40:677, 1969.
32. Uhley HN, Rivkin LM: Electrocardiographic patterns following interruption of the main and peripheral branches of the canine left bundle of His, *Am J Cardiol* 10:41, 1964.
33. Watt TB: Features of fascicular block imposed upon existing right bundle branch block in the dog and baboon, *Am J Cardiol* 39:1000, 1977.

CHAPTER 6

Echocardiography

More than any other technology since the harnessing of x-rays and radiographic imaging, ultrasound imaging of the heart and great vessels (echocardiography) has changed the way in which cardiac anatomy is clinically evaluated. Because ultrasound discriminates fluid and soft tissue structures and radiographs distinguish between air and soft tissue densities, ultrasound images of cardiac structure are complimentary to radiographic images for assessing the anatomy of thoracic structures. In addition, the rapid rate of image acquisition allows evaluation of cardiac motion over time, making it possible to noninvasively evaluate cardiac function. Doppler echocardiography (spectral and color flow Doppler) adds the ability to evaluate blood flow direction and velocity and patterns of blood flow within the heart and great vessels. Because echocardiography can critically evaluate cardiac anatomy, cardiac function, and blood flow patterns it has supplanted cardiac catheterization as the preferred method for critically evaluating the heart in clinical veterinary medicine. Although echocardiography is a powerful diagnostic aid, it should not be used in isolation. Rather, it must be considered as one component of a complete cardiovascular examination.

A firm grasp of cardiac anatomy and the relationships between various cardiac structures is essential to understand echocardiography. Consequently, the reader is referred to Chapter 1 before reading this chapter.

Instrumentation and Equipment

A detailed description of the principles, instrumentation, and safety of ultrasound is beyond the scope of this chapter. Consequently, the reader is referred to other sources.[1,2] Only those principles and instruments important for understanding echocardiography are presented.

Sound is produced by a sounding body vibrating in air or other media. These media transmit the sound at the same frequency, but the intensity becomes attenuated with distance from the source. Ultrasound is sound that occurs at a frequency higher than the human ear can detect, usually greater than 20 kHz (20,000 cycles/sec). In medicine, the frequencies used are much higher, generally between 2 and 10 MHz. For diagnostic imaging, an ultrasound beam is produced by a rapidly oscillating piezoelectric crystal commonly housed with other crystals to form a transducer. Piezoelectric crystals oscillate when a voltage is passed across them. Whereas sound travels in air as waves that disperse in all directions, ultrasound can be focused to travel through soft tissue in a single direction. When an ultrasound beam strikes a structure, some of it is reflected back to the transducer. Transducers usually use pulsed-wave technology, in which the crystal turns on for a short time and then waits for a longer period for the reflected waves to return. When the reflected ultrasound strikes the crystal, it oscillates the crystal. This is turned into a voltage detected by the machine. Ultrasound transmits through soft tissue at a relatively constant velocity (approximately 1540 m/sec). Consequently, it can be aimed at various soft tissue structures, and the ultrasound machine (i.e., the computer) can calculate the distance between the transducer and the structure by measuring the time it takes for the ultrasound beam to travel to the structure and come back to the transducer. By using sophisticated computer technology, an ultrasound machine can detect numerous structures at once, creating a two-dimensional image. Ultrasound is dispersed by air and cannot effectively penetrate bone. Consequently, an ultrasound image cannot be obtained from most regions of the chest. An image can only be obtained from regions where the heart contacts an intercostal region. This region is quite small and is called a *window.* Only transducers with small footprints can be used to access an appropriate window. For this reason, linear array transducers should not be used for echocardiography. Transducers used for echocardiography produce a fan-shaped beam or sector. The beam is formed either by placing numerous crystals in a row (i.e., a phased-array transducer) or by rotating the crystal but only allowing the beam to emerge from one section of the transducer (i.e., a mechanical transducer). High-frequency ultrasound (e.g., 7.5 MHz) is reflected off smaller structures than low-frequency ultrasound (e.g., 2.5 MHz). Because it strikes more structures, more of it is reflected as it travels through soft tissue and its energy is dissipated more rapidly. Consequently, high-frequency ultrasound does not penetrate through soft tissue as well as does low-frequency ultrasound. Also, because it reflects from smaller structures, the resolution of high-frequency ultrasound is better than that of low-frequency ultrasound. This makes high-frequency ultrasound preferable for small patients (e.g., small dogs and cats) and low-frequency ultrasound preferable for larger patients (e.g., horses). Lower frequencies are also required for optimal Doppler echocardiography. Because of the different requirements for imaging and Doppler ultrasound, it may be necessary to use several transducers during one examination. However, many newer machines have transducers that are capable of producing more than one frequency.

Technique

Dogs and cats usually require little preparation for echocardiographic examination. Sedation is not required nor desirable except in very uncooperative patients. If sedation is employed, the potential influence of the drug(s) on heart rate, chamber dimensions, and ventricular motion must be considered in the interpretation. The effects of ketamine hydrochloride, the effects of a combination of xylazine and sodium pentobarbital, and the effects of xylazine with or without glycopyrrolate on the feline M-mode echocardiogram have been studied. Intramuscular ketamine administration in healthy cats significantly increases heart rate and septal and left ventricular (LV) wall thickness, whereas the LV internal dimension in diastole, shortening fraction, and the velocity of circumferential fiber shortening significantly decreases.[3] Intravenous administration of a combination of xylazine and sodium pentobarbital produces a significant depression of indices of LV function, including a decrease in the LV internal dimension in diastole, shortening fraction, and the velocity of circumferential fiber shortening compared with values in awake cats.[4] Both the LV shortening fraction and the velocity of circumferential fiber shortening have been shown to be reduced in cats receiving only sodium pentobarbital.[5] Interestingly, these cats did not show a change in ventricular size. Significant changes in the LV shortening fraction, LV wall amplitude, aortic amplitude, and *E*-point–to–septal separation suggest that xylazine, alone or in combination with glycopyrrolate, produces a significant depression of global LV function.[6] The effects of acepromazine maleate and buprenorphine on the echocardiogram have been reported in dogs. Neither acepromazine nor buprenorphine produced significant changes in echocardiographic measures of left ventricular function (i.e., shortening fraction and aortic blood flow acceleration), despite the fact that both produced small decreases in dP/dt_{max}. Buprenorphine significantly decreased the heart rate.[6a] Although possibly similar, the effects of other sedatives on the two-dimensional examination of dogs and cats have not been reported. Ideally, hair is clipped over the left and right precordial transducer locations.

Dogs and cats may be examined in upright (standing, sitting, sternal) or laterally recumbent positions without substantial alteration of examination technique. However, the image quality is enhanced by positioning the animal in lateral recumbency on a table with an opening that allows transducer manipulation and examination from beneath the animal. This position results in the heart contacting a larger area of the lateral thorax and creates a larger ultrasound window for examination. Satisfactory images can almost always be obtained by parting the hair coat on either side of the chest and by applying a liberal quantity of coupling gel or by first wetting the area and then applying coupling gel. Shaving is sometimes required in dogs or cats with thick hair coats.

Normal Examinations

An echocardiographic examination usually starts with the two-dimensional examination. Two-dimensional echocardiography allows the most comprehensive evaluation of anatomy and spatial relationships. Other imaging modalities (M-mode, contrast, and Doppler echocardiography) are usually guided by the two-dimensional image. However, older units may have dedicated M-mode or Doppler capabilities, and continuous wave Doppler examinations are commonly performed without two-dimensional imaging.

TWO-DIMENSIONAL ECHOCARDIOGRAPHY

Two-dimensional echocardiograms are recorded with either mechanical scanners or electronically controlled phased-array scanners that emit a thin wedge or fan-shaped beam. Real-time motion is achieved by rapidly and continuously updating the image (usually 15 to 30 times a second) during the cardiac cycle. Each type of transducer has advantages and disadvantages, which are reviewed elsewhere.[1,7] Phased-array transducers allow simultaneous M-mode and two-dimensional studies and, with newer machines, simultaneous two-dimensional and Doppler examinations (duplex imaging). The study is generally displayed on a video screen and recorded on videotape. Digital acquisition is also possible, although this methodology is expensive. Individual frames may also be captured and recorded on photographic or x-ray film or photographic paper. Because two-dimensional echocardiography produces real-time, anatomic views of the heart, it provides a realistic, understandable, and complete image of the heart that is easy for most clinicians to recognize.

Several authors have studied the normal two-dimensional echocardiogram in the dog and cat.[8-13] The American Society of Echocardiography (ASE) has made recommendations for standardized two-dimensional echocardiographic study and terminology in humans.[14] Similar recommendations have recently been published for dogs and cats.[15] There are three general transducer locations (windows) that provide access to consistent imaging planes for two-dimensional echocardiography (Figure 6-1). The *right parasternal location* is located between the right third and sixth intercostal spaces (usually fourth to fifth) between the sternum and costochondral junctions. It is most easily located by palpating the right apex beat and placing the transducer at this location. The *left caudal (apical) parasternal location* is located between the left fifth and seventh intercostal spaces, as close to the sternum as possible. It is located by palpating the left apex beat. The *left cranial parasternal location* is located between the left third and fourth intercostal spaces between the sternum and costochondral junctions. The optimum transducer locations vary in individual

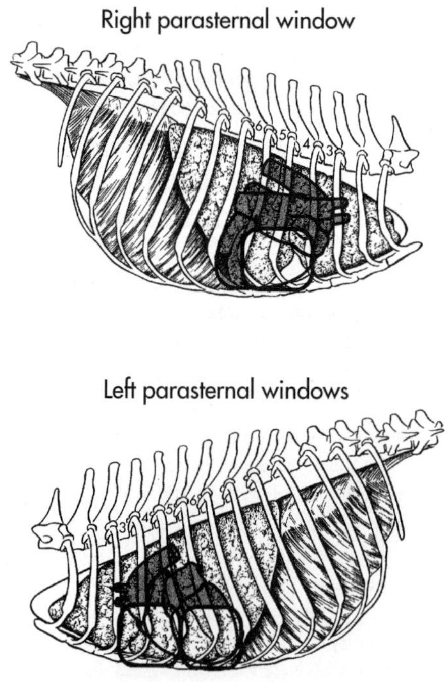

FIGURE 6-1 Schematic diagram of the canine thorax indicating the approximate regions of the optimal transducer "windows" used for echocardiography. (From Kienle RD, Thomas WP: Echocardiography. In Nyland T, Mattoon J, eds: *Veterinary diagnostic ultrasound,* Philadelphia, 1995, WB Saunders.)

animals and must be determined during the examination. Consistently high-quality images can usually be obtained from transducer locations just caudal to the xiphoid (subcostal location) or the thoracic inlet (suprasternal notch location) in humans but not in dogs and cats.

Imaging planes obtained from each transducer location are named with respect to their orientation with the left side of the heart, especially the left ventricle and ascending aorta.[14,15] A plane that transects the left ventricle parallel to the long axis of the heart from apex to base is called a *long-axis (longitudinal) plane.* A plane that transects the left ventricle or aorta perpendicular to the long axis of the heart is called a *short-axis (cross-sectional) plane.* Individual views are further identified by the region of the heart or number of chambers imaged. Variations of standard views may be necessary in individual animals to image some structures optimally.

Two primary imaging planes and one or more views in each plane are defined for each of the three principle transducer locations. The index mark on the two-dimensional transducer (which marks the edge of the imaging plane) is normally placed under the thumb of the operator. It should normally be oriented to indicate the part of the cardiac image that will appear on the right side of the image display.[14,15] The transducer index mark should then be pointed either toward the *base* of the heart (long-axis views) or *cranially* toward the patient's head (short-axis views). The exception to this rule is the left caudal (apical) four-chamber view (see below). In addition, the images should be displayed so that the transducer artifact and near-field echoes appear at the top and the far-field echoes at the bottom of the video display.

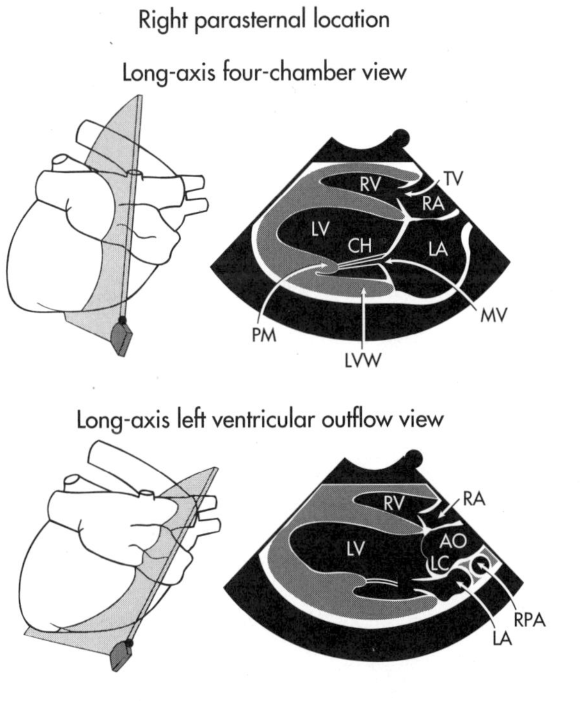

FIGURE 6-2 Schematic representations of the long-axis views obtained from the right parasternal window. The black circle at the top of the sector indicates the index mark. *LV,* Left ventricle; *RV,* right ventricle; *LA,* left atrium; *RA,* right atrium; *VS,* interventricular septum; *AO,* aorta; *PA,* pulmonary artery; *RPA,* right pulmonary artery; *LPA,* left pulmonary artery; *RVO* or *RVOT,* right ventricular outflow tract; *LVO* or *LVOT,* left ventricular outflow tract; *CaVC,* caudal vena cava; *RAu,* right auricle; *MV,* mitral valve; *TV,* tricuspid valve; *AV,* aortic valve; *PV,* pulmonary valve; *LC,* left coronary cusp of the aortic valve; *RC,* right coronary cusp of the aortic valve; *NC,* noncoronary cusp of the aortic valve; *AMV,* anterior mitral valve leaflet; *PMV,* posterior mitral valve leaflet; *CH* or *CT,* chorda tendineae; *PM,* papillary muscle; *APM,* anterior papillary muscle; *PPM,* posterior papillary muscle. (From Keinle RD, Thomas WP: Echocardiography. In Nyland T, Mattoon J, eds: *Veterinary diagnostic ultrasound,* Philadelphia, 1995, WB Saunders.)

The two-dimensional examination usually begins on the right side of the thorax and proceeds to the left caudal and ultimately left cranial views. The following imaging planes can be consistently obtained in most dogs and cats:

Right parasternal location

Long-axis views (Figure 6-2). With the beam plane oriented nearly perpendicular to the long axis of the body, parallel to the long axis of the heart, and with the transducer index mark pointing toward the heart base (dorsal), two views are usually obtained. The first is a four-chamber view with the cardiac apex (ventricles) displayed to the left and the base (atria) to the right. The second, obtained by slight clockwise rotation (when viewed from the bottom of the transducer) of the transducer from the four-chamber view into a slightly more craniodorsal-to-caudoventral orientation, shows the left ventricular outflow tract, aortic valve, aortic root, and proximal ascending aorta.

Short-axis views (Figure 6-3). By rotating the transducer approximately 90 degrees clockwise from the four-chamber view so that the beam plane is oriented close to the long axis of the body and perpendicular to the long axis of the heart and the transducer index mark is pointing cranially (or cranioventrally), a series of short-axis views are obtained. Proper short-axis orientation is identified by the circular symmetry of the left ventricle or aortic root. Short-axis planes are commonly obtained at the level of the left ventricular apex, papillary muscles, chordae tendineae, mitral valve, and aortic valve by angling the beam from the apex (ventral) to the base (dorsal). In most animals, further dorsal angulation and slight rotation allows imaging of the proximal ascending aorta, right atrium, and pulmonary artery branches. The images should be displayed with the cranial part of the image to the right and the right heart encircling the left ventricle and aorta clockwise (the right ventricular outflow tract and pulmonary valve to the right).

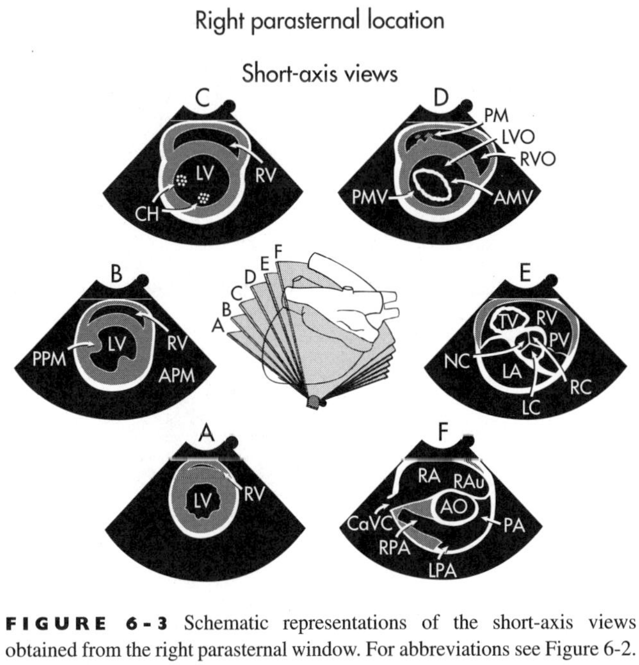

FIGURE 6-3 Schematic representations of the short-axis views obtained from the right parasternal window. For abbreviations see Figure 6-2. (From Kienle RD, Thomas WP: Echocardiography. In Nyland T, Mattoon J, eds: *Veterinary diagnostic ultrasound,* Philadelphia, 1995, WB Saunders.)

Left caudal (apical) parasternal location

Left apical two-chamber views (Figure 6-4). With the beam plane nearly perpendicular to the long axis of the body, parallel to the long axis of the heart, and with the transducer index mark pointing toward the heart base (dorsal), a two-chamber view of the left heart, including left atrium, mitral valve, and left ventricle, is obtained. Slight rotation of the transducer and beam plane into a more craniodorsal-to-caudoventral orientation results in a long-axis view of the left ventricle, outflow tract, aortic valve, and aortic root. This view is commonly used to measure left ventricular outflow tract and aortic root blood flow velocities with Doppler echocardiography (see below) because the transducer can be aligned parallel with blood flow from this position. Both of these views should be displayed with the left ventricular apex to the left and the left atrium or aorta to the right.

Left apical four-chamber views (Figure 6-5). With the beam plane placed into a left-caudal–to–right-cranial orientation and then directed dorsally toward the heart base, and with the transducer index mark pointing caudally and to the left, a four-chamber view of the heart may be obtained. Note that this is the only view in which the transducer index mark is pointing caudally and to the left, opposite the normal convention. Depending on the exact location of the caudal (apical) window, the appearance of this view varies between animals more than other views. The image should show the ventricles in the near field closest to the transducer and the atria in the far field, with the heart oriented vertically. The left heart (the left ventricle, mitral valve, and left atrium) should appear to the right and the right heart to the left on the screen. In some animals, especially cats, the available window allows imaging through the lateral left ventricular wall, rather than the apex, resulting in an image tilted horizontally (apex to the upper left, base to the lower right). Slight cranial tilting of the beam from the four-chamber view brings the left ventricular outflow region into view. In some animals imaging all four cardiac chambers simultaneously is possible, including both atrioventricular valves, the aortic valve, and proximal aorta (sometimes incorrectly called a *five-chamber view*).

Left cranial parasternal location

Long-axis views (Figure 6-6). With the beam plane oriented approximately parallel to the long axis of the body and to the long axis of the heart, and with the transducer index mark pointing cranially, a view of the left ventricular outflow tract, aortic valve, and ascending aorta is obtained. The image is displayed with the left ventricle to the left and the aorta to the right. This view, which is similar to the two-chamber left ventricular outflow view obtained from the left caudal (apical) location, shows the left ventricular outflow tract, aortic valve, and ascending aorta better than the corresponding caudal (apical) view. From this beam orientation, angling of the beam *ventral* to the aorta produces an oblique view of the left ventricle and the right atrium, tricuspid valve, and inflow region of the right ventricle. In this view the left ventricle is displayed to the left and the right auricle to the right. Angling of the transducer and beam plane *dorsal* to the aorta produces a view of the right ventricular outflow tract, pulmonic valve, and main pulmonary artery.

Short-axis view (see Figure 6-8). With the beam plane oriented approximately perpendicular to the long axis of the body and the long axis of the heart, and with the transducer index mark pointing dorsally, an orientation obtained by a 90-degree clockwise beam rotation from the long axis views, a short-axis view of the aortic root

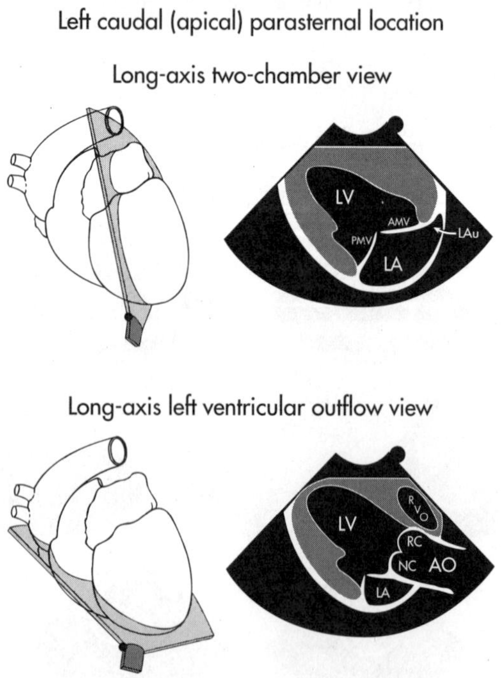

FIGURE 6-4 Schematic representation of the two-chamber views obtained from the left caudal (apical) parasternal window. For abbreviations see Figure 6-2. (From Kienle RD, Thomas WP: Echocardiography. In Nyland T, Mattoon J, eds: *Veterinary diagnostic ultrasound,* Philadelphia, 1995, WB Saunders.)

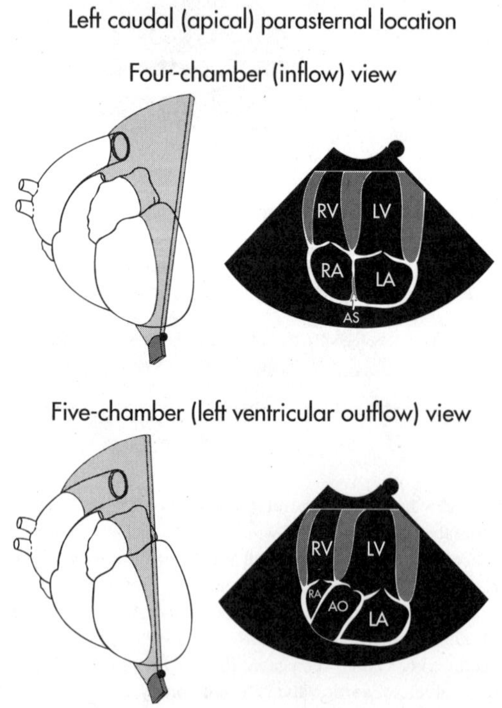

FIGURE 6-5 Schematic representation of the four-chamber views obtained from the left caudal (apical) parasternal window. For abbreviations see Figure 6-2. (From Kienle RD, Thomas WP: Echocardiography. In Nyland T, Mattoon J, eds: *Veterinary diagnostic ultrasound,* Philadelphia, 1995, WB Saunders.)

encircled by the right heart is obtained. The image, which is similar to the short-axis view at the aortic valve level obtained from the right side (see Figure 6-3), is displayed with the right heart encircling the aorta *clockwise,* with the right ventricular inflow tract to the left and the outflow tract and pulmonary artery to the right.

Examples of two-dimensional echocardiographic images from normal dogs and cats are shown in Figures 6-7 through 6-9.

M-MODE ECHOCARDIOGRAPHY

M-mode (motion mode) echocardiography employs a beam from a single ultrasound crystal that pierces the heart much like placing a needle through the heart ("ice-pick view"). Technical aspects of this examination have been described in a previous report.[16] If the transducer is kept in a constant position during the cardiac cycle, the phasic motion of the cardiac structures can be recorded. The M-mode echocardiogram is viewed on a video screen and is recorded either on a strip chart, photographic paper, or videotape. Depth (distance from the transducer) is represented on the vertical axis, and time is represented on the horizontal axis. A simultaneous electrocardiogram serves as a time reference of the cardiac cycle. Cardiac structures are identified by observing characteristic motion relative to the transducer artifact and other cardiac structures (Figure 6-10). Because the vertical axis is calibrated, axial dimensions can be measured and on most ultrasound machines electronic calipers can be used directly to measure cardiac structures on the video screen. Important uses for M-mode echocardiography include the quantification of cardiac chamber sizes and wall thicknesses, wall motion, great vessel dimensions, and valve motion.[8] It should be emphasized that the accuracy of M-mode measurements is directly related to the quality of the tracing and proper positioning of the beam across a structure. The utility of M-mode echocardiography in the diagnosis of cardiovascular disease in dogs and cats has been demonstrated in several reports.[7-9,16,17]

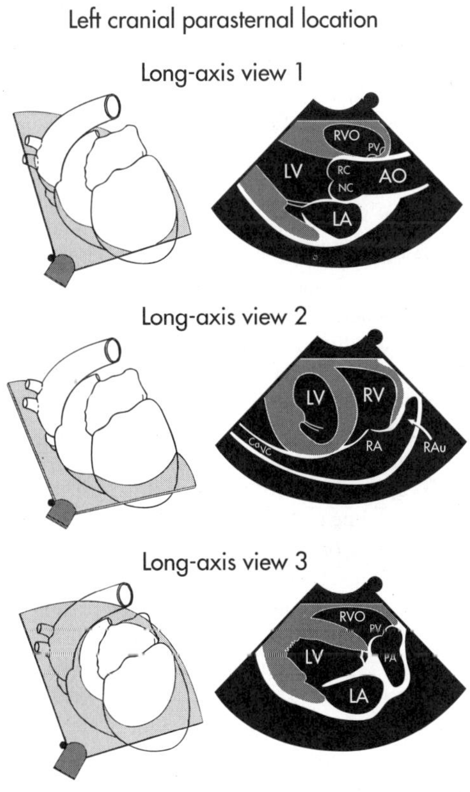

FIGURE 6-6 Schematic representation of long-axis images obtained from the left cranial parasternal window. For abbreviations see Figure 6-2 (From Kienle RD, Thomas WP: Echocardiography. In Nyland T, Mattoon J, eds: *Veterinary diagnostic ultrasound,* Philadelphia, 1995, WB Saunders.)

Unlike two-dimensional examinations, the M-mode echocardiogram is generally only performed from the right parasternal location. The identification of cardiac structures is based on both a preconceived mental image of the expected path of the ultrasound beam and an understanding of normal and pathologic anatomy (see Figure 6-10 and Chapter 1). The former is most easily accomplished by correlating the M-mode structures with two-dimensional images obtained at the right parasternal window (see Figures 6-2 and 6-3) or by using a machine that allows two-dimensional guided M-mode echocardiograms (duplex imaging). A schematic illustration of the standard M-mode echocardiographic positions is illustrated in Figure 6-11, along with the structures commonly measured.[1]

When the ultrasound beam is directed through the heart from the right parasternal position at the level of the left ventricle, the beam sequentially traverses the chest wall, the right ventricular wall, the right ventricular chamber, the interventricular septum, the left ventricular chamber, the posteriolateral left ventricular wall, and the pericardium. The right ventricular chamber is typically quite narrow at this level. The left ventricular free wall may appear falsely thick if a papillary muscle is inadvertently encountered by directing the beam too far ventrally (apically). Systolic ventricular septal motion is usually posterior (left caudal), that is, directed toward the left ventricular free wall and away from the transducer. Normally the interventricular septum and left ventricular free wall move toward each other during systole and away from each other in diastole, mimicking the motion of an accordion. Occasionally, peak motions may not precisely correspond because of slight differences in depolarization and because of movement of the entire heart with respect to the transducer during separate phases of the cardiac cycle.[7] Some reports have said that paradoxic or anteriorly directed (toward the right ventricle) systolic ventricular septal motion suggests a right ventricular volume or pressure overload.[18] It has been our experience that mild paradoxic septal motion may also be seen in normal dogs positioned in lateral recumbency with the examination performed from beneath the animal.

As the transducer is angled dorsally, the mitral valve leaflets appear within the left ventricular chamber. Although both the anterior (the cranial or septal leaflet) and the posterior (the caudal or mural leaflet) leaflets may be imaged, in many cases the posterior leaflet is not well visualized. Occasionally, chordae tendineae are visualized in association with the valve leaflets. A normal mitral valve should impart a discrete, fine-lined excursion. The anterior leaflet typically produces an M-shaped excursion, whereas the posterior leaflet, if visualized, inscribes a smaller, W-shaped image that is a mirror image of the anterior leaflet. Specific points of the mitral valve excursion are labeled as follows: *C,* point of mitral valve systolic closure; *D,* end of systolic closure; *E,* maximal early diastolic separation of the leaflets; *F,* partial closure in middiastole; and *A,* mitral opening as the result of atrial systole. At rapid heart rates, as seen in cats, small dogs, and any patient with a tachyarrhythmia, the *E* point and *A* point merge into a single diastolic opening motion as the diastolic interval decreases. The slope of the line from *D* to *E* is proportional to the rate of blood flow from the left atrium to the left ventricle during early diastolic filling. The middiastolic closure rate of the mitral valve is represented by the *E*-to-*F* slope. In conditions such as mitral stenosis, disorders leading to decreased left ventricular compliance, or pulmonary hypertension, the *E*-to-*F* slope may

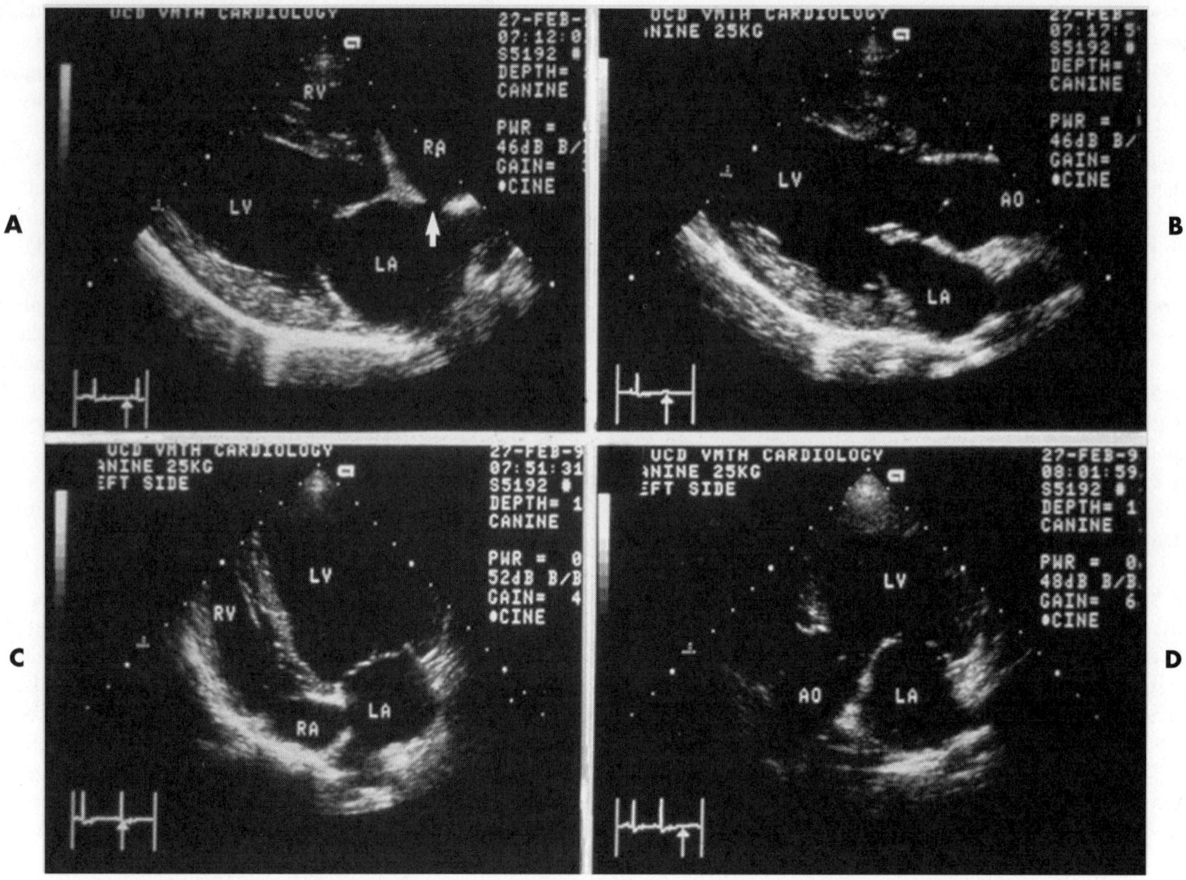

FIGURE 6-7 Long-axis echocardiographic images from a normal dog. **A,** Right parasternal four-chamber view. The arrow identifies the fossa ovalis, which may falsely appear to be a septal defect. **B,** Right parasternal long-axis view. **C,** Left caudal (apical) parasternal four-chamber view. **D,** Left caudal (apical) parasternal long-axis view (five-chamber view). For abbreviations see Figure 6-2. (From Kienle RD, Thomas WP: Echocardiography. In Nyland T, Mattoon J, eds: *Veterinary diagnostic ultrasound,* Philadelphia, 1995, WB Saunders.)

become flatter.[1] In normal individuals the *E* point excursion is greater than the excursion of the *A* point. In situations in which atrial contraction becomes a major contribution to ventricular filling (e.g., with decreased left ventricular compliance), the *A* point excursion may exceed the *E* point excursion. The M-mode of mitral valve motion may be used as a reference in the timing of intracardiac events and in the determination of systolic and diastolic time intervals. The *D* and *C* points of mitral valve motion correspond to mitral valve opening and closure.[19] If the tricuspid valve is imaged, it imparts similar excursions as the mitral valve.

If the transducer is angled further dorsally and slightly cranially, the aortic root and left atrium are brought into view. During a sweep from the mitral valve level to the level of the aorta, the interventricular septum is continuous with the anterior aortic wall and the anterior leaflet of the mitral valve is continuous with the posterior wall of the aorta. The aorta is identified as two parallel lines moving toward the transducer in systole and away in diastole. The left atrium is seen to the left of (below) the aorta. The motion of the aorta occurs because of the systolic ejection of blood from the left ventricle and the motion of the entire heart in systole.[1] The left coronary cusp of the aortic valve is consistently imaged as a thin structure opening toward the posterior wall of the aorta during systole and closing toward the center of the aorta during diastole. A second cusp (either the right coronary or the noncoronary cusp) is less consistently visualized and appears as a mirror image of the left coronary cusp. Aortic valve motion should look like a parallelogram if two cusps are imaged. The posterior wall of the left atrium is continuous with the left ventricular free wall and is distinguished by its decreased motion and thinner appearance.

M-mode and two-dimensional echocardiography are complimentary techniques, each with its own advantages and limitations. The two-dimensional examination is superior for assessing overall anatomy, global patterns of size and motion, and spatial orientation. However, two-dimensional echocardiography is limited by video resolution (especially for small structures), and the slower sampling rate can make real-time motion difficult to measure in animals with very fast heart rates or in structures that move rapidly (e.g., a vibrating portion of a valve). The M-mode has a high sampling rate, allowing for continuous recording of even rapid motion. As a result, the M-mode echocardiogram is more accurate for timing events and tracking subtle or rapid movements. In addition, the resolution of borders is superior on the M-mode, theoretically making measurements easier and more accurate.

Echocardiographic Measurements

Measurements of cardiac structures can be made from either the M-mode or the two-dimensional echocardiogram. Studies have demonstrated a good correlation between measurements made using

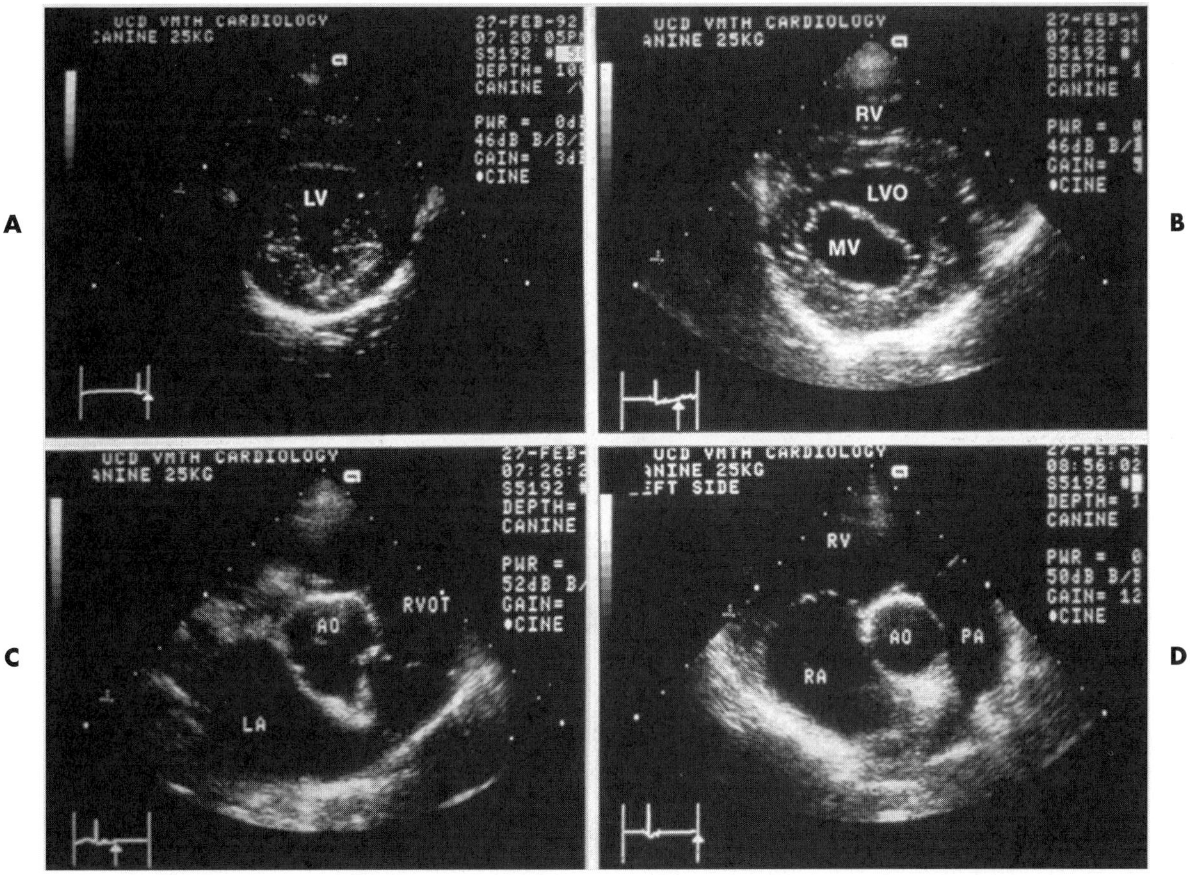

FIGURE 6-8 Short-axis echocardiographic images from a normal dog. **A,** Right parasternal short-axis view at the level of the left ventricular papillary muscles. **B,** Right parasternal short-axis view at the level of the mitral valve. **C,** Right parasternal short-axis view at the level of the aortic valve. **D,** Left cranial parasternal short-axis view at the level of the aortic valve. For abbreviations see Figure 6-2. (From Kienle RD, Thomas WP: Echocardiography. In Nyland T, Mattoon J, eds: *Veterinary diagnostic ultrasound,* Philadelphia, 1995, WB Saunders.)

the two techniques.[20] The most important factors influencing the accuracy of echocardiographic measurements are image quality and consistency of technique and positioning. Recommended procedures for measuring M-mode and two-dimensional echocardiograms have been published for humans.[21,22] These recommendations are generally accepted for veterinary studies (see Figure 6-11). Routine measurements include ventricular internal dimensions, ventricular and septal wall thickness, and aortic and left atrial dimensions. For echocardiographic measurements, it is routine to take end-diastolic measurements at the onset of the QRS complex of the electrocardiogram, although electromechanical delay results in the true end of diastole occurring midway through the QRS complex. End-systolic measurements are taken at the smallest dimension between the interventricular septum and the left ventricular free wall. Measurements should be made at the "leading edge," (the edge closest to the transducer) of a structure, because it denotes a specific interface.[23] Ventricular dimensions and wall thicknesses should be made at the level of the chordae tendineae or tips of papillary muscles just below the tips of the mitral valve, with the beam directed perpendicular to the septum and left ventricular wall. The level of the aortic valve is used for aortic root and left atrial dimensions, and may be used for calculation of systolic and diastolic time intervals (see below). The aortic root is measured at end-diastole, and the left atrium is measured at its maximal anterior (upward) excursion near the end of systole.[1,8,21]

Intracardiac dimensions, ventricular wall thicknesses, other M-mode measurements, and calculations derived from M-mode measurements have been shown to vary with body size, body surface area, breed, and other variables.[24-26] M-mode measurements are also significantly altered by changes in heart rate, loading conditions, and cardiac contractility.[3,27-29] These variables must be taken into account in establishing echocardiographic reference ranges and must be kept in mind when interpreting the M-mode echocardiogram. Normal values for M-mode cardiac measurements have been reported for the dog and the cat[3,5,8,29-37] (Table 6-1). There is greater variation in normal canine measurements because of breed differences than between cat breeds and a much wider range of body size for dogs. To date, no one has acquired echocardiographic variables from enough dogs to make valid conclusions regarding normal values for all dogs. Consequently, although normal data have been published, accepted normal values for dogs have not been established. One of our colleagues has collected values from the literature for 175 to 350 normal dogs ranging in size from 3 to 68 kg and devised regressions of cardiac measurements against body weight (Table 6-2).[38] This table presents only mean values because individual data points have not been reported from the majority of the normal dogs in the reported studies. From our clinical experience, we believe that these data are more accurate than any that we have previously seen published. The estimates of confidence intervals currently in the literature probably overestimate the true intervals, especially in small and large dogs. In our opinion, most dogs should

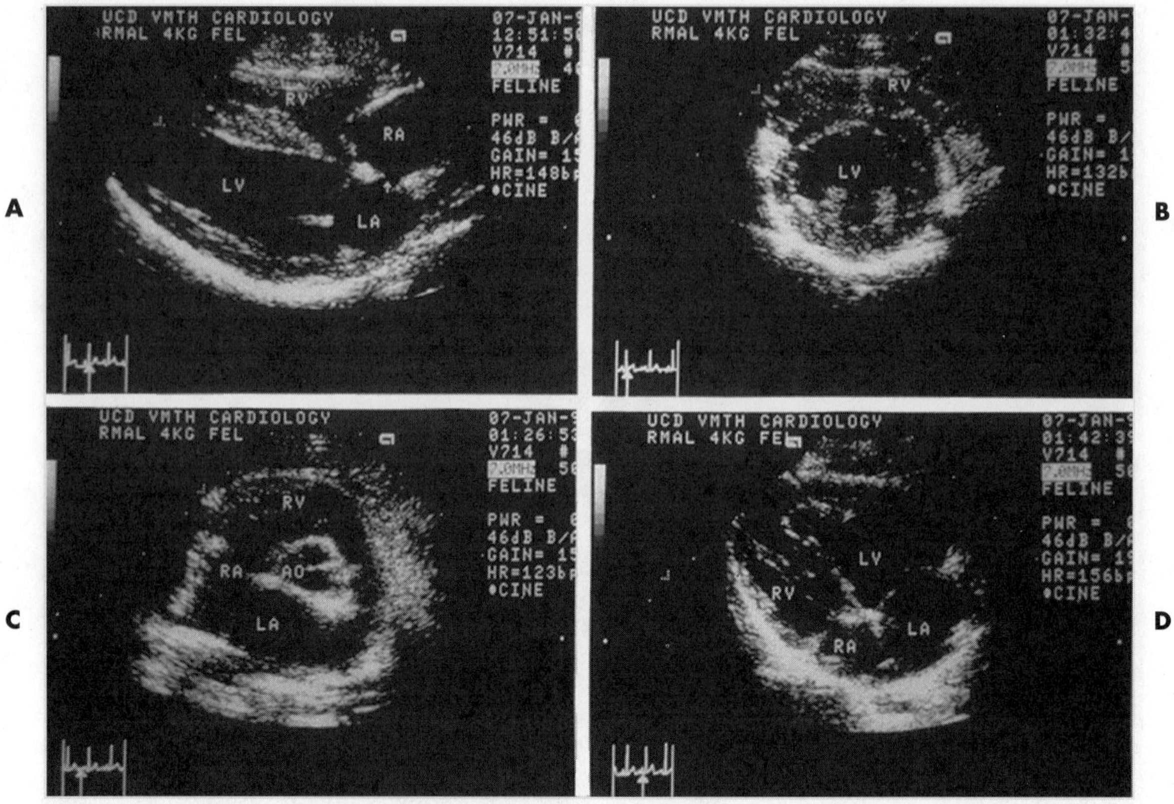

FIGURE 6-9 Two-dimensional echocardiographic images from a normal cat. **A,** Right parasternal four-chamber view. **B,** Right parasternal short-axis view at the level of the left ventricular papillary muscles. **C,** Right parasternal short-axis view at the level of the aortic valve. **D,** Left caudal (apical) parasternal four chamber view. For abbreviations see Figure 6-2. (From Kienle RD, Thomas WP: Echocardiography. In Nyland T, Mattoon J, eds: *Veterinary diagnostic ultrasound,* Philadelphia, 1995, WB Saunders.)

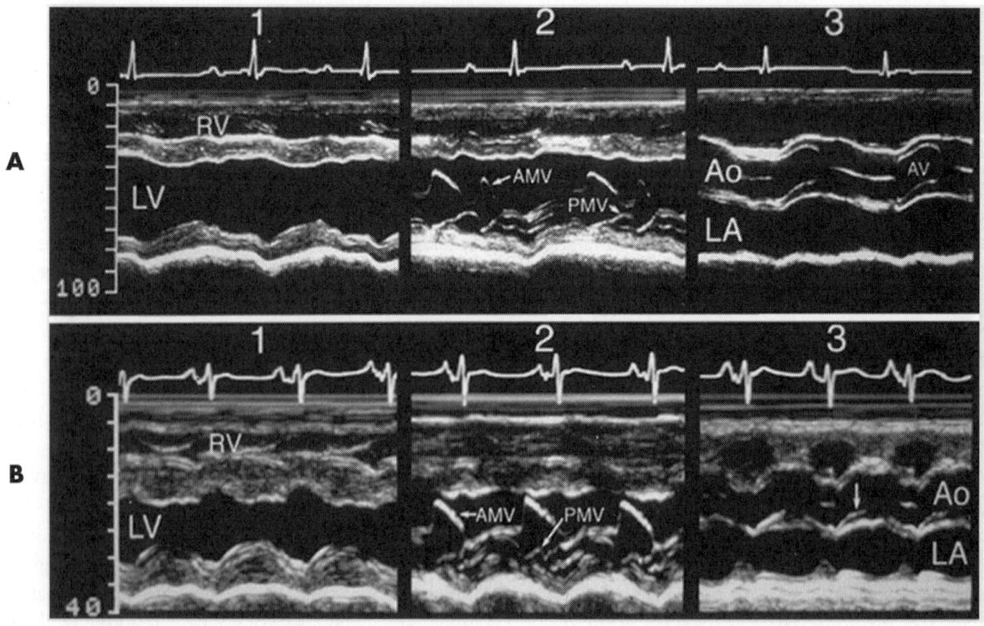

FIGURE 6-10 M-mode echocardiographic images from a normal dog and cat. **A,** Normal canine M-mode echocardiograms recorded at the level of the (1) left ventricle, (2) mitral valve, and (3) aorta and left atrium. **B,** Normal feline M-mode echocardiograms recorded at the same levels as in **A** (arrow indicates the aortic valve). For abbreviations see Figure 6-2. (From Kienle RD, Thomas WP: Echocardiography. In Nyland T, Mattoon J, eds: *Veterinary diagnostic ultrasound,* Philadelphia, 1995, WB Saunders.)

have values for most echocardiographic measures that are within 10% of either side of the mean if the dog is echoed by a skilled individual. Values can vary widely when nonskilled individuals take these measurements.

The ratio of the left atrial diameter to the aortic root diameter is useful in judging the size of the left atrium because judgments based on the absolute size may be inaccurate. In the normal dog and cat, this ratio is usually less than 1.3 and often approaches unity on an M-mode echocardiogram.[8,29-31,36] Values greater than 1.3 suggest left atrial dilation. However, the ultrasound beam passes through the left auricle or cranial portion of the left atrium and not through its main body (as in humans) on most M-mode echocardiograms from dogs and cats. An increased left atrium/aorta ratio suggests left atrial dilation, but a normal ratio does not rule it out. Left atrial size is best evaluated subjectively on the two-dimensional echocardiogram. This provides a more comprehensive examination in multiple planes (Figure 6-12). The left atrial size also can be measured on a two-dimensional echocardiogram. We prefer to place a line at a 45-degree angle from perpendicular that passes through the aorta and the body of the left atrium to measure the diameter of these two structures. Using this measurement, a left atrial to aortic root ratio of greater than 1.5 suggests left atrial enlargement.

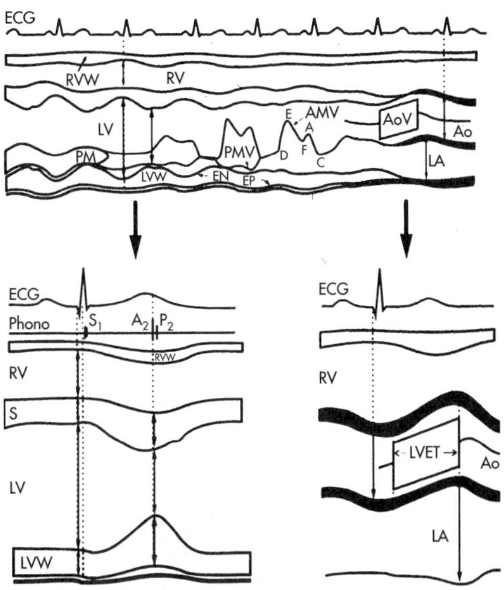

FIGURE 6-11 Recommended methods for echocardiographic measurements from the M-mode echocardiogram. Above is a standard M-mode sweep from the level of the left ventricular papillary muscles to the level of the aorta and left atrium, showing the locations and timing of chamber dimension and wall thickness measurements. For abbreviations see Figure 6-2. (From Kienle RD, Thomas WP: Echocardiography. In Nyland T, Mattoon J, eds: *Veterinary diagnostic ultrasound,* Philadelphia, 1995, WB Saunders.)

Estimation of Cardiac Volume and Mass

Various methods for determining left ventricular volume and mass using both M-mode and two-dimensional echocardiographic measurements have been described. In fact, much of the experimental validation of these methods has been performed in dogs.[39,40] All techniques are limited by geometric assumptions, and their degree of accuracy increases with the number of measurements that make up the calculation. Automatic calculations of these variables, including left ventricular volumes and cardiac output, are commonly generated on newer echocardiographic machines because of the widespread use of electronic calipers and built-in software for these calculations. Extreme attention to detail is required to produce calculations that are close to reality. Most of the data generated from one-dimensional measurements is inaccurate. Information regarding the calculation of cardiac volume and mass is presented in Box 6-1.

TABLE 6-1

Normal echocardiographic values in cats

Mensural	(*n* = 11)[37]	(*n* = 25)[35]	(*n* = 30)[34]	*NG*[8]	(*n* = 30)[29,c]	(*n* = 16)[25,c]
LVEDD (cm)	1.51 ± 0.21[a]	1.48 ± 0.26[a]	1.59 ± 0.19[a]	1.10-1.60[b]	1.40 ± 0.13[a]	0.28 ± 0.17[a]
LVESD (cm)	0.69 ± 0.22	0.88 ± 0.24	0.80 ± 0.14	0.60-1.00	0.81 ± 0.16	0.83 ± 0.15
Ao (cm)	0.95 ± 0.15	0.75 ± 0.18	0.95 ± 0.11	0.65-1.10	0.95 ± 0.11	0.94 ± 0.14
LA (cm)	1.21 ± 0.18	0.74 ± 0.17	1.23 ± 0.14	0.85-1.25	1.03 ± 0.14	0.98 ± 0.17
LA/Ao (mc)	1.29 ± 0.23	—	1.30 ± 0.17	0.80-1.30	1.10 ± 0.18	1.09 ± 0.27
IVSED (cm)	0.50 ± 0.07	0.45 ± 0.09	0.31 ± 0.04	0.25-0.50	0.36 ± 0.08	—
IVSES (cm)	0.76 ± 0.12	—	0.58 ± 0.06	0.50-0.90	—	—
LVWED (cm)	0.46 ± 0.05	0.37 ± 0.08	0.33 ± 0.06	0.25-0.50	0.35 ± 0.08	0.31 ± 0.11
LVWES (cm)	0.78 ± 0.10	—	0.68 ± 0.07	0.40-0.90	—	0.55 ± 0.88
RVED (cm)	0.54 ± 0.10	—	0.60 ± 0.15	—	0.50 ± 0.21	—
LVWA (cm)	0.50 ± 0.07	—	—	—	—	0.32 ± 0.11
EPSS (cm)	0.04 ± 0.07	—	0.02 ± 0.09	—	—	—
AA (cm)	0.36 ± 0.10	—	—	—	—	—
MVEFS (mm/sec)	54.4 ± 13.4	—	87.2 ± 25.9	—	—	83.78 ± 23.81
ΔD% (%)	55.0 ± 10.2	41.0 ± 7.3	49.8 ± 5.3	29-35	42.7 ± 8.1	34.5 ± 12.6
LVWTF (%)	39.5 ± 7.6	—	—	—	—	—
IVSTF (%)	33.5 ± 8.2	—	—	—	—	—
HR (beats/min)	182 ± 22	167 ± 29	194 ± 23	—	255 ± 36	—

[a]Mean ± SD; [b]Normal range; [c]Cats anesthetized with ketamine.

LVEDD, Left ventricular (LV) end-diastolic dimension; *LVESD,* LV end-systolic dimension; *Ao,* aorta; *LA,* left atrium; *LA/Ao,* LA-to-Ao ratio; *IVSED,* interventricular septal thickness in diastole; *IVSES,* interventricular septal thickness in systole; *LVWED,* LV free wall thickness in diastole; *LVWES,* LV free wall thickness in systole; *RVED,* right ventricle in end-diastole; *LVWA,* LV wall amplitude; *EPSS,* E-point–to–septal separation; *AA,* aortic amplitude; *MVEFS,* mitral valve E-F slope; *ΔD%,* LV shortening fraction; *LVWTF,* LV wall thickening fraction; *IVSTF,* interventricular septal thickening fraction; *HR,* heart rate; *NG,* not given.

TABLE 6-2

Normal mean echocardiographic values (cm) in dogs*

BW (kg)	*EDD*	*ESD*	*IVSD*	*LVWD*	*EPSS*	*Ao*	*LA*
3	2.0	1.1	0.5	0.6	0.1	1.1	1.3
5	2.4	1.3	0.6	0.7	0.1	1.3	1.5
10	3.0	1.8	0.7	0.8	0.2	1.6	1.8
15	3.4	2.1	0.8	0.8	0.2	1.9	2.0
20	3.8	2.4	0.9	0.9	0.3	2.1	2.2
25	4.0	2.6	0.9	0.9	0.3	2.2	2.4
30	4.3	2.8	1.0	1.0	0.4	2.4	2.5
35	4.5	3.0	1.0	1.0	0.4	2.5	2.6
40	4.7	3.1	1.0	1.0	0.5	2.6	2.7
45	4.9	3.3	1.1	1.1	0.5	2.7	2.8
50	5.0	3.4	1.1	1.1	0.6	2.8	2.9
55	5.2	3.6	1.2	1.1	0.6	2.9	3.0
60	5.3	3.7	1.2	1.1	0.7	3.0	3.1
65	5.5	3.8	1.2	1.2	0.7	3.1	3.1
Formula	$1.44\ BW^{0.32}$	$0.69\ BW^{0.41}$	$0.36\ BW^{0.29}$	$0.46\ BW^{0.22}$	$0.03\ BW^{0.76}$	$0.72\ BW^{0.35}$	$0.9\ BW^{0.30}$
r value	0.97	0.95	0.89	0.81	0.94	0.96	0.98
Number	350	328	309	309	175	204	204

BW, Body weight; *EDD,* end-diastolic diameter; *ESD,* end-systolic diameter; *IVSD,* interventricular septal thickness in diastole; *LVWD,* left ventricular free wall thickness in diastole; *EPSS,* E-point–to–septal separation; *Ao,* aortic root diameter; *LA,* left atrial diameter. The formula is the formula of the line of best fit for the data. The number represents the number of dogs sampled in the combined studies in the references.
*References 25, 26, 33, 94–103.

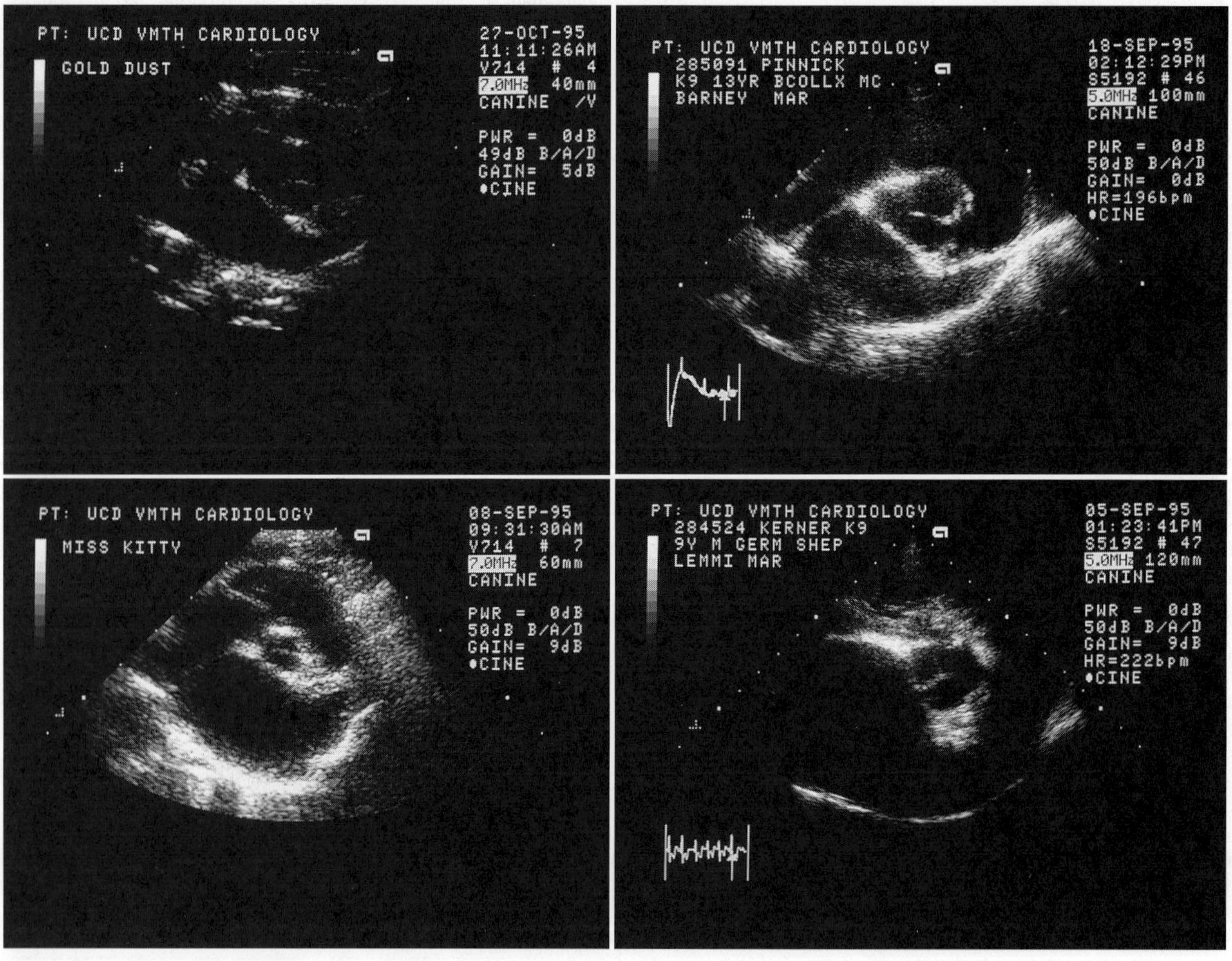

FIGURE 6-12 Two-dimensional echocardiograms from the right parasternal short-axis view from various patients with various diseases showing normal **(A)**, mildly increased **(B)**, moderately increased **(C)**, and severely increased **(D)** left atrial size. Left atrial size is evaluated subjectively by comparing it with the size of the aortic root. (See text for details.)

BOX 6-1

Echocardiographic estimation of cardiac volume and mass

This discussion addresses only those methods commonly used in veterinary practice. Left ventricular (LV) volume can be estimated from the short-axis internal dimensions of the LV at end-diastole and end-systole. Although these methods are relatively simple, they require several geometric assumptions that are not entirely valid. These assumptions are fairly accurate when applied to a heart of normal size and shape, but become increasingly inaccurate as the heart enlarges and changes shape. In lieu of the inherent limitations, various authors, including Pombo, Mashiro, and Teichholz, have proposed formulas for calculating LV volume based on M-mode measurements.[44] The simplest method of estimating LV volume from the M-mode echocardiogram is to cube the internal LV dimensions, as proposed by Pombo and demonstrated by the following equation:

$$LVV_s = ESD^3 \text{ and } LVV_d = EDD^3$$

where LVV_s and LVV_d are *LV* volume at end-systole and end-diastole, *ESD* is end-systolic dimension, and *EDD* is end-diastolic dimension.[44] Dividing this number by 1.5 produces a more accurate estimate of normal ventricular volumes in dogs.[88] The Teichholz formula is a corrected cube formula that attempts to account for the fact that the short axis of the LV widens more than the long axis when the ventricular chamber enlarges. It may be the most accurate of the M-mode methods in humans, but it has generally been inaccurate in dogs in our laboratory. The Teichholz formulas for systolic and diastolic volume are as follows:

$$LVV_s = \frac{7\,(ESD^3)}{2.4 + ESD} \qquad LVV_d = \frac{7\,(EDD^3)}{2.4 + EDD}$$

Estimates of myocardial mass from M-mode methods involve the subtraction of the volume of the LV cavity from the combined volume of the LV cavity, septum, and free wall (usually using diastolic measurements). Several formulas using M-mode measurements of wall thickness have been used for estimating LV mass, but all have important limitations arising from the one-dimensional nature of the techniques.

Because of the inaccuracy of M-mode calculations in enlarged hearts, most quantitative methods currently use two-dimensional methods, which involve more direct measurements and fewer geometric assumptions. Numerous methods for determining two-dimensional LV volume have been proposed. Wyatt et al[39,40] studied the accuracy of these methods in vitro and in vivo in experimental dogs. The American Society of Echocardiography (ASE) recently made recommendations for the quantification of the human left ventricle using two-dimensional echocardiography that are applicable to dogs (and probably cats).[22] With all methods, close attention must be paid to correct image orientation and proper instrument settings to optimize the size and shape of the LV and the endocardial surface. For all measurements, end-diastole is defined as the frame at or before initial mitral valve closure or the first frame in which the QRS complex appears. End systole is identified as the frame just before the initial opening of the mitral valve, or less satisfactory, the smallest visible cavity area. Although not commonly used in practice, high-quality video digitizers and digital frame grabbers combined with dedicated computers for off-line analysis greatly enhance the accuracy of these calculations.

All two-dimensional echo formulas involve the LV long-axis dimension and one or more LV short-axis dimensions or cross-sectional areas. Among the many proposed methods for calculating LV volume from two-dimensional echocardiograms are the single-plane area – length, biplane area – length, bullet formula (Dodge), Simpson's rule, and disc summation (Figure 6-13).[22] The ASE recommends paired orthogonal left apical views (i.e., two-chamber and four-chamber) be used for such measurements. The ASE currently recommends the disc summation method (modified Simpson's rule) as the preferred method of calculating LV volume.[22] With this method, volume is calculated from the summation of areas of a number (usually 20) of parallel slices or cylinders of discs that are proportioned by dividing the LV into 20

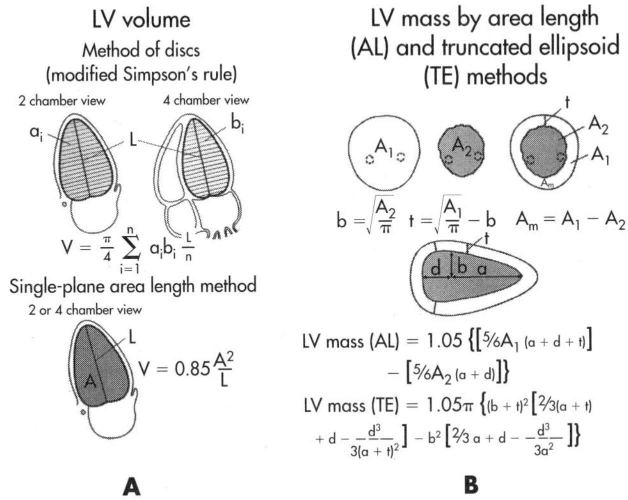

FIGURE 6-13 Methods for measuring left ventricular volume and mass by two-dimensional echocardiography. **A,** Biplane and single-plane algorithms for calculating chamber volume. *Top panel,* Biplane method of discs (modified Simpson's rule), using nearly orthogonal apical two- and four-chamber views. *Bottom panel,* Single-plane area length method, originally developed for angiography, used when only one apical view is obtainable. *V,* Volume; *A,* area; *L,* length; a_i and b_i, diameter of each disc from two-chamber and four-chamber views, respectively. **B,** Methods for measuring left ventricular mass. *Upper panel,* Diagram of left ventricular short-axis views at the level of the papillary muscles, demonstrating epicardial and endocardial perimeters that are traced to calculate myocardial thickness *(t),* short axis radius *(b),* and areas (A_1 and A_2). Both methods of calculating mass use the short-axis in this manner. *Lower panel,* Long-axis view measurements and resulting formulas for left ventricular mass by area length *(AL)* and truncated ellipsoid *(TE)* methods. *a,* Long or semimajor axis from the widest minor axis radius to the apex; *b,* short-axis radius; *t,* myocardial thickness; and *d,* truncated semimajor axis from the widest short-axis diameter to the mitral annulus plane. (From Kienle RD, Thomas WP: Electrocardiography. In Nyland T, Matoon J, eds: *Veterinary diagnostic ultrasound,* Philadelphia, 1995, WB Saunders.)

equal sections obtained from the apical two- and four-chamber views. This method is preferred because it is relatively independent of geometric assumptions. In situations in which only one apical view is available, the single plane area – length method can be used, although it is less accurate.

Two algorithms, both of which have been validated in dogs, are currently being recommended for myocardial mass estimation by the ASE (see Figure 6-13).[22] These formulas are based on the cylinder – ellipse area – length model[89,90] and truncated ellipsoid model.[91,92] Although neither is a superior model, they are both acceptable for clinical use. Both methods use similar measurements to arrive at the calculation. The first step in each method is the determination of the myocardial cross-sectional area from the LV short-axis view at the papillary muscle level. The difference between endocardial and epicardial areas determined by planimetry allows calculation of myocardial area. From this, mean wall thickness can be determined. Both methods then use long-axis dimensions to complete the calculation. The area – length method divides the long axis at the middle of the ventricle, and the truncated ellipse method divides the LV at the base. Values for both methods have been validated in dogs but not in cats.[89-92]

Evaluation of Cardiac Function

The traditional methods for the evaluation of cardiac function (cardiac output, ventricular volumes, ejection fraction, etc.) have used invasive techniques such as the Fick principle, indicator dye or thermodilution principles, or radionuclide angiography. Invasive techniques are impractical for routine clinical use in awake animals. Echocardiography allows many indices of cardiac function to be obtained noninvasively, making these methods more widely acceptable for clinical evaluation.

SYSTOLIC TIME INTERVALS

Before the widespread use of echocardiography, systolic time intervals (STIs) were one of the few noninvasive methods for evaluating left ventricular (LV) performance.[41] Originally, the measurement of STIs involved simultaneous recordings of the ECG, phonocardiogram, and carotid pulse (in humans) or apexcardiogram (in dogs). To measure STIs using echocardiography requires simultaneous recording of the ECG and the M-mode echocardiogram of the aortic valve.

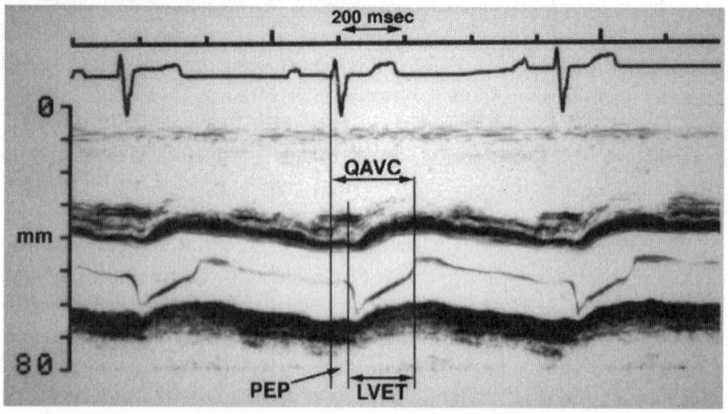

FIGURE 6-14 Simultaneous recording of the electrocardiogram and M-mode echocardiogram of the aortic valve. The method for measuring systolic time intervals is illustrated. *PEP,* Preejection period; *LVET,* left ventricular ejection time; *QAVC,* total electromechanical systole. (See text for details.) (From Kienle RD, Thomas WP: Electrocardiography. In Nyland T, Matoon J, eds: *Veterinary diagnostic ultrasound,* Philadelphia, 1995, WB Saunders.)

Three basic interval measurements are made during systole (Figure 6-14). The preejection period (PEP) is the interval from the onset of ventricular depolarization (the Q wave on the ECG) to the beginning of LV ejection (opening of the aortic valve). It is determined by the amount of electromechanical delay and the time it takes for left ventricular pressure to reach aortic diastolic pressure (the isovolumic contraction time, a correlate of dP/dt). The LV ejection time (LVET) is measured from the opening to the closure of the aortic valve. It is determined by the amount of flow during ejection (i.e., the stroke volume) and the rate of flow. Total electromechanical systole is then defined as the interval from the onset of the QRS complex to the closure of the aortic valve (QAVC) and is the sum of the PEP and the LVET. Fox et al[29] recently evaluated an alternative method for determining the LVET in cats in which the aortic valve is difficult to image. This method uses the duration from the first anterior motion of the LV free wall to its point of peak excursion. The LVET is also used in the calculation of V_{cf} (see below). In assessing LV performance, improvement is characterized by a shortening of the PEP as isovolumic contraction time decreases and a prolongation of the LVET as stroke volume increases. The ratio of PEP to LVET (PEP/LVET) is the most commonly used STI index of performance because it compensates for heart rate variability and because when LV performance improves, PEP shortens and LVET lengthens, making the ratio change more than either PEP or LVET alone. It should be noted that this ratio is purely a mathematical manipulation and has no physiologic basis. The opposite occurs when LV performance worsens.[42] Because STIs are affected by myocardial contractility, heart rate, and loading conditions (preload and afterload), they are not specific indicators of myocardial contractility. Rather, they are nonspecific indicators of global LV performance. Normal values for STIs in dogs and cats have been reported in several studies (Table 6-3).[29,34,35,41,43]

EJECTION PHASE INDICES

The most common clinical methods of assessing cardiac function are the LV ejection phase indices, most of which can be calculated using the same measurements discussed in the previous sections (Table 6-4).[44] None of these indices are measures of LV contractility but instead are measures of global LV performance. As such, they are as easily altered by preload and afterload as they are by contractility.[45]

Several calculations of LV function can be determined from LV dimensions measured from the M-mode or two-dimensional echocardiogram.[1] The most commonly used one-dimensional index is the LV

TABLE 6-3

Normal values for left ventricular systolic time intervals for dogs and cats

	Dog			Cat		
Parameter	*Pipers et al*[43]	*Atkins et al*[41]	*Pipers et al*[35]	*Fox et al*[29]	*Jacobs et al*[34]	*Atkins et al*[41]
n	10	20	25	27	30	6
PEP (msec)	69 ± 8	54 ± 7	N/A	44 ± 9	N/A	45 ± 6
LVET (msec)	256 ± 13	159 ± 15	150 ± 20	116 ± 11	140 ± 20	116 ± 19
LVETI* (msec)	301 ± 10	227 ± 15	217	214	218	206 ± 9
PEP/LVET	0.24 ± 0.09	0.34 ± 0.05	N/A	0.38	N/A	0.40 ± 0.05
QAVC (msec)	324 ± 7	218 ± 18	N/A	160	N/A	162 ± 24
VcF (circ/sec)	N/A	2.48 ± 0.50	2.9 ± 0.8	3.5 ± 0.8	3.7 ± 0.6	4.0 ± 0.9
Heart rate (bpm)	81 ± 7	124 ± 23	167 ± 7	245 ± 36	194 ± 23	226 ± 25

Values presented as mean standard deviation.
*Calculated as LVET + 0.55 (heart rate) for dogs[43] and LVET + 0.40 (heart rate) for cats.[28]
PEP, Preejection period; *LVET,* left ventricular ejection time; *LVETI,* left ventricular ejection time index; *circ,* circumference; *bpm,* beats per minute; *n,* number of animals; *N/A,* not available; *VcF,* velocity of circumferential fiber shortening; *QAVC,* duration from Q wave to aortic valve closure.

fractional shortening, or shortening fraction (FS, SF, or %ΔD). Other indices include the velocity of circumferential fiber shortening (V_{cf}) and the percentage change in septal or LV wall thicknesses (i.e., the thickening fraction).[7,16,43] Fractional changes in dimensions are unitless numbers expressing the percentage change in the dimension from end-diastole to end-systole, and are calculated as the difference between the systolic and the diastolic dimensions divided by the diastolic dimension times 100 (see Table 6-4). Although shortening fraction is the most useful index of LV performance, thickening fraction can be very useful when heterogeneity of myocardial performance is present or when the motion of the entire heart interferes with measurement of wall motion.[16] As explained in Chapter 2, the end-systolic diameter alone is a measure of global left ventricular performance and is a more specific index of myocardial contractility than is fractional shortening although it is also affected by afterload.

The normal shortening fraction in most normal dogs ranges from 25% to 45% and in normal cats from 30% to 55%. Lombard[30] and Boon et al[31] reported the fractional shortening in unsedated dogs to be 27% to 48% and 30% to 50%, respectively. Pipers et al[35] reported the fractional shortening in normal awake cats to be 23% to 56% and Jacobs and Knight[3] reported it to be 50% +/– 5.% (an approximate 95% confidence interval of 40% to 60%). Piper et al's data were obtained before taurine deficiency was recognized as causing myocardial failure. Consequently, their data are probably contaminated with taurine-deficient cats.

The velocity of circumferential fiber shortening (V_{cf}) measures the rate of change in the circumference (circ) of the LV during systole, incorporating both the LV FS and the LVET. Boon et al[31] reported the V_{cf} in normal dogs to be 1.6 to 2.8 circ/sec. Pipers et al[35] reported the V_{cf} in cats to be 1.3 to 4.5 circ/sec, and Jacobs and Knight[3] reported it as 3.6 +/– 0.6 circ/sec.

The distance between the ventricular septum and the maximal initial opening of the MV (*E* point) is inversely related to the volume and rate of LA emptying (LA to LV flow rate) and thus LV stroke volume. This measurement, known as the *mitral E-point–to–septal separation (EPSS)* has been used as a practical and easily reproducible clinical index of LV function.[46] It has been shown in humans that the size of the left ventricle alone does not alter the EPSS unless LV systolic function is also depressed.[46] Although an increased EPSS is a useful indicator of global LV dysfunction, correlation between its magnitude and the degree of impairment has not been established. The EPSS decreases in concert with an increase in shortening fraction in American cocker spaniels treated with taurine and carnitine.[47] Most reports suggest that the normal canine EPSS is less than or equal to 6 mm,[7,48] and the normal feline EPSS is less than 4 to 5 mm.[7,34] Surprisingly, body size has not been reported appear to affect EPSS in dogs; Kirberger[48] reported the EPSS to be the same (3.27 ± 1.29 mm [range 1 to 6 mm]) in 50 normal beagles and German shepherd dogs. However, in the normal values for dogs compiled by Cornell et al,[38] there was a definite increase in EPSS with increasing body size (see Table 6-2).

TABLE 6-4

The ejection phase indices of cardiac function

Ejection fraction	$\frac{EDV - ESV}{EDV} \times 100$
Ejection rate (mean)	$\frac{EDV - ESV}{EDV \times ET}$
Fractional shortening	$\frac{EDD - ESD}{EDD} \times 100$
Mean velocity of circumferential fiber shortening	$\frac{EDD - ESD}{EDD \times ET}$

EDV, End-diastolic volume; *ESV,* end-systolic volume; *EDD,* end-diastolic diameter; *ESD,* end-systolic diameter; *ET,* ejection time.

Because of its simplicity, the LV FS is the most widely used clinical index of LV systolic function in veterinary patients. The V_{cf} may also be easily applied to animals; however, the requirement for LVET makes this calculation more time-consuming, without any known added benefit. Both the LV FS and LV V_{cf} decrease with a reduction in cardiac performance. Consequently, abnormal findings should be considered indicative of one or more categories of disease, rather than a specific condition. We must also remember that the area measured is assumed to be representative of the other regions of the heart. Usually the whole heart is not visualized using M-mode echocardiography, and akinetic, dyskinetic, or hypokinetic areas may be overlooked.

To obtain accurate measures of LV dimensions and fractional shortening, one must be careful to obtain reproducible measurements of the true LV minor axis (i.e., perpendicular to both walls of the LV). To do this requires two-dimensional echocardiographic guidance. Initially, a longitudinal view of the left ventricle should be obtained from the right parasternal position. The M-mode cursor should be placed on the video screen and the image of the left ventricle manipulated until the cursor passes across the left ventricle perpendicular to the interventricular septum and the LV posterolateral wall, at the tips or immediately above the tips of the papillary muscles. At this stage, the image can either be manipulated so that neither papillary muscle is in view or the transducer can be rotated to obtain a cross-sectional view of the LV at the same level and the cursor placed between the tips of the papillary muscles. The M-mode echocardiogram can then be recorded. Respiration moves the heart and produces artifactual motion of the LV walls on almost all echocardiograms, especially in dogs. In humans, patients are asked to hold their breath (often on expiration) to improve the image (decrease lung artifact) and to minimize motion. In dogs, the mouth should be closed and the nares occluded for a brief time while the M-mode is recorded, to eliminate the respiratory artifact. If this is not done, the calculation of shortening fraction becomes especially suspect.

The three-dimensional, volumetric equivalents of LV FS and LV V_{cf} are the ejection fraction and the mean ejection rate, respectively (see Table 6-4). The ejection fraction is a measure of the percentage of the end-diastolic volume ejected with each heart beat. Any of the methods for echocardiographically determining LV volume may be used to calculate the ejection fraction. One must realize that the limitations inherent in the volume measurement effect the accuracy of the calculated ejection fraction and that this inaccuracy is enhanced because two volumes are used in the calculation. The mean ejection rate simply indexes the ejection fraction to the LVET. M-mode and two-dimensional echocardiographic determinations of ejection fraction are less accurate than angiocardiographic techniques.[44] This is particularly true when the heart is irregularly shaped or when regional wall motion abnormalities are present. Improved accuracy may be achieved by using the more reliable models of LV volume (i.e., the disc summation method), as previously described.

Cardiac output (CO) is another measure of global cardiac function, traditionally measured using invasive techniques such as thermodilution. However, CO is a very insensitive indicator of cardiac performance because many compensatory mechanisms act to maintain normal CO even in the face of overt heart failure. CO determination is best used in combination with other invasively and/or noninvasively derived parameters to obtain a complete evaluation of cardiac performance. Serial determination of CO is useful in determining hemodynamic response to acute changes in LV performance.[44] Estimates of stroke volume (SV) and CO can be determined from echocardiographic measurements, using calculated LV volumes to determine the SV (SV = diastolic LV volume − systolic LV volume) and therefore CO (CO = SV × heart rate). As previously stated, these methods require the same geometric assumptions to calculate LV volume and are far less reliable than more direct measurements obtained using invasive techniques. Studies using M-mode methods of determining CO in normal dogs and cats and in dogs under abnormal loading conditions have shown poor correlation with the more direct measures.[49-51] Methods using two-dimensionally derived data to determine CO in dogs and cats have not been evaluated.

Stroke volume and CO can be calculated by measuring blood flow velocity within the great vessels using Doppler echocardiography. Although technically demanding and with a potential for significant errors, most carefully performed studies in humans have reported a good correlation between Doppler-derived CO and values obtained using thermodilution or the Fick method.[52,53] Reports using Doppler echocardiography in dogs have shown a poor-to-good correlation with traditional methods.[54,55]

Because of its complex geometry and increased sensitivity to changes in loading conditions, echocardiographic indices to determine performance of the right ventricle have been more difficult to develop. Clinically useful techniques have not been evaluated in dogs and cats, and the information in humans is limited.

DIASTOLIC FUNCTION

Less attention has been paid to the evaluation of LV diastolic function in veterinary patients. Diastolic properties are more difficult to evaluate echocardiographically because of the subtleties of motion and pressure that distinguish normal from abnormal. In humans, loss of LV compliance and abnormal diastolic filling patterns may create subtle abnormalities of diastolic LV and mitral valve motion.[1] More recently, Doppler echocardiography has been used to characterize diastolic function.[56] When LV compliance diminishes there is an increase in the atrial contribution to ventricular filling and an increased velocity of ventricular inflow during atrial contraction. Thus the *A* wave of LV inflow is increased relative to the early diastolic *E* wave of ventricular inflow (see below). Although this finding has been reported in dogs, it appears to be quite variable and inconsistent in dogs suspected of having abnormal diastolic function.[57,58] In cats, the *E* and *A* waves are commonly not separate because of their relatively fast heart rates, making this technique useless. Recently we and a resident (Brad Gavaghan) have shown that Doppler tissue imaging may be a more accurate means of evaluating diastolic function in cats with cardiac disease.

Contrast Echocardiography

Contrast echocardiography is a noninvasive procedure that uses an injection of multiple microcavitations (microbubbles) trapped in a liquid medium as a vascular contrast medium. Generally, a small amount of the patient's blood is agitated in 0.9% saline, 5% dextrose, or indocyanine green dye to prepare the contrast material. The material is injected as a peripheral intravenous (IV) bolus during M-mode or two- dimensional echocardiographic examination (Figure 6-15).[1,59] Selective injections, via intracardiac catheters, may also be employed in anesthetized patients. The air

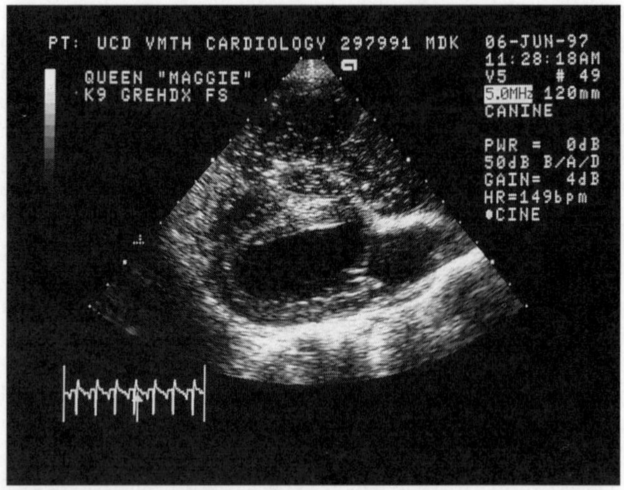

FIGURE 6-15 Right parasternal four-chamber view from a dog taken during an intravenous injection of echocardiographic contrast. Contrast (bubbles) appear as bright dots in the right atrium and ventricle but never appear in the left side of the heart.

in the bubbles reflects ultrasound extremely well, making their detection very easy. Single bubbles can often be detected. On a two-dimensional study the bubbles appear as bright dots. They are recognized as streaks moving over time on an M-mode study.

This technique is most useful for identifying right-to-left intracardiac shunts.[59] In the normal heart, contrast echoes injected intravenously are confined to the right heart chambers and pulmonary arteries, because the bubbles are removed during passage into the pulmonary microcirculation (see Figure 6-15). Documentation of right-to-left cardiac shunting can easily be accomplished by injecting contrast material into any peripheral vein and observing the appearance of any bubbles in the left side of the heart or aorta.[60] Depending on the view obtained and the quality of the echocardiogram, the level of shunting may also be identified by the appearance of the bubbles in the chamber into which blood is shunting or by seeing contrast only in chambers distal to the shunt.

Documentation of a left-to-right cardiac shunt or valvular insufficiency can also be identified by contrast echocardiography. However, the material must be injected into a specific chamber and so cardiac catheterization is usually required. In this case, angiographic evaluation usually prevails. However, with large left-to-right shunts, a negative contrast effect may be produced within right-side chambers following injection of a contrast medium into a peripheral vein.[61] This finding is neither consistent nor very accurate, and nonselective contrast examination should not be considered reliable for diagnosing either of these disorders.

Although partially invasive, contrast echocardiography is considered a safe technique. In a report by the Committee on Contrast Echocardiography for the ASE, the incidence of transient side effects (neurologic and respiratory) was only 0.062% of human patients and no residual complications were observed.[62] Air embolism is the main risk involved. This can generally be prevented if care is taken to avoid the injection of visible amounts of air into patients with large right-to-left shunts or into arterial catheters.

Spontaneous contrast, or echocardiographic "smoke," may be seen in some animals. This is defined as an amorphous, swirling, light gray haze inside the cardiac chambers or great vessels and is generally attributed to conditions of blood stasis.[63] Although this phenomenon may be observed in normal horses and cows, it has not been detected in normal dogs and cats except during prolonged anesthesia.[64] Spontaneous contrast has been shown to result primarily from the interaction of red blood cell clumping and plasma proteins at low-flow and low-shear rate conditions.[65] In humans, its presence is associated with an increased risk of thromboembolism. Although it may be recognized in any case with conditions of low blood flow (e.g., dilated cardiomyopathy), we have most commonly observed spontaneous contrast in the dilated atria of cats with severe myocardial disease.

Doppler Echocardiography

Doppler echocardiography uses the change in frequency of an ultrasound beam that occurs when it reflects from moving blood cellular elements to measure flow velocity. When displayed graphically, this allows noninvasive evaluation of the timing, direction, and character of blood flow within the heart and great vessels.[7,9,66-69] Doppler echocardiography detects abnormal blood flow as a change in direction, velocity, or character (e.g., turbulent blood flow) within a region. It provides direct detection of regurgitant, obstructive, or shunt flow turbulent jets and allows quantitative assessment of certain hemodynamic variables and indices of cardiac performance.

The Doppler Principle, first described by Christian Johan Doppler in 1842, is based on the change, or shift, in reflected sound wave frequency that occurs when sound waves bounce off a moving object (e.g., red blood cells).[66] Ultrasound waves transmitted from the transducer at a known frequency strike red cells and return at a higher frequency (a shorter wavelength) or a lower frequency (a longer wavelength) when they reflect from red blood cells moving toward or away from the transducer, respectively. The difference between the transmitted frequency and the reflected frequency is the Doppler shift. As long as the target is moving directly toward or directly away from the transducer, the magnitude of the shift is directly related to the velocity of the target cells. The Doppler equation used to calculate blood flow velocity is:

$$V = \frac{(\Delta f) \times (C)}{(2) \times (f_o) \times \cos\theta}$$

where V is the flow velocity of blood in meters per second (m/sec), C is the speed of ultrasound in soft tissue (1540 m/sec), Δf is the Doppler shift, f_o is the transmitted frequency, and θ is the intercept angle (i.e., angle between the direction of blood flow and the ultrasound beam).

In contrast to two-dimensional or M-mode echocardiography, which optimize images *perpendicular* to the ultrasound beam, Doppler studies are only accurate when the ultrasound beam is *parallel* or nearly parallel to blood flow, such that the intercept angle (θ) is close to zero degrees. As the intercept angle increases beyond about 20 degrees, the cosine approaches zero, and the perceived frequency shift decreases, significantly underestimating blood flow velocity. With an angle of incidence less than about 20 degrees, the percent error is less than 6%, an acceptable level for most clinical diagnoses.[7,66] Ultrasound machines with Doppler capabilities automatically calculate and display blood flow velocity assuming that θ is zero. Newer machines often provide an electronic protractor that can be used to correct for larger angles.[68]

The different modes of Doppler echocardiography include pulsed-wave spectral (PW), high-pulse-repetition frequency (HPRF) PW spectral, continuous-wave (CW) spectral, and PW color flow (CF) imaging. Each has inherent strengths and weaknesses, and most clinical examinations use a combination of the available modalities.

SPECTRAL DOPPLER

Spectral Doppler recordings (PW, HPRF, and CW) are generally displayed with velocity (m/sec) on the *Y* axis (Figure 6-16) and time on the *X* axis. A simultaneous ECG is also recorded to reference the flow signal to the cardiac cycle. Flow velocity is depicted as pixels of light that move in relation to the baseline. Flow coming toward the transducer produces a signal that is placed above the baseline by convention and flow away from the transducer is placed below the baseline. The intensity of the pixel brightness describes the number of red cells traveling at that dispersion flow velocity within a given location. Pixels shaded with lighter intensities represent small numbers of RBCs, and brighter pixels represent larger numbers of RBCs.[67] Thus the darkest intensities generally represent the modal velocity (i.e., the most common velocity) in any given region of measurement.[68] Many ultrasound units simultaneously display the two-dimensional image, the ECG, and the spectral DE image. The ASE has made recommendations for the standardization of Doppler echocardiographic display and terminology.[70] The Doppler waveform should be calibrated in centimeters or in meters per second with flow toward the transducer displayed above the baseline (positive direction) and flow away from the transducer below the baseline (negative direction), regardless of the direction of the ultrasound beam or area of interrogation. As the Doppler shift is within the audible range (20 to 20,000 Hz), spectral Doppler echocardiography also produces audible signals that can be amplified and sent to a loudspeaker. The audible signal is usually interpreted simultaneously with the graphic display, and the experienced user can generally distinguish normal and abnormal sounding signals.

Pulsed-wave Doppler echocardiography uses a single crystal transducer that acts as both the transmitter and receiver of Doppler information.[67,68] Pulses of ultrasound are sent at a preset interval and the next consecutive pulse is not sent until the previous signal is received. Besides pulsing the signal that is sent, the ultrasound machine only collects returning signals at preset intervals. This allows for interrogation of a distinct area of interest (range gating). This area can be chosen by the operator within the two-dimensional image using the sample volume or gate. The minimum time between pulses, or the maximum pulse repetition frequency (PRF), is determined by the depth of the area being examined and is equal to 2 times the depth divided by the speed of sound in soft tissue (1540 m/sec). The main disadvantage of PW Doppler is its dependence on PRF to determine the maximum velocity (the Nyquist limit) that can be measured without ambiguity (aliasing) (Figure 6-17). It is determined by sample volume depth and the transmitted Doppler frequency and is exceeded if the PRF is less than 2 times the maximal Doppler shift frequency. Thus, as sample volume depth increases, aliasing occurs at progressively lower velocities. The use of lower-frequency transducer, however, produces a lower Doppler shift at any given velocity, and allows higher flow velocities to be measured accurately at any given depth than a higher frequency transducer. Aliasing is described in more detail in Box 6-2.

Aliasing can be minimized by choosing the lowest available transducer frequency that allows adequate imaging, even if this means sacrificing slightly on the two-dimensional image. The area of interest should also be adjusted so that it is as close to the transducer as possible, while maintaining near parallel alignment. In addition the position of the zero baseline can be shifted up or down, allowing increased velocity display in one direction. In many instances, HPRF

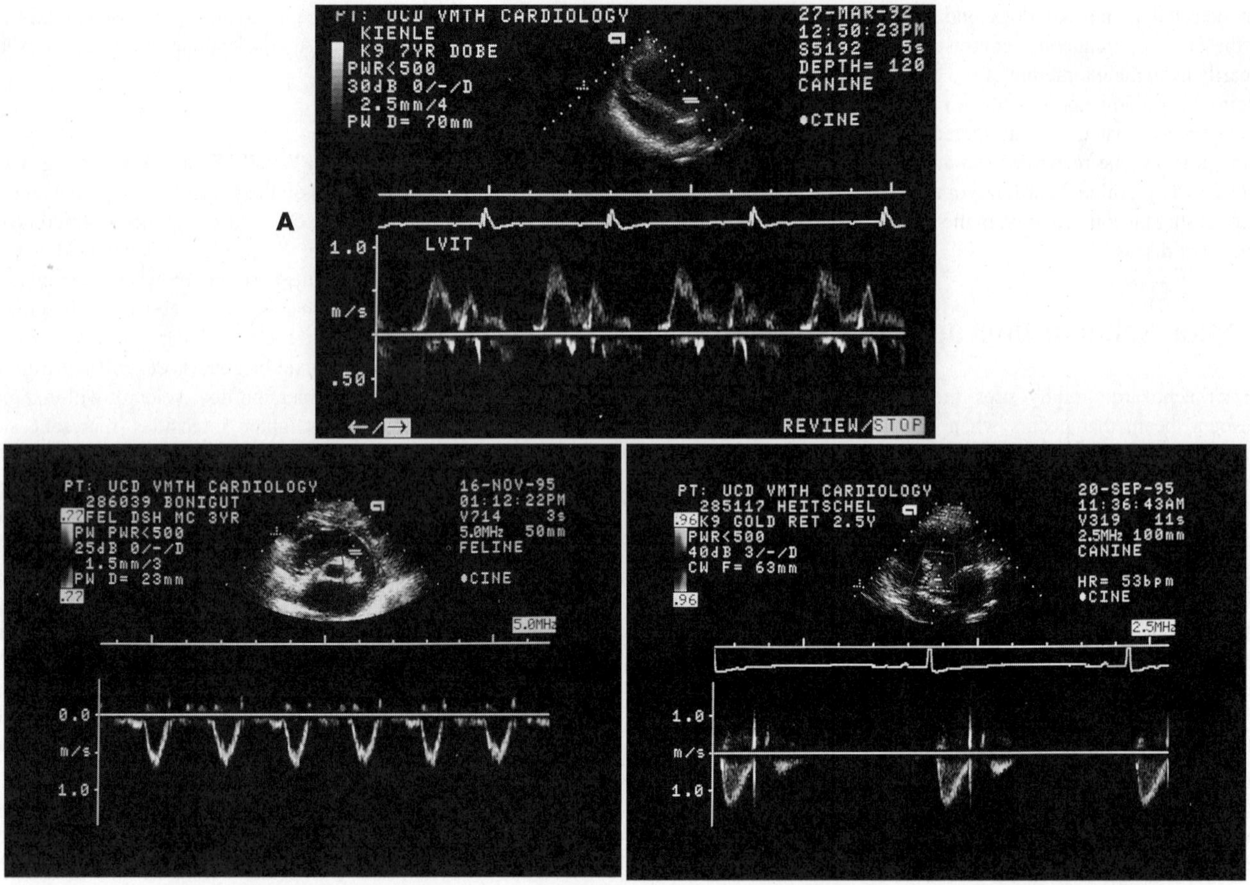

FIGURE 6-16 Spectral Doppler echocardiographic tracings from normal animals. **A,** Pulsed-wave Doppler tracing of the left ventricular inflow tract in a dog, obtained from the left apical position, demonstrating characteristic *E* (early diastolic) and *A* (atrial) waves. This inflow signal is directed toward the transducer and is laminar, as shown by the narrow, discrete envelope of the signal. **B,** Pulsed-wave Doppler tracing of the right ventricular outflow tract from a cat, obtained from the right short-axis position. The systolic outflow signal is directed away from the transducer and is laminar, as shown by the narrow, discrete envelope. **C,** Continuous-wave Doppler tracing of the left ventricular outflow tract, obtained from the left caudal position in a dog. This systolic outflow signal is directed away from the transducer and has the "filled in" appearance characteristic of continuous wave Doppler tracings.

or CW Doppler are necessary to measure blood flow velocity and direction in the area of interest accurately.

Normal blood flow in the heart and great vessels is usually laminar, with most RBCs in any small region moving in the same direction and at similar velocities. If the PW sample volume is placed in the mainstream of flow, a narrow range of velocities is detected as the column of blood accelerates to a peak velocity and then decelerates. This is characterized on the spectral display by a sharp, narrow line that increases to a peak and then decreases back to the baseline (see Figure 6-16).[57,68] The audible signal is usually tonal, because the distribution of frequency shifts is narrow. Disturbed or turbulent flow is characterized by a wide distribution of frequency shifts (i.e., red cell velocities), resulting in the normally clear region within the envelope filling in and the outer envelope disappearing. This is termed *spectral broadening* or *spectral dispersion* (see Figure 6-18). The audible signal is usually polyphonic (harsh or noisy).[57,68] Turbulent flow patterns usually result from increased flow velocity. This is commonly associated with valvular regurgitation, stenotic lesions, and congenital shunts.

High-pulse-repetition frequency Doppler echocardiography, an intermediate between PW and CW, can measure higher velocities than PW Doppler.[67] With this modality, multiple pulses are sent at once, each to a different depth. Thus, three or more sample volumes can be placed simultaneously at these various depths. Although higher velocities may be accurately measured and the quality of flow can often be determined, the exact location of the peak velocity is unknown, although it can commonly be estimated. In most situations, the combination of PW and CW Doppler precludes the need for HPRF Doppler.

Continuous-wave Doppler echocardiography uses two separate crystals, one for transmitting and one for receiving the Doppler information.[67,68] Because continuous signals are employed, the problem of aliasing is not encountered and high velocities can be accurately measured. However, because the information is evaluated along the entire length of the ultrasound beam, selective sampling is not possible and the precise location of the abnormal signal cannot be determined (range ambiguity). The graphic display is similar to that of PW Doppler, but the area under the curve is filled in because

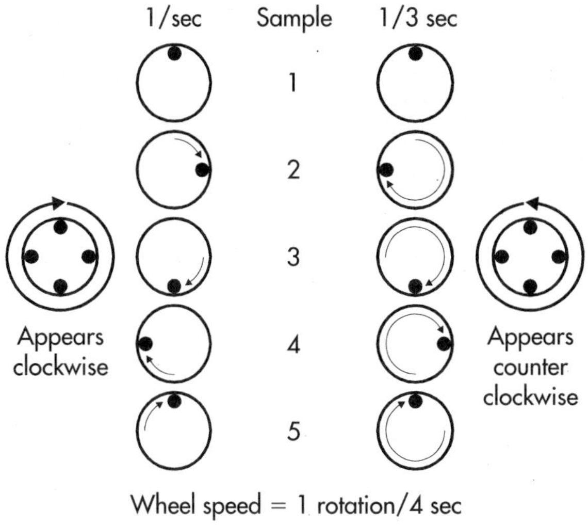

FIGURE 6-17 This schematic illustrates the concept of aliasing. If the wheel rotates one complete revolution every 4 seconds and is filmed at a frame rate of one image per second, the correct clockwise rotation is recorded. If the wheel is filmed at one image per 3 seconds, the wheel appears to turn counterclockwise. Similarly, a pulsed-wave or color Doppler signal will show a false direction and velocity if the blood flow velocity exceeds the frame rate (Nyquist Limit) of the recording.

multiple lower velocities are encountered along the beam, in addition to the higher midstream velocities (see Figure 6-16). This creates spectral broadening whatever the quality of flow, and discrimination between laminar and turbulent flow is not possible. Continuous-wave Doppler is best used to quantify high velocities in areas of abnormal flow initially localized with PW or color flow Doppler.

Early machines could not image and perform CW Doppler simultaneously. Consequently, only "blind" imaging using dedicated pencil (e.g., Piedoff) probes was available. Newer machines have the ability to simultaneously display the two-dimensional image and CW Doppler displays. Consequently, it is possible to "steer" the CW beam within the two-dimensional image (i.e., a steerable CW) allowing the operator to better align the CW beam with the abnormal flow. The quality of both imaging and Doppler information deteriorates when the transducer performs dual imaging. Consequently, optimal velocity information is usually obtained using the dedicated CW transducer.[9,68] Not all jets are consistently directed in a consistent fashion within the internal structures of the heart. Use of the "blind" probe may eliminate bias placed on the operator by the two-dimensional image, thus forcing the operator to "search" for the maximal velocity.

In summary, pulsed-wave Doppler can accurately localize abnormal flow patterns to specific regions of the heart and determine the quality of flow (laminar vs. turbulent), but only low velocities can be measured accurately. CW and HPRF Doppler can measure higher velocities, but the exact location and the quality of flow cannot be determined. Used together, PW and CW Doppler are complimentary, and in situations of abnormal blood flow both modalities are necessary to determine the location, quality, and maximal velocity of the abnormal jet.

When an abnormal flow velocity is identified, spectral Doppler examination can be used to determine the pressure differences between the chambers or vessels in question.[7,57,68] This principle is based on the law of conservation of energy as described by Bernoulli.[71] If a constant volume of fluid flows from one chamber through an obstructed area to another chamber, the flow accelerates and becomes a high-velocity, often turbulent jet in the chamber distal to the obstruction. The pressure difference (gradient) between the chambers is directly related to the velocity difference across the obstruction or opening.[68,72] Energy is conserved because the loss of potential energy (pressure) is made up by an increase in kinetic energy (velocity) at the obstruction. The original equation accounts for convective acceleration, flow acceleration, and viscous friction. If certain assumptions are made, flow acceleration and viscous friction can be ignored and the equation can be simplified for clinical use. This modified Bernoulli equation is shown in the following equation:

$$P_1 - P_2 = 4\,(V_2^2 - V_1^2)$$

where P_1 is the pressure proximal to the lesion, P_2 is the pressure distal to the lesion, V_1 is the velocity proximal to the lesion, and V_2 is the velocity distal to the lesion (Figure 6-19). In most clinical situations V_2 is much larger than V_1 and V_1 is close to 1 m/sec and can then be dropped out of the equation without introducing significant error. Thus the pressure gradient across a flow-restricting

BOX 6-2

Aliasing of the Doppler signal

Aliasing confuses the interpretation of the graphic Doppler signal by introducing ambiguity to the velocity display and therefore must be recognized in order to eliminate erroneous evaluation of flow velocities and direction.

Spectral Doppler

On the display, aliasing appears as a reversal of direction or "wrapping around" of the spectral display (see Figures 6-17, 6-18, and Color Plate 31). This is often coincident with a turbulent appearance to the display. This phenomenon can be explained using the filming of a rotating wheel (see Figure 6-17).[68] If a wheel, with a mark, is turning clockwise at one turn every 4 seconds and a camera filming the event takes 60 frames/sec (1 sample/ sec), the mark is filmed every 90 degrees and the wheel appears to be moving clockwise. If, instead, the camera films the event at 20 frames/sec (1 sample/3 sec), the mark is filmed every 270 degrees and the wheel appears to be moving counterclockwise. Pulsed-wave Doppler is limited in the same manner by its PRF, and aliasing will occur if the PRF is not at least twice the measured velocity. Because of this limitation, PW Doppler is often limited to measuring velocities only in the normal physiologic range.[93]

Color Doppler

When the color flow velocity aliases, the velocity "wraps around" the color display and shifts to a light color shade in the opposite direction. This is characterized on the display as an abrupt change in color from red to blue or vice versa (Color Plate 31). Because of the multi-gated design, color flow Doppler aliasing tends to occur at lower velocities than conventional PW Doppler, usually around 0.6 m/sec.[72] Consequently, although aliasing is a characteristic of high-velocity turbulent flow, it can also occur as an isolated phenomenon. Although one can mistake these isolated color shifts for turbulent flow or variance, closer examination will reveal discriminating characteristics. Turbulent flow typically produces a mosaic pattern of multiple colors. Isolated aliasing, on the other hand, typically produces a gradual progression through consecutive color changes in a concentric fashion within the sample area that ultimately appear to "reverse" direction (see Color Plate 31). Also, on capable systems, turbulence is depicted in the colors coded for variance, and aliased flow is depicted in differing shades of the colors used to depict normal flow patterns. In some instances the velocity distribution results in a central area of aliasing surrounded by more normal flow velocities (Color Plate 31).

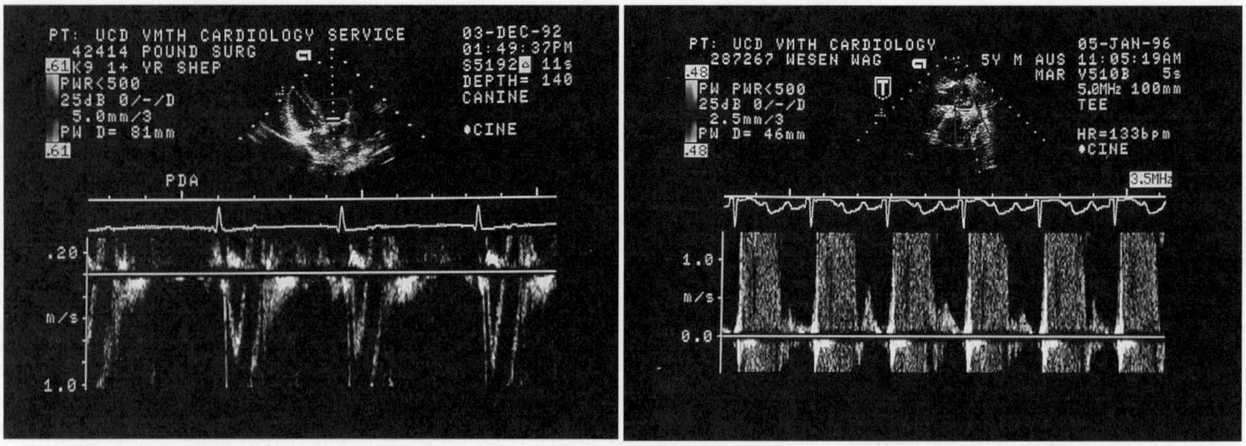

FIGURE 6-18 Examples of spectral Doppler tracings depicting aliased and turbulent flow. **A,** Pulsed-wave Doppler tracing from the left ventricular outflow tract in a dog. This laminar signal (as indicated by the discrete envelop of signals) starts in a downward direction (away from the transducer); however, the peak is "cut off" by the bottom of the display and is instead drawn from the top of the tracing back toward the baseline and through it. This leads to ambiguity in both the true direction and the peak velocity of the signal. **B,** Pulsed-wave Doppler tracing demonstrating turbulence and aliasing. This tracing shows a ventricular septal defect flow jet recorded within the right ventricle. Note that the systolic signal is present both above and below the baseline, resulting in directional ambiguity and the inability to determine peak velocity, and shows a wide band of velocities throughout systole, indicative of turbulent flow or spectral broadening. (See text for details.)

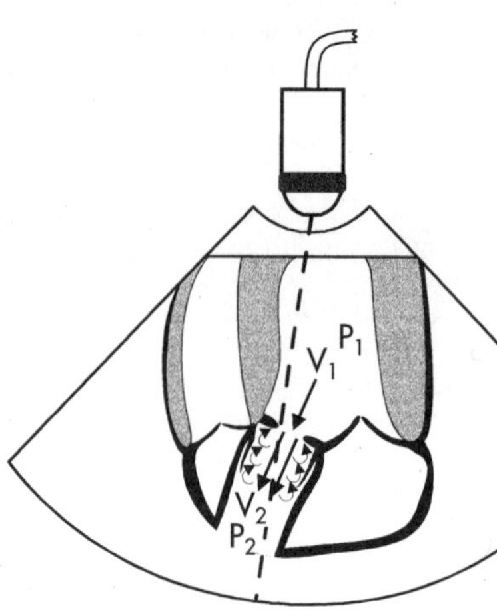

Bernoulli equation

$$P_1 - P_2 = \underbrace{\tfrac{1}{2}\rho\,(V_2^2 - V_1^2)}_{\text{Convective acceleration}} + \underbrace{\rho \int_1^2 \frac{d\vec{V}}{dt}\, d\vec{s}}_{\text{Flow acceleration}} + \underbrace{R(\vec{V})}_{\text{Viscous friction}}$$

$$P_1 - P_2 = \tfrac{1}{2}\rho\,(V_2^2 - V_1^2)$$

If V_2 is much $>V_1$, then ignore V_1

$$\therefore \Delta P = 4V^2$$

FIGURE 6-19 Principle of using the modified Bernoulli equation to measure a pressure difference (gradient) across an obstruction by Doppler echocardiography. The original equation is simplified, as shown, for clinical use. P_1, Pressure proximal to the obstruction; P_2, pressure distal to the obstruction; V_1, velocity proximal to the obstruction; V_2, velocity distal to the obstruction; *P,* pressure difference across the obstruction. (From Kienle RD, Thomas WP: Echocardiography. In Nyland T, Mattoon J, eds: *Veterinary diagnostic ultrasound,* Philadelphia, 1995, WB Saunders.)

lesion (including stenotic lesions, valvular insufficiencies, and shunts) is equal to 4 times the square of the peak velocity in the distal chamber (taken from the spectral Doppler examination). Although the modified Bernoulli equation has largely been used for evaluating stenotic lesions, it can also be used to determine pressure gradients across regurgitant valves and shunts.[73]

It is important to understand that the modified Bernoulli equation only measures the pressure *difference* between two regions of contiguous flow, *not* the absolute pressure of either chamber. However, if the pressure in one chamber can be measured directly or can be estimated indirectly from other diagnostic evaluations (i.e., systemic blood pressure measurement or cardiac catheterization) or can be assumed based on the physiology of the disorder, accurate estimates of absolute pressure can be calculated using the modified Bernoulli equation.[73]

COLOR FLOW DOPPLER

Color flow imaging (two-dimensional Doppler) uses PW technology to build color-coded images of blood flow velocity superimposed over the two-dimensional or M-mode anatomic images of the heart.[74] Instead of using a single sample volume along one sector line, multiple sample sites are simultaneously interrogated along multiple scan lines (Color Plate 29).[68,74] Each sample volume is evaluated for direction, quality (variance), and mean velocity. Different colors are assigned to represent those properties.[72] This color-coded velocity image is then superimposed over the two-dimensional image. A typical image can consist of as many as 250 scan lines and thousands of sample volumes, depending on the sector size and depth of range. Each frame requires individual analysis and 15 to 30 frames/sec are required to provide "real-time" motion.

The colors used to designate the properties of blood flow are arbitrary; however, certain conventions (although not standardized) have been adopted. Red, blue, and green are used by most ultrasound units and can be mixed to produce various shades of yellow, white, and cyan.[72] Newer ultrasound units may offer a variety of other color-coded schemes (maps) to suit individual preferences. Most commonly, flow toward the transducer is coded red and flow away from the transducer is coded blue (Color Plate 30). Increasing velocity of flow is displayed as various shades of the "root" color, with brighter hues representing higher velocity. Velocities below a minimum magnitude or flow directly perpendicular to the ultrasound beam are not assigned colors and are represented by black in the image. Laminar flow is characterized by one homogeneous pattern of flow consisting of similar shades of one color (usually either red or blue) (Color Plate 30).

To display high-velocity turbulent flow, an algorithm is used by the ultrasound machine to test the variation in the frequency shift produced by consecutive bursts along a single scan line.[72] This variability in velocity is displayed as variance that is similar to the spectral broadening shown on the spectral Doppler display, and represents abnormal or turbulent flow. Green or an additional color is added to the shades of red and blue according to the amount of variance detected (Color Plate 29). High-velocity turbulent flow also produces aliasing. With color flow Doppler, this is displayed as a directional change. For example, if flow is toward the transducer it would normally be encoded as red. However, once it exceeds the Nyquist limit, it "wraps" around and becomes blue. If it exceeds twice the Nyquist limit, it "wraps" around again to become red again. The disorganized pattern of velocities and variance that results from turbulent flow produces a so-called mosaic pattern consisting of various shades of multiple colors on the display (Color Plate 31). Aliasing is described in more detail in Box 6-2.

Color flow Doppler offers several advantages over spectral Doppler. First, regions of normal and abnormal flow are identified much faster because color flow Doppler covers a much greater area with each sample, thus increasing the efficiency of the examination. Regurgitant jets and shunts are more rapidly identified and localized. Second, the color display may be used to align the Doppler beam along the center or mainstream of the high-velocity jet, allowing for a more accurate velocity determination than with spectral Doppler echocardiography. Finally, the spatial orientation and real-time display of color flow Doppler are more comprehensible to inexperienced examiners, and therefore is an excellent teaching tool.

Despite its considerable value, color flow Doppler is a PW technique and shares the disadvantages of spectral PW Doppler. Color flow Doppler is subject to aliasing if the measured frequency shift exceeds one half of the systems PRF, or Nyquist limit (Color Plate 31). This is usually more apparent with color flow Doppler because of the low PRF velocities inherent in the technique. Aliasing is commonly observed in animals with completely normal flow patterns and velocities. The other major limitation to color flow Doppler is the relative inability to quantify the displayed velocity signals. Color flow imaging is also limited to available two-dimensional windows and is quite sensitive to both depth of interrogation and malalignment of the ultrasound beam and blood flow.

NORMAL BLOOD FLOW VELOCITIES AND WAVEFORMS

Normal peak flow velocities in systole in the outflow tract regions and the great vessels in dogs and cats are usually around 1 m/sec, with some patients having velocities approaching 2 m/sec. Only rarely will a "normal" patient have flow velocities that exceed 2 m/sec within the heart or great vessels. Flow velocities in diastole are generally lower than systolic velocities. Spectral Doppler velocities and waveforms across normal valves have been reported for dogs (Table 6-5).[75-79] Normal intracardiac blood flow is laminar, although aliasing may occur in normal individuals, depending on system settings, transducer selection, and imaging depth. Most valves are best interrogated using left-side views because they give the best parallel alignment to flow.

The mitral valve is best interrogated from the left apical long-axis views, whereas the tricuspid valve may be examined from both left apical and left cranial views.[75,76,78] Flow across the atrioventricular valves show both passive and active components, resulting in two waves of diastolic flow both directed toward the transducer and above the baseline (see Figure 6-16). The early diastolic wave, or *E* wave, corresponds to passive filling and the late diastolic *A* wave is associated with atrial systole. These waves correspond to the *E*-point and *A*-point on the mitral valve motion seen on an M-mode examination (see Figures 6-10 and 6-11). The *E* wave is normally higher and longer in duration than the *A* wave, and the ratio of the peak *E* wave to peak *A* wave is greater than 1.0. Rapid heart rates shorten diastole, causing merging of the *A* wave and *E* wave into a single diastolic wave. Atrial fibrillation eliminates atrial contraction and the Doppler *A* wave. Many factors, including ventricular compliance and rate of diastolic relaxation (lusitrope), can affect the *E*-to-*A* ratio. Peak velocities across the atrioventricular valves are usually less than 1 m/sec and are almost always somewhat less than the velocities across the semilunar valves in the same patient (see Table 6-5).[75,76,78] Although, the tricuspid valve signal usually looks qualitatively similar to the mitral valve signal, there is greater variation in the tricuspid valve signal because of the influence of respiration and because peak velocities tend to be slightly lower. Physiologic tricuspid valve regurgitation is relatively common (50%), whereas physiologic regurgitation of the mitral valve is uncommon.[75]

TABLE 6-5

Normal Doppler-derived velocities across canine heart valves

Valve	*Brown et al*[77]†	*Gaber*[75]†	*Kirberger et al*[79]†	*Yuill et al*[76]‡
Mitral (cm/sec)	—	—	E 91 ± 15 A 63 ± 13	86.2 ± 9.5
Tricuspid (cm/sec)	—	—	E 86 ± 20 A 58 ± 16	68.9 ± 8.4
Pulmonic (cm/sec)	84.0 ± 17	99.8 ± 30.6	120 ± 20	R 98.1 ± 9.4 L 95.5 ± 10.3
Aortic (cm/sec)	106.0 ± 21	118.9 ± 35.6	157 ± 33	118.1 ± 10.8

Values presented as mean ± standard deviation.
†Velocities measured using pulsed-wave Doppler echocardiography.
‡Velocities measured using continuous-wave Doppler echocardiography.
E, E wave; *A*, A wave; *R*, measured from the right parasternal short-axis view; *L*, measured from the left parasternal long-axis view.

The pulmonary valve is best interrogated from the left cranial position, or in some cases the right parasternal short-axis view. The aortic valve and LVOT are best imaged in the left apical views or from a subcostal approach.[75,76,78] The semilunar valves (aortic and pulmonic) Doppler profile shows a single systolic wave signal away from the transducer and below the baseline, in the views described. Semilunar valve clicks are common and may be heard and displayed as short-duration high-velocity spikes usually occurring at the end of systole. These may be minimized by increasing the wall filter setting, by decreasing the gain settings, or by slightly adjusting the angle of interrogation. However, sometimes they are inevitable. The spectral signal across the aortic valve is slightly different from that of the pulmonary valve, showing slightly higher peak velocities (see Table 6-5), a faster early acceleration (i.e., a steeper slope to the upstroke), and a larger fraction of the stroke output (calculated) during the first half of ejection.[75,77] Mild pulmonic valve regurgitation is detected in more than 50% of normal dogs.[76,77]

Doppler imaging displays the *velocity*, not the actual *volume* of flow. To calculate volumetric flow, the average velocity of the signal (calculated from the spectral display as the velocity – time integral) is multiplied by the cross-sectional area of the region where the velocity was recorded.[44] This is most easily accomplished using the aorta or pulmonary artery but may also be measured from Doppler recordings at the mitral or tricuspid annulus.[80] The significant source of error in these calculations lies in the measurement of the vessel or annulus diameter. A small error in diameter, when squared to determine cross-sectional area, will lead to a large error in volumetric flow calculation. The use of volumetric flow estimates from Doppler recordings have shown only a fair correlation with thermodilution techniques in clinical studies of dogs and cats.[54]

Transesophageal Echocardiography

Transthoracic echocardiography, despite its valuable clinical utility, is limited in some patients by obesity or lung interference, and the distal great vessels are still relatively obscure to adequate imaging in most patients. Transesophageal echocardiography employs ultrasonic transducers mounted at the tip of a flexible, steerable endoscope. This allows imaging of the heart and great vessels from within the esophagus. It has been developed in humans to surmount the technical limitations of transthoracic imaging.[81] Recently, the techniques and clinical applications of transesophageal echocardiography in veterinary patients have been reported in both cats and dogs.[82-86] We primarily use transesophageal echocardiography to interrogate the pulmonic valve anatomy in dogs with pulmonic stenosis before balloon valvuloplasty or to further characterize mass lesions at the base of the heart.

Patterns of Echocardiographic Response to Cardiac Disease

The information in the echocardiogram can be overwhelming. However, in the same way that characteristic patterns simplify radiographic interpretation, defining echocardiographic patterns that characterize different types of cardiovascular disease is possible. To do so requires an understanding of how the heart changes structurally in response to different underlying disorders (a volume overload, a pressure overload, etc.) (see Chapter 2). It is also important to understand the role that echocardiography plays in a comprehensive patient evaluation, without overestimating or underestimating its value. In particular, echocardiography often identifies a pattern of response that identifies a specific condition and its severity only when combined with the information from other sources (history, ECG, radiographs, etc.).

Diminished ventricular contractility causes an increase in the end-systolic dimension of the affected ventricle. Wall motion is reduced, and the percentage change in the lateral dimension (the shortening fraction) or the volume (the ejection fraction) is decreased. The ventricle usually grows larger in response to diminished contractility, resulting in an increase in the end-diastolic dimension of the affected ventricle. Although ventricular eccentric hypertrophy may produce a visual impression of thin walls, they may be normal in thickness or may be thinner than normal when measured.

Leaks (e.g., regurgitation and shunts) result in ventricular volume overload (eccentric) hypertrophy. The end-diastolic dimension is increased and the wall thickness is normal. In many cases, systolic function is maintained, at least initially in the disease course. The result is hyperdynamic or hyperkinetic left ventricular function as identified by an increase in the shortening fraction combined with an exaggerated posterior septal motion during systole. As the myocardium fails, the end-systolic diameter increases, bringing shortening fraction back down to normal range. In contrast, a pressure overload produces concentric hypertrophy. This is most commonly characterized by a normal ventricular dimension and an increase in diastolic wall thickness. The exception is the response of the adult right ventricle to a pressure overload, which usually includes an increase in both chamber size and wall thickness.

The interventricular septum responds to conditions affecting either ventricle. Septal motion and shape reflects the relative systolic and diastolic pressures and volume differences between the two ventricles.[1] The shape of the septum is best evaluated using a two-dimensional short-axis view of the ventricles. As previously discussed, systolic septal motion may be exaggerated in volume overload states. On the other hand, with right ventricular pressure or volume overload septal motion may be reduced or even paradoxic (i.e., in the opposite direction). In a pure right heart failure, septal flattening occurs during diastole because RV diastolic pressure exceeds LV diastolic pressure. With a right ventricular pressure overload the septum may flatten in systole, especially when RV systolic pressure exceeds LV systolic pressure.

The atria dilate in response to both pressure and volume overloads. An atrial volume overload occurs with left-to-right shunts, cardiomyopathies, and atrioventricular valvular abnormalities. An atrial pressure overload without a volume overload most commonly occurs from conditions that reduce ventricular compliance or an obstruction between the atrium and ventricle (e.g., atrioventricular valve stenosis). The atrial septum should be evaluated for continuity and its relationship to other structures. The shape of the atrial septum reflects the relative pressure on either side and tends to bulge away from a chamber with increased pressure.

The size, shape, and position of each of the great vessels are also determined, paying particular attention to the origin of the vessels and their course away from the heart. The main pulmonary artery commonly enlarges with congenital left-to-right shunts, pulmonic stenosis, and pulmonary hypertension and may be smaller than normal with ventricular level right-to-left shunts. The aorta may be dilated with conditions such as aortic stenosis or patent ductus arteriosus.

An evaluation for the presence of pericardial effusion, extracardiac masses, and pleural effusion should follow routine examination of the heart.[7] In cases in which right heart failure is suspected, a cursory abdominal ultrasound examination should be performed to determine the size of the caudal vena cava and liver, to determine the size of the hepatic veins, and to detect ascites.

Echocardiographic Artifacts

To interpret the normal echocardiogram one must be able to identify artifacts and distinguish them from pathologic abnormalities.[87] Artifacts may be secondary to the physical properties of ultrasound, the quality of the ultrasound equipment, improper scanning technique, or improper adjustment of controls. One of the most common artifacts is produced by poor contact. This results in horizontal lines overlying the two-dimensional image or a poor-quality image. It can be avoided in most instances by clipping the hair of thick-coated animals, liberal use of coupling gel, or wetting the hair. Excessive gain will decrease lateral resolution, causing fusion of some indistinct areas and potentially obscuring some hypoechoic or anechoic areas. When the gain is set too low, some structures may not be detected. Lung artifact is common and appears as large areas of "white-out" on the screen. Poor near field resolution is a common problem, especially in smaller patients. This may be more problematic with older ultrasound units and sometimes may be minimized by using a higher-frequency transducer or a standoff pad.[7]

Side lobe artifacts are aberrant echoes caused by crystals on the edges of the transducer whose beams are not oriented along the main beam.[1] This creates faint bands of echoes that reflect off other echogenic structures within the image. They are most commonly encountered with left atrial enlargement and are rarely seen with normal hearts.

Reverberation artifact is another commonly encountered artifact, especially on older ultrasound units.[87] These artifacts are also more commonly encountered when using a standoff pad. They are created when sound waves are reflected off structures causing an echo to form at the transducer face, reenter the patient, and reflect back to the transducer again. This phenomenon causes a second echo to form twice the distance from the original interface. These usually occur at air-fluid interfaces and appear as highly echoic parallel lines recurring at regular intervals. Reverberation artifact is increased by increasing gain and may be minimized by not allowing the depth of field to exceed the limits of the echoed structure.

REFERENCES

1. Feigenbaum H: *Echocardiography,* ed 4, Philadelphia, 1986, Lea & Febiger.
2. Nyland TG, Mattoon JS, Wisner ER: Physical principles, instrumentation, and safety of diagnostic ultrasound. In Nyland TG, Mattoon JS, eds: *Veterinary diagnostic ultrasound,* Philadelphia, 1995, WB Saunders.
3. Jacobs GJ, Knight DH: Changes in M-mode echocardiographic values in cats given ketamine, *Am J Vet Res* 46:1712, 1985.
4. Allen DG, Downey RS: Echocardiographic assessment of cats anesthetized with xylazine-sodium pentobarbital, *Can J Comp Med* 47:281, 1983.
5. Allen DG: Echocardiographic study of the anesthetized cat, *Can J Comp Med* 46:115, 1982.
6. Dunkle N, Moise NS, Scarlett-Kranz J et al: Cardiac performance in cats after administration of xylazine and glycopyrrolate: echocardiographic evaluations, *Am J Vet Res* 47:(10)2212, 1986.

6a. Stepien RL, Bonagura JD, Bednarski RM, et al: Cardiorespiratory effects of acepromazine maleate and buprenorphine hydrochloride in clinically normal dogs, *Am J Vet Res* 56(1):78, 1995 (erratum 56[3]:402, 1995).

7. Moise NS: Echocardiography. In Fox PR, ed: *Canine and feline cardiology,* New York, 1988, Churchill Livingstone.
8. Bonagura JD, O'Grady MR, Herring DS: Echocardiography: principles of interpretation, *Vet Clin North Am Small Anim Pract* 15:1177, 1985.
9. Miller MW, Knauer KW, Herring DS: Echocardiography: principles of interpretation, *Sem Vet Med Surg Small Anim* 4:58, 1989.
10. Thomas WP: Two-dimensional, real-time echocardiography in the dog, *Vet Radiol* 25:50, 1984.
11. O'Grady MR, Bonagura JD, Powers JD et al: Quantitative cross-sectional echocardiography in the normal dog, *Vet Radiol* 27:34, 1986.
12. Yamaga Y, Too K: Diagnostic ultrasound imaging in domestic animals: two-dimensional and M-mode echocardiography, *Jpn J Vet Sci* 46:493, 1984.
13. Le Bobinec G: Bi-dimensional echocardiography in carnivores: practical cases, *Rec Med Vet* 164:151, 1988.
14. Henry WL, DeMaria A, Gramiak R et al: Report of the American Society of Echocardiography Committee on nomenclature and standards in two-dimensional echocardiography, *Circulation* 62:212, 1980.
15. Thomas WP, Gaber CE, Jacobs GJ et al: Recommendations for standards in transthoracic two-dimensional echocardiography in dogs and cats, *J Vet Intern Med* 7:247, 1993.
16. Bonagura JD: M-mode echocardiography: basic principles, *Vet Clin North Am Small Anim Pract* 13:299-319, 1983.
17. Pipers FS, Hamlin RL: Clinical use of echocardiography in the domestic cat, *J Am Vet Med Assoc* 176:57, 1980.
18. DeMadron E, Bonagura JD, O'Grady MR: Normal and paradoxical ventricular septal motion in the dog, *Am J Vet Res* 46:1832, 1985.
19. Pohost GM, Dinsmore RE, Rubenstein JJ et al: The echocardiogram of the anterior leaflet of the mitral valve: correlation with hemodynamic and cineroentgenographic studies in dogs, *Circulation* 51:88, 1975.
20. DeMadron E, Bonagura JD, Herring DS: Two-dimensional echocardiography in the normal cat, *Vet Radiol* 26:149, 1985.
21. O'Rourke RA, Hanrath P, Henry WN et al: Report of the joint International Society and Federation of Cardiology/World Health Organization task force on recommendations for standardization of measurements from M-mode echocardiograms, *Circulation* 69:854a, 1984.
22. Schiller NB, Shah PM, Crawford M: Recommendations for quantitation of the left ventricle by two-dimensional echocardiography, *J Am Soc Echocardiogr* 2:358, 1989.
23. Sahn DJ, DeMaria A, Kisslo JA et al: Recommendations regarding quantitation in M-mode echocardiography: results of a survey of echocardiographic measurements, *Circulation* 58:1072, 1978.
24. Jacobs GJ, Mahjoob K: Multiple regression analysis, using body size and cardiac cycle length, in predicting echocardiographic variables in dogs, *Am J Vet Res* 49:1290, 1988.
25. Sisson DD, Schaeffer D: Changes in linear dimension of the heart, relative to body weight, as measured by M-mode echocardiography in growing dogs, *Am J Vet Res*; 52:1591, 1991.
26. Morrison SA, Moise NS, Scarlett J et al: Effect of breed and body weight on echocardiographic values in four breeds of dogs of differing somatotype, *J Vet Intern Med* 6:220, 1992.
27. Moise NS, Horne WA, Flanders JA et al: Repeatability of the M-mode echocardiogram and the effects of acute changes in heart rate, cardiac contractility, and preload in healthy cats sedated with ketamine hydrochloride and acepromazine, *Cornell Vet* 76:241, 1986.
28. Jacobs GJ, Mahjoob K: Influence of alterations in heart rate on echocardiographic measurements in the dog, *Am J Vet Res* 49:548, 1988.
29. Fox PR, Bond BR, Peterson ME: Echocardiographic reference values in healthy cats sedated with ketamine hydrochloride, *Am J Vet Res* 46:1479, 1985.
30. Lombard CW: Normal values of the canine M-mode echocardiogram, *Am J Vet Res* 45:2015, 1984.
31. Boon JA, Wingfield WE, Miller CW: Echocardiographic indices in the normal dog, *Vet Radiol* 24:214, 1983.
32. Dennis MO, Nealeigh RC, Pyle RL et al: Echocardiographic assessment of normal and abnormal valvular function in beagle dogs, *Am J Vet Res* 39:1591, 1978.

33. Mashiro I, Nelson RR, Cohn JN et al: Ventricular dimensions measured noninvasively by echocardiography in the awake dog, *J Appl Physiol* 41:953, 1976.
34. Jacobs GJ, Knight DH: M-mode echocardiographic measurements in nonanesthetized healthy cats: effects of body weight, heart rate, and other variables, *Am J Vet Res* 46:1705, 1985.
35. Pipers FS, Reef VB, Hamlin RL: Echocardiography in the domestic cat, *Am J Vet Res* 40:882, 1979.
36. Soderberg SF, Boon JA, Wingfield WE et al: M-mode echocardiography as a diagnostic aid for feline cardiomyopathy, *Vet Radiol* 24:66, 1983.
37. Moise NS, Dietze AE: Echocardiographic, electrocardiographic, and radiographic detection of cardiomegaly in hyperthyroid cats, *Am J Vet Res* 47:1487, 1986.
38. Cornell C: Regression for EDD and ESD vs. body weight in dogs, personal communication 1997.
39. Wyatt HL, Meerbaum S, Heng MK et al: Cross-sectional echocardiography. III. Analysis of mathematical models for quantifying volume of symmetric and asymmetric left ventricles, *Am Heart J* 100:821, 1980.
40. Wyatt HL, Haendchen RV, Meerbaum S et al: Assessment of quantitative methods for 2-dimensional echocardiography, *Am J Cardiol* 52:396, 1983.
41. Atkins CE, Snyder PS: Systolic time intervals and their derivatives for evaluation of cardiac function, *J Vet Intern Med* 6:55, 1992.
42. Weissler AM, Harris WS, Schoenfeld CD: Bedside techniques for the evaluation of ventricular function in man, *Am J Cardiol* 23:577, 1969.
43. Pipers FS, Andrysco RM, Hamlin RL: A totally noninvasive method for obtaining systolic time intervals in dogs, *Am J Vet Res* 39:1822, 1978.
44. Sisson DD: The clinical evaluation of cardiac function. In Ettinger SJ, ed: *Textbook of veterinary internal medicine,* ed 3, Philadelphia, 1989, WB Saunders.
45. Benzing G, Stockert J, Nave E et al: Evaluation of canine left ventricular contractility, *Cardiovasc Res* 8:313, 1974.
46. Child JS, Krivokapich J, Perloff JK: Effect of LV size in mitral E point to ventricular septal separation in assessment of cardiac performance, *Am Heart J* 101:797, 1981.
47. Kittleson MD, Pion PD, Keene BW et al: Results of the multicenter spaniel trial (MUST): taurine and carnitine responsive dilated cardiomyopathy in American cocker spaniels with decreased plasma taurine, *J Vet Intern Med* 11:204, 1997.
48. Kirberger RM: Mitral valve E point to ventricular septal separation in the dog, *J S Afr Vet Med Assoc* 62:163, 1991.
49. Atkins CE, Curtis MB, McGuirk SM et al: The use of M-mode echocardiography in determining cardiac output in dogs with normal, low, and high output states: comparison to thermodilution method, *Vet Radiol Ultrasound* 33:297, 1992.
50. Dyson DH, Allen DG, McDonell WN: Comparison of three methods of cardiac output determination in cats, *Am J Vet Res* 46:2546, 1985.
51. Allen DG, Nymeyer D: A preliminary investigation on the use of thermodilution and echocardiography as an assessment of cardiac function in the cat, *Can J Comp Med* 47:112, 1983.
52. Fisher DC, Sahn DJ, Freidman MJ et al: The mitral valve orifice method for noninvasive two-dimensional echo Doppler determination of cardiac output, *Circulation* 67:872, 1983.
53. Nishimura RA, Callahan MJ, Schaff HV et al: Noninvasive measurement of cardiac output by continuous-wave Doppler echocardiography: initial experience and review of the literature, *Mayo Clinic Proc* 59:484, 1984.
54. Rishniw M, Golder F, Wolf D et al: Transthoracic and transesophageal pulsed-wave Doppler echocardiographic estimates of cardiac output in anesthetized healthy adult dogs: comparison with thermodilution, *J Vet Intern Med* 11:146, 1997 (abstract).
55. Uehara Y, Koga M, Takahashi M: Determination of cardiac output by echocardiography, *J Vet Med Sci* 57:401, 1995.
56. Nishimura RA, Housmans PR, Hatle LK et al: Assessment of diastolic function of the heart: background and current applications for Doppler echocardiography. I. Physiologic and pathophysiologic features, *Mayo Clinic Proc* 64:71, 1989.
57. Darke PG: Doppler echocardiography, *J Small Anim Pract* 33:104, 1992.
58. Moise NS: Doppler echocardiographic evaluation of congenital heart disease, *J Vet Intern Med* 3:195, 1989.
59. Bonagura JD, Pipers FS: Diagnosis of cardiac lesions by contrast echocardiography, *J Am Vet Med Assoc* 182:396, 1983.
60. Boehrer JD, Lange RA, Willard JE et al: Advantages and limitations of methods to detect, localize, and quantitate intracardiac right-to-left and bidirectional shunting, *Am Heart J* 125:215, 1993.
61. Boehrer JD, Lange RA, Willard JE et al: Advantages and limitations of methods to detect, localize, and quantitate intracardiac left-to-right shunting, *Am Heart J* 124:448, 1992.
62. Bommer WJ, Shah PM, Meltzer R et al: The safety of contrast echocardiography: report of the committee on contrast echocardiography for the American Society of Echocardiography, *J Am Coll Cardiol* 3:6, 1984.
63. Daniel WG, Nellessen U, Schroeder E, et al: Left atrial spontaneous echo contrast in mitral valve disease: an indicator for an increased thromboembolic risk, *J Am Coll Cardiol* 11:1204, 1988.
64. Garcia-Fernandez MA, Lopez-Sendon J, Coma-Canella I et al: Echocardiographic detection of circulating blood in normal canine hearts, *Am J Cardiol* 56:834, 1992.
65. Merino A, Hauptman P, Badimon L et al: Echocardiographic "smoke" is produced by an interaction of erythrocytes and plasma proteins modulated by shear forces, *J Am Coll Cardiol* 20:1661, 1992.
66. Goldberg SJ, Allen CJ, Marx GR et al, eds: *Doppler echocardiography,* Philadelphia, 1985, Lea & Febiger.
67. Kirberger RM: Doppler echocardiography: facts and physics for practitioners, *Compend Contin Educ Pract Vet* 13:1679, 1991.
68. Gaber CE: Doppler echocardiography, *Probl Vet Med* 3:479, 1991.
69. Knight DH, ed: Doppler echocardiography: theoretical considerations and clinical applications in veterinary cardiology, *Proc 4th ACVIM Forum* 9:43, 1986.
70. Sahn D, Baker DW, DeMaria A: Recommendations for terminology and display for Doppler echocardiography, *J Am Soc Echocardiogr* 1-12, 1984.
71. Hatle LK, Angelsen B: *Doppler ultrasound in cardiology: physics, principles and clinical applications,* ed 2, Philadelphia, 1985, Lea & Febiger.
72. Missri J: *Clinical Doppler echocardiography: spectral and color flow imaging,* New York, 1990, McGraw-Hill.
73. Snider AR: Prediction of intracardiac pressures and assessment of ventricular function with Doppler echocardiography, *Echocardiography* 4:305, 1985.
74. Feigenbaum H: Doppler color flow imaging. In Braunwald E, ed: *Heart disease: a textbook of cardiovascular medicine,* ed 3, Philadelphia, 1988, WB Saunders.
75. Gaber CE: Normal pulsed Doppler flow velocities in adult dogs, *Proc ACVIM Forum* 1987, p 923 (abstract).
76. Yuill CD, O'Grady MR: Doppler-derived velocity of blood flow across the cardiac valves in the normal dog, *Can J Vet Res* 55:185, 1991.
77. Brown DJ, Knight DH, King RR: Use of pulsed-wave Doppler echocardiography to determine aortic and pulmonary velocity and flow variables in clinically normal dogs, *Am J Vet Res* 52:543, 1991.
78. Kirberger RM, Bland-van den Berg F, Grimbeck RJ: Doppler echocardiography in the normal dog. II. Factors influencing blood flow velocities and a comparison between left and right heart blood flow, *Vet Radiol Ultrasound* 33:380, 1992.
79. Kirberger RM, Bland-van den Berg F, Grimbeck RJ: Doppler echocardiography in the normal dog. I. Velocity findings and flow patterns, *Vet Radiol Ultrasound* 33:370, 1992.
80. Valdez-Cruz LM, Horowitz S, Sahn DL et al: A simplified mitral valve method for 2D echo Doppler cardiac output, *Circulation* 68:230, 1983 (abstract).
81. Fisher EA, Stahl JA, Budd JH et al: Transesophageal echocardiography: procedures and clinical application, *J Am Coll Cardiol* 18:1333, 1991.
82. Kienle RD, Thomas WP, Rishniw M: Biplane transesophageal echocardiography in the cat: technique, anatomy and image quality, *J Vet Intern Med* 9: 1995 (abstract).

83. Thomas WP: Clinical applications of transesophageal echocardiography, *Proc 12th ACVIM Forum,* 1994, p 312.
84. Kramer GA: Transesophageal echocardiography, *Proc 10th ACVIM Forum,* 1992, p 618.
85. Loyer C, Thomas WP: Transesophageal echocardiography in the dog, *Proc 10th ACVIM Forum,* 1992, p 621.
86. Loyer C, Thomas WP: Biplane transesophageal echocardiography in the dog: technique, anatomy and imaging planes, *Vet Radiol Ultrasound* 35:1, 1994.
87. Herring DS, Bjornton G: Physics, facts and artifacts of diagnostic ultrasound, *Vet Clin North Am Small Anim Pract* 15:1107, 1985.
88. Wyatt HL, Heng MK, Meerbaum S et al: Cross-sectional echocardiography. II. Analysis of mathematical models for quantifying volume of the formalin-fixed left ventricle, *Circulation* 61:1119, 1980.
89. Stack RS, Ramage JE, Bauman RP et al: Validation of in vivo two-dimensional echocardiographic dimension measurements using myocardial mass estimates in dogs, *Am Heart J* 113:725, 1987.
90. Wyatt HL, Heng MK, Meerbaum S et al: Cross-sectional echocardiography. I. Analysis of mathematic of mathematic models for quantifying mass of the left ventricle in dogs, *Circulation* 60:1104, 1979.
91. Schiller NB, Skiôldebrand CG, Schiller EJ et al: Canine left ventricular mass estimation by two-dimensional echocardiography, *Circulation* 68:210, 1983.
92. Coleman B, Cothran LN, Ison-Franklin EL et al: Estimation of left ventricular mass in conscious dogs, *Am J Physiol* 251:H1149, 1986.
93. Durell M: Doppler instrumentation. In Nanda NC, ed: *Doppler echocardiography,* New York, 1985, Igaku-Shion.
94. Snyder PS, Sato T, Atkins CE: A comparison of echocardiographic indices of the nonracing healthy greyhound to reference values from other breeds, *Vet Radiol Ultrasound* 36:387, 1995.
95. Bayon A, Fernandez del Palacio J, Montes AM et al: M-mode echocardiography study in growing Spanish mastiffs, *J Small Anim Pract* 35:473, 1994.
96. Herrtage M: Echocardiographic measurements in the normal boxer, *Proc Eur Soc Vet Internal Med Ann Cong,* 1994, p 172.
97. Crippa L, Ferro E, Melloni E et al: Echocardiographic parameters and indices in the normal beagle dog, *Lab Anim* 26:190, 1992.
98. Haggstrom J, Hamlin RL, Hanson K et al: Heart rate variability in relation to severity of mitral regurgitation in Cavalier King Charles spaniels, *J Small Anim Pract* 37:69, 1996.
99. Gooding JP, Robinson WF, Mews GC: Echocardiographic assessment of left ventricular dimensions in clinically normal English cocker spaniels, *Am J Vet Res* 47:296, 1986.
100. Page A, Edmunds G, Atwell RB: Echocardiographic values in the greyhound, *Aust Vet J* 70:361, 1993.
101. Calvert CA, Brown J: Use of M-mode echocardiography in the diagnosis of congestive cardiomyopathy in Doberman pinschers, *J Am Vet Med Assoc* 189:293, 1986.
102. Koch J, Pederson HD, Jensen AL et al: M-mode echocardiographic diagnosis of dilated cardiomyopathy in giant breed dogs, *J Vet Med* 43:297, 1996.
103. DeMadron E: Update on normal M-mode echocardiographic values in the dog, *Pract Med Chir Anim Comp* 30:647, 1995.

CHAPTER 7

Cardiac Catheterization

The diagnosis of cardiovascular disease is dependent on identifying physiologic and anatomic abnormalities within the cardiovascular system. Before the advent of echocardiography, specific anatomic identification and measurement of intracardiac variables (pressure, blood flow, etc.) required invasive catheterization and angiocardiography. Although invasive techniques are no longer relied upon as heavily for clinical diagnosis, they still play a key role in the diagnosis and therapy of some patients with heart disease and are still considered by many to be the gold standard in cardiovascular research. For some hemodynamic variables, such as cardiac output, an accurate and widely accepted noninvasive counterpart has not been developed. For these reasons, cardiac catheterization and angiocardiography are still an integral part in the overall evaluation of cardiovascular disease, although the degree of usefulness and the justifiable indications have decreased in recent years. It is important for those involved in small animal practice to have a basic understanding of the availability, usefulness, and limitations of cardiac catheterization so that appropriate cases can be referred for proper diagnosis and therapy when circumstances dictate.

This chapter focuses on the techniques used for obtaining and interpreting physiologic and anatomic data by cardiac catheterization and angiography. Cardiac catheterization data and techniques specific to diseases are discussed in detail in later chapters. Although few reports discuss the clinical application of cardiac catheterization in dogs and other domestic animals, extensive scientific cardiovascular research is available in domestic animals.[1-3] The techniques in animals are similar to those used in humans and useful information can also be obtained from detailed human reports.[4,5]

General Principles

HISTORICAL PERSPECTIVE

Cardiac catheterization was first performed in 1844 by Claude Bernard, on equine subjects, using the jugular vein and carotid artery to access the left and right ventricles.[4] Following was an era of numerous cardiac catheterization studies in animals, which led to many of the cardiovascular physiologic principles and catheterization techniques still used today. In 1929, Werner Forssman was the first to successfully pass a catheter into the heart of a living human.[5] Surprisingly, his first subject was himself. Over the next few decades, multiple investigations into the catheterization of living human hearts were performed. Notable achievements in this period were the discovery of oxygen saturation as an evaluation of pulmonary blood flow and the discovery and application of pulmonary capillary wedge pressure.[5]

After 1950, further developments came rapidly. Retrograde left heart catheterization was first performed by Zimmerman in 1950, and the Seldinger technique for percutaneous vascular access was introduced in 1953.[6] Selective coronary artery catheterization, initially described by Sones in 1959, was perfected over the ensuing years.[4] One of the most influential developments was the balloon-tipped, flow-guided catheter introduced by Swan and Ganz in 1970.[7] In more recent years, the focus of investigators has been toward the therapeutic potential of cardiac catheterization, including angioplasty, valvuloplasty, and the placement of intravascular stents.[5]

INDICATIONS

The decision to proceed with cardiac catheterization is based on the balance between the relative risk of the procedure vs. the anticipated benefit of the results. In some instances the decision is easily made because noninvasive options are not available. However, in other situations noninvasive alternatives may be sought. In veterinary medicine, the expense of the procedure must be weighed carefully. Because of the need for specialized equipment and general anesthesia, invasive techniques are generally more costly than other methods. In general, cardiac catheterization should only be pursued when the results are expected to alter the management of the animal's suspected condition, when a better determination of an animal's prognosis can be made, or when a noninvasive alternative is not available. The following indications should be used as guidelines when considering cardiac catheterization in a clinical patient.[2-4]

1. *Diagnostic catheterization:* Since the advent of echocardiography, the need for cardiac catheterization in veterinary patients has diminished substantially, as many more conditions can be well defined and categorized in a noninvasive fashion. However, situations may arise in which invasive diagnosis of a disease process is necessary, especially when other means of diagnosis are inadequate or unavailable. In some instances, more detailed information regarding the anatomy or physiology of a disorder may become important, especially if it is anticipated to alter patient management or prognosis. Cardiac catheterization is generally recommended when there is a need to confirm the presence of or determine the severity of a condition that is suspected from other clinical data but is not clearly and adequately defined.[4] This indication applies most often to young animals with complex congenital defects or patients in which echocardiographic data are not sensitive enough to discriminate between normal and

disease (e.g., restrictive cardiomyopathy). In some cases, confirmatory information is necessary to determine the breeding soundness of an individual.[8]

2. *Presurgical evaluation:* In humans there is little argument that consideration for cardiovascular surgery is an adequate justification for catheterization.[4,5] The argument, although medically sound, may be financially more difficult to justify in veterinary patients. With the exception of isolated patent ductus arteriosus, however, catheterization in patients considered for cardiac surgery may provide the surgical team with a more complete anatomic and functional characterization of the disorder and should be considered. This is especially important when dealing with congenital defects in which the nature and severity of the lesion are critical in determining its operability. In addition, associated but clinically silent lesions (such as small atrial or ventricular septal defects) that might alter the surgical approach may be further characterized.
3. *Therapeutic intervention:* Currently, the most widely justified indication for cardiac catheterization in veterinary patients is therapeutic intervention. Many congenital diseases are not responsive to medical therapy and require surgical intervention. With the current emphasis on less invasive interventions in human cardiology, more catheterization interventions will become available to veterinary patients. Currently, only balloon valvuloplasty has gained widespread acceptance as a standard of therapy for obstructive conditions, especially congenital pulmonic stenosis.[9]
4. *Clinical research:* Much of the current knowledge of heart disease, in both human and veterinary medicine, has been gained from studies of naturally occurring and artificially induced disease in animals. The use of clinical patients, with the proper informed consent of the owner, to continue the advancement of fundamental cardiovascular principles remains a justifiable indication for cardiac catheterization. Because there may be no direct benefit to the individual, patients selected for clinical research should not be subjected to undue risk and owners should be fully informed about the inherent risks that are involved.

CONTRAINDICATIONS

With the current anesthetic protocols and sophisticated monitoring techniques, there are no absolute contraindications to cardiac catheterization when performed by experienced individuals. However, some relative contraindications should be understood, to minimize the development of preventable complications in patients selected for cardiac catheterization.[4,5] Metabolic abnormalities, infectious conditions, or drug toxicities that might compromise a patient during anesthesia or exacerbate the development of ventricular irritability should be corrected before proceeding with an elective catheterization. Likewise, any decompensated cardiac condition should be stabilized before catheterization. Uncontrollable ventricular arrhythmias (presumably related to the underlying condition) may increase the risk of ventricular catheterization as a result of the induction of potentially life-threatening arrhythmias that may also interfere with the interpretation of the hemodynamic or angiographic data. Bleeding disorders may disrupt hemostasis at the sites used for vascular access, resulting in excessive blood loss or hematoma formation. Coagulopathies may also lead to increased device-induced thrombosis related to catheters. Although not well documented in veterinary patients, idiosyncratic reactions to contrast agents is potential and dogs known to have had prior reactions to radiographic contrast should be dealt with accordingly.

EQUIPMENT

Cardiac catheterization requires specialized monitoring and recording equipment. The use of substandard or inadequate equipment significantly adds to the risk of the procedure and diminishes the benefit of the results. The placement and positioning of catheters and other instruments is generally performed with fluoroscopic guidance, using image intensification to reduce radiation exposure to the operator. Most fluoroscopes allow images to be displayed on television monitors and recorded on videotape or photographic film for archiving. Depending on the procedure performed, an easily moveable table is advantageous so that patient positioning may remain constant during the procedure. This may be further facilitated using a C-arm type of fluoroscope, to allow multiple imaging planes without the need to reposition the patient.

Patient monitoring and recording of hemodynamic data are accomplished using multichannel physiologic recorders. Many types of physiologic recorders are available. The important features are the ability to continuously display updated data (such as the electrocardiogram and systemic arterial pressure) and to record several variables simultaneously. Angiocardiograms are generally recorded on videotape or on 35-mm cinematic film. A variety of cardiac catheters should be sterile and ready for use, and a standard pack of surgery instruments is necessary for vascular access. Other specialized studies may require specific equipment for proper recording (e.g., a cardiac output computer).

Ancillary equipment to ensure the safety of the patient is also beneficial. Proper anesthetic equipment is necessary to maintain an adequate and safe level of restraint and a direct-current defibrillator should be readily available. Drugs used for cardiac emergencies and cardiopulmonary resuscitation should be available at all times during the procedure.

PREPARATION AND ANESTHESIA

Proper preparation of the patient and facilities and developement of a well-thought-out plan before the procedure are essential for completing a successful study. All patients considered for cardiac catheterization should have a thorough diagnostic workup, with a detailed history and physical examination, a complete cardiovascular evaluation, and any necessary adjunct evaluations to ensure safe anesthesia. Each patient must be considered individually and the sequence of studies and materials needed planned accordingly. Monitoring and recording equipment must be set up and calibrated, and all ancillary supplies (catheters, pressure transducers, contrast material, etc.) should be placed in a convenient location before the induction of anesthesia. Complications can occur during catheterization, and the clinician must be flexible enough to alter the procedure as necessary. With a proper precatheterization routine, delays and complications can be minimized.

General anesthesia is required for the majority of catheterization procedures, although some procedures (e.g., endomyocardial biopsy, Swan-Ganz catheterization) can be performed with no or light sedation and physical restraint. Proper preanesthetic evaluation should be pursued in each patient. In general, withholding medications before and during catheterization, which is common practice in human medicine, is not necessary.

Several anesthetic protocols are currently available for patients with cardiovascular disease.[10-13] Most sedatives and anesthetic agents affect cardiac output and blood pressure. Consequently, an attempt should be made to keep the plane of anesthesia as light as possible to minimize the hemodynamic effects. Because cardiac catheterization is a minor surgical procedure, light anesthesia sufficient to provide immobilization, and desensitization of the patient usually will suffice except during dissection of the neck musculature for carotid artery isolation. Endotracheal intubation usually is necessary, because most anesthetic protocols used in clinical patients involve inhalation anesthesia with either halothane or isoflurane. Likewise, equipment for positive-pressure ventilation and oxygen administration are highly recommended. The electrocardiogram should be monitored closely throughout the anesthetic period.

Cardiac catheterization is a minor surgical procedure and an effort must be made to maintain a sterile environment. All catheters, surgical instruments, drapes, and other equipment should be sterilized using accepted methods. However, caps and masks often are not used in human cardiac catheterization laboratories when permanently implanted materials are not used and may be optional in veterinary catheterization laboratories. Routine use of antibiotics during or after cardiac catheterization is probably inappropriate. We have yet to see an instance of infection following cardiac catheterization with or without antibiotic administration.

Technique

VASCULAR ACCESS

Recording of hemodynamic data, blood sampling, and contrast injections require the placement of needles or catheters into selective or nonselective positions within the heart and great vessels. Two general methods of obtaining vascular access, with numerous variations, are commonly used: direct vascular exposure (surgical cutdown) and percutaneous (needle) puncture.[5] In veterinary patients, vascular cutdown is used more often, because the animals are generally anesthetized for the procedure.

Direct vascular exposure. The most rapid means of gaining vascular access is to surgically expose the vessel and place catheters directly into the vessel lumen through a small incision in the vessel (Color Plate 32). With the patient under general anesthesia, the procedure is usually performed in the neck region to access the external jugular vein or carotid artery. The femoral vessels on the proximal and medial aspect of the pelvic limb may also be used. The hair is clipped on the lateral cervical area over the jugular vein and the skin is surgically prepared. A 1- to 1.5-inch incision is made over the jugular vein. Care is taken not to lacerate the jugular vein by pulling the skin dorsal to the vein while making the incision. After the initial skin incision, all dissection is performed bluntly, using either forceps or scissors. In cats, lidocaine without epinephrine must be placed on an exposed vessel at least 5 minutes before manipulation to prevent intense vasoconstriction.

The external jugular vein is easily isolated through blunt dissection. It is maintained in an exterior position by securing it with rubber bands, umbilical tape, or nonabrasive suture material both proximal and distal to the intended venotomy site. A small venotomy is made in a convenient location using vascular scissors. The occluding bands provide hemostasis once the venotomy is performed. When the catheter is introduced into the vessel through the venotomy, the proximal occluding band is tightened around the vessel and catheter combination.

The carotid artery lies deep, beneath the neck musculature, along the dorsolateral aspect of the trachea. To gain access to the carotid artery, the deep muscle tissue and fascia just medial to the jugular vein is separated in blunt fashion to gain access to the trachea and associated fascia. The carotid pulse is digitally located, and the carotid sheath is "hooked" with a hemostat, in a blind fashion, and exteriorized. The vagosympathetic trunk is then bluntly separated from the carotid artery and returned to its internal position. The most common reason for failure to identify the carotid artery is failure to dissect deep enough in the neck. All muscle and fascial tissues between the subcutaneous layer and the trachea must be fully dissected to allow proper access to the carotid sheath. Once exteriorized, the carotid artery is maintained in a similar fashion as the jugular vein and a small arteriotomy is performed using vascular scissors to allow catheter access. Rubber bands generally should not be used to secure a carotid artery because they can break. Loss of an incised carotid artery can result in fatal hemorrhage because the carotid artery often is impossible to find once it has been dropped.

Once the procedure is completed, the vessel can either be sacrificed or the incision in the vessel sutured closed. The success rate of producing a patent vessel after suturing is variable.

Percutaneous (needle) puncture. Although effective, vascular cutdown procedures often result in loss of the vessel for future studies. The percutaneous (Seldinger) procedure is quick for experienced operators, requires a minimum of surgical instruments, and in most situations can be performed in awake or sedated patients. The technique can be used for arterial or venous access and in dogs and cats primarily is used for accessing the jugular vein or femoral artery.[14,15] The carotid artery is not accessible via a percutaneous approach. Although it is possible to gain percutaneous access to the femoral vein, the inability to confidently palpate this structure makes the technique difficult in this location.

A wide area around the puncture site is clipped, scrubbed, and draped in a sterile fashion (Color Plate 33). The vessel is located by means of digital palpation (usually the jugular vein must be compressed near the thoracic inlet to allow digital palpation), and the skin and subcutaneous tissues over the vessel are anesthetized with 1% lidocaine unless the patient is under general anesthesia. A small puncture incision is made with a no. 11 scalpel to facilitate catheter or sheath passage through the skin. A vascular cannula (with stylet) or 18-gauge vascular needle is inserted into the vessel initially. Venous access produces a slow insidious flow of dark blood in the needle. Arterial access produces strong pulsatile flow that may literally shoot several inches past the hub of the needle. If present, the stylet is removed, and a flexible guidewire is inserted through the cannula or needle into the vessel. The needle is then removed, leaving the wire in place. If direct catheter placement is desired, a flexible guidewire, long enough to extend from within the vessel to the distal end of the catheter, must be used. The absolute length of the wire will vary with catheter length. An end-hole catheter is then guided over the wire into the vessel, the guidewire is removed, and the catheter is flushed with heparinized saline. If multiple catheter changes are anticipated or excessive catheter manipulation will be necessary, the placement of an introducer sheath may be advantageous. For the placement of an introducer sheath, a shorter guidewire long enough to extend from within the vessel out the distal end of the dilator (obturator) is used. After the guidewire has been placed 10 to 15 cm within the vessel, an introducer sheath with an appropriate-size obturator is placed into the vessel over the guidewire. The sheath should be inserted with a gentle twisting, forward motion. The guidewire and obturator are removed, and the sheath is flushed with heparinized saline. Catheters may then be passed through the sheath directly into the vascular system.

One common complication of percutaneous needle puncture is postoperative hematoma formation at the insertion site, especially following arterial puncture. Continuous and direct pressure (20 to 30 minutes for arterial puncture) must be applied following catheter or sheath removal, and the leg must remain immobile.

CATHETER SELECTION

Catheter selection is based largely on availability, the studies to be performed, the sites to be catheterized, and operator experience and preference. A variety of cardiac catheters are commercially available, all of which are radiopaque. Many catheters are designed for specific purposes, whereas others have a wider range of utility. The catheter most suited to easily and accurately completing the planned study should be used. The characteristics and uses of the most common catheters used in veterinary medicine are presented in Table 7-1.

TABLE 7-1

Commercial catheters used for cardiac catheterization

Type	*Description*	*Use*
NIH angiographic	Rigid catheter; closed tip with six round side holes within first centimeter	Angiography, primarily LV and Ao; pressure measurement
Nycor-Pigtail	Semirigid catheter; tightly curved tip with end hole; multiple side holes	Angiography, primarily LV; pressure measurement in LV
Berman angiographic	Flexible catheter; closed tip with multiple side holes; inflatable balloon tip	Angiography, primarily RV and PA
Lehman ventriculographic	Semirigid catheter; flexible tapered closed tip with four side holes	Pressure measurement, primarily LV and Ao; pullback pressure recordings; LV angiography
Cournand	Flexible catheter; end hole only	Pressure measurement, primarily LV and Ao; blood sampling
Goodale-Lubin	Flexible catheter; open tip with two side holes close to tip	Pressure measurement, primarily LV and Ao; blood sampling
Balloon wedge	Flexible catheter; end hole only; inflatable balloon tip	Pressure measurement, primarily PCWP, PA, RV, and RA; blood sampling
Swan-Ganz	Flexible catheter; inflatable balloon tip with end hole, thermistor at tip, proximal side hole 15-30 cm from tip	Pressure measurement, primarily PCWP, RV, RA, and PA; thermodilution cardiac output measurement; blood sampling

LV, Left ventricle; *Ao,* aorta; *RV,* right ventricle; *PA,* pulmonary artery; *PCWP,* pulmonary capillary wedge pressure; *RA,* right atrium.

When deciding on catheter type, a few guidelines apply. For pressure measurement or angiography of the right heart chambers, inflatable balloon-tip catheters facilitate catheter placement into the right ventricle and pulmonary artery. The aortic valve may be difficult to cross with a catheter, especially in small patients or patients with aortic stenosis. Catheters specifically designed to facilitate passage through the aortic valve while minimizing trauma to the surrounding structures, such as the Lehman ventriculography catheter or the Nycor-pigtail catheter, should be used if available. An end-hole catheter is essential if the use of a guidewire is anticipated. Several different types of catheters should be available in the event the initial catheter selection does not allow successful completion of the study.

For pressure measurement, catheters with either side holes, end holes, or both may be used. However, side holes are preferred whenever blood flow toward the catheter is anticipated, because the kinetic energy of the blood flow will falsely increase pressure. For measurement of the pulmonary capillary wedge pressure (discussed below) an end-hole only catheter is necessary. For angiography, a stiff, closed-tip catheter is preferred for several reasons. Side holes allow dispersion of the energy of injection (and so minimize catheter recoil) and provide uniform dispersion of the contrast medium. They also reduce the risk of intramyocardial injection of contrast medium.

Catheters used for dogs and cats are usually 4- to 8-French outside diameter and 50 to 120 cm in length. The largest catheter that can be easily introduced and manipulated to the desired position is preferred.

RIGHT HEART CATHETERIZATION

Right heart catheterization may be accomplished via either a femoral vein or an external jugular vein. However, it is easier to pass a catheter into the right ventricle or pulmonary artery from a cervical (jugular vein) approach. The positioning of the patient (usually right or left lateral recumbency) depends on operator preference. However, in dogs with a persistent left cranial vena cava, the right jugular vein must be used to gain access to the right ventricle.

Catheterization of the right heart with semirigid catheters requires fluoroscopic guidance and substantial skill. These catheters increase the risk of cardiac puncture. Abnormal positions of the heart chambers and right ventricular hypertrophy increase the difficulty, even for experienced cardiologists. These problems have been largely surmounted by the use of balloon-tipped flow-directed catheters, which allow rapid and safe catheterization of the pulmonary artery with or without fluoroscopy. The inflated latex balloon protrudes beyond the tip of the catheter and protects the tip from damaging or puncturing the myocardium, making it easier to guide the catheter around the right ventricular apex and into the right ventricular outflow tract. Most balloon-tipped catheters are constructed from soft polyvinyl chloride that further softens at body temperature. The balloon-tip flow-directed catheters most commonly used in veterinary medicine are the Swan-Ganz thermodilution catheter, the Berman angiographic catheter, and the balloon wedge catheter (see Table 7-1).

From the jugular vein, the catheter is guided down the jugular vein, into the cranial vena cava, and into the right atrium (Figure 7-1). Occasionally the catheter will preferentially go into the azygous vein rather than the right atrium because of the slight curvature of the catheter. Keeping the tip directed ventrally and slightly rotating the catheter at the junction of the cranial vena cava and right atrium usually will allow the tip to be directed into the right atrium. When using a balloon-tipped catheter, the balloon may be inflated with air once the catheter is in the right atrium or right ventricle. The tip is directed caudally and ventrally across the tricuspid valve into the main body of the right ventricle. If the catheter is directed too far caudally or dorsally, the catheter may be misdirected into the coronary sinus or caudal vena cava. Preforming the catheter with a gentle curvature at the tip will aid placement into the right ventricle. Within the right ventricle, the balloon is inflated and the catheter tip manipulated around the apex and into the right ventricular outflow tract. From there it is advanced into the pulmonary artery (Figures 7-1 and 7-2).

From the femoral vein, the catheter is advanced through the caudal vena cava into the right atrium. The multiple side branches of the caudal vena cava may pose difficulty when passing flexible, curved catheters. The use of a guidewire, slow and careful advancement, and fluoroscopic observation assist the placement of the catheter into the right atrium. Positioning of the catheter into the right ventricle and pulmonary artery is similar to the cervical approach. However, the maneuver is more difficult because of the catheter's tendency to move into the cranial right atrium and right auricle rather than across the tricuspid valve. A large, sweeping bend or S-curve at the catheter tip may be helpful.

From either approach, the pulmonary "wedge" position is achieved by advancing the catheter as far as possible into the pulmonary circulation and wedging it into a small vessel, thereby occluding flow through the vessel. Alternatively, using a balloon-tipped catheter, the balloon can be inflated in one of the main branches, allowing flow to carry the balloon and catheter tip into a wedged position (see Figure 7-2). When an end-hole catheter is in the wedged position, regional pulmonary flow is occluded and the catheter measures pulmonary capillary pressure rather than pulmonary arterial pressure.

A B

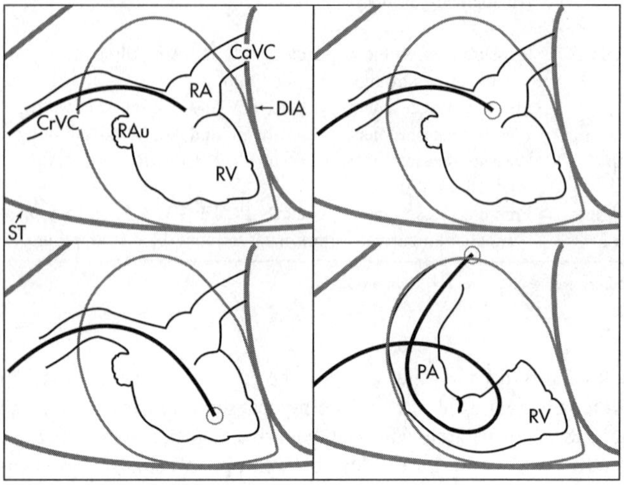

C D

FIGURE 7-1 Schematic representation of right heart catheterization from the jugular vein. The diagrams illustrate the placement of a balloon-tipped catheter into the right atrium, right ventricle, and pulmonary artery. The schematics represent how the heart chambers relate to the cardiac silhouette as it appears under fluoroscopy in the lateral projection. **A,** The catheter is generally placed from the jugular vein into the right atrium. **B,** Once in the right atrium, the balloon may be inflated. **C,** With or without the balloon inflated, the tip of the catheter is guided across the tricuspid valve. **D,** Further advancement with the balloon inflated allows the tip of the catheter to bounce off the right ventricular wall, turn toward and cross the pulmonary valve, and advance into the main pulmonary artery. *CrVC,* cranial vena cave; *CaVC,* caudal vena cava; *RA,* right atrium; *RAu,* right auricle; *RV,* right ventricle; *PA,* pulmonary artery; *DIA,* diaphragm; *ST,* sternum.

LEFT HEART CATHETERIZATION

Left heart catheterization may be accomplished via either a femoral or a carotid artery. From the carotid artery, the catheter is advanced into the brachiocephalic trunk and aortic arch (Figure 7-3). Directing the tip dorsally advances the catheter into the descending aorta, whereas directing the tip ventrally places the catheter into the ascending aorta and aortic root. In the aortic root, the catheter tip tends to deflect off the aortic valve leaflets and snag in the sinuses of Valsalva. Repeated, gentle, to-and-fro movements and timing catheter advancement with ventricular systole aids passage of the catheter through the aortic valve. The flexible tip of the Lehman ventriculographic catheter is designed to flip into the ventricle from the sinuses of Valsalva. The tight curve of the pigtail catheter, which must be placed into the ascending aorta using a guidewire, usually passes easily into the left ventricle. Alternatively, when using a rigid catheter, a very flexible guidewire can be looped across the aortic valve and into the left ventricle. The catheter is then advanced over the guidewire. Placement of the catheter into the left atrium, a relatively difficult procedure, is not routinely performed. However, the left atrium can be catheterized with a flexible or slightly curved catheter by an experienced operator. Alternatively, the left atrium (and left ventricle) can be catheterized using a transseptal approach from the right atrium.[16]

From the femoral artery, the catheter is directed from the descending aorta into the aortic root. Because of the curvature of the aortic arch, the catheter tends to pass into the brachiocephalic trunk or left subclavian artery. This obstacle is overcome by using a slightly curved catheter tip or a flexible guidewire. Passage of the catheter across the aortic valve is the same as for the carotid artery, although catheter manipulations may be more difficult as a result of the greater distance, which reduces catheter control.

Hemodynamic Studies

PRESSURE MEASUREMENT

The force generated by the myocardium is transmitted through the fluid medium of blood as a pressure wave. The measurement and analysis of these waveforms, generated by the various cardiac

A

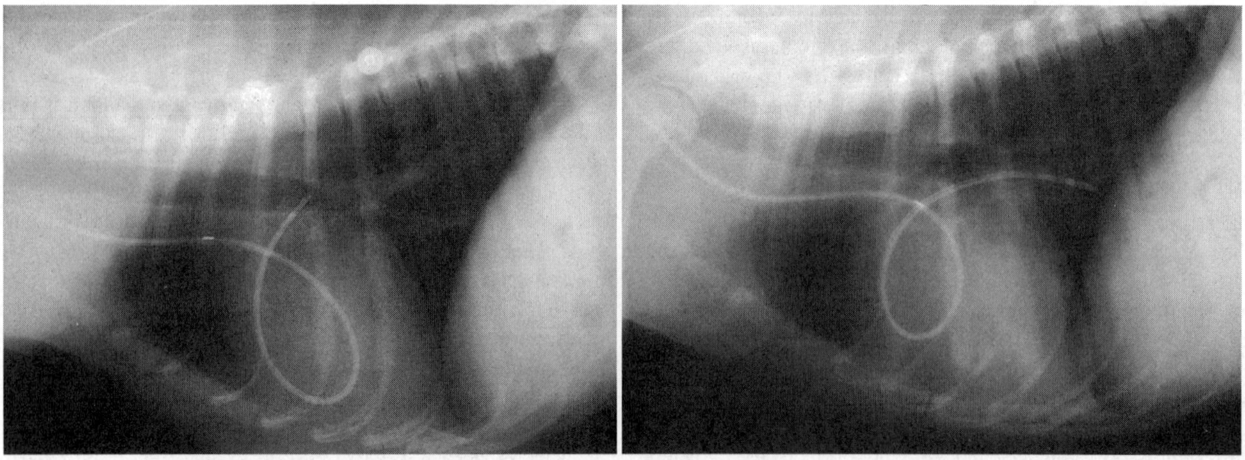

B

FIGURE 7-2 Thoracic radiographs from a dog with a balloon-tipped catheter placed in the pulmonary artery from the jugular vein. **A,** The tip of the catheter is in one of the main pulmonary arterial branches. Notice the catheter comes from the cranial cervical region (jugular vein), enters the right atrium through the cranial vena cava, crosses the tricuspid valve, is looped through the right ventricle, and crosses the pulmonary valve. **B,** The same catheter and placement as in **A.** The balloon has been inflated, and the pulmonary blood flow has advanced the tip of the catheter into a wedged position. (See text for details.)

chambers, is probably the most important focus of cardiac catheterization. The pressure waveform is complex. It is a mathematical summation of simple sine waves of differing frequencies and amplitudes.[17] The frequency response of a system is defined as the ratio of the output amplitude to the input amplitude over a range of frequencies of the input wave. To achieve accurate recordings, the system must respond such that the frequency response is close to 1.[17] In reality, this is rarely the case. The frequency response reflects the interaction of the natural forces and the degree of damping by the system. The output amplitude is exaggerated as the frequency of the signal approaches that of the natural frequency of the system. Optimal damping dissipates the energy, thereby maintaining a nearly flat frequency response curve.

Pressure measurements can be recorded using either fluid-filled catheter systems coupled with an external strain-gauge transducer or high-fidelity micromanometer-tipped catheters.[4,18] Fluid-filled systems are the most popular because of their ease of use and low relative cost. With fluid-filled systems, an external pressure transducer connected to the catheter is used to detect changes in pressure that are transmitted through the fluid column in the system. The intracardiac catheter is usually connected to the transducer by a three-way stopcock and a short piece of extension tubing (jumper). The transducer chamber and jumper are filled with sterile water or saline, so that when the stopcock is closed to room air, a fluid chamber exists between the tip of the catheter and the transducer diaphragm. Deformation of the diaphragm, created by changes in intravascular pressure at the catheter tip, produces a proportional change in the electrical resistance of the transducer. The resistors are coupled to a Wheatstone bridge type of circuit that converts changes in electrical resistance created by deformation of the diaphragm into electrical potentials that are amplified and sent to the output device (usually an oscilloscope or a heat-sensitive strip chart recorder).

A B

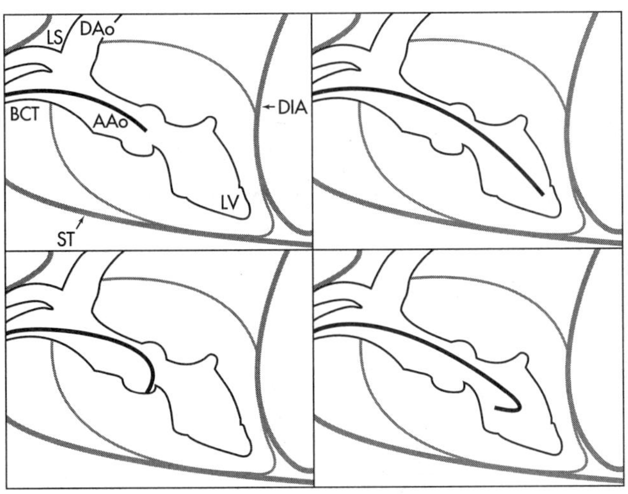

C D

FIGURE 7-3 Schematic representation of left heart catheterization from the carotid artery. The diagrams illustrate the placement of a catheter into the aorta and left ventricle. The schematics represent how the heart chambers relate to the cardiac silhouette as it appears under fluoroscopy in the lateral projection. **A,** Placement of a catheter into the ascending aorta. **B,** The catheter is guided across the aortic valve into the left ventricle. **C,** If the catheter is difficult to place across the valve, the catheter can be advanced gently into one of the sinuses of Valsalva. Further advancement then produces a loop in the ascending aorta. **D,** The loop has prolapsed into the left ventricle. The catheter is then withdrawn to eliminate the loop (**B**). *DAo,* descending aorta; *AAo,* ascending aorta; *LV,* left ventricle; *BCT,* brachiocephalic trunk; *LS,* left subclavian artery; *DIA,* diaphragm; *ST,* sternum.

Before the procedure, the pressure transducer is calibrated using a mercury manometer. The transducer chamber is exposed to several known pressures while amplifier gain is adjusted to give the desired deflection on the recorder and to ensure linearity in the systems response. The calibration settings should be periodically checked electronically during the procedure. The transducer is placed at the level of the heart and opened to room air. The recorder is then calibrated to record zero pressure at atmospheric pressure. This is known as the *zero reference point* and indicates that a fluid-filled catheter exposed to atmospheric pressure will register 0 mm Hg when its tip is at the same level as the transducer. In veterinary patients, the transducer is usually placed at the midthoracic level in a laterally recumbent animal. The catheter tip and the transducer must be at the same level to avoid the influence of gravity (especially when measuring low pressures). A relative pressure of 1 mm Hg is imparted to the transducer for every 1.36 cm of height difference from the catheter tip (1 mm Hg = 1.36 cm H_2O).[18] Pressures measured inside the heart do not necessarily correspond to exact transmural forces because of normal intrathoracic pressure.

The accuracy of pressure recordings obtained with fluid-filled systems is affected by several factors.[17,18] Blood clots or air bubbles may overdamp the system, thereby decreasing the high-frequency components of the waveform. Leaks in the system may produce the same effect. The system must have a flat frequency response in the range of 10 to 12 Hz because of low-frequency resonance associated with the small fluid movements. The natural, or resonant, frequency of the system should be significantly higher to avoid accentuation of the output signal. To avoid inaccuracies, the largest and shortest catheter possible, as few stopcocks and jumpers as necessary, and small volume-displacement transducers should be used. Even when the system is appropriate and properly set up, distortions and artifacts that hamper interpretation may occur. Motion of the catheter within the heart (catheter whip) accelerates the fluid column and may produce unavoidable superimposed waves of ±10 mm Hg, especially when recording pressure form the pulmonary arteries. If pressures appear to be erroneous, the catheter-transducer-recorder system should be examined and calibrated. Common causes of falsely low pressure recordings include the presence of a clot, loose connections in the system, kinked catheters, entrapment of the catheter tip within the heart, and air bubbles in the tubing or transducer. Catheter systems are commonly underdamped, resulting in accentuation of reflected waves within the cardiovascular and catheter systems. This commonly results in false elevations of systolic pressures, especially in the left and right ventricles. Whereas the top of these pressure waveforms should be quite flat, underdamping produces waveforms that are peaked. This can significantly increase a pressure gradient in a patient with a stenotic lesion. It may be necessary to introduce a small air bubble into a catheter system to damp the system in this situation.

Micromanometer-tipped catheters minimize artifacts associated with low-frequency resonance, catheter whip, and excessive damping. These catheters have a high fidelity pressure transducer mounted at the tip, which can be placed directly in the chamber in which the pressure is to be measured. Manometer-tipped catheters should be used when exact pressure measurements are required, which usually is only necessary in research. Recordings obtained with micromanometer-tipped catheters are often distinctly different from those obtained with fluid-filled systems (Figure 7-4).[18] Recordings made from fluid-filled systems tend to undershoot pressure in early diastole, overshoot pressure in early systole, and impart a 30- to 40-ms delay in the recording. More optimal damping and natural frequency characteristics of the fluid-filled system can minimize these artifacts but not eliminate them. Disadvantages of micromanometer-tipped catheters include: fragility, delicate calibration, drift of the frequency response curve, rigid design, and a high relative cost. They are generally only available in large sizes, although smaller sizes may be custom-ordered from some suppliers.[18]

In the course of a normal catheterization study, a record is made of the pressure waveform from each chamber that is entered during the procedure. Care should be taken to keep the catheter tip free in the lumen to prevent erroneous readings from occlusion of the holes. The catheter tip should be placed in a position that allows the tip to remain as stable as possible, so that catheter whip artifact can be avoided. When the desired position is attained, the catheter is flushed, the balance and calibration are checked, and the pressure is recorded.

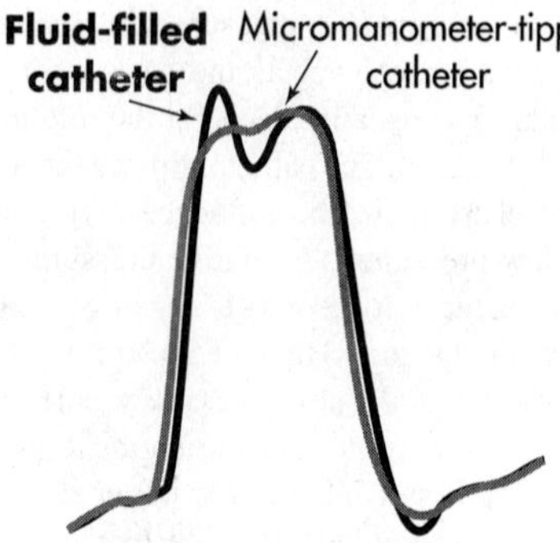

FIGURE 7-4 Schematic left ventricular pressure tracings obtained with standard fluid-filled catheter and a micromanometer (catheter-tip pressure manometer). (See text for details.)

Normal pressure waveforms. An understanding of both normal and abnormal pressure waveforms is based on a thorough knowledge of the cardiac cycle (see Chapter 2). Normal waveforms from each of the cardiac chambers are shown in Figures 7-5 and 7-6. The normal values for intracardiac pressures in dogs and cats are shown in Table 7-2. The actual pressures measured during cardiac catheterization depend on the hardware used (inherent accuracy of the system) and the physiologic state of the subject, which may be influenced by disease and anesthetic depth. In general, systolic pressures measured under general anesthesia underestimate the same pressures measured in awake animals. In some cases, measurements made in awake or lightly sedated animals overestimate the true pressures because of excitement and apprehension.[19]

The right atrial, left atrial, and pulmonary capillary wedge pressure pulses consist of two major positive waves (*a* and *v* waves), each followed by a negative descent (*x* and *y*). A small positive deflection, the *c* wave, may also be seen on the downslope of the *a* wave at the onset of ventricular systole on the left and right atrial pressure pulses. The *a* wave is the result of atrial systole and follows

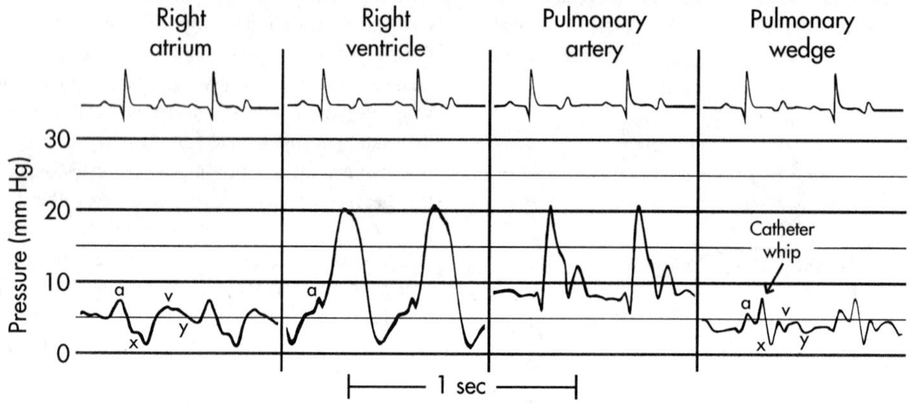

FIGURE 7-5 Schematic pressure tracings from the right side of a normal heart. *a, a* wave; *v, v* wave; *x, x* descent; *y, y* descent. (See text for details.)

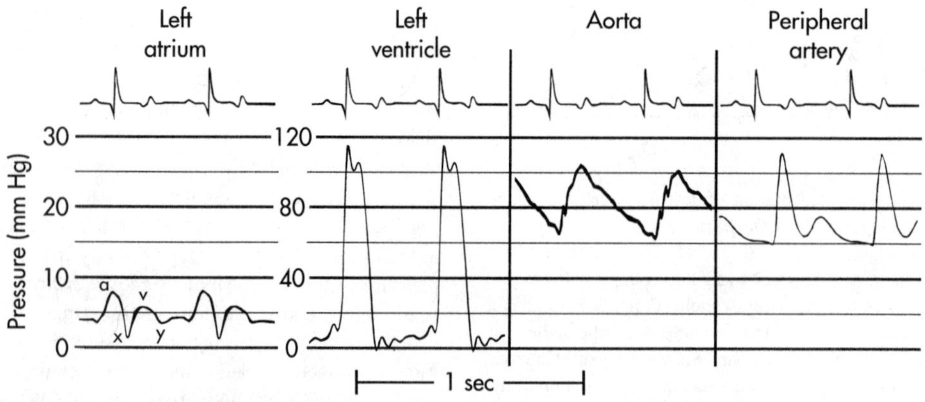

FIGURE 7-6 Schematic pressure tracings from the left side of a normal heart. *a, a* wave; *v, v* wave; *x, x* descent; *y, y* descent. (See text for details.)

the *P* wave of the electrocardiogram. The *c* wave is produced at the beginning of ventricular systole as the closed valve bulges into the atrium. The *x* descent coincides with the reduction of atrial pressure because of atrial relaxation and the descent of the atrioventricular ring during ventricular contraction. Full atrial relaxation occurs at the nadir of the *x* descent. The *v* wave corresponds to the rise in atrial pressure with continued atrial filling against a closed valve and occurs during ventricular systole. The *v* wave reaches its peak as the atrioventricular valve opens. After the mitral or tricuspid valve opens the pressure again falls as the atrium empties into the ventricle and the recorder inscribes the *y* descent. The pressure is measured at the peak of the *a* and *v* waves. The mean pressure is determined electronically.[4]

Left and right atrial pressures are similar but are not identical. The mean left atrial pressure is normally higher than the mean right atrial pressure. The *v* wave is usually dominant on the left atrial pressure tracing, and the *a* wave is dominant on the right atrial pressure tracing.[17] The pulmonary capillary wedge pressure tracing is similar to the left atrial tracing except it lacks a *c* wave, is damped, and is delayed as much as 50 to 70 ms by transmission through the capillary bed.[18] Pulmonary capillary wedge pressure is a direct measure of pulmonary capillary pressure and is used to estimate pulmonary venous and left atrial pressure in patients in which the left atrium will not or cannot be catheterized directly.

The ventricular pressure pulse can be divided into two phases, systole and diastole. The diastolic phase of the ventricular pressure waveform consists of an early rapid filling wave, a slow filling period (diastasis), and an atrial systolic wave (*a* wave). At the onset of ventricular systole, the atrioventricular valve closes and the ventricular pressure rises abruptly. The systolic phase includes isovolumic contraction, ejection, and protodiastole.[17] Isovolumic contraction occurs from the closure of the atrioventricular valve at end-diastole and ends with the opening of the semilunar valve. Ejection occurs from semilunar valve opening until semilunar valve closure. Two pressures are usually measured from the ventricular pressure pulse: the peak systolic pressure and the end-diastolic pressure immediately following the *a* wave.[4]

The pulmonary artery pressure and aortic pressure waveforms consist of a systolic pressure pulse owing to blood flow into the artery during ventricular contraction. There is an initial, steep rise in pressure with the onset of ventricular ejection, followed by a gradual rise to a rounded peak. There is a subsequent gradual decline to the dicrotic notch, which marks semilunar valve closure, and a slow diastolic descent to end-diastole. Pressure is normally measured at peak systole and at end-diastole, and mean pressure is determined electronically.[4] Aortic and pulmonary arterial pressure waveforms are similar, although aortic pressures are appreciably higher than those recorded from the pulmonary artery in a normal subject.

Pressure pulses recorded from a peripheral artery are similar to aortic pressure waveforms, except the dicrotic notch is missing. There is usually an anacrotic notch in early ejection corresponding to semilunar valve opening. As the pulse moves toward the periphery, the peak pressure increases and the ascending limb becomes steeper. There is also a proportional decrease in diastolic and mean pressures. The change in the pressure waveform as it travels away from the heart is largely the result of reflected waves which are presumably reflected from the aortic bifurcation, arterial branch points, and small peripheral vessels.[20]

TABLE 7-2

Normal intracardiac and intravascular pressures in dogs (mm Hg)*

Site	*Systolic*	*Diastolic*	*Mean*
Right atrium	4-6	0-4	2-5
Right ventricle	15-30	<5	—
Pulmonary artery	15-30	5-15	8-20
Pulmonary wedge	6-12	4-8	5-10
Left atrium	5-12	<8	<10
Left ventricle	95-150	<10	—
Aorta	95-150	70-100	80-110
Systemic arteries	110-160	80-110	90-120

*Many variables influence pressure measurements. The values presented here are "expected" ranges in dogs and cats under general anesthesia.

CARDIAC OUTPUT

Of the number of techniques developed and evaluated over the years to measure cardiac output, only two have gained widespread acceptance in the cardiac catheterization laboratory: the Fick oxygen method and the indicator-dilution technique.[4,21]

Fick oxygen method. The Fick principle states that the total uptake or release of any substance by an organ is the product of blood flow to the organ and the arteriovenous concentration difference of the substance. Pulmonary blood flow can be estimated by measuring the arteriovenous oxygen difference across the pulmonary capillaries and determining the rate of oxygen uptake by the blood. If no intracardiac shunt is present, pulmonary blood flow is virtually equal to systemic blood flow, such that:

$$\text{Cardiac output (L/min)} = \frac{\text{Oxygen consumption (mL } O_2\text{/min)}}{\text{Arteriovenous oxygen difference (mL } O_2\text{/L blood)}}$$

In actual practice, the rate of oxygen uptake from room air by the lung is measured, not the rate of oxygen uptake by the blood, because under steady-state conditions the two are equal. Two methods are commonly used in human medicine, both of which are technically demanding and fraught with inaccuracy if not performed properly. Neither method is easily modified for use in animals, especially in the clinical setting. The polarographic method uses a metabolic rate meter, and the Douglas bag method uses a breathing bag to collect expired air. The O_2 consumption in milliliters per minute is usually indexed to square meters of body surface area. Normal in humans is 110 to 150 mL O_2/min/m^2. In animals, oxygen consumption is difficult to determine and is estimated from body surface area.

The arteriovenous oxygen difference across the lungs is determined as the difference in oxygen content between the pulmonary arterial blood (considered mixed venous) and the systemic arterial blood (considered pulmonary venous). However, it is understood that the systemic arterial blood oxygen content is actually 2 to 5 mL/L lower than pulmonary venous blood because of affluence from the bronchial and Thebesian veins. Thus a small overestimation, albeit insignificant, generally results. In practice, direct measurement of oxygen saturation and hemoglobin are easier and faster than the methods available to determine oxygen content. The oxygen content can be calculated by multiplying the oxygen saturation by the theoretic oxygen-carrying capacity of normal hemoglobin and adding the influence of dissolved oxygen. The following formula is used for approximating the oxygen carrying capacity.

$$O_2 \text{ capacity (mL } O_2\text{/L blood)} = \text{Hemoglobin (g/dL)} \times 1.36 \text{ (mL } O_2\text{/g hemoglobin)} \times 10 \text{ (dl/L)}$$

Blood oxygen saturation is most commonly measured by reflectance oximetry. Alternatively, blood oxygen tension can be determined and

BOX 7-1

Formulae for calculating cardiac output by the Fick oxygen method

Arterial O_2 content: $CaO_2 = (Hgb \times SaO_2 \times 1.36 \times 10) + (PaO_2 \times 0.003)$
Venous O_2 content: $CvO_2 = (Hgb \times SvO_2 \times 1.36 \times 10) + (PvO_2 \times 0.003)$
$C_{(A-V)}O_2 = CaO_2 - CvO_2$
Cardiac output: $CO = VO_2 \div AV\ O_2$ difference
Oxygen delivery: $DO_2 = CO \times CaO_2$

CaO_2, CvO_2, Oxygen content of systemic arteries and mixed venous blood, respectively (mL O_2/L blood); *SaO_2, SvO_2*, oxygen saturation of systemic arteries and mixed venous blood (%), respectively; *PaO_2, PvO_2*, oxygen tension of systemic arteries and mixed venous blood, respectively (mm Hg); *VO_2*, oxygen consumption (mL O_2/min/m^2); *$C_{(A-V)}O_2$*, difference in arteriovenous O_2 content (mL O_2/L blood); *CO*, cardiac output (L/min); *DO_2*, oxygen delivery to the tissues (mL O_2/min); *Hgb*, hemoglobin (g/dL). 1.36 is a constant and denotes the amount of oxygen carried per gram of Hgb (mL O_2/g Hgb).

converted to oxygen saturation using a nomogram for oxygen dissociation from hemoglobin at different temperatures. Once the oxygen consumption is estimated and oxygen saturations are known, the calculations presented in Box 7-1 can be made.

The Fick oxygen method assumes that oxygen consumption and cardiac output are constant during the period of measurement. Consequently, the animal should be maintained at a stable level of anesthesia and manipulation of the catheter should be minimal. Potential errors include (1) improper calculation or estimation of oxygen consumption, (2) changes in mean pulmonary volume, (3) inaccuracies in blood oxygen saturation determination, and (4) improper collection of blood samples. Overall, the average error with this method in human laboratories is about 10%. The Fick method is most accurate in patients with low cardiac output, in whom the arteriovenous oxygen difference is wide. An example of the Fick method of cardiac output determination is demonstrated in Box 7-2.

Indicator-dilution method. The indicator-dilution method is a variation of calculating a volume of a container by placing a known quantity of an indicator (e.g., a dye) in a fluid, stirring, and measuring the concentration. In this technique, volume (L) = quantity of indicator (mg) divided by concentration (mg/L). In the circulatory system, instead of calculating volume, flow (volume per unit time) is calculated by injecting an indicator and measuring its average concentration over time. The Fick method is also an indicator-dilution method. In the Fick oxygen method, the indicator is oxygen, which is injected into the pulmonary circulation by continuous infusion from the lungs. Because pulmonary artery blood is not devoid of oxygen, the content of oxygen in the pulmonary artery must be subtracted. There are two general types of indicator-dilution methods—one in which the indicator is injected as a single bolus and one in which it is injected as a continuous infusion. The single-injection method is most widely used. The fundamental requirements of the single-injection method of indicator-dilution are as follows:

1. A nontoxic indicator substance that mixes completely with blood and whose concentration can be readily and accurately measured must be used.
2. The indicator substance can neither be added nor subtracted from the blood during passage from site of injection to site of sampling.
3. The majority of the indicator substance must pass the sampling site before recirculation.
4. The indicator substance must pass through a portion of the central circulation, where mixing of all of the blood of the body occurs.

BOX 7-2

Example of the Fick method of cardiac output determination

A 7-year-old male Doberman pinscher presents with clinical signs of forward (low output) heart failure. Based on the following values calculate his cardiac output and oxygen delivery to the tissues.

Temp = 37°
PaO_2 = 95 mm Hg
PvO_2 = 21 mm Hg
Hgb = 15 gm/100 mL
Estimated oxygen consumption (VO_2) = 200 mL O_2/min

Step 1: Determine the oxygen saturation from a nomogram.
Arterial O_2 saturation (SaO_2) = 97.2%
Venous O_2 saturation (SvO_2) = 35.0%

Step 2: Calculate oxygen content of arterial and mixed venous blood.

CaO_2 (mL O_2/L of blood) = (Hgb)(SaO_2)(1.34)(10) + (PaO_2)(0.003)
= (15)(.972)(1.34)(10) + (95)(0.003)
= 195.4 + 0.3
= 195.7 (mL O^2/L of blood)

CvO_2 (mL O_2/L of blood) = (Hgb)(SvO_2)(1.34)(10) + (PvO_2)(0.003)
= (15)(0.35)(1.34)(10) + (21)(0.003)
= 70.4 + 0.06
= 70.5 (mL O_2/L of blood)

Step 3: Calculate cardiac output (CO).

CO (L/min) = VO_2/(CaO_2 − CvO_2)
= 200/(195.7 − 70.5)
= 200/125.2
= 1.6 L/min (Normal = 3-5 L/min)

Step 4: Calculate arterial oxygen delivery (DO_2)

DO_2 (mL O_2/min) = (CO)(CaO_2)
= 1.6 × 195.7
= 313 mL O_2/min (normal = 600-700/min)

If we assume that all of the indicator substance passes the site of the sampling, then:

$$\dot{Q} \text{ or } CO = \frac{I \times 60}{\int_0^\infty C(t)dt}$$

where $\dot{Q}$ = flow, *CO* = cardiac output (L/min), *I* = amount of indicator (mg), *60* = 60 sec/min, *C* = concentration of indicator at the sampling site (mg/L), *t* = time (seconds), and the integral of *C(t)dt* is the area under the deflections time curve following the injection of the indicator.

Numerous indicators have been used successfully, but only two have gained widespread acceptance. Indocyanine green has enjoyed long-standing acceptance in both clinical and research settings. However, thermodilution is now used almost exclusively (Figure 7-7, *A*). The indocyanine green dye method uses a spectrophotometric measurable dye, whereas thermodilution uses temperature ("cold" units), as the indicator (Figure 7-7, *B*). For a more detailed description of the thermodilution method see Box 7-3.

SHUNT DETECTION AND QUANTIFICATION

The localization and quantification of shunts can be determined with precision during cardiac catheterization using several methods. In most cases, the presence of a shunt is suspected on the basis of clinical and echocardiographic evaluations. However, in some cases shunts are not suspected until data obtained at cardiac catheterization alert the operator. These may include unexplained arterial desatura-

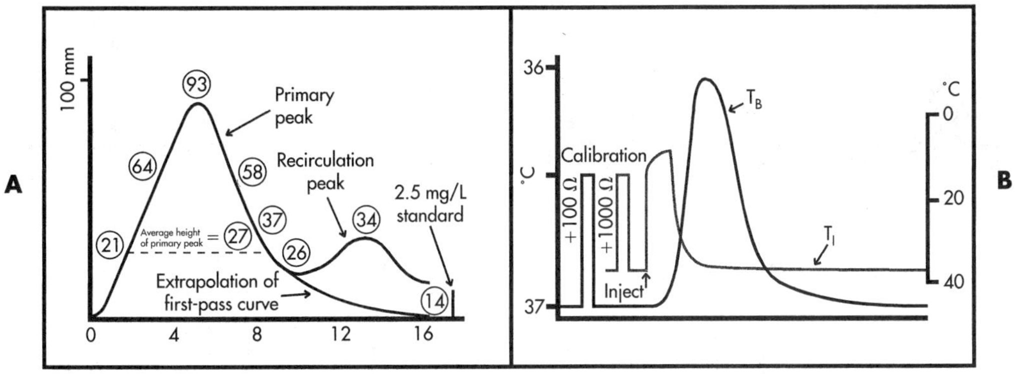

FIGURE 7-7 **A,** Schematic representation of a green dye curve. Five milligrams of dye was injected into the venous system. At time 0 it is detected by the densitometer; it peaks at about 5 seconds, and the recirculation curve begins to appear at 9 seconds. The gray line is the extrapolation of the primary curve back to the baseline. The numbers in the circles indicate the height of the dye curve in millimeters. **B,** Schematic of a representative thermodilution curve for cardiac output determination. The curve labeled T_I was recorded within the lumen of the catheter for determination of mean injectate temperature. The curve labeled T_B was recorded in the pulmonary artery and represents the mean temperature change, over time, of the pulmonary arterial blood. (See text for details.)

BOX 7-3

Thermodilution method for estimating cardiac output

The thermodilution method of cardiac output determination has become widely accepted in both clinical and research medicine since the availability of the Swan-Ganz thermodilution catheter. With this application of the indicator-dilution method, a thermal indicator (e.g., cold saline or 5% dextrose in water) of known temperature is injected into the right atrium and the resultant change in blood temperature is continuously recorded by a thermal sensor (thermistor) mounted at the tip of a catheter at a point downstream, usually in the pulmonary artery. Initially, two thermistors were used, one at the site of injection and a second downstream thermistor. Two thermistors allow accurate measurement of injectate temperature (TI) and the temperature of the downstream blood (TB). Most thermodilution systems now use a single downstream thermistor, and assume the injectate temperature (measured in a bowl outside the patient) is warmed by a predictable amount during injection. The thermodilution equation is multiplied by an empiric correction factor to correct for catheter warming. The Swan-Ganz thermodilution catheter has a thermistor at the tip of a flexible balloon-tipped flow-directed catheter for easy insertion into the pulmonary artery. A proximal port is placed 15 to 30 cm proximal to the tip for positioning within the right atrium and there is a built in connector for use with cardiac output computers.

The injectate temperature compared with the core temperature of the patient is used to determine the "concentration" of temperature as it passes the thermistor. Using an application of the basic indicator-dilution equation, the cardiac output is given as the following:

$$CO_{TD} = \frac{V_I \rho_I C_I (T_B - T_I) \times 0.825 \times 60}{\rho_B C_B \times \int_0^{\infty} \Delta T_B(t)dt}$$

where *CO* = cardiac output (L/min); V_1 = injectate volume (mL); T_1 = injectate temperature (C); T_B = blood temperature (°C); ΔT_B = the temperature of blood injectate mixture at the distal thermistor; ρx and Cx are the specific gravity and heat of the blood (B) and injectate (I), respectively; *60* = 60 sec/min; and *0.825* = empirical correction factor for catheter warming. The expression ($\rho_1 \times C_1$ / $\rho_B \times C_B$) is a constant that is related to the type of injectate. For 5% dextrose it is equal to 1.08 and for saline it is equal to 1.0. The expression equals the area under the curve and is the mean indicator concentration in °C × seconds.

A curve relating the change in temperature over time is recorded by the cardiac output computer (Figure 7-7, *B*). Manual computation of the cardiac output using the thermodilution method is tedious and time-consuming. Several types of analog computers facilitate the calculation, all based on the assumption that the downslope of the temperature curve has an exponential decay following a curved peak.

Most laboratories agree, that when CO is normal or elevated, there is good agreement between indicator-dilution methods and other independent methods of measurement. The error of these methods are greatest when CO is low, there is valvular insufficiency, or there are intracardiac shunts. When carefully performed, indicator dilution methods have an inherent error of 5% to 10%. The values obtained from both the indocyanine green dye and thermodilution methods correlate well with those calculated by the Fick method.

---

tion, unexpectedly increased pulmonary oxygen content or oxygen saturation, and data that do not completely confirm the suspected lesion.

A variety of methods are used to detect both left-to-right and right-to-left intracardiac shunts.[22,23] The methods vary in sensitivity, type of indicator, and equipment required. Only oximetry and angiography are commonly used in veterinary medicine, and they are discussed here.

Normally pulmonary blood flow (Q_P) is equal to systemic blood flow (Q_S). That is, all of the blood that enters the right atrium is ultimately conveyed to the pulmonary circulation. From there it enters the left heart to be ejected into the systemic circulation. The blood ejected from the left ventricle in turn ultimately reaches the right atrium. In the presence of an intracardiac shunt, this equality is disrupted. With left-to-right shunts, Q_P is greater than Q_S because a portion of the systemic blood flow is shunted to the right side of the heart or pulmonary circulation before it reaches the systemic capillaries. Conversely, with right-to-left shunts the amount of blood shunted from the right heart to the left heart is added to that returning from the lungs and is ejected into the systemic circulation, such that Q_S is greater than Q_P. Effective pulmonary blood flow (Q_{EP}) is defined as that portion of the venous blood that carries desaturated blood from the systemic capillaries to the pulmonary capillaries to be oxygenated. Normally, Q_{EP} is equal to both Q_P and Q_S. In the presence of an intracardiac shunt, Q_{EP} is equal to the blood flow through the side of the heart where the shunt originates, such that in

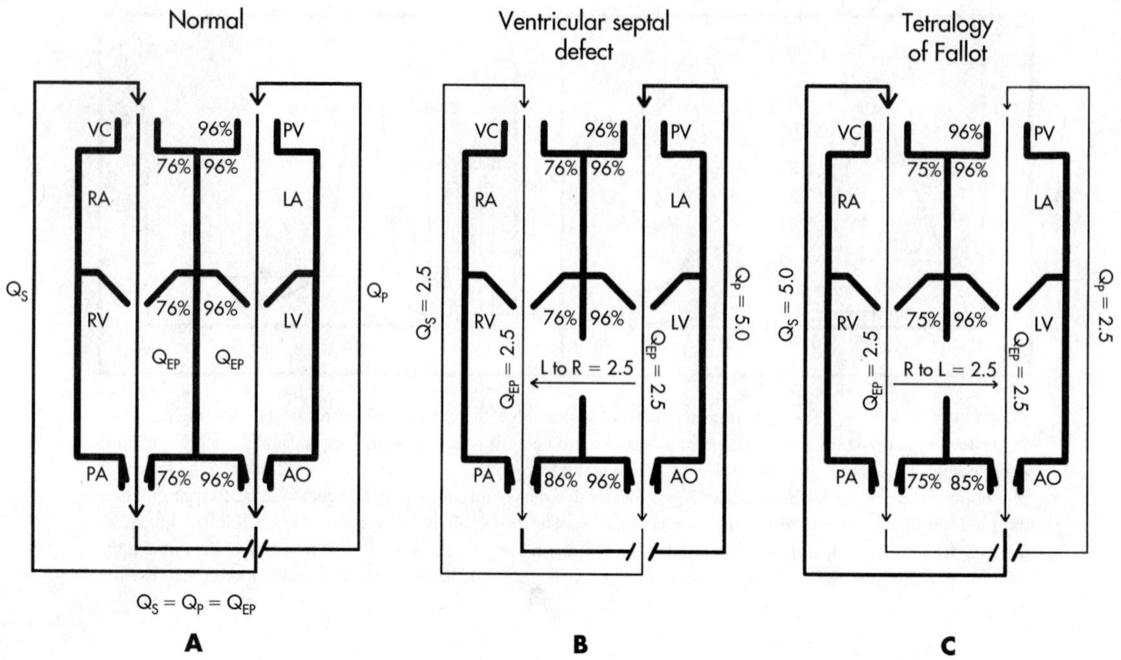

FIGURE 7-8 Using oximetry to calculate cardiovascular shunts. **A,** Normal oximetric values. Normally, $Q_S = Q_P = Q_{ES}$. **B,** Representative oximetric values from a dog with ventricular septal defect. With a left-to-right shunt $Q_P > (Q_S = Q_{EP})$. **C,** Representative oximetric values from a dog with tetralogy of Fallot. With a right-to-left shunt $Q_S > (Q_P = Q_{ES})$. *VC,* vena cava; *RA,* right atrium; *RV,* right ventricle; *PA,* pulmonary artery; *PV,* pulmonary vein; *LA,* left atrium; *LV,* left ventricle; *Ao,* aorta; Q_S, systemic blood flow; Q_P, pulmonary blood flow; Q_{EP}, effective pulmonary blood flow. (See text for details.)

a left-to-right shunt Q_{EP} equals Q_S and in a right-to-left shunt Q_{EP} equals Q_P. Therefore the following relationships can be derived:

$$\text{Left–to–right shunt} = Q_P - Q_{EP}$$
$$\text{Right–to–left shunt} = Q_S - Q_{EP}$$

Shunt detection involves identifying the discrepancy between Q_P and Q_S. To specifically localize the shunt requires the ability to identify a physiologic difference between specific heart chambers and the severity of a shunt is based on calculating absolute values for Q_P, Q_S, and Q_{EP}. In the clinical setting, shunt severity is primarily described as the ratio of pulmonary blood flow to systemic blood flow (Q_P/Q_S). It is always calculated with the denominator as 1. Normally, Q_P/Q_S equals 1 (or 1/1); left-to-right shunts produce Q_P/Q_S ratios greater than 1 (e.g., 2/1, 3/1, etc.), and right-to-left shunts produce Q_P/Q_S ratios less than 1 (e.g., 0.6/1, 0.5/1, etc.).

Left-to-right shunts

Oximetry. In oximetry, the oxygen content, or percent saturation, is measured in blood samples drawn from multiple sites within both left and right heart chambers. Left-to-right shunts are usually detected by determining and localizing a step-up (increase) in oxygen content or saturation in one of the right heart chambers. This occurs as oxygenated blood flows from a left heart chamber into the deoxygenated blood of a right heart chamber. By taking samples from the inferior and superior vena cavae, the right atrium, the main body, and outflow tract of the right ventricle, and the main, right, and left pulmonary arteries, the exact location of the shunt can often be identified (Figure 7-8).

Quantification of shunt severity using oximetry is based on the Fick principle described for cardiac output determination. As previously stated, if the shunt is unidirectional, the degree of shunting is proportional to the difference between systemic and pulmonary blood flow. Systemic, pulmonary, and effective pulmonary blood flows can be calculated from oximetry data (Boxes 7-4 and 7-5).

BOX 7-4

Formulae for calculating shunt severity using oximetric data

$$\dot{Q}_P = \frac{\dot{V}O_2}{C_{PV}O_2 - C_{PA}O_2} = \frac{\dot{V}O_2}{(S_{PV}O_2 - S_{PA}O_2)(O_2\ \text{capacity})}$$

$$\dot{Q}_S = \frac{\dot{V}O_2}{C_AO_2 - C_{MV}O_2} = \frac{\dot{V}O_2}{(S_AO_2 - S_{MV}O_2)(O_2\ \text{capacity})}$$

$$\dot{Q}_{EP} = \frac{\dot{V}O_2}{C_{PV}O_2 - C_{MV}O_2} = \frac{\dot{V}O_2}{(S_{PV}O_2 - S_{MV}O_2)(O_2\ \text{capacity})}$$

$$\dot{Q}_P/\dot{Q}_S = \frac{\dfrac{\dot{V}O_2}{(S_{PV}O_2 - S_{PA}O_2)(O_2\ \text{capacity})}}{\dfrac{\dot{V}O_2}{(S_AO_2 - S_{MV}O_2)(O_2\ \text{capacity})}} = \frac{S_AO_2 - S_{MV}O_2}{S_{PV}O_2 - S_{PA}O_2}$$

$$L \rightarrow R\ \text{shunt} = \dot{Q}_P - \dot{Q}_{EP}$$

$$R \rightarrow L\ \text{shunt} = \dot{Q}_S - \dot{Q}_{EP}$$

$$\text{Net shunt} = (L \rightarrow R\ \text{shunt}) - (R \rightarrow L\ \text{shunt})$$

$$\text{Theoretical } O_2 \text{ capacity (m}10_2\text{/L)} = 1.36 \times \text{g Hgb/dL} \times 10$$

VO_2, Oxygen consumption (mL O_2/min/m^2). $C_{PV}O_2$, $C_{PA}O_2$, C_AO_2, and $C_{MV}O_2$ = O_2 content (mL O_2/L blood) of pulmonary veins, pulmonary arteries, systemic arteries, and mixed venous blood, respectively; $S_{PV}O_2$, $S_{PA}O_2$, S_AO_2, $S_{MV}O_2$, pulmonary venous, pulmonary arterial, systemic arterial, and mixed venous O_2 saturations (%), respectively; Q_P, pulmonary blood flow; Q_S, systemic blood flow; Q_{EP}, effective pulmonary blood flow. All blood flows are measured in liters of blood per minute.

The O_2 content of blood contains both dissolved O_2 and the O_2 combined with hemoglobin. While breathing room air the amount of dissolved O_2 is negligible and can be ignored. If the inspired O_2 concentration is increased, the dissolved O_2 may become significant and can be calculated as $PO_2 \times 0.003$.

In the clinical setting Q_P/Q_S is the primary means of determining the magnitude of a shunt. By comparing the complete formulae for Q_P and Q_S, it can be seen that the oxygen consumption and oxygen capacity cancel out, so that only oxygen saturations are needed to complete the calculation.

BOX 7-5

Oximetric shunt quantification (refer to Box 7-4 for formulae)

Schematic diagrams of a normal dog and the two examples are provided in Figure 7-8.

Example 1. A dog with a ventricular septal defect has the following oximetric values:

Systemic arterial saturation, 96%	Pulmonary venous saturation, 96%
Pulmonary arterial saturation, 86%	Mixed venous saturation, 76%
Hemoglobin, 14 g/dL	O_2 consumption = 95.2 mL $O_2/min/m^2$

$$Q_P = \frac{95.2}{(0.96 - 0.86)\,(14 \times 13.6)} = 5.0 \text{ L/min}$$

$$Q_S = \frac{95.2}{(0.96 - 0.76)\,(14 \times 13.6)} = 2.5 \text{ L/min}$$

$$Q_{EP} = \frac{95.2}{(0.96 - 0.76)\,(14 \times 13.6)} = 2.5 \text{ L/min}$$

Left-to-right shunt = 5.0 – 2.5 = 2.5 L/min

$$Q_P/Q_S = 5.0/2.5 = 2.0/1$$

Example 2. A dog with tetralogy of Fallot has the following oximetric data:

Systemic arterial saturation, 85%	Pulmonary venous saturation, 95%
Pulmonary arterial saturation, 75%	Mixed venous saturation, 75%
Hemoglobin, 14 g/dL	O_2 consumption = 95.2 mL $O_2/min/m^2$

$$Q_P = \frac{95.2}{(0.95 - 0.75)\,(14 \times 13.6)} = 2.5 \text{ L/min}$$

$$Q_S = \frac{95.2}{(0.95 - 0.75)\,(14 \times 13.6)} = 5.0 \text{ L/min}$$

$$Q_{EP} = \frac{95.2}{(0.95 - 0.75)\,(14 \times 13.6)} = 2.5 \text{ L/min}$$

Right-to-left shunt = 5.0 – 2.5 = 2.5 L/min

$$Q_P/Q_S = 2.5/5.0 = 0.5/1$$

Few laboratories still measure O_2 content. Instead, O_2 saturation is measured by reflectance oximetry (see above). Oxygen saturation is the amount of oxygen combined to hemoglobin divided by the oxygen capacity, as in the following equation:

$$O_2 \text{ saturation} = \frac{(O_2 \text{ content} - \text{dissolved } O_2) \times 100}{O_2 \text{ capacity}}$$

A significant atrial step-up in oxygen content is considered to be an increase in atrial O_2 content of 20 mL O_2/L or greater compared with the CaVC and CrVC. A significant step-up at the ventricular level is present if the highest right ventricular sample is equal to or greater than 10 mL O_2/L higher than the atrial sample. A significant step-up at the level of the pulmonary artery requires an O_2 content equal to or greater than 5 mL O_2/L higher than the right ventricular sample. Using averaged O_2 saturation, a significant step-up at the atrial level is a 7% increase, and a significant step-up at the ventricular or great vessel level is an increase of equal to or greater than 5%. One limitation to the use of oximetry to localize intracardiac shunts is its low degree of sensitivity. Small shunts are not easily detected because of the normal variability in O_2 saturation and content.

Oximetry is easy, provides immediate results, and can identify the site of the shunt. Usually, the location of a shunt is known before catheterization, so oximetry is more commonly used to quantitate the size of the shunt. However, the calculations can only be considered estimates of the true values. The other limitation is that the percent inspired oxygen must not be 100%, because this floods the system with oxygen. We either use room air to provide 21% FIO_2 or use nitrous oxide as part of the anesthetic protocol, with 3 parts nitrous oxide to 1 part oxygen to give an FIO_2 of 25%.

The saturations in the pulmonary artery, right ventricle, and systemic arteries are easily determined. Determining the oxygen saturation of mixed venous blood, on the other hand, is more difficult. The mixed venous blood is the sum of all blood leaving the systemic circulation that enters the heart (right atrium). In reality, complete mixing of venous return does not occur until the pulmonary artery. Thus the oxygen saturation of pulmonary arterial blood is often used as the mixed venous sample in patients without a left-to-right shunt. In the presence of a left-to-right shunt, the oxygen saturation of the venous blood in the chamber proximal to the shunt must be used. In the case of an atrial septal defect, various methods of averaging the oxygen saturations from the caudal and cranial vena cavae have been advocated. One commonly used method is (3 × CrVC O_2 content + CaVC O_2 content) ÷ 4. Another difficulty is obtaining blood samples from the left atrium and pulmonary veins. In the absence of a right-to-left shunt, systemic O_2 content may be substituted for pulmonary venous O_2 content. In the presence of a right-to-left shunt, pulmonary venous O_2 content is assumed to be 98% of oxygen carrying capacity.

Calculation of shunt flow itself equals the difference in blood crossing the pulmonary or systemic capillaries (Shunt = $Q_S - Q_P$). One can use Q_S and Q_P or use Q_{EP}. Using only Q_S and Q_P, a left-to-right shunt gives a positive number. With a right-to-left shunt the number is negative. In a patient with bidirectional shunting a more complicated formula must be used (see Box 7-4).

Alternatively, if just a systemic to pulmonary blood flow ratio is desired, the Q_P/Q_S ratio can easily be calculated using the following formula:

$$\dot{Q}_P/\dot{Q}_S = \frac{\dfrac{\dot{V}O_2}{(S_{PV}O_2 - S_{PA}O_2)(O_2 \text{ capacity})}}{\dfrac{\dot{V}O_2}{(S_AO_2 - S_{MV}O_2)(O_2 \text{ capacity})}} = \frac{S_AO_2 - S_{MV}O_2}{S_{PV}O_2 - S_{PA}O_2}$$

This calculation does not require the oxygen consumption to be known or oxygen capacity to be calculated because they cancel out of the equation. Therefore the ratio is more accurate, although absolute numbers are not available. For examples of the oximetry method for determining shunt severity see Box 7-5.

Angiography. If a contrast agent is introduced into a left-side chamber, its movement into a right-side chamber may be directly visualized in a left-to-right shunt. The converse is true with a right-to-left shunt. Because angiographic demonstration of abnormal cardiac anatomy has become a routine part of cardiac catheterization, the role of other methods for detecting intracardiac shunts have been largely superseded. The reliability of angiography depends on the exact location of the defect and the obliquity in which the angiogram is performed.

The technique is easy and the results are immediately available. It can detect and localize shunts at the ventricular and great vessel level. However, it cannot reliably localize shunting at the atrial level using standard projections. Angiography does not allow for quantification of the defect and cannot replace the important physiologic measurements that do allow shunt quantification (e.g., oximetry).

Right-to-left and bidirectional shunts

Oximetry. The concept is the same as that for left-to-right shunts, except a decrease in oxygen content, or saturation, is identified in left-side chambers. Blood samples should be obtained from accessible left-side chambers, the vena cavae, right ventricle, right atrium, and pulmonary artery. If a pulmonary venous sample is not obtainable, it is assumed to be 98% saturated. Specific criteria for a significant step-down have not been defined.

A left-side saturation of less than 95% is considered abnormal and may be the result of intracardiac shunting, diffusion abnormalities, V/Q mismatch, or hypoventilation. To determine the cause of the desaturation, the patient is allowed to breath 100% oxygen for 10 minutes and the sampling is repeated. If the cause of the desaturation is right-to-left shunting, it will not correct with oxygen inhalation.

The technique is easy and the results are immediately available. This technique also may allow the location to be determined, and the magnitude of the shunt may be estimated. The use of oximetry for the quantification of right-to-left shunts is limited by the absence of specific criteria, the technical difficulty of obtaining samples from the left atrium and pulmonary ventricles, the limited ability to detect small shunts, and the difficulty in differentiating intracardiac and intrapulmonary shunting. In human medicine, this technique is often combined with the indocyanine green dye technique for greater sensitivity.

Oximetry is the only technique available for accurate quantification of bidirectional shunting. It is most accurate when the arteriovenous oxygen saturation differences are wide and should only be used in patients with right-to-left shunts that result in arterial desaturation. Quantification of right-to-left shunts is identical to that discussed above with left-to-right shunts.

Endomyocardial Biopsy

Obtaining biopsies from the myocardium may be important in the initial diagnosis of a condition and for serial measurement of biochemical, structural, and ultrastructural abnormalities. Most myocardial biopsy techniques carry high morbidity and/or mortality and are not applicable for routine diagnostic use. On the other hand, the practicality, safety, and capability of using a biopsy catheter (bioptome) for the transvenous acquisition of myocardial samples is widely accepted.[24] Transvenous endomyocardial biopsy is an important component of the invasive evaluation of patients with known or suspected myocardial disease; however, its use in human medicine is controversial and varies from center to center and its use in veterinary medicine is limited by several factors.[24]

INDICATIONS

Most human patients who undergo cardiac biopsy are suspected of having myocardial disease, and the most frequent histologic abnormalities are consistent with idiopathic cardiomyopathy.[24] Endomyocardial biopsy may be helpful in the diagnosis of veterinary patients with myocardial dysfunction of unknown etiology. However, the lack of experienced pathologists and the lack of studies involving large numbers of dogs limit the clinical usefulness in this setting. Endomyocardial biopsy has also been used to document the presence of myocardial carnitine deficiency in a small number of dogs, but the relationship of myocardial carnitine deficiency to clinical myocardial disease is still controversial.[25] The serial monitoring of patients undergoing chemotherapy with doxorubicin to circumvent the development of doxorubicin-induced cardiomyopathy is another potential indication that is neither proven nor widely accepted in dogs.[26,27]

TECHNIQUE

Although right and left ventricular myocardial biopsy techniques have proved to be safe and easily performed in humans, right ventricular endomyocardial biopsy through the jugular vein is more widely used in dogs and cats.[26,28-30] The procedure may be performed via vascular cutdown under general anesthesia or patients may be awake or lightly sedated for percutaneous access.[26,29,30] Original reports described placing the dog in dorsal recumbency. However, a modified technique with the dog in lateral recumbency to minimize respiratory- and anesthetic-related complications is now more widely employed.[29]

Two types of bioptomes are in common use—the Stanford bioptome and disposable biopsy forceps.[29,30] The disposable forceps are used in conjunction with a long introducing sheath that extends across the tricuspid valve to protect the structures from the bioptome. The Stanford bioptome is modified by creating a 70-degree bend near the tip to facilitate taking the specimen from the interventricular septum. Under fluoroscopic control, the bioptome is guided through the cranial vena cava and into the right atrium in a fashion similar to intracardiac catheters. Once inside the atrium, the tip is rotated 90 degrees and the forceps are advanced across the tricuspid valve and into the right ventricular apex. The forceps are then rotated approximately 60 degrees counterclockwise to position the bioptome toward the right ventricular septum. The jaws are opened and the bioptome is gently advanced, pushing the jaws into the endocardial surface. The jaws are closed and the bioptome is immediately withdrawn with a gentle tug. The procedure is repeated as many times as necessary to obtain the required number of samples (usually 6 to 12 repititions are necessary).[29]

COMPLICATIONS

Complications in dogs are remarkably uncommon or minor in nature with the use of proper technique. Reported complications and complications we have encountered include cardiac tamponade, arrhythmias, and vascular damage at the access site.[26,29,30] Ventricular arrhythmias are common with isolated complexes, couplets, or brief runs of ventricular tachycardia occurring when the specimens are taken. Sustained rhythm disturbances requiring intervention are infrequent in dogs with healthy hearts but may be problematic in dogs with dilated cardiomyopathy and may warrant aborting the procedure.[29] Atrial fibrillation may also develop. However, it often resolves spontaneously shortly after completion of the procedure. Cardiac tamponade, which is more common in cats than in dogs, is the most severe complication and is presumably the result of ventricular rupture. Cardiac tamponade resulting from endomyocardial biopsy of the right ventricle requires immediate pericardiocentesis.[29] In our experience, further hemorrhage usually stops spontaneously within minutes of catheter placement within the pericardial sac.

Interventional Techniques

The use of interventional cardiac catheterization as a therapeutic modality has recently gained wide acceptance in human cardiovascular medicine.[31] Although most interventional techniques would find clinical application in veterinary medicine, the cost of the procedures, the need for specialized equipment, and the lack of clinical experience make the routine use of many of these procedures largely impractical.

Balloon valvuloplasty, or angioplasty, involves the dilation of stenotic valves or vessels with large-diameter balloon catheters introduced percutaneously or by way of vascular cutdown. Balloon valvuloplasty is widely employed for the treatment of canine congenital pulmonic stenosis (discussed in detail in Chapter 16) and also has been used in the therapy of tricuspid stenosis and cor triatriatum dexter in dogs.[9,32-35]

Percutaneous catheter occlusion of patent ductus arteriosus is currently undergoing evaluation as an alternative to thoracotomy and ductal ligation.[36,37] The technique potentially eliminates the need for thoracotomy, and the cost, postoperative discomfort, and postoperative recovery period are decreased. The major complications, beyond those inherent to cardiac catheterization, include migration of the occlusion device into the pulmonary circulation and incomplete occlusion of the ductus.[36] In spite of several studies involving animals and humans, the present occlusion devices still have shortcomings, including limited indications, large vascular sheaths, complicated delivery mechanisms, residual leaks, and device-related embolizations.[37] Improvement in occlusion devices is needed and may increase the number of defects that can be successfully treated without surgery when available.

Complications

With proper technique and precaution, serious complications during or after cardiac catheterization are relatively uncommon. Animals with more serious underlying conditions are, in general, at greater risk of complications than those with uncomplicated and asymptomatic disorders. As with any invasive procedure, there are inherent risks associated with general anesthesia, which also increase with increasing severity of the underlying condition (see above). Most complications encountered during catheterization are transient and minor. However, the potential for serious, even life-threatening, complications exists.

ARRHYTHMIAS

The most common transient complication is the development of arrhythmias. Most commonly, atrial or ventricular ectopic tachyarrhythmias develop as a result of irritation of the endocardium by the catheter tip. These consist of either single beats or short runs of tachycardia that subside when the catheter is repositioned. The right ventricular outflow tract appears to be specially sensitive to catheter irritation, and it is quite common to create arrhythmias when attempting to position a catheter across the pulmonic valve. Rarely, a catheter-induced ventricular arrhythmia may progress suddenly to ventricular fibrillation. Emergency drugs and a defibrillator should always be present and ready for immediate use.

Another electrocardiographic finding commonly associated with right heart catheterization is right bundle branch block. This conduction disturbance occurs most commonly during balloon valvuloplasty of the pulmonic valve. It is apparently caused by catheter-induced trauma to the right bundle branch as it courses from the interventricular septum to the right ventricular free wall in the moderator band. Although this may persist for several days, it is rarely a permanent or clinically important sequela.

INTRACARDIAC DAMAGE

Vigorous manipulation of the catheter may result in perforation of the heart or a large vessel, leading to severe hemorrhage or cardiac tamponade. The catheter should never be forced against excessive resistance. Preforming the catheter for the anticipated placement plus continued withdrawal and gentle rotation usually will allow uncomplicated passage beyond most obstacles. Occasionally, in small animals or in patients with severe anatomic obstructions, catheter positioning is impossible without threatening the well-being of the patient. In this situation, the procedure should be aborted.

Vigorous catheter manipulation may also lead to perforation or tearing of a cardiac valve. Care and finesse are required to gently cross the aortic valve without force. Furthermore, catheters specifically designed for retrograde passage across the aortic valve (i.e., Lehman ventriculography catheter) may facilitate left ventricular catheterization. The tricuspid valve is especially prone to damage during manipulation of balloon valvuloplasty catheters within the right ventricle.

MISCELLANEOUS COMPLICATIONS

Complications at the incision site may include hemorrhage or hematoma formation, infection, or seroma formation, which may require medical attention. Proper closure or ligation of vessels, proper control of dead space during closure, and appropriate postoperative bandaging (vascular cutdown) or the proper use of direct pressure (percutaneous access) should greatly minimize complications at the access site.

Occasional complications are associated with angiocardiography, most commonly, intramyocardial injection of contrast medium. This generally occurs when using an end-hole catheter and can be substantial if power injectors are used. Usually no severe clinical complications occur, but regional myocardial dysfunction or ectopic arrhythmias may ensue. Using a closed tip, side-hole catheter and checking the position of the catheter tip by a small test injection usually will prevent this complication.

Catheters are frequently reused in veterinary medicine because of financial limitations and therefore should be carefully inspected for cracks and splits, especially near the tip, before use. Use of defective catheters may lead to breakage during catheterization and foreign body embolization. Care must also be taken during catheter manipulation not to tangle the catheter onto itself, forming a knot, or around any cardiac structures (e.g., atrioventricular valve apparatus), because removal of the catheter may then require thoracotomy and open heart recovery.

Blood clots that may form at the catheter tip may be inadvertently flushed into the animal. This can be avoided by frequently flushing or slowly dripping heparinized saline through the catheter and by routinely aspirating blood back into the flushing syringe before flushing the catheter. Care must be taken not to overhydrate the animal with saline injections or contrast media, because acute congestive heart failure either during or following the procedure may be precipitated in patients with already severely compromised cardiac function.

Aftercare and Recovery

At the completion of planned studies, catheters are removed to avoid the danger of clot formation. Free bleeding should occur from both proximal and distal portions of the incised vessels (unless they were ligated). Unlike as is true of humans, there is little danger in ligating the jugular vein, carotid artery, femoral artery, or femoral vein in animals, because sufficient collateral vessels are present. In larger dogs, the vessel incisions may be carefully sutured with fine silk or similar suture. The skin incision is closed routinely, taking particular care to control dead space.

After recovery from anesthesia, previous medications can be resumed and the animal allowed sufficient water to compensate for the diuretic effect of any contrast medium used. The incision is given routine care. Unless obvious contamination occurred or permanent foreign objects were implanted during the procedure, postoperative antibiotic therapy is not routinely administered. Discharge from the hospital may be from several hours to several days postoperatively, depending on the animal's anesthetic recovery and the patient's clinical status.

REFERENCES

1. Ettinger SJ, Suter PF: Cardiac catheterization and angiocardiography. In Ettinger SJ, Sutter PF, eds: *Canine cardiology.* Philadelphia, 1970, WB Saunders.
2. Knight DH: Principles of cardiac catheterization. In Kirk RW, ed: *Current veterinary therapy,* ed 5, Philadelphia, 1974, WB Saunders.
3. Wood GL, Suter PF: Principles of cardiac catheterization. In Kirk RW, ed: *Current veterinary therapy,* ed 6, Philadelphia, 1977, WB Saunders.
4. Grossman W: Cardiac catheterization. In Braunwald E, ed: *Heart disease: a textbook of cardiovascular medicine,* ed 4, Philadelphia, 1992, WB Saunders.
5. Grossman W, Baim DS: *Cardiac catheterization: angiography and intervention,* ed 4, Philadelphia, 1991, Lea & Febiger.
6. Seldinger SI: Catheter replacement of the needle in percutaneous arteriography: a new technique, *Acta Radiol* 39:368, 1953.
7. Swan HJC, Ganz W, Forrester J et al: Catheterization of the heart in man with use of a flow directed balloon-tipped catheter, *N Engl J Med* 283:447, 1970.
8. Patterson DF: Genes and the heart: congenital heart disease, *Proc Acad Vet Cardiol* 1991, p 13.
9. Martin MWS, Godman M, Fuentes VL et al: Assessment of balloon pulmonary valvuloplasty in six dogs, *J Small Anim Pract* 33:443, 1992.
10. Bednarski RM: Anesthetic concerns for patients with cardiomyopathy, *Vet Clin North Am Small Anim Pract* 22:460, 1992.
11. Evans AT: Anesthesia for severe mitral and tricuspid regurgitation, *Vet Clin North Am Small Anim Pract* 22:465, 1992.
12. Haskins SC, Klide AM: Anesthesia for very old patients, *Vet Clin North Am Small Anim Pract* 22:467, 1992.
13. Wilson DV: Anesthesia for patients with severe systemic debilitation, *Vet Clin North Am Small Anim Pract* 22:491, 1992.
14. Henderson RA, Dillon AR, Brawner WR et al: Technique for percutaneous pulmonary arterial catheterization in conscious dogs, *Am J Vet Res* 46:1538, 1985.
15. Bellucci M, Battistacci M, Crivellini L: Radiography of the arterial system of the dog, using Seldinger's method, *Clinica Veterinaria* 101:74, 1978.
16. Baim DS, Grossman W: Percutaneous approach, including transseptal catheterization and apical left ventricular puncture. In Grossman W, Baim DS, eds: *Cardiac catheterization: angiography and intervention,* ed 4, Philadelphia, 1991, Lea & Febiger.
17. Yang SS, Bentivoglio LG, Maranhao V et al: Basic measurements and calculations. In Yang SS, Bentivoglio LG, Maranhao V, eds: *From cardiac catheterization data to hemodynamic parameters,* ed 2, Philadelphia, 1978, FA Davis.
18. Vargo TA: Cardiac catheterization: hemodynamic measurements. In Garson A Jr, Bricker JT, McNamara DG, eds: *The science and practice of pediatric cardiology,* Philadelphia, 1990, Lea & Febiger.
19. Gross DR: Normal cardiovascular parameters from intact, awake animals. In Gross DR, ed: *Animal models in cardiovascular research,* ed 2, Boston, 1994, Kluwer.
20. Grossman W: Pressure measurement. In Grossman W, Baim DS, eds: *Cardiac catheterization: angiography and intervention,* ed 4, Philadelphia, 1991, Lea & Febiger.
21. Grossman W: Blood flow measurement: the cardiac output. In Grossman W, Baim DS, eds: *Cardiac catheterization: angiography and intervention,* ed 4, Philadelphia, 1991, Lea & Febiger.
22. Boehrer JD, Lange RA, Willard JE et al: Advantages and limitations of methods to detect, localize, and quantitate intracardiac right-to-left and bidirectional shunting, *Am Heart J* 125:215, 1993.
23. Boehrer JD, Lange RA, Willard JE et al. Advantages and limitations of methods to detect, localize, and quantitate intracardiac left-to-right shunting, *Am Heart J* 124:448, 1992.
24. Levine MJ, Baim DS: Endomyocardial biopsy. In Grossman W, Baim DS, eds: *Cardiac catheterization: angiography and intervention,* ed 4, Philadelphia, 1991, Lea & Febiger.
25. Keene BW, Panciera DP, Atkins CE et al: Myocardial L-carnitine deficiency in a family of dogs with dilated cardiomyopathy, *J Am Vet Med Assoc* 198:647, 1991.
26. Burk RL, Tilley LP, Henderson M et al: Endomyocardial biopsy in the dog, *Vet Clin North Am Small Anim Pract* 13:355, 1983.
27. Henderson BM, Dougherty WJ, James VC: Safety assessment of a new anticancer compound, mitoxanthrone, in beagle dogs: comparison with doxorubicin. I. Clinical observations, *Cancer Treat Rep* 66:1139, 1982.
28. Burk RL, Tilley LP, Henderson BM et al: Endomyocardial biopsy in the dog, *Am J Vet Res* 41:2106, 1980.
29. Keene BW, Kittleson MD, Atkins CE et al: Modified transvenous endomyocardial biopsy technique in dogs, *Am J Vet Res* 51:1769, 1990.
30. Rush JE, Keene BW, Eicker SW: Endomyocardial biopsy in cats, *Am J Vet Res* 51:1765, 1990.
31. Allen HD, Drescill DJ, Fricker FJ: Guidelines for pediatric therapeutic cathererization, *Circulation* 84:2248, 1991.
32. Sisson DD, MacCoy DM: Treatment of congenital pulmonic stenosis in two dogs by balloon valvuloplasty, *J Vet Intern Med* 2:92, 1988.
33. Stern A, Fallon RK, Aronson E: Cor triatriatum dexter in a dog, *Compend Contin Educ Pract Vet* 8:411, 1986.
34. Miller MW, Bonagura JD, DiBartola SP et al: Budd-Chiari-like syndrome in two dogs, *J Am Anim Hosp Assoc* 25:277, 1989.
35. Brown WA, Thomas WP: Balloon valvuloplasty of tricuspid stenosis in a Labrador retriever, *J Vet Intern Med* 9:419, 1995.
36. Miller MW, Bonagura JD, Meurs KM et al: Percutaneous catheter occlusion of patent ductus arteriosus, *Proc ACVIM Forum,* 1995, p 308.
37. Grifka RG, Miller MW, Frischmeyer KJ et al: Transcatheter occlusion of a patent ductus arteriosus in a Newfoundland puppy using the Gianturco-Grifka vascular occlusion device, *J Vet Intern Med* 10:42, 1996.

CHAPTER 8

Classification of Heart Disease by Echocardiographic Determination of Functional Status

There are several ways to classify diseases of the cardiovascular system, including presence or absence of the disease at birth (e.g., congenital vs. acquired), duration (e.g., chronic vs. acute), anatomic malformation (e.g., septal defects), clinical status (e.g., left heart failure), and etiology (e.g., infections, inherited). Although these classification schemes are helpful from a standpoint of conferring with colleagues and describing population statistics and trends, they are not always the most beneficial way to approach an individual patient. Therapeutic strategies and prognosis should be outlined individually in each patient and tailored to the specific alterations of the cardiovascular system that are present, regardless of the terminology used to classify them.

As with any other disease system, the proper management of heart disease requires a rational and logical thought process and a thorough, systematic diagnostic strategy. The goal of a cardiovascular workup should be to (1) define the etiology (if possible), anatomy, and underlying pathophysiology of the disorder; (2) define the duration of the condition (acute vs. chronic); (3) define the clinical severity of the condition; (4) define the associated clinical syndrome(s) (e.g., congestive heart failure), if present; (5) predict the clinical course and prognosis of the disorder; and (6) recommend appropriate medical or surgical therapy. Often a true etiologic diagnosis (e.g., myocardial failure secondary to dietary taurine deficiency) cannot be made. More often, the result of a workup is the identification of a morphologic diagnosis (e.g., degenerative mitral valve disease) or a functional abnormality (see below). The fact that a true etiology cannot be defined should not be thought of as a failure; instead it should be considered a limitation of current medical technology and knowledge. Fortunately, specific and often effective therapy can be formulated based on either a functional classification or a morphologic diagnosis.

Functional Classification(s) of Heart Disease

The cardiovascular system responds in a limited number of ways to various insults imposed upon it. It is possible to define clinically important echocardiographic patterns that characterize different functional types of cardiac disease (Table 8-1). There are several well-recognized cardiovascular disorders for which a morphologic or descriptive diagnosis is based primarily on a functional abnormality. A skilled echocardiographer uses these functional alterations to guide the diagnostic ultrasound examination. First, the two-dimensional examination is performed, and note is made of any increases or decreases in chamber dimensions or wall thicknesses. Differential diagnoses for the identified abnormalities are then devised and each one ruled in or ruled out based on careful two-dimensional and Doppler examination. These patients are then treated according to established guidelines. There are many situations in which defining the abnormal anatomy and/or functional alterations is all that can be reliably accomplished. Although standard guidelines may not be established, therapy often can be tailored to manipulate these morphologic and functional alterations using detailed echocardiographic findings as a guide (see Chapter 6).

SYSTOLIC MYOCARDIAL FAILURE

Many types of functional abnormalities may lead to global ventricular dysfunction whereby the ability for the ventricle to maintain normal cardiac output is reduced. Myocardial failure strictly implies a generalized reduction in myocardial contractility. Other causes of reduced ventricular performance are classified elsewhere. Myocardial failure may be further subdivided into primary or secondary types. Primary myocardial failure is of unknown etiology and is otherwise known as *dilated cardiomyopathy* (see Chapter 20). Many causes of secondary myocardial failure have been identified (see Table 8-1). Diminished ventricular contractility (myocardial failure) results in an increase in end-systolic diameter and end-systolic volume. It usually results in a compensatory increase in end-diastolic diameter and end-diastolic volume (volume overload or eccentric hypertrophy). The percentage change in volume (the ejection fraction) or the lateral dimension (the shortening fraction) is decreased, with the appearance of decreased contractions (wall motion) and diminished atrioventricular valve motion. The ventricular enlargement may produce the visual impression of thinning of the ventricular walls, but the wall thicknesses are often normal or only mildly decreased in thickness (eccentric hypertrophy). Treatment strategies for patients with myocardial failure generally include inotropic support of the failing ventricle and management of the associated clinical syndrome (usually congestive heart failure) with diuretics and angiotensin-converting enzyme inhibitors.

TABLE 8-1

Common cardiovascular disorders classified by functional alteration

Functional classification	*Morphologic classification*	*Examples*
Primary systolic myocardial failure		Dilated cardiomyopathy
Secondary systolic myocardial failure	Infectious myocarditis	Bacterial, fungal, viral, protozoal
	Drugs, chemicals, toxins	Doxorubicin (Adriamycin), alcohol
	Physical damage	Heat stroke, electric shock, trauma
	Nutritional	Taurine deficiency
	Ischemic	Atherosclerosis
	Infiltrative	Neoplasia, metabolic (amyloid)
	Other cardiac disorders	Valvular insufficiency, shunts
Pressure overload	Hypertension	Systemic or pulmonary hypertension
	Anatomic outflow obstruction	Aortic stenosis, pulmonic stenosis
	Dynamic outflow obstruction	Hypertrophic obstructive cardiomyopathy
Primary volume outflow	Valvular insufficiency	Mitral insufficiency
	Left-to-right shunt	Patent ductus arteriosus, ventricular septal defect
	High-output states	Hyperthyroidism, atrioventricular fistula, anemia
Impedance to cardiac inflow	Pericardial disease	Pericardial effusion, constrictive pericarditis
	Diastolic dysfunction	Hypertrophic and restrictive cardiomyopathy
	Atrioventricular valvular obstruction	Mitral and tricuspid stenosis
	Space-occupying lesions	Atrial mass lesions, right ventricular outflow tract tumors, Budd-Chiari syndrome

EXCESS VENTRICULAR WORKLOAD

Pressure overload. A pressure overload is imposed when there is a chronic increase in systolic wall stress because of an increase in systolic pressure within the affected ventricle (see Chapter 2). Pressure overloads are the result of either stenotic lesions (e.g., subaortic stenosis and pulmonic stenosis) or increases in vascular resistance or flow causing an increase in arterial pressure (e.g., systemic arterial hypertension and pulmonary arterial hypertension). The typical response to a pressure overload is a secondary increase in wall thickness (concentric hypertrophy) of the affected chamber in an attempt to return wall stress to normal. The exception to this general rule is the response of the adult right ventricle to acquired pressure overload, which usually includes both increased chamber size and increased wall thickness (see Chapter 26). The only other thing that causes concentric hypertrophy is hypertrophic cardiomyopathy. Hypertrophic cardiomyopathy is a form of primary concentric hypertrophy and is almost always a disease confined to the left ventricle. When a pressure overload is moderate to severe, the increase in wall thickness is readily apparent on an echocardiogram.

Once a pressure overload is identified by seeing the increase in wall thickness on an echocardiogram, the first thing to do is determine whether or not a stenotic lesion is present. Stenotic lesions almost always produce a heart murmur. Consequently, if a heart murmur is not present, it is unlikely that a stenotic lesion is causing the concentric hypertrophy. Stenotic lesions can also be ruled out by measuring the velocity of the blood flow across the appropriate valve (e.g., the pulmonic valve region in a dog with right ventricular concentric hypertrophy). If right ventricular concentric hypertrophy is present and a stenotic lesion has been ruled-out, pulmonary hypertension is invariably present. This can be confirmed by measuring the velocity of a tricuspid or pulmonic regurgitant jet, using the modified Bernoulli equation to calculate the pressure gradient across the valve and estimating the right ventricular systolic pressure or pulmonary artery pressure (see Chapter 6). If a stenotic lesion and hypertension are not present and left ventricular concentric hypertrophy is present, hypertrophic cardiomyopathy is the usual diagnosis.

Treatment of a pressure overload is generally aimed at reducing the systolic wall stress. In most situations this involves the physical removal of an obstruction to blood flow (in the case of a stenotic lesion) or the use of medications to decrease vascular resistance (in the case of hypertension).

Volume overload. A primary volume overload is characterized by an increase in left ventricular chamber volume or diameter with a relatively normal wall thickness (eccentric hypertrophy) that is the result of a regurgitant or shunting lesion. Volume overload or eccentric hypertrophy occurs whenever it is advantageous for the ventricle to increase the total stroke volume of the ventricle for any given amount of contraction. Volume overload or eccentric hypertrophy occurs secondary to myocardial failure to compensate for reduced contraction. Primary volume overloads commonly occur secondary to lesions that produce blood flow leaks in the cardiovascular system, such as valvular insufficiencies (e.g., mitral, tricuspid, or aortic regurgitation) or cardiovascular shunts (e.g., patent ductus arteriosus, ventricular septal defect, and arteriovenous fistula). The initial insult is usually a leak that results in an increase in venous return to a ventricle, resulting in an increase in ventricular end-diastolic volume and pressure. For example, with a patent ductus arteriosus, blood shunts from the aorta to the pulmonary artery. The blood flows through the pulmonary vasculature to the left atrium and left ventricle. The left ventricle grows larger (i.e., eccentric hypertrophy occurs) to accommodate the increased flow of blood into it in diastole and to pump a larger stroke volume in systole to compensate for the leak. The increase in chamber size and volume is advantageous because the larger heart is able to eject more blood for any given amount of contraction and is also able to normalize or near normalize end-diastolic pressure despite the often marked increase in diastolic volume. In some cases, systolic function is maintained, with normal or near normal end-systolic ventricular volume and dimension. The result is the appearance of hyperdynamic or hyperkinetic left ventricular motion, with an increased shortening fraction (exaggerated wall motion) during systole. In others, myocardial failure results, causing an increase in end-systolic volume and diameter. This often brings the shortening fraction back down to within the normal range. Treatment is directed at reducing diastolic volume and pressure, either by the use of diuretic agents and vasodilators or by reducing the amount of blood that flows through the leak by the use of arteriolar dilators or surgical closure.

IMPEDANCE TO CARDIAC INFLOW (DECREASED PRELOAD)

In this group of disorders caused by impedance to cardiac outflow, acute or chronic reductions in ventricular filling lead to acute or chronic reductions in ventricular volume that may lead to a decrease in cardiac output. This may be caused by external compression or constriction of the heart (e.g., as with a pericardial effusion) or an anatomic obstruction to ventricular filling (e.g., as with mitral stenosis and cor triatriatum). In an obstructive lesion, the diastolic pressure proximal to the obstruction is elevated and may lead to signs of congestion and edema (i.e., heart failure). On an echocardiogram, the motion of the affected valve is reduced in the case of atrioventricular valve stenosis and the ventricular chamber may be decreased in size (i.e., the end-diastolic diameter is reduced). In cor triatriatum dexter, a skilled echocardiographer can identify the obstructing lesion in the right atrium. Ventricular diastolic pressures are increased with external compression, also leading to heart failure, usually right heart failure. Echocardiography can readily identify pericardial effusion if it is present. With constrictive pericarditis, right heart failure is present but the heart appears normal, making the diagnosis difficult. Diastolic ventricular dysfunction, usually a result of reduced ventricular compliance, may also lead to increased diastolic pressures caused by impaired ventricular filling. This occurs with severe hypertrophy, as in hypertrophic cardiomyopathy, or with myocardial or endocardial fibrosis, as in restrictive cardiomyopathy.

Treatment of obstructive lesions is generally directed at normalizing ventricular filling by alleviating the underlying condition and is most often surgical or interventional (e.g., balloon valvuloplasty) in nature. Pericardial lesions resulting in compression or constriction require either pericardiocentesis to relieve the compression or surgery to relieve the constriction (see Chapter 25). In cases of diastolic dysfunction or in situations in which the obstruction is not physically correctable, medical therapy of the associated clinical syndrome (i.e., congestive heart failure) may be beneficial. Medical therapy is sometimes effective at improving myocardial relaxation (e.g., diltiazem in hypertrophic cardiomyopathy).

ATRIAL ENLARGEMENT

Unlike the ventricles, the atrial chambers increase in size (i.e., grow to a larger chamber size) in response to both volume and pressure overloads. Consequently, when an enlarged atrium is identified on an echocardiogram, one cannot differentiate a pure increase in atrial pressure from a pure increase in atrial volume from a combination of the two. To make this differentiation one usually must identify the primary abnormality that is causing the increase in atrial pressure or volume. For example, when an enlarged left atrium is identified in a cat, the left ventricle and mitral valve must be examined carefully. If the left ventricular walls are markedly increased in thickness, hypertrophic cardiomyopathy is most likely causing severe left ventricular diastolic dysfunction with resultant increases in left ventricular diastolic and left atrial pressures. If the left ventricular chamber is increased in size, wall motion is normal or hyperdynamic, and the mitral valve leaflets are thickened, then mitral regurgitation is most likely causing a left atrial volume overload. This can usually be confirmed using color flow Doppler. One general statement can be made regarding left atrial size in relationship to left ventricular size when differentiating atrial pressure from volume overload. That is that the atria in volume overloads due to atrioventricular valve regurgitation are generally larger than the corresponding ventricle when the regurgitation is severe. This general rule can be used to make a preliminary differentiation when identification of the primary abnormality is in doubt. For example, in a dog with an enlarged left ventricle and a normal–to–mildly reduced shortening fraction, the left atrium is often but not always larger than the left ventricle in a dog that has primary mitral regurgitation and secondary myocardial failure. In a dog with primary myocardial failure (i.e., dilated cardiomyopathy) and secondary mitral regurgitation, the left atrium is almost always similar in size to the left ventricle.

VENTRICULAR WALL MOTION

The motion of ventricular walls on echocardiography can also be used to make a preliminary judgment as to the type of functional alteration. Although reduced wall motion can occur secondary to myocardial failure, an acute increase in afterload, or decreased preload, the vast majority of the time it is due to myocardial failure in clinical cases. The reduced wall motion in this situation is always due to an increase in end-systolic diameter. Occasionally, a marked reduction in preload, most commonly because of severe dehydration or hypovolemia, will result in a decrease in end-diastolic diameter without a compensatory decrease in end-systolic diameter. This also results in decreased wall motion. Compensation for chronic increases in afterload, in the form of concentric hypertrophy, almost always brings wall motion back to normal.

Increased wall motion occurs most commonly either because the end-diastolic diameter is increased and the end-systolic diameter is normal to mildly increased or because end-diastolic diameter is normal and end-systolic diameter is decreased. The former occurs in primary volume overloads, as described above. The latter occurs in response to inotropic stimulation. Clinically, the former is most commonly identified in patients with shunts such as patent ductus arteriosus and ventricular septal defect or in patients with valvular regurgitation such as mitral and aortic regurgitation. The latter can be seen during the administration of a positive inotropic agent such as dobutamine but is most commonly seen clinically in dogs with mild mitral regurgitation in which endogenous catecholamine stimulation is apparently present.

Occasionally, regional changes in wall motion are observed. This is most commonly seen in large dogs with severe mitral regurgitation. In these dogs, the left ventricular free wall motion is commonly reduced, and the motion of the interventricular septum is often increased. Wall motion is sometimes heterogeneous in dogs with dilated cardiomyopathy. Rarely, myocardial infarction produces regions of hypokinesis (i.e., reduced wall motion), akinesis (i.e., no wall motion), or dyskinesis (i.e., systolic bulging of the wall). Absolute akinesis and dyskinesis are rare in abnormalities other than myocardial infarction.

CHAPTER 9

Pathophysiology of Heart Failure

Definitions of Heart Disease and Heart Failure

Heart *disease* is any abnormality of the heart, encompassing everything from valvular regurgitation to a persistent left cranial vena cava. Heart *failure* is the end result of severe heart disease and is a clinical syndrome seen as congestion and edema, poor peripheral perfusion, and/or systemic hypotension. Heart disease is always present when heart failure is present. However, heart disease can be present and never lead to heart failure.

The cardiovascular system is responsible for maintaining normal systemic arterial blood pressure, normal perfusion (blood flow to tissues), and normal venous and capillary pressures. Heart failure occurs when heart disease becomes so severe that the cardiovascular system can no longer maintain one or more of these normal functions. To make the diagnosis of heart failure, one must document the presence of moderate-to-severe (usually severe) heart disease accompanied by increased capillary or venous pressures, low cardiac output, and/or low blood pressure.

Heart failure is commonly defined as an abnormality of cardiac function that results in the failure of the heart to pump blood at a rate commensurate with the requirements of metabolizing tissues.[1] It has also been defined as the inability of the heart to pump sufficient blood to meet the metabolic needs of the body at normal filling pressures, provided the venous return to the heart is normal.[2] These are incomplete definitions in that they only describe the situation in which systolic dysfunction results in signs of heart failure. They also only describe the inability of the heart to pump blood in a forward direction, into the aorta (commonly termed *a decrease in cardiac output* or *forward heart failure*). These definitions ignore diseases such as hypertrophic cardiomyopathy in cats, in which cardiac output may never be decreased and a thickened and stiff left ventricle causes diastolic dysfunction that results in congestion and edema. This problem with definitions has occurred because it is unusual for human patients with heart failure to have only diastolic dysfunction creating heart failure, although this type of abnormality alone or in combination with systolic dysfunction is becoming more frequently recognized.[3-6]

For this discussion we will define heart failure as a clinical syndrome caused by a heart disease that results in systolic and/or diastolic cardiac dysfunction severe enough to overwhelm the cardiovascular system's compensatory mechanisms. This produces clinical signs referable to congestion/edema (pulmonary edema, ascites, pleural effusion, etc.) and/or decreased peripheral perfusion (low cardiac output) either at rest or with exercise. Therefore some abnormality in heart function must cause heart failure (as opposed to, for example, the decrease in cardiac output observed in hypovolemic shock) and for practical purposes should result in clinical signs recognizable to an owner or veterinarian. Subtle changes in cardiac function can be detected by more sophisticated means, such as cardiac catheterization and cardiac ultrasound, but unless clinical signs result they should be characterized as a type of disease or dysfunction (e.g., myocardial failure when myocardial contractility is decreased) rather than heart failure.

It should be noted that many other circulatory abnormalities can cause congestion/edema and decreased perfusion. Hypovolemia from dehydration or hemorrhage commonly causes a low cardiac output. Such diverse abnormalities as decreased plasma oncotic pressure and altered capillary endothelium commonly cause edema. Appropriate diagnostic testing must distinguish heart failure from these other types of circulatory failure.

For this discussion, abnormalities in cardiac function are limited to those abnormalities that affect the left heart. Because of the shape of the right heart, its function is difficult to study, and the pathophysiology of right heart disease is more difficult to explain. For the most part, however, we can assume that the pathophysiology of a certain type of disease of the right heart will be similar to the pathophysiology of a similar disease of the left heart (e.g., the pathophysiology of tricuspid regurgitation will be similar to the pathophysiology of mitral regurgitation).

Causes of Heart Failure

Heart failure is the end-result of many different cardiac and pericardial diseases. It can result from several distinct and very different abnormalities of cardiac function. These include but are not limited to myocardial failure (decreased myocardial contractility [weak heart muscle], a type of systolic dysfunction), valvular regurgitation (a leak in a valve and a type of systolic dysfunction), and increased myocardial stiffness (a form of diastolic dysfunction).[2]

MYOCARDIAL FAILURE

Myocardial failure is the classic type of cardiac dysfunction that clinicians usually think of when they think of heart failure. It can lead to signs of heart failure or can be present without signs of heart failure. Dogs with dilated cardiomyopathy apparently have myocardial failure for years before showing clinical evidence of heart failure.[7] We have watched experimental cats live for years with taurine deficiency and mild-to-moderate myocardial failure without signs of heart failure.[8] Myocardial failure without heart failure can be detected by echocardiogram and is seen as an increase in end-systolic left ventricular diameter and decreased excursions of the left ventricular free wall and interventricular septum from diastole to systole (decreased wall motion). Myocardial failure is always severe in dogs and cats with dilated cardiomyopathy at the time clinical signs become obvious. Myocardial failure can occur secondary to other chronic diseases that affect the left ventricle, such as aortic regurgitation or patent ductus arteriosus. It is usually less severe in these instances when heart failure becomes evident.

OTHER CAUSES OF HEART FAILURE

Myocardial failure is frequently not present in other left ventricular diseases, although the patient has clinical signs of heart failure. Feline hypertrophic cardiomyopathy is the classic example in veterinary medicine. Cats with this disease can have heart failure but apparently have normal myocardial contractility and enhanced left ventricular performance because of an increase in myocardial mass. Signs of heart failure occur in this disease because the heart muscle is extremely thick and therefore stiff, causing an increase in the left ventricular diastolic pressure. Small dogs with mitral regurgitation are another example of a disease in which myocardial failure is not the prevalent problem.[9] In this disease the major factor leading to the signs of heart failure is massive regurgitation (leakage) of blood into the left atrium rather than a decrease in myocardial contractility. Patent ductus arteriosus does not result in clinically significant myocardial failure in very young dogs but can cause signs of heart failure. Myocardial failure develops if the lesion is left untreated for months to years. The pathophysiology of each of these diseases is discussed in the appropriate chapter. This chapter, however, compares the pathophysiology of heart failure secondary to severe myocardial failure as a result of dilated cardiomyopathy with heart failure secondary to a shunting lesion (patent ductus arteriosus).

Signs of Heart Failure

Signs of heart failure are divided into those referable to congestion and edema (congestive, or backward, heart failure), to inadequate blood flow (low output, or forward, heart failure), or to markedly decreased blood flow and low blood pressure (cardiogenic shock).[2,10] Cardiogenic shock is rare in patients with chronic heart failure, although it can occur in patients treated vigorously with diuretics that stop eating and drinking and become markedly dehydrated. Cardiogenic shock is more commonly identified in patients with acute heart failure.

CONGESTIVE LEFT HEART FAILURE

Congestion and edema in heart failure occur because of an increase in capillary hydrostatic pressure.[2] In left heart failure, increased diastolic pressure in the left ventricle (and consequently an increase in diastolic left atrial pressure, because the left ventricle and the left atrium are essentially one chamber during diastole when the mitral valve is open) and/or high systolic and diastolic pressures in the left atrium and pulmonary veins result in increased pulmonary capillary hydrostatic pressure, leading to pulmonary edema (Figures 9-1 through 9-4 and Color Plate 34). In other words, the high diastolic pressures in the left ventricle and/or left atrium "back up" into the pulmonary veins and capillaries, causing transudation of fluid from the capillaries into the pulmonary interstitium and alveoli (pulmonary edema). Increased left ventricular diastolic pressure is generally caused either by a marked increase in blood volume and venous return to the left heart that overwhelms the ability of the heart to distend or by a stiff left ventricle that cannot accept a normal venous return at a normal pressure or by both. Signs of congestive left heart failure are tachypnea, orthopnea, dyspnea, and coughing, usually secondary to pulmonary edema.

When capillary hydrostatic pressure is increased, fluid leaks from the capillaries according to Starling's law of edema formation, or ultrafiltration.[11] This law states that fluid movement across a membrane results from hydrostatic and osmotic pressure differences across that membrane and is dependent on the characteristics of the membrane. The formula for this law is as follows:

$$FM = K(P_c + \pi_i - P_i - \pi_c)$$

where *FM* is fluid motion, *K* is filtration coefficient, P_c is capillary hydrostatic pressure, π_i is colloid osmotic pressure of the interstitial

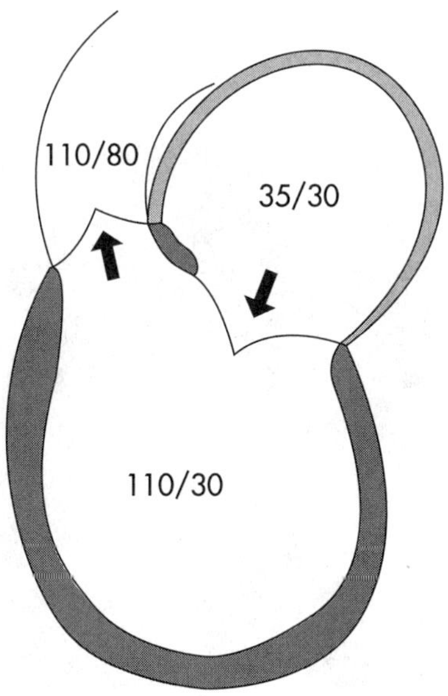

FIGURE 9-1 Schematic drawing of a failing left heart. The left ventricular end-diastolic pressure (LVEDP) is increased to 30 mm Hg. The increase in the LVEDP results in an increase in the left atrial pressure that "backs-up" into the pulmonary veins and capillaries to produce pulmonary edema.

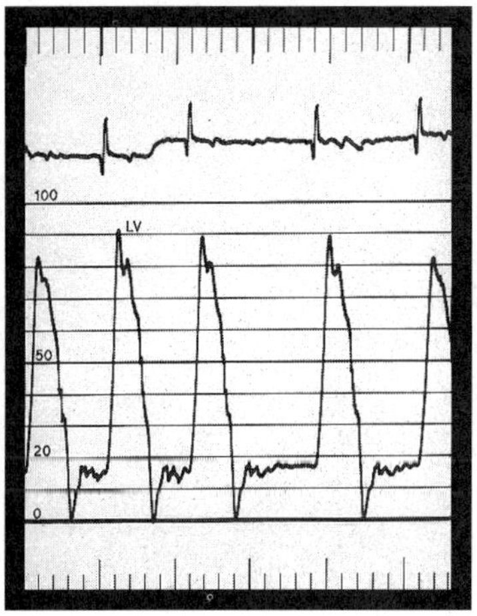

FIGURE 9-2 Left ventricular (LV) pressure tracing from a dog with mild left heart failure secondary to mitral valve dysplasia. The left ventricular end-diastolic pressure (immediately before the left ventricular systolic pressure upstroke) is increased to approximately 18 mm Hg.

fluid, P_i is interstitial hydrostatic pressure, and π_c is colloid osmotic pressure in the capillary. The filtration coefficient varies between capillary beds with the coefficient in glomerular capillaries much higher than in skeletal muscle capillaries. This coefficient is apparently less in hepatic sinusoids than in pulmonary capillaries because ascites forms at a lower pressure than does pulmonary edema. The capillary hydrostatic pressure is approximately the same as the venous pressure. It is relatively high compared with interstitial hydrostatic pressure, ranging from zero to 12 mm Hg, depending on the capillary bed. Capillary hydrostatic pressure forces fluid across the capillary membranes into the interstitium. The interstitial hydrostatic pressure is probably near zero in normal conditions but may increase substantially when edema is present. The colloid osmotic pressure of the plasma is primarily determined by plasma albumin concentration, which draws fluid into the vascular space. Plasma albumin concentration is high in the blood compartment (2.5 to 3.5 g/dL). Colloid osmotic pressure in the interstitial space is low. The net result is that hydrostatic pressure forces fluid out of the vascular space into the interstitium while colloid osmotic pressure draws fluid into the vascular space. The net motion of fluid is out of the vascular space into the interstitium. The lymphatics function to clear this fluid and route it back into the vascular space. The lymphatics have a flow reserve such that at mild elevations of capillary hydrostatic pressure, edema fluid does not accumulate. For example, the upper limit for normal pulmonary capillary pressure is 12 mm Hg. Yet patients with pulmonary capillary pressures in the 15- to 20-mm Hg range may not accumulate pulmonary edema fluid because the lymphatics can increase flow and "drain" the excess fluid back to the vascular space.

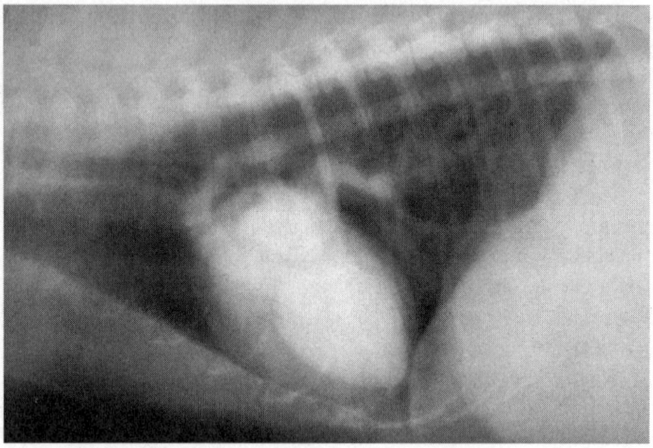

FIGURE 9-3 Lateral thoracic radiograph taken after the injection of a contrast agent into a jugular vein of a cat with left heart failure as a result of dilated cardiomyopathy. The contrast agent has passed through the right heart and pulmonary arterial circulation and is now in the pulmonary veins and the left heart. The pulmonary veins are distended and tortuous because of the increase in pulmonary vein pressure (pulmonary venous hypertension). The left atrial and left ventricular chambers are enlarged.

In humans, increased pulmonary vein pressure (left heart failure) can also cause pleural effusion, probably because the visceral pleural veins drain into the pulmonary veins.[12,13] Visceral pleural veins (the veins on the surface of the lung) also drain into the pulmonary veins in cats and dogs.[14] In fact, this has been known since 1907.[15] Consequently, it is logical that increased pulmonary vein pressure as a result of left heart failure can lead to the formation of pleural effusion. Cats appear to develop pleural effusion with left heart failure much more readily than dogs, based on our clinical experience. Parietal pleural veins drain into the systemic venous circuit, so right heart failure may also cause pleural effusion. A combination of left heart failure and right heart failure is the most efficient means of producing pleural effusion.

CONGESTIVE RIGHT HEART FAILURE

In congestive right heart failure, increased right ventricular diastolic pressure and/or increased right atrial, systemic venous, and systemic capillary pressures cause ascites, pleural effusion, and/or peripheral edema, depending on the species (Figure 9-5).[13] Ascites occurs when the hepatic sinusoidal pressure is increased, resulting in fluid weeping from the capsular surface of the liver into the peritoneal space. Jugular vein distension may or may not be present (see Color Plate 27).

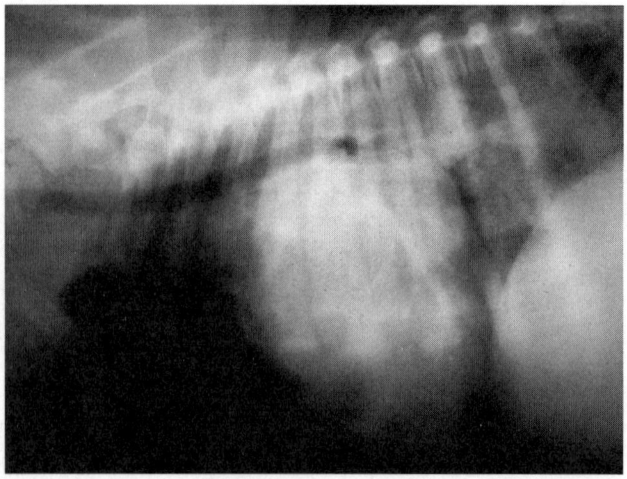

FIGURE 9-4 Lateral radiograph taken from a 6-month-old great Dane with dilated cardiomyopathy and left heart failure. There is a heavy interstitial/alveolar lung pattern in the caudodorsal lung fields that is caused by pulmonary edema.

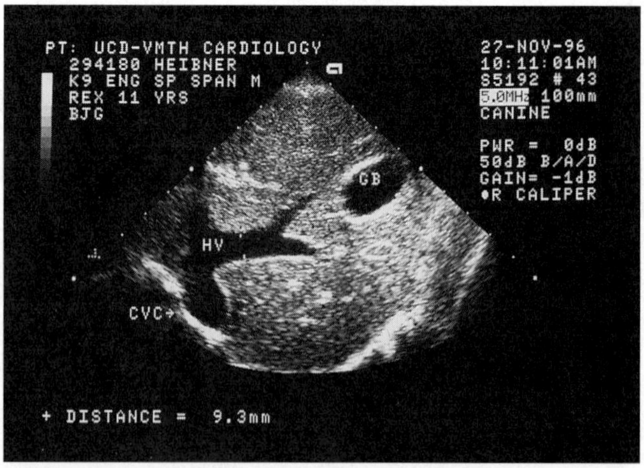

FIGURE 9-5 Ultrasound examination of the liver from an 11-year-old English springer spaniel with tricuspid and mitral regurgitation and ascites. The hepatic veins *(HV)* and caudal vena cava *(CVC)* are distended. The dog's mean right atrial (central venous) pressure was 14 mm Hg. *GB*, Gallbladder.

Identification of distended hepatic veins using ultrasound is a more sensitive means of identifying elevated right heart diastolic pressures. Measuring right atrial pressure from a jugular catheter is the definitive means of identifying congestive right heart failure.

LOW-OUTPUT, OR FORWARD, HEART FAILURE

A poor cardiac output (blood flow into the aorta per unit time) results in poor tissue perfusion and can be caused by a myriad of abnormalities that affect the ability of the ventricle to pump properly. Examples of these abnormalities are presented later in this discussion. Poor tissue perfusion caused by a decreased cardiac output causes clinical signs of fatigue, weakness, poor exercise tolerance, cold extremities, slow capillary refill time, poor mucous membrane color, and hypothermia.[2] All of the signs except exercise tolerance will not become evident until forward heart failure becomes severe. Laboratory evidence of forward failure consists of a decreased cardiac output, a widened arteriovenous oxygen difference (arterial – venous oxygen content), a decreased venous oxygen tension in a patient that is not hypoxemic or anemic, and azotemia and lactic acidosis if the cardiac output is severely depressed.[10] Decreased cardiac output results in decreased tissue oxygen delivery (tissue oxygen delivery = arterial oxygen content × cardiac output). Arterial oxygen content (mL O_2/100 mL blood) is [Hgb](g/100 mL of blood) × O_2 saturation (%) × 1.34 (mL O_2/g Hgb). This indicates the number of milliliters of oxygen carried in a given quantity of blood. At rest, if resting tissue oxygen consumption remains stable, the actively metabolizing cells in the body must extract more oxygen from the bloodstream to meet their needs for oxygen when cardiac output is reduced, as seen in Chapter 2, Figure 2-24. This results in a decreased amount of oxygen and partial pressure of oxygen at the end of a capillary bed and on the venous side. The oxygen tension at the end of the capillary bed is the critical factor that determines oxygen delivery to the mitochondria.[16] In animals the normal value for end-capillary or venous oxygen tension is greater than 30 mm Hg.[16] If oxygen delivery decreases enough at rest because of a decreased cardiac output, this can result in the end-capillary or venous oxygen tension decreasing below a critical level of 20 to 24 mm Hg. When end-capillary Po_2 is less than 20 to 24 mm Hg, oxygen delivery to mitochondria becomes inadequate. At this stage, cells must start relying on anaerobic metabolism, resulting in lactic acid production.[10,16,17] If the patient is exercising, lactic acid production in skeletal muscle results in the feeling of fatigue and forces the patient to stop exercising. Therefore signs of forward heart failure are best identified in a patient that has mild or moderate heart failure either by exercising the patient and measuring blood lactate concentration or venous oxygen tension from blood draining working skeletal muscle or by obtaining a history of the patient's exercise capabilities.[18] Patients with severe heart failure may have evidence of forward heart failure at rest.

ORDER OF PRESENTATION

As a rule, patients with chronic heart failure exhibit signs of congestion and edema before signs of low cardiac output. Signs of low cardiac output are generally only seen together with signs of edema.[19] Systemic arterial blood pressure is usually maintained within normal range or only mildly decreased even in severe chronic heart failure. As an example, in a study of dogs with chronic heart failure as a result of mitral regurgitation, mean aortic blood pressure was normal (104 mm Hg), cardiac index (cardiac output/body surface area) was moderately reduced (2.92 L/min/m^2), and mean pulmonary capillary pressure was severely increased (40 mm Hg).[20] This occurs because of the cardiovascular system's prioritization of its functions.[19]

Functions of the Cardiovascular System

As stated previously, the cardiovascular system performs the following three basic functions: (1) maintains normal systemic arterial pressure, (2) maintains normal tissue blood flow, and (3) maintains normal systemic and pulmonary capillary pressures.[19] Elaborate control mechanisms are present throughout the body to maintain these functions within normal limits. When the heart fails, however, all functions cannot be maintained. During evolution, the cardiovascular system was given a choice in chronic heart failure—either to allow each function to deteriorate at a rate similar to the rate of deterioration of the other functions or to allow one or two functions to deteriorate more rapidly so that the second or third could be maintained. Clinical and experimental evidence, as referred to above, proves that the latter occurs in chronic heart failure. Certainly, the high-pressure baroreceptors responsible for maintaining normal systemic arterial blood pressure predominate over the low-pressure atrial receptors responsible for maintaining normal venous pressures in mammals.[21-24]

PRIORITY OF FUNCTIONS

First and second priorities: systemic blood pressure and blood flow. In our view, the cardiovascular system, when the heart is chronically failing, works within a framework of priorities. Because chronic heart failure is much more common in veterinary medicine, this discussion is limited to chronic heart failure. Maintaining systemic arterial blood pressure is the cardiovascular system's first priority, and it will maintain blood pressure even at the expense of the other functions. As an example, if myocardial contractility is decreased suddenly (e.g., a large section of myocardium is infarcted, resulting in a decrease in stroke volume), cardiac output (stroke volume × heart rate) will decrease. Because of the decrease in the amount of blood pumped into the arterial system, the systemic arterial pressure also decreases, as long as arteriolar tone and therefore peripheral vascular resistance stay the same (blood flow × peripheral vascular resistance = arterial pressure). The cardiovascular system must make a choice at this time whether to increase blood pressure by increasing arteriolar tone and therefore the resistance to blood flow or to decrease arteriolar tone, reduce resistance to blood flow, and consequently increase cardiac output (blood flow). It chooses to increase blood pressure, although this results in cardiac output decreasing further. This prioritization of pressure over flow persists in chronic heart failure. In most patients with chronic severe heart failure that we have studied, systemic arterial blood pressure has been normal or only mildly decreased, whereas cardiac output has been decreased.[20,25]

Second and third priorities: blood flow and capillary pressure. The cardiovascular system's second priority is to maintain a normal cardiac output, and its third and last priority is to maintain normal capillary pressures. As an example, a dog with chronic mitral regurgitation and mild heart failure suffers a ruptured chorda tendineae. This results in an increase in blood flow into the left atrium and consequently an increase in left atrial pressure and a decrease in forward blood flow into the aorta (cardiac output). The cardiovascular system must choose between retaining sodium and water to increase end-diastolic volume to increase cardiac output back toward normal or to decrease sodium and water retention to decrease the left atrial pressure and consequently reduce pulmonary edema. The body always chooses to chronically increase renal sodium and water retention to increase cardiac output at the expense of increasing the left atrial pressure.

Order of clinical presentations. Because of this system of priorities, animals with chronic heart failure usually present first with signs referable to congestion and edema because the cardiovascular system chooses to allow venous pressures to rise in an attempt to maintain pressure and flow. Later these animals have signs referable to poor tissue perfusion. Patients that present with severe chronic heart failure may have signs of both; however, it is unusual to see a patient that has not been treated that has just signs of forward heart failure at rest.

Because of this system of priorities, the body continues to try to increase cardiac output by retaining sodium and water as long as the cardiac output is decreased, although this fluid retention aggravates any edema present. Also because of this system of priorities, systemic arterial blood pressure is maintained within normal limits or only mildly decreased until extremely late in the course of heart failure. This occurs even though the arteriolar constriction required to maintain normal pressure contributes to poor tissue perfusion.

Reasons for prioritization. Why is the system set up in this fashion? One can only speculate, but most likely there are teleologic (teleology is the philosophic study of evidence of design in nature) reasons for it. Normal or adequate blood pressure is required for the perfusion of the three "critical" vascular beds in the body: the brain, the heart, and the kidneys. All three vascular beds have high innate resistances to blood flow. Consequently, they need high pressures to force blood flow through them.[26] These are the vascular beds that demand that mean systemic arterial blood pressure be greater than 50 to 60 mm Hg. The other vascular beds would function normally with systemic arterial blood pressure well below 50 to 60 mm Hg. Without adequate blood flow to these critical vascular beds, death comes about rapidly, hence the high priority assigned to blood pressure. Systemic blood pressure also has a large reserve built in. Normal mean systemic arterial blood pressure is 100 to 110 mm Hg, whereas a mean blood pressure of only 50 to 60 mm Hg is required.

With a decreased cardiac output, the vascular system can compensate for poor blood flow to the critical vascular beds by constricting blood vessels in other regions of the body, shifting blood flow to the critical beds.[27] If blood flow becomes inadequate to the other regions of the body, however, oxygen delivery to the body becomes inadequate, resulting in anaerobic metabolism, lactic acidosis, cell death, and, finally, death of the patient. Inadequate blood flow results in poor exercise performance. Consequently, during evolution the organism could not escape predators. Possibly because of this, maintaining blood flow takes priority over maintaining normal capillary pressures.

Elevated capillary pressures cause edema, resulting in poor organ function. The rapidity with which this abnormality kills the patient depends on the organ involved. Peripheral edema of skin and subcutaneous tissue does not cause death or markedly affect exercise performance, whereas fulminant pulmonary edema can cause rapid death. Receptors in the left atrium are present in the normal animal to prevent increased left atrial pressure. However, these receptors become desensitized in chronic heart failure, allowing pressure to increase unchecked.[28] The receptors in the body regulating blood pressure and flow remain functional in heart failure, again proving the relative priorities in heart failure.

The lesson to be learned by this is that the cardiovascular system is set up so that death is delayed as long as possible. In other words, Mother Nature prefers slow death to quick death. This logic allows compensation for cardiovascular disease to keep the patient alive for relatively long periods. In dilated cardiomyopathy and mitral regurgitation, for example, patients live for years before the cardiovascular disease becomes severe enough to overwhelm the compensatory mechanisms. Veterinarians usually see patients in the last stages of their disease, when the compensatory mechanisms are contributing to the problems. We aim much of our therapy at counteracting the compensatory mechanisms. Consequently, these mechanisms appear to be detrimental to the patient and at the time we see the patient they probably are. We must remember, however, that these mechanisms have kept the patient clinically normal and alive for a long time before signs of heart failure developed. Therefore these mechanisms are not inappropriate and are not excessive. They are necessary and beneficial.

What occurs in heart failure to create these abnormalities? It depends on the disease that is present. The best way to explain how the body responds to a "failing" heart and how signs of heart failure are generated is to present an example of a disease process and examine how this disease produces changes from the early stages of the disease to the very end stage. For this purpose, the pathophysiology of dilated cardiomyopathy is presented.

Heart Failure Secondary to Dilated Cardiomyopathy (Primary Idiopathic Myocardial Failure)

DEFINITION OF MYOCARDIAL FAILURE

Myocardial failure is defined as a decrease in myocardial contractility.[2] It can be primary or secondary. Primary idiopathic myocardial failure is generally called *dilated cardiomyopathy.*

PATHOPHYSIOLOGY OF DILATED CARDIOMYOPATHY

Acute insult. To illustrate the changes seen in dilated cardiomyopathy we can postulate an acute cardiac insult that results in a sudden decrease in left ventricular contractility (Figure 9-6). A sudden decrease in contractility of this magnitude is unusual in veterinary medicine and is presented in this manner only for illustrative purposes. More commonly, the contractility decreases slightly and continuously over several years.[29] The decrease in myocardial contractility results in decreased myocardial fiber shortening, if afterload and preload are constant. The decreased myocardial fiber shortening results in a larger end-systolic volume (ESV) and larger end-systolic diameter (ESD) (the chamber does not eject as much of its contents because of the weaker heart muscle). Decreased ejection fraction, shortening fraction, and stroke volume result because of the increase in ESV and ESD. Consequently, EDV stays normal in this scenario at 53 mL/m^2 (EDD [end-diastolic diameter] = 4.3 cm/m^2), whereas ESV increases to 27 mL/m^2 (ESD = 3.4 cm/m^2), ejection fraction decreases to 49%, shortening fraction decreases to 20%, and stroke volume decreases to 26 mL/m^2. Note that this ventricle looks identical to the ventricle at end-diastole and end-systole in Chapter 2, Figure 2-15, in which afterload was increased suddenly by increasing systolic intraventricular pressure.

Acute compensation. The decrease in stroke volume results in an initial decrease in systemic arterial blood pressure. This occurs because a smaller quantity of blood is ejected into the aorta and impedance and resistance are still normal (i.e., the systemic arterioles have not constricted at this time). Systolic intraventricular pressure subsequently decreases, producing an initial decrease in afterload.

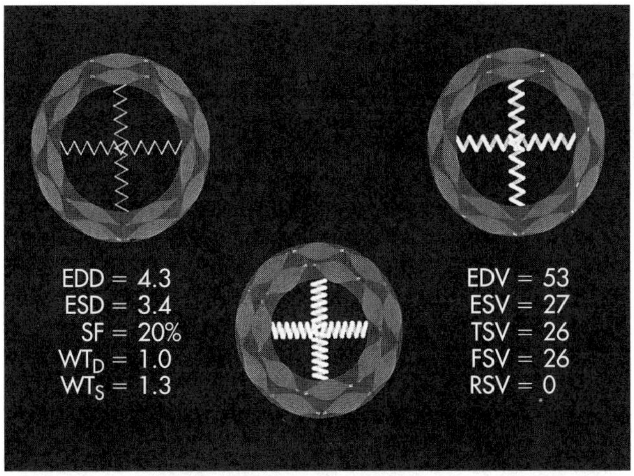

FIGURE 9-6 Schematic drawing of cross-sections of a left ventricle from a 28-kg (lm^2 body surface area) dog with mild myocardial failure and no compensation. The figure is similar to the drawings in Chapter 2, Figures 2-13 through 2-17. Note that the end-systolic diameter has increased from a normal size of 2.9 cm to 3.4 cm, and end-systolic volume has increased from a normal size of 16 mL to 27 mL. End-diastolic variables are normal, and stroke volume is decreased. *EDD,* End-diastolic diameter (cm/m^2); *ESD,* end-systolic diameter (cm/m^2); *SF,* shortening fraction (%); WT_D, wall thickness in diastole (cm/m^2); WT_S, wall thickness at end-systole (cm/m^2); *EDV,* end-diastolic volume (mL/m^2); *ESV,* end-systolic volume (mL/m^2); *TSV,* total stroke volume (mL/m^2); *FSV,* forward stroke volume (mL/m^2); *RSV,* regurgitant stroke volume (mL/m^2).

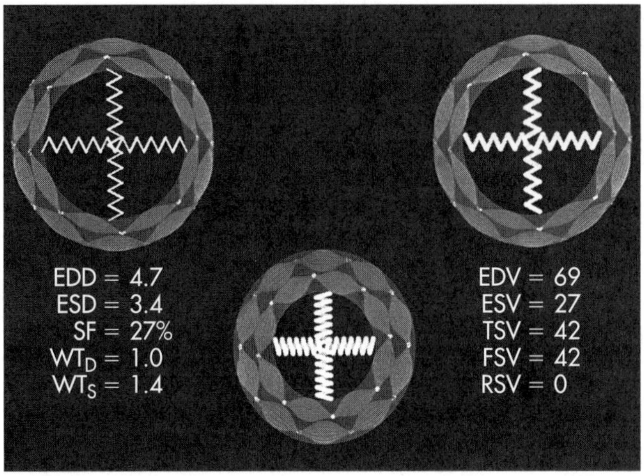

FIGURE 9-7 Cross-sections of a left ventricle with mild myocardial failure and mild volume overload (eccentric) hypertrophy. Note that the number of contractile elements (muscles) in the outside row of the ventricular wall has increased from the normal value of 9 to 10 to increase the end-diastolic diameter and end-diastolic volume. The end-systolic diameter is the same as in Figure 9-6. Total and forward stroke volumes are normal and diastolic pressure is normal. Shortening fraction (the amount of wall motion or contraction) is decreased but has increased from Figure 9-6, without a change in myocardial contractility because of the increase in end-diastolic diameter. Abbreviations are as in Figure 9-6.

The body suddenly senses, through the arterial baroreceptors, a decrease in systemic blood pressure. It also probably senses a decrease in blood flow and tissue perfusion. The body's initial response is to produce constriction of systemic arterioles. Several factors produce vasoconstriction. The large number of factors again underscores the importance the body places on maintaining systemic arterial blood pressure. Arteriolar constriction is produced by increased circulating concentrations of norepinephrine (α_1-receptor stimulation), angiotensin II, vasopressin, and endothelin and by increasing sympathetic nervous system discharge.[30-33] Angiotensin II formation is controlled by renin secretion. Renin secretion is controlled by several factors, including distal tubule sodium delivery and sympathetic input to the juxtaglomerular apparatus. The increased sympathetic drive and circulating concentrations of catecholamines also increase contractility by stimulating β_1 receptors and increase the heart rate. The increases in contractility and heart rate bring stroke volume back toward normal, and the arteriolar constriction increases resistance and so aortic input impedance. The increase in blood flow into the aorta and the increase in resistance returns blood pressure to normal. The subsequent increase in afterload opposes the influence of contractility to decrease end-systolic volume.

With everything brought back into homeostasis one would expect that compensation would be complete and additional compensatory mechanisms would not be required. However, the heart protects itself from long-term catecholamine stimulation and within 24 to 72 hours after this initial compensation takes place, the β_1 receptors on the heart undergo a process called *down-regulation.* Consequently, catecholamine release can no longer stimulate them to the same degree.[34-36] Therefore contractility decreases again, albeit partially. At this time the cardiovascular system must identify another means of increasing stroke volume.

Chronic compensation. The only other means the cardiovascular system has to decrease end-systolic volume is to decrease afterload. The only practical means to do this is to dilate the peripheral arterioles and decrease afterload. This has been done experimentally by administering an angiotensin-converting enzyme (ACE) inhibitor to dogs undergoing induction of heart failure with chronic rapid ventricular pacing.[37] This resulted in better cardiac output and lower left ventricular filling pressure in the dogs receiving ACE inhibitors compared with the dogs not receiving them. However, systemic arterial blood pressure also decreased. Without intervention, the body is set up so that decreasing blood pressure is the last thing it will do.[38] The baroreceptors are set to keep systemic arterial pressure at a fixed point. Therefore natural arteriolar dilation in this situation is not a viable option. The body instead chronically elevates circulating catecholamine, angiotensin II, vasopressin, and endothelin concentrations in congestive heart failure to maintain vasoconstriction and therefore systemic blood pressure.[39] Therefore the only other thing that can be done to increase stroke volume (EDV − ESV) is to increase EDV, initially to take advantage of Starling's law and chronically by producing eccentric hypertrophy. Therefore the kidneys are stimulated to retain more sodium and water, and the patient is stimulated to drink more water and eat more salt. This results in an increase in blood volume and venous return to the left ventricle.

Chronic mild-to-moderate myocardial failure. The increase in venous return to the heart caused by sodium and water retention and subsequent increase in blood volume results in an increase in end-diastolic wall stress. The increased stretch placed on the myocardium forces it to grow larger via volume overload (eccentric) hypertrophy (Figure 9-7). With time, EDV increases to 69 mL/m^2 (EDD = 4.7 cm/m^2), ESV stays at 27 mL/m^2 (ESD = 3.4 cm/m^2), and ejection fraction and shortening fraction increase to values of 61% and 27% respectively (note that shortening fraction increases with an increase in EDD). Stroke volume and therefore cardiac output and heart rate are normal. Note that the number of muscles in both rows encircling the chamber has increased by one. This hyperplasia of contractile elements results in the heart weight increasing from the normal 120 g to 138 g. Myocardial failure is mild at this point, and there are no clinical signs of heart failure. If no further myocardial damage occurs, everything stays stable at this point. This generally does not happen, however. Instead, myocardial failure progresses over the following months to several years.

As the myocardial disease progresses, the myocardial failure eventually becomes moderate in severity (Figure 9-8). We will assume that there is no mitral regurgitation at this time. At this midpoint, ESV is 46 mL/m^2 (EDD = 4.1 cm/m^2), EDV is 83 mL/m^2 (EDD = 5 cm/m^2), ejection fraction is 45%, and shortening fraction is 18%. Note that stroke volume is normal in this scenario. No clinical signs of heart failure are present at rest. However, cardiac function is probably compromised enough at this point to be inadequate to support heavy exercise (the dog cannot run a sled dog race). As a result, oxygen delivery is inadequate for the amount of oxygen consumed by tissues during exercise and early fatigue and lactate production result. The weight of the left ventricle increases from a normal value of 120 g to 152 g (hypertrophy), although wall thickness is normal.

Severe myocardial failure and heart failure

Dogs and cats with heart failure as a result of myocardial failure are presented for clinical signs of heart failure when the myocardial failure is severe.[40] As seen in Figure 9-9, at this time it is common for the ESV to be 95 mL/m^2 (ESD = 5.2 cm/m^2), the EDV 130 mL/m^2 (EDD = 5.8 cm/m^2), shortening fraction 10%, and the stroke volume 35 mL/m^2. The left ventricular diastolic pressure, however, is increased, which causes pulmonary edema. Note that the stroke volume is normal even though the shortening fraction is markedly reduced. Also note that this has occurred because of volume overload hypertrophy. The hemodynamics presented assume that there is no mitral regurgitation. Mitral regurgitation often occurs in dilated cardiomyopathy and can complicate the hemodynamics in this disease.[41] However, the mitral regurgitation generally is mild. If significant mitral regurgitation is present, the stroke volume going into the aorta will be less because some percentage of it will go into the left atrium. Consequently, the heart failure could be more severe at this stage. Heart weight in this example is 195 g, an increase of about 60% from normal. Wall thickness is still normal, and additional contractile elements are depicted.

In Figure 9-10 the shortening fraction is only 5%, and so wall motion on an echocardiogram is barely perceptible. Stroke volume has decreased even without mitral regurgitation. Left ventricular diastolic pressure is increased, resulting in pulmonary edema. In this example of severe dilated cardiomyopathy, the left ventricular chamber diastolic volume has tripled and the left ventricular weight has almost doubled to 213 g. Note also that the number of muscles (contractile elements in these illustrations) encircling the chamber in the outside row has increased from a normal of 9 to 12 and wall

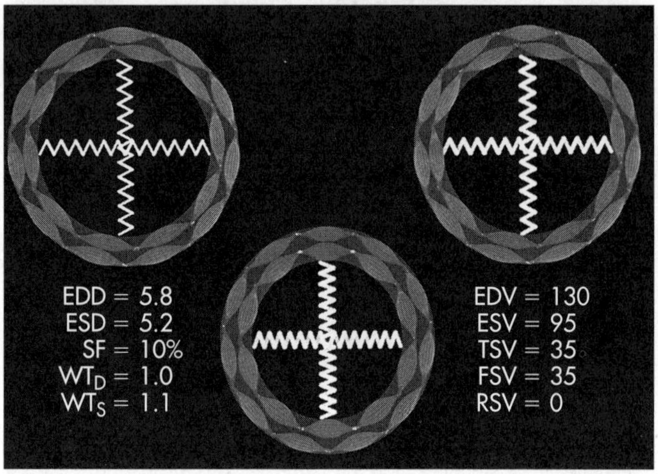

FIGURE 9-9 Cross-sections of a left ventricle from a dog with severe myocardial failure (marked increase in end-systolic diameter and volume). Severe volume overload hypertrophy is present. Note the increase in thickness of the spring in diastole. This represents a moderate increase in end-diastolic pressure. Stroke volume is still normal. Abbreviations are as in Figure 9-6.

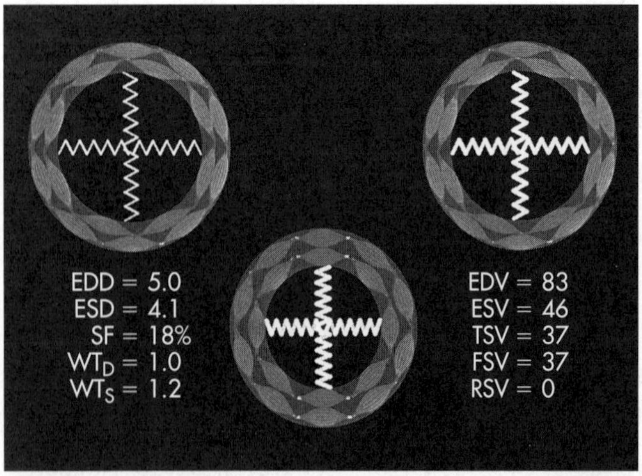

FIGURE 9-8 Cross-sections of a ventricle from a dog with moderate myocardial failure and moderate volume overload hypertrophy. The end-systolic diameter and volume are greater than in Figure 9-7. Systolic intraventricular pressure remains normal. The systolic wall stress, however, should be increased because of the increase in chamber radius. Stroke volume and diastolic pressure are still normal. Abbreviations are as in Figure 9-6.

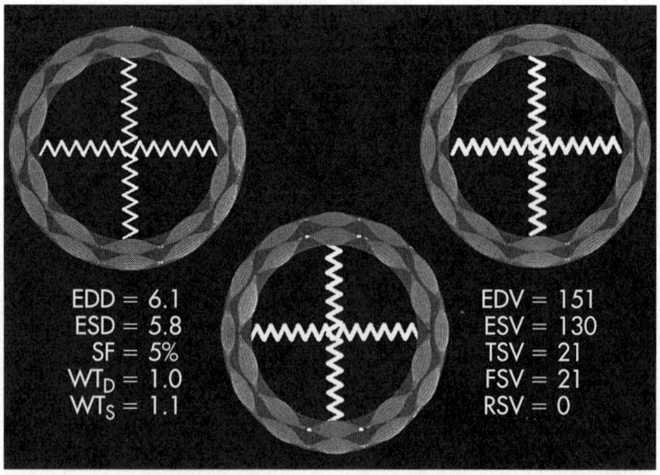

FIGURE 9-10 Cross-sections of a ventricle from a dog with very severe myocardial failure. Note the marked volume overload hypertrophy shown as a larger end-diastolic volume and an increased number of contractile elements (12 in the outside row). The diastolic pressure is severely increased and stroke volume is decreased. Abbreviations are as in Figure 9-6.

thickness is normal. This scenario holds true for some dogs but not others (i.e., in some dogs wall thickness is normal, and in others it is thinner than normal). True ventricular dilation does appear to occur in some patients with end-stage disease. Slippage of myofibrils occurs histologically, and the left ventricular wall becomes thinner, both evidence of dilation. However, ventricular dilation is probably a very late event in dilated cardiomyopathy. It probably occurs when the diastolic pressure in the left ventricle becomes severely increased. Mild-to-moderate increases in diastolic pressure stimulate myocardial growth. When the diastolic pressure in the left ventricle is greater than 25 mm Hg, however, it seems reasonable to expect chamber distension to occur. When the wall thins, this contributes to an increase in systolic wall stress (afterload). This contributes to the decrease in left ventricular function.[42,43] A ventricle that is markedly enlarged and has a smaller-than-normal wall thickness now takes on some characteristics of a "dilated" ventricle. However, there is also still a marked hypertrophy present (i.e., these ventricles weigh much more than normal when placed on a scale at a postmortem examination). Note that the systolic springs are still the same thickness in Figure 9-10. This means that the systolic intraventricular pressure is still normal, indicating that systemic arterial blood pressure is still normal, as documented in canine patients with severe dilated cardiomyopathy.[38]

In Figure 9-11, wall stress–volume loops are drawn from a normal dog and a dog with dilated cardiomyopathy. The line representing contractility (E_{max}) has flattened and shifted to the right. Marked volume overload hypertrophy has occurred to increase the end-diastolic volume. The end-systolic volume has increased markedly because of the decrease in contractility and somewhat because of the increase in afterload caused by the increase in the chamber radius.

PLASMA VOLUME EXPANSION

From this example one can readily appreciate that the formation of volume overload hypertrophy causing an increase in EDV of the left ventricle is the major compensatory mechanism present in dilated

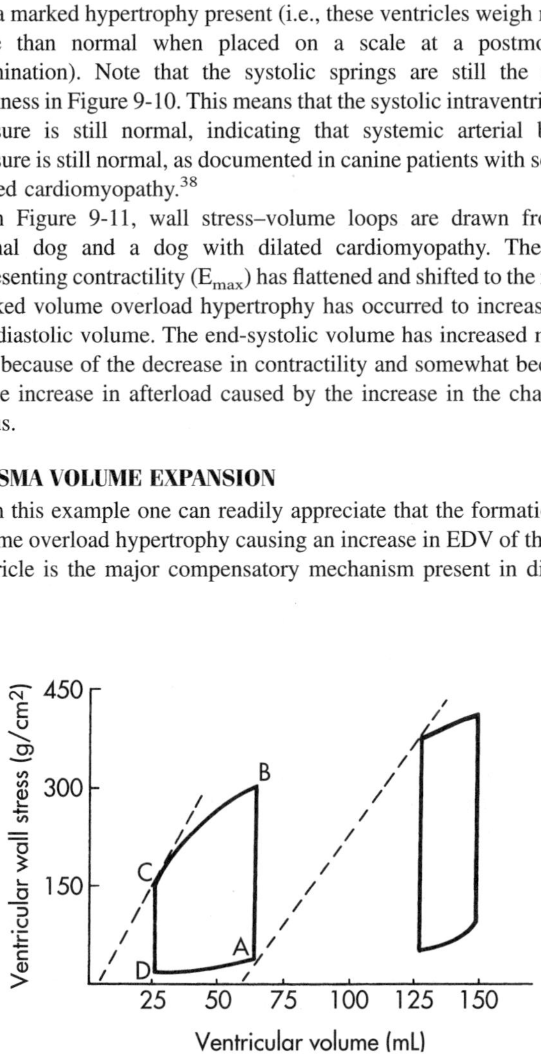

FIGURE 9-11 Wall stress–volume loops from a normal dog and a dog with dilated cardiomyopathy, similar to the dog in Figure 9-9. The end-systolic wall stress–volume relationship *(dashed lines)* for the dog with dilated cardiomyopathy is severely shifted to the right because of the severe decrease in myocardial contractility. Diastolic wall stress is increased because of the increase in diastolic pressure. *A,* End of diastole and onset of isovolumic systole where the mitral valve closes; *B,* end of isovolumic systole where the aortic valve opens; *C,* end of systole and the onset of isovolumic relaxation where the aortic valve closes; *D,* end of isovolumic relaxation and the onset of ventricular filling where the mitral valve opens.

cardiomyopathy. Without it, patients with myocardial failure and many other cardiac diseases would die much earlier in their disease. At this point let us examine the mechanisms present in the body that are activated to cause sodium and water retention and as a result stimulate volume overload hypertrophy.

Renal retention of sodium and water is extremely important in heart failure. It helps the heart compensate, so that it can increase cardiac output by increasing end-diastolic volume. Renal retention of sodium and water also produces many of the clinical signs usually seen in the end stages of chronic cardiac disease. In experimental dogs with rapid ventricular pacing–induced myocardial failure, sodium excretion and urine volume decrease precipitously once rapid ventricular pacing is started.[44] These reductions occur even before plasma concentrations of renin and aldosterone increase.

The renin-angiotensin-aldosterone system

The renin-angiotensin-aldosterone system (RAAS) is probably the best-explained system for sodium and water retention in heart failure. It also may be the most important, as evidenced in one study of human patients with heart failure in which plasma renin activity was increased 5 to 6 times normal and plasma vasopressin concentration was increased to twice normal.[45] However, one should be aware that edema of cardiac origin can occur without apparent renin and aldosterone secretion.[46] Many different mechanisms stimulate renin release by the juxtaglomerular apparatus. Sympathetic nervous fibers innervate the juxtaglomerular apparatus, and β-receptor stimulation causes the release of renin.[47] Stretch receptors also apparently lie in the media of the afferent renal arterioles (the arterioles entering the glomerulus). They detect decreases in afferent arteriolar blood pressure and stimulate renin release.[48] The macula densa is a region of specialized tissue in the distal tubule. It plays a role in the modulation of renin secretion, by which a decrease in sodium and/or chloride load at the macula densa increases renin release.[49] In addition, many humoral factors (sodium and potassium, circulating angiotensin II, and vasopressin concentrations) also affect renin release.[45,49] In cardiac disease, renin is secreted in response to a decrease in cardiac output. The decrease in cardiac output results initially in a decrease in renal perfusion pressure and chronically results in decreased sodium and chloride delivery to the distal tubule. As long as cardiac output is reduced, renin will continue to be elaborated in an attempt to bring systemic blood flow back to normal.

Renin is an enzyme that converts angiotensinogen, a polypeptide formed in the liver, to angiotensin I.[50] A converting enzyme, found predominantly in endothelial cells of the lung, converts angiotensin I in turn to angiotensin II. Angiotensin II is a potent vasoconstrictor that also stimulates thirst and aldosterone secretion.

Angiotensin II, plasma potassium concentration, and, to a lesser degree, adrenocorticotropic hormone control aldosterone secretion.[51] Aldosterone is a primary mediator in the RAAS system. Its major action is to promote sodium reabsorption and potassium excretion in the distal tubules of the kidney. Plasma aldosterone concentration is elevated in dogs, cats, and humans with heart failure.[52,53] The elevation in plasma aldosterone concentration is higher in dogs and humans when the clinical signs of heart failure are more severe. It is not unusual to have a plasma aldosterone concentration 3 to 10 times normal in a patient with severe heart failure. In addition to effects on salt and water retention, angiotensin II and aldosterone probably also increase salt appetite in patients with congestive heart failure.[54]

In addition to the circulating RAAS, it has been suggested that there is a role for the tissue renin-angiotensin system in heart failure.[55] It is not uncommon for plasma concentrations of renin, angiotensin II, and aldosterone to be within normal range during stable stages of heart failure (although relatively elevated because

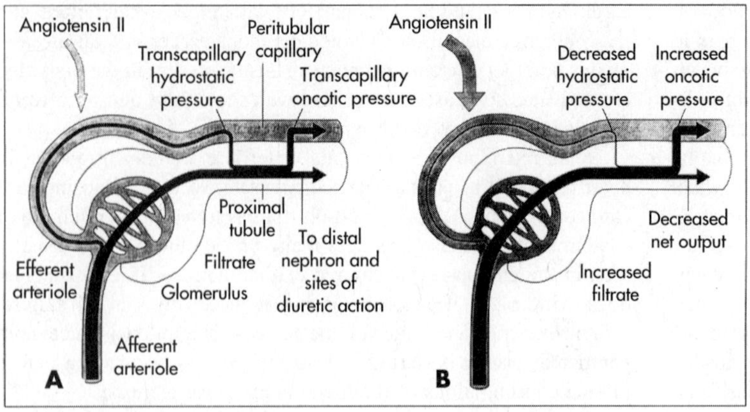

FIGURE 9-12 Schematic drawings of a glomerulus and proximal tubule from a normal dog **(A)** and a dog with heart failure **(B).** In **B,** the plasma concentration of angiotensin II is increased, resulting in efferent arteriolar constriction. Constriction of this vessel increases the percentage of serum filtered from the blood into the proximal tubule (increased filtration fraction). This results in an increase in the oncotic pressure in the peritubular capillary. The decrease in peritubular capillary flow results in a decrease in hydrostatic pressure in this vessel. The combination of the decrease in hydrostatic pressure and the increase in oncotic pressure results in increased reabsorption of filtrate back into the peritubular capillary.

serum concentrations should be decreased in this situation).[53] It has been postulated that the plasma RAAS is activated primarily when cardiac status is actively changing, whereas the tissue renin-angiotensin system may be activated primarily during stable stages of heart failure.[55]

Along with the altered RAAS, changes in renal blood flow distribution, proximal tubular fluid reabsorption, and circulating vasopressin concentration aid in the retention of sodium and water in heart failure. When cardiac output decreases in humans and dogs, renal blood flow distribution changes so that an increased percentage of the renal blood flow goes to the juxtamedullary nephrons, away from the cortical nephrons.[27,56] Because the juxtamedullary nephrons travel deeper into the renal medulla, they are able to conserve larger quantities of sodium.

When cardiac output decreases, renal blood flow decreases. This decrease is probably disproportionately high compared with other organs because of afferent (the arteriole entering the glomerulus) renal arteriolar constriction, which occurs secondary to sympathetic stimulation.[27] In humans, renal blood flow is normally 20% of the cardiac output, whereas in heart failure it can fall to 10%.[27] The net effect of the decrease in renal blood flow is a decrease in glomerular filtration rate and an increase in blood urea nitrogen and serum creatinine concentration. To increase filtration back to or toward normal, the efferent arteriole leaving the glomerulus constricts secondary to angiotensin II stimulation (Figure 9-12).[57,58] The afferent arteriole, although constricted, remains relatively dilated compared with the efferent arteriole. This increases the pressure back to or above normal within the glomerular capillaries, which increases the percentage of filtrate squeezed from the blood (the filtration fraction increases). This increase maintains a normal glomerular filtration rate, whereas total renal blood flow is reduced. When renal blood flow is severely compromised in heart failure, this mechanism becomes overwhelmed and glomerular filtration becomes reduced, resulting in an increase in serum urea nitrogen and creatinine concentrations.

The increase in filtration fraction that occurs when renal blood flow is reduced results in the blood within the efferent arteriole and peritubular capillaries being relatively dehydrated or hyperosmolar compared with normal.[50] The plasma protein concentration (oncotic pressure) within these vessels is increased, and the hydrostatic pressure is decreased. Therefore, as blood traverses the peritubular capillaries, a greater percentage of fluid is resorbed back into the vascular space from the proximal tubules (see Figure 9-12). This helps increase blood volume.

The RAAS has been studied in canine clinical patients with dilated cardiomyopathy and with mitral regurgitation. In dogs with dilated cardiomyopathy, the plasma renin activity is marginally increased in those dogs with myocardial failure but no evidence of heart failure.[59] In dogs in heart failure the plasma concentration of renin is mildly increased in dogs with mild-to-moderate heart failure and markedly increased in dogs with severe heart failure. Plasma aldosterone concentration is not increased in dogs with no evidence of heart failure but is mildly increased in dogs with mild-to-moderate heart failure and markedly increased in dogs with severe heart failure. In dogs with mitral regurgitation, plasma renin activity and plasma aldosterone concentration are marginally increased before heart failure is evident.[60] One study has suggested that plasma aldosterone concentration decreases in Cavalier King Charles spaniels with mitral regurgitation once heart failure becomes evident.[61] There was tremendous overlap in values in these dogs before decompensation and after decompensation. It is unlikely that this finding is meaningful, although it is interesting in this breed that the aldosterone concentration did not increase further with the onset of heart failure.

Other hormonal systems. Plasma vasopressin (ADH) concentration can also be elevated in patients with congestive heart failure.[62] This increase can be stimulated by the sympathetic nervous system.[63] Vasopressin aids in water retention, and in terminal heart failure it can be present in a concentration high enough to cause dilutional hyponatremia.[31,64] Vasopressin also stimulates thirst in patients with heart failure, which helps increase intravascular volume. The increase in vasopressin concentration in heart failure does not suppress normally with ethanol administration in humans.[65] Vasopressin also contributes to vasoconstriction in some human patients with heart failure.[28]

A hormone that promotes renal sodium loss (atrial natriuretic factor [ANF] hormone, or peptide) is present in normal animals. This hormone is stored in granules, primarily in the atria. It is secreted into the circulation via the coronary sinus to promote diuresis, vasodilation, and inhibition of the RAAS when atrial pressures increase, resulting in increased stretch of the atrial myocytes.[66] These effects are produced by ANF interacting with specific receptors termed *NPR-A* and *NPR-B* and are mediated by cGMP. Clearance of ANF from plasma is rapid (half-life is several minutes) and is carried out by interaction with a third receptor *(NPR-C)* or enzymatic degradation by neutral endopeptidase. The plasma concentration of ANF is increased in patients with heart failure but its effects are blunted, and it apparently cannot overcome the other effects causing sodium and water retention.[38,67,68] Although ANF is ineffectual in patients with heart failure, it does increase with increasing severity of disease and failure.[61] Consequently, it may be a marker of disease and failure severity.

Cardiopulmonary baroreceptors are also present in the atria that produce increased urine flow and sodium excretion when blood volume is increased independent of atrial natriuretic factor. These baroreceptors are also present in the ventricles and are less responsive to stimuli in dogs with chronic heart failure.[28,69]

In addition to the factors that are known to produce volume expansion, other unknown factors may contribute significantly to sodium and water retention and intake. A recent study of human patients compared hemodynamics, fluid intake and output, body weight, respiratory function, and neurohormonal status in patients that received a bolus dose of furosemide with the same factors in patients who lost a similar amount of fluid through ultrafiltration of their blood.[70] The researchers found similar acute responses to these interventions but also found that the beneficial effects of ultrafiltration lasted for 3 months after the one-time intervention. The beneficial effects of furosemide lasted less than 4 days. Ultrafiltration removes many small proteins from the bloodstream and may have removed an important but unidentified factor in these patients.

Fluid retention: good and bad. In summary, with chronic heart failure, renal retention of sodium and water, increased thirst, increased salt appetite, and systemic venoconstriction cause increases in intracardiac diastolic volumes. This increase in volume stretches the myocardium (preload), which enables it to contract more forcefully and eject a larger stroke volume. The increased preload stimulates volume overload hypertrophy, increasing end-diastolic volume. The increase in diastolic volume is beneficial to the systolic pumping properties of the heart in that it increases the amount of blood ejected during systole for any amount of contraction.

The fluid retention, however, can also be harmful. It causes no harm in mild-to-moderate heart disease, in which it is very beneficial. When the disease becomes severe, however, the heart reaches a point where it apparently can enlarge no further. At this time, cardiac output is still depressed and consequently all of the mechanisms for sodium and water retention are still stimulated and blood volume continues to increase. Because the heart is relatively stiff and cannot enlarge at this stage, the increased blood volume pushed back into the heart during diastole results in an increase in the diastolic pressure in the ventricle. Because the mitral valve is open during diastole, the left ventricle, left atrium, pulmonary veins, and pulmonary capillaries are essentially one chamber. As a result, whatever pressure is present in the left ventricle in diastole is also present in the pulmonary capillaries. An increase in the hydrostatic pressure in the pulmonary capillaries causes an increase in the transudation of fluid into the lungs (pulmonary edema).

Magnitude of hormonal change. Of what magnitude are the changes in circulating hormone concentrations in patients with heart failure? In one study of human patients with dilated cardiomyopathy and severe heart failure, plasma aldosterone concentration was increased 6.4 times normal, plasma renin activity 9.5 times normal, and atrial natriuretic factor 14.3 times normal.[71] Renal plasma flow was 29% of control, and glomerular filtration was 65% of control. This decrease in glomerular filtration rate resulted in only mild increases in serum urea concentration (43 mg/dL) and serum creatinine concentration (1.6 mg/dL). Obviously, filtration fraction was markedly increased. These changes resulted in a 32% increase in extracellular volume, a 34% increase in plasma volume, a 22% increase in blood volume, a 16% increase in body water, and a 37% increase in exchangeable sodium. Patients with lesser degrees of heart failure would be expected to have milder changes in these variables. The aldosterone concentration in dogs and cats with severe heart failure has been measured and is comparably elevated to that seen in humans.[52]

In a study performed in dogs, heart failure was produced via rapid ventricular pacing.[30] In this study plasma aldosterone concentration rose over the first 7 days to values approximately 7 times baseline, and plasma renin concentration increased to approximately 10 times baseline. Norepinephrine concentration also increased to approximately 3 times baseline. Although it did have some effect on arteriolar constriction, it did not appear to be the primary factor in producing the constriction.

In a study performed in canine patients with heart failure, blood volume was increased in dogs with class III and class IV heart failure but not in dogs with class II heart failure.[38] Blood volume, on average, was increased 18% in the dogs with class III heart failure and 32% in dogs with class IV heart failure. Plasma volume was increased similarly. Plasma concentration of atrial natriuretic factor was increased in patients in class III and IV heart failure, increasing to 5 times control in class III patients and 9 times control in the patients with class IV heart failure. With blood volume expansion and edema, body weight increases. However, this increase is probably less than 10% and may be offset by loss of fat and muscle.[61] Hematocrit and plasma protein concentration may decrease with fluid expansion, but the changes often are small.[61]

VASOCONSTRICTION

Venoconstriction. In addition to sodium and water retention causing an increase in intracardiac blood volumes in cardiac disease, systemic venoconstriction also takes place.[2] This constriction results in a redistribution of blood volume from the peripheral circuit (the abdominal torso and limbs) to the central circuit (the heart and pulmonary vasculature) and aids in increasing venous return and producing volume overload hypertrophy. The constriction of the veins occurs secondary to catecholamine and angiotensin II stimulation.[2]

Arteriolar constriction. Systemic arterial blood pressure is maintained, often within the normal range, in patients with chronic heart failure via constriction of systemic arterioles. Constriction of systemic arterioles increases systemic vascular resistance. This increase in resistance is often interpreted as being inappropriate or excessive. However, once one realizes that maintenance of systemic blood pressure is the cardiovascular system's number one priority it becomes readily apparent that constriction of systemic arterioles is appropriate in patients with a low cardiac output as a result of heart failure. Several factors contribute to the constriction of systemic arterioles. Stimulation of α_1 receptors by circulating catecholamines and sympathetic nerves is one primary means. Angiotensin II and endothelin are also potent constrictors of systemic arterioles. Plasma concentrations of norepinephrine, angiotensin II, and endothelin are all increased in dogs with heart failure.[33]

Heart Failure Secondary to Patent Ductus Arteriosus

Patent ductus arteriosus is an example of another disease that commonly results in heart failure. Although myocardial failure plays a role in this disease, volume overload as a result of the shunt is the predominate mechanism by which this disease causes heart failure in young dogs and cats.

Patent ductus arteriosus, aortic regurgitation, and arteriovenous fistulas are viewed similarly by the left ventricle. In each disease the left ventricle is forced to eject a larger-than-normal quantity of blood into the high-pressure aorta to compensate for a leak in the high-pressure systemic arterial system, a physically demanding task. Over time this is more likely to result in myocardial failure than

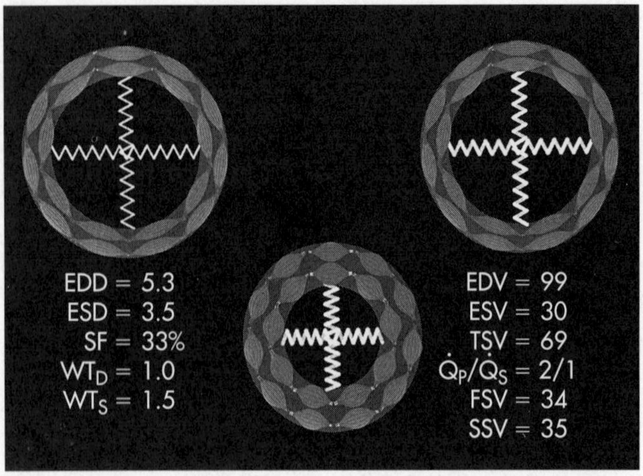

FIGURE 9-13 Cross-sections of a left ventricle from a dog with a moderate-size patent ductus arteriosus and moderate volume overload hypertrophy. Note the increase in end-systolic volume as a result of the increase in systolic wall stress (afterload). The stroke volume is normal and diastolic pressure is normal. Abbreviations as in Figure 9-6.

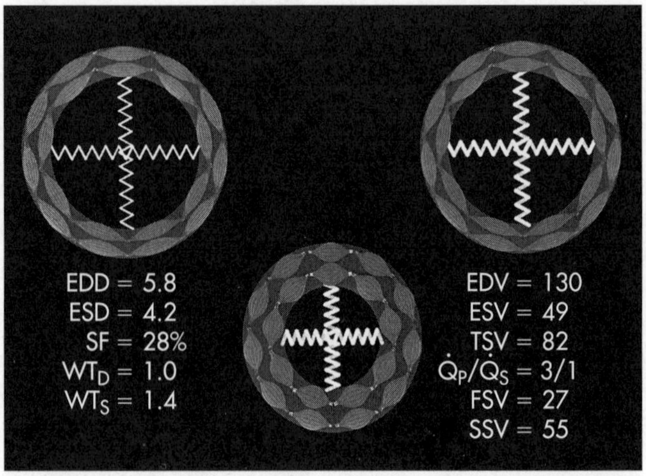

FIGURE 9-14 Cross-sections of a left ventricle from a dog with a large patent ductus arteriosus, marked volume overload hypertrophy, and myocardial failure. Despite the increase in afterload and the decrease in contractility producing the moderate increase in the end-systolic diameter, the shortening fraction is only mildly decreased. The shortening fraction is maintained by the increase in end-diastolic diameter. Abbreviations as in Figure 9-6.

is a comparable degree of mitral regurgitation in which the left ventricle ejects into the low-pressure left atrium.

In patent ductus arteriosus a quantity of the left ventricular stroke volume is lost through the patent ductus. The quantity of blood that leaks into the pulmonary artery then flows through the lungs and back into the left heart. This increase in venous return to the left heart results in left ventricular volume overload hypertrophy. Because there is a lesser quantity of blood flowing through the systemic circulation (because of the loss of blood through the shunt), the RAAS and other hormonal systems are turned on to force the kidneys to retain sodium and water in order to increase blood volume and increase venous return back to the heart. This also stimulates volume overload hypertrophy.

The changes that occur in a dog with a moderately large patent ductus arteriosus are depicted in Figure 9-13. The EDV has increased to 99 mL/m^2 (EDD = 5.3 cm/m^2). The ESV has also increased to 30 mL/m^2 (ESD = 3.6 cm/m^2). The increase in ESD and ESV is primarily the result of the increase in afterload seen in this stage of the disease. In a study of experimental aortocaval fistulas in dogs in which a shunt of comparable size to the illustration provided here was produced, myocardial contractility was not decreased.[37] The increase in chamber radius without an increase in wall thickness results in an increase in systolic wall stress. The shortening fraction is normal at 33%. Total stroke volume of the left ventricle is 69 mL/m^2. Of this total, 34 mL/m^2 goes down the aorta past the patent ductus and 35 mL/m^2 goes through the shunt. Right ventricular stroke volume has to be 34 mL/m^2 also, so the ratio of pulmonary blood flow (including the amount going through the patent ductus) to the systemic flow is 2:1, which is comparable with a regurgitant fraction of approximately 50%. One would not expect this dog to be in heart failure.

In Figure 9-14 is a depiction of a left ventricle from a dog with a very large patent ductus arteriosus. This dog has an EDV that is increased to 130 mL/m^2 (EDD = 5.8 cm/m^2) and ESV increased to 49 mL/m^2 (ESD = 4.2 cm/m^2). Again the ESD and ESV have increased. The increase at this stage probably has occurred because of the further increase in afterload and a mild decrease in contractility. In the same study cited for the previous example, dogs with large shunts, comparable to the shunt size in the example in Figure 9-14, did have a decrease in myocardial contractility.[37] Shortening fraction is mildly depressed at 28% in Figure 9-14. The left ventricle now ejects 82 mL/m^2 into the proximal aorta, but 55 mL/m^2 leaks through the patent ductus arteriosus. The ratio of pulmonary to systemic blood flow is 82/27 or 3/1. This is comparable to a regurgitant fraction of 67%. Because this shunt size is so large it overwhelms the capability of the left heart to compensate for the disease and the dog is in congestive heart failure. This is depicted again as a thicker diastolic spring. The heart weight is 195 g because of the increased number of contractile elements.

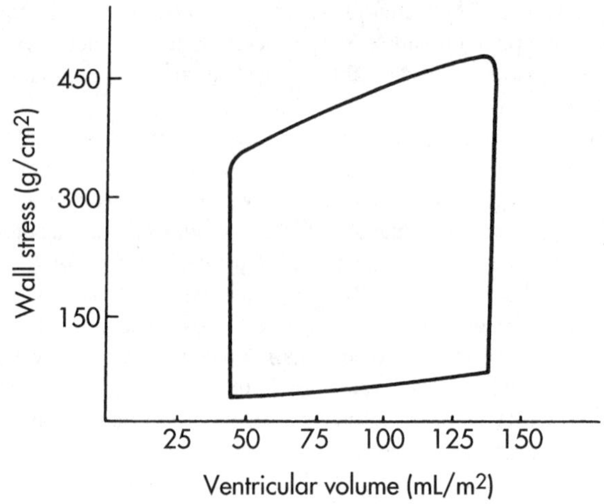

FIGURE 9-15 Wall stress–volume loop from a dog with a large patent ductus arteriosus. Systolic wall stress (afterload) is increased (compare with normal in Figure 9-11) because the ventricle must achieve a normal systolic pressure with an increased chamber radius and normal wall thickness. The end-diastolic volume is approximately 135 mL and the end-systolic volume is approximately 45 mL. Consequently, the total stroke volume is approximately 90 mL.

A wall stress–volume loop from a dog with a similar shunt to the dog described in Figure 9-14 is seen in Figure 9-15. In this situation isovolumic systole still exists, because the ventricle must eject all of its stroke volume into the high-pressure aorta. Subsequently, in contrast to mitral regurgitation, systolic wall stress is increased above normal. This results in an increase in end-systolic volume and a decrease in stroke volume.

REFERENCES

1. Braunwald E: Pathophysiology of heart failure. In Braunwald E, ed: *Heart disease: a textbook of cardiovascular medicine,* Philadelphia, 1980, WB Saunders.
2. Schlant RC, Sonnenblick EH: Pathophysiology of heart failure. In Hurst JW, Schlant RC, Rackley CE et al, eds: *The Heart,* ed 7, New York, 1990, McGraw-Hill.
3. Eichhorn P, Grimm J, Koch R et al: Left ventricular relaxation in patients with left ventricular hypertrophy secondary to aortic valve disease, *Circulation* 65:1395, 1982.
4. Bonow RO, Bacharach SL, Green MV et al: Impaired left ventricular diastolic filling in patients with coronary artery disease: assessment with radionuclide angiography, *Circulation* 64:315, 1981.
5. Hanrath P, Mathey DG, Siegert R et al: Left ventricular relaxation and filling pattern in different forms of left ventricular hypertrophy: an echocardiographic study, *Am J Cardiol* 45:15, 1980.
6. Hirota Y: A clinical study of left ventricular relaxation, *Circulation* 62:756, 1980.
7. Calvert C: Long-term ambulatory electrocardiographic (Holter) monitoring as an aid in the diagnosis of occult cardiomyopathy in Doberman pinschers, *Proc Ann Vet Med Forum,* 1991, p 691.
8. Pion PD, Kittleson MD, Rogers QR: Cardiomyopathy in the cat and its relation to taurine deficiency. In Kirk RW, Bonagura JD, eds*: Current veterinary therapy: small animal practice,* ed 10, Philadelphia, 1989, WB Saunders.
9. Kittleson MD, Eyster GE, Knowlen GG et al: Myocardial function in small dogs with chronic mitral regurgitation and severe congestive heart failure, *J Am Vet Med Assoc* 184:455, 1984.
10. Weber KT, Janicki JS: Pathophysiology of cardiac failure, *Am J Cardiol* 56:3B, 1985.
11. Foldi M, Lehotai L: Starling's law of oedema production: its mathematical analysis from haemo-lymphodynamic aspects, *Acta Med Acad Sci Hung* 23:371, 1967.
12. Wiener-Kronish JP, Matthay MA, Filly RA et al: Relationship of pleural effusions to pulmonary hemodynamics in patients with congestive heart failure, *Am Rev Respir Dis* 132:1253, 1985.
13. Mellins RB, Levine OR, Fishman AP: Effect of systemic and pulmonary venous hypertension on pleural and pericardial fluid accumulation, *J Appl Physiol* 29:564, 1970.
14. McLaughlin RF, Tyler WS, Canada RO: A study of the subgross pulmonary anatomy in various mammals, *Am J Anat* 108:149, 1961.
15. Miller WS: The vascular supply of the pleura pulmonalis, *Am J Anat* 7:389, 1907.
16. Clemmer TP: Oxygen transport, *Int Anesthesiol Clin* 19:21, 1981.
17. Simmons DH, Alpas AP, Tashkin DP et al: Hyperlactatemia due to arterial hypoxemia or reduced cardiac output, or both, *J Appl Physiol* 45:195, 1978.
18. Kittleson MD, Johnson LE, Pion PD: Submaximal exercise testing using lactate threshold and venous oxygen tension as endpoints in normal dogs and in dogs with heart failure, *J Vet Intern Med* 10:21, 1996.
19. Kittleson MD: Cardiovascular physiology and pathophysiology. In Slatter DH, ed: *Textbook of small animal surgery,* Philadelphia, 1985, WB Saunders.
20. Kittleson MD, Johnson LE, Oliver NB: Acute hemodynamic effects of hydralazine in dogs with chronic mitral regurgitation, *J Am Vet Med Assoc* 187:258, 1985.
21. Goetz KL, Bond GC, Bloxham DD: Atrial receptors and renal function, *Physiol Rev* 55:157, 1975.
22. Schrier RW, Berl T: Mechanism of effect of alpha adrenergic stimulation with norepinephrine on renal water excretion, *J Clin Invest* 52:502, 1973.
23. Anderson RJ, Pluss RG, Berns AS et al: Mechanism of effect of hypoxia on renal water excretion, *J Clin Invest* 62:769, 1978.
24. Anderson RJ, Cadnapaphornchai P, Harbottle JA et al: Mechanism of effect of thoracic inferior vena cava constriction on renal water excretion, *J Clin Invest* 54:1473, 1974.
25. Kittleson MD, Johnson LE, Pion PD: The acute hemodynamic effects of milrinone in dogs with severe idiopathic myocardial failure, *J Vet Intern Med* 1:121, 1987.
26. Braunwald E: Regulation of the circulation. II. *N Engl J Med* 290:1420, 1974.
27. Mason DT, Tonken MJ: *Management of fluid and electrolyte disturbances in congestive heart failure,* New York, 1975, Science and Medicine.
28. Zucker IH, Earle AM, Gilmore JP: The mechanism of adaptation of left atrial stretch receptors in dogs with chronic congestive heart failure, *J Clin Invest* 60:323, 1977.
29. Calvert CA, Brown J: Use of M-mode echocardiography in the diagnosis of congestive cardiomyopathy in Doberman pinschers, *J Am Vet Med Assoc* 189:293, 1986.
30. Riegger GA, Liebau, Holzschuh M et al: Role of the renin-angiotensin system in the development of congestive heart failure in the dog as assessed by chronic converting-enzyme blockade, *Am J Cardiol* 53:614, 1984.
31. Creager MA, Faxon DP, Cutler SS et al: Contribution of vasopressin to vasoconstriction in patients with congestive heart failure: comparison with the renin-angiotensin system and the sympathetic nervous system, *J Am Coll Cardiol* 7:758, 1986.
32. Margulies KB, Hildebrand FL, Lerman A et al: Increased endothelin in experimental heart failure, *Circulation* 82:2226, 1990.
33. Cavero PG, Miller WL, Heublein DM et al: Endothelin in experimental congestive heart failure in the anesthetized dog, *Am J Physiol* 259:F312, 1990.
34. Bohm M, Beuckelmann D, Brown L et al: Reduction of beta-adrenoceptor density and evaluation of positive inotropic responses in isolated, diseased human myocardium, *Eur Heart J* 9:844, 1988.
35. Bristow MR: Myocardial beta-adrenergic receptor downregulation in heart failure, *Int J Cardiol* 5:648, 1984.
36. Vatner DE, Vatner SF, Fujii AM et al: Loss of high affinity cardiac beta adrenergic receptors in dogs with heart failure, *J Clin Invest* 76:2259, 1985.
37. Legault F, Rouleau JL, Juneau C et al: Functional and morphological characteristics of compensated and decompensated cardiac hypertrophy in dogs with chronic infrarenal aorto-caval fistulas, *Circ Res* 66:846, 1990.
38. Vollmar AM, Montag C, Preusser U et al: Atrial natriuretic peptide and plasma volume of dogs suffering from heart failure or dehydration, *J Vet Med Assoc* 41:548, 1994.
39. Ware WA, Lund DD, Subieta AR et al: Sympathetic activation in dogs with congestive heart failure caused by chronic mitral valve disease and dilated cardiomyopathy, *J Am Vet Med Assoc* 197:1475, 1990.
40. Calvert CA, Chapman WL, Toal RL: Congestive cardiomyopathy in Doberman pinscher dogs, *J Am Vet Med Assoc* 181:598, 1982.
41. Levisman JA: Echocardiographic diagnosis of mitral regurgitation in congestive cardiomyopathy, *Am Heart J* 93:33, 1977.
42. Feild BJ, Baxley WA, Russell RO et al: Left ventricular function and hypertrophy in cardiomyopathy with depressed ejection fraction, *Circulation* 47:1022, 1973.
43. Hood WP, Rackley CE, Rolett EL: Wall stress in the normal and hypertrophied human left ventricle, *Am J Cardiol* 22:550, 1968.
44. Sisson D, Thomas WP, Miller M: The effects of neutral endopeptidase inhibition in a rapid ventricular pacing model of heart failure in dogs, *Proc Ann Vet Med Forum,* 1997, p 209.
45. Goldsmith SR, Francis GS, Cowley AW et al: Increased plasma arginine vasopressin levels in patients with congestive heart failure, *J Am Coll Cardiol* 1:1385, 1983.
46. Chonko AM, Bay WH, Stein JH et al: The role of renin and aldosterone in the salt retention of edema, *Am J Med* 63:881, 1977.

47. Francis GS: The relationship of the sympathetic nervous system and the renin-angiotensin system in congestive heart failure, *Am Heart J* 118:642, 1989.
48. Davis JO, Freeman RH: Mechanisms regulating renin release, *Physiol Rev* 56:1, 1976.
49. Linden RJ: Neurocirculatory control of sodium and water excretion. In Dickenson CJ, Marks J, eds: *Developments in cardiovascular medicine,* Baltimore, 1978, University Park Press.
50. Cannon PJ: The kidney in heart failure, *N Engl J Med* 296:26, 1977.
51. Nicholls MG, Espiner EA, Donald RA et al: Aldosterone and its regulation during diuresis in patients with gross congestive heart failure, *Clin Sci Mol Med* 47:301, 1974.
52. Knowlen GG, Kittleson MD, Nachreiner RF et al: Comparison of plasma aldosterone concentration among clinical status groups of dogs with chronic heart failure, *J Am Vet Med Assoc* 183:991, 1983.
53. Dzau VJ, Colucci WS, Hollenberg NK et al: Relation of the renin-angiotensin-aldosterone system to clinical state in congestive heart failure, *Circulation* 63:645, 1981.
54. Sakai RR, Nicolaidis S, Epstein AN: Salt appetite is suppressed by interference with angiotensin II and aldosterone, *Am J Physiol* 251:R762, 1986.
55. Hirsch AT, Pinto YM, Schunkert H et al: Potential role of the tissue renin-angiotensin system in the pathophysiology of congestive heart failure, *Am J Cardiol* 66:22D, 1990.
56. Sparks HV, Kopald HH, Carriere S et al: Intrarenal distribution of blood flow with chronic congestive heart failure, *Am J Physiol* 223:840, 1972.
57. Ichikawa I, Kon V, Pfeffer MA et al: Role of angiotensin II in the altered renal function of heart failure, *Kidney Int Suppl* 20:S213, 1987.
58. Packer M, Lee WH, Kessler PD: Preservation of glomerular filtration rate in human heart failure by activation of the renin-angiotensin system, *Circulation* 74:766, 1986.
59. Koch J, Pedersen HD, Jensen AL et al: Activation of the renin-angiotensin system in dogs with asymptomatic and symptomatic dilated cardiomyopathy, *Res Vet Sci* 59:172, 1995.
60. Pedersen HD, Koch J, Poulsen K et al: Activation of the renin-angiotensin system in dogs with asymptomatic and mildly symptomatic mitral valvular insufficiency, J *Vet Intern Med* 9:328, 1995.
61. Haggstrom J, Hansson K, Karlberg BE et al: Effects of long-term treatment with enalapril or hydralazine on the renin-angiotensin-aldosterone system and fluid balance in dogs with naturally acquired mitral valve degeneration, *Am J Vet Res* 57:1645, 1996.
62. Pruszczynski W, Vahanian A, Ardaillou R et al: Role of antidiuretic hormone in impaired water excretion of patients with congestive heart failure, *J Clin Endocrinol Metab* 58:599, 1984.
63. Schrier RW: Pathogenesis of sodium and water retention in high-output and low-output cardiac failure, nephrotic syndrome, cirrhosis, and pregnancy, *N Engl J Med 3*19:1065, 1988 (erratum 320[10]:676, 1989).
64. Szatalowicz VL, Arnold PE, Chaimovitz C et al: Radioimmunoassay of plasma arginine vasopressin in hyponatremic patients with congestive heart failure, *N Engl J Med* 305:263, 1981.
65. Goldsmith SR, Dodge D: Response of plasma vasopressin to ethanol in congestive heart failure, *Am J Cardiol* 55:1354, 1985.
66. Goetz KL, Wang BC, Geer PG et al: Atrial stretch increases sodium excretion independently of release of atrial peptides, *Am J Physiol* 250:R946, 1986.
67. Haggstrom J, Hansson K, Karlberg BE et al: Plasma concentration of atrial natriuretic peptide in relation to severity of mitral regurgitation in Cavalier King Charles spaniels, *Am J Vet Res* 55:698, 1994.
68. Cody RJ, Atlas SA, Laragh JH et al: Atrial natriuretic factor in normal subjects and heart failure patients: plasma levels and renal, hormonal, and hemodynamic responses to peptide infusion, *J Clin Invest* 78:1362, 1986.
69. Hirsch AT, Dzau VJ, Creager MA: Baroreceptor function in congestive heart failure: effect on neurohumoral activation and regional vascular resistance, *Circulation* 75:IV36, 1987.
70. Agostoni P, Marenzi G, Lauri G et al: Sustained improvement in functional capacity after removal of body fluid with isolated ultrafiltration in chronic cardiac insufficiency: failure of furosemide to provide the same result, *Am J Med* 96:191, 1994.
71. Anand IS, Ferrari R, Kalra GS et al: Edema of cardiac origin: studies of body water and sodium, renal function, hemodynamic indexes, and plasma hormones in untreated congestive cardiac failure, *Circulation* 80:299, 1989.

CHAPTER 10

Management of Heart Failure

General Principles

The primary aim of treating heart failure is to reduce the formation of edema and effusion. A second goal is to increase cardiac output. Almost all heart failure treatments are palliative rather than curative. Consequently, most patients that develop heart failure die from heart failure, often within a relatively short time. No studies have been performed in veterinary medicine to determine if any cardiovascular drug prolongs life. Certainly, diuretics prolong life. Without their administration, most patients with severe heart failure would die before leaving the hospital. Angiotensin converting enzyme (ACE) inhibitors have been shown to prolong life in humans with heart failure. However, this prolongation is modest, usually being measured in months rather than years. Digoxin has recently been shown not to prolong life in humans with heart failure.[1] Often of more importance is the effect cardiovascular drugs have on the quality of a patient's life. Diuretics and ACE inhibitors definitely improve quality of life in dogs and cats with heart failure. When patients become refractory to these drugs, other drugs may help reduce edema formation and improve perfusion and so reduce clinical signs and increase comfort.

In human medicine, heart failure is often staged and therapy altered depending on the stage or class of heart failure. The New York Heart Association (NYHA) developed a classification scheme that has been used in human medicine for decades. This classification scheme is primarily based on exercise limitation and ranges from class I (no exercise limitation) to class IV (inability to carry on any activity without symptoms). Exercise limitation is not the primary clinical abnormality that is noted by most owners of animals with heart failure. Instead, they most commonly note tachypnea, dyspnea, and coughing with left heart failure, ascites with right heart failure, or combinations of these plus respiratory difficulty resulting from pleural effusion with left and right heart failure. Consequently, the use of the NYHA scheme in dogs and cats is not useful. For the purposes of deciding drug therapy and drug doses, we prefer to categorize our patients simply into those with mild, moderate, or severe disease and mild, moderate, severe, fulminant, or refractory heart failure (Table 10-1). All patients with heart failure have severe disease. We further subdivide heart failure into acute and chronic heart failure. Most patients with acute heart failure present in severe or fulminant heart failure and require intensive therapy with intravenously administered furosemide or nitroprusside with or without dobutamine. Chronic left heart failure is graded based on the severity of the pulmonary edema on thoracic radiographs, and chronic right heart failure is based on hepatic vein size on an ultrasound examination and the amount of ascites present clinically or ultrasonographically. Increasing severity of chronic heart failure is treated with escalating doses of furosemide, whereas an ACE inhibitor is administered at a fixed dose. Digoxin may also be used, depending on the underlying disease and the stage of heart failure. Refractory heart failure is treated by adding a thiazide diuretic or a vasodilator, such as hydralazine or a nitrate, depending on the underlying disease and monitoring capabilities.

STANDARD THERAPY

Most human patients with heart failure are treated with the combination of three drug classes: digitalis glycosides, diuretics, and angiotensin converting enzyme (ACE) inhibitors. In 1994, a panel was convened to examine all of the large clinical studies pertaining to heart failure therapy in humans performed between 1966 and 1993.[2] A summary of their recommendations is as follows:

> ACE inhibitors should be given to all patients unless specific contraindications exist. Diuretics should be used judiciously early in treatment to prevent excessive diuresis that could prevent titration of ACE inhibitors to target doses. Digoxin has not been shown to affect the natural history of heart failure and should be reserved for patients who remain symptomatic after treatment with ACE inhibitors and diuretics. Isosorbide dinitrate and hydralazine should be tried in patients who cannot tolerate ACE inhibitors or who have refractory symptoms.

These recommendations are appropriate for many canine and feline patients with heart failure. However, this is not universally true. For example, the digitalis glycosides are generally considered to be contraindicated in patients with hypertrophic cardiomyopathy. As another example, there does not appear to be any primary indication for the digitalis glycosides in small canine patients with primary mitral regurgitation, although there may be secondary indications. Although many patients are treated with these three standard drug classes, there are certain situations in which the addition of other drugs is beneficial to the patient.

DRUG EFFICACY

It should be stressed that the efficacies of drugs that are used to treat heart failure vary considerably from drug class to drug class, from drug to drug, and from patient to patient. The efficacy of drugs when used for treating acute heart failure may be very different from when they are used for chronic therapy and vice versa. In general, the diuretics are the most efficacious of any drug class, and the loop diuretics are the most efficacious diuretic type. Although self-evident, no controlled studies have been performed to prove this. Tables 10-2 and 10-3 list our opinions of the efficacy of various drugs or drug types for acute and chronic therapy of heart failure in dogs and cats. The scale is from 1 to 10, with 10 being the best, representing the ideal heart failure drug ("idealamide"). Idealamide would decrease ventricular filling pressures while increasing cardiac

TABLE 10-1

Suggested drug regimens for treating heart failure caused by the three most common acquired cardiac diseases in dogs and cats

Type of heart failure	*Mitral regurgitation: dog*	*Dilated cardiomyopathy: dog*	*Hypertrophic cardiomyopathy: cat*
Chronic mild (mild pulmonary edema, ascites, and/or mild pleural effusion)	1. Furosemide: 1-2 mg/kg q12h-48h PO 2. ACEI	1. Furosemide: 1-2 mg/kg q12h-48h PO 2. ACEI 3. Digoxin	1. Furosemide: 3-6 mg/cat q12h-48h PO 2. Diltiazem or β-blocker
Chronic moderate (as above but moderate)	1. Furosemide: 1-2 mg/kg q8h-12h PO 2. ACEI 3. +/– Digoxin	1. Furosemide: 1-2 mg/kg q8h-12h PO 2. ACEI 3. Digoxin	1. Furosemide: 6-12.5 mg/cat q12-24h PO 2. Diltiazem or β-blocker
Chronic severe (as above but severe)	1. Furosemide: 2-4 mg/kg q8h-q12h PO 2. ACEI 3. +/– Low-salt diet 4. +/– Digoxin	1. Furosemide: 2-4 mg/kg q8h-q12h PO 2. ACEI 3. Digoxin 4. +/– Low-salt diet	1. Furosemide: 12.5 mg/cat q8h-q12h 2. Diltiazem and/or β-blocker 3. +/– Low-salt diet 4. +/– ACEI
Acute severe (severe pulmonary edema or pleural effusion)	1. Furosemide: 4-6 mg/kg q1h-q4h IV 2. Oxygen 3. +/– Nitroprusside 4. +/– Hydralazine 5. +/– Nitroglycerin	1. Furosemide: 4-6 mg/kg q1h-q4h IV 2. Oxygen 3. +/– Nitroprusside 4. +/– Dobutamine	1. Pleurocentesis 2. Furosemide: 2-4 mg/kg q2h-q4h IV or IM 3. Oxygen 4. Do not stress
Acute fulminant (massive pulmonary edema or pleural effusion with severe dyspnea)	1. Furosemide: 6-8 mg/kg q1h-q2h IV 2. Oxygen 3. +/– Nitroprusside 4. +/– Hydralazine 5. +/– Nitroglycerin	1. Furosemide: 6-8 mg/kg q1h-q2h IV 2. Oxygen 3. +/– Nitroprusside 4. +/– Dobutamine 5. +/– Nitroglycerin	1. Pleurocentesis 2. Furosemide: 2-4 mg/kg q1h-q2h IV or IM 3. Oxygen 4. Do not stress
Chronic refractory (signs of heart failure despite the administration of adequate doses of standard drugs)	1. Furosemide: 4 mg/kg q8h PO 2. ACEI 3. Low-salt diet 5. +/– Thiazide diuretic 6. +/– Hydralazine 7. +/– A nitrate	1. Furosemide: 4 mg/kg q8h PO 2. ACEI 3. Low-salt diet 4. Digoxin 5. +/– Thiazide diuretic 6. +/– A nitrate	1. Furosemide: 12.5-18.5 mg/cat q8h-q12h 2. Diltiazem and/or β-blocker 3. Low-salt diet 4. ACEI 5. +/– Thiazide diuretic 6. +/– A nitrate

The drugs and drug dosages in this table are presented as guidelines only. Choices of drugs and drug choices must be tailored to the individual patient. *Acute,* Patients that have usually been showing clinical signs for 24 hours or less that are not on current medications; *Chronic,* patients showing clinical signs usually for days to weeks or patients that are being treated and are now representing with clinical signs; +/–, the drug may be used in this situation; *ACEI,* angiotensin converting enzyme inhibitor

TABLE 10-2

Efficacy of drugs used acutely to treat heart failure

Drug	*Efficacy score*
Idealamide	10
Furosemide	8
Intravenous nitroprusside or nitroglycerin	7
Dobutamine/dopamine	4
Topical nitroglycerin	3
Digoxin	2
Angiotensin converting enzyme inhibitors	2
Hydralazine	6 (for MR); 2 (for DCM)

MR, Mitral regurgitation; *DCM,* dilated cardiomyopathy.

TABLE 10-3

Efficacy of drugs used chronically to treat heart failure

Drug	*Efficacy score*
Idealamide (e.g., taurine)	10
Furosemide	8
Angiotensin converting enzyme inhibitors	5
Digoxin	3
Hydralazine	6 (for MR); 2 (for DCM)
Topical nitroglycerin	3
Orally administered nitrates	Unknown, but may be as high as 4

MR, Mitral regurgitation; *DCM,* dilated cardiomyopathy.

output and would produce no change nor decrease systemic arterial blood pressure. In patients with myocardial failure, idealamide would produce these changes by increasing contractility without increasing myocardial oxygen consumption. Idealamide would not be arrhythmogenic. The only ideal heart failure "drug" identified in veterinary medicine is taurine in cats with taurine deficiency-induced myocardial failure (dilated cardiomyopathy). No other agent produces a response that is close to the response observed in these cats. Until the causes of the common cardiovascular diseases are identified in other species, therapy of heart failure will remain palliative and ultimately futile in most situations. Surgical therapy can be curative in some congenital heart abnormalities, such as patent ductus arteriosus.

Most patients that have clinical signs referable to heart failure, and most patients that die of heart failure do so because of severe edema or effusion. Consequently, drugs that reduce edema formation are generally considered more efficacious than drugs that primarily increase cardiac output. In human patients with severe chronic heart failure, inability to return pulmonary capillary pressure to normal with drug therapy is an independent predictor of mortality, whereas cardiac output and blood pressure are not.[3]

The efficacy of drugs to treat heart failure in human patients has been established by physicians performing large clinical trials that usually include more than 1000 patients. These types of clinical trials will never be conducted in veterinary medicine because of the expense involved and because there are too few qualified veterinarians able to conduct these sophisticated trials. Consequently, treatment of heart failure in veterinary medicine will probably always be based on the results of small clinical trials, on the opinions of "experts," and on extrapolation of data from human medicine. Expert opinion is based on clinical experience and biased by theory that has been garnered from the research and human clinical literature. One must always remember that theoretic mechanisms don't necessarily translate into clinical benefit. For a drug to be approved by the Food and Drug Administration (FDA) for use in humans in the United States, it must have a firm theoretic basis for its use (i.e., its use must be biologically plausible), a strong database of clinically meaningful benefit without significant complications or side effects, and statistically credible data in its support. Too often in veterinary medicine, recommendations for treating a disease are based on theory alone. This has been especially true in veterinary cardiovascular medicine. One must always be careful when taking the advice of an "expert" to make sure that individual is basing his or her advice on experience and not on theory alone.

Even in human medicine, results from large clinical trials only provide a physician with knowledge about how the average patient will respond. They provide only limited information about how an individual patient will respond and how that patient should be treated. Consequently, individual physicians must still rely on their own clinical experience and that of more experienced physicians to treat most patients. In many situations, physicians, like veterinarians, must rely on administering a drug or drugs to a patient and then evaluating and reevaluating the patient to determine the response and to plot a new strategy. As in all medical disciplines, there is an art to treating and caring for patients. Although some of this art can be taught, much of it must be learned by each individual through his or her own experience. The art of medical practice is best learned by working one-on-one with an experienced individual. That is why residency programs produce skilled individuals so quickly. Most veterinarians, however, do not have the luxury of learning in this type of environment. Working with a skilled veterinary practitioner, reading, practicing, and attending continuing education seminars are other ways of learning the art of medicine.

AGGRESSIVE TREATMENT OF SEVERE HEART FAILURE

Treating dogs and cats with mild-to-moderate heart failure is generally straightforward and rewarding. More skill is required to treat dogs and cats with severe heart failure. In our experience, these patients generally require aggressive therapy with high-dose furosemide administration in conjunction with other drugs. Less aggressive management is often less successful and often results in the patient's arguably premature death. This lack of success sometimes is rationalized by telling the owner and oneself that the patient had severe heart disease and could not be expected to live. However, in our experience, most of these patients do survive if treated aggressively, albeit for a finite time. In human medicine, Dr. Lynne Warner Stevenson is the cardiologist who has written the most recently about treating this type of patient. Her treatment style is very aggressive and very successful. She treats human patients that are referred for cardiac transplantation. Because there are always more patients than there are organs, she has a large population base of adults with severe heart failure that need aggressive therapy. In human medicine, this type of patient almost always has severe myocardial failure (ejection fraction less than 20%, which is comparable to a shortening fraction of less than 7%) and severe heart failure (average pulmonary capillary pressure is 35 mm Hg [normal is less than 12 mm Hg] and average cardiac index is 1.6 L/min/m^2 [normal is 3 to 4 L/min/m^2]). Her initial goal is to decrease pulmonary capillary pressure to normal (less than 15 mm Hg) and to decrease systemic vascular resistance to less than 1200 dynes $\times s \times cm^{-5}$ while maintaining systolic systemic blood pressure greater than 80 mm Hg.[4] She does this initially primarily by administering either nitroprusside or nitroglycerin and furosemide intravenously.[5] If necessary, she also administers dobutamine or dopamine intravenously. In a few patients, amrinone or milrinone administration is also required. Once the aforementioned hemodynamic goals are achieved (within 24 to 48 hours), she weans her patients off of the intravenous drugs while titrating them onto oral drugs. To maintain the same hemodynamic variables, she uses combinations of furosemide, ACE inhibitors, oral nitrates (usually isosorbide dinitrate), hydralazine, and digoxin. She uses ACE inhibitors at higher doses than those generally used by most physicians. For captopril, she will often administer 50 mg q6-8h. This is comparable to the dose of 0.5 to 1.0 mg/kg q8h recommended for dogs and cats. She rarely can produce her desired hemodynamic effect with ACE inhibitors and furosemide alone and almost always must administer isosorbide dinitrate in conjunction with the ACE inhibitor.[4] She does not hesitate to administer hydralazine in combination with the other drugs but presumably titrates the dose of this drug carefully to an effective endpoint. She advocates keeping patients very dry and feels this predicts her success.[6] In patients who drink fluids excessively she even advocates restricting their water intake. With this regimen, she improves the quality of her patients' lives to such a degree that their quality of life rivals that of patients who have received heart transplants.[7] She has also reported that the survival rate of her patients is much better than that of comparable patients who have been treated in large clinical trials.[6] Conventional wisdom would say that decreasing left ventricular filling pressure (pulmonary capillary pressure) to this degree in a patient with heart failure would result in a further decrease in cardiac output because of the decrease in preload and could result in harm to the patient. Dr. Stevenson has documented that stroke volume actually increases in her patients when left ventricular filling pressure is normalized.[8] This is probably the result of a decrease in the amount of mitral regurgitation that occurs as the left ventricle is decreased in size.[9] The decrease in left ventricular size probably results in a decrease in the size of mitral valve annulus and more appropriate papillary muscle orientation.

Because of the general lack of hemodynamic monitoring in veterinary medicine, administration of nitroprusside or nitroglycerin intravenously is generally not practical. Consequently, we teach students to administer high-dose (4 to 8 mg/kg) furosemide intravenously to achieve similar initial results to patients with severe or fulminant heart failure. Aggressive maintenance therapy with furosemide, ACE inhibitors, thiazide diuretics, and hydralazine is then used to maintain a normal respiratory rate. Drug doses are listed in Table 10-4. Unfortunately, veterinarians have little experience with the orally-active nitrates such as isosorbide dinitrate.

TABLE 10-4

Doses of drugs used in treating heart failure

Drug (trade name)	Species	Route	Dose
Angiotensin converting enzyme inhibitors			
Captopril (Capoten)	Both	PO	0.5-2.0 mg/kg q8h
Enalapril (Vasotec, Enacard)	Both	PO	0.5 mg/kg q12h
Lisinopril (Prinivil, Zestril)	Dog	PO	0.5 mg/kg q24h
Benazepril (Lotensin)	Both	PO	0.25-0.5 mg/kg q24h
Diuretics			
Furosemide (Lasix)	Dog	PO	1-4 mg/kg q8-24h, depending on need
Furosemide (Lasix)	Cat	PO	0.5-2 mg/kg q8-24h in most cases (may be increased if needed and the cat is eating and drinking normally)
Furosemide (Lasix)	Dog	IV, IM	2-8 mg/kg q1-6h (short-term emergency therapy)
Furosemide (Lasix)	Cat	IV, IM	1-4 mg/kg q1-6h (short-term emergency therapy)
Hydrochlorothiazide (many)	Dog	PO	2-4 mg/kg q12h
Spironolactone (many)	Dog	PO	2-4 mg/kg q12h
Positive inotropes			
Amrinone (Inocor)	Dog	IV	1-3 mg/kg (loading dose); 10-100 μg/kg/min (constant-rate infusion; start low; titrate)
Milrinone (Primacor)	Dog	IV	30-300 μg/kg (loading dose); 1-10 μg/kg/min (constant-rate infusion; start low; titrate)
Digoxin (Lan-/Cardoxin)	Dog	PO	Dog <15 kg: 0.006-0.011 mg/kg q12h; dog >15 kg: 0.22 mg/m^2 body surface area q12h
Digoxin (Lanoxin)	Dog	IV	0.0025 mg/kg q1h × 4 hr (total 0.01 mg/kg)
Digoxin (Lan-/Cardoxin)	Cat	PO	Cat 2-3 kg: ¼ of 0.125-mg tab q48h; cat 4-6 kg: ¼ of 0.125-mg tab q24h; cat >6 kg: ¼ of 0.125-mg tab q12-24h
Digitoxin (Crystodigin)	Dog	PO	0.02-0.03 mg/kg q8h
Dobutamine (Dobutrex)	Dog	IV	2.5-20 μg/kg/min (constant-rate infusion)
Dobutamine (Dobutrex)	Cat	IV	2-10 μg/kg/min (constant-rate infusion)
Dopamine (Intropin)	Dog	IV	2.5-15 μg/kg/min (constant-rate infusion)
Dopamine (Intropin)	Cat	IV	2-10 μg/kg/min (constant-rate infusion)
Vasodilators			
Hydralazine (Apresoline)	Dog	PO	0.5-3 mg/kg q12h (start low; titrate)
Hydralazine (Apresoline)	Cat	PO	2.5-10 mg/cat q12h (start low; titrate)
Nitroglycerin ointment (many)	Dog	Topical	4-15 mg q6-12h (1 inch = 15 mg)
Nitroglycerin ointment (many)	Cat	Topical	3-4 mg q6-12h
Nitroprusside (Nipride)	Dog	IV	2.0-10 μg/kg/min (constant-rate infusion; start low; titrate)
Prazosin (Minipress)	Dog	PO	Small dog: 0.5-1.0 mg q8h, begin with 0.5 mg; medium to large dog: 1-2 mg; begin with 1 mg

Drugs Used in Treating Heart Failure

A summary of drugs, including manufacturers and supply information, used in treating heart failure in veterinary patients is presented in Table 10-5.

DIURETICS

In veterinary medicine, diuretics, especially the loop diuretics, are the most important and efficacious class of drugs used for treating heart failure. Most patients with heart failure, if left untreated, would die of severe edema. Death from poor systemic blood flow would be extremely uncommon. Consequently, the primary goal in these patients is to control edema formation. Although other agents, such as ACE inhibitors, nitrates, and low-salt diets, are used for this purpose, their ability to control edema formation is at least one order of magnitude less than that of the loop diuretics.

In many patients with heart failure, edema is the direct consequence of an increase in blood volume. Blood volume may be increased by as much as 30% in patients with severe heart failure.[10] Diuretics decrease edema formation by decreasing this excess blood volume. The decrease in blood volume results in decreases in diastolic intraventricular and capillary pressures.

Furosemide is the most commonly used diuretic in small animal veterinary medicine. This particular drug has many advantages. It is potent and so generally will produce a response. It can be administered over a wide dose range so the dose can be tailored to the individual patient's needs. It can be administered per os or parenterally and so can be used for chronic administration or for emergency therapy. In dogs and cats, as long as the patient is eating and drinking normally and the drug is used judiciously, the side effects are few.

Because diuretics have been used for decades to treat patients with heart failure and because their mechanism of action is relatively simple, diuretics are often taken for granted. It is common for a veterinarian to administer furosemide and an ACE inhibitor to a patient with severe congestive heart failure and then ascribe the

TABLE 10-5

Drugs used in treating heart failure

Drug	*Trade name*	*Manufacturer*	*Address*	*Supply*
Milrinone	Primacor IV	Sanofi Winthrop Pharmaceuticals	New York, N.Y.	10- and 20-mL vials (1 mg/mL)
Amrinone	Inocor	Sanofi Winthrop Pharmaceuticals	New York, N.Y.	20-mL ampules (5 mg/mL)
Dobutamine	Dobutrex	Eli Lilly and Co.	Indianapolis, Ind.	250 mg white powder; 20-mL vial
Dopamine	Intropin	DuPont Critical Care	Waukegan, Ill.	Ampules, vials, and syringes at concentrations from 40 mg/mL to 160 mg/mL
Digoxin capsules	Lanoxicaps	Burroughs Wellcome Co.	Research Triangle Park, N.C.	Capsules containing 0.05, 0.1, and 0.2 mg digoxin in 8% alcohol
Digoxin elixir	Lanoxin Elixir	Burroughs Wellcome Co.; Bausch & Lomb, Inc.; Halsey Drug Co.; Roxane Laboratories, Inc.	Research Triangle Park, N.C.; Rochester, N.Y.; Brooklyn, N.Y.; Columbus, Ohio	Liquid preparation containing digoxin in 10% alcohol containing 0.05 or 0.15 mg/mL
Digoxin tablets	Lanoxin	Burroughs Wellcome Co.	Research Triangle Park, N.C.	0.125-, 0.250-, and 0.5-mg tablets
Injectable digoxin	Lanoxin Injection Pediatric	Burroughs Wellcome Co.	Research Triangle Park, N.C.	Solution containing 0.1 mg/mL
Digitoxin	Crystodigin	Eli Lilly and Co.	Indianapolis, Ind.	0.05-, 0.1-, 0.15-, and 0.2-mg tablets
Spironolactone	Aldactone	Searle Laboratories	Chicago, Ill.	25-mg tablets and 25-, 50-, and 100-mg film-coated tablets
Spironolactone/ hydrochlorothiazide	Aldactazide	Searle Laboratories	Chicago, Ill.	Tablets containing 25 mg spironolactone and 25 mg hydrochlorothiazide or as film-coated tablets containing 25 mg spironolactone and 25 mg hydrochlorothiazide or 50 mg spironolactone and 50 mg hydrochlorothiazide
Triamterene	Dyrenium	SmithKline Beecham	Philadelphia, Pa.	50- and 100-mg capsules
Triamterene/ hydrochlorothiazide	Dyazide	SmithKline Beecham	Philadelphia, Pa.	50-mg triamterene and 25-mg hydrochlorothiazide tablets
Amiloride	Midamor	Merck Sharpe & Dohme	West Point, Pa.	5-mg tablets
Amiloride/ hydrochlorothiazide	Moduretic	Merck Sharpe & Dohme	West Point, Pa.	5-mg amiloride and 50-mg hydrochlorothiazide tablets
Bumetanide	Bumex	Roche Laboratories	Nutley, N.J.	0.5-, 1-, and 2-mg tablets
Furosemide (veterinary formulation)	Lasix	Hoechst-Roussell Pharmaceuticals	Somerville, N.J.	12.5- and 50-mg tablets, 10-mg/mL oral solution, and 50-mg/mL solution for injection
Furosemide	Fumide, Lasix, Luramide	Everett Laboratories; Hoechst-Roussell Pharmaceuticals; Major Pharamaceutical	East Orange, N.J.; Somerville, N.J.; San Diego, Calif.	20-, 40-, and 80-mg tablets

marked beneficial response to the ACE inhibitor. This is rarely the correct assessment. Rather, marked beneficial responses in patients with severe heart failure are much less common with any other type of drug. We have observed dramatic responses to only a few specific drugs in patients with congestive heart failure. Approximately 90% of these observations have occurred following furosemide administration (Figure 10-1). The other 10% have occurred following hydralazine administration to dogs with mitral or aortic regurgitation (Figure 10-2), following experimental chronic oral milrinone administration to dogs with dilated cardiomyopathy or mitral regurgitation, following nitroprusside administration to dogs with mitral regurgitation or dilated cardiomyopathy, and, occasionally, following ACE inhibitor administration. Milrinone is not available for chronic administration. Hydralazine is not commonly used because of its side effects and the difficulty that veterinarians have in titrating it to an effective endpoint. Nitroprusside is rarely used in veterinary practice because it must be titrated and because of the requirement for hemodynamic monitoring. ACE inhibitors produce dramatic responses less than 10% of the time. Consequently, furosemide is the only commonly used cardiovascular drug that frequently produces dramatic clinical responses in patients with heart failure. Most other drugs produce a lesser response and should be considered as adjunct therapy. These other drugs are still valuable to help fine-tune the therapeutic regimen and help stabilize the patient in many cases. They also are very helpful in patients that are refractory to furosemide administration.

Diuretics have been used for decades to treat a variety of cardiovascular disorders in humans. The organic mercurials were originally used to treat syphilis and it was in this context that their diuretic action was noted. Furosemide first became available to the veterinary profession in the late 1960s.[11,12]

Renal tubule physiology and diuretic actions. To understand the action of diuretics, it is necessary to understand basic renal tubule physiology. The proximal tubule resorbs 50% to 60% of the filtered

A

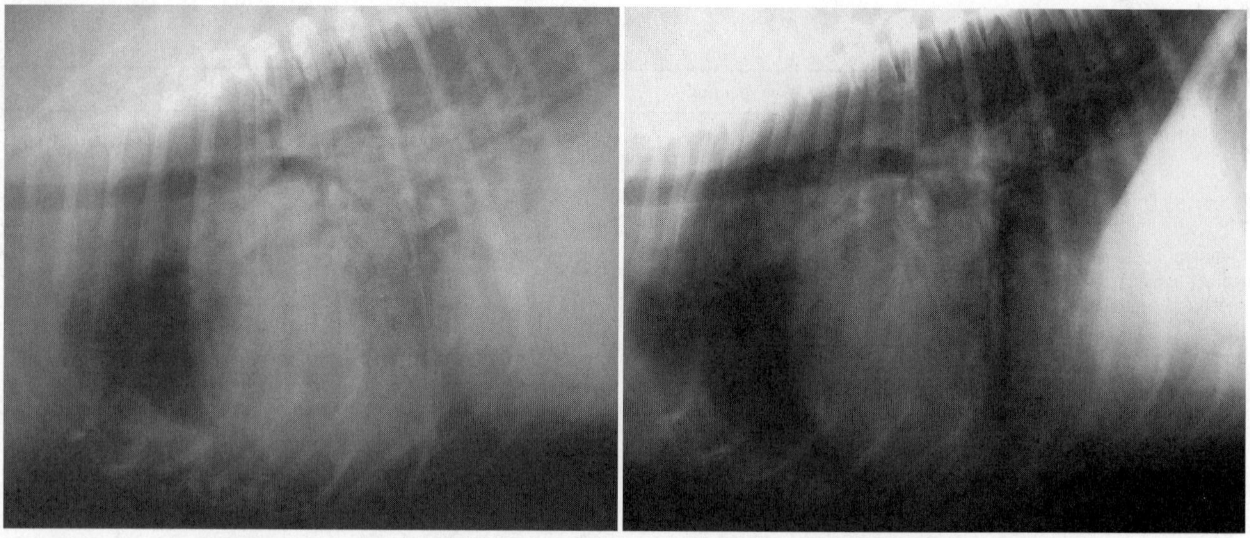

B

FIGURE 10-1 Lateral radiographs from a 9-year-old male Doberman pinscher with severe dilated cardiomyopathy taken before **(A)** and 24 hours after **(B)** starting high-dose furosemide therapy. In **A** there is severe pulmonary edema. The dog was administered approximately 8 mg/kg furosemide IV q1-2 hours for 6 hours. The dose was then reduced to 4 mg/kg q6 hours. The day after initiating therapy **(B)** the edema has resolved. The dog's respiratory rate decreased from 84 breaths/min to 48 breaths/min within the first 8 hours and its dyspnea resolved.

A

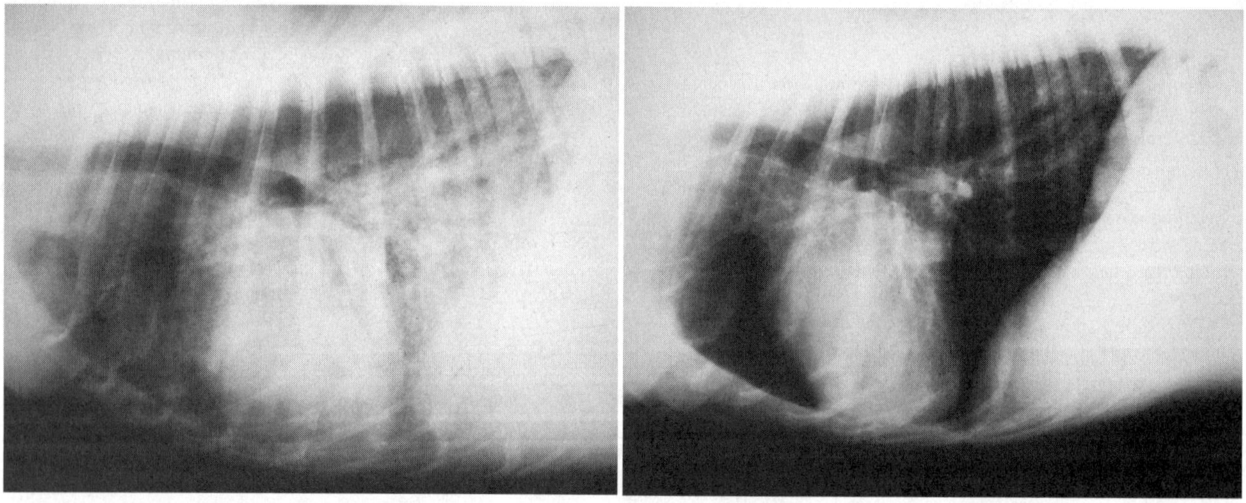

B

FIGURE 10-2 Lateral radiographs from a 6-year-old Doberman pinscher with acute bacterial endocarditis of the aortic valve leading to severe aortic regurgitation. The radiographs were taken before **(A)** and 24 hours after **(B)** hydralazine administration. Before drug administration there is severe pulmonary edema. After hydralazine administration, the pulmonary edema has resolved. The cardiac silhouette does not appear to be enlarged because of the acute nature of this dog's illness.

sodium and water. Sodium is initially transported across the cell membrane in exchange for a hydrogen ion by a protein called the *Na^+/H^+ antiporter.*[13] Sodium is then transported out of the cell into the interstitium and into the blood at the basolateral membrane by a sodium pump and the $Na^+/3HCO_3^-$ cotransporter.[14] Sodium transport in the proximal tubule is regulated by glomerular filtration rate, the sympathetic nervous system, angiotensin II, atrial natriuretic factor, and peritubular hemodynamics.[15] The brush border of the proximal tubule contains a vast quantity of carbonic anhydrase, an enzyme that catalyzes the reaction between carbon dioxide and water to form carbonic acid. Drugs that inhibit carbonic anhydrase constitute the major class of diuretics that act in the proximal tubule. Acetazolamide is the only carbonic anhydrase inhibitor available in the United States. It is not useful in patients with heart failure primarily because the remaining portion of the nephron can reabsorb sodium. As a consequence, carbonic anhydrase inhibitors can only cause the excretion of modest amounts of sodium, approximately 3% to 5% of the filtered load.

About 25% to 30% of the filtered sodium is reabsorbed in the loop of Henle. The thin descending loop of Henle is impermeable to sodium but permeable to water. Sodium and chloride transport into the interstitium occurs in the thick ascending loop of Henle. The sodium transport in this region is the basis for the countercurrent exchange mechanism. The amount of sodium reabsorbed is regulated by the amount of sodium delivered to the thick ascending loop, the sympathetic nervous system, the osmolality of the filtrate, and prostaglandins. Loop diuretics act by inhibiting the $Na^+/K^+/2Cl^-$ transporter on the luminal surface of the thick ascending loop of Henle.[16] Because this transporter is present only on the luminal surface, loop diuretics must be delivered to the tubule by blood flow and then secreted into the lumen of the nephron to be effective. Loop diuretics are the most potent natriuretic drugs available. They are capable of causing excretion of 15% to 20% of filtered sodium. This potent effect is possible because loop diuretics act in a region of the nephron where significant sodium transport occurs and at a site where only limited sodium reabsorption can occur distal to the site of action.

Approximately 5% to 8% of filtered sodium is reabsorbed in the early distal convoluted tubule. The proximal portion of the distal tubule is an extension of the thick ascending loop of Henle. It contains an electroneutral sodium chloride cotransporter. Sodium chloride reabsorption is impaired in this region by the thiazide diuretics. Very little is known about the NaCl transport system that is inhibited by thiazides.

Only about 2% to 3% of filtered sodium is reabsorbed in the terminal portion of the distal tubule and the collecting tubule. At these sites, a specialized transport mechanism causes the reabsorption of sodium in exchange for potassium and hydrogen ions. This transport system is subdivided into a portion that is influenced by aldosterone and a portion that is independent of mineralocorticoid influence. Spironolactone antagonizes the effect of aldosterone at this site, resulting in mild natriuresis. Amiloride also acts in this site, but blocks the independent sodium channel.[16] Triamterene's mode of action is not well understood but it is probably similar to that of amiloride.[16]

Diuretics increase urine flow by increasing renal plasma flow or altering nephron function. Diuretics that increase renal plasma flow by expanding plasma volume (e.g., mannitol, glucose) are contraindicated in patients with heart failure because they increase venous and capillary pressures and thus increase edema formation. Agents that alter nephron function increase urine production by interfering with ion transport or the action of aldosterone or antidiuretic hormone (ADH) within the nephron (Color Plate 35). Because the goal of diuretic therapy in heart failure is promotion of sodium and water loss, agents that cause only water loss by interfering with ADH are not generally indicated for use.

Agents that interfere with ion transport do so by altering (1) intracellular ionic entry, (2) energy generation and utilization for ion transport, or (3) ion transfer from the cell to the peritubular capillaries through the antiluminal membrane.[17] Agents that interfere with ion transport also differ as to their site of action within the nephron. In general, agents that act on the loop of Henle are the most potent.

Three classes of diuretics are used clinically in dogs to treat heart failure: thiazide diuretics, loop diuretics, and potassium-sparing diuretics. They differ in their ability to promote sodium and water excretion and in mechanism of action. Thiazide diuretics are mildly to moderately potent agents.[18] They are most commonly used in conjunction with a loop diuretic in patients with severe congestive heart failure that are refractory to loop diuretics. The loop diuretics are the most potent and can be used in small doses in patients with mild-to-moderate heart failure and in higher doses in patients with severe heart failure. They can be administered orally for chronic administration or can be administered parenterally to patients with acute, severe heart failure. The use of potassium-sparing diuretics is reserved for those patients that become hypokalemic with other diuretics and for patients refractory to other agents because of an elevated plasma aldosterone concentration. In the latter situation, potassium-sparing diuretics are administered in conjunction with another diuretic, usually a loop diuretic.

Loop diuretics (e.g., furosemide) are the diuretics of choice in cats, but thiazides are occasionally employed. Potassium-sparing agents are rarely used in cats.[19]

Thiazide diuretics

Actions. The thiazides act primarily by reducing membrane permeability in the distal convoluted tubule to sodium and chloride.[18] They promote potassium loss at this site and produce large increases in the urine sodium concentration but only mild-to-moderate increases in urine volume. Consequently, only mild-to-moderate renal sodium loss is promoted. Thiazide diuretics increase renal sodium excretion from a normal value of about 1% to 5% up to 8% of the filtered load. Thiazide-induced renal sodium excretion is only one third that achieved with the loop diuretics. Thiazide diuretics also inhibit carbonic anhydrase in the proximal tubules, but this effect varies considerably among the various agents. The thiazides are ineffective when renal blood flow is low, which may explain their lack of efficacy in patients with severe heart failure.

Thiazide diuretics decrease the glomerular filtration rate, which may explain their lack of efficacy in patients with renal failure. It is unknown whether this effect is due to a direct effect on renal vasculature or is secondary to decrease in intravascular fluid volume.

In addition to their effects on sodium and chloride, the thiazides also increase potassium excretion because of the increased sodium that reaches the distal tubular site of sodium-potassium exchange. Thiazides also increase bicarbonate excretion. Long-term thiazide administration can result in mild metabolic alkalosis associated with hypokalemia and hypochloremia in human patients. The effects in dogs and cats are less clear. Plasma renin concentration is increased by thiazide administration. This probably is due to the decrease in plasma volume.

Pharmacokinetics and dosage. In dogs, the thiazides are well absorbed after oral administration. The action of chlorothiazide begins within 1 hour, peaks at 4 hours, and lasts 6 to 12 hours. The dosage is 20 to 40 mg/kg q12h. Hydrochlorothiazide has an onset of action within 2 hours, peaks at 4 hours, and lasts 12 hours. The oral canine dose is 2 to 4 mg/kg q12h; cats are administered 1 to 2 mg/kg q12h. The newer, more lipid-soluble thiazides (trichlormethiazide, cyclothiazide) have not been studied in the dog or cat.

Indications. Our most common use of the thiazide diuretics is in patients that are refractory to furosemide administration. Use of a thiazide diuretic in combination with furosemide in such patients commonly results in restoration of diuresis, decreased edema formation, and clinical improvement. Side effects are more common with this combination.

Supply. Chlorothiazide (Diachlor, Major Pharmaceutical, San Diego, Calif.; Diurigen, Goldline Laboratories, Fort Lauderdale, Fla.; Diuril, Merck Sharp & Dohme, West Point, Pa.) is supplied as 250- and 500-mg tablets and as a 50-mg/mL oral suspension. Hydrochlorothiazide is supplied as 25- and 50-mg tablets by numerous manufacturers (Esidrex, Ciba Pharmaceutical, Summit, N.J.; HydroDIURIL, Merck Sharp & Dohme, West Point, Pa.; Hydro-T, Major Pharmaceutical, San Diego, Calif.; Oretic, Abbott Laboratories, North Chicago, Ill.; Thiuretic, Warner-Chilcott Labs, Morris Plains, N.J.).

Loop diuretics (furosemide, bumetanide). The loop diuretics include furosemide, ethacrynic acid, and bumetanide. Furosemide is the most commonly used diuretic for treating heart failure in the dog and cat. Ethacrynic acid is rarely used. Bumetanide is a new agent that is 40 to 50 times as potent as furosemide and may offer some clinical advantages.[20] No one in veterinary medicine in the United States has much clinical experience with this drug. All loop diuretics inhibit sodium, potassium, and chloride reabsorption in the thick portion of the ascending loop of Henle.[21] In so doing, they inhibit sodium and obligatory water reabsorption in the nephron. The loop diuretics are capable of increasing the maximal fractional excretion of sodium to 15% to 25% of the filtered load, making them the most powerful natriuretic agents available.[22]

Actions. Furosemide is a sulfonamide type of loop diuretic. Furosemide inhibits the reabsorption of electrolytes in the thick ascending loop of Henle. Furosemide also decreases reabsorption of sodium and chloride in the distal renal tubule. Furosemide diuresis results in enhanced excretion of sodium, chloride, potassium, hydrogen, calcium, magnesium, and, possibly, phosphate. Chloride excretion is equal to or exceeds sodium excretion.[23,24] In one study, furosemide at a dose of 1 mg/kg to normal anesthetized dogs increased sodium excretion from a baseline average of 144 μEq/min to 2419 μEq/min, approximately a 17-fold increase.[24] Potassium excretion is much less affected in dogs.[23,25] In this same study, potassium excretion did not change (112 μEq/min at baseline and 110 μEq/min following 1 mg/kg furosemide IV).[24] In another study, a 1-mg/kg dose doubled potassium excretion.[26] In one study, magnesium excretion increased from 12.3 μEq/min to 51.9 μEq/min.[24] Calcium excretion increased from 24 μg/min to 1169 μg/min. The effect on calcium excretion makes furosemide particularly useful in patients with hypercalcemia. The natriuretic effect of furosemide is attenuated by aspirin administration in dogs.[27] Aspirin and furosemide are commonly administered together in cats with cardiomyopathies. This practice should be reexamined. Enhanced hydrogen ion excretion without a concomitant increase in bicarbonate excretion can result in metabolic alkalosis in normal dogs.[23] This effect is rarely clinically significant, although it could be beneficial in dogs with preexisting metabolic acidosis as a result of poor perfusion. Despite the increase in net acid excretion, urinary pH falls slightly after furosemide administration.[23] Urine specific gravity generally decreases into the 1.006 to 1.020 range.

In addition to its diuretic effects, furosemide acts as a venodilator, decreasing venous pressures before diuresis takes place (especially after intravenous administration).[28] The venodilation requires the presence of the kidneys (does not occur in anephric dogs or humans), meaning this effect is probably an indirect one.[28,29] Furosemide decreases renal vascular resistance; thus it acutely increases renal blood flow (on the order of 50%) without changing glomerular filtration rate.[30-33] Indomethacin and aspirin completely inhibit this increase in renal blood flow in dogs.[33] Furosemide's effects on intrarenal distribution of blood flow in dogs is controversial. Distribution has been reported to increase to the inner cortical region in one study and not to change in another.[33,34]

Furosemide increases thoracic duct lymph flow in dogs.[35] This effect is independent of renal function because it occurs in nephrectomized animals and animals with bilateral ureteral ligation. However, this effect is only observed following high doses (8 to 10 mg/kg IV) and not after doses of 1 to 2 mg/kg. The basis for this effect is unexplained.

Furosemide acts as a bronchodilator in humans, horses, and guinea pigs.[36-38] It can be administered as an inhalant in humans with asthma. Its effects in dogs and cats are unknown. If it does have bronchodilating effects in cats and dogs, it could have beneficial effects in cats with asthma, in dogs with chronic bronchitis, and, possibly, in dogs with pulmonary edema secondary to left heart failure.[39] The importance of bronchoconstriction in humans with heart failure ("cardiac asthma") is unknown. A recent review article in the human literature on the subject states, "Patients with left ventricular failure are commonly treated with bronchodilator drugs, but the basis for this approach needs further clarification."[40] Producing bronchodilation is probably of less importance in dogs than in humans because airway responsiveness (e.g., bronchoconstriction) in dogs is less than that observed in humans.

Renin secretion is increased by furosemide administration.[41] This occurs via two mechanisms. There is an early and rapid increase in renin secretion following furosemide administration that is not prevented by β-blocker administration or ureterovenous anastomosis to prevent volume depletion. Consequently, this increase is a direct effect of the drug on the macula densa.[42] There is also a later (6 hours) increase in renin secretion that is prevented by β-blocker administration and ureterovenous anastomosis. Consequently, this increase is due to volume depletion and secondary sympathetic stimulation. Renin secretion with subsequent aldosterone secretion should result in sodium and water retention. This effect is obviously easily overcome by furosemide's more potent actions on the nephron.

Pharmacokinetics. Furosemide is highly protein bound (86% to 91%).[26,43] The ratio of kidney to plasma concentration is 5:1.[44] A small amount of furosemide (1% to 14%) is metabolized to a glucuronide derivative in dogs, but this metabolism does not take place in the liver.[26,43] However, about 45% of furosemide is excreted in the bile and 55% is excreted in the urine in dogs.[45] After intravenous administration, furosemide has an elimination half-life of approximately 1 hour.[25] Intravenously, furosemide's onset of action is within 5 minutes, peak effects occur within 30 minutes, and duration of effect is 2 to 3 hours.[25] Also after intravenous administration, about 50% of the drug is cleared from the body within the first 30 minutes, 90% is eliminated within the first 2 hours, and almost all is eliminated within 3 hours.[45] Furosemide is rapidly but incompletely absorbed after oral administration, with a bioavailability of 40% to 50%.[46] The terminal half-life after oral administration is biexponential, with an initial phase that has a half-life of approximately 30 minutes and a second phase with a half-life of approximately 7 hours.[46] The initial disposition phase has the most effect on plasma concentration, with plasma concentration decreasing from therapeutic to subtherapeutic range within the first 4 to 6 hours after oral administration. After oral administration, onset of action occurs within 60 minutes, peak effects occur within 1 to 2 hours, and duration of effect is approximately 6 hours.[46] In normal dogs, a dose of 2.5 mg/kg furosemide intramuscularly results in maximum natriuresis (beyond that dose there is no further increase in sodium excretion). This occurs at a plasma concentration of approximately 0.8 μg/mL.[33] Because the diuretic effect of furosemide is dependent on its delivery to the kidney by blood flow, patients with decreased renal blood flow (e.g., patients with heart failure) need a higher plasma concentration and higher doses to produce the same effect observed in normal dogs.

Experimentally-induced renal failure (BUN = 70 +/– 26; creatinine = 2.4 +/– 0.9) approximately doubles the serum half-life of furosemide in dogs and decreases renal clearance to 15% of control.[45] Experimentally induced renal failure also markedly attenuates the diuretic effect of the drug to approximately one third of control. Consequently a higher serum concentration of furosemide is required to produce the same diuretic effect in dogs with renal failure. However, the relationship between the rate of urinary furosemide excretion and diuresis remains constant. Consequently, the decrease in diuresis in dogs with renal failure appears to be due to a decrease in delivery of furosemide to the nephron. In canine patients with renal failure, two discordant effects interact on the diuretic effects of furosemide. First, the prolongation in half-life increases the serum concentration for any given chronically administered dose. This increases diuresis. Second, the diuretic effect for any given serum concentration is reduced. This complex interaction makes it much more difficult to determine an effective dose for furosemide in a patient with renal failure.

Very few studies have examined the effects of furosemide in cats. Cats may be more sensitive to furosemide than dogs. In one study, the increase in urine volume was comparable between normal cats and normal dogs in doses from 0.625 to 10 mg/kg IM.[47] However, sodium excretion was between 1.3 and 2.2 times (average, 1.7 times) that seen in dogs at each dosage. The slope and x-axis intercept of the regression equation between furosemide dose and sodium excretion (mmole/kg) for cats were both about twice that for dogs. In another study, fractional excretion of sodium increased from an average of 1.5% at baseline to 23% with a dose of 5 mg/kg furosemide IV.[48] Even with a dose of 1 mg/kg fractional excretion of sodium was 18%, indicating that the effect of furosemide starts to plateau somewhere between 1 and 5 mg/kg IV in cats. Clinically, cats commonly require no more than 2 mg/kg q8-12h PO chronically for the treatment of pulmonary edema.[19] However, as stated previously, higher doses may be needed in feline patients with severe heart failure because of reduced renal blood flow.

Administration and dosage. The canine oral dose for furosemide for treating chronic heart failure ranges from 1 mg/kg every other day for very mild heart failure to 4 mg/kg q8h for severe heart failure. The oral furosemide dose in cats ranges from 1 mg/kg every 2 to 3 days to 2 mg/kg q8-12h in most cases.[19] We, however, have used doses as high as 7 mg/kg q12h and have administered 6 mg/kg every other day to cats that are difficult to pill. Owners must be warned that high-dose diuretic therapy can produce profound dehydration in patients that are not drinking or that stop drinking adequate quantities of water.

Severe pulmonary edema requires immediate intensive intravenous or intramuscular administration in dogs and cats, using doses up to 8 mg/kg every 1 to 2 hours in dogs and up to 4 mg/kg every 1 to 2 hours in cats. High-dose furosemide administration generally should be continued until the respiratory rate decreases and/or respiratory character improves. Such intensive dosing may result in mild hypokalemia (serum K^+ concentration between 3.0 and 3.5 mEq/L), mild-to-moderate hyponatremia (serum Na^+ concentration between 135 and 145 mEq/L), and mild dehydration. These may need to be addressed after the life-threatening pulmonary edema has been controlled. However, in dogs, electrolyte disturbances and dehydration are usually corrected when the dog feels good enough to eat and drink once the pulmonary edema has resolved. In addition, the electrolyte abnormalities and dehydration are usually not clinically significant unless severe overdosing has occurred. Consequently, aggressive fluid therapy for these abnormalities is not required and often is contraindicated because such fluid therapy can result in recrudescence of the heart failure. In cats, judicious administration of fluids may be required to rehydrate the patient after intensive diuresis, because cats often do not start to eat and drink as readily as dogs. Clinically significant electrolyte disturbances and dehydration are rare in dogs that are chronically being administered furosemide unless maximal doses are employed and anorexia is present.[49] These abnormalities may be more common in cats.

An alternative to bolus injection of high doses of furosemide to patients with severe heart failure is continuous infusion of furosemide. This method has been employed in human medicine. The same dose administered continuously over 24 hours produces greater natriuresis and diuresis than bolus administration.[50]

Adverse effects. Furosemide can produce adverse effects in dogs and cats. Those adverse effects shared with other diuretics are presented below. Furosemide has the potential for ototoxicity. However, when administered as the sole agent, doses in excess of approximately 20 mg/kg IV are required to produce any loss in hearing ability in dogs.[51] Doses in the 50- to 100-mg/kg range produce profound loss of hearing. Furosemide can potentiate the ototoxic effects of other drugs, such as the aminoglycosides. Furosemide also potentiates the nephrotoxic effects of the aminoglycosides in the dog.[52] This may occur because furosemide accelerates the accumulation of gentamicin in renal cells.[53] Furosemide does not have any nephrotoxic effects when administered by itself. Prerenal azotemia can occur if moderate-to-severe dehydration is produced in an animal with heart failure. Theoretically, primary renal failure can occur if severe dehydration is produced in a patient with heart failure, resulting in a marked and prolonged decrease in renal perfusion.

Formulation. Furosemide injection contains the sodium salt of furosemide that is formed by the addition of sodium hydroxide during manufacturing. It should be stored at a temperature of 15° to 30° C and protected from light. Injections with a yellow color have degraded and should not be used. Exposure of furosemide tablets to light may cause discoloration and should not be used. Furosemide injection can be mixed with weakly alkaline and neutral solutions having a pH of 7 to 10, such as 0.9% saline or Ringer's solution. A precipitate may form if the injection is mixed with strongly acidic solutions, such as those containing ascorbic acid, tetracycline, epinephrine, or norepinephrine. Furosemide injection also should not be mixed with most salts of organic bases including local anesthetics, alkaloids, antihistamines, and morphine.

Supply. The veterinary formulation of furosemide (Lasix, Hoechst-Roussell Pharmaceuticals, Somerville, N.J.) is supplied as 12.5- and 50-mg tablets, a 10-mg/mL oral solution, and a 50-mg/mL solution for injection. Furosemide (Fumide, Everett Laboratories, East Orange, N.J.; Lasix, Hoechst-Roussell Pharmaceuticals, Somerville, N.J.; Luramide, Major Pharmaceutical, San Diego, Calif.) is also supplied as 20-, 40-, and 80-mg tablets.

Bumetanide. Bumetanide is a potent, sulfonamide type of loop diuretic that is structurally related to furosemide. It is approximately 25 to 50 times as potent as furosemide in the dog.[54] This increased potency is due to a more potent effect on sodium transport in the ascending loop of Henle and to a threefold greater renal uptake of the drug compared with furosemide.[26,44] Bumetanide is more potent in the dog than in rabbits, mice, or rats because metabolism to inactive metabolites is less in the dog.[55] Approximately 67% of bumetanide in dogs is recovered as unchanged drug in the urine and feces. Most of the remaining drug is conjugated in the liver to form an alkali-labile acyl glucuronide metabolite.[55]

Similar to furosemide, bumetanide produces pronounced natriuresis and chloruresis, with chloride excretion being more pronounced in the dog. In normal anesthetized dogs, bumetanide increases sodium and chloride excretion 25- to 50-fold while increasing potassium excretion only 3- to 5-fold.[24] Also, like furosemide, bumetanide increases renal blood flow through renal artery dilation.[42] This effect is also abolished by administration of prostaglandin synthetase inhibitors (e.g., indomethacin).[44] In dogs, it redistributes blood flow to the midcortical and juxtamedullary regions of the kidney. Bumetanide also increases renin secretion, presumably through direct and indirect effect.[44]

After oral administration of bumetanide to experimental dogs, urine volume and sodium excretion increase within the first hour, peak effects are observed within 2 hours, and duration of effects is 4 to 5 hours. After intravenous administration, peak effect occurs in the first hour and the duration of effect is 3 to 4 hours.[44,56]

There are no reports in the veterinary literature of the use of bumetanide in dogs or cats with heart failure. The effects of bumetanide in human patients with heart failure appears to be comparable to those observed with furosemide.[57] Consequently, it is questionable if there are any distinct advantages of this drug over furosemide. Based on the comparisons of potency that have been done between bumetanide and furosemide in dogs, the oral dose of bumetanide should be approximately 1⁄50 of furosemide. This means the dose should be in the range of 0.02 to 0.1 mg/kg administered 2 to 3 times a day.

Bumetanide (Bumex, Roche Laboratories, Nutley, N.J.) is supplied in 0.5-, 1-, and 2-mg tablets. It is also supplied as a 1% solution for parenteral injection at a concentration of 0.25 mg/mL.

Potassium-sparing diuretics (spironolactone, triamterene, amiloride)

Actions. The potassium-sparing class of diuretics acts by inhibiting the action of aldosterone on distal tubular cells or blocking the entry of sodium in the latter regions of the distal tubule and collecting tubules.[16] In normal animals, plasma aldosterone concentration is relatively low, hence the effect of these diuretics is mild. In normal dogs, they can only increase the maximal fractional excretion of sodium to 2% of the filtered load.[58] In dogs with heart failure and increased plasma aldosterone concentration, the effect of these diuretics may be greater. However, potassium-sparing diuretics are rarely used as sole agents in patients with heart failure. When potassium-sparing diuretics are administered with other diuretics, potassium loss is decreased. Consequently, they can be administered to patients that become hypokalemic because of the administration of other diuretic agents.

Spironolactone. Spironolactone is structurally similar to aldosterone and binds competitively to aldosterone's binding sites in the distal tubule. Its onset of action is slow in dogs and peak effect does not occur until 2 to 3 days after administration commences.[59] The drug is extensively and rapidly metabolized to canrenone and other metabolites in plasma, which are pharmacologically active but much less so than the parent compound. The duration of effect for spironolactone is 2 to 3 days after cessation of drug administration.[59] The dose of spironolactone for dogs is 2 to 4 mg/kg/day.

Triamterene. Triamterene is a potassium-sparing diuretic that is structurally related to folic acid. It acts directly on the distal tubule to depress reabsorption of sodium and decrease the excretion of potassium and hydrogen.[60] It does not competitively inhibit aldosterone. Its action begins within 2 hours, peaks at 6 to 8 hours, and lasts 12 to 16 hours.[59] The oral canine dose of triamterene is 2 to 4 mg/kg/day.

Amiloride. Amiloride is another potassium-sparing diuretic that has some structural similarities to triamterene. It also acts directly on the distal renal tubule to inhibit sodium-potassium exchange. Amiloride has actions in addition to producing diuresis in experimental dogs. It prolongs action potential duration and refractory period and also produces vasodilation.[61,62] We were unable to identify any studies of the pharmacokinetics of amiloride in dogs or cats. An effective dose and dosing interval are not known.

Supply. Spironolactone (Aldactone, Searle Laboratories, Chicago, Ill.) is supplied as 25-mg tablets and as 25-, 50-, and 100-mg film-coated tablets. It is also supplied in a fixed combination with hydrochlorothiazide (Aldactazide, Searle Laboratories, Chicago, Ill.). This combination is supplied as tablets containing 25 mg spironolactone and 25 mg hydrochlorothiazide or as film-coated tablets containing 25 mg spironolactone and 25 mg hydrochlorothiazide or 50 mg spironolactone and 50 mg hydrochlorothiazide. Triamterene (Dyrenium, SmithKline Beecham, Philadelphia, Pa.) is supplied as 50- and 100-mg capsules. It is also supplied in a fixed combination with hydrochlorothiazide (Dyazide, SmithKline Beecham, Philadelphia, Pa.) containing 50 mg triamterene and 25 mg hydrochlorothiazide. Amiloride (Midamor, Merck Sharpe and Dohme, West Point, Pa.) is supplied as 5-mg tablets. It is also supplied in a fixed combination with hydrochlorothiazide (Moduretic, Merck Sharpe and Dohme, West Point, Pa) containing 5 mg amiloride and 50 mg hydrochlorothiazide.

Adverse effects of diuretics. Diuretic therapy has the potential of causing undesirable effects, primarily electrolyte disturbances, and dehydration. It appears that these undesirable effects are less common in dogs and cats than they are in humans. However, these effects can occur in canine and feline patients, especially in those patients that are not eating and/or drinking or in patients that are being administered acute, high-dose therapy. Cats appear to be more susceptible to becoming electrolyte-depleted and dehydrated with diuretic therapy than dogs. This may be due to a species difference in drug effect but more likely is due to the fact that cats tend to stop eating and drinking more readily when they are sick.

Electrolyte abnormalities. Hypokalemia is one of the more common undesirable effects. However, the incidence of hypokalemia in dogs being administered furosemide chronically is low.[49,63] In one study of 23 canine patients with heart failure being administered furosemide at doses of 2.87 to 19.7 mg/kg/day (mean = 8.77), serum potassium concentration ranged from 3.9 to 5.2 mEq/L (normal = 3.5 to 5.5 mEq/L). None of these dogs were being administered ACE inhibitors. All were outpatients that were eating and drinking normally. In another study, serum potassium concentration was not different in control dogs and in dogs with heart failure treated with furosemide +/– digoxin and an ACE inhibitor.[64] In an experimental study, it has been documented that although sodium and chloride excretion doubled in response to a dose of 1.5 to 2.0 mg/kg furosemide q8h, potassium excretion only increased by 25%.[65]

Hyponatremia may also occur in patients on high-dose diuretic therapy. Patients with severe heart failure may also become hyponatremic as a result of antidiuretic hormone secretion and resultant water retention. It may be impossible to distinguish between these two causes in some patients with heart failure.

Hypomagnesemia may be identified in human patients with heart failure.[66] The incidence of hypomagnesemia in dogs with heart failure that are administered diuretics is very low. In one study, there was no significant difference in serum magnesium concentration between control dogs and dogs with heart failure treated with diuretics +/– digoxin.[64] In another study of 113 dogs with heart failure, only four had a low serum magnesium concentration.[49]

Dehydration. Dehydration is probably common in patients with severe heart failure that require maximum doses of diuretics to treat their heart failure. Usually the dehydration is subclinical. At times, however, patients will be mildly dehydrated on physical examination and in some patients, prerenal azotemia will be present. If the patient is clinically affected (e.g., not eating), the diuretic dose must be reduced, and, in some cases, judicious fluid therapy must be employed. Patients that are not clinically affected by their dehydration and azotemia, however, often need the dose of diuretic they are receiving. In those cases, the prerenal azotemia can be safely ignored if the azotemia is not severe (e.g., BUN greater than 100 mg/dL).

Diuretic resistance. Numerous factors determine the response to diuretic therapy. These include the potency of the drug, the dosage administered, the duration of action of the drug, the route of administration, renal blood flow, glomerular filtration rate, and nephron function. For example, furosemide must be delivered to its site of action in the loop of Henle to produce its effect. The number of molecules of furosemide that reach the site of action depends on the concentration of the drug in plasma and renal blood flow. The plasma concentration depends on the route of administration (intravenous administration produces a higher concentration than oral administration) and the dose. The duration of effect also determines the total diuretic effect produced in a certain period.

Patients with congestive heart failure may become refractory to furosemide as a result of decreased delivery of the drug to the nephron because of decreased renal blood flow and because of hormonal stimulus for sodium and water retention. Drug delivery can be increased by administering a drug that increases renal blood flow, such as hydralazine.[67,68] Delivery can also be increased by increasing plasma concentration. This is most readily accomplished by administering the drug intravenously or increasing the dose. Administering the drug as a constant rate infusion increases nephron delivery over a longer period than does bolus administration.[50] Heart failure and diuretic administration stimulate the renin-angiotensin-aldosterone system, resulting in a marked increase in plasma aldosterone concentration. Aldosterone counteracts the effects of a diuretic and may contribute to diuretic resistance. Consequently, the administration of an ACE inhibitor is often beneficial. Furosemide administration produces hypertrophy of the distal convoluted tubular cells and increases ion transport capacity in this region in rats.[69] This shifts the dose-response to the right and downward in humans.[70] If this also occurs in cats and dogs, it may also contribute to diuretic resistance.

It is possible that bioavailability of furosemide is decreased in patients with right heart failure. Gastrointestinal edema is the reputed offender in this scenario. However, it was recently documented in humans that massive fluid accumulation as a result of heart failure does not alter the pharmacokinetics of furosemide.[71]

We most commonly treat resistance to furosemide administration by adding another diuretic into the therapeutic plan. Most commonly we add a thiazide diuretic. This results in drug effects at two different sites in the nephron, which enhances diuresis. Although this type of treatment can cause dangerous complications in humans, serious complications in dogs with severe heart failure appear to be less common with this approach; however, we have identified severe electrolyte disturbances and dehydration on occasion. We have only attempted this approach rarely in cats.

DIGITALIS GLYCOSIDES

The digitalis glycosides are primarily used to treat patients with heart failure as a result of systolic dysfunction and to slow the heart rate, especially in patients with atrial fibrillation. The means by which they improve cardiovascular function in patients with heart failure patients is multifactorial. Digitalis glycosides act as positive inotropic agents. They also alter baroreceptor sensitivity and directly alter autonomic function. In so doing, they increase vagal efferent nerve traffic to the heart and tend to decrease sympathetic nervous tone, when present in therapeutic concentrations. They may also directly produce diuresis and natriuresis and directly decrease renin release.[72]

History. Digitalis glycosides have been used for centuries. The foxglove plant, *Digitalis purpurea*, was mentioned under the name "foxes glofa" in the "Meddygon myddmai," an early pharmacopoeia in Wales around the year 1200.[73] In 1785, William Withering published a paper describing his 10 years of experience using the purple foxglove (*Digitalis purpurea,* or purple fingers) to treat ascites (dropsy) and peripheral edema in human patients.[74] He described the actions of this digitalis glycoside (gitaloxin and digitoxin) as that of a diuretic and used it to treat not only patients with heart failure but other conditions that produced ascites, such as hepatic failure. William Ferrier published a treatise 14 years later in which he ascribed the beneficial effects of digitalis to an action on the heart.

Efficacy. Ever since these original clinical studies, the digitalis glycosides have been embroiled in controversy regarding their use, mechanisms of action, and efficacy. During the nineteenth century, the digitalis glycosides fell out of favor because of toxicity. At the beginning of the twentieth century, their ability to slow the heart rate in atrial fibrillation was discovered.[75] In the 1920s and later, documentation of the positive inotropic effects and efficacy in treating patients with heart failure in sinus rhythm was provided.[76] It wasn't until 1953, however, that the mechanism responsible for the positive inotropic effect of this class of drugs was identified.[77] Since that time, the digitalis glycosides have become the most studied of all cardiac drugs. Still, controversy exists, especially pertaining to their efficacy in treating myocardial failure. The human literature is replete with reports documenting the efficacy and lack of efficacy of digitalis in the treatment of patients with heart failure.[78-85] More recent studies using blinded and placebo-controlled trials have more strongly suggested that digoxin is efficacious for treating human patients in sinus rhythm.[86-88] The issue of efficacy has remained controversial, however. Recently, a large clinical trial designed to answer the question of digoxin's efficacy in human patients was completed.[1,89] This trial enrolled 7788 human patients with heart failure. About 6800 had a low ejection fraction (less than 45%). Most (80% to 90%) were being treated with a diuretic and an ACE inhibitor at presentation. About 50% of the patients were in class II (mild) heart failure, and about 30% were in class III (moderate) heart failure. Patients were randomized to receive either placebo or digoxin. The serum digoxin concentration was in the 0.5- to 1.0-ng/mL range in approximately 60% of patients and in the 1.0- to 1.5-ng/mL range in approximately 20%. Patients were followed by measuring ejection fraction, measuring the cardiothoracic ratio on a chest radiograph, recording hospitalizations, and recording death. There was no difference in deaths from cardiovascular causes between the two groups. Consequently, it was concluded that digoxin has no impact on survival in human patients with heart failure. However, there was a trend toward a significant decrease in deaths caused by heart failure. This was offset by a higher incidence of other types of cardiac death (sudden death, acute myocardial infarction, bradyarrhythmias, low output states, and surgery) in the digoxin group. The digoxin group had significantly fewer hospitalizations; however this effect was small. For the average physician, only nine hospitalizations would be avoided for every 1000 patients treated each year.[90] In general, the effect of digoxin in this clinical trial can be described, for the average human patient, as underwhelming. As one editorial stated, "Digoxin's inability to substantially influence morbidity or mortality eliminates any ethical mandate for its use and effectively relegates it to be prescribed for the treatment of persistent symptoms after the administration of drugs that do reduce the risk of death and hospitalization."[90]

In small animal veterinary medicine, the question of digoxin efficacy will probably never be answered. There is no reason to believe that results of studies examining digoxin's efficacy in human patients can be directly extrapolated to digoxin's efficacy in dogs or cats. Consequently, extrapolating data from human medicine to veterinary medicine should be enthusiastically discouraged. A small clinical trial in dogs has suggested that a minority of dogs with myocardial failure have a clinically significant response to digoxin, whereas the majority do not.[91] The response in those dogs that did respond in this trial was small. To document the efficacy of a drug that produces little or no response in clinical patients requires carefully examining several thousand patients. Nothing requiring this type of cooperation and expense has ever been attempted in veterinary medicine and it is unlikely that it ever will be, especially considering the fact that digoxin is inexpensive and has been marketed for decades. Consequently, controversy regarding the efficacy of digoxin in dogs and cats probably will continue until better means of dealing with severe cardiac disease are identified.

As with any cardiovascular drug, it is our opinion that individual response to digoxin is highly variable. Although the majority of dogs and cats have no-to-minimal response to the drug, some patients have a mild-to-moderate response. The only way to identify this type of patient is to administer the drug and monitor the response. We believe that digoxin should be administered to any patient that has severe myocardial failure. The patient then should be monitored clinically for any signs of improvement and monitored echocardiographically, if possible. If no response is identified, the drug can be continued if there are no untoward effects identified or discontinued.

Efficacy could depend on dose. It is often thought that if a low dose of digoxin is ineffective, then a larger dose may be beneficial. This is not necessarily true and may be false. A recent study in humans suggests that patients who receive a moderate dose of digoxin (0.25 mg q24h) and have a moderate serum digoxin concentration (1.5 ng/mL) have no more benefit than patients that receive a low dose of digoxin (0.125 mg q24h) and a lower serum digoxin concentration (0.8 ng/mL).[92] In this study, increased contractility and decreased heart rate were the primary endpoints. Another human study suggests that a serum digoxin concentration greater than 1 ng/mL was associated with greater mortality than a serum concentration less than 1 ng/mL.[93]

Chemistry and structure. *Cardiac glycosides, digitalis glycosides,* and *digitalis* are terms used to identify a spectrum of compounds that are steroid derivatives that have the ability to increase myocardial contractility and elicit characteristic electrophysiologic responses. These compounds are usually of plant origin.[94] The most frequently used compounds are digoxin, an extract from the leaf of the *Digitalis lanata* plant, and digitoxin, which is extracted from the *Digitalis purpurea* plant. Both are types of foxglove plants.

A cardiac glycoside consists of a steroid nucleus combined with a lactone ring and a series of sugars linked to the carbon 3 of the nucleus. The steroid nucleus and the lactone ring are termed an *aglycone.* The number of sugar moieties is a major determinant of drug half-life. For example, in humans, digitoxin, which has three sugar moieties, has a half-life of 134 hours, bis-digitoxoside with two sugars has a half-life of 15 hours, and the monodigitoxoside of digitoxigenin has a half-life of 30 minutes. The only difference between digoxin and digitoxin is a hydroxyl group at position 12. Because the half-life of digitoxin in dogs is approximately one third that of digoxin, this difference also has a profound effect on half-life. The lactone ring is crucial for inotropic activity.

Actions

Positive inotropic effects. The digitalis glycosides increase contractility in normal myocardium and may also do so in failing myocardium. However, their ability to increase contractility in normal myocardium is only about one third that of the sympathomimetics (e.g., dopamine, dobutamine) and bipyridine compounds (e.g., amrinone, milrinone).[95] This translates into a lesser inotropic response in clinical patients.[96] The ability to increase contractility is species- and age-dependent. Guinea pig and rabbit myocardium responds about one order of magnitude less to digitalis glycosides compared with human, dog, cat, cow, and sheep myocardium.[97] Aged (12 to 14 years of age) beagles have about one half the inotropic response of young beagles.[96]

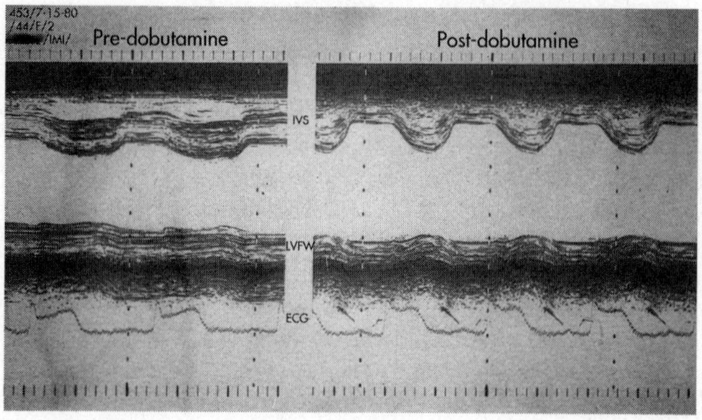

FIGURE 10-3 M-mode echocardiograms from an experimental dog with infarction of the left ventricular free wall. The echocardiograms were recorded before and after the administration of 10 μg/kg/min dobutamine. Before dobutamine administration, the motion of the interventricular septum is normal and the free wall motion is severely reduced. After dobutamine administration, septal motion is hyperkinetic, whereas the motion of the free wall is only mildly increased from baseline. This demonstrates the reduced responsiveness of failing myocardium to a positive inotropic agent.

The positive inotropic effect of digitalis is thought to be caused by the effect of digitalis on the Na^+,K^+-ATPase pumps located on myocardial cell membranes (see Chapter 2, Figures 2-10 and 2-11).[85] Digitalis competitively binds to the site at which potassium normally attaches and effectively stops pump activity.[98] A therapeutic concentration of digoxin "poisons" approximately 30% of the Na^+,K^+-ATPase pumps in the myocardium. Thus the cell loses some of its ability to extrude sodium from the intracellular space during diastole, resulting in an increase in intracellular sodium concentration. This leads to increased intracellular osmolality. The cell counters by exchanging the intracellular sodium for extracellular calcium via the Na^+/Ca^{++} cation exchanger or by reducing the exchange of intracellular calcium for extracellular sodium. The net result is an increase in the number of calcium ions within the cell. In a normal cell, these excess calcium ions are bound by the sarcoplasmic reticulum during diastole. They are subsequently released onto the contractile proteins during systole, causing increased contractility (see Chapter 2, Figure 2-9).[99] This mechanism also works in failing myocardium if the sarcoplasmic reticulum is able to bind the increased calcium. However, the effects of positive inotropic agents are usually reduced in the presence of myocardial failure (Figure 10-3). Our clinical impression is that the positive inotropic effects of digoxin are severely reduced in most patients with severe myocardial failure.

Diuretic effects. Most investigators have focused on the positive inotropic effects of the digitalis glycosides in their use in heart failure. However, digitalis glycosides may have other beneficial effects unrelated to their positive inotropic action. It is intriguing to read William Withering's original paper from 1785 and his descriptions of what happened to his 163 patients.[74] At the time he was treating his patients, he had no sophisticated methods for distinguishing ascites resulting from heart failure from that resulting from portal hypertension or intraabdominal neoplasia. Consequently, he treated them all with "foxglove tea." He attributed all of his observations to the diuretic actions of the drug and so used it in any patient with fluid accumulation. He also did not have any other efficacious drugs to use on his patients, so he was able to evaluate the effects of digitalis without confounding his results with other, more powerful drugs. He noted that ovarium dropsy, which we interpret to have developed from ovarian cancer in his patients, did not respond to foxglove. Hydrocephalus was also resistant to its effects. However, scattered throughout his paper are descriptions of patients who clearly had end-stage liver disease and portal hypertension but still responded to the use of digitalis. For example, case LIX that he saw on January 3 was a Mrs. B., who presented with "ascites, anasarca, and jaundice. After a purge of calomel and jallup, was ordered the Infusion of Digitalis: it acted kindly as a diuretic, and greatly reduced her swellings. Other medications were then administered, with a view to her other complaints, but to no purpose, and she died about a month afterwards." He ascribed all of the effects that he saw to a diuretic effect, and, after reading about some of his cases, it is difficult to disagree with him. There is no apparent reason why a patient with ascites not resulting from heart failure would respond to an agent that only produced a positive inotropic effect. Only recently, investigators have examined the renal effects of a digitalis glycoside (ouabain) and found it to have diuretic properties.[72] There are Na^+,K^+-ATPase pumps present on the basolateral aspect of renal tubular epithelial cells that may promote renal tubular reabsorption of sodium. There appears to be an up-regulation of pump activity in the proximal tubule in heart failure.[100] These pumps appear to be regulated by prostaglandins. Indomethacin decreases prostaglandin synthesis and increases Na^+,K^+-ATPase activity and renal sodium retention. Prostaglandin administration, on the other hand, results in natriuresis. Digitalis had a similar effect in one study, increasing sodium excretion up to 284% above the baseline in experimental dogs with rapid ventricular–induced pacing heart failure.[100] This same study documented decreased renal renin release when digitalis was injected directly into the renal artery. It is also interesting to note that in one study of children with ventricular septal defects that digoxin administration improved signs of congestive heart failure in 12 of 21 infants but only produced a clinically significant inotropic effect in six, which suggests that it affected the other six infants by some other mechanism.[101]

Baroreceptor effects. In addition to the aforementioned effects, the digitalis glycosides also have effects on vascular baroreceptors. Baroreceptor function is reduced in human patients and experimental dogs with heart failure.[102,103] This results in decreased vagal tone to the heart and increased sympathetic activity. This is clearly a compensatory mechanism, although it is commonly construed to be a primary abnormality.[103] This compensatory mechanism, however, can be detrimental in patients with heart failure. The digitalis glycosides clearly have the ability to increase baroreceptor function in normal cats, dogs, and humans.[104-106] The digitalis glycosides decrease plasma catecholamine concentrations, directly recorded sympathetic nerve activity, and plasma renin activity, which may all be related to increased baroreceptor activity.[107,108] In addition, the increase in vagal tone observed with digitalis administration is due in part to this effect.

Antiarrhythmic effects. The digitalis glycosides are used as antiarrhythmic agents, mostly for controlling supraventricular tachyarrhythmias. These agents increase parasympathetic nerve activity to the sinus node, atria, and atrioventricular (AV) node when the digitalis serum concentration is within the therapeutic range.[109] By so doing, they decrease the sinus rate and are capable of abolishing supraventricular premature depolarizations and supraventricular tachycardia. The latter arrhythmias are most commonly a result of reentry, and the AV node is commonly part of the reentrant pathway. Digitalis glycosides increase vagal tone to the AV node and so prolong the conduction time and refractory period of the AV node, which commonly interrupts the reentrant pathway. Cardiac glycosides also produce direct effects that help slow AV nodal conduction and prolong the AV nodal refractory period. The direct and indirect effects of the digitalis glycosides on the AV node are most commonly used to slow the ventricular response to atrial flutter and fibrillation. Dogs with atrial fibrillation have atrial rates that are in the 500- to 700-beats/min range. The AV node, because of its long refractory period, filters out most of these depolarizations so that they never reach the ventricles. In dogs that are in heart failure, circulating catecholamine concentrations are increased and sympathetic tone to the heart is increased. Sympathetic stimulation of the AV node shortens its refractory period and increases the conduction velocity through it. This usually results in approximately one third of the atrial depolarizations reaching the ventricles and a ventricular rate of 200 to 240 beats/min. Digitalis glycosides are administered in this situation to prolong AV nodal refractoriness and slow conduction. The net result is a decrease in the number of depolarizations that traverse the AV node and a decrease in the ventricular rate.

Although digitalis may be effective in controlling some ventricular arrhythmias, other drugs are preferred. Digitalis should be used with extreme caution for this purpose in patients with myocardial failure. In one study in humans, 45% of patients had improved rhythms after administration of acetylstrophanthidin, a short-acting cardiac glycoside, whereas 26% showed no change and 28% had worse ventricular arrhythmias.[110] There were no clinical or hemodynamic features that predicted which patients would respond to the drug. The antiarrhythmic effect appeared to be separate from any positive inotropic action. Proarrhythmic effects of digitalis (resulting from enhanced cellular calcium overload) in the setting of heart failure and ventricular arrhythmias must always be a clinical concern.

Effects on diaphragmatic muscle. Digoxin increases diaphragmatic muscle function in experimental dogs and in human patients.[111,112] This effect may be of benefit in canine patients that have chronic respiratory failure or that have acute respiratory failure with muscle fatigue and resultant hypercapnia. Drugs such as dopamine and theophylline have similar effects, and theophylline appears to be a more relevant choice.[113,114] Of course, chronically stimulating fatigued diaphragmatic muscle may also be detrimental to the muscle.

Indications. The digitalis glycosides are indicated for the treatment of myocardial failure and supraventricular tachyarrhythmias. Myocardial failure is always present in patients with dilated cardiomyopathy or a long-standing (longer than 5 years) moderate-size patent ductus arteriosus. It is usually present in patients with heart failure secondary to chronic severe aortic regurgitation and in large dogs with severe mitral regurgitation. Myocardial function is usually not clinically significantly depressed in small dogs with heart failure secondary to severe mitral regurgitation, although it may become apparent (on an echocardiogram) by the time a dog has become refractory to conventional medical therapy. The use of digitalis in small dogs with mitral regurgitation and no myocardial failure is not contraindicated, but other drugs are more beneficial. Myocardial failure is never present in hypertrophic cardiomyopathy or pericardial disease. Digitalis is contraindicated in hypertrophic cardiomyopathy, because increased contractility can worsen systolic anterior motion of the mitral valve and increase the outflow tract gradient. It is not contraindicated in pericardial diseases, but beneficial effects should not be expected.

In dogs with myocardial failure, digitalis does not routinely result in a clinically significant increase in myocardial contractility. Of 22 dogs with dilated cardiomyopathy in one study, only five responded to digoxin.[91] All five dogs lived longer than 6 months after their response. Dogs with dilated cardiomyopathy that respond to digoxin live significantly longer than do those that do not respond.[115] Consequently, we treat all of our patients with myocardial failure with digoxin. However, we are not hesitant to take a dog off of digoxin if there has been no apparent response and complications of digoxin therapy have occurred.

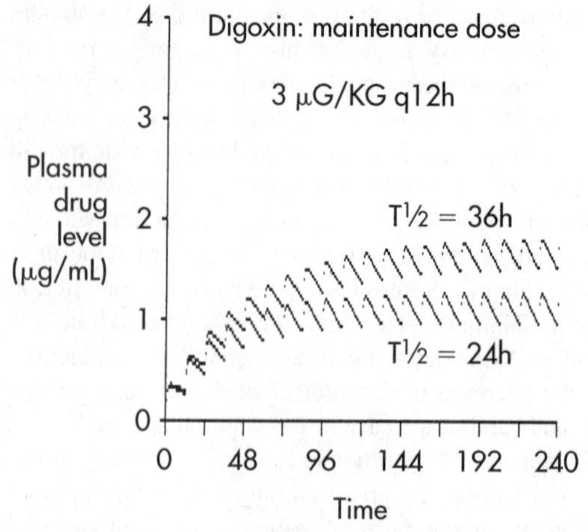

FIGURE 10-4 Theoretic graph of the serum concentration of digoxin over time following the administration of 11 μg/kg digoxin PO to a dog. The graph was generated using a pharmacokinetic computer program. The bioavailability was assumed to be 60%, so that the dose that reached the body was 7 μg/kg. The volume of distribution was set at 8 L/kg and absorption half-life at 30 minutes. Two elimination half-lives are depicted (twenty-four and thirty-six hours).

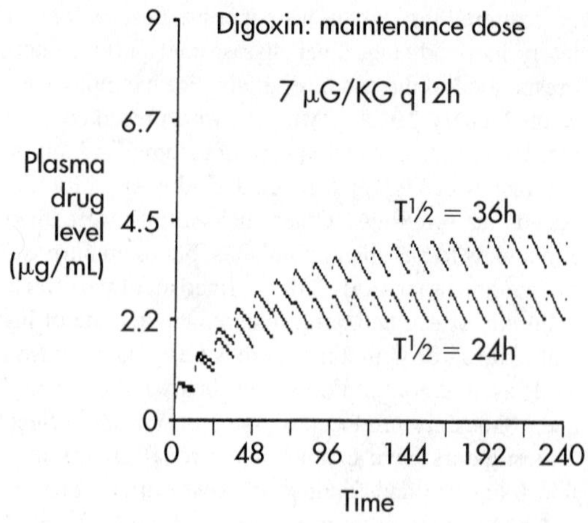

FIGURE 10-5 Theoretic graph of the serum concentration of digoxin over time following the administration of 5 μg/kg digoxin PO to a dog, as in Figure 10-4.

The digitalis glycosides are used to treat supraventricular tachyarrhythmias. They are generally regarded as moderately effective in controlling supraventricular premature depolarizations and supraventricular tachycardia and moderately effective for controlling the ventricular rate in atrial fibrillation. In veterinary patients with atrial fibrillation, digoxin may produce a minimal decrease, a moderate decrease, or an adequate decrease in the ventricular rate. If the decrease is inadequate (ventricular rate greater than 160 beats/min), another drug, either a β-adrenergic blocking drug or diltiazem must be added into the therapeutic regimen to produce the desired decrease in heart rate.

Pharmacokinetics. The pharmacokinetics of the two most commonly used digitalis glycosides, digoxin and digitoxin, are remarkably different despite their similar molecular structures.

Digoxin. Digoxin is well absorbed after oral administration. Approximately 60% of the tablet is absorbed, whereas about 75% of the elixir is absorbed. There is very little hepatic metabolism, so that almost all of the drug that is absorbed reaches the serum. In the serum, an average of 27% of digoxin is bound to albumin.[116] The volume of distribution is 12 to 15 L/kg.[117]

In the dog, serum half-life of digoxin is 23 to 39 hours.[118] Much interpatient variability exists. With a drug whose half-life exceeds the dosing interval (digoxin is usually administered every 12 hours in the dog), drug accumulation occurs until a steady-state serum concentration is reached. It takes one half-life to achieve 50% of the steady-state serum concentration, two half-lives to reach 75%, three half-lives to reach 87.5%, and so on. Theoretically, it takes about five half-lives to reach steady state, and so it is commonly thought that five half-lives are required to achieve therapeutic serum concentrations. However, this is not the case. Serum concentrations of digoxin between 1.0 and 2.5 ng/mL are generally considered to be within the therapeutic range.[119] The canine maintenance dose of digoxin (0.005 to 0.011 mg/kg q12h) generally achieves serum concentrations of 1.5 to 2.0 ng/mL. Serum concentrations after two half-lives (75% of steady state) should be 1.1 to 1.5 ng/mL and after three half-lives (87.5% of steady state) should be 1.3 to 1.75 ng/mL (Figures 10-4 and 10-5). Consequently, maintenance doses should theoretically achieve a therapeutic serum concentration within 2 to 4.5 days. In one study of dogs given 0.022 mg/kg digoxin every 24 hours, the serum concentration was within therapeutic range by the second day.[120] Based on these data, maintenance doses of digoxin in dogs should be used to achieve therapeutic serum concentrations in almost all situations. Loading doses designed to achieve therapeutic concentrations within a shorter period should only be used for emergencies, and then with caution, because loading dose schedules more often produce toxic serum concentrations. Other positive inotropic agents, such as dobutamine and amrinone, are safer and more efficacious and are preferred for acute short-term inotropic support. Other drugs, such as the calcium channel blockers and β-blockers, are preferred for the acute management of supraventricular tachycardia. If digoxin is used parenterally in an emergency situation, it must be administered slowly over at least 15 minutes, because rapid intravenous administration results in peripheral vasoconstriction and increased afterload.[121]

Most of a digoxin dose is excreted in the urine via glomerular filtration and renal secretion. About 15% is metabolized in the liver. Bile duct ligation increases the half-life of digoxin from an average of 26 hours to 35 hours in experimental dogs.[122] Renal failure reduces renal clearance, total body clearance, and volume of distribution, resulting in increased serum digoxin concentrations (Figure 10-6).[123] Digoxin should be avoided in dogs with renal failure, if possible. If a digitalis glycoside is required, digitoxin may be used instead or a much lower dose of digoxin administered and serum concentration monitored closely. Formulas have been devised to calculate the reduction in digoxin dosage needed to achieve therapeutic serum concentrations in humans with renal failure.[124] There is no correlation between the degree of azotemia and serum digoxin concentrations in dogs or cats, so such formulas cannot be used.[125,126] Digitoxin is not a viable option for cats because of its long half-life in that species. Consequently, in cats with renal failure that are administered digoxin, the dosage should be markedly reduced and serum concentration monitored.

The pharmacokinetics of digoxin in the cat are controversial. The half-life is extremely variable from cat to cat, ranging from 25.6 to 50.6 hours in one study (mean = 33.5 hours) and 39.4 to 78.8 hours in another report (mean = 57.8 hours).[118,127] In a more recent study, the half-life in a group of six normal cats ranged from 30 to 173 hours, with a mean half-life of 82 hours. The first study reported that

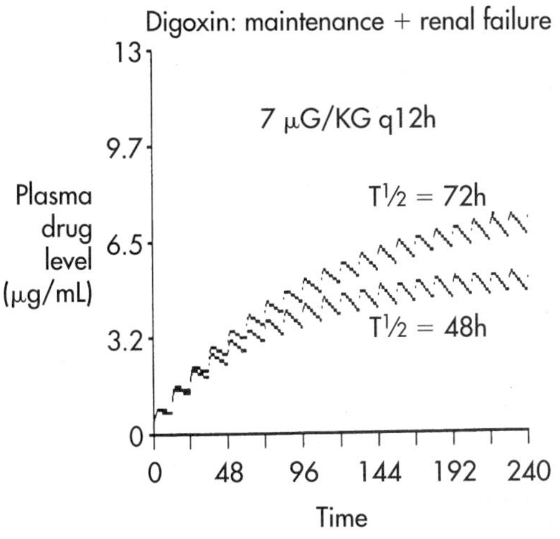

FIGURE 10-6 Theoretic graph of the serum concentration of digoxin over time following the administration of 11 µg/kg digoxin PO to dogs with mild and moderate renal failure, as in Figure 10-4. Half-lives have prolonged to 48 hours and 72 hours, respectively.

the half-life of digoxin increased dramatically to an average of 72.7 hours after prolonged oral administration. The elixir form results in serum concentrations approximately 50% higher than the tablet.[128] However, cats generally dislike the taste of the alcohol-based elixir. When digoxin tablets are administered with food to cats, serum concentration is reduced by about 50% compared with the concentration without food.[128]

Digitoxin. Digitoxin (Crystodigin, Eli Lilly and Co., Indianapolis, Ind.) has superior pharmacokinetic properties in the dog compared with digoxin.[129] Its half-life is only 8 to 12 hours. Therapeutic serum concentration can be achieved more rapidly than with digoxin, and serum concentration decreases more quickly if a dog becomes toxic; 95% to 100% of tincture of digitoxin is absorbed. About 90% of the drug is bound to serum protein, so a higher dose of digitoxin is needed relative to digoxin. Digitoxin is excreted by the liver and can therefore be used safely in dogs with renal failure. Bile duct ligation in experimental dogs increases the half-life of digitoxin from an average of 10 hours to 31 hours.[122]

In cats, the half-life of digitoxin is greater than 100 hours.[130] Consequently, this drug should be avoided in cats. Digoxin is the only recommended digitalis glycoside for this species.[19]

Dosing: digoxin

Starting dose: dogs. Because of the variability in pharmacokinetics from animal to animal, digoxin administration to any animal should be viewed as a pharmacologic experiment. An initial dose should be chosen, that dose administered, and a serum concentration measured 3 to 5 days after starting administration to determine if the chosen dose has resulted in a therapeutic serum concentration. The initial starting dose of digoxin in normal small dogs weighing less than 20 kg can be based on body weight at 0.005 to 0.011 mg/kg administered per os every 12 hours. In dogs weighing more than 20 kg, this dose cannot be safely used. Instead, the dosage should be based on body surface area (i.e., 0.22 mg/m^2 of body surface area q12h PO).[130] These doses result in a serum concentration in the therapeutic range by the second day of administration. If more rapid digitalization is required, the maintenance dose can be doubled for the first one or two doses. This method results in a therapeutic serum concentration within the first day.

Starting dose: cats. The starting dose for normal cats is one fourth of a 0.125-mg tablet administered every other day for cats weighing less than 3 kg, one fourth of a tablet every day for cats weighing 3 to 6 kg, and one fourth of a tablet every day to q12h for cats weighing more than 6 kg.[19] Tablets are better tolerated than the alcohol-based elixir.

Factors that alter the dose. Commonly, the initial starting dose of a digitalis glycoside must be modified because of factors that alter the pharmacokinetics of the drug. In a study in which digoxin dose (0.005 to 0.23 mg/kg/day) was plotted against serum concentration in dogs with heart failure, the correlation coefficient was only 0.39 (1.0 is a perfect correlation).[131] This weak correlation was statistically significant. The drug dosage is therefore a factor determining serum concentration, but it is only one factor among a number of other variables to consider when administering digoxin.

Because most of a digitalis glycoside is bound to skeletal muscle, dogs or cats that have lost a significant muscle mass (decreased volume of distribution) have an increased serum concentration for any given dose. Consequently, for patients that are cachectic, the dose must be reduced. Older dogs commonly have decreased muscle mass and impaired renal function, so dosing digoxin in these patients must be performed cautiously.

Digoxin is poorly lipid-soluble. Consequently, dosing should be based on a lean body weight estimate. Lean body weight is an estimate of the weight that an obese patient should weigh. Conversely, digitoxin is lipid-soluble, so no change in the dosage is required for lean or obese dogs.

Digoxin does not distribute well into ascitic fluid. Consequently the dose of digoxin must be reduced in patients with ascites if total body weight is used to calculate the dose.[132] In general, patients with mild ascites should have their dose reduced by 10%. Patients with moderate ascites require a 20% dose reduction, and patients with severe ascites need a 30% reduction in the dose.

The administration of other drugs along with digitalis may affect the serum concentration. Quinidine displaces digoxin from skeletal muscle binding sites and reduces its renal clearance, resulting in an increased serum digoxin concentration.[133] Quinidine probably also displaces digoxin from myocardial binding sites.[134,135] This may lessen the direct cardiac toxicity of digoxin and decrease its positive inotropic effect. In general, the combination of digoxin and quinidine should be avoided. If both drugs must be used together, the rule of thumb in human medicine is to reduce the digoxin dosage by 50%.[133] Because serum digoxin concentration approximately doubles following quinidine administration in dogs, this recommendation appears to be valid in veterinary patients.[134] No interaction between digitoxin and quinidine exists in the dog.[136] In humans, there are reports of numerous other drugs that increase the serum concentration of digoxin. These include oral aminoglycosides (neomycin), amiodarone, anticholinergics, captopril, diltiazem, esmolol, flecainide, ibuprofen, indomethacin, nifedipine, tetracycline, and verapamil.[137-139]

Drugs that alter hepatic microsomal enzymes may affect digoxin pharmacokinetics, because about 15% of digoxin is metabolized in the liver.[140] Drugs that induce hepatic microsomal enzymes, such as phenylbutazone and the barbiturates, may have a tendency to increase digoxin clearance, whereas such drugs as chloramphenicol and tetracycline, which inhibit hepatic enzymes, should increase the serum digoxin concentration. However, one study has documented that chloramphenicol decreases serum digoxin concentration in dogs.[141] The effects of these drugs on digitoxin elimination are unknown.

Hypokalemia predisposes to digitalis myocardial toxicity. Digitalis and potassium compete for the same binding site on the membrane Na^+,K^+ -ATPase pumps.[97] Hypokalemia leaves more binding sites available for digitalis. Hyperkalemia displaces digitalis from the myocardium. Hypercalcemia and hypernatremia potentiate the positive inotropic and toxic effects of digitalis, whereas hypocalcemia and hyponatremia reduce these effects.

Hyperthyroidism increases the myocardial effects of digitalis.[123] It may be necessary to decrease the dose in this situation. Although hypothyroidism has been reported to reduce renal clearance of digoxin in humans, this does not appear to be the case in dogs.[123] In one study, acute and chronic digoxin pharmacokinetics were measured in dogs before and after experimental induction of hypothyroidism.[142] There was no difference between the groups. Consequently, it is not necessary to adjust the digoxin dose in hypothyroid dogs.

Myocardial failure increases the sensitivity of the myocardium to the toxic effects of digitalis. Failing myocardial cells are usually thought to be overloaded with calcium. Digitalis may cause further calcium loading. Calcium-overloaded cells may become electrically unstable, resulting in tachyarrhythmias.[143] Digitalis should be administered cautiously in these patients, and loading doses should not be used.

Hypoxia increases the sensitivity of the myocardium to the toxic effects of digitalis. The mechanism is unexplained but digitalis should be used carefully in hypoxemic patients.

Digoxin pharmacokinetics are not significantly altered in cats with compensated heart failure that are being administered furosemide and aspirin.[126] This is despite increases in serum urea and creatinine concentrations.

Strategy. Patients should be evaluated carefully before digoxin is administered. Factors that alter the dosage should be noted and an initial dose chosen. The patient should be monitored during the initial course of therapy for signs of toxicity or improvement. A decrease in heart rate or resolution of an arrhythmia are documentable benefits in patients with tachycardia or arrhythmia. Clinical responsiveness as a result of improved hemodynamics in patients with heart failure is the desired endpoint of digitalis administration but can be difficult to identify for several reasons. First, other drugs are generally administered with digitalis, so it may be impossible to identify the beneficial drug. Second, many dogs do not respond to digoxin, so clinical resolution may never occur. The dosage in the latter case should not be increased unless the serum concentration has been measured and documented to be subtherapeutic (i.e., less than 0.5 to 1.0 ng/mL). Each case should have a serum digoxin concentration measured 2 to 7 days (usually 3 to 5 days) after initiating therapy. The serum sample should be acquired 6 to 8 hours after the last dose and sent to a laboratory for analysis. Therapeutic range for serum digoxin concentration is somewhat controversial but can generally be considered to be between 1 and 2 ng/mL. A serum concentration greater than 2.5 ng/mL should be considered toxic. If such an elevation is identified in a patient, digoxin administration should be discontinued until the serum concentration is less than 2.5 ng/mL. The dosage should be reduced accordingly.

Dosing: digitoxin. The starting dose of digitoxin in dogs is 0.033 mg/kg administered q8-12h PO.[129] In general, small dogs should receive the dose q8h and large dogs q12h. The cumulative daily dose in small dogs would be greater than that for large dogs on a per-weight basis but similar on a per-body-surface-area basis.

Toxicity. Therapeutic endpoints for digitalis in patients with heart failure include clinical improvement or attainment of therapeutic serum concentration. Progressive dosing until signs of toxicity occur or until the PR interval on the ECG increases is not justified.[144] By the time gastrointestinal signs of toxicity are present in dogs with myocardial failure, myocardial toxicity may be present and may be fatal. Dogs without myocardial failure (e.g., small dogs with mitral regurgitation) tolerate digitalis toxicity better than do those with myocardial failure (i.e., myocardial toxicity occurs at a higher serum concentration) and generally show signs of anorexia and vomiting before exhibiting electrocardiographic evidence of myocardial toxicity.

In normal beagles, a serum concentration of digoxin that exceeds 2.5 ng/mL generally produces clinical signs of toxicity.[145] However, dogs and cats may show clinical evidence of toxicity at a serum concentration less than 2.5 ng/mL, and occasionally a dog will show no clinical signs of toxicity at a serum concentration greater than 2.5 ng/mL.

The incidence of digoxin toxicity in human medicine is estimated to be between 13% and 23%.[146] At the same time, 11% to 36% of patients have been identified as underdigitalized. The incidence in veterinary medicine is less clear. In one canine study, 25% of dogs receiving digoxin had a serum concentration in the toxic range, whereas 24% had a subtherapeutic concentration. In dogs receiving digitoxin, 5% were found to be toxic and 19% to be in the subtherapeutic range.[129] In our experience, clinically significant digitalis toxicity is rare if the drug is used judiciously and the serum concentration is monitored. Toxicity occurs most frequently when an owner becomes overzealous with drug administration when the patient is not responding, when the pet develops renal failure while on digoxin, and during the initial stages of digoxin administration. Owners should always be warned not to administer more of a digitalis glycoside if their pet does not appear to be improving on medication.

Clinical signs. Problems from digitalis intoxication fall into three general classes—those referable to the central nervous system, those to the gastrointestinal system, and those to the myocardium.[145] Most dogs that are intoxicated with digoxin appear depressed. Humans experience malaise and drowsiness and have headaches.[97] Anorexia and vomiting are common manifestations of digitalis intoxication and are probably due to the direct effect of the digitalis molecule on the chemoreceptor trigger zone (CTZ) located in the area postrema in the medulla.[147] In one study, normal dogs with a serum concentration of digoxin in the 2.5- to 6.0-ng/mL range decreased their food intake to about half of normal while maintaining a normal water intake, whereas dogs with a serum concentration greater than 6 ng/mL stopped eating, decreased their water intake to less than one third of normal, and vomited.[145] In clinical practice, a serum concentration of digoxin greater than 3 to 4 ng/mL usually produces anorexia and vomiting. In dogs without myocardial failure, gastrointestinal signs of toxicity generally occur well before signs of myocardial toxicity. This may not be true in the patient with myocardial failure in which myocardial toxicity may appear first. Also, signs of anorexia may go unnoticed in the hospitalized patient, especially if the animal was not eating a normal quantity before digitalis administration. In addition to the aforementioned clinical signs, body temperature decreases in digitalis intoxication. In one study of healthy beagles, body temperature decreased by approximately 1° C in dogs with moderate toxicity and 1° to 3° C in dogs with severe toxicity.[145]

Autonomic manifestations. Autonomic tone to the heart is increased with digitalis toxicity. Increased vagal tone can result in a decrease in sinus node rate and altered atrioventricular (AV) nodal conduction and refractoriness. Increased sympathetic tone can counter these effects. Sinus node rate is variable in dogs with digitalis intoxication. In one study of normal dogs administered toxic doses of digoxin for 2 weeks, the heart rate initially decreased from baseline values of 90 to 130 beats/min to 50 to 90 beats/min after intravenous administration of digoxin but returned to baseline by 24 to 48 hours after dosing.[145] Despite continued administration of toxic doses, the heart rate remained at baseline values or was mildly decreased. During the periods of most severe toxicity, the heart rate increased to 130 to 190 beats/min. Increased vagal tone predominates at the AV nodal level. First-degree AV block is a common finding in dogs with digoxin toxicity. Second-degree AV block may also occur, especially after prolonged intoxication.[145] Third-degree AV block is rare.

Myocardial toxicity. Myocardial toxicity is the most serious complication of digitalis administration. Toxic serum concentrations disrupt the normal electric activity of the heart in several ways. Sympathetic nerve activity to the heart is increased through the effects of digitalis on the CTZ, resulting in increased normal automaticity.[148,149] In dogs, blockade of the sympathetic nervous system increases the dose of digitalis required to produce arrhythmias.[97] However, in cats it has been shown that cardiac toxicity occurs at the same dosage with or without destruction of the area postrema.[150] Digitalis also slows conduction and alters the refractory period, making it easier for re-entrant arrhythmias to develop. Triggered activity appears to be the most important reason for the development of arrhythmias in digitalis intoxication. The classic cellular event produced by digitalis intoxication is the formation of late afterdepolarizations in which the diastolic membrane potential oscillates, eventually reaches threshold potential, and depolarizes the cell.[143] The ECG counterpart of this depolarization is a premature beat. Late afterdepolarizations are attributed to cellular calcium overload and are more easily induced in myocardium that has been stretched (analogous to a ventricle with an increased end-diastolic pressure) and in a hypokalemic environment. It is speculated that calcium overload results in oscillatory calcium movements between the sarcoplasmic reticulum and the myocyte cytoplasm.[97] Myocyte calcium overload occurs when too many Na^+,K^+-ATPase pumps are poisoned. Digitalis cardiotoxicity occurs when 60% to 80% of Na^+,K^+-ATPase pumps are inhibited.[97]

Clinically, myocardial toxicity can take the form of almost every known rhythm disturbance. In the dog, ventricular tachyarrhythmias and bradyarrhythmias are most common. The ventricular tachyarrhythmias consist of ventricular premature depolarizations, ventricular bigeminy and trigeminy, and ventricular tachycardia. The common bradyarrhythmias are second-degree AV block, sinus bradycardia, and sinus arrest that occur because of increased vagal tone. Digitalis can also induce supraventricular premature depolarizations and tachycardia, junctional tachyarrhythmias, and other arrhythmias. At times it may be difficult or impossible to distinguish whether an arrhythmia is due to digitalis or to the underlying heart disease. Arrhythmias characterized by tachycardia with impaired conduction are highly suggestive of digitalis-induced problems. Ventricular tachyarrhythmias and AV nodal conduction disturbances that appear in a dog or cat being administered digitalis should generally be regarded as digitalis-induced until proved otherwise.

Digitalis intoxication also appears to produce abnormal myocardial function and myocyte damage. In isolated hearts, digitalis intoxication results in an increase in diastolic tension (diastolic dysfunction) and a decrease in developed (systolic) tension (myocardial failure).[97] In normal dogs, severe digoxin toxicity results in an increase in serum CPK concentration and histologic evidence of myocardial degeneration and necrosis.[145]

Renal toxicity. Digoxin toxicity also causes renal damage. In one study, there was hydropic degeneration and epithelial necrosis in the proximal tubule and in the medullary collecting ducts.[145] This resulted in increases in serum concentrations of urea nitrogen and creatinine. There was a direct correlation between the degree of elevation in serum concentration and the severity of the tubular damage.

Electrolyte abnormalities. A digitalis overdose can produce hyperkalemia and hyponatremia.[151] In one study, moderate toxicity (serum digoxin concentration = 2.5 to 6.0 ng/mL) resulted in serum concentrations of sodium between 130 and 145 mEq/L, with a normal serum potassium concentration. Severe toxicity (serum digoxin concentration greater than 6 ng/mL) produced serum sodium concentrations in the 110- to 130-mEq/L range and serum concentrations of potassium anywhere from 3.2 to 7.7 mEq/L. These electrolyte abnormalities are probably caused by digitalis inhibition of the $Na,^+K^+$-ATPase pumps throughout the body.

Treatment of digitalis intoxication. The mainstay of treating digitalis intoxication is discontinuing drug administration. Because the half-life of digoxin in a normal dog is between 24 and 36 hours, it should take one to one and one-half days for the serum concentration to decrease to one half the original concentration. Half-life is commonly prolonged in older animals and diseased animals. Consequently, the time to reach one half the original concentration is prolonged. Theoretically, one can estimate the time to discontinue digoxin administration by knowing the serum concentration at the time of presentation. If the original serum concentration is 8 ng/mL and the desired serum concentration is 2 ng/mL one should wait two half-lives (one half-life to achieve a serum concentration of 4 ng/mL and another half-life to achieve a serum concentration of 2 ng/mL). If the animal is otherwise normal, discontinuing drug administration for 3 days might be adequate. Similarly, one can theoretically determine the dose required to maintain a therapeutic concentration based on the presenting serum concentration. If an owner was administering 0.5 mg of digoxin to the patient with a serum concentration of 8 ng/mlL, then, theoretically, the owner can be instructed to administer one fourth that dose to maintain a serum concentration of 2 ng/mL. We have used this rationale in clinical patients and have generally failed to predict the correct outcome. Consequently, this section is included to warn veterinarians against relying on this type of logic. Instead, serum concentration should be measured every day or two to actually determine the desired outcome.

Gastrointestinal signs related to a digitalis overdose are treated by drug withdrawal and correction of fluid and electrolyte abnormalities. Conduction disturbances and bradyarrhythmias usually require only digitalis withdrawal, although atropine administration is occasionally necessary.[152] Ventricular tachyarrhythmias are generally treated aggressively, especially when ventricular tachycardia is present. It is estimated that two thirds of human patients with ventricular tachycardia secondary to digitalis intoxication will not survive, despite therapy.[153]

Lidocaine is the drug of choice for treating ventricular tachyarrhythmias caused by digitalis intoxication.[152] It decreases sympathetic nerve traffic and can abolish reentrant arrhythmias and late afterdepolarizations.[154,155] Lidocaine usually has little effect on sinus rate or atrioventricular nodal conduction, so it does not usually exacerbate these problems. It is safe in the dog, can readily be administered intravenously, and has a rapid onset of action. It may be administered as an initial bolus (2 to 4 mg/kg IV over 1 to 2 minutes) followed by continuous infusion of 30 to 100 µg/kg/min for arrhythmia control. Cats are more sensitive to the neurotoxic effects of lidocaine, so the dose must be reduced and the drug used with caution (0.25 to 1 mg/kg IV over 5 minutes).

Phenytoin (diphenylhydantoin) is the second drug of choice for the treatment of digitalis-induced toxicity in the dog. It has similar properties to lidocaine. When administered intravenously, the drug vehicle can produce hypotension and exert a depressant effect on the myocardium.[156] The total intravenous dose is 10 mg/kg, given in 2-mg/kg increments over 3 to 5 minutes. Phenytoin can also be administered orally either to treat a digitalis-induced ventricular tachyarrhythmia or to prevent these tachyarrhythmias.[129] The oral dose is 35 mg/kg administered q8h.[157]

Serum potassium concentration should always be determined in patients intoxicated with digitalis. If serum potassium is less than 4 mEq/L, potassium supplements should be administered, preferably in intravenous fluids. Potassium competes with digitalis for binding sites on the $Na,^{+}K^{+}$-ATPase pumps and provides a more suitable environment for the antiarrhythmic agents to work.

Other drugs may be administered in digitalis intoxication. Propranolol may be useful for digitalis-induced ventricular tachyarrhythmias, but not when the patient exhibits conduction blocks. Quinidine increases the serum concentration of digoxin and should not be used to treat digitalis intoxication. Procainamide is less effective than other drugs in treating digitalis-induced arrhythmias.

Orally administered activated charcoal avidly binds digoxin and is useful after accidental ingestion or administration of a large oral dose. It decreases digoxin absorption up to 96%.[158] Cholestyramine, a steroid-binding resin, may also be useful early after digoxin ingestion but only decreases absorption 30% to 40%.[158] Cholestyramine is more useful in digitoxin toxicity.[159] Cholestyramine binds digitalis in the intestinal tract. Digitoxin undergoes enterohepatic circulation and so can be bound by this resin. Digoxin undergoes minimal enterohepatic circulation so cholestyramine administration is only useful soon after an accidental overdose with this drug.

Cardiac glycoside-specific antibodies are used in humans to bind digitalis glycosides in the bloodstream and thus remove them from myocardial binding sites.[160] A commercial product, digoxin immune Fab (ovine) (Digibind, Burroughs Wellcome Co., Research Triangle, N.C.), is available This product may be a useful means of treating life-threatening digitalis intoxication in veterinary medicine, but it is very expensive. There has been one report of its use in a dog.[161] It cost $1200 to treat this 23-kg Labrador retriever. Digoxin immune Fab (ovine) is produced by immunizing sheep with digoxin bound to human albumin. After purification, papain is used to cleave the antibody into a Fab fragment and an Fc portion. The Fab fragment diffuses more rapidly and is cleared more rapidly than the whole antibody molecule. It binds with the antigenic epitope on the digoxin molecule. This complex cannot bind to $Na,^{+}K^{+}$-ATPase pumps and is cleared by glomerular filtration. These effects result in rapid resolution of clinical signs. In one report of its use in humans, the median time to initial response was 19 minutes with 75% of the patients having evidence of response within 1 hour.[162] In this same report, 80% to 90% of patients had resolution of all clinical signs and symptoms of digitalis intoxication. The measured serum concentration of digoxin may increase or decrease after administration of digoxin immune Fab (ovine), depending on the type of assay used.[163] This appears to occur primarily because some assays measure total serum digoxin concentration and some measure primarily free serum concentration. Serum concentration of free digoxin decreases rapidly to very low concentrations after administration of digoxin immune Fab (ovine). Most digoxin is bound to tissues, however. The concentration gradient between the extracellular space and tissue is decreased by digoxin immune Fab (ovine) binding the extracellular free digoxin, resulting in diffusion of digoxin from the tissues to the extracellular space, where it is bound by digoxin immune Fab (ovine). Consequently, the total serum concentration of digoxin (free plus digoxin bound to Fab) increases to 10 to 20 times the baseline after administration of digoxin immune Fab (ovine). The dose of digoxin immune Fab (ovine) can be calculated if either the dose of digoxin ingested or the serum digoxin concentration is known. The body load of digoxin (mg) is calculated by one of the following two methods:

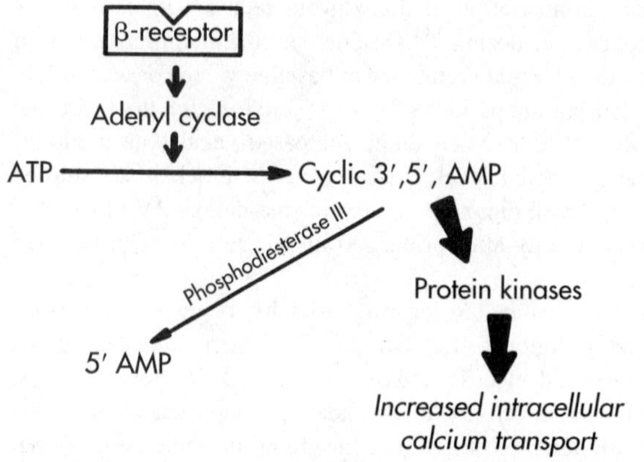

FIGURE 10-7 The cascade of events that follow β-adrenergic receptor stimulation by a sympathomimetic drug. Phosphodiesterase III is an enzyme responsible for the breakdown of cAMP within the cell. Protein kinases phosphorylate intracellular proteins, such as phospholamban, that increase intracellular calcium transport. The resultant increased systolic intracellular calcium concentration causes an increase in myocardial contractility.

1. Amount of ingested digoxin (mg) × bioavailability of digoxin = mg × 0.6
2. $\frac{\text{Serum concentration (ng/mL)} \times \text{volume of distribution (12 L/kg)} \times \text{weight (kg)}}{1000}$

The dose of digoxin immune Fab (ovine) is then calculated as follows:

1. $\frac{\text{MW Fab (50,000)}}{\text{MW digoxin (781)}} = 64 \times (\text{body load [mg]}) = \text{Fab dose (mg)}$

Each vial of digoxin immune Fab (ovine) (Digibind) contains 40 mg of Fab fragments, so the number of vials is calculated by dividing the Fab dose by 40. For example, a 25-kg dog is presented with a serum digoxin concentration of 7.5 ng/mL and the owner thinks that he ingested ten 0.25 mg tablets. Using serum concentration, the body load is 2.25 mg. Using the owner's information, the body load is 2.5 mg. Using the serum concentration to calculate the body load gives a Fab dose of 144 mg, or 3.6 vials. The four vials will cost approximately $1000.

Supply. Digoxin is supplied in several forms. Digoxin liquid-filled capsules (Lanoxicaps, Burroughs Wellcome Co., Research Triangle Park, N.C.) are supplied as capsules containing 0.05, 0.1, and 0.2 mg digoxin in 8% alcohol. Digoxin elixir (Lanoxin Elixir Pediatric, Burroughs Wellcome Co., Research Triangle Park, N.C.; Digoxin Elixir, Bausch & Lomb, Inc., Rochester, N.Y.; Digoxin Elixir, Halsey Drug Company, Brooklyn, N.Y.; Digoxin Elixir, Roxane Laboratories, Inc., Columbus, Ohio) is a liquid preparation containing digoxin in 10% alcohol containing 0.05 or 0.15 mg/mL. Digoxin tablets (Lanoxin, Burroughs Wellcome Co., Research Triangle Park, N.C.) are supplied in 0.125-, 0.25-, and 0.5-mg tablets. Injectable digoxin is supplied as a solution containing 0.1 mg/mL (Lanoxin Injection Pediatric, Burroughs Wellcome Co., Research Triangle Park, N.C.) and 0.25 mg/mL (Digoxin Injection, Elkins-Sinn, Inc., Cherry Hill, N.J.; Digoxin Injection, Wyeth-Ayerst, Philadelphia, Pa.; Lanoxin, Burroughs Wellcome Co., Research Triangle Park, N.C.).

Digitoxin (Crystodigin, Eli Lilly and Co., Indianapolis, Ind.) is supplied as 0.05-, 0.1-, 0.15-, and 0.2-mg tablets.

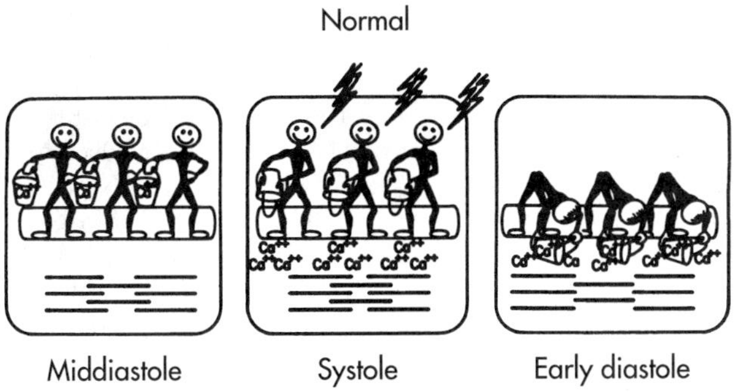

FIGURE 10-8 Cartoon of a cardiac myocyte, the sarcoplasmic reticulum (SR), and the contractile proteins throughout the cardiac cycle. The smiling-face figures represent the calcium-binding proteins of the SR (e.g., calsequestrin). In middiastole the figures have full buckets of calcium. In systole, electrical activity and calcium entry into the cell stimulate the figures to "dump" the calcium from their buckets into the cytoplasm of the cell, stimulating contraction. In early diastole, the figures retrieve the calcium from the cytoplasm, resulting in relaxation.

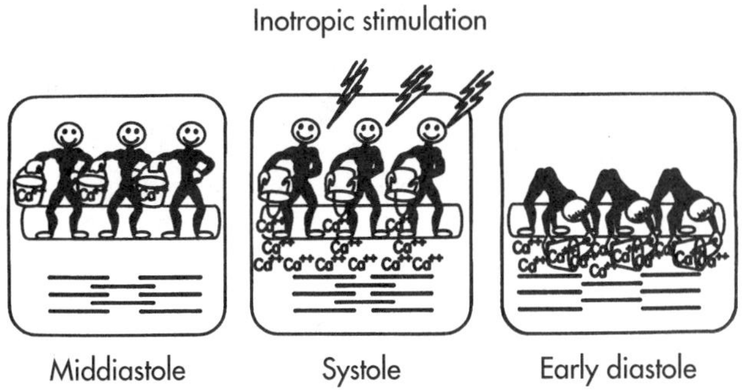

FIGURE 10-9 Similar cartoon to the one in Figure 10-8. A β-adrenergic agonist agent, such as dobutamine, has been administered. The phosphorylation of intracellular proteins has resulted in enhanced calcium uptake by the sarcoplasmic reticulum. This is depicted as larger figures carrying larger buckets. The figures now have more calcium to release in systole. The net result is an increase in myocardial contractility.

SYMPATHOMIMETICS

Sympathomimetic amines increase contractility, conduction velocity, and heart rate by binding to cardiac β-adrenergic receptors (Figure 10-7). The increase in contractility is brought about by activation of adenyl cyclase within the cell. Adenyl cyclase cleaves adenosine triphosphate (ATP) to cyclic adenosine monophosphate (cAMP), which stimulates a cellular protein kinase system. Protein kinases phosphorylate intracellular proteins, such as phospholamban on the sarcoplasmic reticulum, allowing it to bind more calcium during diastole and thereby release more calcium during systole (Figures 10-8 and 10-9).[164] Cyclic AMP also affects L- type calcium channels, to increase calcium entry into the cell during systole.

Most sympathomimetics have the ability to increase contractility about 100% above baseline, but many are unsuitable for treating heart failure because of other drug properties. Sympathomimetics can stimulate both α- and β-adrenergic receptors. The degree to which each type of receptor is stimulated depends on the specific sympathomimetic and the dose administered.[165] Isoproterenol is a pure β-adrenergic–stimulating agent. It increases contractility but also increases the heart rate, stimulates the formation of arrhythmias, and may decrease blood pressure through β-receptor mediated vasodilation. Norepinephrine increases contractility but also stimulates peripheral α-adrenergic receptors, causing systemic arteriolar constriction and increased systemic vascular resistance and blood pressure. Epinephrine also produces tachycardia and is arrhythmogenic. All three of these drugs are therefore unsuitable for treating heart failure. Newer sympathomimetics, such as dopamine and dobutamine, are less arrhythmogenic, produce a smaller heart rate increase, and are more suitable for heart failure therapy.[166] The arrhythmogenic potential for all catecholamines is increased when dogs are anesthetized with drugs such as thiamylal and halothane. In this setting, the arrhythmogenic potential of epinephrine, dopamine, and dobutamine is similar.[167]

All currently available sympathomimetics have very short half-lives (1 to 2 minutes). When administered orally they are metabolized extensively and rapidly by the liver before they reach the circulation.[168] Consequently, they must be administered intravenously, usually as a constant-rate infusion.

One of the major limitations of using sympathomimetics to treat patients with heart failure is the major alterations that occur in β-receptor density and sensitivity during subacute-to-chronic stimulation by endogenous or exogenous catecholamines. Typically, the inotropic response to sympathomimetics decreases to 50% of baseline after a day or two of constant stimulation because of the decrease in β-receptor number and sensitivity. Therefore the efficacy of sympathomimetics decreases rapidly once therapy is initiated. Consequently, one should generally not consider using a sympathomimetic longer that 2 or 3 days for inotropic support.

Dopamine

Actions. Dopamine is the precursor of norepinephrine. It stimulates cardiac β_1- adrenergic receptors, as well as peripherally located dopaminergic receptors.[169] The latter appear to be located most prevalently in the renal and mesenteric vascular beds, where they produce vasodilation. Dopamine increases portal vein blood flow but decreases hepatic arterial blood flow.[170] Dopamine administration to a patient with acute heart failure should improve contractility and thereby increase cardiac output. The renal and mesenteric vasodilation should cause preferential blood flow to these areas. In humans, dopamine administration to patients with chronic heart failure can cause increased ventricular filling pressures and edema formation.[171] However, in one study of experimental heart failure in dogs induced by creating an aorta–left atrial shunt, dopamine decreased ventricular filling pressures.[172] Consequently, the effects of dopamine may be more advantageous in dogs than in humans. The effects of dopamine become attenuated with time. In one study, the hemodynamic effects of dopamine and dobutamine were indistinguishable, except for the increase in renal and mesenteric flow produced with dopamine following a 15 minute infusion.[172] However, after a 5-hour infusion, the mesenteric/renal vasodilation was lost, and the increase in contractility was attenuated.

Indication. In cardiovascular medicine, dopamine is recommended for short-term use in animals with myocardial failure. It has many other but similar indications in critical care and anesthetized patients.

Administration and dosage. The dosage for dopamine in dogs is 1 to 10 μg/kg/min IV. Doses higher than 10 μg/kg/min can be used but result in norepinephrine release and increased peripheral vascular resistance and heart rate.[173] An initial dose of 2 μg/kg/min may be started and titrated upward to obtain the desired clinical effect (improved hemodynamics).

Supply. Dopamine is supplied as a liquid in ampules, vials, and syringes at concentrations ranging from 40 mg/mL to 160 mg/mL (Dopamine HCl, various manufacturers; Dopamine HCl, Abbott Laboratories, North Chicago, Ill.; Intropin, DuPont Critical Care, Waukegan, Ill.). The liquid must be diluted in solutions suitable for intravenous administration. The solution is stable at room temperature for a minimum of 24 hours. Dopamine is inactivated when mixed with sodium bicarbonate or other alkaline IV solutions. The solution becomes pink or violet. The product should not be used if it is discolored.

Dobutamine

Actions. Dobutamine is a synthetic catecholamine. It stimulates β_1-adrenergic receptors, increasing myocardial contractility. In so doing it decreases end-systolic volume, increases stroke volume, and increases cardiac output. It also weakly stimulates peripheral β_2- and α_1-adrenergic receptors. As this response is balanced, systemic arterial blood pressure is usually unchanged after dobutamine administration.[174] Dobutamine is less arrhythmogenic than most of the other sympathomimetics in awake animals. In vagotomized experimental dogs under anesthesia, dobutamine is as arrhythmogenic as dopamine and epinephrine.[167] In one study of dogs with experimental myocardial infarction, dobutamine did not increase the frequency of premature ventricular ectopic beats.[175]

Dobutamine's hemodynamic effects have been studied in normal conscious and normal anesthetized dogs.[173,174] It has also been examined in conscious and anesthetized dogs following myocardial infarction.[176] In each situation, dobutamine produced dose-related increases in myocardial contractility, cardiac output, stroke volume, and coronary blood flow, with no change in systemic arterial blood pressure. When administered to a patient with acute or chronic myocardial failure, it should increase contractility and cardiac output and decrease ventricular diastolic pressures, leading to a decrease in edema formation. This has been poorly documented in dogs and cats with chronic myocardial failure but has been well documented in human patients.[177,178] In one canine study, dogs were placed on cardiopulmonary bypass with their aortas cross-clamped for 1 hour and studied after surgery.[179] Comparisons were made between a group treated with dobutamine (5 μg/kg/min) and a group that received no treatment. Dobutamine administration resulted in an increased stroke volume, a decreased heart rate, an increase in blood pressure toward normal, and improved survival (75% vs. 37.5%). There was no increase in arrhythmias.

Dobutamine's effects on heart rate are generally less than that of other catecholamines. When studied in normal dogs and in dogs with experimental myocardial infarction, the heart rate did not increase at infusion rates less than 20 μg/kg/min.[174,176] Dobutamine, however, does increase heart rate in a dose-dependent manner in dogs that are anesthetized.[173,176]

Indications. In clinical situations, dobutamine can be used to treat acute heart failure resulting from myocardial failure until inotropic support is no longer needed or until other longer-acting positive inotropic agents (e.g., digoxin) have taken effect. It can also be used to treat acute exacerbations of chronic heart failure requiring acute inotropic support. There is some evidence in human medicine to suggest that intermittent administration (3-day infusion every 2 to 4 weeks) of dobutamine to patients with chronic myocardial failure can result in continued improvement in cardiac function.[180] There is no confirmation of this effect in veterinary patients, however, and the effect in humans is very small (comparable with an increase in shortening fraction of 2%).

Pharmacokinetics. Dobutamine must be administered as a constant-rate infusion. A plateau plasma concentration is achieved within approximately 8 minutes of starting the infusion.[168] Upon cessation of the infusion, dobutamine rapidly clears from the plasma with a terminal half-life of 1 to 2 minutes. The rapid clearance is due primarily to degradation of the drug by catechol O-methyltransferase.

Administration. The dosage of dobutamine is 5 to 40 μg/kg/min IV. Doses of 5 to 20 μg/kg/min are generally adequate for dogs. Infusion rates of greater than 20 μg/kg/min may produce tachycardia.[176] Cats may be administered 5 to 15 μg/kg/min. The positive inotropic effect is dosage-dependent.

Adverse effects. Dobutamine can exacerbate existing arrhythmias, especially ventricular arrhythmias. It can also produce new arrhythmias and increase heart rate.

Supply. Dobutamine (Dobutrex, Eli Lilly and Co., Indianapolis, Ind.) is supplied as 250 mg of a white powder in a 20-mL vial for reconstitution with sterile water or 5% dextrose. Once in solution, dobutamine is only stable for approximately 6 hours at room temperature and for 48 hours when refrigerated. The solution should not be frozen, because crystallization can occur. Reconstitution with alkaline products should be avoided because it causes more rapid deterioration. The reconstituted solution must be further diluted into at least 50 mL of a solution suitable for intravenous administration. Once in an intravenous solution, the compound is stable at room temperature for 24 hours. Dobutamine should not be mixed with bicarbonate, heparin, hydrocortisone sodium succinate, cephalothin, penicillin, or insulin.

BIPYRIDINE COMPOUNDS (AMRINONE AND MILRINONE). Bipyridine compounds increase myocardial contractility and produce mild systemic arteriolar dilation. Milrinone is about 30 to 40 times as potent as amrinone. Both compounds are active after oral administration, although only intravenous formulations are available commercially.

Actions. Bipyridine compounds primarily act as inhibitors of phosphodiesterase fraction III.[181] Phosphodiesterase fraction III is an intracellular enzyme that specifically breaks down (hydrolyzes) cAMP in myocardial and vascular tissue. When phosphodiesterase III is inhibited, intracellular cAMP concentration increases. This increase results in the same type of inotropic effect in the myocardium produced by sympathomimetics (see Figure 10-7). The major difference is that bipyridine compounds "bypass" the β receptors, and so there is no decrement in inotropic effect over time. Consequently, bipyridine compounds can be used to chronically increase contractility in patients. At high doses, alterations in calcium transport may contribute to the increase in contractility seen with amrinone and milrinone.[181] Bipyridine compounds also produce systemic arteriolar dilation, probably also mediated by phosphodiesterase inhibition. Increased cAMP decreases calcium uptake in vascular smooth muscle, which results in muscle relaxation and vasodilation. There is a direct correlation between decreased phosphodiesterase fraction III activity and smooth muscle relaxation.[182] Milrinone also increases left ventricular relaxation and distensibility in human patients with heart failure.[183]

Cardiovascular effects of the bipyridine compounds are species-dependent. Myocardial contractility increases to a similar degree as that observed following the administration of a β agonist in dogs and cats (i.e., approximately 100% above baseline). Myocardial contractility increases only about 50% above baseline in nonhuman primates and, presumably, humans.[184] When amrinone is administered to rats, contractility only increases about 25% above baseline.[185] Because of this marked species difference, data obtained from human patients administered amrinone or milrinone cannot be extrapolated to dogs or cats.

Amrinone. In normal anesthetized dogs, an intravenous bolus of amrinone (1 to 3 mg/kg) causes contractility to increase 60% to 100%, systemic arterial blood pressure to decrease 10% to 30%, and heart rate to increase 5% to 10%.[186] The maximal contractility increase occurs within 5 minutes after injection and decreases 50% by 10 minutes. Effects are dissipated within 20 to 30 minutes. This short duration of effect necessitates administering the drug by constant intravenous infusion following the initial bolus injection. Infusion rates of 10 to 100 μg/kg/min in anesthetized experimental dogs increases contractility 30% to 90% and in unanesthetized dogs, 10% to 80% above baseline. In anesthetized dogs, an infusion of 10 μg/kg/min does not decrease systemic blood pressure, whereas 30 μg/kg/min decreases it 10% and 100 μg/kg/min decreases it 30%. Heart rate does not increase at 10 μg/kg/min but elevates 15% at 30 μg/kg/min and increases 20% at 100 μg/kg/min. In anesthetized dogs with drug-induced myocardial failure, amrinone infusions increase contractility 40% to 200% above baseline and increase cardiac output by 80%. Constant infusions in dogs take about 45 minutes to reach peak effect. In experimental cats, amrinone infused at 30 μg/kg/min causes contractility to increase 40% above baseline. Peak effect occurs 90 minutes after starting an infusion.

Studies have not been performed to determine the hemodynamic changes brought about by amrinone administration in dogs or cats with naturally occurring heart failure. Based on the information from normal dogs, however, clinical recommendations can be made. The drug has a wide margin of safety, and the risk of toxicity is low. With milrinone (which has similar toxic effects in dogs as amrinone), exacerbation of ventricular arrhythmias may occur in about 5% of dogs treated for heart failure. In humans, amrinone can cause thrombocytopenia and flulike symptoms in a small percentage of patients, but these signs have not been noted in drug studies involving amrinone and normal dogs.[187] Amrinone is marketed only as a solution for intravenous administration and so is useful only for short-term administration. The initial dose should be 1 to 3 mg/kg administered as a slow intravenous bolus followed by a constant-rate infusion of 10 to 100 μg/kg/min. One half of the initial bolus may be administered 20 to 30 minutes after the first bolus. The same regimen may be effective in the cat.

Milrinone. Milrinone is a bipyridine compound with pharmacologic effects that are almost identical to amrinone. Milrinone is currently marketed for intravenous administration only. No clinical studies of the effects of intravenous milrinone administration for acute myocardial failure in dogs or cats have been performed. Clinical studies of the effects of chronic oral administration have been performed, but this form of the drug has not been approved for veterinary use. The results of the veterinary clinical trials of chronic milrinone administration per os in dogs with heart failure have been reviewed.[188]

In normal anesthetized dogs, milrinone dosed at 30 to 300 μg/kg intravenously increases contractility 40% to 120% while decreasing diastolic blood pressure 10% to 30%.[189] Peak effect occurs within 1 to 2 minutes and is reduced to 50% of maximum in 10 minutes, and effects essentially are gone in 30 minutes. Constant rate intravenous infusions (1 to 10 μg/kg/min) increase contractility 50% to 140%, with peak effect in 10 to 30 minutes. In the normal unanesthetized dog, the oral administration of 0.10 mg/kg milrinone increases contractility 30% above baseline, 0.30 mg/kg increases contractility 50% above baseline, and 1 mg/kg increases contractility more than 80% above baseline. Systemic arterial blood pressure is essentially unchanged at these doses, whereas heart rate increases up to 30% at the 1-mg/kg dose. In the normal anesthetized cat, a constant-rate infusion of 1 μg/kg/min increases contractility about 40%, with peak effect occurring within 30 minutes.

Dogs with myocardial failure (predominantly from idiopathic dilated cardiomyopathy) display improved echocardiographic parameters with milrinone dosed at 0.5 to 1.0 mg/kg q12h per os during a 4-week treatment regimen.[190] Ventricular arrhythmias worsen in a small percentage of dogs.

In another study of the oral administration of milrinone to dogs with dilated cardiomyopathy, cardiac index increased 54%, stroke volume index increased 40%, and pulmonary capillary pressure (the pressure that determines whether or how much pulmonary edema is produced) decreased 50%.[191] Mean arterial blood pressure did not change. Heart rate increased 11%. The end-systolic diameter (measured from the M-mode echocardiogram) decreased 9%, whereas blood pressure remained constant. This suggested an increase in E_{max} or a decrease in V_o (i.e., an increase in contractility).

Milrinone has been scrutinized by numerous investigators for chronic oral administration to human patients with heart failure. In 1991, the results of a large clinical trial (approximately 1100 patients) were reported.[93] The investigators in this study found that chronic administration of milrinone to patients with heart failure resulted in an increased risk of sudden death. Consequently, the request for a new drug approval was removed from consideration with the Food and Drug Administration (FDA). Largely because of this event, the drug company that manufactures milrinone lost interest in pursuing approval for milrinone's chronic oral use in dogs. This is despite the fact that milrinone appears to be a better drug in dogs than it is in humans for the treatment of heart failure.

Supply. Amrinone (Inocor, Sanofi Winthrop Pharmaceuticals, New York, N.Y.) is supplied in 20-mL ampules in a concentration of 5 mg/mL for administration as supplied or for dilution in 0.9% or 0.45% saline. Amrinone is reportedly incompatible with dextrose. The drug is prepared with the aid of lactic acid as a sterile solution of the drug in water. The commercially available injection is a clear yellow solution that is stable for 2 years from the date of manufacture. When the drug is diluted, it is stable for up to 24 hours at room temperature or at 2° to 8° C under usual lighting conditions. Amrinone is chemically incompatible with furosemide. If furosemide is injected into the tubing of an amrinone infusion, a precipitate forms.

Milrinone lactate (Primacor IV, Sanofi Winthrop Pharmaceuticals, New York, N.Y.) is supplied in 10- and 20-mL single-dose vials containing 1 mg/mL. It can be diluted in 0.45% and 0.9% sodium chloride and 5% dextrose in water. Milrinone is also chemically incompatible with furosemide.

PURE VASODILATORS

Vasodilator therapy was first introduced in human medicine in the early 1970s after it was noted that the acute administration of nitroprusside resulted in marked improvement in hemodynamics.[192] The first reports of vasodilator use in veterinary medicine were published in the late 1970s and early 1980s.[193-196]

Actions. In patients with heart disease, systemic arterioles are constricted so that a normal blood pressure can be maintained when cardiac output is reduced. In addition, systemic veins are constricted so that blood volume is shifted from the peripheral to the central compartment to increase ventricular preload, produce volume overload hypertrophy, and, in so doing, increase stroke volume and cardiac output. In patients with heart failure, these compensatory mechanisms become detrimental. Although vasoconstriction of systemic arterioles is able to maintain a normal systemic blood pressure, it increases resistance to blood flow and contributes to producing an increased afterload. The normal systemic blood pressure and increased afterload decreases the effective transfer of mechanical energy into blood propulsion into the aorta.[197] The net result is a decrease in stroke volume and an increase in energy consumption by the heart. Systemic venoconstriction in patients with heart failure contributes to the increase in central blood volume. In these patients, the ventricular chambers are unable to grow larger in response to this increase in volume. Consequently, the increase in central blood volume and venoconstriction contribute to the increase in ventricular diastolic pressures and hence to edema formation.

Vasodilators are drugs that act on arteriolar or venous smooth muscle to cause vasodilation. Their effects depend on the vascular beds they influence, as well as relative drug potency. The effect of these drugs on the pulmonary vasculature is erratic or insignificant. This discussion is therefore limited to the systemic vascular beds.

Vasodilators are generally classified as arteriolar dilators, venodilators, or combination (i.e., balanced) arteriolar and venodilators. Arteriolar dilators relax the smooth muscle of systemic arterioles, decreasing peripheral vascular resistance and impedance (Color Plate 36). This usually results in decreased systemic arterial blood pressure, systolic intraventricular pressure, and systolic myocardial wall stress (or afterload). Thus the force that opposes myocardial fiber shortening is reduced. This allows the heart muscle to shorten further and increase stroke volume. Arteriolar dilators are especially useful in patients with mitral regurgitation, aortic regurgitation, ventricular septal defect, and patent ductus arteriosus. In mitral regurgitation and ventricular septal defects, the left ventricle pumps blood in two directions—forward into the systemic circulation and backward, either through a defect in the mitral valve or through a defect in the interventricular septum. In these situations, the percent of blood pumped into the systemic circulation vs. the percent pumped through the defect depends on the relative resistances to blood flow. If resistance to blood flowing into the left atrium (e.g., 1000 dynes sec cm^{-5} m^2) is one half of systemic vascular resistance (e.g., 2000 dynes sec cm^{-5} m^2), twice as much blood will be ejected into the left atrium in systole as is ejected into the aorta (i.e., 66.6% of the stroke volume will be ejected into the left atrium, and 33.3% will be ejected into the aorta). Resistance to blood flow into the systemic circulation depends primarily on the cross-sectional area of the systemic arterioles. Resistance to blood flow through a defect depends on the size of the defect. Defect size is fixed, and therefore resistance to regurgitant or shunt flow is fixed. Systemic vascular resistance, however, is labile and can be manipulated with drugs. If an arteriolar dilating drug is administered to a patient with mitral regurgitation, the decrease in systemic vascular resistance will result in an increase in forward flow into the aorta and systemic circulation. This will result in a decrease in backward flow into the left atrium (Figure 10-10). For example, if systemic vascular resistance is reduced (e.g., 1000 dynes sec cm^{-5} m^2) such that resistance to blood flowing into the left atrium is equal to the systemic vascular resistance, 50% of the total left ventricular stroke volume will be ejected into the left atrium and 50% will be ejected into the aorta and systemic circulation. The decreased backward, or regurgitant, flow will decrease left atrial volume, which will result in a decrease in left atrial pressure, pulmonary capillary pressure, and pulmonary edema formation. Similarly, in aortic regurgitation and patent ductus arteriosus, a decrease in systemic vascular resistance will result in increased forward flow and decreased flow through the aortic valve or the patent ductus arteriosus in diastole.

To illustrate this concept in a more intuitive manner, pretend that you own some land that has a river on it. This river branches into two rivers on your property. On each branch, beavers have built a dam. The river branches are of equal width and depth, and the beaver dams are not complete. One branch goes by your living room window and the other goes through a field. The dam on the branch that goes through the field has a large hole in it. The dam on the branch that goes by your house has a smaller hole such that only one fourth as much water goes through it as goes through the field branch. There is so much water going through the field branch that is has resulted in flooding in that field (i.e., field edema). You decide you want more water flowing by your house and less water flowing into the flooded field. You also decide that you don't want to make the hole in the dam to the field smaller. Consequently, you go out and widen the hole in the dam that is blocking flow to the branch of the river by your house. This results in increased flow through that branch and a decrease in flow through the other branch. This is comparable to administering an arteriolar dilator to a patient with mitral regurgitation where you want more flow going into the aorta (the branch by your house) and less flow into the left atrium (the field river branch).

Venodilators relax systemic venous smooth muscle, effectively redistributing some of the blood volume into the systemic venous reservoir, decreasing cardiac blood volume and reducing pulmonary congestion. The net result is reduced ventricular diastolic pressures, decreased pulmonary and systemic capillary pressures, and diminished edema formation. Consequently, venodilators are used in the same situations as diuretics and low-sodium diets.

Vasodilators are also classified according to their mechanism of action (Table 10-6). Angiotensin converting enzyme inhibitors not only produce vasodilation, they also decrease plasma aldosterone concentration, which results in less sodium and water retention.

Therapeutic endpoints. The therapeutic endpoint of vasodilator therapy is reduction in edema (reduced pulmonary capillary pressure and venous pressures) for venodilators and improved forward perfusion (elevation of cardiac output) for arteriolar dilators in patients with diseases such as dilated cardiomyopathy. When regurgitation or left-to-right shunting is present, arteriolar dilators reduce edema formation and improve forward flow. Although it may not be feasible to measure these parameters directly, close monitoring of clinical signs and radiographic appearance of the lungs is realistic. Therapeutic response is seen as a decrease in coughing, return of normal respiratory rate and effort, improved capillary refill time and color (sometimes hyperemic), improved distal extremity perfusion and temperature, improved attitude and possibly exercise tolerance, resolution of ascites, and radiographic resolution of the pulmonary edema or pleural effusion. Blood lactate concentration and venous

TABLE 10-6

Vasodilator drugs commonly used in veterinary medicine

Vasodilator	*Type (mechanism)*	*Route*	*Dose: dogs*	*Dose: cats*
Hydralazine	Arteriolar [↑ PGI_2 (?)]	PO	0.5-3 mg/kg q12h	2.5-10 mg/cat q12h
Prazosin	Combination [α_1 blocker]	PO	0.5-2 mg/dog q8h-q12h	
Nitroglycerin	Venous [cGMP formation]	Cutaneous	¼ inch per 5 kg q6h-q8h	¼ inch/cat q6h-q8h
Nitroprusside	Combination [cGMP formation]	IV	2-10 μg/kg/min	
Captopril	Combination [ACE inhibitor]	PO	0.5-2 mg/kg q8h	3-6 mg/cat q8h-12h
Enalapril	Combination [ACE inhibitor]	PO	0.5 mg/kg q12h-q24h	0.5 mg/kg q12h-q24h

ACE, Angiotensin converting enzyme.

oxygen tension should improve if they were initially abnormal following arteriolar dilator therapy. Mean or systolic systemic arterial blood pressure is usually reduced by 10 to 40 mm Hg after the administration of an arteriolar dilator. Mean systemic arterial blood pressure should be maintained at approximately 70 mm Hg or above.

Adverse effects. Although vasodilators enable one to achieve better therapeutic results, with their use comes the potential for adverse effects. These drugs are often used in critically ill canine or feline patients or patients with multiple problems who may be on several medications at the time of evaluation or during the course of treatment. These patients, in general, are at greater risk for experiencing adverse effects from a drug. To avoid adverse events and to use these drugs wisely one must have a working knowledge of the mechanism of action, dosages, side effects, drug interactions, and patient risks before their use. If adverse effects occur, one must be cognizant of what constitutes a life-threatening adverse event vs. a relatively benign complication and how to deal with the more serious complications of drug therapy. One must have an accurate diagnosis before institution of therapy. Complications can be expected to be more frequent if the patient is treated before establishing an accurate diagnosis. In cardiovascular medicine, thoracic radiographs, an electrocardiogram, and an echocardiogram are frequently required to establish the diagnosis before therapy.

The primary major adverse effect of vasodilator therapy is hypotension. This usually occurs as an isolated event following administration of the first doses of the drug or during titration of the dose and may only warrant a decrease in the dose rather than discontinuation of the drug. The additive effects of a diuretic and a vasodilator may be a factor in producing hypotension. In our clinical experience, this generally only occurs if the patient is clinically dehydrated and severely volume-depleted. Hypotension is more common and often more severe when two arteriolar dilators are administered concurrently.

It is important to recognize systemic arterial hypotension. If it is misinterpreted as incomplete response to medication or progression of the disease, further doses could result in added complications. Acute-onset weakness and lethargy following drug administration are the most common clinical signs of hypotension.

Hypotension is defined in Webster's dictionary as an abnormally low blood pressure. Hypotension is poorly defined in the medical literature or defined as any systemic arterial blood pressure less than normal. However, in clinical patients hypotension probably should not denote a mild-to-moderate decrease in blood pressure. For this discussion hypotension is defined as systemic arterial blood pressure low enough to result in clinical signs. To produce clinical signs, systemic arterial blood pressure must decrease to a point that blood will not flow through particular vascular beds. When mean systemic arterial blood pressure decreases to less than approximately 50 to 60 mm Hg, flow becomes compromised to renal, myocardial, and cerebral vascular beds. Normal mean arterial blood pressure is 100 to 110 mm Hg. Therefore there is a blood pressure reserve of about 50 mm Hg. Arteriolar dilators take advantage of this reserve in patients with heart failure and cause mild-to-moderate decreases in blood pressure as a therapeutic effect. In patients with heart failure it is common to decrease mean systemic arterial blood pressure to 70 to 80 mm Hg. This is an expected and therapeutic effect and causes no clinical signs of hypotension. On the contrary, clinical signs are generally improved because of the increase in systemic blood flow brought about by the decrease in afterload.

Hydralazine

Actions. Hydralazine directly relaxes the smooth muscle in systemic arterioles, probably by increasing the prostacyclin concentration in the systemic arterioles.[198,199] It also increases aortic compliance. Hydralazine has no effect on systemic venous tone.[200] Hydralazine decreases vascular resistance in renal, coronary, cerebral, and mesenteric vascular beds more than in skeletal muscle beds.[201] Hydralazine also reflexly increases myocardial contractility. This is most likely secondary to hydralazine-induced histamine release resulting in norepinephrine release.[202]

Hydralazine is a very potent arteriolar dilator.[203] In dogs it is able to decrease systemic vascular resistance to less than 40% of baseline compared with captopril, which can only decrease systemic vascular resistance by about 25%.[194,204] Hydralazine's potency can be both beneficial and detrimental to its use. Its potency is of benefit because it results in good-to-profound improvement in the majority of patients in which it is indicated. Its potency can be detrimental if it results in hypotension.

In small dogs with severe mitral regurgitation refractory to the administration of furosemide, regurgitant flow may constitute 80% to 90% of cardiac output.[205] Left ventricular contractile function is usually normal or only mildly depressed.[206] Consequently, the major hemodynamic abnormalities are caused by marked regurgitant flow through an incompetent mitral valve. The ideal treatment would be mitral valve repair, but this is not technically feasible at this time. Consequently, the theoretic treatment of choice is arteriolar dilator administration. Angiotensin converting enzyme (ACE) inhibitors are usually the first choice for achieving mild arteriolar dilation. Hydralazine is more potent and is reserved for patients that are refractory to ACE inhibitors. Hydralazine decreases regurgitant flow, increases forward aortic flow and venous oxygen tension, and decreases radiographic evidence of pulmonary edema (Figures 10-2 and 10-10).[195,207] A therapeutic dosage decreases mean arterial blood pressure from 100 to 110 mm Hg to 60 to 80 mm Hg (Figure 10-11). These effects improve the quality of life and seem to prolong survival time.

In dogs with dilated cardiomyopathy, hydralazine also improves cardiac output but does not usually appreciably reduce edema formation. Consequently, the drug does not seem to improve the

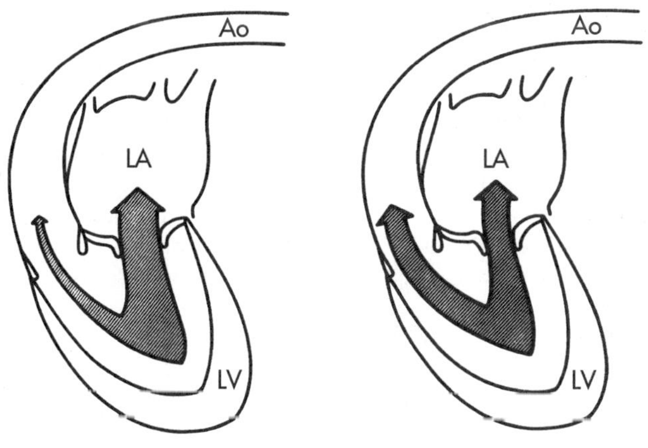

FIGURE 10-10 Drawings of the left heart from a dog with severe mitral regurgitation before *(left)* and after *(right)* hydralazine administration. Before drug administration, approximately 80% of the left ventricular *(LV)* total stroke volume is ejected into the left atrium. Following hydralazine administration, systemic vascular resistance has decreased, forward (aortic *[Ao]*) flow has increased, and backward (regurgitant) flow has decreased. The decrease in regurgitant blood flow results in a decrease in left atrial *(LA)* pressure and resolution of pulmonary edema, as seen in Figure 10-2.

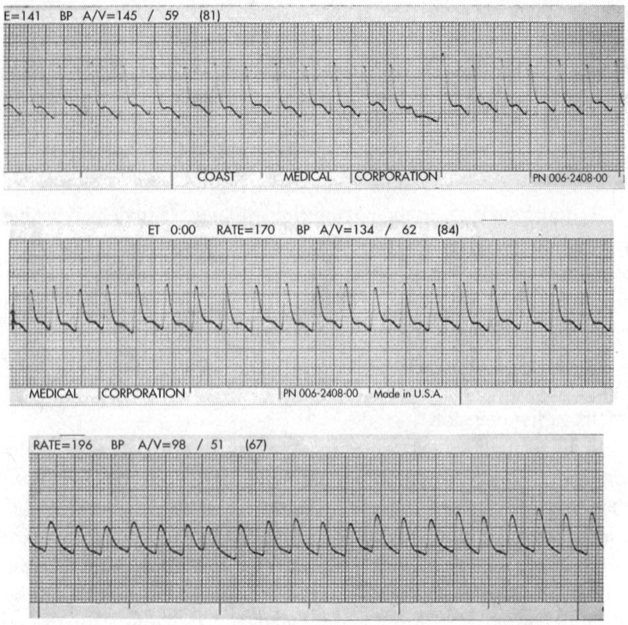

FIGURE 10-11 Systemic blood pressure tracings from a dog before hydralazine administration *(top),* 1 hour after 1 mg/kg hydralazine administered PO *(middle),* and 1 hour after a second 1 mg/kg dose *(bottom).* The cumulative 2-mg/kg PO dose resulted in a decrease in mean, systolic, and diastolic blood pressures in the bottom tracing.

quality of life for the patient nor does it usually result in appreciable prolongation of life.

Indications. The primary indication for hydralazine administration in veterinary medicine is severe mitral regurgitation that is refractory to conventional therapy.[194,195] Hydralazine is also very effective for treating canine and feline patients with severe aortic regurgitation and patients with a large ventricular septal defect. Hydralazine can also be used to decrease systemic blood pressure in dogs with systemic hypertension. Administration of a β-adrenergic blocking drug is frequently required when the drug is used to treat systemic hypertension to block the reflex increase in cardiac output brought about by the increase in contractility and heart rate.

Administration and dosage. The oral route of hydralazine administration has been studied in dogs.[194,207] The effective dose is 0.5 to 3.0 mg/kg q12h PO. This dose must be titrated, starting with a low dose and titrating upward to an effective endpoint. Hydralazine is well absorbed from the gastrointestinal tract but undergoes first-pass hepatic metabolism by acetylation.[208] Presumably, variations from dog to dog in their ability to acetylate hydralazine explain the wide dose range required to produce a response. Although hydralazine is not excreted by the kidney, its biotransformation is affected by renal failure, which may increase serum concentration. The vasodilating effect of hydralazine occurs within 30 minutes to 1 hour after oral administration and peaks within 3 hours. The effect is then stable for the next 8 to 10 hours, after which it rapidly dissipates. The net duration of effect is about 12 hours.[194]

In dogs that are not being administered ACE inhibitors, the starting dose of hydralazine should be 1 mg/kg. This can then be titrated up to as high as 3 mg/kg if no response is observed at lower doses. Titration in these animals can be performed with or without blood pressure measurement. If blood pressure cannot be monitored, titration is performed more slowly and clinical and radiographic signs are monitored. Baseline assessments of mucous membrane color, capillary refill time, murmur intensity, cardiac size on radiographs, and severity of pulmonary edema are made. A dose of 1 mg/kg is administered q12h PO, and repeat assessments are made in 12 to 48 hours. If no response is identified, the dose is increased to 2 mg/kg and then to 3 mg/kg if no response is seen at the previous dose. Mucous membrane color and capillary refill time become noticeably improved in about 50% to 60% of dogs (Color Plate 37). In most dogs with heart failure as a result of mitral regurgitation, the severity of the pulmonary edema will improve within 24 hours. In many of these dogs the size of the left ventricle and in some the size of the left atrium will decrease. In some dogs, improvement will not be great enough to identify with certainty. In those dogs the titration may continue with the realization that some dogs will be mildly overdosed and clinical signs of hypotension may become evident. Owners should be warned to watch for signs of hypotension and notify the clinician if they are identified. If a dog becomes weak and lethargic following hydralazine administration, the dog should be rechecked by a veterinarian, but in almost all situations the dog should only be observed until the drug effect wears off 11 to 13 hours later. The drug dose should then be reduced. In the rare event that signs of shock become evident, fluids and vasopressors may be administered. In human medicine, there has never been a death recorded that was secondary to the administration of hydralazine alone. The dosage record is 10 g. We have observed dogs become very weak following an overdose of hydralazine but have never observed a serious complication when the drug was not administered in conjunction with another vasodilator, such as an ACE inhibitor.

More rapid titration can be performed if systemic blood pressure monitoring is available. In this situation, baseline blood pressure is measured and 1 mg/kg hydralazine administered. Blood pressure measurement should then be repeated 1 to 2 hours later. If blood pressure (systolic, diastolic, or mean) has decreased by at least 15 mm Hg, the dose administered (1 mg/kg) is effective and should be administered q12h from then on. If no response is identified, another 1-mg/kg dose should be administered (cumulative dose of 2 mg/kg) and blood pressure measured again 1 to 2 hours later. This can continue until a cumulative dose of 3 mg/kg has been administered within a 12-hour period. The resultant cumulative dose then becomes the dose administered q12 hours.

When used in dogs that are already being administered an ACE inhibitor, the addition of hydralazine must be performed with caution. ACE inhibition depletes the body's ability to produce angiotensin II in response to hydralazine-induced vasodilation. Severe hypotension can occur if the hydralazine dose is not titrated carefully. In general, the dosage should start at 0.5 mg/kg, and the dose should be titrated at 0.5 mg/kg increments until a response is identified. Blood pressure monitoring is strongly encouraged in this situation. Referral to a board certified cardiologist or internist is also encouraged.

In dogs with acute, fulminant heart failure as a result of severe mitral regurgitation that are not already receiving an ACE inhibitor, hydralazine titration can be more aggressive. An initial dose of 2 mg/kg may be administered along with intravenous furosemide. This dose should produce a beneficial response in more than 75% of dogs. This dose may produce hypotension but the hypotension is rarely fatal, whereas fulminant pulmonary edema is commonly fatal.

Adverse effects. Common side effects include first-dose hypotension and anorexia, vomiting, and diarrhea. Anorexia and/or vomiting occur in approximately 20% to 30% of patients. They are often intractable as long as the drug is being administered. Consequently, discontinuation of the drug may be necessary. Reducing the dose to 0.25 to 0.5 mg/kg q12h for 1 to 2 weeks and then increasing the dose to its therapeutic range may be effective in some cases. The most serious adverse effect is hypotension, indicated by signs of weakness and depression. In most cases, this does not require treatment and the signs will abate within 10 to 12 hours after the last dose of hydralazine. The dose should then be reduced. We have observed dogs with clinical signs of hypotension and counseled owners over the telephone that have had dogs with clinical signs of hypotension and have only rarely observed clinically significant sequela.

When hydralazine is used as the only agent in patients with hypertension and normal cardiac function, hydralazine induces a reflex increase in sympathetic nervous system tone. The increased sympathetic drive increases myocardial contractility and heart rate. Consequently, cardiac output increases dramatically, offsetting the effect of the arteriolar dilation. The net result is no change in systemic arterial blood pressure. When a β-adrenergic receptor blocker is added to the therapeutic regime, the reflex effect is blocked and systemic arterial blood pressure decreases. Although hydralazine is not commonly used to treat hypertension in veterinary medicine, this same response would be expected in a patient that is misdiagnosed and receives hydralazine when it is not in heart failure. Reflex sympathetic tachycardia is not as common in patients with heart failure as in patients with systemic hypertension. However, in one study, heart rate in dogs with mild-to-moderate heart failure increased from an average of 136 beats/min to 153 beats/min following hydralazine administration.[209] In patients with heart failure, the sympathetic nervous system is already activated, but the heart's ability to respond to the sympathetic nervous system is blunted or abolished. In fact, the heart's ability to respond to any type of stimulus is overwhelmed. Therefore, when hydralazine is administered to a patient with heart failure, systemic arterial blood pressure does decrease and a less profound increase in systemic blood flow is produced than that observed when the drug is administered to patients with systemic hypertension. Reflex tachycardia may require the addition of β-adrenergic blocking drugs or digoxin to control.

Rebound increases in renin and aldosterone secretion and decreased sodium excretion occurs following hydralazine administration.[209] This is generally not a clinical problem, however. The beneficial effect on regurgitant fraction usually outweighs these effects. One should remember that drugs such as furosemide also increase renin release and so increase plasma aldosterone concentration.[209] In humans, systemic lupus erythematosus, drug fever, and peripheral neuropathy have been reported.

In human medicine, hydralazine is used in only about 5% of patients with heart failure. It is our impression that hydralazine may also be this unpopular in veterinary medicine. This view of hydralazine is probably the result of adverse effects of the drug observed in certain patients by individual clinicians. Certainly, intractable anorexia and vomiting in a patient warrants discontinuing the drug in that patient. It does not warrant not using the drug in subsequent patients. Producing hypotension during drug titration in a patient can be of concern to the client and the clinician. The clinician must be cognizant of the fact that hypotension in this situation is reversible and generally without sequela, unless the patient is also being administered an ACE inhibitor. Warning the clients of this possible side effect, explaining that this is almost never a lethal side effect (when an ACE inhibitor is not present), and explaining how to deal with it should allay their concerns if signs of hypotension become evident. Again, observing this side effect in a patient does not warrant not using this drug subsequently in the same or other patients.

Drug interactions. Hydralazine administration may have beneficial effects on the pharmacokinetics and pharmacodynamics of other drugs. The increased renal blood flow produced by hydralazine administration can increase the glomerular filtration rate (if initially depressed) and thereby enhance digoxin excretion.[210] The increased renal blood flow also improves furosemide delivery to the nephron.[68] This increases furosemide's renal effects (increases natriuresis and diuresis), especially in patients that are refractory to furosemide administration because of decreased renal flow as a result of decreased cardiac output.

Summary. In summary, hydralazine is a potent and very effective drug for treating dogs and cats with mitral regurgitation, aortic regurgitation, and left-to-right shunts refractory to conventional therapy. Side effects are relatively common, and dosage titration may be difficult. The effectiveness of the drug, however, may warrant its use despite difficulties associated with its administration.

Supply. Hydralazine (Apresoline, Ciba, Summit, N.J.) is available as 10-, 25-, 50-, and 100-mg tablets. We have witnessed a lack of response to some generic hydralazine products and do not recommend their use.

Nitrates: general statement. The organic nitrates, such as nitroglycerin, are esters of nitric oxide. Nitroprusside is a nitric oxide–containing compound without an ester bond. There are important differences in the biotransformation of these compounds, but it is generally accepted that they share a common final pathway of nitric oxide (endothelium-derived relaxing factor) production and a common therapeutic effect.[211] Organic nitrates, such as nitroglycerin, are explosive. They are rendered nonexplosive by diluting the compound with an inert recipient, such as lactose.

Nitrates relax vascular smooth muscle. They do this through a complex series of events. Nitrates are denitrated in smooth muscle cells to form nitric oxide (NO), which binds with the heme moiety on the enzyme guanylate cyclase.[211-213] This causes activation of guanylate cyclase, which enzymatically forms cGMP from GTP. Cyclic GMP activates a serine/threonine protein kinase that phosphorylates myosin light chains, resulting in smooth muscle relaxation.[211,214] Cyclic GMP also stimulates calcium efflux and uptake by intracellular proteins and may inhibit calcium influx.[211] Nitrates are metabolized in the liver by nitrate reductase to two active major metabolites, 1-2 and 1-3 dinitroglycerols. Although less active than their parent compounds, they have longer half-lives and are present in substantial plasma concentrations. Consequently they may be responsible for some of the pharmacologic effect.

Nitrates have been advocated as agents to produce systemic venodilation in dogs and cats with heart failure.[215] Few studies have been performed to document the pharmacodynamics or establish the therapeutic dosage of the nitrates in dogs or cats. Nitrates can be administered orally, intravenously, or transcutaneously to patients with heart failure. When administered transcutaneously or orally to humans, low plasma concentrations are achieved. Nitrates act primarily as venodilators at low plasma concentrations. When administered intravenously, higher concentrations are achieved and arteriolar dilation may also occur. Intravenous nitroglycerin is a potent venodilator with moderate arteriolar dilating properties.

Nitrates are well absorbed from the gastrointestinal tract but are rapidly metabolized by hepatic organic nitrate reductase. Consequently, bioavailability of orally administered nitrates is very low, typically less than 10%. That nitrates are absorbed across the skin (transcutaneously) in humans has been known for decades. Munitions workers exposed to nitroglycerin in the 1940s commonly developed headaches secondary to exposure.[216] In humans, the duration of effect after transcutaneous administration is 3 to 8 hours.

Nitrate tolerance. The phenomenon of nitrate tolerance dates back to the 1940s.[216] Munitions workers exposed to nitroglycerin commonly developed a headache on Monday that abated over the week as they developed tolerance. Over the weekend, their tolerance abated, and, on Monday, reexposure again resulted in headache.

Tolerance to the organic nitrates is a common problem in human patients, occurring in up to 70% of individuals exposed to intravenous infusions of nitroglycerin.[217] The exact mechanism is poorly understood.[218] There are two proposed mechanisms. The most popular theory is that sulfhydryl groups (thiols) are depleted with repeated exposure. This theory is supported by evidence that the tolerance can be reversed by repletion of sulfhydryl groups using *N*-acetylcysteine.[219] One study, however, has not identified tolerance reversal in patients to *N*-acetylcysteine administration or to the administration of captopril, a sulfhydryl-containing angiotensin converting enzyme inhibitor.[220] In addition, *N*-acetylcysteine may reverse tolerance by mechanisms other than sulfhydryl repletion.[221] The second theory is neurohormonal activation resulting in vasoconstriction and increased renal sodium retention. In human patients with heart failure, plasma renin concentration and body weight increase and hematocrit decreases with continuous intravenous nitroglycerin infusion.[219,222]

Intermittent administration of nitrates prevents tolerance in human patients. However, this approach is limited by the fact that the hemodynamic benefit is interrupted. Concurrent administration of hydralazine with a nitrate appears to prevent nitrate tolerance in human patients with heart failure.[223] Hydralazine also prevents tolerance in a rat model of heart failure and in vitro in rat aortas rendered tolerant to nitrate in vivo.[224,225] The results of the in vitro experiment suggest that the effect was due to inhibition of a pyridoxyl-dependant reaction, such as the catabolism of cysteine and methionine, which could enhance the availability of sulfhydryl groups. Others have suggested a beneficial hemodynamic effect. Nitrates are known to decrease renal blood flow, which may explain their ability to increase renin secretion. Hydralazine increases renal blood flow. Consequently, one group of investigators has proposed that hydralazine counteracts the neurohormonal effects of the nitrates.[224] This seems unlikely, however, because hydralazine administration also routinely results in activation of the neurohormonal axis.

Nitroglycerin. Nitroglycerin is an organic nitrovasodilator that possesses a nitrate ester bond. The biotransformation of nitroglycerin to nitric oxide is complex and not completely understood. Thiols (compounds containing sulfhydryl groups) appear to be important as intermediary structures.[211]

Nitroglycerin is diluted with lactose, dextrose, alcohol, propylene glycol, or another suitable inert excipient, so that the medical grade material usually contains about 10% nitroglycerin. It appears as a white powder when diluted with lactose or as a clear, colorless or pale yellow liquid when diluted with alcohol or propylene glycol. Nitroglycerin ointment should be stored in tight containers at 15 to 30° C. Owners should be instructed to tightly close the container immediately after each use. Intravenous nitroglycerin solutions should be stored only in glass bottles because nitroglycerin migrates readily into many plastics. About 40% to 80% of the total amount of nitroglycerin in a diluted solution for intravenous administration is absorbed by the polyvinyl chloride (PVC) tubing of intravenous administration sets. Special non-PVC–containing administration sets are available.

Nitroglycerin has a very short half-life of 1 to 4 minutes.[226] It is metabolized to 1,3- glyceryl dinitrate, 1,2-glyceryl dinitrate, and glyceryl mononitrate. The parent compound is approximately 10 to 14 times as potent as the dinitrate metabolites. The mononitrate metabolite is inactive. The onset of action with the transdermal route of administration is delayed and the duration of effect prolonged. Transdermal systems are designed to provide continuous, controlled release of nitroglycerin to the skin, from which the drug undergoes absorption. The rates of delivery and absorption of the drug to the skin vary with the specific preparation. Individual manufacturers' information for a drug should be consulted for this information. However, one must remember that this information pertains to human skin and probably does not translate into the actual rate of delivery for a dog or a cat.

In human patients with heart failure, transdermal administration of nitroglycerin primarily results in systemic venodilation. This effect results in a redistribution of blood volume from the central to the peripheral vascular compartments, resulting in a decrease in diastolic intraventricular pressures and a reduction in the formation of edema fluid.[227,228] Systemic vascular resistance is lowered to a lesser degree.[227] The dosage required to produce a beneficial effect is highly variable from patient to patient, and some patients are refractory to the drug. Tolerance develops quickly, within 18 to 24 hours.[227] A rebound increase in systemic vascular resistance is observed when nitroglycerin is withdrawn, which results in a decrease in cardiac output.[227] There is no rebound effect on ventricular diastolic and atrial pressures.

Transdermal administration of nitroglycerin has been advocated for use in dogs and cats with heart failure.[215] All references in the veterinary literature to the use of nitroglycerin, including dosing, are anecdotal. Nitroglycerin is usually administered in conjunction with furosemide, most commonly to patients with severe heart failure. Beneficial effects in this situation cannot be directly ascribed to nitroglycerin because it is well known that furosemide by itself can produce dramatically beneficial effects in these patients. Anecdotal reports of the skin in the region of administration turning beet red certainly suggests that there is local vasodilation but does not directly translate into systemic vasodilation. In our clinic, transdermal nitroglycerin is only rarely used in patients with heart failure. However, we have on occasion observed beneficial effects in dogs that were not responding or had become unresponsive to other cardiovascular drugs. Consequently, we believe that there may be a limited role for this drug in veterinary patients. We do not believe that nitroglycerin is a very effective drug and would never administer it as the sole agent to a patient with moderate-to-severe heart failure.

We compared the effects of nitroglycerin ointment and petrolatum ointment in four dogs with dilated cardiomyopathy instrumented with a Swan-Ganz and an arterial catheter. Ointments were applied to a large, shaved area on the lateral thorax. Cardiac output, pulmonary capillary wedge pressure and systemic arterial blood pressure were monitored periodically for 24 hours, at doses up to 4 times the recommended dose. There was no change in any measured variable with either ointment, and the blinded investigator was unable to distinguish the effects of one from the other. It may be that cutaneous absorption from this area on the body in dogs is different from humans or that the drug was placed in an area that is less than optimal. More recently, another investigator has examined splenic weight and diameter in anesthetized dogs following transcutaneous administration of nitroglycerin ointment (1 inch per 10 kg), inside the pinna of the ear. He found that splenic weight and size increased significantly, starting within 10 minutes and peaked within the first 20 minutes. (RL Hamlin, personal communication)

Supply. Nitroglycerin ointment (Nitro-Bid Ointment, Marion Merrell Dow, Kansas City, Mo.; Nitrol, Savage Laboratories, Melville, N.Y.) is available in a 2% formulation to be spread on the skin for absorption into the systemic circulation.[229] It is also supplied in a transcutaneous patch preparation by numerous manufacturers.[227] In dogs and cats, 2% nitroglycerin cream has been used (½ inch per

2.5 kg body weight q12h for dogs, ⅛ to ¼ inch q4-6h for cats), but efficacy has not been documented.[215] If transcutaneous nitroglycerin cream is used, it should be applied on a hairless area (usually inside the ear flap), using gloves, because transcutaneous absorption will occur in the clinician or owner, as well as in the patient. Cutaneous absorption in a human can cause a profound headache and a very unhappy client. Transdermal patches have been used successfully in large dogs with dilated cardiomyopathy.[230]

When nitroglycerin (Nitro-BID IV, Marion Merrell Dow, Kansas City, Mo.; Nitroglycerin Injection, Abbott Laboratories, North Chicago, Ill.; Tridil, DuPont Pharmaceuticals, Wilmington, Del.) is administered intravenously it acts as a potent arteriolar dilator and venodilator. The onset of action after intravenous administration is similar to nitroprusside. Duration of effect is minutes so the drug must be administered by constant-rate infusion. The recommended administration rate to start with *in humans* is 5 μg/min (*not* μg/kg/min). This dose is increased in increments of 10 to 20 μg/min until an effect is identified. There is no fixed optimum dose. Effective doses in small animals have not been identified. To use this drug, a low starting dose would have to be identified and titrated upward as blood pressure was monitored.

Limited experience with a slow-release form of orally available nitroglycerin has been conveyed to the authors.[231] The extended-release preparations are supplied as 2.5-, 6.5-, 9.0-, and 13.0-mg capsules (Nitroglyn, Kenwood Laboratories, Inc., Fairfield, N.J.) or as 2.6- and 6.5-mg scored tablets (Nitrong, Sanofi Winthrop, New York, N.Y.). In cats and dogs, extended-release nitroglycerin can be used to treat refractory heart failure alone or in conjunction with other vasodilators. The most experience has been garnered in dogs and cats with refractory ascites or pleural effusion. Anecdotal evidence suggests that the time between fluid removal can be increased by several weeks and, in some cases, the procedure eliminated altogether. The dose should be titrated, starting at 2.5 mg q12h orally in cats, up to a maximum of 6.5 mg q8h PO. Small dogs can be treated the same as cats. In medium-to-large dogs, the dose is started at 6.5 mg q12h PO. The maximum dose is 9 mg q8h PO.

Isosorbide dinitrate. Isosorbide dinitrate is an organic nitrate that can be administered orally. Its efficacy in dogs and cats has not been studied. Isosorbide mononitrate has been studied in experimental dogs. In one study, a dose of 30 mg q12h PO to dogs weighing 17 kg +/− 3 kg (approximately 1 to 2 mg/kg PO) subjected to transmyocardial direct-current shock produced acute hemodynamic effects that lasted only 2 hours. However, this dose, when administered over days, resulted in a chronic decrease in pulmonary capillary wedge pressure and a decrease in left ventricular volume and mass compared with control dogs.[232] The dose of isosorbide dinitrate is probably similar to isosorbide mononitrate.

Isosorbide dinitrate is supplied as 5-, 10-, 20-, 30-, and 40-mg tablets (Major Pharmaceutical, San Diego, Calif.; Wyeth-Ayerst, Philadelphia, Pa.; ICI Pharma, Wilmington, Del.).

Nitroprusside. Nitroprusside (sodium nitroferricyanide) produces nitric oxide in vascular smooth muscle. Unlike the organic nitrates, nitroprusside releases nitric oxide when it is nonenzymatically metabolized directly via one-electron reduction.[233] This may occur on exposure to numerous reducing agents and tissues such as vascular smooth muscle. The major difference between nitroprusside and the organic nitrates is that tolerance to nitroprusside does not develop.

Nitroprusside is rapidly metabolized after intravenous administration, with a half-life of a few minutes. Consequently, no loading dose is required, and any untoward effects of the drug can be rapidly reversed by discontinuing drug administration. When nitroprusside is metabolized, cyanogen (cyanide radical) is produced. This is converted to thiocyanate in the liver by the enzyme thiosulfate sulfurtransferase (rhodanese).

Nitroprusside is a potent venodilator and potent arteriolar dilator.[200] It may also increase left ventricular compliance.[234] It is administered intravenously and is used only for short-term treatment of dogs with severe or fulminant heart failure. In one study in normal dogs, nitroprusside (25 μg/kg/min) decreased systemic arterial blood pressure by 23% and increased cardiac output by 39%.[235] This effect became attenuated over time. Because tolerance does not occur with nitroprusside, this attenuation of effect probably was due to reflex changes. The decrease in systemic blood pressure did result in a reflex increase in sympathetic discharge, as evidenced by increases in heart rate and myocardial contractility. As expected, left ventricular end-diastolic and end-systolic diameters decreased in this study, as did left ventricular end-diastolic pressure.

Nitroprusside is beneficial in dogs with experimentally induced acute mitral regurgitation (comparable to a patient with a ruptured chorda tendineae). In one study, a dose of 5 μg/kg/min reduced left ventricular systolic pressure 16% and decreased left ventricular end-diastolic pressure from 23 mm Hg to a normal value of 10 mm Hg.[236] Left atrial pressure, left atrial diameter, and left ventricular diameter also decreased. The left atrial *v* wave decreased from 41 mm Hg to 16 mm Hg. Nitroprusside is also beneficial in human patients with mitral regurgitation.[237]

In humans with severe heart failure, nitroprusside can produce beneficial effects that are as good as or better than administration of intravenous furosemide.[238] In one study, nitroprusside reduced pulmonary capillary pressure from 31 mm Hg to 16 mm Hg while increasing the cardiac index from 2.33 L/min/m^2 to 3.62 L/min/m^2.[239] Furosemide (200 mg IV) in these same patients decreased pulmonary capillary pressure to 27 mm Hg, whereas the cardiac index did not change. Consequently, it appears that nitroprusside may be a preferred drug for treating patients with acute, severe heart failure. Unfortunately, nitroprusside generally is not a practical drug to use in clinical practice because blood pressure monitoring is required.

Nitroprusside, in combination with dobutamine, has been shown to be effective in dogs with severe heart failure as a result of dilated cardiomyopathy.[240] Otherwise, all information is anecdotal. We have had success with nitroprusside in a limited number of dogs with severe heart failure and have heard from others of similar successes. We have also heard that in some cases it may be difficult to wean a dog off of nitroprusside after the initial response is achieved. To this end, it should be remembered that nitroprusside only produces a temporary improvement that is readily reversible. When administration is discontinued, vasodilation will rapidly disappear and a rebound increase in vasoconstriction, above that observed before drug administration, may occur.[235] In human patients, when nitroprusside is discontinued after 24 to 72 hours, pulmonary capillary and systemic arterial pressures return to pretreatment values within 5 minutes.[238] This occurs despite increases in urine volume and sodium excretion while on the drug. Consequently, other, more long-acting drugs must be administered while patients are weaned off of the nitroprusside in order to maintain the improvement in hemodynamics.

The dose of nitroprusside is highly variable from patient to patient. In addition, the hemodynamic response can be varied depending on the amount of change in filling pressures and cardiac output desired. Consequently, the dosage range is large. Doses from 2 to 25 μg/kg/min reduce systemic arterial blood pressure in a dose-dependent manner in experimental dogs.[241] However, the decrease in blood pressure with 25 μg/kg/min is only about 5 mm Hg more than that observed with 10 μg/kg/min. Consequently, it does not appear that doses greater than 10 μg/kg/min provide much more benefit than those less than 10 μg/kg/min. In humans, the dosage rarely exceeds 10 μg/kg/min.[226]

Adverse effects of nitroprusside are hypotension and cyanide toxicity. Nitroprusside-induced hypotension can be rapidly (1 to 10 minutes) reversed by discontinuing drug administration. Sodium nitroprusside infusions in excess of 2 μg/kg/min generate cyanogen in amounts greater than can be effectively buffered by the normal quantity of methemoglobin in the body. Deaths caused by cyanogen toxicity can result when this buffering system is exhausted. In humans, this has only been reported in patients receiving total continuous infusion doses greater than 10 mg/kg.[226] However, increased circulating cyanogen concentration, metabolic acidosis, and clinical deterioration have been observed at infusion rates within the therapeutic range. In humans, it has been recommended that an infusion rate of 10 μg/kg/min should not last for longer than 16 hours.[226] Cyanogen toxicity can be manifest as venous hyperoxemia (bright red blood resulting from the inability of oxygen to dissociate from hemoglobin), lactic acidosis, and dyspnea. Administration of thiosulfate and hydroxocobalamin have been reported to prevent cyanide toxicity.[226,242] In the presence of thiosulfate, cyanogen is converted to thiocyanate, which is excreted in the kidneys. Thiocyanate toxicity can occur, especially in patients that have a decreased glomerular filtration rate, are on prolonged infusions, or are receiving thiosulfate. Neurologic signs occur in humans at serum concentrations of 60 μg/mL, and death can occur at concentrations greater than 200 μg/mL.[226] As for other hypotensive agents, nitroprusside increases plasma renin activity.[243]

Sodium nitroprusside (Nitropress, Abbott Laboratories, North Chicago, Ill.; Nitropress ADD-Vantage, Abbott Laboratories, North Chicago, Ill.; Sodium Nitroprusside Sterile, Elkins-Sinn, Cherry Hill, N.J.) is supplied as vials containing 50-mg of lyophilized dry powder for dilution in 5% dextrose in water.[244] Sodium nitroprusside is sensitive to light, heat, and moisture. Exposure to light causes deterioration, which may be observed as a change in color from brown to blue caused by reduction of the ferric ion to ferrous ion. If not protected from light, approximately 20% of the drug in solution in glass bottles will deteriorate every 4 hours when exposed to fluorescent light. The drug deteriorates even faster in plastic containers. Consequently, sodium nitroprusside should be protected from light by wrapping the bottle with aluminum foil. When adequately protected from light, the solution is stable for 24 hours. Nitroprusside reacts with minute quantities of a variety of agents, including alcohol, forming blue, dark red, or green products. The solution should be discarded if this occurs.

Prazosin. Prazosin is an arteriolar and venous dilating agent. It acts primarily by blocking α_1-adrenergic receptors but also peripherally inhibits phosphodiesterase.[245] Because prazosin does not block α_2-adrenergic receptors, norepinephrine release is still controlled via negative feedback. Reflex tachycardia is generally not seen. The vasodilating effects of prazosin become attenuated after the first dose in humans and in rats.[246,247] This problem has markedly limited its use in human medicine. In rats, it is thought that this effect is brought about by stimulation of the renin-angiotensin-aldosterone system. Elimination and metabolism are primarily hepatic, and no adjustment is made for renal insufficiency. Prazosin is effective in reducing mean arterial blood pressure in some dogs with renal hypertension. It may cause first-dose hypotension, anorexia, vomiting, diarrhea, and syncope.

The hemodynamic effects of prazosin have not been documented in the dog or cat. In humans with heart failure, its administration decreases right and left ventricular filling pressures, edema, and congestion, and increases stroke volume and cardiac output.[248] The starting dose in dogs is 1 mg q8h PO for dogs weighing less than 15 kg and 2 mg q8h PO for dogs weighing more than 15 kg. The dose then should be titrated upward if the initial dose is ineffective or reduced if hypotension occurs.

Prazosin is supplied as capsules containing 1, 2, and 5 mg of drug (Minipress, Pfizer Laboratories, New York, N.Y.). This preparation is not amenable for use in cats.

ANGIOTENSIN CONVERTING ENZYME (ACE) INHIBITORS

Actions. The renin-angiotensin-aldosterone system plays an important role in regulating cardiovascular homeostasis in normal individuals and patients with heart failure. Renin is released from the juxtaglomerular apparatus in response to sympathetic stimulation and to decreased sodium flux by the macula densa (see Chapter 9, Figure 9-14). In the plasma, renin is a protease that acts on the glycoprotein angiotensinogen to form the polypeptide angiotensin I. Angiotensin converting enzyme (ACE) cleaves two amino acids from the decapeptide angiotensin I to form the octapeptide angiotensin II. This conversion primarily occurs in the vascular endothelium of the lung, although other vascular beds are involved.

ACE inhibitors bind to the same site on angiotensin converting enzyme as angiotensin I, effectively arresting its action. This site contains a zinc ion, and ACE inhibitors contain a sulfhydryl, carboxyl, or phosphoryl group that interacts with this site. The relative potency of these compounds depends on the affinity of the compound for the active site. ACE inhibitors that are more tightly bound to the active site tend to be more potent. They also tend to have a longer duration of effect. The effects of ACE inhibitors occur as a result of the decreased concentration of circulating angiotensin II. Angiotensin II has the following important effects in patients with heart failure: (1) it is a potent vasopressor, (2) it stimulates the release of aldosterone from the adrenal gland, (3) it stimulates vasopressin (ADH) release from the posterior pituitary gland, (4) it facilitates the central and peripheral effects of the sympathetic nervous system, and (5) it preserves glomerular filtration when renal blood flow is decreased. ACE inhibitors have several effects in patients with heart failure. Arteriolar and venous dilation occur as a direct result of the decreased concentration of angiotensin II. Consequently, ACE inhibitors are generally classified as vasodilators. One must remember, however, that ACE inhibitors also decrease plasma aldosterone concentration. This may, in fact, be their most important role. When the stimulus for aldosterone secretion is lessened, Na^+ and water excretion are enhanced and edema is lessened.

The effects of ACE inhibitors become evident at different times following the onset of administration. Arteriolar dilation is observed after the first dose is administered, whereas the lessening of sodium and water retention takes days to become clinically significant.[204] Because most dogs presenting for severe heart failure are dying from pulmonary edema, the ACE inhibitors are poor emergency heart failure drugs.

The ability of ACE inhibitors to decrease plasma aldosterone secretion may become attenuated or lost with time. In one study of Cavalier King Charles spaniels with severe mitral regurgitation, enalapril significantly decreased plasma aldosterone concentration after 3 weeks of administration.[209] However, 6 months later the plasma aldosterone concentration was increased to an even higher level than at baseline. These dogs were also on furosemide at 6 months, which may have contributed to the increase.

ACE inhibitors act acutely and chronically as arteriolar dilators. In most canine patients, however, this effect is relatively mild compared with the more potent arteriolar dilators such as hydralazine and nitroprusside. In general, ACE inhibitors can decrease systemic vascular resistance by 25% to 30%, whereas hydralazine can decrease it by 50%. This explains the reduced number of hypotensive events observed with ACE inhibitors. This probably also explains why the effect of ACE inhibitors on edema formation and cardiac output in dogs with mitral regurgitation is usually not as profound as with hydralazine.

There are several methods of evaluating the pharmacodynamic effects of ACE inhibitors. None of these methods are perfect. One method is to determine plasma ACE activity in serum and the effects of an ACE inhibitor on ACE activity over time. It is generally thought that any enzyme system must be suppressed by greater than 90% to produce a pharmacologic effect. Consequently, suppression of ACE to greater than 90% should equate with a pharmacologic effect. A more direct means of measuring a pharmacologic effect of disrupting ACE activity is to administer angiotensin I intravenously and measure the increase in vascular resistance before and after the administration of an ACE inhibitor over time. This is probably the most accurate means of determining the ability of an ACE inhibitor to prevent vasoconstriction at a given dose and over a certain time. It does not predict the amount of vasodilation that will be produced in a patient and does not address the effects of blocking the renin-angiotensin-aldosterone system on aldosterone secretion. Plasma aldosterone concentration can be measured in patients with heart failure to document this effect. Lastly, hemodynamic effects of the drug can be measured in patients with heart failure.[204] Unfortunately, the hemodynamic effects of these drugs are often small, making it difficult to accurately determine the appropriate dose, the duration of effect, and the clinical benefit.

Benefits. The clinical benefits of ACE inhibitors in heart failure are reasonably good in human and canine studies. In general, ACE inhibitors improve clinical signs and improve quality of life in dogs with heart failure resulting from diverse causes.[249,250] The improvement in clinical signs is primarily due to reduction in capillary pressure and edema formation and increased perfusion of vascular beds. ACE inhibitors are one of the few drug types used to treat heart failure that has been proven to both improve symptoms and prolong life in humans.[251,252] One must be cognizant that similar survival studies have not been performed using diuretics. Several large clinical trials have documented that captopril and enalapril significantly improve the quality of life and significantly increase survival time in human patients with heart failure.[252-254] A combination of hydralazine and isosorbide dinitrate has also been shown to prolong survival time in humans.[255] Vasodilator therapy is still palliative, however, and even in humans, death still occurs at a relatively rapid pace despite intervention with ACE inhibitors.

In addition to their effects on hemodynamics, ACE inhibitors also appear to have direct or indirect effects on several other cardiovascular variables. Increases in plasma aldosterone and angiotensin II concentrations increase myocardial collagen synthesis and decrease myocardial collagen degradation.[256-258] Angiotensin II–mediated increases in collagen synthesis are mediated by stimulation of AT_1 receptors that are coupled to G proteins that are coupled to multiple signaling pathways, including phospholipase C, protein kinase C, and tyrosine kinases.[258] Administration of spironolactone or captopril prevents fibrosis. Angiotensin II also appears to be cardiotoxic, causing myocyte necrosis and secondary fibrosis.[256] This effect could theoretically be reduced by the administration of an ACE inhibitor. Any effect that ACE inhibitors might have in reducing collagen deposition in dog and cat hearts with cardiovascular disease are theoretic. The amount of fibrosis in most veterinary cardiovascular diseases is unknown. It is presumed that subaortic stenosis is associated with significant subendocardial fibrosis. It is theoretically possible that an ACE inhibitor would be beneficial in this situation because of its effects on collagen deposition. The amount of fibrosis in dogs with volume overloads is unknown. However, in one study of dogs with experimentally-induced left and right heart volume overload as a result of surgically induced aortocaval fistulas, no increase in collagen deposition was identified.[259] This suggests that the ACE inhibitors may not be beneficial in this regard in dogs with valvular valve regurgitation or left-to-right shunts.

Angiotensin II induces myocardial hypertrophy.[260] ACE inhibitors reduce myocardial hypertrophy in several different settings and species. This has been studied most avidly in models of myocardial infarction and in human patients with myocardial infarction in whom ACE inhibitors have a beneficial effect on left ventricular remodeling and survival.[261-265] ACE inhibitors reduce hypertrophy in human patients with systemic hypertension.[266] They also reduce hypertrophy and left ventricular remodeling in dogs after the induction of myocardial failure via intracoronary injections of microspheres.[267] ACE inhibitors can even reduce hypertrophy in rats with experimentally induced aortic stenosis.[268] Whether reduction in hypertrophy can be produced and is beneficial or detrimental to ventricular function and survival probably depends on the disease process and the species involved. There has been no-to-little indication that the ACE inhibitors have any moderate-to-marked benefit on left ventricular size and function in dogs with dilated cardiomyopathy. Presumably, in such a disease, the inherent disease process in the myocardium is unaffected and the disease process progresses at its inherent rate, resulting in continued progression of myocardial dysfunction leading to death. If hypertrophy regression did occur in this situation, it could theoretically be beneficial or detrimental to the heart and to the patient. If myocardial function remained unchanged, reduction in hypertrophy and in left ventricular size would result in a reduction in chamber volume and so a decrease in stroke volume. If, however, myocardial function improved at the same time, then the decrease in ventricular size could increase ventricular efficiency and potentially prolong survival.[197] There is evidence that ACE inhibitors can positively affect myocardial performance.[268,269] To illustrate this point, a study has been performed in rats with experimentally induced aortic stenosis.[197] In this study, aortic stenosis was created by placing steel clips on the ascending aorta to produce a left ventricular pressure of approximately 230 mm Hg (left ventricular systolic pressure in the control group was approximately 100 mm Hg). One group of rats received an ACE inhibitor starting 6 weeks after surgery. Over the next 15 weeks, 31% of the rats in the control group died, and 3% of the rats on the ACE inhibitor died. Left ventricular hypertrophy regressed in the group on the ACE inhibitor. This theoretically should result in a depression in left ventricular function. However, in the rats on the ACE inhibitor, myocardial function improved, resulting in no change in global left ventricular function. In contrast, the control group of rats experienced a decline in myocardial function and a decline in global left ventricular function, despite the increase in myocyte mass. In contrast to progressive myocardial diseases, diseases characterized by acute myocardial insult (e.g., myocardial infarction) where there is no immediate inherent progression of disease (at least not until the next infarct is produced), appear to be benefited by ACE inhibitor administration.

Exactly how ACE inhibitors decrease hypertrophy is controversial. The circulating concentration of angiotensin II is decreased by

ACE inhibitor administration and may be beneficial in decreasing hypertrophy. A renin-angiotensin-aldosterone system has been identified at the myocyte level.[270] Theoretically, ACE inhibitors could interrupt this system. However, a non-ACE tissue chymase has been localized within myocardium, which converts angiotensin I to angiotensin II.[271] This enzyme may be responsible for as much as 80% of the angiotensin II generation in myocardium.[272] If so, ACE inhibition would have to work via another mechanism for reducing hypertrophy, because chymase is unaffected by ACE inhibitors. There is some evidence to suggest that bradykinin may be an inhibitor of myocardial hypertrophy, and ACE inhibitors are known to increase circulating bradykinin concentration.[273]

In veterinary medicine, the primary studies that have documented clinical benefit have been performed using enalapril. These benefits are outlined in the discussion of enalapril (see pp. 180-182).

Adverse effects. The risks of interfering with angiotensin II formation lie in its role of preserving systemic blood pressure and glomerular filtration rate (GFR) as renal flow decreases.[274] Blocking its action on peripheral arterioles can result in hypotension that leads to cerebral hypoperfusion. Dizziness is seen in 15% of humans taking ACE inhibitors. The incidence of clinically significant hypotension in dogs appears to be much less, probably because dogs do not walk upright. The second risk is seen in patients that are very dependent on angiotensin II to maintain GFR. Glomerular efferent arteriolar constriction maintains normal GFR in mild-to-moderately severe heart failure when renal blood flow is reduced.[275] The primary stimulus for this vasoconstriction is increased plasma angiotensin II concentration, which is elaborated in response to the decrease in renal blood flow.[276] Glomerular capillary pressure provides the force for filtration, and glomerular capillary pressure is determined by renal plasma flow and efferent arteriolar resistance. When renal plasma flow is low (such as in heart failure), angiotensin II causes efferent arterioles to vasoconstrict, increasing glomerular capillary pressure. GFR is preserved despite the decrease in flow, and normal blood urea nitrogen (BUN) and serum creatinine concentrations are maintained. The filtration fraction (ratio of GFR to renal plasma flow) is increased. When an ACE inhibitor is administered, efferent arteriolar dilation must occur. In some patients this dilation appears to be excessive, resulting in a moderate-to-marked reduction in GFR and subsequent azotemia. Those human patients that are at greatest risk for developing azotemia include patients with high plasma renin activity, low renal perfusion pressure, hyponatremia, and excessive volume depletion.[277-279] When angiotensin II concentration is decreased in at-risk patients, GFR becomes decreased and azotemia results. The azotemia is generally mild but occasionally can be severe in both human and canine patients. Functional azotemia can occur secondary to the administration of any ACE inhibitor. However, the long-acting agents (e.g., enalapril) may more frequently produce azotemia in human patients than the short-acting agents (e.g., captopril).[280] However, in one study in rats, captopril produced a marked reduction in GFR, whereas perindopril did not.[281] Treatment consists of reducing the diuretic dose or stopping the administration of the ACE inhibitor.

A decrease in GFR and an increase in BUN and serum creatinine concentration is seen in 35% of human patients receiving ACE inhibitors. In most cases the increase in BUN is mild. In dogs, the incidence of clinically significant azotemia appears to be low. In fact, studies suggest that there are no differences between populations of dogs on placebo and furosemide and dogs on an ACE inhibitor.[249] However, our clinic has enough documented cases in which severe azotemia (BUN greater than 100 mg/dL) developed after initiating ACE inhibitor therapy in a canine patient on a stable dose of furosemide to suggest that ACE inhibitor–induced functional renal insufficiency still occurs frequently enough that any veterinarian using these drugs should be aware of the potential occurrence of azotemia. Also in our experience, mild-to-moderate increases in BUN (BUN between 35 and 60 mg/dL) occur with some frequency. In these patients, BUN may increase without a concomitant increase in serum creatinine concentration or the increase in creatinine may be milder. As long as these patients continue to eat and act normally, our tendency is to ignore these changes and to maintain the administration of the ACE inhibitor and the dose of diuretic in those patients that require these doses to treat their heart failure.

Recommended guidelines for ACE inhibitor therapy with regard to azotemia based on human studies and guidelines include the following: (1) identify high-risk patients (patients with moderate-to-severe dehydration, hyponatremia) before therapy; (2) ensure that the patient is not clinically dehydrated and ensure adequate oral fluid intake throughout therapy; (3) evaluate renal function at least once within 1 week after commencing therapy; (4) decrease the dose of furosemide if moderate azotemia develops or discontinue the ACE inhibitor if the azotemia is severe or if a reduction in furosemide dose does not improve renal function.[277,279,282] The prescribing information for Enacard states that if azotemia develops, the dose of diuretic should be reduced, and that if azotemia continues, the dose should be reduced further or discontinued. This sounds as if diuretic administration should be discontinued permanently. Recommendations to permanently discontinue furosemide therapy in a patient with a clear history of moderate-to-severe heart failure are not tenable. In human medicine, the recommendation is to discontinue diuretic therapy for 24 to 48 hours if needed, not permanently.[277] We would also like to stress that azotemia may develop in a canine patient that appears to have no risk factors other than heart failure (Box 10-1). Consequently, it is important to warn owners of the clinical signs of severe azotemia (usually anorexia and other gastrointestinal signs) and to measure serum creatinine concentration and BUN within the first week of initiating ACE inhibitor therapy. If a patient develops severe azotemia, we generally discontinue the use of the ACE inhibitor and make sure the patient is not moderately to severely dehydrated. If dehydration is moderate to severe, we reduce the furosemide dose or discontinue its administration for 1 to 2 days and administer intravenous fluids cautiously. Once the dog is stable, we reassess the need for an ACE inhibitor. In many cases, the ACE inhibitor was being administered because of its potential benefits and the patient did not require its administration. In that case we do attempt to readminister the ACE inhibitor. If the patient is refractory to furosemide administration we feel we have several options. One is to readminister the ACE inhibitor but at a lower dose and then try to gradually titrate the dose into the therapeutic range. A second option is to use a short-acting ACE inhibitor, such as captopril, if a longer-acting agent, such as enalapril, lisinopril, or benazepril, was administered initially. A third option is to add a thiazide diuretic, and a fourth is to add hydralazine or, possibly, amlodipine (see p. 185).

Drug interactions. It should be noted that the arteriolar dilating effect of enalapril, and probably other ACE inhibitors, is attenuated by the concomitant administration of aspirin in humans. Angiotensin converting enzyme inhibitors also decrease the breakdown of bradykinin, which stimulates prostaglandin synthesis.[283,284] The predominant effect of prostaglandins in the systemic circulation is vasodilation. In one study in humans, the normal decrease in systemic vascular resistance induced by an ACE inhibitor was blocked by the concomitant administration of aspirin.[285] However, a study has been performed in experimental dogs with heart failure in which

BOX 10-1

Example of ACE-inhibitor-induced azotemia

A 6-year-old terrier mix, weighing 4 kg was presented as an emergency because of severe respiratory distress (12/31/93). The dog's respiratory rate was 84 breaths/min. Severe pulmonary edema was present on the thoracic radiographs. The dog was placed in an oxygen cage, and 8 mg (2 mg/kg) of furosemide was administered intravenously by an internal medicine resident at 4:30 AM. Blood was withdrawn for a CBC and chemistry panel. This subsequently revealed that the hematocrit was 45%, the total serum protein concentration was 6.4 g/dL, the serum albumin concentration was 2.6 g/dL, the serum bicarbonate concentration was 26 mM/L, the BUN was 24 mg/dL, and the serum creatinine concentration was 0.9 mg/dL. At 9:00 AM the dog was still very dyspneic. A flail mitral valve leaflet as a result of a ruptured chorda tendineae and severe mitral regurgitation were identified on an echocardiogram. The cardiology resident then administered 30 mg (7.5 mg/kg) of furosemide intravenously at 10:00 AM. The dog's respiratory rate was still greater than 70 breaths/min at noon. Consequently, doses of 22 mg (5.5 mg/kg) of furosemide were administered at 12:30 PM and at 3:30 PM. By 5:00 PM the dog's respiratory rate was 54 breaths/min, and so the furosemide dose was decreased to 15 mg every 8 hours. The following day (1/1/94) the dog's respiratory rate was less than 30 breaths/min and she was drinking water but not eating. She was 5% to 6% dehydrated clinically. The next day (1/2/94) she was much "brighter," she was drinking water, and she ate some cooked turkey. Chest radiographs revealed that the pulmonary edema was resolved. The dose of furosemide was decreased to 8 mg IV q8h. Repeat blood work revealed that the hematocrit was 40%, the total serum protein concentration was 6.9 g/dL, and the BUN was 30 to 40 mg/dL. The dog was hyponatremic (serum sodium concentration = 139 mEq/L) and hypokalemic (serum potassium concentration = 3 mEq/L). The dog was not showing any clinical signs referable to her electrolyte abnormalities. Consequently, no therapy for the electrolyte disturbances was administered. On the following day (1/3/94), the dog was eating dog food and drinking normally. The BUN was 38 mg/dL, and the serum creatinine concentration was 0.75 mg/dL. Serum sodium concentration was normal (144 mEq/L), and serum potassium concentration was 2.9 mEq/L. Serum albumin concentration was 2.8 g/dL. The albumin concentration was similar to the value obtained at entry and indicated that the dog was not or only minimally dehydrated at this stage. Furosemide administration was continued at 8 mg IV q8h. The next day (1/4/96), the dog was doing well, and the owner was scheduled to take the dog home that evening on the same furosemide dose plus 2.5 mg enalapril q12h and a potassium supplement. The owner failed to arrive, and the new medications were started that evening. The following morning (1/5/96), the dog was less active and would not eat. Blood work was repeated. The BUN was 89 mg/dL, the serum creatinine concentration was 3.2 mg/dL, and the serum phosphate concentration was 14.3 mg/dL. The serum albumin concentration was 2.9 mg/dL, again demonstrating no-to-mild dehydration. The diuretic dose was decreased to 6.25 mg PO q12h, and intravenous fluids were administered at a rate of 15 mL/hour. The dose of enalapril was maintained. The following morning, the dog appeared a little "brighter" and she ate some turkey. However, her BUN was 149 mg/dL and her serum creatinine concentration was 5.5 mg/dL. Serum albumin concentration was 2.2 g/dL, indicating that dehydration and subsequent prerenal azotemia were not the problems. At this time, the enalapril was discontinued and furosemide and fluid therapy continued. By the following day she was feeling better and eating. Her BUN had decreased to 109 mg/dL and her serum creatinine concentration had decreased to 3.8 g/dL. Serum albumin concentration was 2.5 g/dL. At this time the intravenous fluid administration was discontinued and she was sent home on furosemide at the same dose.

The dog was presented to another emergency clinic 2 weeks later for dyspnea. At that time her BUN was 42 mg/dL, her serum creatinine concentration was 1.2 mg/dL, and her total serum protein concentration was 6.8 g/dL. Her furosemide dose was increased. She remained stable for the next 14 months and then was euthanized. The azotemia in this case was attributed to ACE inhibitor-induced vasodilation of the efferent glomerular arterioles.

low-dose aspirin produced no decrease in hemodynamic response to enalaprilat.[286]

It should also be noted that not all the effects of ACE inhibitors are beneficial in patients with heart failure. One study of human patients with heart failure has documented that captopril acutely decreases the natriuretic and diuretic effects of furosemide.[287] In this study, furosemide increased sodium excretion 623% above baseline, whereas captopril plus furosemide only increased it 242% above baseline. Urine volume increased 225% above baseline with furosemide but only increased 128% above baseline in patients receiving both furosemide and captopril. This was an acute study. The chronic effects of administering captopril to patients stabilized on furosemide are unknown. This finding suggests that an ACE inhibitor should not be administered to a patient with severe, acute heart failure that needs the diuretic effect of furosemide to maintain life.

There are four ACE inhibitors that have been used in dogs and cats: captopril, enalapril, lisinopril, and benazepril. Enalapril is approved by the FDA for use in dogs. Generally these drugs have similar effects. The primary difference is in duration of effect. Captopril is short-acting, lasting less than 3 to 4 hours. Enalapril's effects last 12 to 14 hours. Lisinopril is thought to be the longest-acting and is advocated for once-a-day use in humans. In general, the ACE inhibitors have very similar effects on hemodynamics.

Captopril

Actions. Captopril prevents the conversion of angiotensin I to angiotensin II by competing with angiotensin I for the active site of angiotensin converting enzyme. Captopril's affinity for ACE is approximately 30,000 times greater than that of angiotensin I.[226]

Administration of captopril results in arteriolar and venous dilation and decreased circulating plasma aldosterone concentration.[288] Decreased arteriolar tone reduces systemic blood pressure and afterload. This permits a greater stroke volume, which increases cardiac output. Decreased venous tone coupled with the reduced aldosterone concentration decrease diastolic ventricular, atrial, venous, and capillary pressures and edema formation in patients with congestive heart failure.

The primary effect of captopril in the dog following its first dose is arteriolar dilation.[204] Little change in pulmonary capillary pressure and thus edema formation is noted following the first dose. In addition, in human patients with heart failure, acute captopril administration decreases the natriuretic and diuretic effects of furosemide.[287] Consequently, captopril is not a good emergency drug in dogs with severe pulmonary edema. The effect of reducing edema appears to take more than 48 hours to develop. After that time clinically significant reductions in pulmonary capillary pressure can be noted.

Pharmacokinetics. Captopril has a half-life in dogs of about 3 hours.[289] It is about 75% bioavailable in fasted dogs. This decreases to about 30% to 40% in dogs that are fed.[290] Captopril is metabolized in the liver, but almost all of the captopril and its metabolites are eliminated by the kidneys. Biliary excretion is negligible. Renal excretion of captopril occurs principally via tubular secretion. In patients with decreased renal function, a decrease in dose interval or dose is recommended. The average total body clearance and the renal clearance of captopril are 605 mL/kg in the dog. The volume of distribution of captopril in the dog is 2.6 L/kg;

the volume of the central compartment is about 0.5 L/kg. Captopril is 40% protein bound.

Indications. In dogs with acquired mitral regurgitation, some display marked improvement following captopril administration; others have no change or reduced cardiac output.[115] These variable effects may be explained by differences in baseline aldosterone concentration, but this remains to be studied. In dogs with dilated cardiomyopathy, clinical improvement is usually noted, although this improvement may be short-lived. In humans, captopril is thought to be an effective drug for treating all stages of heart failure in which therapy is required. The drug produces mild-to-moderate reductions in blood pressure, improves exercise tolerance, and prolongs life in human patients.[229] Improvement in survival time has not been documented in veterinary medicine.

A small study has been performed in large (20 to 30 kg) dogs to examine the effects of captopril on mitral regurgitation before the onset of heart failure.[291] In this study, 10 dogs with induced mitral regurgitation were randomly assigned to placebo or captopril (2 mg/kg q8h). These dogs had moderate mitral regurgitation, with an average regurgitant fraction of approximately 57%. They were not in heart failure. The significant findings from this study were that forward ejection fraction (1 − regurgitant fraction) decreased significantly in the dogs administered placebo but did not change in the dogs administered captopril. This was accompanied by a significant decrease in total peripheral resistance. Unexpectedly, the significant increase in forward ejection fraction was not accompanied by a significant decrease in regurgitant fraction. However, this appeared to be due to the marked variability from dog to dog and the small number of dogs studied.

Administration and dosage. The recommended dosage for captopril is 0.5 to 1.0 mg/kg q8h PO. Doses of 3 mg/kg q8h have been associated with glomerular lesions and renal failure in experimental dogs and in clinical canine patients. In a study performed by one of the authors, the onset of activity of captopril was within 1 hour following the first dose.[204] Drug effect lasted less than 4 hours. A dose of 1 mg/kg produced slightly greater effects than a dose of 0.5 mg/kg. A dose of 2 mg/kg produced no additional benefit. Doses in excess of 2 mg/kg q8h can produce renal failure and therefore should be avoided. The dose of captopril in cats, determined from clinical experience, is 0.5 to 1.5 mg/kg q8-12h. Anorexia is a common side effect.[292]

Adverse effects. Captopril is generally well tolerated in most patients. However, side effects can occur and include anorexia, vomiting, diarrhea, azotemia, and hypotension. Gastrointestinal side effects appear to be more common in dogs administered captopril than in dogs administered other ACE inhibitors. In human patients, captopril produces fewer instances of azotemia and hypotension than do the longer-acting ACE inhibitors.[280]

Captopril (Capoten, E.R. Squibb & Sons, Princeton, N.J.) is supplied as 12.5-, 25-, 50-, and 100-mg tablets.

Enalapril

Actions. Enalapril is the ethyl ester of enalaprilat.[226] It has little pharmacologic activity until it is hydrolyzed in the liver to enalaprilat. Enalapril is available commercially as the maleate salt. Enalapril maleate is absorbed better from the gastrointestinal tract than enalaprilat in dogs.[293] Enalapril is structurally and pharmacologically similar to captopril but contains a disubstituted nitrogen rather than the sulfhydryl group. The lack of the sulfhydryl group may result in decreased risk of certain side effects in humans, such as taste disturbances and proteinuria. These adverse effects have not been documented in dogs or cats administered ACE inhibitors.

Enalaprilat prevents the conversion of angiotensin I to angiotensin II by binding competitively to the angiotensin I binding sites on ACE. The affinity for enalaprilat is approximately 200,000 times that of ACE.[226]

Pharmacokinetics. In dogs, enalapril maleate achieves peak concentration within 2 hours of administration.[293] Bioavailability is approximately 60%. Enalapril is metabolized to enalaprilat. Peak serum concentration of this active form occurs 3 to 4 hours after an oral dose. The half-life of accumulation is approximately 11 hours and duration of effect is 12 to 14 hours. Steady-state serum concentration is achieved by the fourth day of administration. Excretion of enalapril and enalaprilat is primarily renal (40%), although 36% is excreted in the feces.[293] Approximately 85% of an oral dose is excreted as enalaprilat.

The pharmacodynamics of enalapril have been examined in experimental dogs.[294] A dose of 0.3 mg/kg administered per os results in approximately 75% inhibition of the pressor response to angiotensin I. This effect lasts for at least 6 hours and is completely dissipated by 24 hours after administration. A dose of 1 mg/kg produces only slightly better inhibition (approximately 80%) for at least 7 hours. About 15% inhibition is still present 24 hours after oral administration.

Administration and dosage. Dose ranging has been performed with enalapril in dogs with surgically induced mitral regurgitation and heart failure.[295] In these dogs, a dose of 0.5 mg/kg enalapril PO acutely produced a greater decrease in pulmonary capillary pressure than a dose of 0.25 mg/kg. A dose of 0.75 mg/kg produced no better response. After 21 days of administration, the 0.5-mg/kg q24h dose produced a significant decrease in heart rate, whereas the 0.25 mg q24h dose did not. Consequently, the enalapril dose is 0.5 mg/kg. Whether this dose should be administered once a day or twice a day is debatable. The package insert recommends starting with once-a-day dosing, increasing to twice-a-day dosing if the clinical response is inadequate. Based on the pharmacodynamics presented in the previous paragraph, we generally start the drug by administering it twice a day to dogs in heart failure, approximately 12 hours apart.

Adverse effects. The adverse effects of enalapril are the same as for all ACE inhibitors, as outlined above. Chronic enalapril toxicity appears to be confined to the kidneys.[296] In healthy dogs administered doses up to 15 mg/kg/day over 1 year, drug-induced renal lesions are not seen.[296] High-dose (30 to 60 mg/kg/day) enalapril administration to dogs results in dose-related renal toxicity. At 30 mg/kg/day, increasing degrees of renal damage are observed that are shown to be a direct nephrotoxic response of enalapril itself on proximal tubular epithelium. This damage is permanent only when potentiated by marked hypotension. The damage is confined to the proximal tubules, primarily to the juxtamedullary regions of the cortex, where necrosis of the tubular cells but not the basement membrane is present. Dogs that survive the initial insult to the proximal tubules undergo regeneration. Doses of 90 to 200 mg/kg/day is rapidly lethal as a result of renal failure.[226] The renal toxicity appears to be due to a direct nephrotoxic effect of the drug and to an exaggerated decrease in systemic blood pressure. Saline administration ameliorates the toxicity.

Efficacy and safety. Studies of enalapril's efficacy in dogs with dilated cardiomyopathy and in dogs with primary mitral regurgitation with heart failure have been completed and reported. In one study, 58 dogs were enrolled for study at seven different centers.[250] This study was identified by the acronym IMPROVE (Invasive Multicenter Prospective Veterinary Evaluation of Enalapril Study). Of the 58 dogs, 35 had dilated cardiomyopathy, 22 had primary mitral regurgitation, and one had aortic regurgitation. Dogs were randomly assigned to be administered enalapril (n = 31) or a placebo (n = 27). The enalapril dose was 0.5 mg/kg q12h. Physical examinations, electrocardiograms, echocardiograms, and thoracic radiographs were obtained before and 2 (range = 1-4) and 20 (range = 17 to 28) days after starting placebo or drug administration. In addition, a Swan-Ganz catheter was placed to monitor pulmonary capillary pressure, right atrial pressure, and cardiac output, and an arterial catheter was placed to measure systemic arterial blood pressure intermittently for the first 24 hours (baseline and 4, 8, 12, and 24 hours after drug administration). Forty-one dogs (19 placebo-treated and 22 enalapril-treated) completed the study. The acute (first 24 hours) hemodynamic effects of enalapril were not spectacular. Heart rate decreased significantly only at the 4-hour period. Mean systemic arterial blood pressure decreased significantly only at the 8-hour period. Pulmonary capillary pressure decreased significantly at the 8-hour period. Cardiac output and right atrial pressure did not change at all. Clinical response over the 20 days was better. Overall the dogs on enalapril improved clinically and had increased mobility compared with dogs on the placebo (7 of 24 dogs on the placebo improved clinically, whereas 19 of 27 dogs on enalapril experienced an overall clinical improvement). Of the dogs administered enalapril, 26% were classified as greatly improved, and 44% were classified as improved. No dog that was administered the placebo was classified as greatly improved, but 29% were classified as improved. This overall clinical improvement was significant only for dogs with dilated cardiomyopathy, not for dogs with primary mitral regurgitation. There were no significant changes in activity, attitude, cough, appetite, demeanor, respiratory effort, or murmur intensity. Radiographic evidence of pulmonary edema was decreased in 40% of the dogs treated with enalapril on day 2, and 56% were improved on day 20. This is compared with 15% of dogs treated with the placebo on day 2 and 17% on day 20. There was no significant change in any echocardiographic variable. A significantly greater number of enalapril-treated dogs also improved clinically based on class of heart failure compared with placebo-treated dogs.

A second study was performed and identified by the acronym COVE (Cooperative Veterinary Enalapril study group).[249] In this study, 211 dogs were studied at 19 centers. Of these, 141 dogs had primary mitral regurgitation and 70 had dilated cardiomyopathy as the primary diagnosis. All except one dog was being administered furosemide with (approximately 75%) or without digoxin on entry into the study. Dogs were assigned to be administered either placebo or enalapril based on a randomized allocation schedule. The study was blinded so that neither the investigator nor the client knew which treatment the dog was receiving. Dogs with renal failure, other terminal disease, or uncorrected hypothyroidism were excluded from the study. Dogs that had been administered calcium antagonists or nonnitrate vasodilators within 4 days before entering the study were also excluded. Clinical evaluations of each dog were performed at baseline and 2 and 4 weeks later. Dogs were evaluated by physical examination, electrocardiography, thoracic radiography, CBC, serum chemistry profile, urinalysis, and serum digoxin concentration at each time point. Echocardiography was performed at baseline to confirm the diagnosis. Fourteen subjective clinical variables were assessed by each investigator with the aid of the owner at each time point. The investigators had the option of removing a dog from study at any point if they thought that continuation in a blinded study placed the dog at risk or if the dog was not improving adequately. Furosemide and digoxin doses did not change significantly during the study in either group. Significantly more enalapril-treated dogs (32%) completed the study than placebo-treated dogs (15%). More dogs in the placebo group died of heart failure (7 vs. 0) or were removed from the study because of progression of heart failure (16 vs. 7). In dogs with dilated cardiomyopathy, there was significant improvement in class of heart failure, overall evaluation, mobility, activity, and amount of pulmonary edema on both days 14 and 28. By day 28, there was further improvement, as evidenced by significant improvement in demeanor, cough, and appetite. In dogs with mitral regurgitation, there was no significant clinical improvement on day 14, but by day 28 there was significant improvement in activity, mobility, overall evaluation, and cough. Renal function tests were abnormal in approximately 45% of the dogs in both groups at baseline. They did not change significantly in either group.

A long-term efficacy study has also been completed. The acronym for this study is LIVE (Long Term Investigation of Veterinary Enalapril study).[297,298] Dogs (n = 148) from the COVE and IMPROVE studies were continued on either the placebo (n = 71) or enalapril (n = 77) and studied in an identical manner to the COVE study for up to 15.5 months. Dogs remained in the study until they developed intractable heart failure (n = 48), died of heart failure (n = 17), died suddenly (n = 10), died of a noncardiac cause (n = 4), dropped out of the study for other reasons (n = 48), or the study ended (n = 21). Dogs administered enalapril remained in the study significantly longer (169 days) than dogs administered the placebo (90 days). Most of this benefit occurred in the first 60 days. After that, dogs in both groups either developed intractable heart failure or died at a similar rate. When divided into dogs with mitral regurgitation and those with dilated cardiomyopathy, the dogs with dilated cardiomyopathy that were administered enalapril remained in the study significantly longer (158 days) than those that were administered the placebo (58 days). Dogs with mitral regurgitation administered enalapril, however, did not remain in the study significantly longer (172 days) than those administered the placebo (110 days).

The three aforementioned studies are the result of one of the largest efforts ever put forth to document drug efficacy in small animal veterinary medicine. The results are quite clear. Enalapril, despite the fact that it produces minimal hemodynamic change, results in clinical improvement in dogs with heart failure resulting from mitral regurgitation or dilated cardiomyopathy. It appears to perform better in dogs with dilated cardiomyopathy but is clearly efficacious in many dogs with mitral regurgitation. However, in general and in both diseases, the clinical response is not profound. Rather, in most cases the drug results in mild and gradual improvement that helps to stabilize the clinical course of the patient and improve the quality of life. Therefore enalapril is a good adjunctive agent for treating patients with heart failure. It may be effective as the sole agent in some dogs with very mild heart failure but in most cases must be administered in conjunction with a more effective drug, usually furosemide. The drug's effects on survival are less clear. No true survival study has been performed. However, a study (LIVE) of the time to treatment failure or death has been performed. The data from this study may translate into increased survival, but this is not assured. The ability of enalapril to prolong the life of dogs with heart failure secondary to primary mitral regurgitation is questionable.

Enalapril has been shown to be beneficial in dogs with mitral regurgitation but of less benefit for the group as a whole than possibly expected. In our clinical experience, some dogs with mitral regurgitation have dramatic responses to an ACE inhibitor, many improve clinically, and a significant number have little response.

In the IMPROVE study, which included 22 dogs with mitral regurgitation, enalapril did not significantly improve any clinical variable.[250] Almost no echocardiographic variable was significantly altered. Hemodynamic variables were statistically significantly altered, with mean systemic arterial blood pressure decreasing an average of approximately 5 mm Hg, and pulmonary capillary wedge pressure (the pressure that determines the amount of pulmonary edema) decreasing approximately 3 to 5 mm Hg. The decrease in systemic blood pressure is clinically insignificant because cardiac output did not increase significantly. The decrease in pulmonary capillary wedge pressure is very small and probably clinically insignificant for the group. Almost assuredly there were some dogs within this group that did experience a more clinically significant decrease in pulmonary capillary pressure, however. In the LIVE study, dogs with mitral regurgitation ($n = 88$) were treated with either placebo ($n = 41$) or enalapril ($n = 47$).[297] Treatment was continued until the investigator thought the dog's heart failure was not adequately responding to treatment (at which time the investigator was unblinded as to whether the dog was receiving placebo or enalapril and switched to enalapril if on placebo), the patient died, the patient was dropped from the study for other reasons, or the study was terminated. Time until treatment failure was not significantly different between these two groups that had mitral regurgitation. A survival study using clinical patients with mitral regurgitation has not been conducted. In the COVE study, dogs with mitral regurgitation were enrolled, but the exact number has not been published. A total of 190 dogs were enrolled, the vast majority with either mitral regurgitation or dilated cardiomyopathy. In this study, more dogs with mitral regurgitation receiving enalapril experienced improvement in class of heart failure than dogs on placebo.[299] The overall evaluation also improved in more dogs on enalapril than in dogs on placebo. These data underscore the clinical impression that the clinical response to ACE inhibitors can be quite varied (some dogs have dramatic responses, and some have no response, but most have mild-to-moderate improvement). They also underscore the fact that clinical improvement with these drugs is commonly more dramatic than the hemodynamic or echocardiographic response.

Early intervention. Studies have been performed in humans to determine if starting ACE inhibitor therapy with enalapril in patients with left ventricular dysfunction but without evidence of heart failure is beneficial. *Benefit* has been defined as reduction in mortality, reduction in the incidence of heart failure, and reduction in the hospitalization rate. In a study of human patients with chronic cardiac disease, 4228 patients with ejections fractions less than 35% (comparable to a shortening fraction less than 15%) were randomized to receive either placebo or enalapril.[251] They were followed clinically for an average of 37 months. During this time there was no reduction in mortality associated with enalapril administration. There was a reduction in the incidence of heart failure and in hospitalizations for heart failure (the drug delayed the onset of heart failure). These latter findings should be expected. Any efficacious heart failure drug should prolong the time until heart failure is evident if it is administered before the onset of heart failure to a patient with cardiac disease. Almost assuredly, the same or better results could be obtained with a diuretic.

Because of findings in humans, recommendations have been made to administer enalapril to canine patients with cardiac disease but without heart failure.[297] Many veterinary cardiologists recommend that an ACE inhibitor be administered to dogs with mitral regurgitation when there is severe left atrial enlargement but no evidence of pulmonary edema. There are certainly theoretic grounds for doing this, but there is no proof that this tactic is beneficial. Presently, we do not follow this approach and instead administer ACE inhibitors, usually in conjunction with furosemide, when there is evidence of heart failure. Because there is no proof that either approach is superior, each veterinarian must use his or her own judgment on how to approach this type of case. A few veterinary cardiologists recommend initiating ACE inhibitor therapy when mild-to-moderate mitral regurgitation is present. We oppose this approach for several reasons. First and foremost, many dogs with mild-to-moderate mitral regurgitation will never progress to develop heart failure. If these dogs are administered an ACE inhibitor, it condemns the owner to years of expensive treatment. Second, there is no clinical proof and no experimental evidence to suggest that administering an ACE inhibitor this early in the course of the disease is beneficial. Third, ACE inhibitors are not without side effects. Administering a drug that has the potential of producing side effects to a dog that does not need the drug (presuming the patient will never develop heart failure) is questionable medical practice. Currently, a study is in progress to determine if enalapril administration to dogs with severe mitral regurgitation but without heart failure is beneficial. Until the results of that study are known, recommendations to start enalapril before the onset of heart failure are premature. If the results of this trial show a true increase in survival time, there will be no doubt that administration of an ACE inhibitor to dogs with severe cardiac disease but without heart failure is warranted. If, however, it only shows that the onset of heart failure is delayed, then early administration of such drugs should only be undertaken after detailed consultation with the client, primarily because of the cost of these drugs. If this scenario comes to pass, there undoubtedly will be clients that will opt for early therapy because they want to delay seeing their pet with any degree of respiratory distress regardless of cost. There also, however, undoubtedly will be clients that do not want to spend several dollars a day just to delay the inevitable.

There is experimental evidence in dogs that enalapril helps preserve left ventricular function and stabilize the severity of functional mitral regurgitation in a model of dilated cardiomyopathy. In one study, enalapril was administered to dogs with global myocardial failure produced by injecting latex microspheres into the coronary circulation.[300] In a control group of dogs, end-diastolic and end-systolic volumes increased over 3 months and the ejection fraction decreased. In dogs treated with enalapril, chamber volumes and the ejection fraction did not change. In this same study, metoprolol, a β-adrenergic blocking drug produced the same results as enalapril, whereas digoxin was unable to lessen the progression of disease. In another study, the same model was used and the amount of mitral regurgitation was quantified using color flow Doppler mapping.[301] In the control group, the regurgitant fraction increased from an average of 14% to 23% in control dogs and did not change in dogs administered enalapril.

This may not be the case in dogs with naturally occurring mitral regurgitation. One study has examined the short- and long-term effects of enalapril on left ventricular size and function in Cavalier King Charles spaniels with myxomatous mitral valve degeneration and mild-to-moderate heart failure.[209] In this study, enalapril did not result in a decrease in left ventricular size after 3 weeks of drug administration. After this time, furosemide was administered in conjunction with enalapril. Six months later the left ventricular size actually increased. In a comparable group administered hydralazine and furosemide, the left ventricular size remained the same. End-systolic diameter did not change at any time in either group, suggesting that afterload and myocardial function were not significantly altered.

Supply. The veterinary formulation of enalapril maleate (Enacard, Merck & Co., Rahway, N.J.) is supplied as 1-, 2.5-, 5-, 10-, and 20-mg tablets. The human formulation (Vasotec, Merck Sharp & Dohme, West Point, Pa.) is supplied as 2.5-, 5-, 10-, and 20-mg tablets. There is also a formulation of enalapril maleate and hydrochlorothiazide that contains 10 mg enalapril maleate and 25 mg hydrochlorothiazide in one tablet (Vaseretic 10-25, Merck Sharp & Dohme, West Point, Pa.). Enalaprilat (Vasotec IV, Merck Sharp & Dohme, West Point, Pa.) is available for intravenous injection as enalaprilat in 0.9% alcohol at a concentration of 1.25 mg of anhydrous enalaprilat per milliliter.

Lisinopril

Actions. Lisinopril is a lysine derivative of enalaprilat. It does not require hydrolysis to become active. It has a higher affinity for ACE than either captopril or enalapril.

Pharmacokinetics. Lisinopril's bioavailability is 25% to 50%.[290,294] Feeding does not affect bioavailability. Peak plasma concentration occurs 4 hours after oral administration in dogs.[294] Peak inhibition of the pressor response to angiotensin I occurs 3 to 4 hours after oral administration. Peak ACE inhibition occurs 6 to 8 hours after administration. Elimination half-life of lisinopril in dogs is about 3 hours.

Lisinopril's effects last for 24 hours but are quite attenuated 24 hours after oral administration in dogs.[294] A dose of 0.3 mg/kg per os to dogs results in approximately 75% inhibition of the pressor response to angiotensin I 3 hours after administration. This response decreases to about 60% inhibition by 6 hours and to approximately 10% at 24 hours. When a dose of 1 mg/kg is administered per os, greater than 90% inhibition of the pressor response to angiotensin I is achieved 4 hours after drug administration. This response is still approximately 90% inhibition at 6 hours after administration and is still approximately 40% at 24 hours after administration.

Administration and dosage. A clinically effective dose of lisinopril has not been identified in dogs or cats. We and others generally use a dose of 0.5 mg/kg q24h PO. From the pharmacodynamic data just presented, a dose of 0.25 to 0.5 mg/kg q12h or a dose of 1 mg/kg q24h may be more effective. The primary benefit of lisinopril is cost. Cost to treat a dog per day is often half that of other ACE inhibitors if a dose of 0.5 mg/kg q24h is used. The major factor that retards its use is the fact that the studies to document its pharmacodynamics and efficacy have not been performed.

Indications and adverse effects. The indications for and the adverse effects of lisinopril are the same as the other long-acting ACE inhibitors.

Supply. Lisinopril (Prinivil, Merck Sharp & Dohme, West Point, Pa.; Zestril, Zeneca Pharmaceuticals, Wilmington, Del.) is supplied in 5-, 10-, 20-, and 40-mg tablets.

Benazepril

Actions. Benazepril is a nonsulfhydryl ACE inhibitor. Like enalapril, it is a prodrug that is converted to benazeprilat by esterases, mainly in the liver. Benazeprilat is approximately 200 times more potent as an ACE inhibitor than benazepril. The conversion of benazepril to benazeprilat is incomplete, and other metabolites are formed in the dog.[302]

Pharmacokinetics. Benazeprilat is poorly absorbed from the gastrointestinal tract, whereas benazepril hydrochloride is well absorbed in the dog.[302] Bioavailability increases by about 35% with repeated dosing.[303] Following the administration of oral benazepril, plasma benazeprilat concentration reaches peak concentration in plasma within 1 to 3 hours. Benazeprilat is rapidly distributed to all organs except the brain and placenta. Benazeprilat is excreted approximately equally in the bile and the urine in dogs. Less dependence on renal excretion may make it safer to use in dogs with preexisting renal failure. The terminal half-life is approximately 3.5 hours. There may be an additional slow terminal elimination phase in dogs, which may have a half-life between 55 and 60 hours.[303]

The pharmacodynamics of benazepril have been studied in dogs by measuring plasma ACE activity before and after various doses of the drug. A dose of 0.125 mg/kg benazepril q24h appears to be too low. It only inhibits plasma ACE activity to approximately 80% of baseline. A dose of 0.25 mg/kg decreases plasma ACE activity to less than 10% of baseline within 3 hours of administration. This effect lasts for at least 12 hours. By 16 hours, plasma ACE activity is back to 20% of baseline, and by 24 hours it is approximately 30% of baseline. Doses of 0.5 and 1.0 mg/kg cause the greater than 90% suppression to last at least 16 hours. When benazepril is administered chronically, doses from 0.25 mg/kg to 1.0 mg/kg produce indistinguishable effects at the time of peak effect, 2 hours after oral administration. The same can be said for dosage effects on plasma ACE activity 24 hours (trough) after oral administration. From these data it can be concluded that the benazepril dose that will be effective clinically will probably be between 0.25 and 1.0 mg/kg PO and that once-a-day administration will probably be clinically effective in dogs.

Indications and adverse effects. Benazepril can be used in dogs or cats with heart failure as with any other ACE inhibitor. However, no clinical studies have been performed to document safety and efficacy. Anticipated adverse effects would be the same as for other long-acting ACE inhibitors. Benazeprilat has been studied in dogs with experimentally induced heart failure.[304] In this study, acute left heart failure was produced by injecting microspheres into the left coronary circulation. This resulted in an increase in left ventricular end-diastolic pressure (LVEDP) and a decrease in cardiac output. Benazeprilat (30 μg/kg IV) decreased LVEDP by approximately 15%, peripheral resistance by approximately 30%, and aortic pressure by 30%. Cardiac output did not increase in these anesthetized dogs.

Supply. Benazepril (Lotensin, Ciba-Geigy Corp., Summit, N.J.) is supplied as 5-, 10-, and 20-mg tablets.

DILTIAZEM

Diltiazem is a calcium channel blocker commonly used to treat heart failure resulting from hypertrophic cardiomyopathy. It improves myocardial relaxation, reduces myocardial contractility, and may reduce heart rate in cats with hypertrophic cardiomyopathy. The improvement in myocardial relaxation may help decrease left ventricular diastolic pressure and so reduce pulmonary edema formation. The reduction in myocardial contractility may reduce systolic anterior motion of the mitral valve. Heart rate reduction may be beneficial in cats with sinus tachycardia or atrial fibrillation. A complete discussion of this drug and its use is presented in Chapter 21.

Diltiazem is also commonly used to decrease the ventricular rate in patients with atrial fibrillation, a common sequela to severe heart disease. Rapid heart rates induce myocardial failure in dogs. Consequently, rate reduction with diltiazem may be viewed as producing myocardial protection. Digoxin and β-blockers are used for this same purpose. For a complete discussion of the treatment of atrial fibrillation see Chapter 29.

NEW OR EXPERIMENTAL HEART FAILURE DRUGS

Because there is no cure for most cardiovascular diseases that result in heart failure, there are always new drugs being developed to treat cardiac disease and heart failure. Some drugs eventually make it to the marketplace, while others fall by the wayside during any phase of drug development. This section presents a few drugs that may become useful for treating heart failure in the future.

β-Adrenergic blockers. There is an impressive amount of data that suggests that the administration of β-adrenergic blocking drugs to human patients with myocardial failure and heart failure results in improved myocardial function, improved exercise capabilities, and, in some studies, improved survival. This effect is counterintuitive because β-blockers are generally considered to be negative inotropic agents, and negative inotropic agents are generally contraindicated in myocardial failure.

Waagstein in 1973 first noted that one of his patients, a woman with refractory dilated cardiomyopathy and resting tachycardia, improved following the intravenous administration of practolol and the subsequent oral administration of alprenolol.[305] This experience prompted him to examine the effects of oral practolol on six more patients and report his findings in 1975.[306] His patients improved clinically, and their left ventricular function improved (shortening fraction increased). In 1979, he and his coinvestigators reported the results of an additional 24 patients that were compared with 13 historical controls.[307] They reported that the patients treated with β-blockers survived longer. As expected, this novel approach was not immediately embraced by human cardiologists. However, over the past 15 years, data from blinded and placebo-controlled trials have documented that β-blockers do have a significant effect in human patients with myocardial failure.[308-310] This effect, however, is relatively mild. Ejection fraction commonly increases in the range of 10 to 15 percentage points. This is comparable to shortening fraction increasing 4% to 7%. Exercise tolerance usually improves. Survival time generally does not improve.[308,310] There are no reports of physicians being able to wean their patients off of other cardiovascular drugs.

When β-adrenergic blocking drugs are used in human patients with myocardial failure, a small test dose is administered orally to determine if the patient can tolerate any negative inotropic effects of the drug. If the patient does not deteriorate on this small test dose, the dose is gradually increased over the next 1 to 3 months, with the dose being doubled weekly. Eventually doses 4 to 15 times the starting dose are administered. β-Adrenergic blocking drugs that have been used include metoprolol, labetalol, carvedilol, bisoprolol, and bucindolol. Starting doses for adult humans range from 1.25 mg PO for bisoprolol to 6.25 mg PO for metoprolol.[311] The target dose ranges from 5 to 10 mg PO for bisoprolol to 50 mg to 100 mg PO for labetalol and bucindolol.

There are a limited number of studies of the use of β-adrenergic blocking drugs in normal dogs or dogs with experimental heart disease. In normal dogs, atenolol has no significant effects on the structural or functional properties of the myofibril.[312] One study has examined the effect of metoprolol on the progression of myocardial failure after production of acute myocardial failure using intracoronary injections of microspheres.[300] In this study, severe myocardial failure (ejection fraction = 30% to 40%) was produced in two groups of dogs. The dogs were allowed to stabilize for 3 weeks. They were then randomly assigned to receive either placebo or metoprolol (25 mg q12h). In the control group, left ventricular function deteriorated (ejection fraction decreased from an average of 36% to 26%). In the group that was administered metoprolol, ejection fraction did not improve but did remain the same. This suggests that β-blocker therapy may have a 'protective' effect in dogs. In another study, atenolol was administered to large dogs with experimentally induced mitral regurgitation.[313] As opposed to the last study, left ventricular myocardial function and myocyte function improved in these dogs.

There is an ongoing interest in this approach to therapy in veterinary medicine. We have tried to administer β-adrenergic blocking drugs for this purpose to several canine patients with severe dilated cardiomyopathy in our clinic. We have been uniformly unsuccessful. The patients have generally worsened rather than improved during the titration phase. At least one other veterinary cardiologist has had similar experiences.[314] This individual was funded to examine this issue in dogs and was unable to complete the study because of the poor response. There are several potential reasons for this lack of success. First, it is possible that the disease is different in dogs and that β-receptor blockade specifically alters a biochemical abnormality in the myocardium of humans with myocardial failure. This seems unlikely because β-receptor blockade has been shown to improve myocardial and myocyte function in large dogs with experimentally induced mitral regurgitation.[313] Second, and more likely, the disease in dogs may be more severe and progress at a more rapid rate, resulting in an inability to produce significant results with a drug regimen that appears to take some time to develop. In humans, patients considered to be candidates for β-blocker therapy are those that have mild-to-moderately severe heart failure (NYHA class II, class III, or early class IV).[311] Most of the canine patients we see with dilated cardiomyopathy have severe heart failure at presentation. It takes 4 to 10 weeks before any improvement is noted in humans following the initiation of β-blocker therapy.[311] This is the survival time for many dogs with dilated cardiomyopathy.

Exactly how chronic β blockade improves myocardial function in patients with myocardial failure is unknown. The most popular theory seems to be that up-regulation of β receptors occurs, which results in increased contractile performance. β-Receptor up-regulation in these patients has been documented.[315] It seems unlikely that this can be a primary mechanism, because the additional β receptors that are present should be blocked by the β-adrenergic blocking drug. However, in one study of humans with dilated cardiomyopathy, β-receptor density increased and responsiveness to catecholamine administration did improve, despite the fact that the patients were still receiving β-blocker therapy.[316] Heart rate control does not appear to be the mechanism because beneficial effects are present in patients in whom the heart rate is maintained by atrial pacing.[317] Improved diastolic function and afterload reduction also have been suggested as reasons for the improved ventricular function.[318] The fact that innate myocyte function and myofibrillar density increase in dogs with experimentally induced mitral regurgitation after chronic β-adrenergic blockade suggests that most of these mechanisms do not clearly explain the underlying beneficial effect of these drugs in myocardial failure. Rather, there seems to be some protective effect of the drugs against chronic β-receptor stimulation.[313] Authors have argued that β blockade may protect against the myocardial toxicity seen with high levels of catecholamines.[317,318] There is one study that strongly suggests that this is true.[319] In this study, isolated cardiocytes were exposed to various concentrations of norepinephrine. Concentration-dependent toxicity was identified, and this toxicity could be mimicked by selectively stimulating β-receptors on the cardiocytes. The toxic effect appeared to be due to cellular calcium overload that was cAMP-mediated and required L-type calcium channels to produce toxicity.

One study suggests that myocardial function improves in dogs with experimentally induced mitral regurgitation.[313] This has stimulated interest in administering β-adrenergic blocking drugs to clinical canine patients with mitral regurgitation. We believe that this is a rational step to take in large dogs with mitral regurgitation, because myocardial failure is clearly a significant component of this disease. Myocardial failure does not appear to be nearly as important in small dogs with primary mitral regurgitation, and so β-adrenergic blockade may not be rational for this group of dogs unless controlled clinical trials document a benefit. Cats do not appear to develop myocardial dysfunction with volume overload, and so β-adrenergic blockade for this purpose in this species may not be warranted.[320]

Vesnarinone. Vesnarinone is a positive inotropic and vasodilating agent that has not been approved for use in the United States. It acts primarily as a phosphodiesterase-III inhibitor, although it has other properties, including direct effects on myocyte L-type calcium channels.[321] It has a marked positive inotropic effect in dogs.[322] One clinical trial in humans has suggested that vesnarinone administered at a dose of 60 mg per day PO to patients with heart failure improves the quality of the patient's life and increases survival time.[323] A dose of 120 mg per day PO in this same study, however, increased the mortality of patients with heart failure. However, a more recent study has suggested that the 60-mg dose produces no clinical benefit and increases the risk of sudden death.[324] This trial is also examining a 30-mg dose. Results were not available at time of publication. If vesnarinone is as effective in dogs as milrinone, it may be a viable agent to treat heart failure in dogs with myocardial failure if it is approved for use in humans.

Losartan. Losartan is an angiotensin II receptor blocker formulated to treat systemic hypertension and congestive heart failure in humans. It blocks only one type of angiotensin II receptor (AT1) and does not potentiate bradykinin activity like the ACE inhibitors. Despite this, hemodynamic and clinical benefits in humans with heart failure appear to be similar to the ACE inhibitors.[325] This drug was primarily developed to avoid the coughing that ACE inhibitors produce in humans, which is not a problem in dogs. Clinical use of this drug will probably be limited to those patients that cannot tolerate ACE inhibitors.

Amlodipine. Amlodipine is a calcium channel blocker that affects primarily the calcium channels in vascular smooth muscle, specifically in systemic arteriolar smooth muscle. Amlodipine is similar to nifedipine. Both drugs have primarily arteriolar dilating properties, although amlodipine has even fewer negative inotropic effects than its parent compound.[326] Amlodipine therefore should be able to impart benefits similar to hydralazine to patients with mitral regurgitation. These benefits can probably be realized without the reflex tachycardia seen with hydralazine, and the drug appears to be better tolerated by the gastrointestinal tract.[327] Nifedipine decreases systemic vascular resistance and systemic blood pressure while increasing cardiac output and decreasing regurgitant fraction in human patients with aortic regurgitation, as expected.[328]

Amlodipine probably will never be examined in-depth in human patients with mitral regurgitation because those patients are amenable to surgical correction. Consequently, studies should be performed in veterinary medicine to determine if this drug will be effective in this setting. Amlodipine, however, has already been studied in human patients with dilated cardiomyopathy and with myocardial failure secondary to ischemic heart disease in a large prospective clinical trial.[329] Deaths were reduced in the patients with dilated cardiomyopathy but not in the patients with ischemic heart disease. The use of amlodipine in dogs is discussed further in Chapter 26.

Potassium channel activators. Drugs that act specifically on vascular smooth muscle outward K^+ conductance have been formulated. The decrease in potassium conductance results in cell hyperpolarization and muscle relaxation. Minoxidil is the classic potassium channel activator. It has many side effects. A newer potassium channel activator, nicorandil, has been studied in humans with heart failure.[330] Acute intravenous administration to humans produces very similar effects to intravenous nitroglycerin. Consequently, the drug appears to be both an arteriolar dilator and a venodilator. Tolerance to the drug did not develop in this study within the first 24 hours.

Calcium-sensitizing drugs. Calcium-sensitizing agents increase the rate and extent of myocardial force development for any given intracellular concentration of calcium. As such they primarily act as positive inotropic agents. They may, however, also have effects on myocardial relaxation. Of the calcium-sensitizing drugs examined in human clinical trials to date, both have had significant effects on type III phosphodiesterase, giving them similarities to the bipyridine compounds. Pimobendan and sulmazole have increased the quality of life for human patients but have decreased survival time.[331]

Endothelin receptor antagonists. The plasma concentration of endothelin-1 (ET-1) is increased in human patients with heart failure.[332] A precursor of ET-1, big-ET-1, is increased in dogs with heart failure.[333,334] Recently, ET_A receptor antagonists have been formulated.[335,336] One such antagonist has been administered to rabbits with rapid pacing–induced heart failure. It resulted in an increase in shortening fraction, a decrease in end-diastolic diameter, and improved myocyte function. Although these drugs are experimental, they may be useful for treating heart failure in the future.

Neutral endopeptidase inhibitors. Atrial natriuretic factor (ANF) is a peptide hormone of cardiac origin that increases sodium and water excretion, inhibits the renin-angiotensin-aldosterone system and produces vasodilation. It is elaborated in response to increased stretch placed on myocardium, especially atrial myocardium. Consequently, it is elaborated in response to increased ventricular diastolic and atrial pressures (filling pressures). Although the plasma concentration of this hormone is increased in patients with heart failure, other factors overwhelm its effects, resulting in sodium and water retention and increased filling pressures. In addition, the effects of ANF are blunted in heart failure.[337] Neutral endopeptidase (NEP) is an enzyme that is present in many tissues of the body but is concentrated in renal tissue in microvilli of the brush border of the proximal tubules. It is responsible for rapidly degrading ANF, as well as enkephalins, bradykinin, and substance P. Within the last 10 years, inhibitors of NEP have been formulated and examined in human patients and experimental dogs with heart failure.[338-340] In dogs with rapid ventricular pacing–induced heart failure, one NEP inhibitor has been shown to acutely increase the plasma concentration of ANF and increase the fractional excretion of sodium.[340,341] In humans, short-term administration of another NEP inhibitor has resulted in significant natriuresis and a significant decrease in pulmonary capillary pressure.[338] Yet another NEP inhibitor has been studied in experimental dogs with heart failure secondary to rapid ventricular pacing.[342] In these dogs, the compound (ecadotril) produced significant clinical and hemodynamic improvement and increased survival.[342] When combined with an ACE inhibitor, NEP inhibition potentiates the renal and hemodynamic responses to ACE inhibition.[340] Compounds are being formulated that inhibit both NEP and ACE or NEP and endothelin converting enzyme. When combined with furosemide in experimental dogs with heart failure, NEP inhibitors enhance the actions of furosemide and prevent the activation of the renin-angiotensin-aldosterone system normally observed following furosemide administration.[343]

Supplementation

TAURINE

Taurine supplementation is indicated for the treatment of taurine deficiency–induced myocardial failure in cats and dogs. In the past, taurine deficiency was a common cause of dilated cardiomyopathy in cats. Almost all cat foods are currently supplemented with an adequate quantity of taurine. Consequently, dilated cardiomyopathy is rare in cats. Cats currently diagnosed with dilated cardiomyopathy are generally not taurine-deficient. However, plasma taurine concentration should be determined on any cat with dilated cardiomyopathy, or supplementation should be tried for at least 3 months. The dose is 250 mg/cat q12h. Cats on nontraditional diets (e.g., dog food, boiled chicken, vegetarian diets) are most likely to be deficient in taurine.

American cocker spaniels are also taurine-deficient and respond to taurine or taurine and carnitine supplementation. They are supplemented with 500 mg taurine and 1 g carnitine q12h PO. For further discussion see Chapter 20.

CARNITINE

Carnitine deficiency is a potential cause of dilated cardiomyopathy. A family of boxers has been reported with dilated cardiomyopathy and carnitine deficiency.[344] Not all of these dogs had a low plasma carnitine concentration, and some responded to supplementation. Consequently, we recommend that boxers with severe myocardial failure be supplemented with 2 to 3 g carnitine q12h PO for 2 to 4 months to determine if they respond to supplementation. Although myocardial concentration of carnitine is often low in other dogs with dilated cardiomyopathy, this does not appear to be a primary abnormality and most do not have a clinically demonstrable response to supplementation. For further discussion see Chapter 20.

Ancillary Therapy

LOW-SODIUM DIET

A diet low in sodium is another means of reducing circulating blood volume in patients with heart failure. Sodium is retained in these patients by a variety of mechanisms, including activation of the renin-angiotensin-aldosterone system. Diuretic and ACE inhibitor therapy as therapeutic modalities for reducing total body sodium and blood volume has previously been discussed.

Patients with severe heart failure that are refractory to diuretic administration have the greatest need for a low-sodium diet. Patients with early and mild heart failure generally do not need marked salt restriction. However, foods high in sodium content should be avoided during these stages. There is no evidence that feeding a diet low in sodium to a patient with cardiac disease but with no evidence of heart failure is beneficial. Consequently, there is no need to place such a patient on a prescription diet and no reason to subject the owner to the increased cost of such a diet or the increased aggravation of switching to a less palatable food.

All nonprescription commercial dog and cat foods have much more sodium chloride added than is required. Commercial canned dog foods commonly have close to 20 times (1.13% dry matter) the minimum sodium allowance for adult maintenance (0.06% dry matter). Dry dog foods have 6 to 7 times the minimum allowance (0.41% dry matter). Presumably this excess quantity of sodium chloride is added by the manufacturers to increase palatability. Cats have a higher minimum allowance (0.20% dry matter), and the sodium content of cat food is the same as dog food. One means of decreasing sodium intake in a patient is to switch from a canned food to a dry food. Foods formulated for older dogs and prescription diets formulated for dogs or cats with renal failure have a lower sodium content (0.20 to 0.25% dry matter) and can be used for moderate sodium restriction. Sodium-restricted diets formulated for dogs with heart failure are very low in sodium (0.10% of dry matter) but are still above the minimum requirement. Low-sodium diets formulated for cats with heart failure have sodium contents that are similar to foods formulated for cats with renal failure (0.28% dry matter).

Palatability can be a problem with low-sodium diets. Dogs prefer canned foods that are higher in sodium content. Palatability enhancers probably overshadow the taste effects of sodium chloride in dry dog foods. Consequently, it may be easier to switch a dog from a commercial dry food to a low-sodium dry food than from a commercial canned food to a low-sodium canned food. However, most hospitalized dogs will accept a low-sodium diet within 3 days of switching foods.[345] In cats, we have the most experience with Purina's CV-Formula diet. The cats to which we have fed this liver-based diet have eaten it readily and sometimes preferred it to their regular diet.

OXYGEN THERAPY

Dogs and cats with severe pulmonary edema develop life-threatening hypoxemia. The hypoxemia is primarily due to the decreased ability of oxygen to diffuse from the alveoli into the pulmonary capillaries.[346] Increasing the inspired concentration of oxygen increases the pressure gradient of oxygen from the alveoli to the capillaries, resulting in an increase in arterial oxygen tension. Consequently, dogs and cats with severe pulmonary edema and respiratory distress should have supplemental oxygen administered while they are treated for the pulmonary edema. In general, the percent inspired oxygen should be increased from the normal 21% to between 40% to 50%. This can best be achieved by placing the patient in an oxygen cage or administering oxygen via a nasal cannula (nasal insufflation). It can also be achieved with a tight-fitting mask. Masks should only be used if the patient will tolerate their placement without struggling. Oxygen cages must have a mechanism for removing carbon dioxide and for cooling the environment. Cages or enclosures contrived from plastic bags or boxes are dangerous and can cause death from hyperthermia or hypercarbia unless the flow rate for oxygen is high enough to wash out the carbon dioxide and the temperature is controlled by some means. Patients in extreme respiratory distress may benefit from sedation or anesthesia, endotracheal intubation, controlled ventilation, and 100% oxygen administration. These patients usually have copious amounts of pulmonary edema fluid spew forth from the endotracheal tube. Postural drainage and suction must be used to remove this fluid.

THORACENTESIS

Dyspneic patients with pleural effusion benefit from withdrawal of the fluid from their pleural space. Pleural effusion is a common cause of severe respiratory distress in cats. Any dyspneic cat suspected of having cardiac disease should undergo a pleurocentesis to determine if pleural effusion is the cause of the respiratory distress at the time of initial examination. This can usually be performed with the cat in sternal recumbency with a butterfly catheter. Fluid removal often results in prompt and dramatic improvement in both dogs and cats.

ABDOMINOCENTESIS

Dogs with severe right heart failure develop a large quantity of ascites that commonly makes them feel uncomfortable and often places enough pressure on the diaphragm to cause breathing difficulties. This fluid is readily amenable to drainage. Abdominocentesis can be performed periodically in these patients, usually at or near the midline, and most of the fluid safely removed. Although concerns regarding the loss of protein produced by this approach have been voiced, we have only rarely noted a clinically significant decrease in serum albumin concentration, even following months of draining ascitic fluid every couple of weeks. Consequently, we believe this is a safe and effective approach to managing the patient with severe right heart failure.

ANXIOLYTIC THERAPY

Dogs and cats with severe respiratory distress may become severely anxious and may benefit from sedation. However, most patients with respiratory distress in our hospital are not sedated.

Morphine is commonly recommended for its analgesic and antianxiety effects in humans with respiratory distress secondary to heart failure.[347] Morphine also has venodilating properties that may be beneficial. Morphine is generally not used in cats because they may become aggressive and agitated following its administration. In dogs, the dose is 0.1 to 0.25 mg/kg subcutaneously. The dose is repeated as necessary to achieve the desired effect. The primary adverse effect of morphine is respiratory depression. This can be a fatal complication in a hypoxemic animal so this drug must be used carefully.

Phenothiazine tranquilizers may be used to produce similar effects. Acepromazine is the tranquilizer we use most commonly in patients with heart failure with severe respiratory distress. It reduces the agitation in these patients and does not depress respiration. Acepromazine is also an α-adrenergic blocker that decreases peripheral vascular resistance, which may be beneficial, especially in patients with mitral regurgitation (see Chapter 19). The dose is 0.01 to 0.2 mg/kg IM or IV. This drug can cause cardiovascular collapse in boxers and probably should not be used in this breed. Acepromazine should not be used in combination with an opioid in animals with respiratory distress because of enhanced respiratory depression.[348]

BRONCHODILATOR THERAPY

Bronchodilators, such as theophylline and aminophylline, are occasionally prescribed for use in patients with heart failure. As discussed under the section on furosemide, attempting to produce bronchodilation in patients with heart failure has been called into question in human medicine and is less likely to be of benefit in dogs. Aminophylline and theophylline are nonspecific phosphodiesterase inhibitors. Consequently, they do have positive inotropic effects and may also act as diuretics. However, these effects are extremely mild and probably of little benefit. In general, we reserve these drugs for use in dogs with chronic airway disease.

COUGH SUPPRESSANTS

Cough suppressants are contraindicated in patients that have cough secondary to pulmonary edema. Consequently, pulmonary edema must be ruled out before initiating these drugs in a coughing patient. This usually can be done by obtaining a thoracic radiograph. In some dogs with mild edema, a trial of furosemide administration may be required to exclude pulmonary edema as a possible cause of a cough. In dogs with cough secondary to airway compression by an enlarged left atrium, hydrocodenone bitartrate with homatropine (Hycodan, DuPont, Wilmington, Del.) and butorphanol (Torbutrol, Fort Dodge Laboratories, Fort Dodge, Iowa) are generally the most effective drugs. Butorphanol recently has been reclassified a controlled substance in most states. Hycodan is supplied as 5-mg tablets. The oral dose in dogs is 2.5 to 10 mg/dog q6h-q12h or 0.25 mg/kg q6h-q12h. Torbutrol is supplied as 1-, 5-, and 10-mg tablets. The dose in dogs is 0.55 to 1.1 mg/kg q6h-q12h PO. Dextromethorphan (various preparations and manufacturers), as an over-the-counter drug, may also be effective in some situations. A dose has not been defined. We generally base the dose on a pediatric dose compared with the size of the dog.

REFERENCES

1. The effect of digoxin on mortality and morbidity in patients with heart failure. The Digitalis Investigation Group, *N Engl J Med* 336:525, 1997 (see comments).
2. Baker DW, Konstam MA, Bottorff M et al: Management of heart failure. I. Pharmacologic treatment, *JAMA* 272:1361, 1994 (see comments).
3. Saxon LA, Stevenson WG, Middlekauff HR et al: Predicting death from progressive heart failure secondary to ischemic or idiopathic dilated cardiomyopathy, *Am J Cardiol* 72:62, 1993.
4. Fonarow GC, Chelimsky-Fallick C, Stevenson LW et al: Effect of direct vasodilation with hydralazine versus angiotensin-converting enzyme inhibition with captopril on mortality in advanced heart failure: the Hy-C trial, *J Am Coll Cardiol* 19:842, 1992.
5. Stevenson LW: Advanced congestive heart failure: inpatient treatment and selection for cardiac transplantation, *Postgrad Med* 94:97, 1993.
6. Cody RJ, Leier CV, Stevenson LW: Optimal management of severe congestive heart failure, audio tape of the Forty-Fifth Annual Scientific Session of the American College of Cardiology, 1996.
7. Walden JA, Stevenson LW, Dracup K et al: Extended comparison of quality of life between stable heart failure patients and heart transplant recipients, *J Heart Lung Transplant* 13:1109, 1994.
8. Stevenson LW, Tillisch JH: Maintenance of cardiac output with normal filling pressures in patients with dilated heart failure, *Circulation* 74:1303, 1986.
9. Stevenson LW, Bellil D, Grover-McKay M et al: Effects of afterload reduction (diuretics and vasodilators) on left ventricular volume and mitral regurgitation in severe congestive heart failure secondary to ischemic or idiopathic dilated cardiomyopathy, *Am J Cardiol* 60:654, 1987.
10. Vollmar AM, Montag C, Preusser U et al: Atrial natriuretic peptide and plasma volume of dogs suffering from heart failure or dehydration, *J Vet Med Assoc* 41:548, 1994.
11. Baker J: Clinical experiences with a new diuretic: furosemide, *Vet Med* 62:879, 1967.
12. Becker W, Zuschek F, Smith GB: Report on a new diuretic-saluretic agent: furosemide, *Vet Med* 62:760, 1967.
13. Aronson PS: Mechanisms of active H^+ secretion in the proximal tubule, *Am J Physiol* 245:F647, 1983.
14. Skou JC: The Na,K-pump, *Methods Enzymol* 156:1, 1988.
15. Windhager EE, Lewy JE, Spitzer A: Intrarenal control of proximal tubular reabsorption of sodium and water, *Nephron* 6:247, 1969.
16. Puschett JB: Pharmacological classification and renal actions of diuretics, *Cardiology* 84(suppl)2:4, 1994.
17. Grantham JJ, Chonko AM: The physiologic basis and clinical use of diuretics. In Brenner BM, Steinm JH, eds: *Contemporary issues in nephrology,* vol 1, *Sodium and water homeostasis,* New York, 1978, Churchill Livingstone.
18. Kunau RT, Weller DR, Webb HL: Clarification of the site of action of chlorothiazide in the rat nephron, *J Clin Invest* 56:401, 1975.
19. Pox P: Feline myocardial diseases. In Kirk RW, ed: *Current veterinary therapy,* ed 8, Philadelphia, 1983, WB Saunders.
20. Brater DC: Disposition and response to bumetanide and furosemide, *Am J Cardiol* 57:20A, 1986.
21. Puschett JB: Clinical pharmacologic implications in diuretic selection, *Am J Cardiol* 57:6A, 1986.
22. Puschett JB: Sites and mechanisms of action of diuretics in the kidney, *J Clin Pharmacol* 21:564, 1981.
23. Bosch JP, Goldstein MH, Levitt MF et al: Effect of chronic furosemide administration on hydrogen and sodium excretion in the dog, *Am J Physiol* 232:F397, 1977.
24. White MG, van Gelder J, Eastes G: The effect of loop diuretics on the excretion of Na^+, $Ca2^+$, $Mg2^+$, and Cl^-, *J Clin Pharmacol* 21:610, 1981.
25. Hirai J, Miyazaki H, Taneike T: The pharmacokinetics and pharmacodynamics of furosemide in the anaesthetized dog, *J Vet Pharmacol Ther* 15:231, 1992.
26. Cohen MR, Hinsch E, Vergona R et al: A comparative diuretic and tissue distribution study of bumetanide and furosemide in the dog, *J Pharmacol Exp Ther* 197:697, 1976.

27. Berg KJ, Loew D: Inhibition of furosemide-induced natriuresis by acetylsalicylic acid in dogs, *Scand J Clin Lab Invest* 37:125, 1977.
28. Bayne EJ, Williamson HE: Effect of furosemide on peripheral venous compliance following ureteral ligation in the adult dog, *Res Commun Chem Pathol Pharmacol* 25:399.
29. Mukherjee SK, Katz MA, Michael UF et al: Mechanisms of hemodynamic actions of furosemide: differentiation of vascular and renal effects on blood pressure in functionally anephric hypertensive patients, *Am Heart J* 101:313, 1981.
30. Fernando ON, Newman SP, Hird VM et al: Enhancement of renal blood flow in transplanted dog kidneys following perfusion with furosemide, *Scott Med J* 19(suppl)1:50, 1974.
31. Ludens JH, Heitz DC, Brody MJ et al: Differential effect of furosemide on renal and limb blood flows in the conscious dog, *J Pharmacol Exp Ther* 171:300, 1970.
32. Burke TJ, Duchin KL: Glomerular filtration during furosemide diuresis in the dog, *Kidney Int* 16:672, 1979.
33. Data JL, Rane A, Gerkens J et al: The influence of indomethacin on the pharmacokinetics, diuretic response and hemodynamics of furosemide in the dog, *J Pharmacol Exp Ther* 206:431, 1978.
34. Carriere S, Desrosiers M, Friborg J et al: The effect of furosemide on the intrarenal blood flow distribution in the dog, *Can J Physiol Pharmacol* 50:774, 1972.
35. Szwed JJ, Kleit SA, Hamburger RJ: Effect of furosemide and chlorothiazide on the thoracic duct lymph flow in the dog, *J Lab Clin Med* 79:693, 1972.
36. Rubie S, Robinson NE, Stoll M et al: Flunixin meglumine blocks furosemide-induced bronchodilation in horses with chronic obstructive pulmonary disease, *Equine Vet J* 25:138, 1993.
37. Stevens EL, Uyehara CF, Southgate WM et al: Furosemide differentially relaxes airway and vascular smooth muscle in fetal, newborn, and adult guinea pigs, *Am Rev Respir Dis* 146:1192, 1992.
38. Bianco S, Pieroni MG, Refini RM et al: Inhaled loop diuretics as potential new anti-asthmatic drugs, *Eur Respir J* 6:130, 1993.
39. Padrid P: Chronic lower airway disease in the dog and cat, *Probl Vet Med* 4:320, 1992.
40. Snashall PD, Chung KF: Airway obstruction and bronchial hyperresponsiveness in left ventricular failure and mitral stenosis, *Am Rev Respir Dis* 144:945, 1991.
41. Imbs JL, Schmidt M, Velly J et al: Comparison of the effect of two groups of diuretics on renin secretion in the anaesthetized dog, *Clin Sci Mol Med* 52:171, 1977.
42. Corsini WA, Hook JB, Bailie MD: Control of renin secretion in the dog: effects of furosemide on the vascular and macula densa receptors, *Circ Res* 37:464, 1975.
43. Verbeeck RK, Gerkens JF, Wilkinson GR et al: Disposition of furosemide in functionally hepatectomized dogs, *J Pharmacol Exp Ther* 216:479, 1981.
44. Cohen M: Pharmacology of bumetanide, *J Clin Pharmacol* 21:537, 1981.
45. Miyazaki H, Hirai J, Taneike T: The pharmacokinetics and pharmacodynamics of furosemide in anesthetized dogs with normal and experimentally decreased renal function, *Jpn J Vet Sci* 52:265, 1990.
46. Yakatan GJ, Maness DD, Scholler J et al: Plasma and tissue levels of furosemide in dogs and monkeys following single and multiple oral doses, *Res Commun Chem Pathol Pharmacol* 24:465, 1979.
47. Klatt P, Muschaweck R, Bossaller W et al: Method of collecting urine and comparative investigation of quantities excreted by cats and dogs after administration of furosemide, *Am J Vet Res* 36:919, 1975.
48. Friedman PA, Roch-Ramel F: Hemodynamic and natriuretic effects of bumetanide and furosemide in the cat, *J Pharm Exp Therapeut* 203:82, 1977.
49. Edwards NJ: Serum potassium concentration in dogs administered furosemide, personal communication, 1996.
50. Dormans TPJ, van Meyel JJM, Gerlag PGG et al: Diuretic efficacy of high dose furosemide in severe heart failure: bolus injection versus continuous infusion, *J Am Coll Cardiol* 28:376, 1996.
51. Brown RD: Comparative acute cochlear toxicity of intravenous bumetanide and furosemide in the purebred beagle, *J Clin Pharmacol* 21:620, 1981.
52. Raisbeck MF, Hewitt WR, McIntyre WB: Fatal nephrotoxicosis associated with furosemide and gentamicin therapy in a dog, *J Am Vet Med Assoc* 183:892, 1983.
53. Nakahama H, Fukuhara Y, Orita Y et al: Furosemide accelerates gentamicin accumulation in cultured renal cells (LLC-PK1 cells), *Nephron* 53:138, 1989.
54. Frey HH: Pharmacology of bumetanide, *Postgrad Med J* 51(suppl 6):14, 1975.
55. Schwartz MA: Metabolism of bumetanide, *J Clin Pharmacol* 21:555, 1981.
56. Ostergaard EH, Magnussen MP, Nielsen CK et al: Pharmacological properties of 3–butylamino-4-phenoxy-5-sulfamylbenzoic acid (Bumetanide), a new potent diuretic: *Arzneimittelforschung* 22:66, 1972.
57. Dixon DW, Barwolf-Gohlke C, Gunnar RM: Comparative efficacy and safety of bumetanide and furosemide in long-term treatment of edema due to congestive heart failure, *J Clin Pharmacol* 21:680, 1981.
58. Brater DC, Their SO: *Renal disorders,* New York, 1978, MacMillan.
59. Muir WW, Sams R: Pharmacodynamics of cardiac drugs, monograph, The Ohio State University, 1979.
60. Crosley AP, Ronquillo LM, Strickland WH et al: Triamterene, a new natriuretic agent, *Ann Intern Med* 56:241, 1962.
61. Duff HJ, Lester WM, Rahmberg M: Amiloride: antiarrhythmic and electrophysiological activity in the dog, *Circulation* 78:1469, 1988.
62. Haddy FJ, Pamnani MB, Swindall BT et al: Sodium channel blockers are vasodilator as well as natriuretic and diuretic agents, *Hypertension* 7:I121, 1985.
63. Edwards NJ: Magnesium and congestive heart failure, *Proc Annu Vet Med Forum* 1990, 679.
64. O'Keefe D, Sisson DD: Serum electrolytes in dogs with congestive heart failure, *J Vet Intern Med* 7:118, 1993 (abstract).
65. Kahn T, Albertini B, von, Goldstein M et al: Effect of increased NaCl or KCl intake on response to chronic furosemide administration (dog), *Am J Physiol* 238:F509, 1980.
66. DeCarli C, Sprouse G, LaRosa JC: Serum magnesium levels in symptomatic atrial fibrillation and their relation to rhythm control by intravenous digoxin, *Am J Cardiol* 57:956, 1986.
67. Nomura A, Yasuda H, Minami M et al: Effect of furosemide in congestive heart failure, *Clin Pharmacol Ther* 30:177, 1981.
68. Nomura A, Yasuda H, Katoh K et al: Hydralazine and furosemide kinetics, *Clin Pharmacol Ther* 32:303, 1982.
69. Ellison DH, Velazquez H, Wright FS: Adaptation of the distal convoluted tubule of the rat: structural and functional effects of dietary salt intake and chronic diuretic infusion, *J Clin Invest* 83:113, 1989.
70. Brater DC, Chennavasin P, Seiwell R: Furosemide in patients with heart failure: shift in dose-response curves, *Clin Pharmacol Ther* 28:182, 1980.
71. Gottlieb SS, Khatta D, Wentworth D et al: Massive fluid accumulation does not affect the pharmacokinetics of the loop diuretics furosemide and torsemide in patients with heart failure, *J Am Coll Cardiol* 29:370A, 1997 (abstract).
72. Lloyd MA, Sandberg SM, Edwards BS: Role of renal Na^{+},$K^{(+)}$-ATPase in the regulation of sodium excretion under normal conditions and in acute congestive heart failure, *Circulation* 85:1912, 1992.
73. Greeff K: *Cardiac glycosides.* I. Berlin, 1981, Springer.
74. Withering W: An account of the foxglove and some of its medical uses, with practical remarks on dropsy, and other diseases. In Willis FA, Keys TE, eds: *Classics of cardiology,* New York, 1941, Henry Schuman.
75. MacKenzie J: Digitalis, *Heart* 2:253, 1911.
76. Wiggers CJ, Stimson B: Studies on the cardiodynamic actions of drugs. III. The mechanism of cardiac stimulation by digitalis and γ-strophanthin, *J Exp Med* 30:251, 1927.

77. Schatzman HJ: Herzglykoside als Hemmstoffe fur den aktiven Kalium und Natriumtransport durch die Erythocytenmembran, *Helv Physiol Pharmacol Acta* 11:346, 1995.
78. Dobbs SM, Kenyon WI, Dobbs RJ: Maintenance digoxin after an episode of heart failure: placebo-controlled trial in outpatients, *Br Med J* 1:749, 1977.
79. Kleiman JH, Ingels NB, Daughters G II et al: Left ventricular dynamics during long-term digoxin treatment in patients with stable coronary artery disease, *Am J Cardiol* 41:937, 1978.
80. Arnold SB, Byrd RC, Meister W et al: Long-term digitalis therapy improves left ventricular function in heart failure, *N Engl J Med* 303:1443, 1980.
81. Mulrow CD, Feussner JR, Velez R: Reëvaluation of digitalis efficacy: new light on an old leaf, *Ann Intern Med* 101:113, 1984.
82. Gheorghiade M, Beller GA: Effects of discontinuing maintenance digoxin therapy in patients with ischemic heart disease and congestive heart failure in sinus rhythm, *Am J Cardiol* 51:1243, 1983.
83. Taggart AJ, Johnston GD, McDevitt DG: Digoxin withdrawal after cardiac failure in patients with sinus rhythm, *J Cardiovasc Pharmacol* 5:229, 1983.
84. McHaffie D, Purcell H, Mitchell-Heggs P et al: The clinical value of digoxin in patients with heart failure and sinus rhythm, *Q J Med* 47:401, 1978.
85. Hougen TJ, Smith TW: Inhibition of myocardial monovalent cation active transport by subtoxic doses of ouabain in the dog, *Circ Res* 42:856, 1978.
86. Gheorghiade M, Zarowitz BJ: Review of randomized trials of digoxin therapy in patients with chronic heart failure, *Am J Cardiol* 69:48G, 1992 (discussion p 62G).
87. Uretsky BF, Young JB, Shahidi FE et al: Randomized study assessing the effect of digoxin withdrawal in patients with mild to moderate chronic congestive heart failure: results of the PROVED trial. PROVED Investigative Group, *J Am Coll Cardiol* 22:955, 1993 (see comments).
88. Packer M, Gheorghiade M, Young JB et al: Withdrawal of digoxin from patients with chronic heart failure treated with angiotensin-converting-enzyme inhibitors. RADIANCE study, *N Engl J Med* 329:1, 1993 (see comments).
89. Ruskin JN, Goldstein S, Bittl JA et al: The major clinical trials: bringing results to practice, audio tape of the Forty-Fifth Annual Scientific Session of the American College of Cardiology, 1996.
90. Packer M: End of the oldest controversy in medicine. Are we ready to conclude the debate on digitalis? *N Engl J Med* 336:575, 1997 (editorial; comment).
91. Kittleson MD, Eyster GE, Knowlen GG et al: Efficacy of digoxin administration in dogs with idiopathic congestive cardiomyopathy, *J Am Vet Med Assoc* 186:162, 1985.
92. Slatton ML, Irani WN, Hall SA et al: Does digoxin provide additional hemodynamic and autonomic benefit at higher doses in patients with mild to moderate heart failure and normal sinus rhythm? *J Am Coll Cardiol* 29:1206, 1997.
93. Packer M, Carver JR, Rodeheffer RJ et al: Effect of oral milrinone on mortality in severe chronic heart failure. The PROMISE Study Research Group, *N Engl J Med* 325:1468, 1991 (see comments).
94. Hollman A: Plants and cardiac glycosides, *Br Heart J* 54:258, 1985.
95. Mahler F, Karliner JS, O'Rourke RA: Effects of chronic digoxin administration on left ventricular performance in the normal conscious dog, *Circulation* 50:720, 1974.
96. Goldstein RA, Passamani ER, Roberts R: A comparison of digoxin and dobutamine in patients with acute infarction and cardiac failure, *N Engl J Med* 303:846, 1980.
97. Akera T, Brody TM: Pharmacology of cardiac glycosides. In Sperelakis N, ed. *Physiology and pathophysiology of the heart,* ed 3, Boston, 1995, Kluwer.
98. Caprio A, Farah A: The effect of the ionic milieu on the response of rabbit cardiac muscle to ouabain, *J Pharmacol Exp Ther* 155:403, 1967.
99. Mason DT, Zelia R, Amsterdam EA: Unified concept of the mechanism of action of digitalis: influence of ventricular function and cardiac disease on hemodynamic response to fundamental contractile effect. In Marks BH, Weissler AM, eds: *Basic and clinical pharmacology of digitalis,* St Louis, 1972, Mosby.
100. Wald H, Scherzer P, Popovtzer MM: Na,K-ATPase in isolated nephron segments in rats with experimental heart failure, *Circ Res* 68:1051, 1991.
101. Berman WJ, Yabek SM, Dillon T et al: Effects of digoxin in infants with congested circulatory state due to a ventricular septal defect, *N Engl J Med* 308:363, 1983.
102. Higgins CB, Vatner SF, Eckberg DL et al: Alterations in the baroreceptor reflex in conscious dogs with heart failure, *J Clin Invest* 51:715, 1972.
103. Creager MA, Creager SJ: Arterial baroreflex regulation of blood pressure in patients with congestive heart failure, *J Am Coll Cardiol* 23:401, 1994.
104. Ferrari A, Gregorini L, Ferrari MC et al: Digitalis and baroreceptor reflexes in man, *Circulation* 63:279, 1981.
105. Reing CM, Thibodeaux H, Gillis RA et al: Influence of baroreceptor reflexes on cardiovascular responses of the dog to acetylstrophanthidin, *J Pharmacol Exp Ther* 184:641, 1973.
106. McLain PL: Effects of ouabain on spontaneous afferent activity in the aortic and carotid sinus nerves of cats, *Neuropharmacology* 9:399, 1970.
107. Ferguson DW, Berg WJ, Sanders JS et al: Sympathoinhibitory responses to digitalis glycosides in heart failure patients: direct evidence from sympathetic neural recordings, *Circulation* 80:65, 1989.
108. Covit AB, Schaer GL, Sealey JE et al: Suppression of the renin-angiotensin system by intravenous digoxin in chronic congestive heart failure, *Am J Med* 75:445, 1983.
109. Moe GK, Farah AE: Digitalis and allied cardiac glycosides. In Goodman LS, Gilman A, eds: *Pharmacological basis of therapeutics,* ed 4, New York, 1970, MacMillan.
110. Lown B, Graboys TB, Podrid PJ et al: Effect of a digitalis drug on ventricular premature beats, *N Engl J Med* 296:301, 1977.
111. Aubier M, Murciano D, Viires N et al: Effects of digoxin on diaphragmatic strength generation in patients with chronic obstructive pulmonary disease during acute respiratory failure, *Am Rev Respir Dis* 135:544, 1987.
112. Aubier M, Viires N, Murciano D et al: Effects of digoxin on diaphragmatic strength generation, *J Appl Physiol* 61:1767, 1986.
113. Aubier M, Murciano D, Menu Y et al: Dopamine effects on diaphragmatic strength during acute respiratory failure in chronic obstructive pulmonary disease, *Ann Intern Med* 110:17, 1989.
114. Aubier M: Effect of theophylline on diaphragmatic muscle function, *Chest* 92:27S, 1987.
115. Kittleson MD: Positive inotropic agents and captopril, *Proceedings of the Ninth Annual Kal Kan Symposium,* Vernon, Calif, Kal Kan Foods, Inc, 1986, p 19.
116. Baggot JD, Davis LE: Plasma protein binding of digitoxin and digoxin in several mammalian species, *Res Vet Sci* 15:81, 1973.
117. Button C, Gross DR, Johnston JT et al: Pharmacokinetics, bioavailability, and dosage regimens of digoxin in dogs, *Am J Vet Res* 41:1230, 1980.
118. Weidler DFJ, Jazladd NS, Movahhed HS: Pharmacokinetics of digoxin in the cat and comparisons with man and the dog, *Res Commun Chem Pathol Pharm* 19:57, 1987.
119. Rick AD, Belpaire FM, Bogaert MG et al: Plasma concentrations of digoxin and digitoxin during digitalization of healthy dogs and dogs with cardiac failure, *Am J Vet Res* 39:811, 1978.
120. Pedersoli WM: Serum digoxin concentrations in healthy dogs treated without a loading dose, *J Vet Pharm Ther* 1:279, 1978.
121. DeMots H, McAnulty JH, Porter GA: Effects of rapid and slow infusion of ouabain on systemic and coronary vascular resistance in patients not in clinical heart failure, *Circulation* 52:II, 1975 (abstract).
122. Miyazawa Y, Sato T, Kobayashi K et al: Influence of induced cholestasis on pharmacokinetics of digoxin and digitoxin in dogs, *Am J Vet Res* 51:605, 1990.

123. Smith TW, Haber E: Digitalis. III. *N Engl J Med* 289:1063, 1973.
124. Doherty JE: Digitalis glycosides: pharmacokinetics and their clinical implications, *Ann Intern Med* 79:229, 1973.
125. Gierke KD, Perrier D, Mayersohn M et al: Digoxin disposition kinetics in dogs before and during azotemia, *J Pharmacol Exp Ther* 205:459, 1978.
126. Atkins CE, Snyder PS, Keene BW et al: Effects of compensated heart failure on digoxin pharmacokinetics in cats, *J Am Vet Med Assoc* 195:945, 1989.
127. Bolton GR, Powell W: Plasma kinetics of digoxin in the cat, *Am J Vet Res* 128:1994, 1982.
128. Erichsen DF, Harris SG, Upson DW: Plasma levels of digoxin in the cat: some clinical applications, *J Am Anim Hosp Assoc* 14:734, 1978.
129. Hamlin RL: Basis for selection of a cardiac glycoside for dogs, *Proc Symp Vet Pharm Ther* 1978, p 83.
130. Kittleson MD: Drugs used in the management of heart failure. In Kirk RW, ed: *Current veterinary therapy,* ed 8, Philadelphia, 1983, WB Saunders.
131. Bonagura JD, Ware WA: Atrial fibrillation in the dog: clinical findings in 81 cases, *J Am Anim Hosp Assoc* 22:111, 1986.
132. Button C, Gross DR, Allert JA: Application of individualized digoxin dosage regimens to canine therapeutic digitalization, *Am J Vet Res* 41:1238, 1980.
133. Bigger JT: The quinidine-digoxin interaction, *Mod Concepts Cardiovasc Dis* 51:73, 1982.
134. Warner NJ, Barnard JT, Leahey EB et al: Myocardial monovalent cation transport during the quinidine-digoxin interaction in dogs, *Circ Res* 54:453, 1984.
135. Warner NJ, Leahey EB, Hougen TJ et al: Tissue digoxin concentrations during the quinidine-digoxin interaction, *Am J Cardiol* 51:1717, 1983.
136. Peters DN, Hamlin RL, Powers JD: Absence of pharmacokinetic interaction between digitoxin and quinidine in the dog, *J Vet Pharmacol Ther* 4:271, 1981.
137. Klein HO, Lang R, Weiss E et al: The influence of verapamil on serum digoxin concentration, *Circulation* 65:998, 1982.
138. In: Amsterdam EA, ed: *Cardiology drug facts,* New York, 1989, JB Lippincott, p 341.
139. Lesko LJ: Pharmacokinetic drug interactions with amiodarone, *Clin Pharmacokinet* 17:130, 1989.
140. Breznock EM: Effects of phenobarbital on digitoxin and digoxin elimination in the dog, *Am J Vet Res* 36:371, 1975.
141. Pedersoli WM: Serum digoxin concentration in dogs before and after concomitant treatment with chloramphenicol, *J Am Anim Hosp Assoc* 16:839, 1980.
142. Snyder PS, Panciera DL, Volk L: Digoxin pharmacokinetics in dogs with experimental hypothyroidism, *Proc Annu Vet Med Forum,* 1993, p 950 (abstract).
143. Karagueuzian HS, Katzung BG: Relative inotropic and arrhythmogenic effects of five cardiac steroids in ventricular myocardium: oscillatory afterpotentials and the role of endogenous catecholamines, *J Pharmacol Exp Ther* 218:348, 1981.
144. Gross DR, Hamlin RL, Pipers FS: Response of P-Q intervals to digitalis glycosides in the dog, *J Am Vet Med Assoc* 162:888, 1973.
145. Teske RH, Bishop SP, Righter HF et al: Subacute digoxin toxicosis in the beagle dog, *Toxicol Appl Pharmacol* 35:283, 1976.
146. Smith TW: Digitalis toxicity: epidemiology and clinical use of serum concentration measurements, *Am J Med* 58:470, 1975.
147. Borison HL, Borison R, McCarthy LE: Role of the area postrema in vomiting and related functions, *Fed Proc* 43:2955, 1984.
148. Gillis RA: Digitalis: a neuroexcitatory drug, *Circulation* 52:739, 1975.
149. Somberg JC, Smith TW: Localization of the neurally mediated arrhythmogenic properties of digitalis, *Science* 204:321, 1979.
150. Thron CD, Riancho JA, Borison HL: Lack of protection against ouabain cardiotoxicity after chronic ablation of the area postrema in cats, *Exp Neurol* 85:574, 1984.
151. Citrin D, Stevenson IH, O'Malley K: Massive digoxin overdose: observations on hyperkalaemia and plasma digoxin levels, *Scott Med J* 17:275, 1972.
152. Smith TW, Willerson JT: Suicidal and accidental digoxin ingestion: report of five cases with serum digoxin level correlations, *Circulation* 44:29, 1971.
153. Dreifus LS, McKnight EH, Katz M et al: Digitalis intolerance, *Geriatrics* 18:494, 1963.
154. Hoffman BF, Rosen MR: Cellular mechanisms for cardiac arrhythmias, *Circ Res* 49:1, 1981.
155. Peon J, Ferrier GR, Moe GK: The relationship of excitability to conduction velocity in canine Purkinje tissue, *Circ Res* 43:125, 1978.
156. Rall TW, Schleifer LS: Drugs effective in the therapy of the epilepsies. In Gilman AG, Goodman LS, Gilman A, eds: *The pharmacological basis of therapeutics,* ed 6, New York, 1980, MacMillan.
157. Sanders JE, Yeary RA: Serum concentrations of orally administered diphenylhydantoin in dogs, *J Am Vet Med Assoc* 172:153, 1978.
158. Neuvonen PJ, Kivisto K, Hirvisalo EL: Effects of resins and activated charcoal on the absorption of digoxin, carbamazepine and furosemide, *Br J Clin Pharmacol* 25:229, 1988.
159. Caldwell JH, Greenberger NJ: Interruption of the enterohepatic circulation of digitoxin by cholestyramine. I. Protection against lethal digitoxin intoxication, *J Clin Invest* 50:2626, 1971.
160. Smith TW, Butler VP, Haber E et al: Treatment of life-threatening digitalis intoxication with digoxin-specific Fab antibody fragments: experience in 26 cases, *N Engl J Med* 307:1357, 1982.
161. Senior DF, Feist EH, Stuart LB et al: Treatment of acute digoxin toxicosis with digoxin immune fab (ovine), *J Vet Intern Med* 5:302, 1991.
162. Antman EM, Wenger TL, Butler VP et al: Treatment of 150 cases of life-threatening digitalis intoxication with digoxin-specific Fab antibody fragments: final report of a multicenter study, *Circulation* 81:1744, 1990.
163. Rainey PM: Effects of digoxin immune Fab (ovine) on digoxin immunoassays, *Am J Clin Pathol* 92:779, 1989.
164. Katz AM: Congestive heart failure: role of altered myocardial cellular control, *N Engl J Med* 293:1184, 1975.
165. Adams HR: New perspectives in cardiopulmonary therapeutics: receptor-selective adrenergic drugs, *J Am Vet Med Assoc* 185:966, 1984.
166. Maekawa K, Liang CS, Hood WB: Comparison of dobutamine and dopamine in acute myocardial infarction: effects of systemic hemodynamics, plasma catecholamines, blood flows and infarct size, *Circulation* 67:750, 1983.
167. Bednarski RM, Muir WW: Catecholamine infusion in vagotomized dogs during thiamylal-halothane and pentobarbital anesthesia, *Cornell Vet* 75:512, 1985.
168. Murphy PJ, Williams TL, Kau DL: Disposition of dobutamine in the dog, *J Pharmacol Exp Ther* 199:423, 1976.
169. McNay JL, McDonald RH, Goldgern LI: Direct renal vasodilation produced by dopamine in the dog, *Circ Res* 16:510, 1965.
170. Kinoshita G, Washizu M, Murata N et al: The selective effects of dopamine and dobutamine on liver circulation in the dog, *J Vet Med Sci* 57:293, 1995.
171. Loeb HS, Bredakis J, Gunner RM: Superiority of dobutamine over dopamine for augmentation of cardiac output in patients with chronic low output cardiac failure, *Circulation* 55:375, 1977.
172. MacCannell KL, Giraud GD, Hamilton PL et al: Haemodynamic responses to dopamine and dobutamine infusions as a function of duration of infusion, *Pharmacology* 26:29, 1983.
173. Robie NW, Goldberg LI: Comparative systemic and regional hemodynamic effects of dopamine and dobutamine, *Am Heart J* 90:340, 1975.
174. Vatner SF, McRitchie RJ, Braunwald E: Effects of dobutamine on left ventricular performance, coronary dynamics, and distribution of cardiac output in conscious dogs, *J Clin Invest* 53:1265, 1974.
175. Tuttle RR, Mills J: Dobutamine: development of a new catecholamine to selectively increase cardiac contractility, *Circ Res* 36:185, 1975.
176. Willerson JT, Hutton I, Watson JT et al: Influence of dobutamine on regional myocardial blood flow and ventricular performance during acute and chronic myocardial ischemia in dogs, *Circulation* 53:828, 1976.

177. Akhtar N, Mikulic E, Cohn JN et al: Hemodynamic effect of dobutamine in patients with severe heart failure, *Am J Cardiol* 36:202, 1975.
178. Andy JJ, Curry CL, Ali N et al: Cardiovascular effects of dobutamine in severe congestive heart failure, *Am Heart J* 94:175, 1977.
179. Eyster GE, Anderson LK, Bender G et al: Effect of dobutamine in postperfusion cardiac failure in the dog, *Am J Vet Res* 36:1285, 1975.
180. Unverferth DV, Magorien RD, Lewis RP et al: Long-term benefit of dobutamine in patients with congestive cardiomyopathy, *Am Heart J* 100:622, 1980.
181. Braunwald E: A symposium: amrinone—introduction, *Am J Cardiol* 56:1B, 1985.
182. Evans DB: Overview of cardiovascular physiologic and pharmacologic aspects of selective phosphodiesterase peak III inhibitors, *Am J Cardiol* 63:9A, 1989.
183. Piscione F, Jaski BE, Wenting GJ et al: Effect of a single oral dose of milrinone on left ventricular diastolic performance in the failing human heart, *J Am Coll Cardiol* 10:1294, 1987.
184. Keister DM: *A summary of phase IV clinical data on milrinone (Wincardin), a canine cardiotonic, protocol H,* New York, 1988, Sterling-Winthrop.
185. Emmert SE, Stabilito II, Sweet CS: Acute and subacute hemodynamic effects of enalaprilat, milrinone and combination therapy in rats with chronic left ventricular dysfunction, *Clin Exp Hypertens [A]* 9:297, 1987.
186. *A summary of laboratory and clinical data on Inocor (brand of amrinone),* New York, 1980, Sterling-Winthrop.
187. Treadway G: Clinical safety of intravenous amrinone, *Am J Cardiol* 56:39B, 1985.
188. Kittleson MD: The efficacy and safety of milrinone for treating heart failure in dogs, *Vet Clin North Am Small Anim Pract* 21:905, 1991.
189. Alousi AA, Canter JM, Montenaro MJ et al: Cardiotonic activity of milrinone, a new and potent cardiac bipyridine, on the normal and failing heart of experimental animals, *J Cardiovasc Pharmacol* 5:792, 1983.
190. Kittleson MD, Pipers FS, Knauer KW et al: Echocardiographic and clinical effects of milrinone in dogs with myocardial failure, *Am J Vet Res* 46:1659, 1985.
191. Kittleson MD, Johnson LE, Pion PD: The acute hemodynamic effects of milrinone in dogs with severe idiopathic myocardial failure, *J Vet Intern Med* 1:121, 1987.
192. Cohn JN, Mathew KJ, Franciosa JA et al: Chronic vasodilator therapy in the management of cardiogenic shock and intractable left ventricular failure, *Ann Intern Med* 81:777, 1974.
193. Atwell RB: The use of alpha blockade in the treatment of congestive heart failure associated with dirofilariasis and mitral valvular incompetence, *Vet Rec* 104:114, 1979.
194. Kittleson MD, Hamlin RL: Hydralazine pharmacodynamics in the dog, *Am J Vet Res* 44:1501, 1983.
195. Kittleson MD, Eyster GE, Olivier NB et al: Oral hydralazine therapy for chronic mitral regurgitation in the dog, *J Am Vet Med Assoc* 182:1205, 1983.
196. Kittleson MD, Hamlin RL: Hydralazine therapy for severe mitral regurgitation in a dog, *J Am Vet Med Assoc* 179:903, 1981.
197. Asanoi H, Kameyama T, Ashizaka S et al: Energetically optimal left ventricular pressure for the failing human heart, *Circulation* 93:67, 1996.
198. Greenwald JE, Wong LK, Alexander M et al: In vivo inhibition of thromboxane biosynthesis by hydralazine, *Adv Prostaglandin Thromboxane Res* 6:293, 1980.
199. Maekawa K, Liang CS, Tsui A et al: Vasodilative effect of hydralazine in awake dogs: the roles of prostaglandins and the sympathetic nervous system, *Circulation* 70:908, 1984.
200. Tabrizchi R, Pang CC: Effects of drugs on body venous tone, as reflected by mean circulatory filling pressure, *Cardiovasc Res* 26:443, 1992.
201. Spokas EG, Wang HH: Regional blood flow and cardiac responses to hydralazine, *J Pharmacol Exp Ther* 212:294, 1980.
202. Khatri I, Uemura N, Notargiacomo A et al: Direct and reflex cardiostimulating effects of hydralazine, *Am J Cardiol* 40:39, 1977.
203. Yamamoto J, Trippodo NC, Ishise S et al: Total vascular pressure-volume relationship in the conscious rat, *Am J Physiol* 238:H823, 1980.
204. Kittleson MD, Johnson LE, Pion PD et al: The acute haemodynamic effects of captopril in dogs with heart failure, *J Vet Pharmacol Ther* 16:1, 1993.
205. Brown WA, Kittleson MD: Color flow Doppler estimation of mitral regurgitation using the proximal flow convergence method in dogs with chronic degenerative valve disease, *J Vet Intern Med* 8:143, 1994 (abstract).
206. Kittleson MD, Eyster GE, Knowlen GG et al: Myocardial function in small dogs with chronic mitral regurgitation and severe congestive heart failure, *J Am Vet Med Assoc* 184:455, 1984.
207. Kittleson MD, Johnson LE, Oliver NB: Acute hemodynamic effects of hydralazine in dogs with chronic mitral regurgitation, *J Am Vet Med Assoc* 187:258, 1985.
208. Koch-Weser J: Hydralazine, *N Engl J Med* 295:320, 1976.
209. Haggstrom J, Hansson K, Karlberg BE et al: Effects of long-term treatment with enalapril or hydralazine on the renin-angiotensin-aldosterone system and fluid balance in dogs with naturally acquired mitral valve degeneration, *Am J Vet Res* 57:1645, 1996.
210. Cogan JJ, Humphreys MH, Carlson CJ et al: Acute vasodilator therapy increases renal clearance of digoxin in patients with congestive heart failure, *Circulation* 64:973, 1981.
211. Anderson TJ, Meredith IT, Ganz P et al: Nitric oxide and nitrovasodilators: similarities, differences and potential interactions, *J Am Coll Cardiol* 24:555, 1994.
212. Gruetter CA, Gruetter DY, Lyon JE et al: Relationship between cyclic guanosine 3':5'-monophosphate formation and relaxation of coronary arterial smooth muscle by glyceryl trinitrate, nitroprusside, nitrite and nitric oxide: effects of methylene blue and methemoglobin, *J Pharmacol Exp Ther* 219:181, 1981.
213. Ignarro LJ, Lippton H, Edwards JC et al: Mechanism of vascular smooth muscle relaxation by organic nitrates, nitrites, nitroprusside and nitric oxide: evidence for the involvement of S-nitrosothiols as active intermediates, *J Pharmacol Exp Ther* 218:739, 1981.
214. Tzeng TB, Fung HL: Pharmacodynamic modeling of the in vitro vasodilating effects of organic mononitrates, *J Pharmacokinet Biopharm* 20:227, 1992.
215. Hamlin RL: Evidence for or against clinical efficacy of preload reducers. In Hamlin RL, ed: *The veterinary clinics of North America,* vol 21, ed 5, Philadelphia, 1991, WB Saunders.
216. Schwartz AM: The cause, relief, and prevention of headache arising from contact with dynamite, *N Engl J Med* 235:541, 1946.
217. Abrams J: Tolerance to organic nitrates, *Circulation* 74:1181, 1986.
218. Fung HL: Solving the mystery of nitrate tolerance. A new scent on the trail? *Circulation* 88:322, 1993 (editorial; comment).
219. Packer M, Lee WH, Kessler PD et al: Prevention and reversal of nitrate tolerance in patients with congestive heart failure, *N Engl J Med* 317:799, 1987.
220. Dupuis J, Lalonde G, Lemieux R et al: Tolerance to intravenous nitroglycerin in patients with congestive heart failure: role of increased intravascular volume, neurohumoral activation and lack of prevention with N-acetylcysteine, *J Am Coll Cardiol* 16:923, 1990 (see comments).
221. Fung HL, Chong S, Kowaluk E et al: Mechanisms for the pharmacologic interaction of organic nitrates with thiols: existence of an extracellular pathway for the reversal of nitrate vascular tolerance by N-acetylcysteine, *J Pharmacol Exp Ther* 245:524, 1988.
222. Lis Y, Bennett D, Lambert G et al: A preliminary double-blind study of intravenous nitroglycerin in acute myocardial infarction, *Intensive Care Med* 10:179, 1984.
223. Gogia H, Mehra A, Parikh S et al: Prevention of tolerance to hemodynamic effects of nitrates with concomitant use of hydralazine in patients with chronic heart failure, *J Am Coll Cardiol* 26:1575, 1995.
224. Bauer JA, Fung HL: Concurrent hydralazine administration prevents nitroglycerin-induced hemodynamic tolerance in experimental heart failure, *Circulation* 84:35, 1991.

225. Unger P, Berkenboom G, Fontaine J: Interaction between hydralazine and nitrovasodilators in vascular smooth muscle, *J Cardiovasc Pharmacol* 21:478, 1993.
226. American Hospital Formulary Service, AHFS Drug Information, 1995.
227. Packer M, Medina N, Yushak M et al: Hemodynamic factors limiting the response to transdermal nitroglycerin in severe chronic congestive heart failure, *Am J Cardiol* 57:260, 1986.
228. Cohn JN, Franciosa JA: Vasodilator therapy of cardiac failure. I. *N Engl J Med* 297:27, 1977.
229. Ader R, Chatterjee K, Ports T et al: Immediate and sustained hemodynamic and clinical improvement in chronic heart failure by an oral angiotensin-converting enzyme inhibitor, *Circulation* 61:931, 1980.
230. Ware WA: Management of congestive heart failure. In Nelson RW, Couto CG, eds: *Essentials of small animal internal medicine,* St Louis, 1992, Mosby.
231. Braunwald E: Hypotension and syncope. In Braunwald E, ed: *Heart disease: a textbook of cardiovascular medicine,* ed 4, Philadelphia, 1992, WB Saunders.
232. McDonald KM, Francis GS, Matthews J et al: Long-term oral nitrate therapy prevents chronic ventricular remodeling in the dog, *J Am Coll Cardiol* 21:514, 1993.
233. Harrison DG, Bates JN: The nitrovasodilators: new ideas about old drugs, *Circulation* 87:1461, 1993.
234. Brodie BR, Grossman W, Mann T et al: Effects of sodium nitroprusside on left ventricular diastolic pressure-volume relations, *J Clin Invest* 59:59, 1977.
235. Pagani M, Vatner SF, Braunwald E: Hemodynamic effects of intravenous sodium nitroprusside in the conscious dog, *Circulation* 57:144, 1978.
236. Sasayama S, Takahashi M, Osakada G et al: Dynamic geometry of the left atrium and left ventricle in acute mitral regurgitation, *Circulation* 60:177, 1979.
237. Goodman DJ, Rossen RM, Holloway EL et al: Effect of nitroprusside on left ventricular dynamics in mitral regurgitation, *Circulation* 50:1025, 1974.
238. Guiha NH, Cohn JN, Mikulic E et al: Treatment of refractory heart failure with infusion of nitroprusside, *N Engl J Med* 291:587, 1974.
239. Franciosa JA, Silverstein SR: Hemodynamic effects of nitroprusside and furosemide in left ventricular failure, *Clin Pharmacol Ther* 32:62, 1982.
240. Keene BW: Unpublished observations on the use of nitroprusside and dobutamine in dogs with severe congestive heart failure due to dilated cardiomyopathy, 1996, personal communication.
241. Finegan BA, Chen HJ, Singh YN et al: Comparison of hemodynamic changes induced by adenosine monophosphate and sodium nitroprusside alone and during dopamine infusion in the anesthetized dog, *Anesth Analg* 70:44, 1990.
242. Cottrell JE, Casthely P, Brodie JD et al: Prevention of nitroprusside-induced cyanide toxicity with hydroxocobalamin, *N Engl J Med* 298:809, 1978.
243. Kaneko Y, Ikeda T, Takeda T et al: Renin release during acute reduction of arterial pressure in normotensive subjects and patients with renovascular hypertension, *J Clin Invest* 46:705, 1967.
244. Palmer RF, Lasseter KC: Drug therapy: sodium nitroprusside, *N Engl J Med* 292:294, 1975.
245. Lowenstein J, Steele JM: Prazosin, *Am Heart J* 95:262, 1995.
246. Packer M, Meller J, Gorlin R et al: Hemodynamic and clinical tachyphylaxis to prazosin-mediated afterload reduction in severe chronic congestive heart failure, *Circulation* 59:531, 1979.
247. Smith RD, Tessman DK, Kaplan HR: Acute tolerance to prazosin in conscious hypertensive rats: involvement of the renin-angiotensin system, *J Pharmacol Exp Ther* 217:397, 1981.
248. Awan NA, Miller RR, DeMaria AN et al: Efficacy of ambulatory systemic vasodilator therapy with oral prazosin in chronic refractory heart failure: concomitant relief of pulmonary congestion and elevation of pump output demonstrated by improvements in symptomatology, exercise tolerance, hemodynamics and echocardiography, *Circulation* 56:346, 1977.
249. The COVE Study Group: Controlled clinical evaluation of enalapril in dogs with heart failure: results of the Cooperative Veterinary Enalapril Study Group, *J Vet Intern Med* 9:243, 1995.
250. The IMPROVE Study Group: Acute and short-term hemodynamic, echocardiographic, and clinical effects of enalapril maleate in dogs with naturally acquired heart failure: results of the Invasive Multicenter PROspective Veterinary Evaluation of Enalapril study, *J Vet Intern Med* 9:234, 1995.
251. The SOLVD Investigators: Effect of enalapril on mortality and the development of heart failure in asymptomatic patients with reduced left ventricular ejection fractions, *N Engl J Med* 327:685, 1992 (see comments) (erratum 327(24):1768, 1992).
252. The SOLVD Investigators: Effect of enalapril on survival in patients with reduced left ventricular ejection fractions and congestive heart failure, *N Engl J Med* 325:293, 1991 (see comments).
253. Pfeffer MA, Braunwald E, Moye LA et al: Effect of captopril on mortality and morbidity in patients with left ventricular dysfunction after myocardial infarction: results of the survival and ventricular enlargement trial. The SAVE investigators, *N Engl J Med* 327:669, 1992 (see comments).
254. The CONSENSUS Trial Study Group: Effects of enalapril on mortality in severe congestive heart failure: results of the Cooperative North Scandinavian Enalapril Survival Study (CONSENSUS), *N Engl J Med* 316:1429, 1987.
255. Cohn JN, Johnson G, Ziesche S et al: A comparison of enalapril with hydralazine-isosorbide dinitrate in the treatment of chronic congestive heart failure, *N Engl J Med* 325:303, 1991 (see comments).
256. Weber KT, Brilla CG: Pathological hypertrophy and cardiac interstitium: fibrosis and renin-angiotensin-aldosterone system, *Circulation* 83:1849, 1991.
257. Weber KT, Brilla CG, Janicki JS et al: Myocardial fibrosis: role of ventricular systolic pressure, arterial hypertension, and circulating hormones, *Basic Res Cardiol* 86(suppl)3:25, 1991.
258. Booz GW, Baker KM: Molecular signaling mechanisms controlling growth and function of cardiac fibroblasts, *Cardiovasc Res* 30:537, 1995.
259. Weber KT, Pick R, Silver MA et al: Fibrillar collagen and remodeling of dilated canine left ventricle, *Circulation* 82:1387, 1990.
260. Parker TG: Molecular biology of myocardial hypertrophy and failure: gene expression and trophic signaling, *New Horiz* 3:288, 1995.
261. Kramer CM, Ferrari VA, Rogers WJ et al: Angiotensin-converting enzyme inhibition limits dysfunction in adjacent noninfarcted regions during left ventricular remodeling, *J Am Coll Cardiol* 27:211, 1996.
262. Sigurdsson A, Swedberg K: Left ventricular remodeling, neurohormonal activation and early treatment with enalapril (CONSENSUS II) following myocardial infarction, *Eur Heart J* 15(suppl B):14, discussion p 26, 1994.
263. van Wijngaarden J, Pinto YM, van Gilst WH et al: Converting enzyme inhibition after experimental myocardial infarction in rats: comparative study between spirapril and zofenopril, *Cardiovasc Res* 25:936, 1991.
264. Jugdutt BI, Khan MI, Jugdutt SJ et al: Effect of enalapril on ventricular remodeling and function during healing after anterior myocardial infarction in the dog, *Circulation* 91:802, 1995.
265. Jugdutt BI, Schwarz-Michorowski BL, Khan MI: Effect of long-term captopril therapy on left ventricular remodeling and function during healing of canine myocardial infarction, *J Am Coll Cardiol* 19:713, 1992 (see comments).
266. Raman VK, Lee YA, Lindpaintner K: The cardiac renin-angiotensin-aldosterone system and hypertensive cardiac hypertrophy, *Am J Cardiol* 76:18D, 1995.
267. Goldstein S, Sharov VG, Cook JM et al: Ventricular remodeling: insights from pharmacologic interventions with angiotensin-converting enzyme inhibitors, *Mol Cell Biochem* 147:51, 1995.
268. Weinberg EO, Schoen FJ, George D et al: Angiotensin-converting enzyme inhibition prolongs survival and modifies the transition to heart failure in rats with pressure overload hypertrophy due to ascending aortic stenosis, *Circulation* 90:1410, 1994.

269. Nascimben L, Friedrich J, Liao R et al: Enalapril treatment increases cardiac performance and energy reserve via the creatine kinase reaction in myocardium of Syrian myopathic hamsters with advanced heart failure, *Circulation* 91:1824, 1995.
270. Sadoshima J, Xu Y, Slayter HS et al: Autocrine release of angiotensin II mediates stretch-induced hypertrophy of cardiac myocytes in vitro, *Cell* 75:977, 1993.
271. Urata H, Boehm KD, Philip A et al: Cellular localization and regional distribution of an angiotensin II-forming chymase in the heart, *J Clin Invest* 91:1269, 1993.
272. Urata H, Hoffmann S, Ganten D: Tissue angiotensin II system in the human heart, *Eur Heart J* 15(suppl D):68, 1994.
273. McDonald KM, Mock J, D'Aloia A et al: Bradykinin antagonism inhibits the antigrowth effect of converting enzyme inhibition in the dog myocardium after discrete transmural myocardial necrosis, *Circulation* 91:2043, 1995.
274. Packer M: Converting-enzyme inhibition in the management of severe chronic congestive heart failure: physiologic concepts, *J Cardiovasc Pharmacol* 10(suppl 7):S83, 1987.
275. Hollenberg NK: Control of renal perfusion and function in congestive heart failure, *Am J Cardiol* 62:72E, 1988.
276. Packer M, Lee WH, Kessler PD: Preservation of glomerular filtration rate in human heart failure by activation of the renin-angiotensin system, *Circulation* 74:766, 1986.
277. Packer M, Lee WH, Medina N et al: Functional renal insufficiency during long-term therapy with captopril and enalapril in severe chronic heart failure, *Ann Intern Med* 106:346, 1987.
278. Lee WH, Packer M: Prognostic importance of serum sodium concentration and its modification by converting-enzyme inhibition in patients with severe chronic heart failure, *Circulation* 73:257, 1986.
279. Packer M, Lee WH, Kessler PD et al: Identification of hyponatremia as a risk factor for the development of functional renal insufficiency during convert ng enzyme inhibition in severe chronic heart failure, *J Am Coll Cardiol* 10:837, 1987.
280. Packer M, Lee WH, Yushak M et al: Comparison of captopril and enalapril in patients with severe chronic heart failure, *N Engl J Med* 315:847, 1986 (erratum 315(17):1105, 1986).
281. Plante GE, Chainey A, Sirois P et al: Angiotensin converting enzyme inhibition and autoregulation of glomerular filtration, *J Hypertens Suppl* 6:S69, 1988.
282. Gottlieb SS, Robinson S, Weir MR et al: Determinants of the renal response to ACE inhibition in patients with congestive heart failure, *Am Heart J* 124:131, 1992.
283. Blaufarb IS, Sonnenblick EH: The renin-angiotensin system in left ventricular remodeling, *Am J Cardiol* 77:8C, 1996.
284. Zusman RM: Effects of converting-enzyme inhibitors on the renin-angiotensin-aldosterone, bradykinin, and arachidonic acid-prostaglandin systems: correlation of chemical structure and biologic activity, *Am J Kidney Dis* 10:13, 1987.
285. Hall D, Zeitler H, Rudolph W: Counteraction of the vasodilator effects of enalapril by aspirin in severe heart failure, *J Am Coll Cardiol* 20:1549, 1992.
286. Evans MA, Burnett JC, Redfield MM: Effect of low dose aspirin on cardiorenal function and acute hemodynamic response to enalaprilat in a canine model of severe heart failure, *J Am Coll Cardiol* 25: 1445, 1995.
287. McLay JS, McMurray JJ, Bridges AB et al: Acute effects of captopril on the renal actions of furosemide in patients with chronic heart failure, *Am Heart J* 126:879, 1993.
288. Vidt DG, Bravo EL, Fouad FM: Captopril, *N Engl J Med* 306:214, 1982.
289. Singhvi SM, Peterson AE, Ross JJ et al: Pharmacokinetics of captopril in dogs and monkeys, *J Pharm Sci* 70:1108, 1981.
290. Fox PR, Sisson DD: Angiotensin-converting enzyme inhibitors. In Bonagura JD, ed: *Current veterinary therapy.* XII. *Small animal practice.* Philadelphia, 1995, WB Saunders.
291. Blackford LW, Golden AL, Bright JM et al: Captopril provides sustained hemodynamic benefits in dogs with experimentally induced mitral regurgitation, *Vet Surg* 19:237, 1990.
292. Fox PR: Feline cardiomyopathy. In Bonagura JD, ed: *Contemporary issues in small animal practice: cardiology,* New York, 1987, Churchill Livingstone.
293. Tocco DJ, deLuna FA, Duncan AE et al: The physiological disposition and metabolism of enalapril maleate in laboratory animals, *Drug Metab Dispos* 10:15, 1982.
294. Sweet CS, Ulm EH: Lisinopril, *Cardiovasc Drug Rev* 6:181, 1988.
295. Benitz AM, Hamlin RL, Ericsson GF: Titration of enalapril dose for dogs with induced heart failure, *Proc Annu Vet Med Forum,* 1991, p 879 (abstract).
296. MacDonald JS, Bagdon WJ, Peter CP et al: Renal effects of enalapril in dogs, *Kidney Int Suppl* 20:S148, 1987.
297. Ettinger SJ, Benitz AM, Ericsson GF: Relationships of enalapril with other CHF treatment modalities, *Proc Annu Vet Med Forum,* 1994, p 251.
298. Fox PR: The effect of drug therapy on clinical characteristics and outcome in dogs with heart failure, *Proc Annu Vet Med Forum,* 1992, p 592.
299. Ettinger SJ, Lusk R, Brayley K: Evaluation of enalapril in dogs with heart failure in a large multicenter study: Cooperative Veterinary Enalapril (COVE) Study Group, *Proc Annu Vet Med Forum,* 1992, 584.
300. Sabbah HN, Shimoyama H, Kono T et al: Effects of long-term monotherapy with enalapril, metoprolol, and digoxin on the progression of left ventricular dysfunction and dilation in dogs with reduced ejection fraction, *Circulation* 89:2852, 1994.
301. Shimoyama H, Sabbah HN, Rosman H et al: Effects of long-term therapy with enalapril on severity of functional mitral regurgitation in dogs with moderate heart failure, *J Am Coll Cardiol* 25:768, 1995.
302. Waldmeier F, Schmid K: Disposition of [14C]-benazepril hydrochloride in rat, dog and baboon: absorption, distribution, kinetics, biotransformation and excretion, *Arzneimittelforschung* 39:62, 1989.
303. King JN, Mauron C, Kaiser G: Pharmacokinetics of the active metabolite of benazepril, benazeprilat, and inhibition of plasma angiotensin-converting enzyme activity after single and repeated administration to dogs, *Am J Vet Res* 56:1620, 1995.
304. Nakazawa M, Sawanobori T, Iwasaki K et al: Hemodynamic effects of benazeprilat in the anesthetized dog with acute left ventricular failure, *Jpn J Pharmacol* 56:369, 1991.
305. Swedberg K: Initial experience with beta blockers in dilated cardiomyopathy, *Am J Cardiol* 71:30C, 1993.
306. Waagstein F, Hjalmarson A, Varnauskas E et al: Effect of chronic beta-adrenergic receptor blockade in congestive cardiomyopathy, *Br Heart J* 37:1022, 1975.
307. Swedberg K, Hjalmarson A, Waagstein F et al: Prolongation of survival in congestive cardiomyopathy by beta-receptor blockade, *Lancet* 1:1374, 1976.
308. CIBIS Investigators and Committees: A randomized trial of beta-blockade in heart failure: The Cardiac Insufficiency Bisoprolol Study (CIBIS), *Circulation* 90:1765, 1994 (see comments).
309. Olsen SL, Gilbert EM, Renlund DG et al: Carvedilol improves left ventricular function and symptoms in chronic heart failure: a double-blind randomized study, *J Am Coll Cardiol* 25:1225, 1995.
310. Waagstein F, Bristow MR, Swedberg K et al: Beneficial effects of metoprolol in idiopathic dilated cardiomyopathy: Metoprolol in Dilated Cardiomyopathy (MDC) Trial Study Group, *Lancet* 342:1441, 1993 (see comments).
311. Eichhorn EJ, Bristow MR: Practical guidelines for initiation of beta-adrenergic blockade in patients with chronic heart failure, *Am J Cardiol* 79:794, 1997.
312. Davies MK, Cummins P, Littler WA: The effects of acute and chronic beta-adrenoceptor blockade on the myofibrillar contractile system in the dog heart, *Clin Sci* 67:259, 1984.
313. Tsutsui H, Spinale FG, Nagatsu M et al: Effects of chronic beta-adrenergic blockade on the left ventricular and cardiocyte abnormalities of chronic canine mitral regurgitation, *J Clin Invest* 93:2639, 1994.
314. Bright JM: Experience with beta blockade to improve myocardial function in dogs with dilated cardiomyopathy, personal communication, 1996.

315. Waagstein F, Caidahl K, Wallentin I et al: Long-term beta-blockade in dilated cardiomyopathy: effects of short- and long-term metoprolol treatment followed by withdrawal and readministration of metoprolol, *Circulation* 80:551, 1989 (see comments).
316. Heilbrunn SM, Shah P, Bristow MR et al: Increased beta-receptor density and improved hemodynamic response to catecholamine stimulation during long-term metoprolol therapy in heart failure from dilated cardiomyopathy, *Circulation* 79:483, 1989.
317. Bashir Y, McKenna WJ, Camm AJ: Beta blockers and the failing heart: is it time for a U-turn? *Br Heart J* 70:8, 1993.
318. Gilbert EM, O'Connell JB, Bristow MR: Therapy of idiopathic dilated cardiomyopathy with chronic beta-adrenergic blockade, *Heart Vessels Suppl* 6:29, 1991.
319. Mann DL, Kent RL, Parsons B et al: Adrenergic effects on the biology of the adult mammalian cardiocyte, *Circulation* 85:790, 1992.
320. Urabe Y, Hamada Y, Sinale FG et al: Cardiocyte contractile performance in experimental biventricular volume-overload hypertrophy, *Am J Physiol* 264:H1615, 1993.
321. Zhang Y, Li H, Lan T et al: [Effects of vesnarinone on L-type single Ca2+ channel current in cultured ventricular myocytes of embryonic chick], *Hua Hsi I Ko Ta Hsueh Hsueh Pao* 26:403, 1995.
322. Du J, Yang Z: [Effect of Chinese-made vesnarinone on experimental heart failure of dog], *Hua Hsi I Ko Ta Hsueh Hsueh Pao* 23:178, 1992.
323. Feldman AM, Bristow MR, Parmley WW et al: Effects of vesnarinone on morbidity and mortality in patients with heart failure. Vesnarinone Study Group, *N Engl J Med* 329:149, 1993 [see comments].
324. Feldman A, Young J, Bourge R et al: Mechanism of increased mortality from vesnarinone in the severe heart failure trial (VesT), *J Am Coll Cardiol* 29:64A, 1997 (abstract).
325. Crozier I, Ikram H, Awan N et al: Losartan in heart failure: hemodynamic effects and tolerability. Losartan Hemodynamic Study Group, *Circulation* 91:691, 1995.
326. Conti CR: Use of calcium antagonists to treat heart failure, *Clin Cardiol* 17:101, 1994 (editorial).
327. Johnson MA, Hamlin RL, Lyons CD: Cardiovascular effects of nifedipine in the dog, *Angiology* 44:791, 1993.
328. Fioretti P, Benussi B, Scardi S et al: Afterload reduction with nifedipine in aortic insufficiency, *Am J Cardiol* 49:1728, 1982.
329. Packer M, O'Connor CM, Ghali JK et al: Effect of amlodipine on morbidity and mortality in severe chronic heart failure. Prospective Randomized Amlodipine Survival Evaluation Study Group, *N Engl J Med* 335:1107, 1996.
330. Tsutamoto T, Kinoshita M, Nakae I et al: Absence of hemodynamic tolerance to nicorandil in patients with severe congestive heart failure, *Am Heart J* 127:866, 1994.
331. Remme WJ, Krayenbuhl HP, Baumann G et al: Long-term efficacy and safety of pimobendan in moderate heart failure: a double-blind parallel 6-month comparison with enalapril. The Pimobendan-Enalapril Study Group, *Eur Heart J* 15:947, 1994.
332. Wei CM, Lerman A, Rodeheffer RJ et al: Endothelin in human congestive heart failure, *Circulation* 89:1580, 1994.
333. Li K, Rouleau JL: Altered responsiveness to endothelin-1 of myocardium from pacing-induced heart failure model in the dog, *Cardiovasc Drugs Ther* 10:107, 1996.
334. Vollmar AM, Preusser U, Gerbes AL et al: Endothelin concentration in plasma of healthy dogs and dogs with congestive heart failure, renal failure, diabetes mellitus, and hyperadrenocorticism, *J Vet Intern Med* 9:105, 1995.
335. Doherty AM, Patt WC, Edmunds JJ et al: Discovery of a novel series of orally active non-peptide endothelin-A (ETA) receptor-selective antagonists, *J Med Chem* 38:1259, 1995.
336. Doherty AM, Patt WC, Repine J et al: Structure-activity relationships of a novel series of orally active nonpeptide ETA and ETA/B endothelin receptor-selective antagonists, *J Cardiovasc Pharmacol* 26(suppl)3: S358, 1995.
337. Cody RJ, Atlas SA, Laragh JH et al: Atrial natriuretic factor in normal subjects and heart failure patients: plasma levels and renal, hormonal, and hemodynamic responses to peptide infusion, *J Clin Invest* 78:1362, 1986.
338. Munzel T, Kurz S, Holtz J et al: Neurohormonal inhibition and hemodynamic unloading during prolonged inhibition of ANF degradation in patients with severe chronic heart failure, *Circulation* 86:1089, 1992.
339. Moe GW, Forster C, De Bold AJ et al: Pharmacokinetics, hemodynamic, renal, and neurohormonal effects of atrial natriuretic factor in experimental heart failure, *Clin Invest Med* 13:111, 1990.
340. Margulies KB, Perrella MA, McKinley LJ et al: Angiotensin inhibition potentiates the renal responses to neutral endopeptidase inhibition in dogs with congestive heart failure, *J Clin Invest* 88:1636, 1991.
341. Cavero PG, Margulies KB, Winaver J et al: Cardiorenal actions of neutral endopeptidase inhibition in experimental congestive heart failure, *Circulation* 82:196, 1990 (see comments).
342. Sisson D, Thomas WP, Miller M: The effects of neutral endopeptidase inhibition in a rapid ventricular pacing model of heart failure in dogs, *Proc Annu Vet Med Forum,* 1997, p 209.
343. Fett DL, Cavero PG, Burnett JC: Low-dose atrial natriuretic factor and furosemide in experimental acute congestive heart failure, *J Am Soc Nephrol* 4:162, 1993.
344. Keene BW, Panciera DP, Atkins CE et al: Myocardial L-carnitine deficiency in a family of dogs with dilated cardiomyopathy, *J Am Vet Med Assoc* 198:647, 1991.
345. Ross JN: Heart failure. In Lewis LD, Morris ML, Hand MS, eds: *Small animal clinical nutrition,* Topeka, Kan, 1987, Mark Morris Institute.
346. Puri S, Baker BL, Dutka DP et al: Reduced alveolar-capillary membrane diffusing capacity in chronic heart failure: its pathophysiological relevance and relationship to exercise performance, *Circulation* 91: 2769, 1995.
347. Committee on Evaluation and Management of Heart Failure: Guidelines for the evaluation and management of heart failure. Report of the American College of Cardiology/American Heart Association Task Force on Practice Guidelines, *J Am Coll Cardiol* 26:1376, 1995.
348. Jacobson JD, McGrath CJ, Smith EP: Cardiorespiratory effects of four opioid-tranquilizer combinations in dogs, *Vet Surg* 23:299, 1994 (erratum 23(5):434, 1994).

CHAPTER 11

The Approach to the Patient with Cardiac Disease

Congenital cardiac disease accounts for less than 10% of the cardiac disease seen in dogs and cats. However, it is the most common type of cardiac disease seen in dogs less than 1 year of age. Documenting the type of disease and the severity of that disease in this type of patient is extremely important because the owner often must decide whether to keep a dog or cat with a cardiac abnormality. Owners that decide to keep an affected animal should be told any therapeutic options, expected complications of the disease, and the long-term prognosis. The practicing veterinarian may be able to provide this information or at least provide the owner with a short list of possible abnormalities and some idea of the prognosis based on the physical examination and the size and configuration of the heart on thoracic radiographs. Often, however, an echocardiogram is required for a definitive diagnosis. This may necessitate referral of the patient or consultation with a veterinary cardiologist. Consequently, the veterinarian must be able to decide when to refer the patient. The diagnosis of congenital heart disease often is challenging. Consequently, the veterinary cardiologist is often eager to examine this type of patient.

Congenital heart disease (CHD) generally refers to a defect in cardiac structure that is present at birth. For many lesions this definition is perfect because they are present at birth and create clinical manifestations that can be identified at birth. Examples include patent ductus arteriosus and pulmonic stenosis. For other lesions, although the propensity to develop the lesion is present at birth, an anatomic lesion does not develop until later in life. The most common example in veterinary medicine is subaortic stenosis. In subaortic stenosis, the lesion is minimal or not present at birth and progressively worsens during the first 6 months to 1 year of life. Despite this variation, subaortic stenosis is considered a congenital abnormality. As molecular biology techniques evolve, diseases that have not been classically described as congenital may need to be reexamined. Familial hypertrophic cardiomyopathy in humans and cats is an example. In humans, numerous mutations in the genes that encode for sarcomere proteins have been identified in families with hypertrophic cardiomyopathy. The affected individual is born with the genetic abnormality but usually does not express the anatomic lesion until adulthood. Consequently hypertrophic cardiomyopathy is classically categorized as an acquired disease, yet the abnormality that leads to the development of the hypertrophy is present at birth. Dilated cardiomyopathy is probably another example in many dog breeds.

CHD can be inherited or occur spontaneously. Spontaneous occurrence can be due to a new (de novo) mutation that the individual will pass on to offspring or to a nongenetic cause. For example, thalidomide can produce ventricular septal defects and other congenital cardiac abnormalities in cats.[1] Certainly other teratogens can produce similar abnormalities. Consequently the presence of CHD does not necessarily mean the patient has heritable disease. The presence of heritable disease can only be established by identifying affected relatives and offspring or by identifying the same gene abnormalities in related individuals. However, we generally recommend that patients with CHD not be bred unless overwhelming extenuating circumstances exist.

CHD that is truly present at birth is really fetal heart disease manifested at birth. If one can extrapolate from human research, most congenital cardiac anomalies are present by 1 week of gestation in dogs and cats (1 month in humans). Some of these abnormalities are lethal and result in spontaneous abortion. Most anomalies that are compatible with 6 weeks of gestational life (6 months in humans) result in live birth. In human medicine, most congenital cardiac abnormalities can now be diagnosed in utero by 20 to 22 weeks of gestation.[2] In human medicine in the United States, almost all babies are examined by a physician immediately after birth. Once the affected infant is identified, skilled care by pediatric cardiologists results in survival of most infants. In contrast, in veterinary medicine it is unusual for a veterinarian to examine a puppy or kitten in the postnatal period. In fact, most small animals are not examined until they are at least 5 to 6 weeks old. Because of this situation it is almost a certainty that most small animals with very serious congenital cardiac defects die or are killed before ever seeing a veterinarian. Consequently, the lesions that veterinarians identify are commonly less life-threatening because the animal has to live for 5 to 6 weeks on its own before its anomaly is identified. Because of this, veterinarians only rarely see complex or very serious congenital cardiac anomalies, such as transposition of the great vessels, critical aortic stenosis, and hypoplastic left heart. Instead veterinarians more commonly identify simple stenotic, regurgitant, and shunting lesions that are compatible with early life. Examples include pulmonic stenosis, mitral valve dysplasia, and patent ductus arteriosus.

TABLE 11-1

Prevalence of congenital cardiac defects at the University of California, Davis, Veterinary Medical Teaching Hospital (8/1/86-8/1/96)

Defect	*Number of cases: dogs*	*Number of cases: cats*
Subaortic stenosis	288	3
Patent ductus arteriosus	215	7
Isolated pulmonic stenosis	181	8
Ventricular septal defect	79	23
Tetralogy of Fallot	19	4
Atrial septal defect	14	15
Mitral valve dysplasia	58	11
Tricuspid valve dysplasia	62	23
Mitral stenosis	12	6
Total	928	100

The number of cases is from a hospital patient population (not visit population) of 68,690 dogs and 20,150 cats during this 10-year period. The UCD VMTH Cardiology Service examined 2493 dogs and 927 cats as primary patients during the same period. The majority of the congenital cardiac defects come from this population. The Service primary population represents about 45% of the patients examined. The other 55% are secondary patients seen on consultation (approximately 3100 dogs and 1200 cats). Consequently, the Service examined approximately 5600 dogs and 2100 cats. Many of these patients were examined more than once so the visit population would be much higher.

TABLE 11-2

Breed predisposition for congenital cardiac disorders

Congenital abnormality	*Breed predisposition*
Patent ductus arteriosus	Toy and miniature poodles, German shepherd, collie, Pomeranian, Shetland sheep dog, Maltese, English springer spaniel, keeshond, Yorkshire terrier, American cocker spaniel, rottweiler
Subaortic stenosis	Newfoundland, rottweiler, golden retriever, boxer
Pulmonic stenosis	English bulldog, terrier, beagle, mastiff, Samoyed, miniature schnauzer, American cocker spaniel, keeshond, West Highland white terrier
Ventricular septal defect	English springer spaniel
Tetralogy of Fallot	Keeshond
Mitral valve dysplasia	Rottweiler; large breeds
Tricuspid valve dysplasia	Labrador retriever; large breeds (>20 kg)
Persistent right aortic arch	German shepherd, Irish setter

Prevalence. Of the congenital cardiac lesions, subaortic stenosis, patent ductus arteriosus, and pulmonic stenosis are by far the most common defects identified in dogs. Prevalence differs between geographic regions. Subaortic stenosis is the most common congenital cardiac abnormality in dogs in our hospital, as it appears to be in others. Between October 1, 1986, and October 1, 1996, subaortic stenosis was definitively diagnosed in 288 canine patients in our hospital (Table 11-1). This is compared with 215 cases of patent ductus arteriosus and 181 cases of isolated pulmonic stenosis in the same period. In comparison, the most common cyanotic congenital defect, tetralogy of Fallot, was diagnosed in only 19 canine patients. CHD is recognized much less frequently in cats. Ventricular septal defect and tricuspid valve dysplasia have been the most common congenital heart abnormalities diagnosed in cats in our hospital. Approximately 3 times as many dogs as cats were identified with these abnormalities. The ventricular septal defects we have seen in cats may or may not be a manifestation of an atrioventricular canal defect. All other congenital cardiac malformations in both species are rare.

GENERAL APPROACH

Signalment. As with all abnormalities, animals suspected of having congenital cardiac disease should first undergo a complete clinical examination. Signalment (species, breed, age, and sex) is particularly important in congenital cardiac disease because specific abnormalities more commonly are identified in specific types of animals. As an example, subaortic stenosis is common in dogs but rare in cats. Pulmonic stenosis is an abnormality most commonly diagnosed in smaller breeds of dogs, whereas subaortic stenosis is more commonly diagnosed in large breeds. The specific breeds most commonly affected with each abnormality are presented in the chapters describing the common abnormalities and are summarized in Table 11-2. One must remember that signalment is like stereotyping—a stereotype is often but not always true. Consequently, one must be careful when evaluating a young animal with a heart murmur and not leap to a diagnosis automatically based on the signalment. Also, breed predilection changes from region to region and is based on the gene pool present in a particular region. As an example, although subaortic stenosis occurs in boxers in the United States, the problem is much more prevalent in Europe. A sex predilection for certain cardiac malformations is not prevalent. However, patent ductus arteriosus does occur more frequently in female dogs, and mitral and tricuspid valve dysplasias are more common in males.

History. The history may or may not be helpful in a dog or cat with CHD. Many animals with congenital cardiac malformations exhibit no clinical signs. Consequently, the owner is unaware of any problems at the time of presentation. Other dogs or cats develop left or right heart failure, have exercise intolerance, are cyanotic either at rest or with exercise, or fail to grow at an expected rate. Patent ductus arteriosus and mitral valve dysplasia, with or without concomitant subaortic stenosis, are the most common abnormalities that produce left heart failure. Left heart failure may also occur with a large ventricular septal defect. Dogs with left heart failure may cough or may exhibit tachypnea and dyspnea. Tricuspid valve dysplasia is the most common abnormality to produce right heart failure. Animals with right heart failure most commonly have ascites. Syncope can also occur, most commonly with subaortic stenosis. This may be an ominous sign, heralding sudden death. Dogs with a right-to-left shunting patent ductus arteriosus may exhibit pelvic limb weakness when exercised. An owner may observe that an animal is cyanotic. Cyanosis, unless associated with extreme exercise, is only seen with right-to-left shunting lesions such as tetralogy of Fallot and Eisenmenger's syndrome (i.e., right-to-left shunting ventricular septal defect or patent ductus arteriosus). Severe right-to-left shunts are the most common abnormalities that produce stunted growth.

Physical examination. The physical examination is often the first clue that an animal has congenital cardiac disease. This occurs most often when a heart murmur is ausculted, often at the time of the first vaccination. A heart murmur in a young animal is often, but not always, due to cardiac disease. Young animals have a larger stroke volume compared with the size of the aorta than do older animals. This can result in an increase in flow velocity to the point of producing turbulence, either in the aorta or in the pulmonary artery. This produces a *flow* (i.e., *physiologic* or *innocent*) heart murmur. The increase in velocity is generally not great in this situation, and

TABLE 11-3

Auscultatory abnormalities in dogs with congenital cardiac disease

Abnormality	*Timing of murmur*	*Quality or murmur*	*Point of maximal intensity*	*Comments*
Aortic regurgitation	Diastolic	Decrescendo; usually soft	Left base	May occur in association with a VSD
Atrial septal defect	Systolic	Soft	Left base	Result of relative pulmonic stenosis
Eisenmenger's syndrome (right-to-left shunting PDA or VSD)	Absent (a systolic murmur may still be present in a PDA with bidirectional shunting)		Left axillary region for a bidirectional PDA	Split second heart sound may be present
Mitral dysplasia	Systolic	Holosystolic or pansystolic; plateau	Left apex	May radiate widely
Left-to-right shunting patent ductus arteriosus (PDA)	Continuous	Wind-tunnel	Cranial to the left base	Peaks in intensity at S_2
Pulmonic stenosis	Systolic	Crescendo-decrescendo	Left base	Possible ejection sound
Subaortic stenosis	Systolic	Crescendo-decrescendo	Left (occasionally right) base (occasionally apex)	May radiate up into carotid arteries
Tetralogy of Fallot	Systolic (rarely absent)	Crescendo-decrescendo	Left base	Murmur may rarely be absent
Tricuspid dysplasia	Systolic	Holosystolic or pansystolic; plateau	Right apex	May be soft or absent in cats with severe disease
Ventricular septal defect (VSD)	Systolic	Holosystolic or pansystolic	Cranial to or at right apex; left base	Second heart sound may be split
VSD and aortic regurgitation	Systolic and diastolic (to-and fro-murmur)	Pansystolic murmur followed by a diastolic decrescendo murmur	Left base or cranial to right apex	May sound as if it is continuous and be confused with the murmur of a PDA

PDA, Patent ductus arteriosus; *VSD,* ventricular septal defect.

so the heart murmur is usually not loud (grade 1 or 2). A flow murmur may increase in intensity with excitement, decrease with rest, or change in intensity when the position of the animal is changed. Flow murmurs usually disappear by 3 to 4 months of age. A soft heart murmur can be heard with some serious cardiac malformations such as a large ventricular septal defect. With subaortic stenosis, the lesion progressively worsens and the murmur may increase in intensity over the first 6 months of the dog's life. Consequently, a soft heart murmur does not totally discount the presence of serious disease. When a soft heart murmur is ausculted in a young dog, the veterinarian must perform a thorough physical examination and discuss with the client the next course of action. In many cases it is reasonable to only reexamine the dog at the time of the next vaccination. However, if the owner is very cautious or demanding or if other physical signs point toward cardiac disease, further diagnostic testing may be warranted.

A murmur that is grade 3 or louder is usually indicative of mild-to-severe cardiac pathology. The location, timing, and quality of the murmur should be noted so that a tentative list of possible diagnoses can be formulated (Table 11-3). Thoracic radiographs should be obtained in these animals. Moderate-to-severe cardiomegaly indicates significant disease. However, significant disease can also be present without significant radiographic signs. For example, a dog with moderate, and sometimes even severe, subaortic stenosis may not have significant apparent cardiomegaly and may not have a visible poststenotic aortic dilation. Consequently, after radiographs have been obtained, one must judge whether or not further diagnostic testing is warranted. This judgment can be made based on the suspected lesion, the clinical signs, and the owner's wishes or demands. Occasionally a dog or cat with severe cardiac disease does not have a heart murmur. This occurs most frequently with a right-to-left shunting patent ductus arteriosus. It may also occur with a right-to-left shunting ventricular septal defect (Eisenmenger's complex) or a tetralogy of Fallot. The murmur can be absent in these lesions because the defect is large and high-velocity flow is not produced or as a result of polycythemia. Polycythemia increases viscosity, and production of turbulence is more difficult in a more viscous fluid (e.g., producing turbulence in molasses is more difficult than it is in water).

The location and timing of the heart murmur often provide clues as to the type of abnormality (Figure 11-1). However, enough overlap exists between lesions and murmurs that it is common for even an experienced individual to be wrong regarding the type of abnormality following auscultation. This is especially true with a loud murmur that radiates clearly to many regions of the chest. The degree of accuracy depends on the type of lesion. A continuous murmur heard best in the left axillary region is almost always due to a patent ductus arteriosus. With most of the other heart murmurs, more room for doubt is present. A left basilar systolic crescendo-decrescendo murmur is most commonly due to a stenotic lesion such as subaortic stenosis, pulmonic stenosis, or tetralogy of Fallot. A large atrial septal defect may cause a soft left basilar murmur. The murmur caused by subaortic stenosis may, however, be heard best at the left apex or at the right base. A left apical systolic plateau murmur most commonly is due to mitral regurgitation and in a young dog to mitral valve dysplasia. However, occasionally the murmur caused by subaortic stenosis is heard best in this region. Similarly, a right apical systolic murmur most commonly is due to tricuspid valve dysplasia. The murmur created by a ventricular septal defect can also be heard best on the right side of the chest in some dogs. It may be more cranial than a tricuspid valve murmur.

Besides heart murmurs, congenital cardiac abnormalities may also affect heart rate, respiratory rate and character, the peripheral

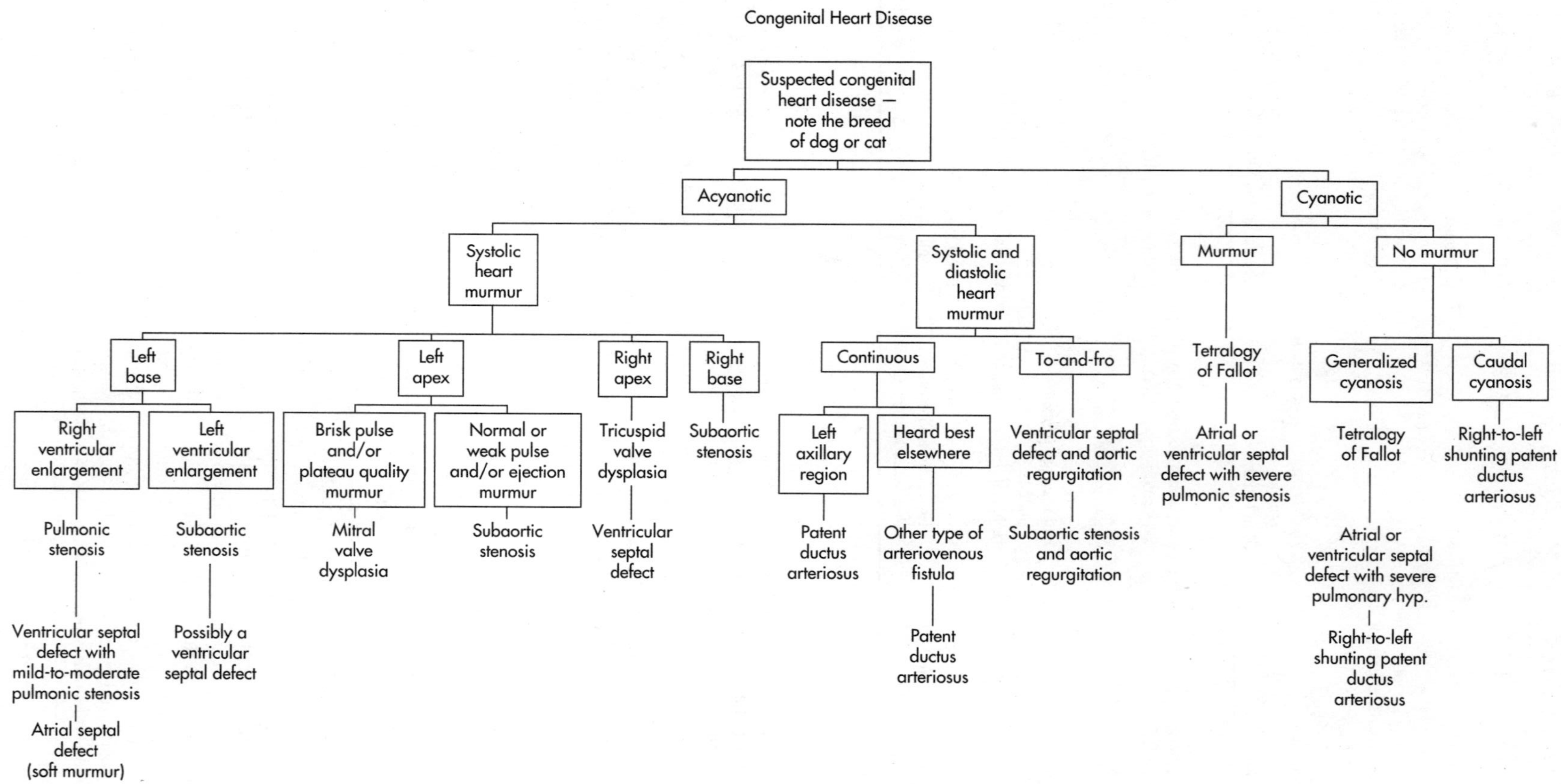

FIGURE 11-1 Algorithm of the initial diagnostic strategy to determine the type of common congenital cardiac disease. An echocardiogram is usually required to make a definitive diagnosis and to determine the severity of a particular lesion.

arterial pulse, mucous membrane color, systemic veins, and the precordium, as described in Chapter 3. Hyperdynamic or hypodynamic pulses, unexplained tachypnea, dyspnea, jugular vein distension or pulsation, unexplained tachycardia, and cyanosis all warrant further investigation because they generally indicate severe disease is present.

Laboratory tests. In most instances, laboratory tests are normal in dogs and cats with CHD. Laboratory tests most commonly are abnormal in patients with right-to-left shunts. Arterial blood gas analysis in these patients reveals hypoxemia. In patients with severe hypoxemia ($Pa0_2$ less than 40 mm Hg), polycythemia is commonly present. This manifests as an increase in the hematocrit in a hydrated animal.

Radiography. Thoracic radiographs reflect the response of the heart and blood vessels to the hemodynamic abnormalities produced by the cardiac abnormality. They usually do not show the defect itself. Thoracic radiographs are often useful to include or preclude moderate-to-severe CHD as a diagnostic possibility. They also may be useful for making a specific diagnosis, usually when used in conjunction with signalment and physical examination findings. For example, if a young terrier breed is presented with a left basilar, ejection-quality heart murmur, has a large right ventricle and a main pulmonary artery bulge on a thoracic radiograph, and is not cyanotic, pulmonic stenosis is by far the most likely diagnosis. Radiographic findings often depend on the severity of the cardiac abnormality. Mild disease usually will not produce radiographic findings, whereas severe disease usually produces radiographic abnormalities. Moderate disease may or may not produce radiographic changes. Common radiographic changes seen with severe disease are outlined in Table 11-4. Specific radiographic findings are defined in the chapters dealing with the specific defects.

Radiographic evidence of a left-to-right shunt may include the presence of enlarged pulmonary arteries and veins (so-called overcirculation). The enlargement is expected to occur because of the increased blood volume flowing through the pulmonary circulation. Of the radiographic abnormalities commonly identified in CHD, pulmonary vasculature changes are the most difficult to assess. This is probably because of the wide variation in size for normal vessels. Consequently, one should never rule out a left-to-right shunt based on the absence of perceived pulmonary overcirculation. Conversely, right-to-left shunting abnormalities may result in a decrease in the size of the pulmonary vasculature because of decreased pulmonary blood flow. However, the pulmonary vasculature may appear normal and occasionally will be larger than normal.

Electrocardiography. The electrocardiogram (ECG) may or may not be useful in a patient with CHD. A normal ECG does not rule out even the presence of severe CHD, although this is lesion-dependent. For example, dogs with severe subaortic stenosis often have a normal ECG, whereas dogs with severe pulmonic stenosis usually have evidence of right ventricular enlargement. If an ECG abnormality is identified, it can be very useful for confirming the presence of cardiac disease and then for helping determine a specific abnormality. Consequently, recording an ECG in a dog with suspected CHD is encouraged, especially if one does not have access to an ultrasound machine or if access is delayed. Congenital cardiac abnormalities that most commonly have associated ECG abnormalities include patent ductus arteriosus (evidence of left ventricular enlargement), pulmonic stenosis (right ventricular enlargement), and tetralogy of Fallot (right ventricular enlargement).

Echocardiography. Echocardiography is usually the diagnostic test of choice for veterinary patients with CHD. It is unusual in our clinic for a definitive diagnosis and prognosis not to be made in a patient with CHD following an echocardiographic examination. The most common patients in which we are unable to make a diagnosis are small puppies and kittens and patients with complex defects. Even in these populations, however, our ability to make a presumptive or definitive diagnosis probably exceeds 80%.

Examples of echocardiographic findings in the various cardiac malformations are provided in the chapters dealing with individual lesions. The common findings in the specific common defects are listed in Table 11-5. The approach to diagnosis in each lesion depends on the lesion and on the type of equipment available. If one only has access to a two-dimensional echocardiograph machine, one must make some assumptions regarding some lesions, depending on the lesion, the ability to see the anatomy, and the compensatory cardiac changes. For a time we only had two-dimensional and M-mode echocardiography available. We estimate that we could make the

TABLE 11-4

Radiographic findings in severe congenital heart disease

Abnormality	*Chamber**	*Great vessel dilation*	*Pulmonary vessels*	*Pulmonary parenchyma*
Aortic regurgitation	Left atrium and *ventricle*	None	+/– Enlarged pulmonary veins	+/– Pulmonary edema
Atrial septal defect	Right atrium and *ventricle*	None	+/– Enlarged pulmonary arteries and veins	Normal
Mitral dysplasia	*Left atrium* and ventricle	None	+/– Enlarged pulmonary veins	+/– Pulmonary edema
Patent ductus arteriosus	Left atrium and ventricle	Descending aortic bulge	+/– Enlarged pulmonary arteries and veins	+/– Pulmonary edema
Pulmonic stenosis	Right ventricle	Main pulmonary artery bulge	Normal	Normal
Subaortic stenosis	Left ventricle	Ascending aortic bulge	Normal	Normal
Tetralogy of Fallot	Right ventricle	Main pulmonary artery bulge	+/– Pulmonary arteries and veins diminished in size	+/– Hyperinflation
Tricuspid dysplasia	*Right atrium* and right ventricle	+/– Caudal vena cava	Normal	Normal
Ventricular septal defect	*Left* and right ventricles	None	+/– Enlarged pulmonary arteries and veins	+/– Pulmonary edema

*The chambers that are predominantly or more frequently enlarged are italicized when more than one chamber is affected.

TABLE 11-5

Echocardiographic findings in congenital heart disease

Abnormality	*Chamber enlargement**	*Anatomic abnormality*	*Color flow Doppler*	*Pulsed-wave Doppler*	*Continuous-wave Doppler*
Aortic regurgitation	Left atrial and *left ventricular* volume overload	Abnormal aortic valve leaflets; presence of a VSD	Diastolic color jet in the left ventricle, originating at the aortic valve	Turbulent diastolic flow in the left ventricular outflow tract (LVOT)	High-velocity (>4 m/sec) diastolic jet in the LVOT
Atrial septal defect	*Right ventricular* and possibly right atrial volume overload	Defect in the atrial septum	Small color jet originating at the atrial septum and projecting into the right atrium	Continuous laminar or turbulent flow on the right side of the interatrial septum	Continuous low-velocity flow that peaks in late systole, early diastole, and with atrial contraction
Mitral dysplasia	*Left atrial* and ventricular volume overload	Abnormal mitral valve leaflets and/or chordae tendineae	Systolic color jet originating at the mitral valve and projecting into the left atrium	Turbulent flow in the left atrium during systole	High-velocity (>4 m/sec) systolic jet recorded when the cursor crosses the left ventricle and left atrium
Patent ductus arteriosus (PDA)	Left atrial and ventricular volume overload	Presence of a PDA	Continuous color jet originating within the PDA and projecting into the main pulmonary artery	Continuous turbulent flow in the main pulmonary artery	High-velocity (>4 m/sec) continuous jet in the main pulmonary artery
Pulmonic stenosis	Right ventricular pressure overload	Thickened valve cusps or subpulmonic constriction	Systolic color jet originating at the pulmonic valve region and projecting into the pulmonary artery	Systolic laminar flow in the right ventricular outflow tract; flow velocity increases and becomes turbulent as the stenotic region is crossed	Increased velocity (2-7 m/sec) systolic signal recorded when the cursor is placed across the right ventricular outflow tract (RVOT) and main pulmonary artery
Subaortic stenosis	Left ventricular pressure overload	Subaortic ridge	Systolic color jet originating at the subaortic region and projecting into the aorta	Systolic laminar flow in the left ventricular outflow tract (LVOT); flow velocity increases and becomes turbulent as the stenotic region is crossed	Increased velocity (2-7 m/sec) systolic signal when the cursor is placed across the LVOT and aorta
Tetralogy of Fallot	Right ventricular pressure overload	Ventricular septal defect; lesions of pulmonic stenosis; aortic override	Laminar flow from the right and left ventricles flowing into the aorta in systole	Same as for pulmonic stenosis	High-velocity jet in the main pulmonary artery
Tricuspid dysplasia	*Right atrial* and ventricular volume overload	Abnormal tricuspid valve leaflets or chordae tendineae	Systolic color jet originating at the tricuspid valve and projecting into the right atrium	Backward flow into the right atrium in systole that is usually turbulent but can be laminar in cats	Usually a low-to-medium–velocity (1.5-3 m/sec) flow signal in the right atrium
Ventricular septal defect (VSD)	Left atrial and *left ventricular* volume overload; possibly right ventricular volume overload	Defect in the ventricular septum, usually immediately below the aortic root	Systolic color jet projecting through a defect in the interventricular septum into the right ventricle	Turbulent systolic flow on the right side of the interventricular septum	Usually a high-velocity jet projecting into the right ventricle

*The chambers that are predominantly or more frequently enlarged are italicized when more than one chamber is affected.

correct diagnosis in greater than 90% of the cases we examined. In nature there is harmony between form and function. This is epitomized in the normal and the abnormal cardiovascular systems. Because of this harmony, logical deduction of changes in function can be deduced by identifying changes in form (structure). The common methods of identifying changes in form are radiographic and two-dimensional echocardiographic examination. These examinations reveal changes in structure that can be deduced to have occurred secondary to a change in function. Because a limited number of means to change cardiac function exist, identification of structural change immediately narrows the list of conditions, usually to two or three possibilities. For example, if a thickened right ventricular wall is identified on an echocardiogram, one can logically deduce that an increase in systolic pressure in the right ventricle is present (i.e., a right ventricular pressure overload). Possible diagnoses for a right ventricular pressure overload include only pulmonary hypertension and pulmonic stenosis. Once this list has been formulated, one often only needs to know if the patient has a heart murmur (pulmonic stenosis) or not (pulmonary hypertension) to further define the abnormality.

Currently we use two-dimensional echocardiography, M-mode echocardiography, spectral Doppler (pulsed- and continuous-wave) echocardiography, and color flow Doppler echocardiography to make diagnoses. Generally a two-dimensional echocardiogram is examined first to note changes in chamber sizes and wall thicknesses and search for anatomic abnormalities. An M-mode echocardiogram is recorded to measure these changes, or measurements are made off the two-dimensional image. Next, color flow Doppler imaging is used to interrogate the cardiac valves and specific regions of the heart (depending on physical examination and two-dimensional echocardiographic findings) to identify any regions of high-velocity, turbulent flow. Once a region or regions of turbulent flow are identified, spectral Doppler is used to further define the origin of turbulence and the peak velocity of the turbulent jet or jets. This allows more accurate quantitation of the severity of the lesion.

Cardiac catheterization. On rare occasions, cardiac catheterization is required either to make a diagnosis or to characterize a lesion or lesions further. The vast majority of the cardiac catheterization procedures we perform are for other reasons, usually for balloon valvuloplasty of pulmonic stenosis. Occasionally cardiac catheterization is performed to quantify the size of a shunt so that the prognosis can be better estimated and decisions regarding surgery can be made. Chapter 7 details the reasons and methods for performing a cardiac catheterization.

SYNTHESIS OF THE DATA

Once data are extracted from each examination, they should be synthesized to make a logical conclusion regarding the diagnosis. The general approach to formulating an initial rule-out list of the common congenital cardiac diseases is shown as an algorithm in Figure 11-1. This approach starts with noting the breed and then examining the patient to determine if cyanosis is present or not. In some patients, cyanosis may only be a historical finding because they do not become cyanotic until they are exercised. Most dogs and cats with CHD are not cyanotic. However, in most patients with CHD, a heart murmur is present. Presence or absence of a heart murmur, the type of heart murmur, and the location of the heart murmur are the next logical points for developing diagnostic strategies for CHD. Cyanotic patients usually either will not have a heart murmur or, more commonly, will have a systolic left basilar murmur as a result of pulmonic stenosis. Of the common acyanotic congenital heart defects, most will have either a systolic heart murmur or a heart murmur that occurs in both systole and diastole. Most of the latter heart murmurs will be continuous. Once a systolic heart murmur is identified, care should be taken to attempt to determine the location where it is heard best (i.e., the point of maximal intensity [PMI]) and the quality of the murmur. The quality of the murmur may be difficult to ascertain, especially in a patient with a fast heart rate. Once the type of murmur is ascertained, radiographs should be evaluated in an attempt to determine if the lesion is primarily affecting the left side or the right side of the heart, especially if a left basilar murmur is present. If this determination cannot be made clearly from the radiograph, an electrocardiogram should be obtained because, in some cases, clear evidence of right or left ventricular enlargement will be identified. In some cases the clinician is still not sure on which side the abnormality lies. Next, other abnormalities of the cardiac silhouette should be noted. Lastly, an attempt should be made to determine if the pulmonary vasculature is normal, increased, or decreased in size. Often, following these determinations, a tentative diagnosis or a list of possible diagnoses can be made. As an example, a continuous heart murmur heard loudest at the left cranial thorax is almost always diagnostic of a patent ductus arteriosus (PDA). Confirmation of this diagnosis is commonly sought, however. Thoracic radiographs often provide evidence of cardiomegaly and a lateral bulge on the proximal descending aortic. Presence of this bulge (i.e., a ductal aneurysm) along with a continuous heart murmur confirms the diagnosis of PDA. Chamber enlargement in PDA is limited to the left ventricle and left atrium. However, the right heart may appear to be enlarged on a thoracic radiograph. This may confuse the examiner making the diagnosis. An ECG may be helpful here because many dogs with a PDA will have evidence of left ventricular enlargement. Some, however, will not. This or other issues may necessitate an ultrasound examination of the heart. Two-dimensional echocardiography can be used to identify the changes that occur secondary to the PDA. These are limited to left ventricular and left atrial volume overloads (i.e., increased diastolic internal dimensions with normal wall thicknesses). This provides suggestive evidence that a continuous heart murmur is due to a PDA and provides more accurate information than the thoracic radiographs and the ECG regarding chamber enlargement. Two-dimensional and color flow Doppler echocardiography can be used specifically to identify the PDA and so confirm the diagnosis. Although rare, the systolic heart murmur created by a ventricular septal defect combined with the diastolic heart murmur of aortic regurgitation can sound like the continuous murmur of a PDA. This combination produces a so-called "to-and-fro" heart murmur that is systolic and diastolic but is not continuous. This usually can be distinguished by a trained individual but can easily fool a veterinary student. Occasionally, a patient with a PDA will also have a concomitant defect. In these patients, the dramatic physical and radiographic findings of the PDA may overshadow findings associated with the other lesion. In this situation, the echocardiogram is helpful for identifying these abnormalities that may alter the prognosis or therapeutic plan in a patient with a PDA.

The Approach to the Older, Chronically Coughing Small-Breed Dog

Older, small-breed dogs are frequently presented to a veterinarian because they have a chronic cough. Many of these dogs have a systolic heart murmur caused by mitral regurgitation. The veterinarian must decipher if the cough is related to the cardiac disease, is related to concomitant respiratory disease, or is caused by both.

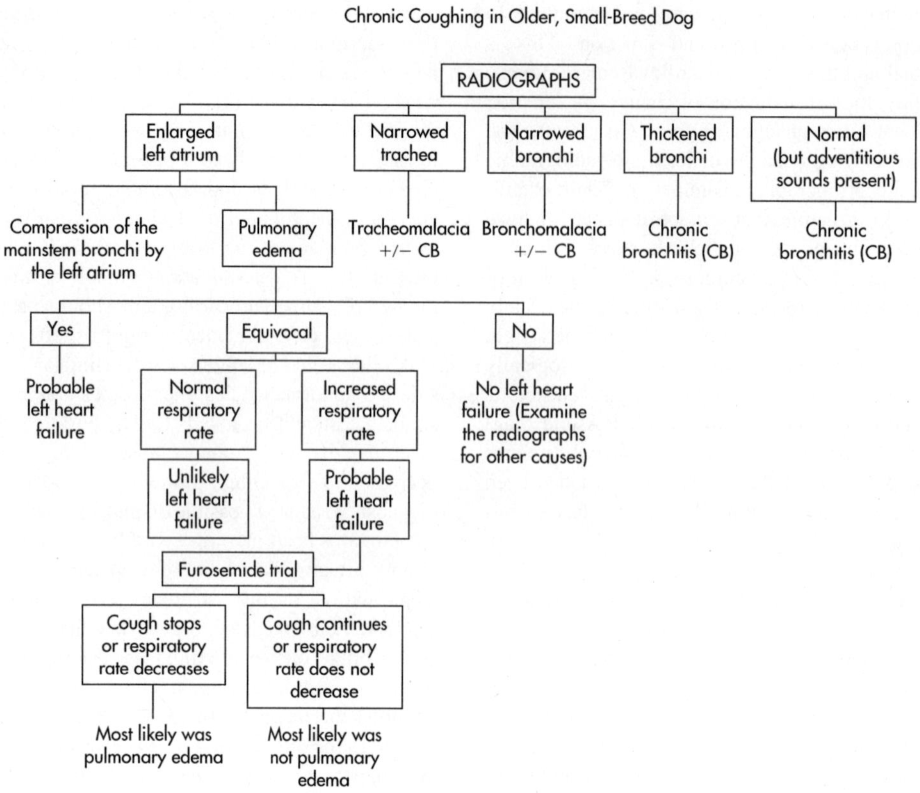

FIGURE 11-2 A general approach to determining the cause of a chronic cough in an older, small-breed dog.

These dogs most commonly have pulmonary edema, tracheomalacia (i.e., a collapsing trachea) and/or bronchomalacia (i.e., collapsing bronchi), chronic bronchitis, or bronchomalacia with compression of the mainstem bronchi by the left atrium causing their cough. Pulmonary neoplasia less commonly produces a chronic cough in an older dog. Heartworm disease should always be ruled out in an endemic area. An algorithm for a general approach to this problem is presented in Figure 11-2.

Tracheal collapse as a result of tracheomalacia is common in older, small-breed dogs. It is characterized by dorsoventral flattening of the trachea, with a wide pendulous dorsal membrane and flattened, weak tracheal cartilage rings.[3] Bronchomalacia with collapsing mainstem bronchi is similar but occurs in the large bronchi. Whenever airway collapse is present, irritation of the airway lining is often present. This irritation leads to coughing. Coughing often causes further irritation, leading to a cycle of increased coughing. Chronic bronchitis is chronic inflammation of the bronchi that results in excessive mucous production leading to coughing.[4] The etiology in dogs is unknown. Dogs with chronic bronchitis may also have collapsing airways, and the increased expiratory effort associated with bronchial narrowing and the coughing may exacerbate airway collapse, especially intrathoracic collapse. Left atrial enlargement can complicate bronchomalacia, collapsing the softened airways and producing irritation.

THE COUGH

A cough is a sudden, forceful expulsion of air that occurs after pressure has been developed in the airways by the animal contracting its rib cage and diaphragm against a closed glottis. The glottis is suddenly opened but kept partially closed during the expulsion to produce high-velocity air flow. This sudden opening of the glottis and the turbulent airflow creates a harsh noise. Coughing occurs either via a reflex or a conscious action. It occurs reflexly when a foreign object, such as water, is aspirated into the airway. Irritation of the pharynx most commonly produces gagging but can also elicit coughing. Irritation of the larynx, tracheobronchial tree, small airways, or pleura can produce a cough, either reflexly or consciously, depending on the severity of the irritation.

Coughing comes in many forms. It can be soft, honking, moist, dry, productive, or nonproductive. It can occur any time during the day or night, more commonly during the day or night, or only after excitement or exercise. Although describing the cough in these terms may be useful, the type of cough seen with different abnormalities is not consistent. Dogs with pulmonary edema commonly have a soft cough, but pulmonary edema can also cause a loud, honking cough, especially in a small dog that has some tracheomalacia. Tracheal collapse as a result of tracheomalacia can produce a dry, honking cough, but a loud productive cough can also be present. Sometimes it produces no cough at all. A productive cough yields material brought up from the lungs. A productive cough is easy to identify in a human because a person can expectorate the material on command. A dog, however, will usually swallow this material. Sometimes an owner will see the swallowing motion and report it. At other times it goes unnoticed. Consequently, although elaborate schemes have been devised to link the type of cough with different diseases, this approach is fraught with error.

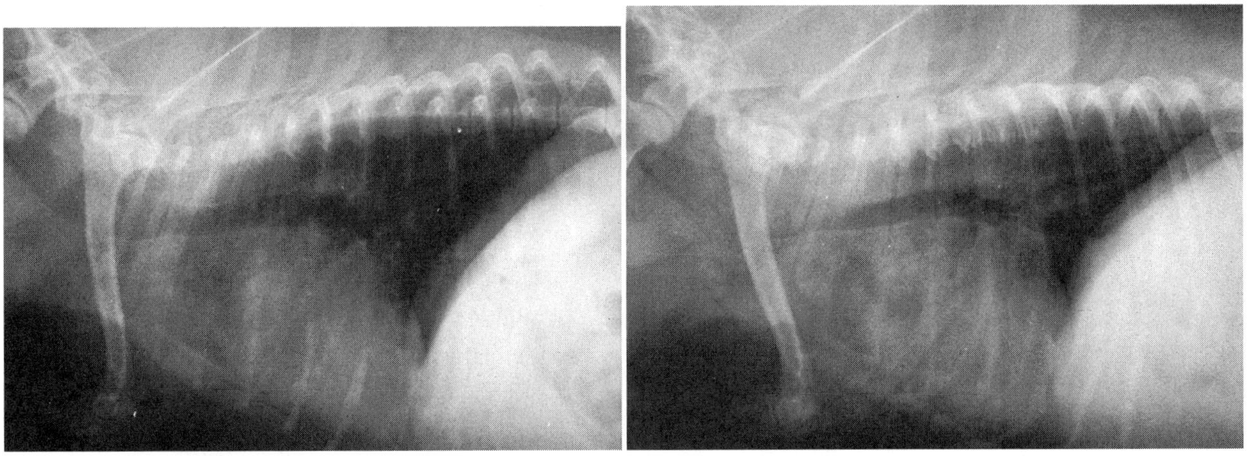

FIGURE 11-3 Lateral thoracic radiographs from a 12-year-old Pomeranian with a chronic cough as a result of a collapsing trachea. **A,** On inspiration, the trachea is distended. **B,** On expiration, the trachea is collapsed with a narrow opening along the ventral aspect of the trachea.

Most older, small-breed dogs that present with a chronic cough have a loud rather than a soft cough. It may sound like a goose honk and may occur once or come in paroxysms. The owner may or may not note that the dog swallows after coughing. A terminal wretch or gag may be present if the cough is productive. This motion is to bring the material coughed into the pharynx forward so that it can be swallowed or, occasionally, expectorated. A dog with a cough that has any or all these characteristics can have pulmonary edema, a collapsing trachea, chronic bronchitis, or bronchial compression. Although it is commonly stated that dogs with pulmonary edema most often cough at night, we commonly examine dogs with heart failure that cough only during the day or primarily after exercise or excitement. We also examine dogs with chronic bronchitis that keep their owners up all night because of their coughing. The type of cough present with each of the common diseases observed in older, small-breed dogs is variable, and the description of the type of cough is often inaccurate for diagnosing the type of disease. Also, dogs with a chronic cough will often have more than one cause (e.g., tracheomalacia and pulmonary edema in a geriatric poodle) and the type of cough may share characteristics of both.

PHYSICAL EXAMINATION

The physical examination may be helpful in distinguishing the type of disease present. However, it usually does not give a definitive diagnosis. After obtaining a history from the client, the cough should be reproduced in the examination room by palpating the cervical trachea. In some dogs, light palpation will stimulate a cough. In others, vigorous palpation is required. One should be able to produce at least one cough in any dog or cat by squeezing the two sides of the trachea together so that they meet in the middle. Cough production allows the veterinarian to reproduce the abnormality for the owners and to observe the cough. When a cough is produced following less-than-vigorous tracheal manipulation, it is often interpreted to mean that the trachea is "sensitive" or irritated. Consequently, many veterinarians interpret this to mean the patient has tracheitis. This is untrue. This is often taken one step further to mean the dog has an infectious tracheitis or "kennel cough." This can be disastrous in the patient with pulmonary edema. *Any dog that is coughing for any reason will cough more easily than a normal dog when its trachea is manipulated.* The only thing this tells the clinician is that the animal truly does have a cough.

The heart and lungs should be carefully ausculted. Dogs with myxomatous mitral valve degeneration and mitral regurgitation severe enough to cause pulmonary edema will almost always have a moderately loud to loud left apical systolic heart murmur. The first heart sound is often louder than normal and sometimes masks the systolic heart murmur. However, in most instances, the lack of a murmur or a soft murmur rules out the presence of severe mitral regurgitation. A loud heart murmur may be heard in a dog with mild-to-moderate mitral regurgitation, however; therefore the presence of a loud heart murmur does not mean that pulmonary edema is causing the cough.

Pulmonary auscultation is also fraught with error. Many dogs with pulmonary edema do not have any auscultatory abnormalities in their lungs except for increased airway sounds as a result of hyperpnea. Some do have adventitious lung sounds (snaps, crackles, pops, and wheezes). Wheezes are less common. Significant respiratory abnormalities are more commonly ausculted in dogs with chronic airway disease. Dogs with chronic bronchitis commonly have crackles and pops on inspiration or expiration and expiratory wheezes.[5] Dogs with collapsing airways may have loud snaps as airways open.

The throat, neck, and thorax should be palpated to identify any abnormalities such as submandibular lymph node enlargement, thoracic malformation, or the presence of a mass. The trachea should be palpated. A very soft cervical trachea can be palpated in some dogs with severe tracheomalacia.

THORACIC RADIOGRAPHY

A thoracic radiograph is usually the most useful diagnostic test and should be evaluated in any dog with a chronic cough. Care should be taken to obtain both an inspiratory and an expiratory lateral film of the cervical (extrathoracic) and intrathoracic trachea to identify tracheal collapse. The intrathoracic trachea usually collapses on expiration as intrathoracic pressure increases and expands on inspiration (Figure 11-3). The extrathoracic trachea does the opposite. This can best be appreciated using fluoroscopy. Tracheal collapse is seen as dorsoventral narrowing of the affected tracheal segment. One must be careful not to interpret an overlying esophagus or *longus colli* muscle as tracheal narrowing.[3]

Dogs with chronic bronchitis often have evidence of thickened bronchial walls, although in some dogs the radiographs will

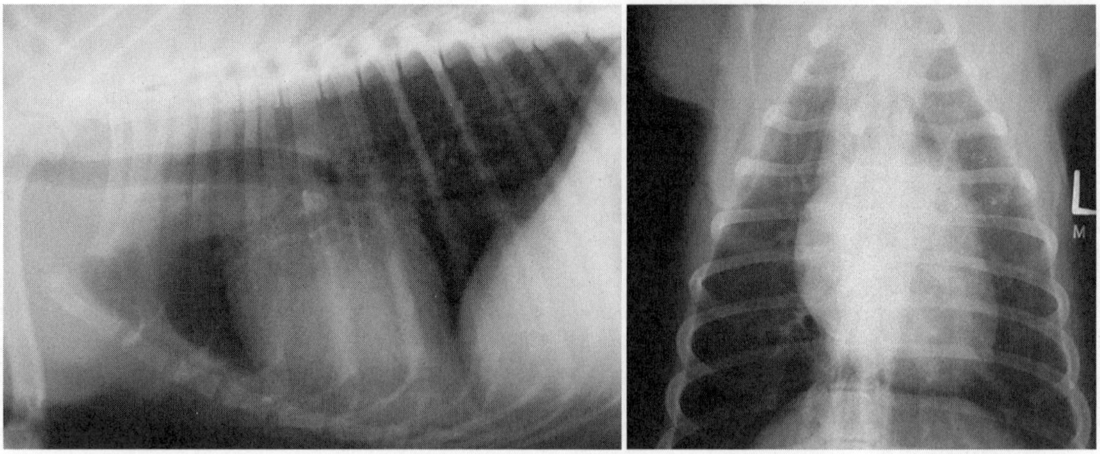

FIGURE 11-4 Radiographs from a 12-year-old terrier with a chronic cough and a systolic left apical murmur as a result of mitral regurgitation. The mitral regurgitation was mild. Consequently, the heart is not enlarged. The radiographs are diagnostic of chronic bronchitis. There are "doughnuts" and obviously thickened bronchial walls seen in longitudinal section in the caudal lung fields on both views.

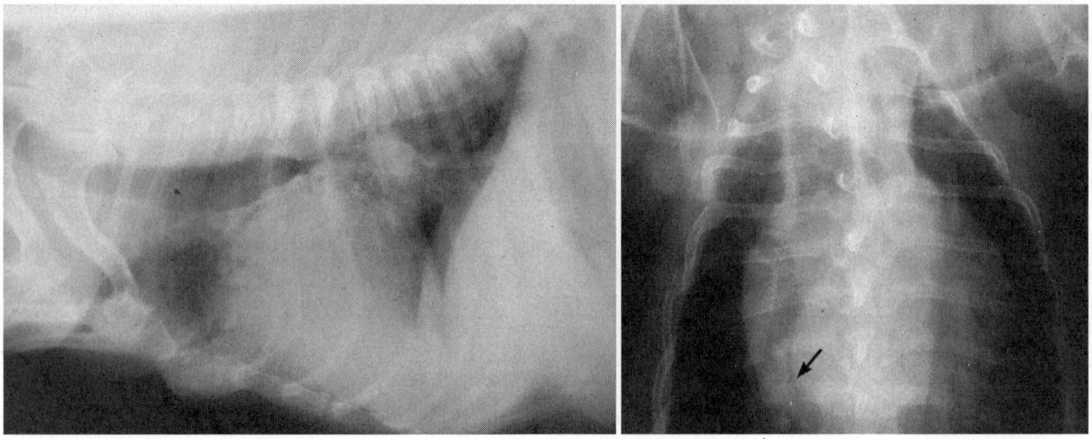

FIGURE 11-5 Radiographs from a dog with mitral regurgitation and subsequent left atrial enlargement. The enlarged left atrium can be appreciated on both views, and the body of the left atrium stands out as a bright, white circle between the mainstem bronchi on the dorsoventral radiograph. The dog also has bronchomalacia and compression of these softened airways by the enlarged left atrium. The collapsed airways can be appreciated on the lateral radiograph, but the exact location cannot be discerned. On the dorsoventral radiograph, the proximal portion of the left mainstem bronchus can be seen, although with some difficulty because the spine and sternum overlie this area. The collapsed accessory lobe bronchus can be clearly seen two rib spaces cranial from the diaphragm, to the right of the vertebrae *(arrow)*.

appear normal and in severe cases bronchiectasis may be present (Figure 11-4).[4] Dogs with normal thoracic radiographs that have audible snaps and crackles on auscultation should be assumed to have chronic bronchitis until proven otherwise. Bronchial thickening appears as "doughnuts" (i.e., thick-walled circles within the lungs) when seen on end or as "tram lines" (i.e., two parallel lines in the lung fields) when seen longitudinally.

The size of the heart and especially the left atrium should be noted. Severe left atrial enlargement may produce coughing by compressing the mainstem bronchi if bronchomalacia is present. It most commonly compresses the left mainstem and accessory lobe bronchi (Figure 11-5).

Although pulmonary edema can be seen without severe left atrial enlargement in a dog with a ruptured chorda tendineae, most dogs with pulmonary edema have severe left atrial enlargement. Whereas moderate-to-severe pulmonary edema is easily recognized, mild pulmonary edema is often difficult to diagnose. It generally occurs in the caudodorsal regions of the lung, next to the left atrium, and usually is centrally located. Many dogs with mild pulmonary edema are older dogs that have pulmonary interstitial densities that have occurred because of age. Small breeds commonly have small thoracic cavities. Many dogs have a large accumulation of intraabdominal fat that pushes the diaphragm forward, making the thoracic cavity even smaller. Most dogs only increase their pulmonary volume by a few milliliters when they inspire, so a radiograph taken on inspiration is little different from an expiratory film. The net result is an increase in the interstitial density of the caudodorsal lungs that makes identification of mild interstitial edema impossible (Figure 11-6). Consequently, it is common to examine a coughing dog with a heart murmur that has a normal trachea and normal bronchi and be unsure whether the dog has pulmonary edema or has chronic lung disease, most commonly chronic bronchitis.

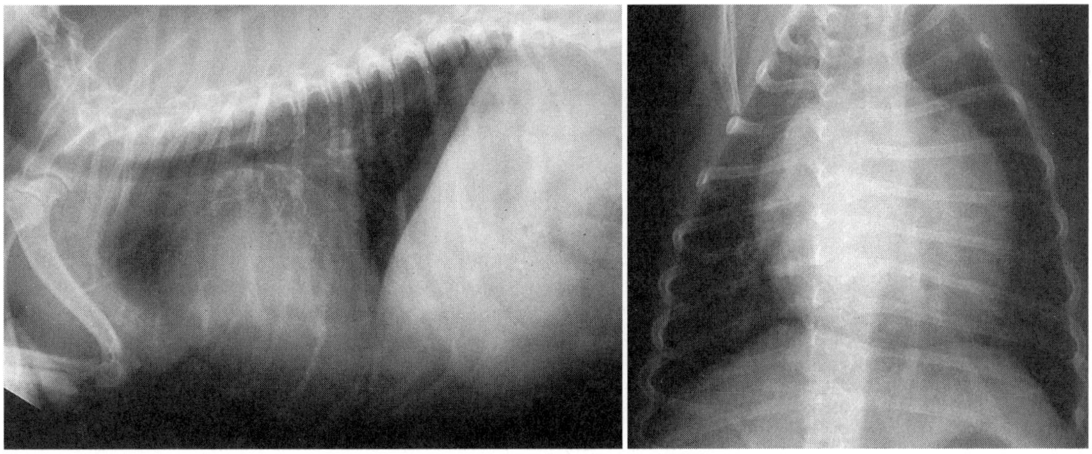

FIGURE 11-6 Radiographs from an 11-year-old Pomeranian presented for coughing. The dog had a loud systolic heart murmur as a result of mitral regurgitation. The radiographs show an enlarged left atrium with increased interstitial density in the caudodorsal lung fields. It was unclear if this was a result of pulmonary edema or a small thoracic cavity and aged lungs. The owner counted the respiratory rate to be 54 breaths/min when the dog was at rest that evening. Furosemide administration resulted in the cough abating, and the respiratory rate decreased to 28 breaths/min. The diagnosis was mild pulmonary edema as a result of left heart failure secondary to severe mitral regurgitation.

OTHER DIAGNOSTIC TESTS

In dogs presenting with cough and a heart murmur without obvious tracheal or bronchial disease, further diagnostic testing may be warranted or a therapeutic trial can be instituted. Dogs with mild pulmonary edema are usually hypoxemic, tachypneic, and hyperpneic. An arterial blood gas can be analyzed; however, if it reveals a lower-than-normal oxygen tension, one cannot be sure whether the hypoxemia is due to pulmonary edema or chronic lung disease. If it is normal, however, clinically significant pulmonary edema can be ruled out. The dog can be sent home with the owner and the owner instructed to count the dog's respiratory rate when it is at rest, or preferably asleep, in a cool environment. If the respiratory rate is less than 30 breaths/min in a dog, clinically significant pulmonary edema can usually be discounted. If the dog is tachypneic at rest, pulmonary edema is more common although chronic lung disease may still be present. Bronchoscopy can be performed if chronic lower airway disease is suspected. Although this procedure usually will not identify the cause of the lower airway disease, the presence of inflamed airways and the presence of mucous accumulations in the airways confirms the diagnosis of chronic bronchitis. Airway collapse can also be documented via bronchoscopy. If the left atrium is contributing to the airway collapse, the region of collapse is often inflamed (i.e., reddened) and the region can be seen to pulsate along with the heart beat. If the left atrial size cannot be adequately evaluated on the radiographs, an echocardiogram will provide a definitive measure of its size.

THERAPEUTIC TRIALS

Therapeutic trials are often used in dogs with chronic coughs. A trial of furosemide administration is often used to determine if a cough is the result of pulmonary edema. Unfortunately, furosemide is also a potent bronchodilator. Consequently, furosemide administration may improve the cough that is due to chronic bronchitis, as well as that due to pulmonary edema. It usually will not completely clear the cough caused by chronic bronchitis, whereas it usually will completely clear mild pulmonary edema and so resolve this cough. The administration of a different diuretic might be more rational in this situation. However, we have no experience with this approach.

Bronchodilators may be administered on a trial basis. Aminophylline and terbutaline are the most commonly used bronchodilators. Although terbutaline and related drugs such as albuterol are β_2-agonists and are supposed to act only as bronchodilators, there is enough crossover and there are enough β_2-receptors in the myocardium that these agents also increase myocardial contractility and heart rate. We know of three dogs that developed acute pulmonary edema within 24 hours after starting albuterol administration, theoretically secondary to mitral chordal rupture. Consequently, we do not recommend administering β_2-agonists to dogs with chronic mitral valve disease. Aminophylline can be very effective in some dogs with chronic bronchitis, but this occurs less than 50% of the time.[4] Although aminophylline has positive inotropic and diuretic effects, these effects are so mild that it is extremely doubtful that it can clear pulmonary edema. Consequently, if aminophylline ameliorates a cough, the cough was most likely due to chronic lower airway disease.

Corticosteroids may also be administered on a trial basis. Most dogs with chronic bronchitis will have a positive response to corticosteroid administration as airway inflammation decreases.[3] Corticosteroids can also have a positive effect in dogs with collapsing airways. One must be careful, however, in dogs with chronic mitral valve disease. Many corticosteroids, including prednisone and prednisolone, have mild mineralocorticoid activity. The resultant increase in sodium retention could exacerbate the pulmonary edema in a dog with severe mitral valve disease. This is unusual in our experience. However, the owner should be instructed to monitor the dog's respiratory rate at home while it is resting or sleeping in a comfortable environment and seek consultation if the respiratory rate increases to greater than 30 breaths/min.

The Approach to the Patient with Left Heart Failure

Left heart failure in dogs and cats develops secondary to several specific diseases of the left heart, including diseases of the myocardium, valves, and great vessels. With chronic disease, the

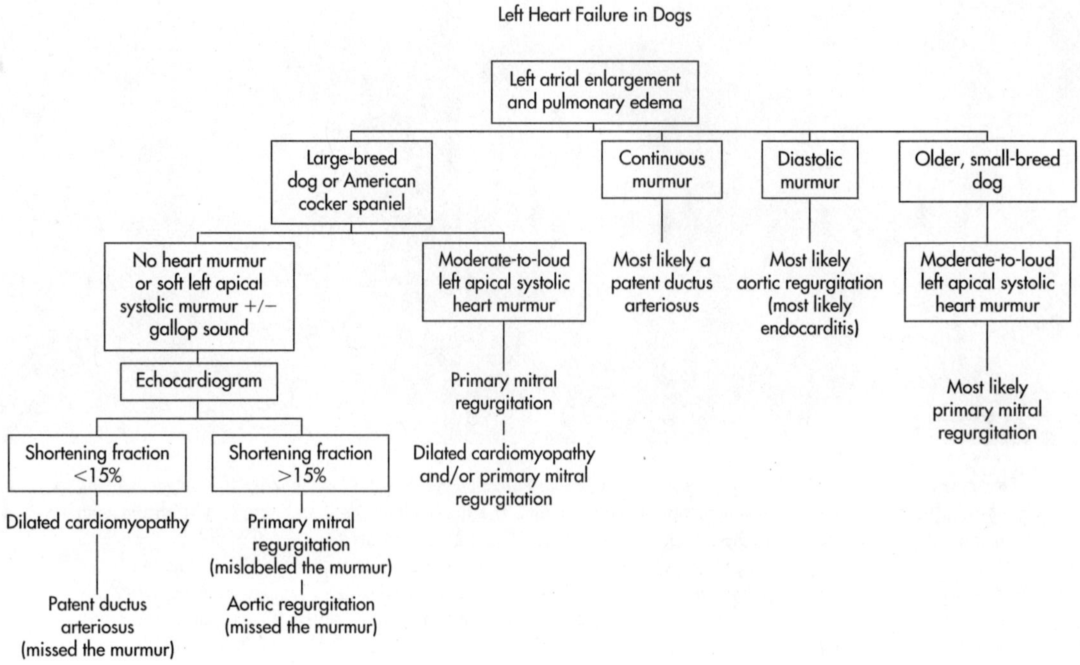

FIGURE 11-7 An algorithm for the diagnosis of the cause of pulmonary edema as a result of left heart failure in dogs.

disease must be severe before left heart failure is evident. Heart failure may be present with moderate heart disease if the cardiac insult is acute.

Left heart failure is not a primary diagnosis. It is a complex of clinical signs that occurs secondary to a primary underlying disease. The specific left heart diseases seen in domestic dogs include mitral regurgitation resulting from either myxomatous degeneration or mitral valve dysplasia, dilated cardiomyopathy, patent ductus arteriosus, or aortic regurgitation (most commonly a result of bacterial endocarditis) (Figure 11-7). In cats, the commonly ruled out diseases include hypertrophic cardiomyopathy, restrictive cardiomyopathy, and unclassified cardiomyopathy (Figure 11-8). Dilated cardiomyopathy, obliterative cardiomyopathy, and myocardial infarction are less common causes of left heart failure in cats. Some of these diseases are more common in certain types of patients. For example, hypertrophic cardiomyopathy is much more common in cats than in dogs. Myxomatous mitral valve degeneration is more common in older small-breed dogs than in younger dogs or large-dog breeds. Dilated cardiomyopathy is more common in dogs than in cats.

The patient with left heart failure most commonly presents with signs referable to the respiratory system. Some present for coughing, some with only tachypnea, some with dyspnea, and some with all three. The severity ranges from mild to severe. These signs are almost always secondary to pulmonary edema in the canine patient with left heart disease unless there is concomitant right heart failure, in which case pleural effusion may be present. In cats, signs may be due either to pulmonary edema or pleural effusion.

Most patients will have a chronic disease and most will have abnormal physical examination findings. Most commonly, auscultation of the heart is abnormal. Auscultation will often provide clues as to the underlying nature of the disease. For example, a dog with left heart failure secondary to myxomatous mitral valve disease will almost always have a grade 3/6 or louder pansystolic murmur heard best at the left apex. Conversely, a dog with left heart failure as a result of dilated cardiomyopathy will often have a softer (grade 2/6 or less) systolic heart murmur at the left apex and may have a soft gallop sound in diastole. A dog with aortic regurgitation will have a soft diastolic heart murmur heard best at the left base. This most commonly is due to bacterial endocarditis. Because this murmur is soft, it may be difficult to auscult, and time must be taken to listen for it in a quiet room. A dog with a patent ductus arteriosus will have a continuous heart murmur heard best in the left axillary region. One must take the time to place the stethoscope in this region and listen.

Most cats with any form of left heart failure secondary to cardiomyopathy will have a systolic heart murmur heard best ventrally, along the sternum at the apex of the heart. The intensity of the murmur is more commonly dynamic in cats with hypertrophic cardiomyopathy than with other forms of cardiomyopathy. The murmur increases in intensity when the cat is excited and decreases in intensity or disappears when the cat is relaxed. This occurs as systolic anterior motion of the mitral valve increases and decreases or comes and goes. Many cats with any form of cardiomyopathy will also have a very distinct gallop sound.

Auscultation of the lungs is often unrewarding in left heart failure. Many dogs and cats with pulmonary edema have only increased bronchovesicular or airway sounds secondary to their hyperpnea. Some, especially those with severe pulmonary edema, will have increased adventitious sounds in their lungs. Cats or dogs with pleural effusion may have absent lung sounds ventrally.

Most patients with left heart failure will have a heart rate that is faster than normal because of increased catecholamine stimulation. Many patients in an examination room have a tachycardia because of excitement, so tachycardia is not a specific indicator of heart failure. Arrhythmias are common in patients with severe heart disease. These

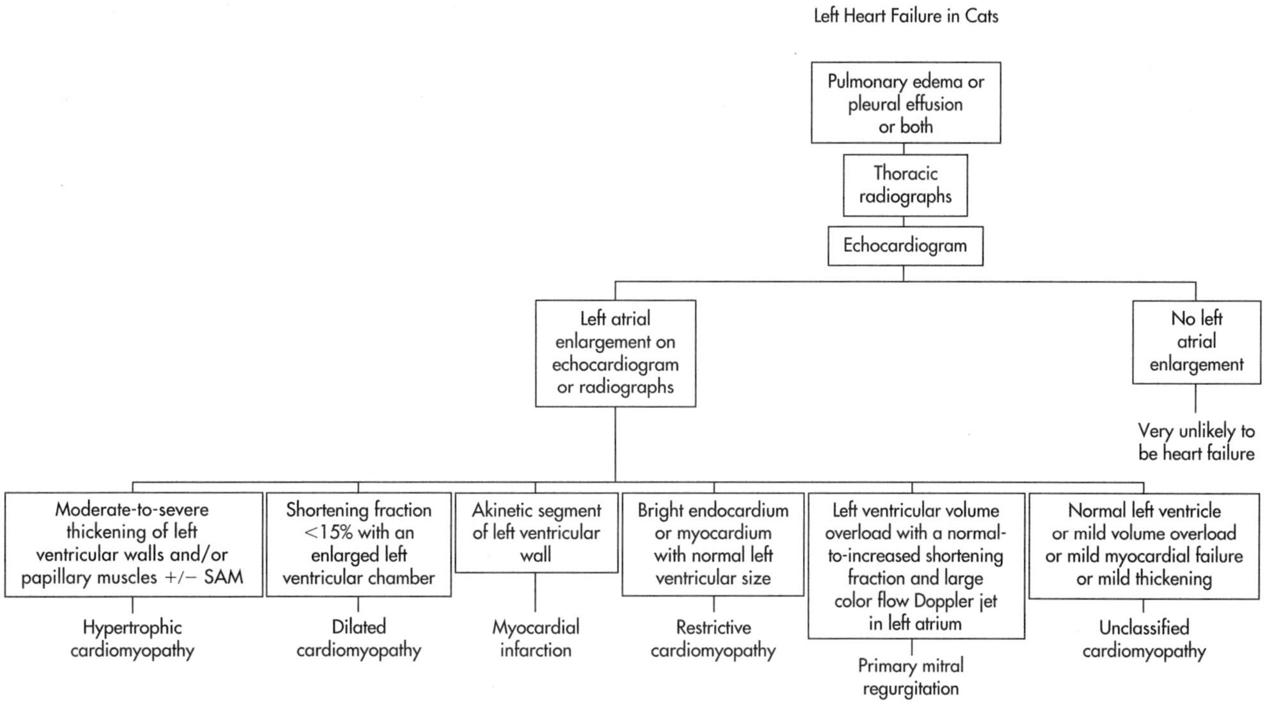

FIGURE 11-8 A diagnostic strategy for determining the cause of left heart failure in cats. An echocardiogram is required in almost all instances to diagnose the type of heart disease that is present in a cat with pulmonary edema and left atrial enlargement. *SAM,* Systolic anterior motion of the mitral valve.

arrhythmias can be ausculted, but an electrocardiographic examination is required for a specific diagnosis.

Pulse quality ranges from exaggerated (e.g., bounding) to weak. Patients with a patent ductus arteriosus or aortic regurgitation commonly have bounding pulses. The pulses of patients with mitral regurgitation are commonly brisk. Dogs with dilated cardiomyopathy may have weak pulses but they may also feel normal.

Thoracic radiographs are used to make the diagnosis of left heart failure and to follow its course, either as the disease progresses or following therapy. They also are used to detect cardiac enlargement (especially left atrial enlargement in chronic severe left heart disease) and to detect complicating diseases, such as thoracic neoplasia. Moderate-to-severe pulmonary edema is readily detected with thoracic radiographs. Mild pulmonary edema may be difficult to detect, especially in an older, obese, and shallow-chested dog. Mild edema is usually present caudodorsal to the heart and is located centrally. Interstitial densities are common in the caudodorsal lung fields in older dogs. They are accentuated when the thoracic cavity is small and the lung is compressed.

The electrocardiogram is primarily used to establish the cardiac rhythm during the time the test is performed. Atrial fibrillation and ventricular tachyarrhythmias are common in patients with left heart failure. Continuous 24-hour recordings of an ECG (Holter recording) are useful to diagnose intermittent arrhythmias and to determine the severity of ventricular tachyarrhythmias in selected patients. The electrocardiogram may also give clues as to chamber enlargement and may reveal conduction abnormalities that are more common in certain types of heart disease (e.g., left axis deviation in cats with hypertrophic cardiomyopathy).

An echocardiographic examination usually provides the definitive diagnosis of the underlying disease. These findings are delineated in the chapters in this book that detail each of the common diseases already mentioned.

Therapy is dependent on the underlying disease. Ligation of a patent ductus arteriosus usually completely alleviates the problem. The dog with dilated cardiomyopathy is treated symptomatically with digoxin, furosemide, an ACE inhibitor, and an appropriate antiarrhythmic drug (e.g., a β-adrenergic blocker or calcium channel blocker for atrial fibrillation). Dogs with mitral regurgitation are treated similarly, although antiarrhythmic therapy is needed less frequently, and arteriolar dilators are efficacious in the patient refractory to standard therapy. Heart failure secondary to aortic regurgitation is also treated similarly but an arteriolar dilator is often used earlier in the disease process. Heart failure secondary to hypertrophic cardiomyopathy is usually treated with a diuretic and a calcium channel blocker (e.g., diltiazem) or a β-adrenergic blocker (e.g., atenolol). An ACE inhibitor may also be beneficial.

The long-term prognosis is also based on the underlying disease. The prognosis is very good for patent ductus arteriosus. On the other end of the spectrum, the long-term prognosis is dismal for dogs with dilated cardiomyopathy, with a median survival time of 80 days. Cats with left heart failure secondary to hypertrophic cardiomyopathy and dogs with aortic regurgitation secondary to infective endocarditis have a slightly better but still poor long-term prognosis. Dogs with severe mitral regurgitation and severe heart failure have a median survival time of about 200 days. This is better than the other noncorrectable lesions but is still short.

If a veterinary cardiologist is available, referral to this specialist should be considered if the diagnosis of the underlying disease is unclear or unknown, if the patient has an arrhythmia that is complicating the disease process and cannot be readily controlled, or if the patient has become refractory to standard drugs. A veterinary cardiologist usually can determine the cause of the heart failure, make appropriate recommendations regarding therapy, and provide a prognosis.

The Approach to the Patient with Right Heart Failure (Usually Ascites)

Right heart failure is most commonly manifested as congestive right heart failure. This most commonly results in ascites in both dogs and cats, although pure right heart failure causing ascites is rare in cats. Dogs may only have a pleural effusion with isolated right heart failure. This is rare in cats. Subcutaneous edema can occur secondary to right heart failure, but this is uncommon in both dogs and cats.

Right heart failure is most commonly secondary to chronic diseases of the right heart, pulmonary vasculature, or pericardium. Left heart failure may occasionally exacerbate moderate-to-severe right heart disease, producing right heart failure. This occurs when the elevated left atrial pressure "backs-up" into the pulmonary capillaries and pulmonary artery to increase the pulmonary artery diastolic pressure. This usually only produces mild-to-moderate pulmonary hypertension in dogs. This does not cause a normal right heart to fail but can complicate moderate-to-severe right heart disease enough to produce right heart failure. Occasionally, severe left heart failure will result in moderate or severe pulmonary hypertension. This can result in right heart failure.

The common diseases that produce right heart failure in dogs are acquired or congenital tricuspid regurgitation, dilated cardiomyopathy, heartworm disease, pericardial tamponade, and pulmonary hypertension resulting from causes other than heartworm disease. Uncommon causes of right heart failure in dogs include cor triatriatum dexter, constrictive pericarditis, and constrictive/effusive pericarditis. Right heart failure with pulmonic stenosis is rare unless the patient also has tricuspid valve dysplasia. However, the right atrium may be mildly enlarged and the right atrial pressure mildly increased in patients with severe pulmonic stenosis. Pure right heart failure is rare in cats and most commonly results from tricuspid valve dysplasia. It most commonly causes ascites in these cats. Right heart failure in conjunction with left heart failure is common in dilated cardiomyopathy in cats. This combination very efficiently produces pleural effusion. Dogs with dilated cardiomyopathy may also have ascites and/or pleural effusion when the right heart fails. All of the other diseases are most commonly seen in dogs, in which they usually cause ascites. A general approach to this problem is presented as an algorithm in Figure 11-9.

The cardiovascular physical examination may reveal several abnormalities in patients with right heart failure. In all forms of congestive right heart failure, the right atrial and central venous pressures are increased. This may result in jugular or other systemic vein distension. This is not always the case. However, the jugular vein usually will distend during abdominal compression (i.e., have a positive hepatojugular reflux test) in those patients in which the jugular vein is not already distended (see pp. 39-40). The liver is commonly enlarged, although this may be difficult to discern, especially in an obese patient. Moderate-to-severe ascites is usually

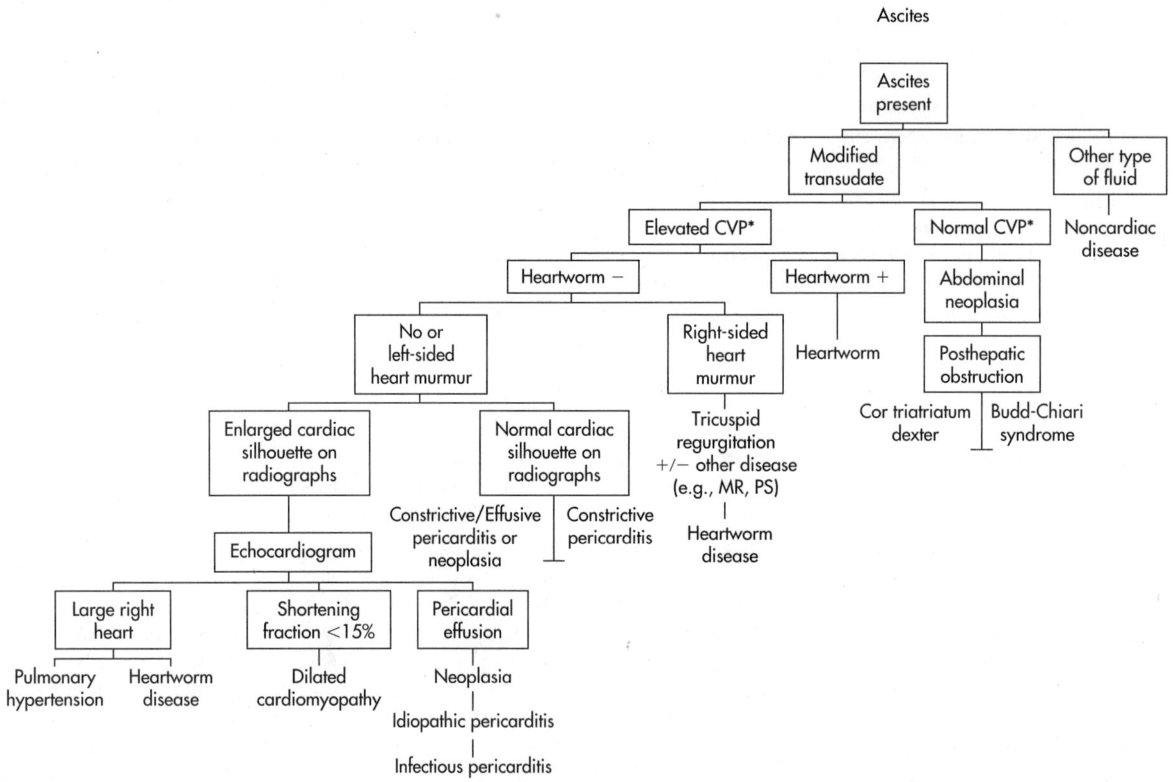

*Elevated central venous pressure (CVP) can be confirmed by identifying distended jugular veins, a positive hepatojugular reflux test, identifying enlarged hepatic veins with ultrasound, or measuring central venous pressure (increased is >5 mm Hg). It is assumed that CVP is measured from a catheter placed in the jugular vein.

FIGURE 11-9 The approach to a patient with ascites. Ascites secondary to right heart failure is rare in cats and is almost always due to tricuspid valve dysplasia. Consequently, this algorithm is primarily for use in dogs.

easy to detect. Sometimes obesity or the pendulous abdomen of a dog with hyperadrenocorticism may be mistaken for ascites. A fluid wave can usually be detected by balloting the abdomen in a patient with ascites. Auscultation may reveal several abnormalities that may help distinguish one disease from another. Dogs or cats with tricuspid valve dysplasia most commonly have a systolic right apical heart murmur. However, some cats with a very large tricuspid valve orifice and resultant severe tricuspid regurgitation may not have a heart murmur. This occurs because the orifice is so large that the flow is laminar. Dogs and cats with dilated cardiomyopathy often have a gallop sound. This sound is often obvious in cats but is usually subtle in dogs. Dogs and cats with dilated cardiomyopathy also commonly have a soft systolic heart murmur, usually heard best over the cardiac apex. In some dogs, neither abnormality is present or identified. Dogs with pericardial effusion may or may not have muffled heart sounds. Dogs with severe heartworm disease often have a right apical systolic heart murmur, but some do not. Consequently, one cannot always distinguish dilated cardiomyopathy from pericardial effusion from heartworm disease on auscultation. The peripheral arterial pulses are often poor in each of these diseases and therefore may not help in distinguishing the cause of the right heart failure. Pericardial tamponade may produce pulsus paradoxus. This is not seen in the other diseases, but it is subtle and commonly missed in patients with pericardial tamponade.

Fluid analysis should be obtained. The fluid that accumulates in the peritoneal space secondary to right heart failure is usually a modified transudate with a specific gravity between 1.018 and 1.025 and a protein content of 2.6 to 6.0 g/dL. The initial fluid that accumulates in the pleural space may be a transudate but usually becomes a modified transudate and in cats may become pseudochylous or chylous. Even when it is a transudate it is usually straw-colored or serosanguinous.

Thoracic radiographs almost always reveal an enlarged cardiac silhouette in a patient with right heart failure. If the cardiac silhouette is not enlarged and right heart failure is still the most likely possibility or has been established via measuring central venous pressure, rare diseases such as cor triatriatum dexter and constrictive pericarditis should be ruled out. Dogs and cats with severe tricuspid regurgitation often have radiographic evidence of predominant right atrial enlargement. The right ventricle is also demonstrably enlarged in many of these patients. Dogs with dilated cardiomyopathy and dogs with severe pericardial effusion may be impossible to distinguish by examining a thoracic radiograph. Pulmonary edema may be present in a patient with dilated cardiomyopathy. An electrocardiogram may also be helpful in this situation. The complexes may be smaller than normal, and electrical alternans may be present with pericardial effusion. The complexes are usually normal to larger than normal in dilated cardiomyopathy, and ventricular and supraventricular arrhythmias are common. Abnormalities of the QRS complex, such as axis deviation and splintering of the QRS complex, are also common with dilated cardiomyopathy.

An ultrasound examination can be used to diagnose right heart failure. It can usually be accurately diagnosed by identifying enlarged hepatic veins. Ascites and/or pleural effusion are usually present and can be definitively identified with ultrasound. The ultrasound examination almost always divulges the reason for the right heart failure. Patients with severe tricuspid regurgitation have a large right atrium that is usually larger than the right ventricular cavity. The tricuspid valve anatomy is usually abnormal. Doppler echocardiography can be used to document the regurgitant jet. Patients with dilated cardiomyopathy have poor ventricular wall motion and enlarged atrial and ventricular cavities. Those with pericardial tamponade usually have a large amount of pericardial effusion. Whenever pericardial effusion is present, an attempt to find the cause must be made. The heart base and the right atrium, auricle, and atrioventricular groove must be examined closely for a tumor. Occasionally, distinguishing pericardial effusion from pleural effusion is difficult. They can usually be distinguished by examining the space between the caudal heart border and the diaphragm. Pleural effusion will usually be present here, and fibrin tags will be floating in the effusion. Fibrin tags are rare in pericardial effusion. The right ventricle and right atrium are similarly enlarged in dogs with right heart failure secondary to heartworm disease or other causes of pulmonary hypertension. In some cases the heartworms can be visualized in the proximal pulmonary arteries. Rarely, they will be identified in the right heart. Pulmonary hypertension and its severity can be documented by measuring the velocity of a tricuspid or pulmonic regurgitation jet, if present.

In any patient with fluid accumulation in which right heart failure is suspected but cannot be proved by other means, the central venous pressure should be measured. This is accomplished by placing a catheter, which is long enough to reach beyond the thoracic inlet, into the jugular vein and laying the patient on its side. The catheter is then attached to a pressure transducer or water manometer that is placed at the level of the right atrium (usually the midthorax). In a normal dog or cat, the central venous pressure should be less than 5 mm Hg, or 7 cm H_2O. In a patient with ascites or pleural effusion secondary to right heart failure, the central venous pressure will be at least 10 mm Hg, or 14 cm H_2O. The most common mistake is to place the catheter in the right ventricle. This results in a falsely high measurement. If a pressure transducer is used, the large pulsations can be seen. A radiograph will confirm the catheter location.

The Approach to the Patient with an Arrhythmia

Arrhythmias are common in dogs and cats with cardiac disease and with many diseases of other organ systems. Although they can be divided in many ways, this section divides them into those that have benign arrhythmias (i.e., those with arrhythmias that are non–life-threatening and produce no clinical signs) and those with malignant arrhythmias (i.e., those that either have a life-threatening arrhythmia or have clinical signs referable to the arrhythmia).

PATIENTS WITH BENIGN ARRHYTHMIAS

The common supraventricular arrhythmias include sinus bradycardia, sinus tachycardia, sinus arrest, atrial standstill, supraventricular premature beats, supraventricular tachycardia, atrial flutter, atrial fibrillation, nodal tachycardia, and isorhythmic atrioventricular dissociation. Of these, sinus tachycardia and supraventricular premature beats are the most common benign arrhythmias. The common ventricular arrhythmias include ventricular premature beats, ventricular tachycardia, accelerated idioventricular rhythm, ventricular flutter, ventricular fibrillation, and idioventricular rhythm. Of these, ventricular premature beats and accelerated idioventricular rhythm are most commonly benign. Conduction abnormalities also cause arrhythmias. These include second- and third-degree atrioventricular blocks and sinoatrial block. Second-degree atrioventricular block is commonly a benign arrhythmia.

Patients with benign arrhythmias are most frequently presented for clinical signs that are referable to something other than the arrhythmia and occur secondary to some other disease process. The disease process is often serious, but often the arrhythmia that occurs secondary to it does not cause clinical problems by itself. Examples include sinus tachycardia secondary to heart failure, hyperthyroidism, pain, supraventricular premature beats secondary to left atrial enlargement in mitral regurgitation, and accelerated idioventricular rhythm secondary to myocardial ischemia following a condition such as gastric-dilatation volvulus.

Benign arrhythmias are most commonly identified during a physical examination, routine electrocardiographic monitoring in the intensive care unit, or anesthesia. Because they cause no clinical signs, it is often impossible to tell how long the arrhythmia has been present in an ambulatory patient. In critically sick or anesthetized animals, the arrhythmia is usually associated with an acute or subacute event. Whenever an arrhythmia is identified, every attempt should be made to identify the type of arrhythmia present. This usually only entails recording a high-quality, diagnostic electrocardiographic recording. Once this is completed, the electrocardiogram must be accurately interpreted. This should most commonly be accomplished by the primary veterinarian interpreting the ECG. However, if the veterinarian does not feel comfortable doing this, the ECG should be interpreted by someone else, such as a mobile veterinary cardiologist or a company or individual that reads transtelephonic or faxed electrocardiograms. Rarely, more complex techniques are required, such as recording intracavitary electrograms.

Because arrhythmias are not usually present in a normal animal, whenever an arrhythmia is identified, its underlying cause should be sought. Sometimes this is obvious. For example, in an animal presented to the clinic for ventricular arrhythmias after being hit by a car, it can be assumed that the arrhythmia has occurred secondary to the traumatic event. In some cases, diagnostic tests for noncardiac diseases will identify an underlying disease process, such as hyperthyroidism. In others cases, cardiovascular diagnostic tests, such as echocardiography, must be performed to rule-out underlying cardiac disease or to identify a subclinical cardiac disease.

The process of evaluating an arrhythmia should follow a standard approach to medicine. The initial evaluation must include a thorough history and physical examination. The signalment should be assessed. A review of the patient's medication history is essential. In many patients a minimum database, including a complete blood count, chemistry panel (including electrolytes), and urinalysis, is warranted, especially in geriatric patients or in patients exhibiting clinical signs referable to another organ system. Thyroid function should be evaluated in any geriatric cat with an unexplained arrhythmia, including sinus tachycardia. Any history of cardiac disease should be reviewed and the cardiovascular system examined carefully. A thoracic radiograph may be helpful in certain situations but is often unrewarding. Even so, it should be included in the database of most geriatric patients. Thoracic neoplasia involving the heart occasionally presents with an arrhythmia as the only physical abnormality. An echocardiogram may be warranted in patients that have no apparent disease of another organ system.

Most benign arrhythmias do not require specific therapy. Treating an underlying disease may result in resolution of the arrhythmia (e.g., treating hyperthyroidism). Completion of an anesthetic event often results in an arrhythmia abating. In some instances, a benign arrhythmia may be a harbinger of a malignant arrhythmia. For example, the presence of frequent supraventricular premature beats or nonsustained supraventricular tachycardia may herald the onset of atrial fibrillation. Or Mobitz type II second-degree atrioventricular block may precede third-degree atrioventricular block. Even here, therapeutic intervention may not be warranted, because early intervention is not known to alter the course of the disease.

PATIENTS WITH MALIGNANT ARRHYTHMIAS

Arrhythmias that cause clinical signs or have the potential of causing clinical signs, including sudden death, are considered malignant and generally warrant therapy. Arrhythmias that commonly cause clinical signs include fast supraventricular tachycardia, fast ventricular tachycardia or ventricular flutter, third-degree atrioventricular block, and sinus arrest. Most of these patients are dogs, and most are presented because of syncopal events, episodes of weakness, or sustained weakness or collapse. Sustained supraventricular tachycardia that depolarizes at a rate of 300 beats/min or greater results in a marked decrease in cardiac output leading to sustained weakness and collapse. Sustained ventricular tachycardia can do the same thing but does so less commonly. More commonly, fast ventricular tachycardia is nonsustained and results in syncope or becomes sustained and degenerates into ventricular fibrillation, causing sudden death. The latter occurs most commonly in Doberman pinschers and boxers with cardiomyopathy and probably in dogs with subaortic stenosis. Patients with third-degree atrioventricular block or sinus arrest most commonly are presented because they have syncopal events.

Syncope is discussed in detail in Chapter 28. An algorithm for the diagnosis of the cause of syncope is presented in Figure 11-10. Any patient that presents for syncope or any other evidence of a malignant arrhythmia should be assessed carefully. A detailed history, especially of any witnessed events, should be obtained. A complete and thorough physical examination should be performed, including careful auscultation. A minimum blood work database, including electrolytes, calcium, and blood glucose concentration, should be obtained. A complete neurologic examination should be performed in an attempt to rule out the presence of neurologic disease as the cause of any event that appears to be syncopal. The cardiovascular examination should include an ECG. The ECG should be monitored for as long as possible in an attempt to identify sporadic arrhythmias. If a bradyarrhythmia is present and especially if periods of sinus arrest or extreme sinus bradycardia are identified, atropine should be administered to determine if the arrhythmia is vagally-mediated. If an arrhythmia is not identified, a Holter monitor or an event recorder should be placed on the animal in an attempt to identify an arrhythmia that is causing the event. An echocardiogram should be performed to identify any underlying cardiac disease. Boxers experiencing syncopal events almost always have a malignant ventricular arrhythmia underlying their signs. Doberman pinschers most commonly also have malignant ventricular arrhythmias, although bradyarrhythmias have also been reported. Both breeds are at risk for sudden death.

Treatment depends on the cause. Dogs with bradyarrhythmias, such as third-degree atrioventricular block and sinus arrest that is unresponsive to atropine administration, respond well to pacemaker implantation. Boxers with ventricular arrhythmias respond well to sotalol administration (see Chapter 20). Lidocaine may be administered acutely and for a short time to dogs with malignant ventricular tachyarrhythmias (see Chapter 29). Mexiletine and amiodarone may be choices for treating Doberman pinschers with dilated cardiomyopathy that are at risk for sudden death.

Sustained fast supraventricular tachycardias such as sustained supraventricular (e.g., atrial) tachycardia or atrial fibrillation can cause myocardial failure. In experimental dogs, pacing the ventricle at rates of 180 beats/min or greater produces myocardial failure severe enough to cause heart failure within 2 to 5 weeks. Consequently, any sustained tachycardia must be treated to prevent this from occurring. Fast atrial fibrillation is the most common

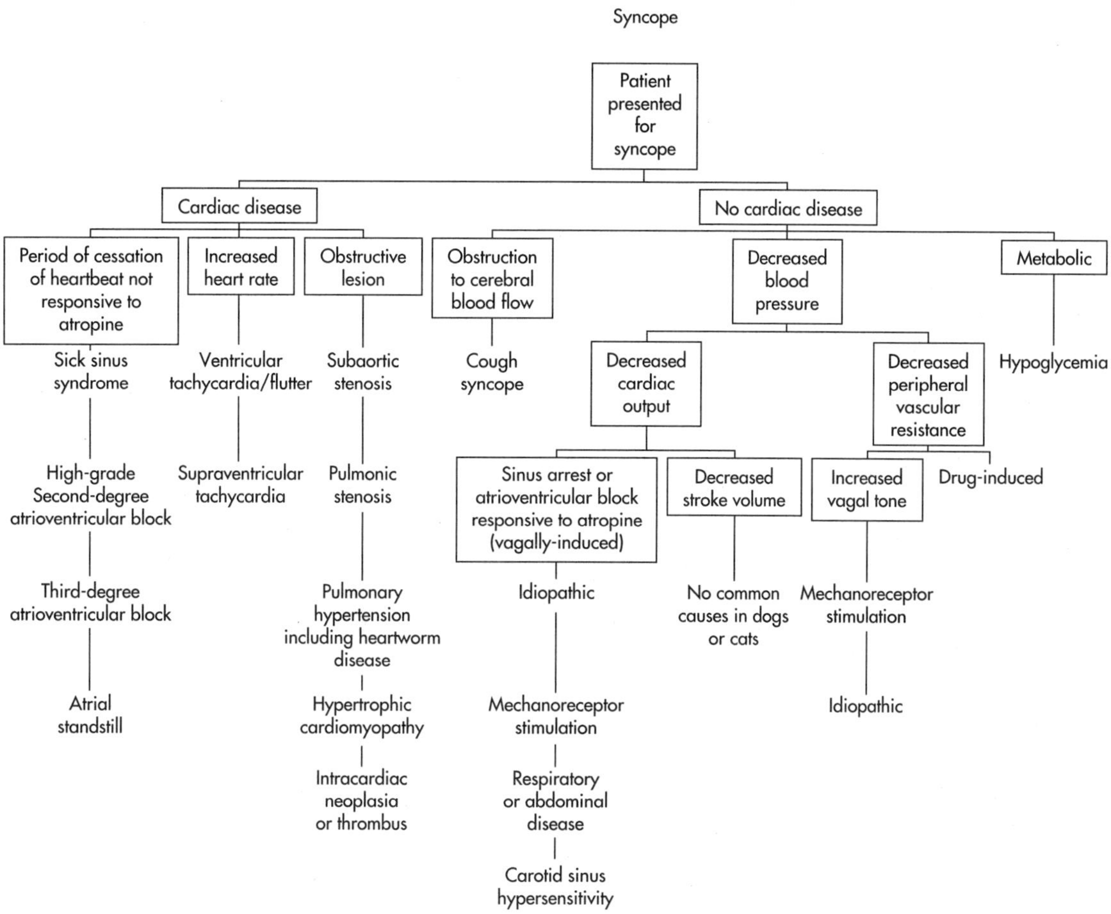

FIGURE 11-10 Algorithm for diagnosing the cause of syncope in a dog. An attempt must first be made to determine if the episode the owner witnesses is a seizure or is syncope. This may not always be possible. The presence of cardiac disease is suggested by the presence of an arrhythmia or a heart murmur. However, a bradyarrhythmia can also be present in a dog without intrinsic cardiac disease. This is usually due to increased vagal tone. Atropine administration differentiates a bradyarrhythmia resulting from high vagal tone from a bradyarrhythmia resulting from intrinsic cardiac disease. The arrhythmias that cause syncope may not be present at the time of an examination and may require a Holter monitor recording to identify the arrhythmia.

arrhythmia that has the potential of causing this complication. Digoxin or a combination of digoxin and either a β-blocker or diltiazem are most commonly used to slow the ventricular rate in patients with this arrhythmia. Digoxin, calcium channel blockers, and β-blockers are most commonly used to control supraventricular tachycardia.

The Approach to the Feline Patient with a Cardiac Auscultatory Abnormality

Systolic heart murmurs and gallop sounds are common auscultatory abnormalities in cats. They are most commonly identified in a cat with no clinical signs during a routine physical examination, during the physical examination of a cat with a disease of another organ system, or in a cat with evidence of heart failure. The systolic heart murmur is most commonly heard best over the cardiac apex, with the stethoscope placed on the sternum. Occasionally a cat will develop dyspnea following routine intravenous or subcutaneous fluid therapy, which heralds the presence of underlying cardiac disease.

THE CAT WITH NO CLINICAL SIGNS AND AN AUSCULTATORY ABNORMALITY

It is common to identify a systolic heart murmur during the routine physical examination of a cat with no other evidence of disease. This auscultatory abnormality may be present in a cat with a normal heart, mild-to-moderate disease, or severe disease. Consequently, identifying the heart murmur does not indicate anything about the underlying status. Because a heart murmur is often the only physical evidence of significant disease, further examinations are usually required. The most accurate means of identifying underlying pathology is to do an ultrasound examination of the heart (i.e., an echocardiogram). Consequently, this is generally the examination method of choice. Unfortunately, this procedure is expensive and many cats will not have significant pathology detected during the examination. Consequently, the veterinarian must talk to a client before this is done, and the client must make the decision whether or not to proceed with the examination. Radiographs are second to echocardiography in accuracy. Severe cardiac enlargement can usually be detected but mild and even sometimes moderate enlargement may be missed, especially if the enlargement is due to increased ventricular wall thickening (e.g., with hypertrophic cardiomyopathy). Thoracic radiographs must be taken in any cat with severe disease, because heart failure may be present. With a client that cannot or does not want to have an echocardiogram, a thoracic radiograph can be obtained to rule out severe disease. This often does not provide a specific diagnosis, even when severe disease is present and does not preclude progression of the disease if the radiograph is normal. Electrocardiography is the least accurate means for detecting cardiac enlargement or for determining the type of enlargement. An electrocardiogram should be evaluated in any cat suspected of having an arrhythmia.

The most common cause of a systolic heart murmur in a cat with a normal heart is turbulence in the right ventricular outflow tract. This usually occurs in a cat with enhanced sympathetic tone that has an elevated heart rate and increased myocardial contractility. Consequently this murmur may be labile, increasing in intensity when the cat is excited and decreasing in intensity or disappearing when the cat is relaxed. If the cat is excited throughout the examination period, the murmur intensity may not change. (Color Plate 28.)

Subclinical hypertrophic cardiomyopathy is the most common cause of a systolic heart murmur in a cat with cardiac disease that is not in heart failure. The disease can range from mild to severe. The severity should be assessed using echocardiography. The cause of the heart murmur in this population of cats is usually systolic anterior motion of the mitral valve. This murmur is also commonly labile, increasing in intensity with excitement and decreasing in intensity or disappearing during relaxation. This abnormality and its severity can also be assessed with echocardiography (see Chapter 21). Subclinical restrictive cardiomyopathy, unclassified cardiomyopathy, dilated cardiomyopathy, and primary mitral regurgitation can also produce a systolic heart murmur in a cat. All of these can be accurately diagnosed using echocardiography, although color flow Doppler is often needed to diagnose primary mitral regurgitation in cats. Subclinical hyperthyroidism may also be a cause of a systolic heart murmur in this population.

Occasionally a gallop sound is heard in a cat that has no other clinical signs of disease. When an echocardiogram is performed, most of these cats have significant underlying cardiac disease and many have hypertrophic cardiomyopathy. The others most commonly have other forms of cardiomyopathy. Rarely, a gallop rhythm is ausculted in a cat with no apparent underlying cardiac pathology. Rarely, a systolic click is mistaken for a gallop sound in a cat and provides the explanation for the auscultatory abnormality. In others the cause is unknown. An older cat with an unexplained auscultatory abnormality should be checked for hyperthyroidism.

THE CAT WITH CLINICAL SIGNS RELATED TO A DISEASE OF ANOTHER ORGAN SYSTEM AND WITH AN AUSCULTATORY ABNORMALITY OR WITH DYSPNEA FOLLOWING FLUID THERAPY

Most cats with a disease of another organ system and an auscultatory abnormality can be approached in the same manner as the cat with no clinical signs. Many of these cats have underlying cardiac disease. Some will have right ventricular outflow tract obstruction. If cardiac disease is present, it can complicate procedures, especially anesthetic procedures, that are required for the management of the other disease. Consequently, it is often mandatory to obtain further information. An echocardiogram is often required to assess the type and degree of cardiac pathology present.

Occasionally a cat will become dyspneic or develop subcutaneous edema following the administration of a standard (i.e., maintenance) dose of intravenous or subcutaneous fluids. This most often is due to significant underlying heart disease. The dyspnea is commonly due to pulmonary edema, but pleural effusion can also develop. A systolic heart murmur or a gallop sound can be ausculted in many of these cats. Any type of underlying cardiac disease can be present. Hypertrophic cardiomyopathy is the most common.

Any cat or dog can develop pulmonary edema or pleural effusion if a volume overload occurs. A volume overload can occur if intravenous fluids are administered too rapidly or in too great a volume. Patients that are oliguric or anuric are already volume-loaded because they cannot excrete a normal urine volume. Consequently, they are especially at risk for developing edema or effusion with fluid administration. On an echocardiogram, all four chambers are enlarged but myocardial function usually appears normal. Mild-to-moderate myocardial failure may develop with a chronic volume overload. Thoracic radiographs may reveal pulmonary edema, pleural effusion, and/or distended pulmonary vasculature (Figure 11-11).

THE CAT WITH DYSPNEA AND AN AUSCULTATORY ABNORMALITY

Cats that present with dyspnea are often medical emergencies that require immediate therapeutic support. A diagnosis should be obtained as quickly as possible in these cats to guide therapy. However, any diagnostic technique that stresses the cat must be postponed until the cat is stable. Dyspneic cats that become stressed often die. A general approach to these cats is presented in the form of an algorithm in Figure 11-12.

Many cats that are presented because they are dyspneic have both a systolic heart murmur and a gallop sound. The presence of either one in a dyspneic cat means that the cat has heart failure until proven otherwise. It also mandates treatment for heart failure. These cats may need to be stabilized before acquiring thoracic radiographs and an echocardiogram. A thoracentesis should be performed initially to determine if pleural effusion or air is present. This should be done with a butterfly catheter, with the cat in sternal recumbency. If fluid is present, the fluid should be analyzed. If the fluid is a purulent exudate, the plan should be changed. If the fluid is a modified transudate or a chylous type of effusion, it is most likely the result of heart failure. One of the common causes of chylothorax in cats is heart failure. As much fluid as possible should be removed. If the patient improves, thoracic radiographs and an echocardiogram should be obtained in an attempt to make a definitive diagnosis (see Figure 11-8). If there is no improvement and the cat is easily stressed, it should be placed in an oxygen-enriched environment and furosemide (4 mg/kg IV or IM) should be administered. If there is no fluid and the cat is severely dyspneic and stressed, furosemide (4 mg/kg IV or IM) again should be administered and the cat placed in an oxygen-enriched environment. A thoracic radiograph can be acquired if the cat will tolerate restraint. Often, only a lateral radiograph is required to make the diagnosis of pulmonary edema and/or pleural effusion. The shape of the cardiac silhouette does not help distinguish one type of heart disease from another in a cat so the dorsoventral view is often not needed at this stage. The cat should not be stretched during the procedure. If the cat appears to become stressed, the procedure should be canceled. An echocardiogram can be performed if the cat will tolerate more prolonged restraint. In some cats, sedation is helpful, especially if the inability to breath places severe stress on the cat. Sometimes anesthesia, intubation, and airway suction are required to treat severe pulmonary edema.

A thoracic radiograph and an echocardiogram are required once the patient is stabilized. This allows one to make a specific diagnosis

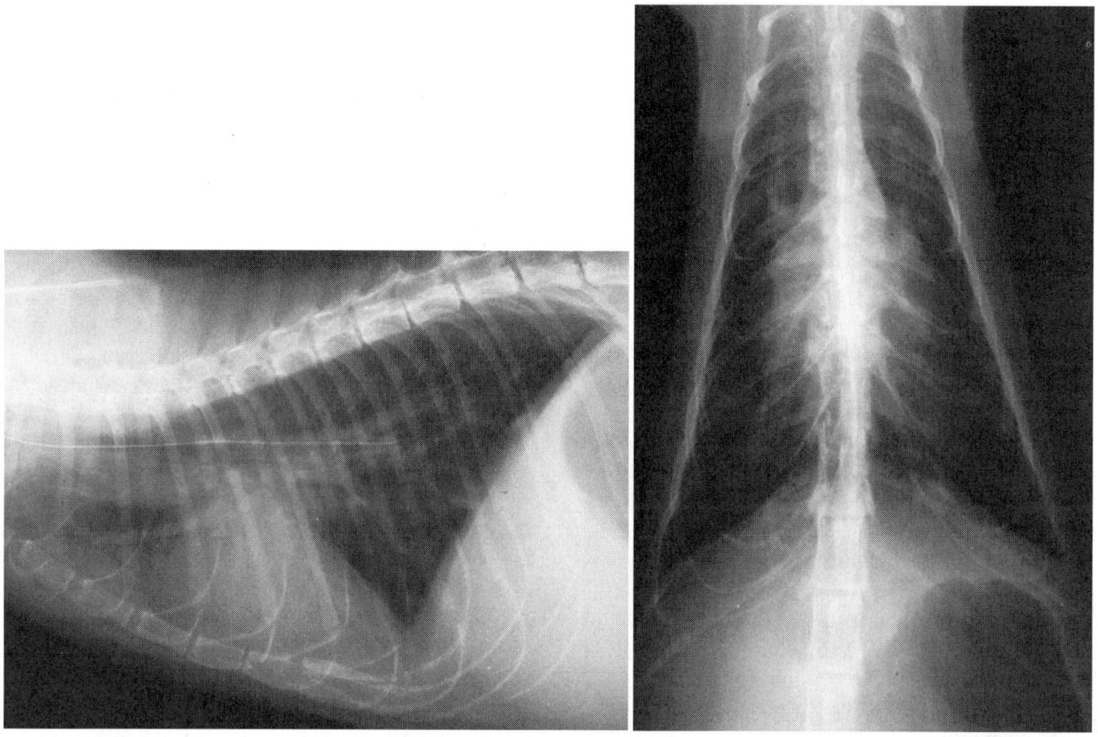

FIGURE 11-11 Thoracic radiographs from a cat with renal failure. The cat became dyspneic following the administration of fluids intravenously. The initial radiographs revealed pulmonary edema. The cat was treated with furosemide. The radiographs in this figure were obtained 12 hours later and show distended pulmonary vasculature. The echocardiogram taken at that time revealed that all four cardiac chambers were enlarged and the left ventricular wall motion was normal to increased, typical of an acute systemic volume overload.

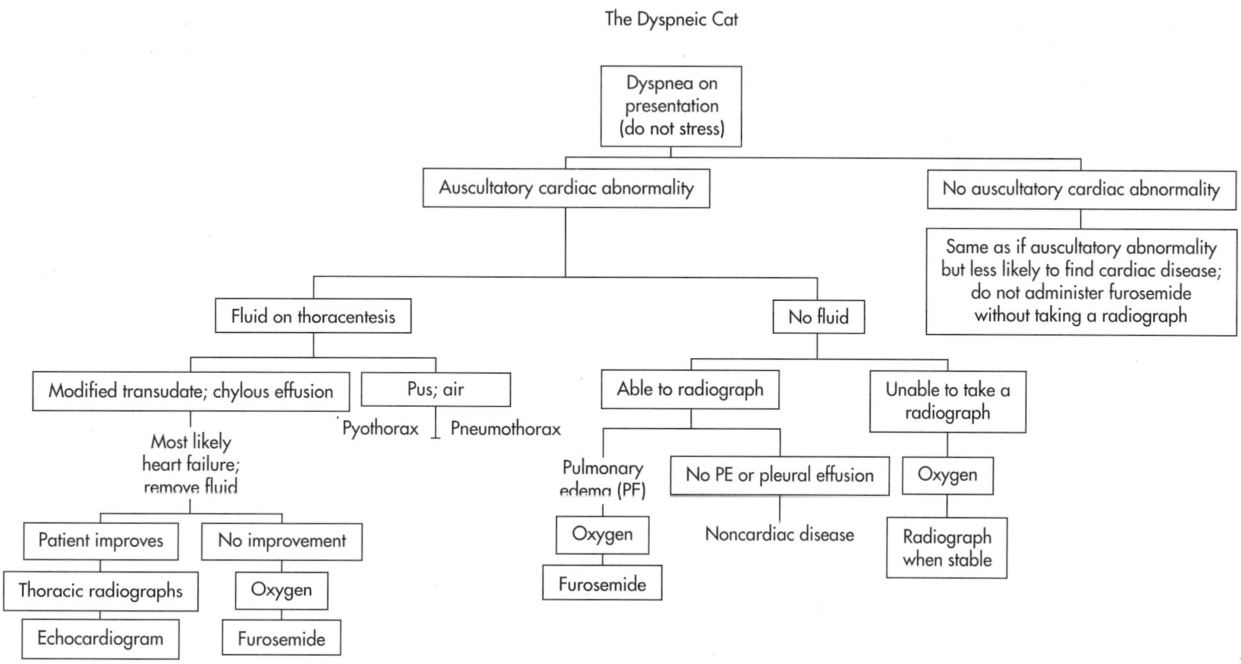

FIGURE 11-12 Algorithm primarily for the approach to a cat with dyspnea and a heart murmur or a gallop sound.

of the underlying cardiac disease and assess the severity. Almost always, severe disease will be present, however. The left atrium should be examined carefully for the presence of spontaneous echo contrast or a thrombus.

The Approach to the Patient with Cyanosis

Cyanosis is seen with diseases other than cardiac disease. It is generally divided into central and peripheral cyanosis, as explained in Chapter 3 and outlined in Figure 11-13. Peripheral cyanosis occurs when blood flow is markedly reduced. Even when heart failure is severe, blood flow is almost never reduced to the point that peripheral cyanosis occurs. Peripheral cyanosis can occur in the terminal stages of acute hypovolemic shock. Peripheral cyanosis more commonly occurs when blood flow to a region is obstructed, most commonly by a thromboembolus. The classic case would be a cat with nonpigmented pads that has a thromboembolus in the terminal aorta. The pads might be blue or might be white in this situation. In most situations the cause of the peripheral cyanosis is obvious.

Central cyanosis is caused by either severe hypoxemia or methemoglobinemia. Congenital methemoglobinemia as a result of methemoglobin reductase deficiency is rare in dogs and cats.[6,7] We have observed one case in the past 15 years. This dog was cyanotic but appeared to be otherwise healthy. Hypoxemia was ruled out by obtaining an arterial blood sample and documenting that the partial pressure of oxygen (PO_2) was normal. The blood methemoglobin concentration was increased, and the blood methemoglobin reductase concentration was reduced. Methemoglobinemia more commonly results from toxicity. It occurs most commonly in dogs following ingestion of onions or large doses (greater than 200 mg/kg) of acetaminophen.[8] Cats are more sensitive to agents that produce methemoglobin because of their unusual metabolism and unique hemoglobin structure. They develop methemoglobinemia most commonly following exposure to methylene blue or acetaminophen. Acetaminophen toxicity is the most common, because as little as one half of a tablet (163 mg) administered by an owner can cause toxicity. It results in both methemoglobinemia and acute hemolytic anemia. Cats with severe toxicity are presented with respiratory distress and mucous membranes that are blue or brown. The blood has a characteristic chocolate brown color. Because these cats are dyspneic and cyanotic, they can resemble a cat with respiratory distress secondary to heart failure. They should not have a heart murmur or a gallop sound. No pulmonary edema or pleural effusion would be present on a radiograph. The arterial oxygen tension would be normal.

Most dogs or cats with cyanosis have severe hypoxemia as the underlying abnormality. These patients can be divided into those that have respiratory disease and those that have right-to-left cardiovascular shunts. Both will have a marked decrease in the arterial oxygen tension on a blood gas analysis. For cyanosis to be apparent clinically, the arterial PO_2 must usually be below 40 mm Hg. Most patients with respiratory disease severe enough to cause extreme hypoxemia will have evidence of a severe abnormality on a thoracic radiograph. These abnormalities include pulmonary edema, pleural effusion, pneumonia, pneumothorax, and neoplasia. They result in impaired ventilation, diffusion impairment, ventilation-perfusion mismatching, and intrapulmonary shunting. Some patients do not have radiographic evidence of disease. These are primarily patients with

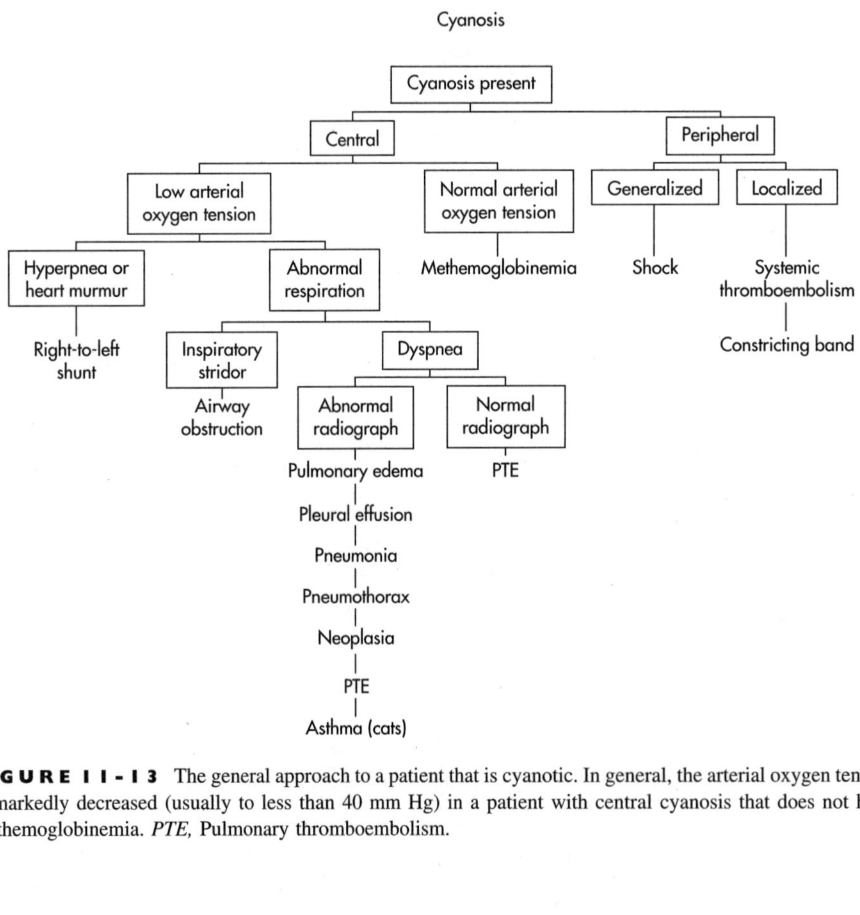

FIGURE 11-13 The general approach to a patient that is cyanotic. In general, the arterial oxygen tension is markedly decreased (usually to less than 40 mm Hg) in a patient with central cyanosis that does not have methemoglobinemia. *PTE,* Pulmonary thromboembolism.

airway obstruction (e.g., laryngeal paralysis or a tracheal foreign body) or pulmonary thromboembolism. Although pulmonary thromboembolism can produce radiographic abnormalities, in many cases it does not. Airway obstruction is often obvious in a cyanotic patient because of the marked stridor. Pulmonary thromboembolism should be the primary consideration in a patient that is tachypneic and dyspneic but without radiographic evidence of pulmonary disease and without stridor.

Patients with cyanosis secondary to right-to-left cardiovascular shunts may have generalized cyanosis or cyanosis confined to the caudal half of the body. Tetralogy of Fallot and Eisenmenger's complex are rare but are the most common causes of a right-to-left shunt and generalized cyanosis. A right-to-left shunting patent ductus arteriosus most commonly causes caudal cyanosis. However, it can also cause generalized cyanosis. Patients with right-to-left shunts may be tachypneic and hyperpneic but usually are not dyspneic. Most patients with a right-to-left shunt severe enough to cause cyanosis will also have polycythemia, whereas many patients with respiratory disease severe enough to cause cyanosis have not had the disease long enough to develop polycythemia. A patient with a right-to-left shunt may or may not have a heart murmur. Most dogs or cats with tetralogy of Fallot will have a murmur. Most with Eisenmenger's syndrome (e.g., a right-to-left shunting ventricular septal defect or patent ductus arteriosus) will not have a heart murmur.

One method touted for differentiating a right-to-left shunt from a ventilation-perfusion mismatch or diffusion abnormality is to administer 100% oxygen and repeat the blood gas. With a right-to-left shunt, the arterial oxygen tension should not increase or should increase slightly. With a respiratory abnormality, the oxygen tension should increase. This has not been universally helpful in our hands. We have seen dogs with severe lung disease not respond to oxygen administration and dogs with a right-to-left shunt have a significant increase in oxygen tension. With lung disease, intrapulmonary right-to-left shunts can develop. This may explain why a dog with severe respiratory disease may not respond to oxygen administration. Inhaled oxygen could cause pulmonary vasodilation and reduced right-to-left shunting in a patient with Eisenmenger's syndrome.

The Approach to Referring a Patient with Cardiac Disease

Although for decades the ability to refer a small animal patient to a specialist has been available to veterinarians who practice close to veterinary schools, it has only been within the past two decades that this service has become available in most large metropolitan areas. Within the past 10 years, the number of specialists in private practice has increased dramatically as residency numbers have increased and the demand for specialists by the pet-owning public has increased. The number of veterinary cardiologists, however, has lagged behind some other specialties. Consequently, some metropolitan areas remain in which no veterinary cardiologists are available. Invariably, whenever a veterinary cardiologist has moved into a new area, he or she has become extremely busy within a very short time. Therefore it appears that general practitioners very quickly see the benefit of having their more complex cases seen by a cardiology specialist, and the public demand for this service is definitely present.

Referral and consultation among veterinarians facilitate optimum care for the patient. However, certain principles and rules of behavior should be observed by both sides. Communication is the key to optimizing the relationship between the referring veterinarian and the specialist. Common courtesy should be expected on both sides of the relationship. During communication, expectations should be enumerated so that reasonable expectations from both parties can be satisfied.

Referrals cover a wide range of services, from phone or computer consultation to complete transfer of a patient. Most veterinary cardiologists consult with general practitioners over the phone, via e-mail or online, or via fax. Some specialists charge for this service and some do not. Many veterinary cardiologists travel from veterinary practice to veterinary practice, carrying their diagnostic equipment with them. They are usually able to provide a diagnosis and prognosis based on their findings. They usually also provide advice regarding therapy and the need and timing for follow-up examinations. However, they cannot provide in-hospital care and may not be able to provide more complex therapeutic interventions, such as pacemaker implantation and cardiac catheterization. Other veterinary cardiologists work within a veterinary practice or veterinary institution where a full line of services is provided. However, they must communicate via telephone and letter, whereas the mobile specialist can communicate in person. This makes the communication effort more difficult, and, consequently, they must be more diligent about maintaining communication.

The reasons to refer are varied and complex. They include help in making a diagnosis or confirmation of a diagnosis, aid in managing a clinical problem, performing a specialty procedure, obtaining a second opinion, reassurance for the client or the veterinarian, pleasing the client, client or veterinary education, and divestiture of responsibility for care. The time to refer is also varied. When a veterinarian is uncomfortable with a situation or unsure of where to go next, referral is always an option if a competent specialist is within the area. If a specialist is not available within the immediate area, the client should be informed of the closest specialist with the necessary skill and equipment. What the referring veterinarian sees as inconvenient is not always so to the client. Ultimately, the client should decide if the distance and inconvenience to get to the nearest specialist are bearable, considering the animal's condition and the expected benefits of the referral. This option should be given to the client and the situation discussed freely. Most clients are very familiar with the concept of referral, having been referred to specialists by their own physicians. Clients are often aware of veterinary specialists in the area and know when the option of referral is not being offered. Some of these clients refer themselves to a specialist, and some seek the advice of a different general practitioner the next time.

Divestiture of responsibility of care is a sensitive issue. It is known as "dumping" by specialists and involves referring a troublesome client or patient or referring a patient with a non-emergency problem after hours to a facility that has residents or interns. Referring a troublesome client may be appropriate if the general practitioner does not have the time to cope with a client that demands special attention. In fact, the act of referring such a client may provide that client with the special attention he or she is seeking, and the referral process will improve the relationship between the client and the veterinarian. On the other hand, referring a client that cannot pay or refuses to pay bills, abuses the veterinary staff, or telephones in the middle of the night and demands attention is poor etiquette.

When in the process to refer a patient can be a difficult question. Most specialists would prefer that the referral occurs before the

BOX 11-1

The five steps of referral

1. The referring veterinarian and the client recognize the need for referral.
2. The referring veterinarian communicates the reason for referral and the clinical information about the patient to the specialist.
3. The specialist evaluates the patient's condition.
4. The specialist communicates the findings and the recommendations to the referring veterinarian.
5. The client, the referring veterinarian, and the specialist decide about continuing care.

terminal stages of the disease when nothing can be done. They would also prefer that the referral occur before numerous "shotgun" approaches to therapy have been tried and have failed, especially if an accurate diagnosis has not been established.

The referral process can be broken down into five steps (Box 11-1).[9] The first step, recognizing the need for the referral, has already been delineated. Once this decision has been made, the referring veterinarian must effectively communicate the reason for the referral to the specialist. This can be done in many ways. A letter may be sent with the client to give to the specialist at the time of the examination. The referring veterinarian may contact the specialist by telephone to convey the same information. Often the combination of a short phone call and a concise referral letter is most effective. When receiving a mobile specialist, the referring veterinarian should set aside a short time to review the case with the specialist and communicate the specific expectations. Sometimes the reason for the referral is obvious and needs no communication (e.g., a young dog with a heart murmur). The clinical information about the patient should be conveyed at the same time. A brief written synopsis is appreciated by all specialists. Photocopies of medical records are generally discouraged as the sole means of presenting the clinical information to the specialist. Handwriting is often illegible, and medical records are often filled with information that is not germane to the referral. Photocopies of blood work and other data are encouraged. In the written synopsis the referring veterinarian should include a list of the current medical problems, the diagnostic test results, the current medications (including dose and frequency), a brief description of the response to these medications, and previous medications that were discontinued and why. The referring veterinarian may also want to tell the specialist his or her desires as to the specific responsibility the specialist should assume and what the client has been told about the referral. Copied or original radiographs should usually be sent with the client. This often saves the client from paying for a second set of radiographs. Radiographs may, however, be repeated if the quality is suboptimal, if different views are required, or if enough time has elapsed between examinations that changes may have occurred.

Once the client arrives at the specialist's office, the consultant must decipher the reason for the referral.[10] If this is not clear from the referral letter, a telephone call to the referring veterinarian is warranted. After reading the referral letter and the provided clinical information, the specialist should look at the material provided, examine the patient, and perform any additional diagnostic tests. The specialist generally examines fewer patients during the day and charges more for his or her services. Consequently, the expectations are greater and it is expected that he or she will take the additional time necessary to obtain a more comprehensive history, perform a more detailed physical examination, and track down additional information that the referring veterinarian may not have had time to do. The specialist should never rely solely on the information provided by the referring veterinarian. Because of his or her additional training, he or she will often recognize significant information overlooked by others. For similar reasons, he or she should not leave it up to the referring veterinarian to explain medications, doses, expected responses, and monitoring procedures to the client. Consequently, the specialist should first verbally communicate with the client. Clients should not be expected to remember information. Written instructions should be provided that include the diagnosis, a brief explanation of the disease process in laymen's terms, the prognosis, the medications and doses, and the need for follow-up, either with the specialist or the referring veterinarian.

The specialist should then answer questions asked by the referring veterinarian and make clear recommendations to the referring veterinarian. This should usually come initially in the form of verbal communication so that a discussion can take place.[11] This should be followed by written communication, which can be in the form of a computerized medical record or a letter. In human medicine, records or letters that contain problem lists with specific recommendations for each problem are preferred to a narrative letter.[12] Major procedures should not be performed until this has been discussed with the referring veterinarian.

Problems can occur at all steps of the referral process. They most commonly occur because of poor communication and misunderstanding of expectations. These can usually be rectified after-the-fact by improving or providing communication. Other issues are more difficult to deal with. Specialists, because they are better trained, sometimes perceive that the referring veterinarian's care was substandard. If this is in any way conveyed to the client, several relationships can be jeopardized. Unless this knowledge is in some way crucial to the care of the patient, this information should not be conveyed or should be dealt with tactfully. An even more awkward situation occurs when the care was obviously substandard. In this situation, the patient's needs must come first. No firm guidelines have been established to deal with this situation unless clear negligence or malpractice are evident. Another awkward situation arises when a client wants to make the specialist the primary veterinarian. This should be discouraged for at least two reasons. First, this compromises the relationship between the referring veterinarian and the specialist, because it often appears as if the specialist is stealing the client. This should be explained to the client. Second, the specialist often has substandard general practice skills. This may also be explained to the client. The schedule for repeat examinations for the current problem must be formulated by the specialist, the client, and the referring veterinarian. Often, follow-up examinations for the current problem are best performed by the specialist, who is more knowledgeable about the natural course of the disease, the medications and their side-effects, and the options available for further therapeutic intervention.

REFERENCES

1. Khera KS: Fetal cardiovascular and other defects induced by thalidomide in cats, *Teratology* 11:65, 1975.
2. Yagel S, Weissman A, Rotstein Z et al: Congenital heart defects: natural course and in utero development, *Circulation* 96:550, 1997.
3. Padrid P, Amis TC: Chronic tracheobronchial disease in the dog, *Vet Clin North Am Small Anim Pract* 22:1203, 1992.

4. Padrid P: Chronic obstructive pulmonary disease in the dog, *Proc Annu Vet Med Forum,* 1989, p 934.
5. Padrid PA, Hornof WJ, Kurpershoek CJ et al: Canine chronic bronchitis: a pathophysiologic evaluation of 18 cases, *J Vet Intern Med* 4:172, 1990.
6. Harvey JW, Ling GV, Kaneko JJ: Methemoglobin reductase deficiency in a dog, *J Am Vet Med Assoc* 164:1030, 1974.
7. Harvey JW, Dahl M, High ME: Methemoglobin reductase deficiency in a cat, *J Am Vet Med Assoc* 205:1290, 1994.
8. Savides MC, Oehme FW, Nash SL et al: The toxicity and biotransformation of single doses of acetaminophen in dogs and cats, *Toxicol Appl Pharmacol* 74:26, 1984.
9. Chosy JJ: Referrals. In Alpert JS, ed: *Cardiology for the primary care physician,* Philadelphia, 1996, Current Medicine.
10. Goldman L, Lee T, Rudd P: Ten commandments for effective consultations, *Arch Intern Med* 143:1753, 1983.
11. Lee T, Pappius EM, Goldman L: Impact of inter-physician communication on the effectiveness of medical consultations, *Am J Med* 74:106, 1983.
12. Lloyd BW, Barnett P: Use of problem lists in letters between hospital doctors and general practitioners, *British Med J* 306:247, 1993.

CHAPTER 12

Patent Ductus Arteriosus

Patent ductus arteriosus (PDA) is one of the three most common congenital heart defects identified in dogs (along with subaortic stenosis and pulmonic stenosis). From 1968 to 1980 the prevalence of PDA was 4.7 dogs per 1000 examined at the University of Pennsylvania.[1] PDA is also observed on occasion in cats. PDA was diagnosed in 0.2 cats per 1000 examined between 1968 and 1980 at the University of Pennsylvania. In our clinic, PDA is the second most commonly diagnosed congenital heart defect in dogs, second only to subaortic stenosis. In one 10-year period (August 1, 1986 to August 1, 1996) we diagnosed PDA in 215 dogs, the vast majority shunting left-to-right (201 left-to-right and 14 right-to-left). This was from a population of 68,690 dogs, for a prevalence of 3.1 dogs per 1000 dogs examined. Consequently, it appears that the prevalence of PDA at our institution and at a different time is less than that reported from the University of Pennsylvania. During that time, our cardiology service examined 3493 dogs as primary patients, meaning about 6% of our primary caseload of dogs was dogs with PDA. However, our caseload consists of approximately 50% consultation examinations, meaning the prevalence of this disease in relationship to our true caseload is much less. In comparison, PDA was diagnosed in only seven cats in the same period, all shunting left-to-right. This was from a population of 20,150 cats, giving an prevalence of 0.3 cats per 1000 cats examined and 0.7% (7/927) of our primary feline caseload. Other defects can be diagnosed in conjunction with PDA, although this is uncommon in dogs. Of the seven cats mentioned previously, two had concomitant defects. One had tetralogy of Fallot and the other had pseudotruncus arteriosus.

PDA is the one common congenital cardiac defect frequently associated with profound hemodynamic alterations that is amenable to surgical repair. Because it can be corrected surgically, it is paramount that this defect is identified when it is present. Differentiating PDA from other cardiac abnormalities is also extremely important.

Embryology

The ductus arteriosus is present during fetal life to allow blood flow to bypass the lung. The lung is not aerated and so is collapsed during fetal development. The amount of blood flow required to maintain pulmonary metabolism and support growth is very small. Consequently, the pulmonary vasculature is markedly constricted, resulting in a very high (suprasystemic) pulmonary vascular resistance.

The ductus arteriosus is a muscular blood vessel that extends from the bifurcation of the pulmonary artery to the ventral aspect of the descending aorta, just beyond the origin of the left subclavian artery in the dog and cat. Its size approximates that of the aorta and pulmonary artery. Consequently, it imposes very little resistance to blood flow. Therefore, blood pumped from both chambers of the heart can traverse both the systemic and pulmonary vascular beds. The amount of blood that flows through each vascular bed depends on the resistance or impedance to flow in that particular vascular bed. During fetal development the vast majority of the blood flow coming from the right ventricle flows through ductus arteriosus and so through the systemic vascular bed because of the very high pulmonary vascular resistance. Only 5% to 8% of the blood that enters the pulmonary artery flows through the lungs.[2] Because the left heart flow should normally go through the systemic circulation and the flow from the right heart should not, this in essence is a right-to-left shunt.

At birth, lung expansion occurs and oxygen tension in the systemic vasculature (PaO_2) increases. The lung expansion decreases pulmonary vascular resistance by allowing the pulmonary vessels to expand. In addition, the increase in oxygen tension produces pulmonary arteriolar dilation. Consequently, pulmonary vascular resistance decreases. This decrease is profound such that the pulmonary vascular resistance goes from being many times systemic vascular resistance to approximately 20% of systemic vascular resistance.

The increase in systemic oxygen tension, besides producing pulmonary arteriolar dilation, also stimulates the musculature in the ductus arteriosus to constrict. The ductus arteriosus is effectively closed via constriction (physiologic closure) within the first minutes to a few hours after birth. The ductal smooth muscle then undergoes degeneration, starting within 48 hours of birth. By 1 month, cytolysis is complete, leaving only the elastic ligamentum arteriosum (anatomic closure).

During fetal development, circulating prostaglandin concentration is high and helps maintain ductal patency. The high concentration is partially due to prostaglandin production by the placenta. Also, prostaglandins are normally metabolized by the lungs. The minimal pulmonary blood flow during fetal development results in minimal prostaglandin metabolism and hence the increased concentration. Closure of the ductus arteriosus is apparently also prostaglandin-mediated. Closure of the ductus can be enhanced or hastened in premature human infants by the administration of aspirin, a prostaglandin synthetase inhibitor.[3,4] This does not occur beyond 36 weeks of gestational age and is attenuated by 34 weeks of gestational age.[5] Administration of prostaglandin synthetase inhibitors to the mammalian fetus results in ductal constriction in utero. Infusion of prostaglandin E_1 prevents closure in infants.

When the ductus arteriosus fails to close at birth, it is termed *persistently patent.* Patency is also a feature of the fetal ductus. For the rest of this discussion, patent ductus arteriosus will refer to patency following birth.

PDA is most commonly hereditary in the dog. In hereditary PDA, the ductal smooth muscle is hypoplastic along the duct in a characteristic pattern. The abnormalities in dogs have been described, and the extent and distribution of muscular hypoplasia have been divided into six types.[6] Grades 1 and 2 lesions lack enough muscle to close the aortic end of the duct but enough muscle at the pulmonary artery end to result in ductal closure. This leaves an aneurysmal dilation of the aorta. This aortic aneurysm can be identified on a dorsoventral radiographic as a bulge in the descending aorta, medial to the region where the main pulmonary artery is located. This is termed a *ductal aneurysm.*[7] Grades 3, 4, and 5 lesions result in a persistently patent ductus of small, medium, and large sizes. In these grades the ductal musculature is absent at the aortic end of the duct, with some muscle along the duct. The most muscle is at the pulmonary artery end of the duct, where there is enough muscle to result in partial closure. The greater the closure (the more muscle that remains), the smaller is the shunt. This distribution of muscle results in the characteristic funnel shape of the typical left-to-right shunting ductus (Color Plate 38). Grade 6 lesions result in virtually no ductal constriction. This leaves the ductus the same size as it was in fetal life. Grade 6 lesions result initially in a large left-to-right shunt and ultimately result in right-to-left shunting, as described below in the discussion of pathophysiology.

Prevalence and Genetics

It has been known for at least 25 years that PDA is hereditary in dogs. Toy and miniature poodles, German shepherds, collies, Pomeranians, Shetland sheep dogs, Maltese, English springer spaniels, keeshonds, and Yorkshire terriers are considered to be predisposed to having a PDA. We have searched the computer database and our echocardiography records at the Veterinary Medical Teaching Hospital at the University of California, Davis, and found that PDA was diagnosed in 215 dogs between October 1, 1986, and October 1, 1996 (approximately 20 cases a year). Out of that population, PDA was diagnosed in 49 mixed-breed dogs. The majority of these dogs were crosses between two small-breed dogs. Of the purebred dogs, PDA was diagnosed most frequently in German shepherds (21), miniature or toy poodles (20), American cocker spaniels (10), poodle crosses (8), Maltese (7), English springer spaniels (6), Pomeranians (5), Shetland sheepdogs (5), rottweilers (5), keeshonds (4), miniature schnauzers (4), and Chihuahuas (4). The remainder were in a large number of different breeds. Of these 215 dogs, 14 had right-to-left shunting PDAs. These also occurred in a number of different breeds, including the toy poodle (4), American cocker spaniel (2), and one each of English springer spaniel, Shetland sheepdog, German shorthaired pointer, Cardigan Welsh corgi, Siberian husky, Australian shepherd, Maltese, and Labrador retriever. German shepherds and cross-bred dogs were noticeably absent from this population. Ages of these dogs at time of diagnosis ranged from 3 months to 6.5 years of age. The majority, however, were between 1 and 3.5 years of age.

The genetics of PDA have been studied in miniature and toy poodles and poodle crosses.[8] The heritability of this defect does not follow simple mendelian genetics. When two dogs with PDA are mated, approximately 80% of the offspring have a PDA or a ductal aneurysm.[9] Of those that have a PDA, approximately 80% have a large patent ductus, resulting either in left heart failure or right-to-left shunting. If a dog with a PDA is mated to a first-degree relative (e.g., a sibling) of a dog with a PDA, approximately 70% of the offspring have a defective ductus. Of those with a PDA, approximately 60% have a large patent ductus. If a dog with a PDA is mated to a normal dog, only 20% of the offspring have an abnormal ductus and only 33% with a PDA have a large PDA. This suggests a quasi-continuous trait, threshold trait, or polygenic trait. Sex is at least a modifying factor in that females outnumber males 2 : 1 to 3 : 1.

Pathophysiology of Left-to-Right Shunts

This section is a general discussion of the pathophysiology of left-to-right shunts. It is placed here because PDA is the first example in this text of a lesion that can result in a left-to-right shunt.

DEFINITION

Normally the systemic and the pulmonary circulations are isolated from each other. When a communication exists between the pulmonary veins, the systemic circulation, or left heart (left) and the right heart, pulmonary circulation, or systemic venous (right) circulations, blood can flow from one side to the other. In a left-to-right shunt, blood flows from the pulmonary veins, the left side of the heart or the systemic circulation into the right side of the heart, the pulmonary circulation, or the systemic venous circulation through the communication. Left-to-right shunting is most common because impedance to blood flow through the right side of the circulation is normally less than the impedance to flow through the left side.

DETERMINANTS OF THE AMOUNT OF SHUNT FLOW

The amount of blood flow through a left-to-right communication is determined by the location of the communication, the size of the communication, and the relative resistances or impedances of the systemic and pulmonary circulations or the relative compliances of the left and right ventricles. It is convenient to divide anatomic locations into pretricuspid lesions and posttricuspid lesions.

The prototype pretricuspid lesion is an atrial septal defect. In a large atrial septal defect, venous return from both circulations is no longer forced to flow into either the left or the right ventricle by the presence of an atrial septum. Rather, flow is determined purely by the impedance to flow into either the right or the left side of the heart. Because resistance to flow across the mitral and tricuspid valves is minimal, the primary variable that determines the direction of flow is the relative compliances of the two ventricles. Normally the right ventricle is a thinner, more compliant (i.e., less stiff) structure, so more blood flows into the right ventricle than into the left ventricle. Consequently blood flows from the left atrium into the right atrium and into the right ventricle.

The prototype posttricuspid lesion is a ventricular septal defect. A PDA is another example. In a posttricuspid valve communication, the amount of blood flow through the communication (relative to the normal left and right heart flows) is determined by the resistance to flow through the communication, the pulmonary vascular resistance, and the systemic vascular resistance. Posttricuspid lesions can be further divided into resistive and nonresistive lesions based on the size of the communication. The size of the communication determines if there is any appreciable resistance to blood flow through the communication. If the size of the communication is as large as or larger than the size of the aortic or pulmonary orifices, little resistance to flow is present. The terms *restrictive* and *nonrestrictive* are also used to describe the features of resistance. These terms are less correct in describing communications between the circulations because there is no hemodynamic term that deals with restriction to flow and because these terms are commonly used to describe whether there is a pressure difference across the communication such that a pressure on the left side is or is not transmitted to the right side. Pressure is a consequence of resistance and flow and is the not the major hemodynamic variable of concern in determining the pathophysiology of a shunt. In other words, pressure is not transmitted across a large ventricular septal defect to produce right ventricular and pulmonary hypertension. Rather, in a large ventricular septal defect that provides no resistance to flow, blood flows through the systemic and pulmonary circulations in relation to the resistances to flow in these circulations. If pulmonary vascular resistance is one fourth of systemic vascular resistance, pulmonary blood flow will be 4 times systemic blood flow. Systemic and pulmonary artery pressures will be the same because the product of flow and resistance are the same in both circulations (pressure = resistance × flow). Right ventricular and left ventricular systolic pressures will also be identical because the pulmonary artery and systemic systolic pressures are identical and there are no stenoses in this scenario. Finding identical pressures in this type of patient indicates only that the septal defect is providing no resistance to flow.

Posttricuspid communications that do provide resistance to flow result in less of an increase in pulmonary blood flow and a lesser pressure increase, assuming pulmonary vascular resistance is not markedly increased. If the resistance to blood flow through a ventricular septal defect is one half that of systemic vascular resistance, twice the amount of blood will be pumped by the left ventricle through the defect than will flow into the aorta. If the ventricle in this type of patient normally pumps 50 mL of blood with each contraction, 100 mL will flow through the defect. The ventricle in this situation will have to grow to a size large enough to be able to pump 150 mL with each beat. The right heart normally pumps 50 mL of its own blood and in this situation pumps the additional 100 mL that the left ventricle pushes through the defect. Consequently, pulmonary blood flow is 150 mL with each beat, and systemic blood flow is 50 mL. This is termed a *3-to-1 shunt* (150/50 = 3).

In posttricuspid lesions, the left ventricle must increase its stroke volume to compensate for the blood "lost" through the communication. In the example above, the left ventricle must pump 150 mL of blood with each beat instead of the normal 50 mL. The blood pumped through the defect flows through the pulmonary circulation and back into the left atrium and left ventricle. The increase in volume coming back into the left ventricle increases the diastolic pressure in the ventricle, placing stretch in the left ventricular myocardium. This increased stretch results in myocardial growth. The net result is an increase in left ventricular end-diastolic volume, which is termed a *volume overload,* as explained in Chapter 2. Consequently, left ventricular volume overload is a characteristic feature of a posttricuspid left-to-right shunt. In general, the size of the left ventricle correlates roughly to the size and clinical significance of the shunt.

Pathophysiology of a Patent Ductus Arteriosus

LEFT-TO-RIGHT SHUNT

Grades 3, 4, and 5 ductal abnormalities result in shunting of blood from the systemic circulation into the pulmonary circulation (left-to-right shunt). Flow occurs in both systole and diastole. Systolic flow occurs as the left ventricle pumps blood into the aorta and produces a systolic pressure (developed energy). Diastolic flow occurs because the pressure developed in the aorta forces blood from the higher-pressure systemic circuit to the lower-pressure pulmonary circuit (kinetic energy). Because the ductus is constricted at the pulmonary artery end, it provides resistance to flow. Consequently, there is a pressure gradient between the aorta and pulmonary artery, and the mean systemic and pulmonary pressures are usually normal. Therefore the consequences of this type of PDA are purely related to the amount of blood flow that crosses the ductus. As can be deduced from the previous section, the amount of flow across a PDA is dependent on the size of the smallest orifice in the PDA and the relative resistances of the systemic and pulmonary circulations. It is not dependent on the pressure gradient per se. Whatever blood flow is "lost" from the systemic circulation through the PDA must be countered by an equal increase in left heart systolic blood flow if systemic flow is to remain normal. Conversely, whatever blood flows through the ductus returns to the left heart and must be pumped out again. The blood that flows from the aorta into the pulmonary artery mixes with normal pulmonary blood flow, traverses the lungs, and returns to the left heart. To accommodate this increased return of diastolic blood flow and to increase the amount of left ventricular systolic blood flow to compensate for the blood shunted through the PDA, the left ventricle grows to a larger size. As discussed in the section on general pathophysiology, this is volume overload or eccentric hypertrophy. In PDA there is an absolute increase in circulating blood volume that is proportionate to the size of the shunt. The net increase in blood volume recirculates within the ductus, pulmonary vasculature, left heart, and proximal aorta. This increase in volume results in increases in the size of all structures involved.

If the ductus has enough smooth muscle to markedly constrict the pulmonary artery end of the ductus, as well as various other portions of the duct (grade 3), resistance to flow is high, resulting in a small shunt. In this case the left ventricle can adapt to the small leak easily through volume overload hypertrophy, resulting in no serious hemodynamic sequelae. If the ductus undergoes moderate constriction at the pulmonary artery end (grade 4), the left ventricle must grow larger to accommodate and pump more blood. No immediate hemodynamic sequelae may be observed. However, the chronic volume overload in this case can lead to myocardial failure over several years. Such a case might then present to a veterinarian at 10 years of age in congestive left heart failure. In a grade 5 ductus, shunt flow is hemodynamically large. A large shunt commonly overwhelms the ability of the left heart to compensate through volume overload hypertrophy (Figure 12-1). Consequently, the increased volume load results in an increase in left ventricular end-diastolic pressure. This results in pulmonary edema (congestive left heart failure). Left heart failure most commonly occurs between a few weeks and 6 months of age.[6]

The presence of a PDA alters left heart function. The left ventricle and left atrium grow in size primarily in proportion to the size of the shunt. In a dog with a large PDA, the end-diastolic diameter and volume are increased maximally, primarily through volume overload hypertrophy. In addition to the increase in end-diastolic diameter, an increase in end-systolic diameter and volume are appreciated on an echocardiogram. Increased afterload or decreased myocardial contractility increase end-systolic diameter. The increase in the chamber radius coupled with the normal intraventricular pressure and wall thickness results in an increase in systolic myocardial wall stress (afterload). This must contribute to the increase in end-systolic size. Myocardial failure also occurs, especially in long-standing cases. The increases in end-diastolic and end-systolic sizes are usually almost equal, resulting in normal myocardial wall motion (shortening

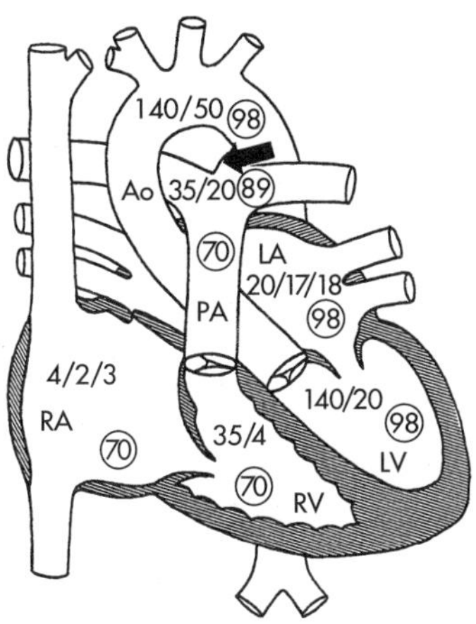

FIGURE 12-1 Schematic drawing of the circulation in a dog with a large left-to-right shunting patent ductus arteriosus (PDA). The shunt results in pulmonary overcirculation and left ventricular volume overload. There is mild systolic pulmonary hypertension. The oxygen saturation in the pulmonary artery beyond the PDA is increased above the oxygen saturation in the right ventricle. Pulmonary blood flow (Q_p) is approximately 3 times systemic blood flow (Q_s). *RA,* Right atrium; *RV,* right ventricle; *LA,* left atrium; *LV,* left ventricle; *PA,* pulmonary artery; *Ao,* aorta. The arrow represents left-to-right flow through the PDA. Pressures are depicted as systolic/diastolic. Oxygen saturations are in circles.

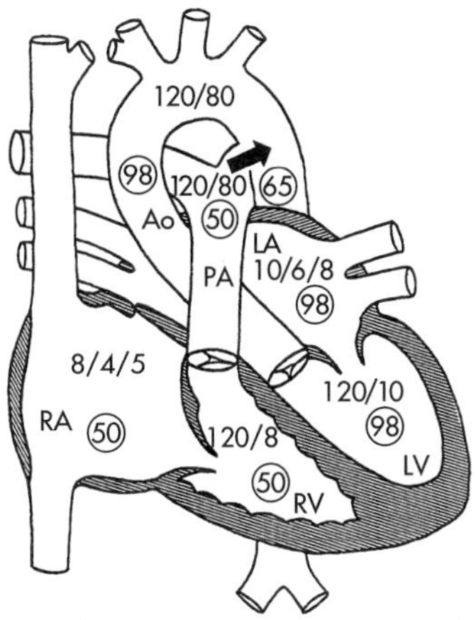

FIGURE 12-2 Schematic drawing of the circulation in a dog with a right-to-left shunting patent ductus arteriosus (PDA). Pulmonary vascular resistance is greater than systemic vascular resistance. Consequently, the shunt is from right-to-left through the PDA *(arrow).* Systemic blood flow is about 1.5 times pulmonary blood flow. Systemic saturation is 65%. This corresponds to a very low oxygen tension of approximately 35 mm Hg. Abbreviations are as in Figure 12-1.

fraction). The increase in chamber size in diastole coupled with normal wall motion results in an increase in stroke volume pumped into the aorta.

RIGHT-TO-LEFT SHUNT

Most dogs with a right-to-left shunting PDA have a large patent ductus that provides no resistance to blood flow. In dogs with a grade 6 PDA, the ductus functionally does not close at all. This results in a communication between the aorta and the pulmonary artery that is the same size as these great vessels (0.83 to 1.25 times the size of the descending aorta).[10] In this situation there is no or very little resistance to blood flow between the aorta and pulmonary artery. Consequently, blood flows from the left and right sides of the heart through both vascular beds in proportion to the resistance to flow in each vascular bed, and pressures in the aorta and pulmonary artery equalize. We would expect pulmonary blood flow to be approximately 5 times systemic flow in this situation because pulmonary vascular resistance is normally about one fifth that of systemic vascular resistance. This amount of flow would result in a massive and overwhelming left heart volume overload shortly after birth. The massive volume overload would result in peracute left heart failure, pulmonary edema, and death. Because these dogs live, pulmonary vascular resistance must not decrease to normal in this situation following birth but must remain partially elevated to prevent massive shunting. That is, the normal maturation of the pulmonary vasculature toward a low-resistance vascular bed does not occur, probably because it is continuously exposed to high pressure and flow after birth.[8] Normally, pulmonary vascular resistance decreases dramatically after birth, as ventilation begins and hypoxic vasoconstriction of the pulmonary vasculature is released. The smooth muscle in the media of the pulmonary arterial resistance vessels is increased during fetal life and gradually thins toward normal adult thickness after birth.[11] This process is delayed in infants with large left-to-right shunts.[12] In sheep with experimentally placed aorticopulmonary shunts (2:1 Q_p/Q_s) placed during late gestational life, the media of the pulmonary vasculature remains increased in thickness at 1 month of age.[13]

With flows matching resistances on both sides of the circulation, blood pressure equalizes in the aorta and the pulmonary artery as a result of the increase in pulmonary blood flow, leading to severe pulmonary hypertension. At this stage, pulmonary vascular resistance is probably only moderately increased, and this increase is not due to pulmonary vascular pathology but rather to vestigial medial hypertrophy and, possibly, reversible vasoconstriction. There is no pulmonary vascular disease. The increase in pulmonary artery pressure combined with the increase in pulmonary blood flow creates pathologic responses in the pulmonary arteries over time. The exact mechanism for this process is unknown but probably involves injury to the endothelial cells that activates growth factors.[12] These factors induce smooth muscle cell hypertrophy and hyperplasia and promote connective tissue protein synthesis. The pathologic response consists primarily of medial hypertrophy and intimal proliferation in the medium and small pulmonary arteries. This narrows the lumina of these vessels, increasing pulmonary vascular resistance. As pulmonary vascular resistance increases, blood flowing from the aorta to the pulmonary artery through the ductus decreases. Systemic and pulmonary arterial pressures remain equalized. As blood flow through the ductus decreases, blood flow velocity decreases. When blood flow velocity approaches 2 m/sec, turbulence disappears and so the murmur disappears. In poodle crosses with grade 6 PDA, a continuous murmur is heard during the first days to weeks of life but disappears before the eighth week of life.[8,9] Presumably by this time pulmonary vascular resistance has increased to the point that left-to-right flow through the ductus has already decreased markedly. Pulmonary vascular resistance continues to increase as pulmonary vascular disease worsens over the dog's life. Generally by the time a dog with a grade 6 lesion is 3 months to 3 years of age, pulmonary vascular resistance exceeds systemic vascular resistance (Figure 12-2). This creates a clinically significant right-to-left shunt.[10] When the shunt is clinically significant, a large amount of deoxygenated blood shunts from the venous circulation (the pulmonary artery) into the aorta. This results in a significant decrease in arterial oxygen tension beyond the region where the ductus joins the aorta, either at rest or with exercise. Caudal body arterial oxygen tension is commonly between 30 and 45 mm Hg at rest in clinically affected dogs and always less than 40 mm Hg with exercise if cyanosis is present. Exercise results in a decrease in systemic vascular resistance whereas pulmonary vascular resistance is fixed because of the pulmonary arterial disease. Consequently, exercise produces an increase in right-to-left shunting and exacerbation of cyanosis.

Another possible scenario exists in dogs born at or living at a high altitude. In these dogs, apparently a smaller ductus with a more common left-to-right shunt can reverse with age. This has not been documented scientifically but the supposition is based on anecdotal reports. This phenomenon also occurs in human patients.[14] We have also observed several puppies with a typical left-to-right shunting PDA that have gone on to develop severe pulmonary hypertension within several weeks before surgery was performed. Histopathology of the pulmonary vasculature has revealed severe, acute necrotizing arteritis in one of these dogs. The mechanism for the pulmonary pathology and hypertension in these dogs is unknown.

Right-to-left shunting PDA results in decreased renal oxygenation with subsequent increased release of erythropoietin. This results in increased erythropoiesis, commonly culminating in polycythemia (increased red cell mass or hematocrit). The polycythemia compensates for the decrease in tissue oxygen delivery caused by the hypoxemia. This is beneficial when the hematocrit is between 55% and 65%. Polycythemia becomes detrimental when the hematocrit increases to a point that the blood becomes hyperviscous. Blood viscosity increases exponentially as hematocrit increases. Viscosity generally becomes clinically significantly increased when hematocrit reaches 70% to 75%. The increased viscosity increases resistance to blood flow. This compromises systemic blood flow and decreases systemic tissue oxygen delivery. In the pulmonary circulation, systemic hypoxemia produces pulmonary vasoconstriction. Increased viscosity produces a further increase in resistance to blood flow, aggravating the pulmonary hypertension.

Diagnosis

MEDICAL HISTORY

Many dogs with a left-to-right shunting PDA have no history of clinical problems. However, many do present in left heart failure and, if left untreated, up to 65% may die of left heart failure within the first year of life.[15] Pulmonary edema can be mild to severe and can produce tachypnea, dyspnea, and cough. Dogs with moderate-to-moderately large left-to-right shunting PDAs that are not diagnosed when the dog is young, may present as adults with signs of left heart failure. Clients most commonly complain that the dogs are dyspneic.

In dogs with right-to-left shunting PDAs, rear limb collapse upon exercise is the most common presenting client complaint. Clinical manifestations resulting from polycythemia may be present. These signs are varied and include lethargy, nonspecific or specific pain, anorexia, and neurologic signs, including collapse and syncope. Clinical signs are probably due to the hyperviscosity resulting in decreased blood flow velocity in small vessels. Decreased blood flow velocity results in red cell aggregation that results in decreased local tissue blood flow. In human medicine, treatment of polycythemic patients is based on relieving symptoms, not on reducing hematocrit for the sake of decreasing the hematocrit.[16] The hematocrit at which a particular patient becomes symptomatic varies significantly; therefore the hematocrit should be followed sequentially and related to clinical signs.

PHYSICAL EXAMINATION

The hallmark of a left-to-right shunting PDA is a continuous heart murmur heard best over the left cranial thorax in the left axillary region (Figure 12-3). The murmur is usually loudest at the time of the second heart sound, decreases in intensity throughout diastole, and then increases in intensity throughout systole. Most commonly the murmur is truly continuous, lasting throughout systole and diastole. At times the murmur may become inaudible in late diastole, especially if the heart rate is slow. The murmur may be of any intensity but is often loud (grade 4 to 6/6). A palpable thrill over the region where the murmur can be heard best is common. The murmur may radiate widely, especially the systolic component, to other regions of the thorax or be localized. The character of the murmur is different from other murmurs and sounds like wind blowing through a tunnel. A separate murmur as a result of mitral regurgitation is often present over the left apex in the presence of a large left-to-right shunting PDA and is due to mitral annular dilation and papillary muscle displacement. This murmur usually disappears within several weeks after surgical ligation of the ductus, as the left ventricle decreases in size.

Occasionally, veterinarians miss the continuous heart murmur of a PDA and so do not diagnose the disease. This usually occurs when the heart murmur is confined to the left cranial thorax and the veterinarian auscults only over the left heart apex and base. All veterinarians should take the time to auscult the left cranial thorax of puppies presented for vaccination. Mistaking systolic murmurs for continuous murmurs is also common. This most commonly occurs in young dogs with fast heart rates in which diastole is short and the murmur is loud. Gaining experience at listening to the murmur of a PDA is the best safeguard against making this mistake, because the murmur is usually very characteristic.

Femoral artery pulse pressure (systolic systemic blood pressure – diastolic systemic blood pressure) is often increased in the patient with a large *left-to-right shunt*. This increase in pulse pressure is often described as a bounding, or water-hammer, pulse. The increase in pulse pressure may be caused by an increase in systolic blood pressure, a decrease in diastolic blood pressure, or both. Systolic

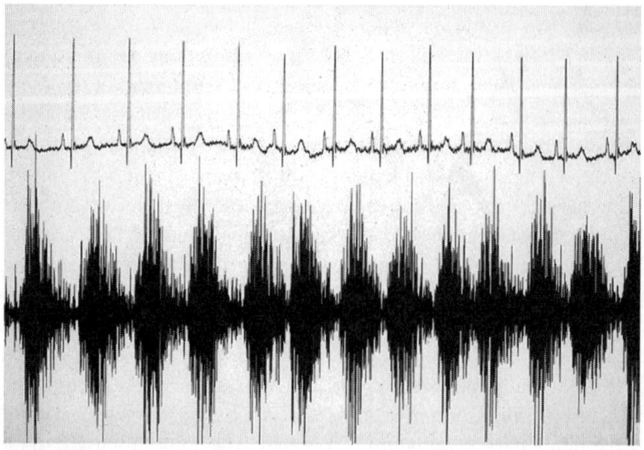

FIGURE 12-3 Lead II electrocardiogram *(top)* and phonocardiogram *(bottom)* from a 6-year-old Maltese with a patent ductus arteriosus. The heart murmur is continuous. Its intensity peaks in late systole and becomes very soft in late diastole.

blood pressure may be increased because of the increase in stroke volume pumped into the aorta. Diastolic blood pressure is almost always decreased because of the rapid runoff of blood through the ductus during diastole.

Dogs with moderate-to–moderately large left-to-right shunting PDAs that present in heart failure in adulthood may or may not have bounding pulses, and the murmur may be difficult to auscult, even when the veterinarian listens in the correct location. Often a veterinarian must be very astute to make this diagnosis on physical examination.

A right-to-left shunting PDA usually has no murmur, although only a systolic murmur may be encountered in a patient whose pulmonary artery pressure has not quite reached systemic pressure or in one that has other cardiac lesions. A common auscultatory abnormality in a patient with a right-to-left shunting PDA is a widely split second heart sound (Figure 12-4).

Differential cyanosis is commonly found at rest or following exercise in dogs with a right-to-left shunting PDA. Deoxygenated (venous) blood enters the aorta after the brachiocephalic trunk and left subclavian arteries (the "head" vessels) exit the aorta and usually flows only to the caudal body. Consequently, the head and front limbs receive oxygenated blood while the caudal portion of the body receives deoxygenated blood. The result is normal oral mucous membrane color and cyanotic preputial, penile, and vulvar mucous membrane color (differential cyanosis) (Color Plate 39). The cyanotic caudal mucous membrane color is exaggerated with and immediately following exercise. Generalized cyanosis can also occur. In one such reported case, radiopaque dye was observed to stream cranially from the PDA into the brachiocephalic trunk.[17] Dogs with cyanosis generally have arterial oxygen tensions between 30 and 40 mm Hg. Occasionally we will see a dog with a right-to-left shunting PDA that is not cyanotic. Presumably these dogs are examined at a time during which pulmonary vascular resistance and systemic vascular resistance are such that only a small-to-moderate amount of right-to-left shunting is occurring. Arterial oxygen tension in these dogs is commonly in the 50- to 70-mm Hg range.

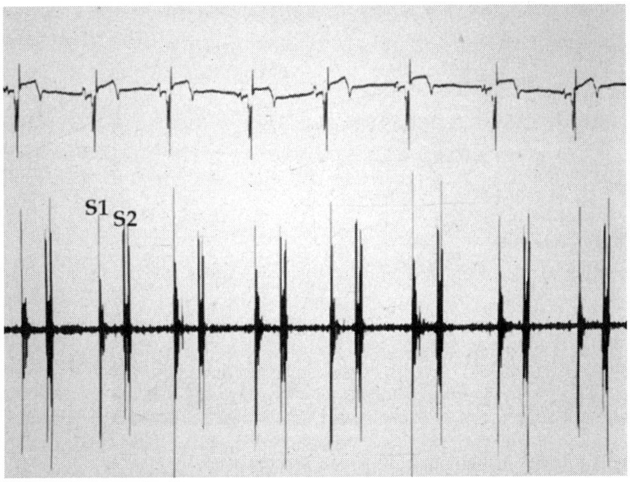

FIGURE 12-4 Lead II electrocardiogram *(top)* and phonocardiogram *(bottom)* from a 2-year-old American cocker spaniel with a right-to-left shunting patent ductus arteriosus. The first heart sound is normal. The second heart sound is split into two separate components. The first component is due to aortic valve closure, and the second component is due to late pulmonic valve closure. The pulmonic valve closes late because pulmonary hypertension causes an increase in right ventricular afterload, prolonging the right ventricular ejection time. The electrocardiogram shows evidence of right ventricular hypertrophy.

LABORATORY FINDINGS

The CBC and chemistry profile in most dogs with a left-to-right shunting PDA are normal. The hematocrit is commonly elevated to greater than 55% (polycythemia) in dogs with a right-to-left shunting PDA. Serum for blood glucose determination from these dogs must be separated from the red cells soon after collection, because the increased number of red cells will result in an increased rate of decline in the glucose concentration.[18]

Analysis of blood gases from femoral arterial blood usually reveals an oxygen tension less than 40 mm Hg in dogs that are symptomatic for a right-to-left shunting PDA. Hypoxemia is also present in dogs with a left-to-right shunting PDA if pulmonary edema is present. However, it is usually greater than 50 mm Hg unless the edema is marked.

RADIOGRAPHY

Radiographic changes depend on the size of the PDA (Figures 12-5 to 12-7). Dogs with a large left-to-right shunting PDA commonly have a long cardiac silhouette on the dorsoventral radiograph. The left ventricular enlargement extends the cardiac silhouette caudally, and the dilated aortic arch extends it cranially. The left heart enlargement is commonly great enough to give the appearance of generalized cardiomegaly. However, right heart enlargement is not present. An aneurysmal bulge in the descending aorta in the region of the ductus origin ("ductal aneurysm") is a common finding on the dorsovental radiograph. Left atrial enlargement may be identifiable on both the dorsoventral and lateral radiographs. An increase in the main pulmonary artery size may be visualized as a bulge at the 2-o'clock position on the dorsoventral radiograph. An increase in pulmonary vascular size ("overcirculation") may be observed. However, the variation in pulmonary vascular size in normal dogs makes this observation difficult. Pulmonary venous enlargement and pulmonary edema are visible in dogs with left heart failure.

Dogs with right-to-left shunting PDAs commonly have the descending aortic bulge visible on the dorsoventral radiograph (Figure 12-8). Evidence of right ventricular enlargement may also be visible. Peripheral pulmonary vasculature may be diminished. Proximal pulmonary vasculature may be diminished or enlarged.

ELECTROCARDIOGRAPHY

In dogs with a large left-to-right shunting PDA the electrocardiogram is often abnormal. The most common abnormality is an increase in *R* wave height in lead II as a result of left ventricular enlargement. This reportedly is present in approximately 50% of cases with left ventricular enlargement.[19] The increase in *R* wave height is frequently impressive, sometimes reaching 5 to 6 mV. A wide *P* wave may also be present, signaling left atrial enlargement. The *P* wave, however, is often normal even when left atrial enlargement is present.

The ECG in dogs with right-to-left shunting PDAs can provide evidence for right ventricular enlargement. A right axis deviation in the limb leads, especially of the terminal forces, is most frequently present. A deep *S* wave in a left chest lead is also commonly present and may be present without changes in the limb leads.

ECHOCARDIOGRAPHY

The echocardiogram provides direct and indirect evidence for the presence and severity of a PDA. In a left-to-right shunting PDA, the

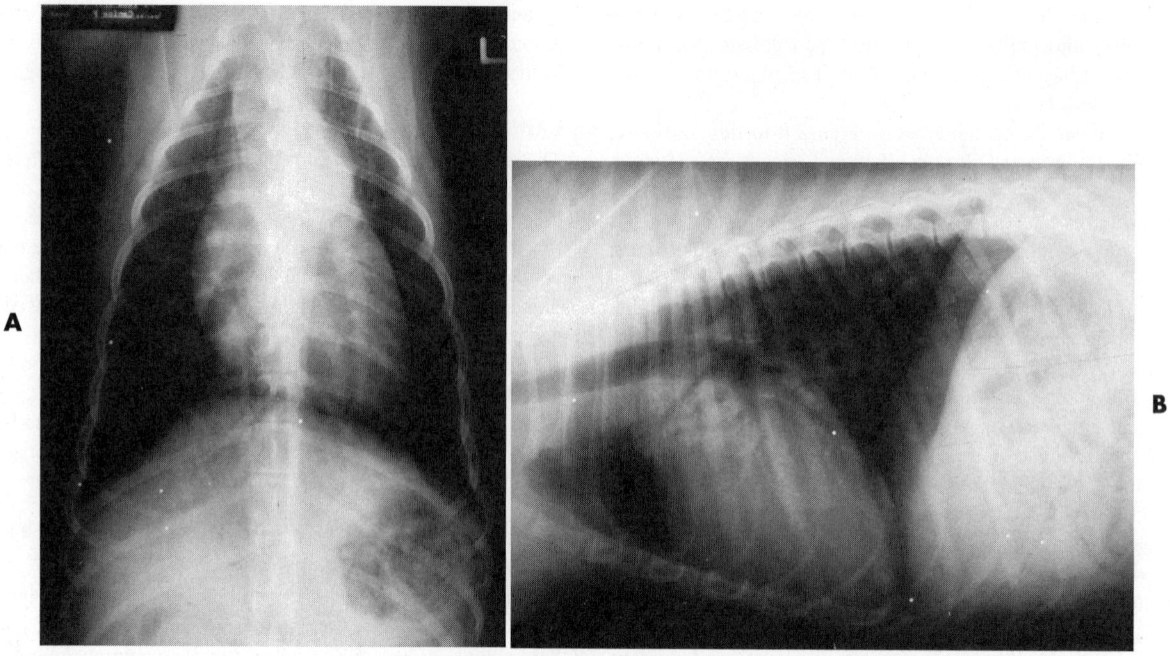

FIGURE 12-5 Dorsoventral (DV) **(A)** and lateral **(B)** radiographs from a 10-month-old Brittany spaniel with a moderate-size patent ductus arteriosus. The left atrium is not enlarged. On the DV radiograph, a ductal aneurysm can be identified on the proximal descending aorta. The left ventricle is closer to the chest wall than the right ventricle on the DV radiograph, indicating that it probably is enlarged. The cardiac silhouette is also somewhat longer than normal on the DV view. The cardiac size, however, is not markedly enlarged. The pulmonary vasculature is normal.

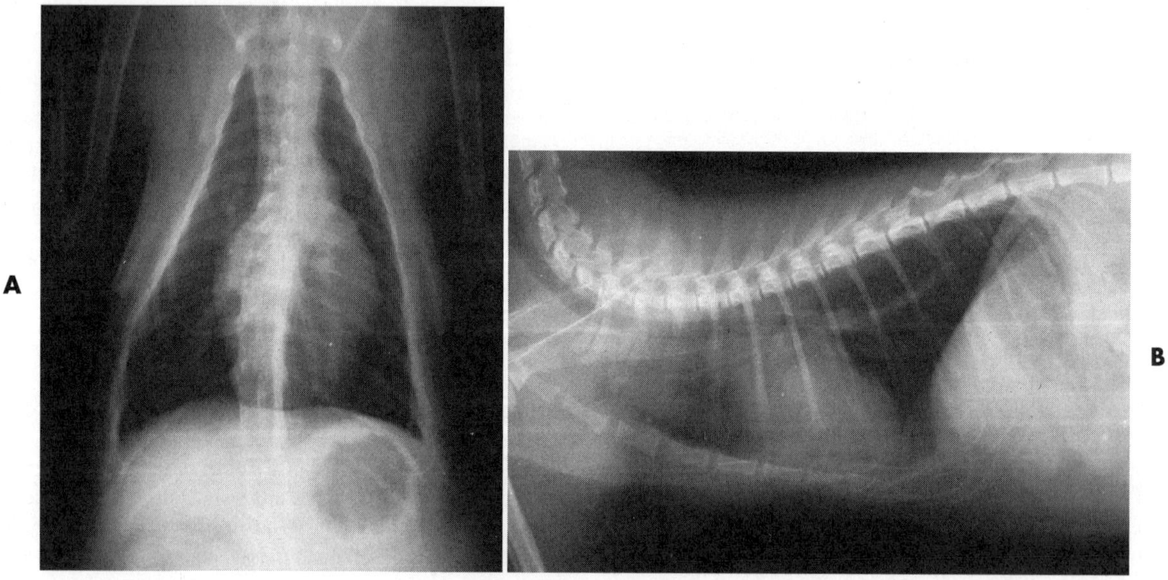

FIGURE 12-6 Dorsoventral **(A)** and lateral **(B)** radiographs from an 8-month-old cat with a patent ductus arteriosus. The cat had moderate left atrial and left ventricular volume overload on an echocardiogram. The radiographs reveal a large ductal aneurysm with moderate cardiomegaly. The pulmonary vasculature is prominent for a young cat.

left ventricular end-diastolic diameter is increased and the left ventricular wall thicknesses are normal. The size of the left ventricle (end-diastolic diameter) generally should correspond to the size of the PDA. Left ventricular end-systolic diameter is normal to increased, and shortening fraction is usually in the normal range (Figure 12-9). End-systolic diameter tends to be normal in young dogs and increased in older dogs. The left atrium is usually enlarged to a similar degree as the left ventricle. The right ventricle and atrium are normal.

Color flow Doppler echocardiography in a left-to-right shunting PDA often reveals a small mitral regurgitant jet. Identifying continuous turbulent flow with spectral or color flow Doppler in the

A

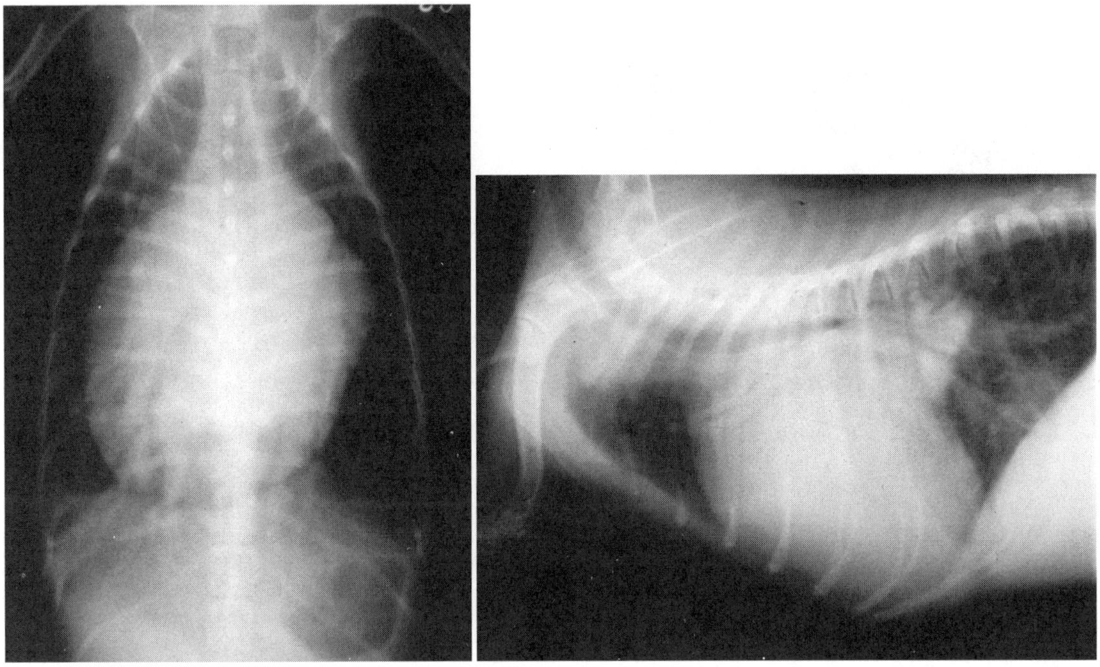

B

FIGURE 12-7 Dorsoventral **(A)** and lateral **(B)** radiographs from a 5-year-old female Maltese with a patent ductus arteriosus. The cardiac silhouette is markedly enlarged. The left atrium is especially prominent. The right heart appears enlarged. However, it was of normal size on an echocardiogram. Pulmonary edema is present, and the echocardiogram reveals severe volume overload hypertrophy and severe myocardial failure.

A

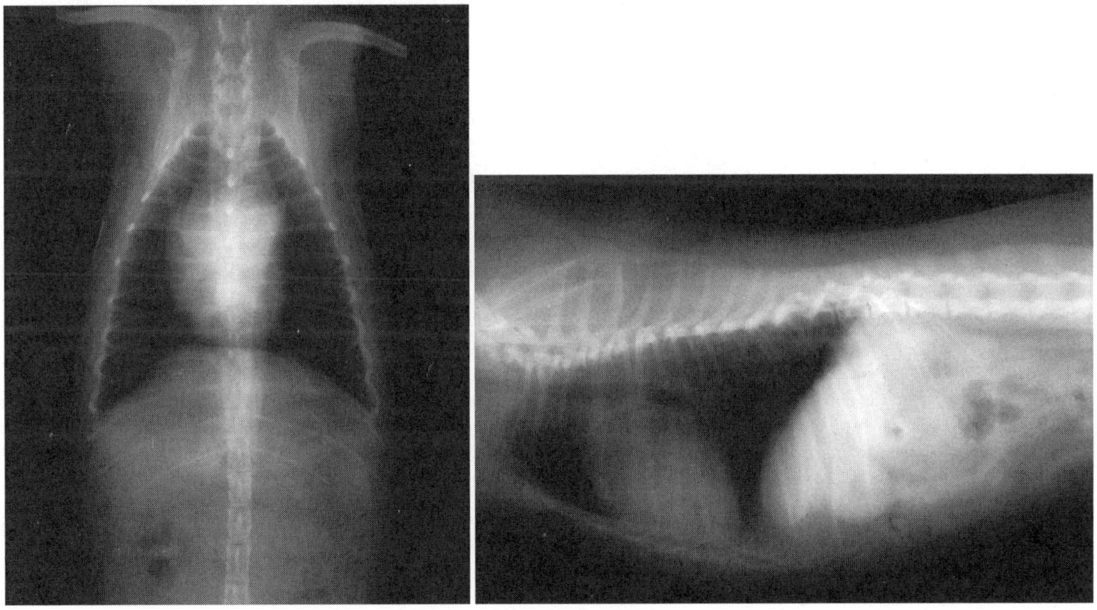

B

FIGURE 12-8 Dorsoventral **(A)** and lateral **(B)** thoracic radiographs from a miniature poodle with a right-to-left shunting patent ductus arteriosus (PDA). On the dorsoventral view, there is a large bulge in the descending aorta between the fourth and fifth ribs where the PDA originates. The cardiac silhouette does not appear to be enlarged. The lung fields are hypovascular.

main pulmonary artery viewed from any position is characteristic of a PDA. The PDA itself can be visualized from a left cranial sternal view using two-dimensional echocardiography (Figure 12-10). The ductal anatomy is characteristic, with the aortic end being wide and the pulmonary artery end narrow, resulting in a funnel shape. Using color flow Doppler markedly simplifies identification of the PDA. The region of the PDA is first identified on two-dimensional echocardiography and then interrogated with color flow Doppler. Laminar flow can be identified proximally to the narrowed region of the PDA. Flow becomes turbulent as it traverses the narrowed region and a large turbulent jet can be observed passing from the narrowed region of the PDA into the pulmonary artery and flowing toward the

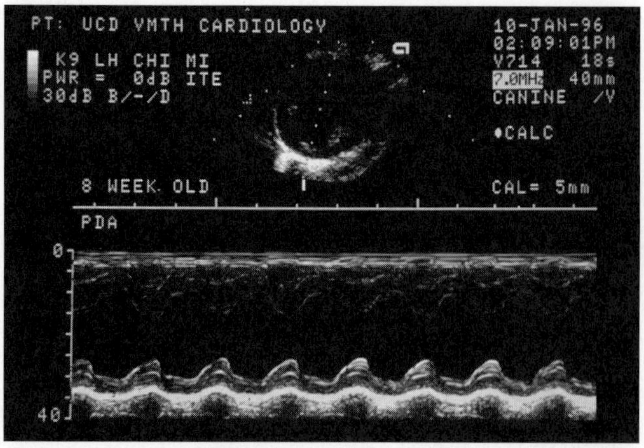

FIGURE 12-9 M-mode echocardiogram from an 8-week-old long-haired Chihuahua with a left-to-right shunting patent ductus arteriosus (PDA). The end-diastolic diameter is increased, and the end-systolic diameter is normal to decreased. The shortening fraction is approximately 40%. This echocardiogram is typical for a young dog with a PDA. Older dogs commonly have an increase in the end-systolic diameter as myocardial contractility decreases.

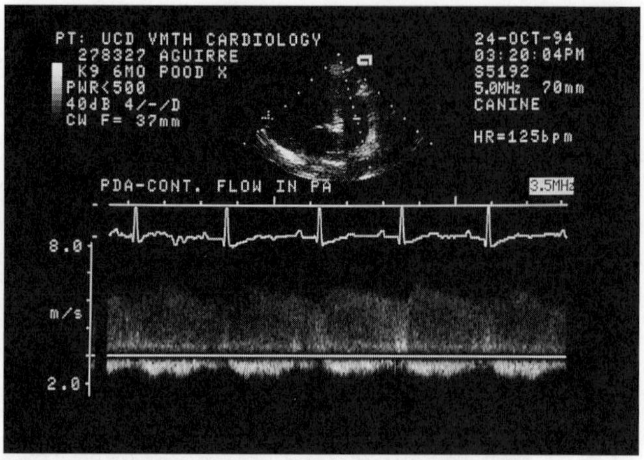

FIGURE 12-11 Continuous-wave Doppler recording of blood flow velocity in the pulmonary artery of a 6-week-old poodle-cross. The ultrasound beam is directed into the high-velocity jet of blood flowing into the main pulmonary artery, toward the transducer. The recording demonstrates that the blood flow is continuous. Peak velocity occurs in mid-to-late systole and is approximately 5 m/sec, consistent with a pressure gradient across the patent ductus arteriosus (between the aorta and pulmonary artery) of 100 mm Hg.

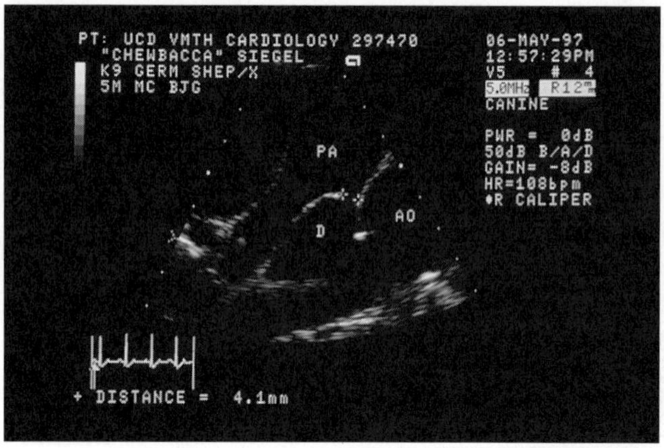

FIGURE 12-10 Two-dimensional echocardiogram from a 5-month-old German shepherd-cross with a left-to-right shunting patent ductus arteriosus (PDA). The echocardiogram was taken from a left cranial view. It shows the PDA *(D)* originating from the aorta *(AO)* and connecting to the pulmonary artery *(PA)*. The PDA is funnel-shaped, with the aortic end wide and the pulmonary artery end narrow (4.1 mm).

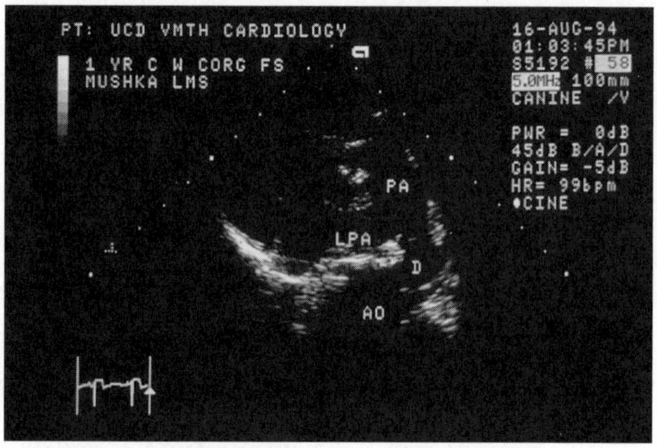

FIGURE 12-12 Two-dimensional echocardiogram from a 1-year-old Cardigan Welsh corgi dog with a right-to-left shunting patent ductus arteriosus (PDA) *(D)*. The view is the same as that in Figure 12-10. In contrast to the echocardiogram in Figure 12-10, the pulmonary artery end of the PDA is not narrowed. Rather, it is as wide as the aortic end, providing a wide-open conduit between the aorta *(AO)* and the main pulmonary artery *(PA)*. *LPA,* Left pulmonary artery.

pulmonic valve (Color Plate 40). The jet frequently strikes the pulmonic valve and wraps back within the pulmonary artery toward the PDA. Spectral Doppler interrogation of the jet shows continuous flow. The flow velocity pattern is analogous to the sound of the murmur, peaking at end-systole and decreasing in velocity throughout diastole (Figure 12-11). Peak velocity is between 4 and 6 m/sec. In a right-to-left shunting PDA, right ventricular concentric hypertrophy is present. The left ventricle and left atrium are normal to small. Ductal anatomy may also be visualized using two-dimensional echocardiography in a right-to-left shunting ductus. The characteristic funnel shape observed with a left-to-right shunting PDA is not seen. Rather, a wide-open conduit between the aorta and pulmonary artery is seen either with transthoracic or transesophageal echocardiography (Figures 12-12 and 12-13). Color flow and spectral Doppler may demonstrate the right-to-left laminar blood flow (Color Plate 41). Presence of an extracardiac right-to-left shunt can be confirmed using contrast echocardiography. Microbubble-laden saline is injected into a peripheral vein and the cardiac image is examined first to document that no intracardiac right-to-left shunt is present. Subsequently the abdominal aorta near the bladder is imaged while the microbubbles are injected. Visualization of microbubbles in the abdominal aorta confirms the presence of a right-to-left shunt (Figure 12-14). Because an intracardiac shunt has already been ruled out, an extracardiac shunt must be present. Pulmonary hypertension can be documented by estimating right ventricular systolic and pulmonary artery pressures using tricuspid regurgitant and pulmonic regurgitant velocities, if regurgitation is present (Figure 12-15).

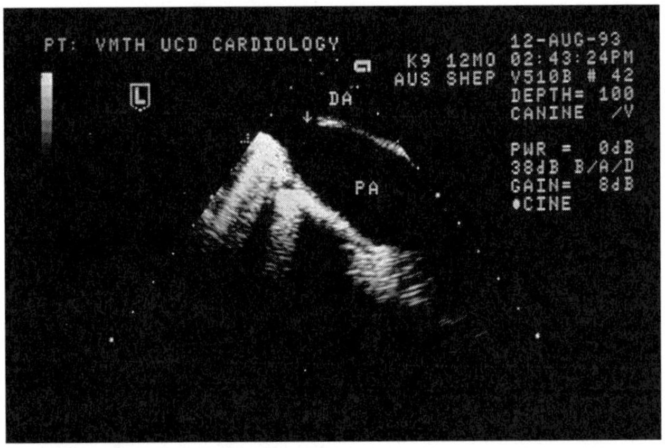

FIGURE 12-13 Transesophageal echocardiogram of a right-to-left shunting patent ductus arteriosus (PDA) from a 1-year-old Australian shepherd. The arrow points to the pulmonary artery (PA) end of the PDA (DA). The pulmonary artery end is not narrowed.

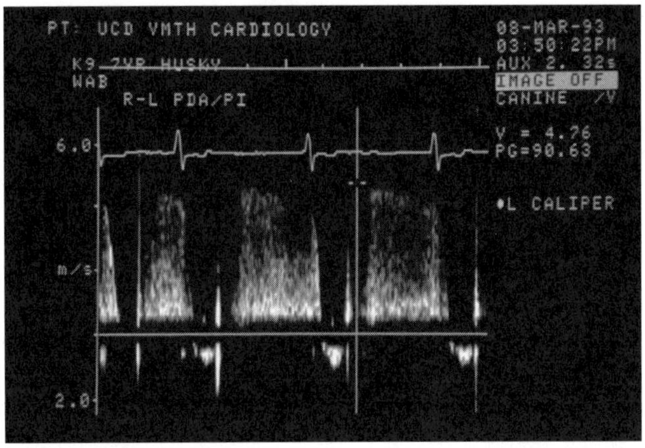

FIGURE 12-15 Continuous-wave Doppler echocardiogram of a pulmonary regurgitation jet from a 7-year-old Siberian husky with a right-to-left shunting patent ductus arteriosus. The jet velocity is increased to 4.8 m/sec, indicating a 91-mm Hg pressure difference (gradient) across the pulmonic valve (from the pulmonary artery to the right ventricle) in diastole. Normal pressure gradient is in the 10- to 15-mm Hg range. This high velocity is diagnostic of severe pulmonary hypertension.

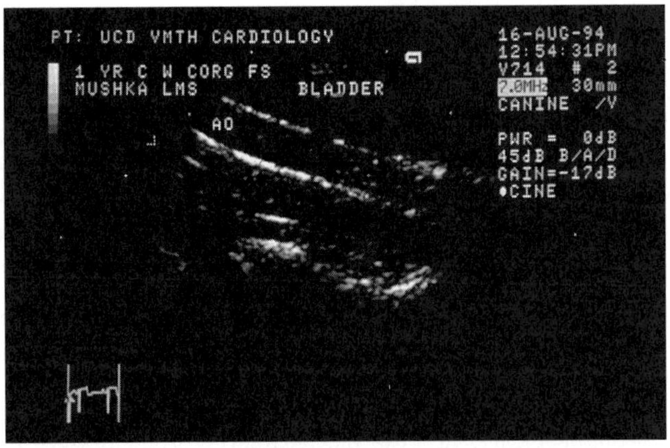

FIGURE 12-14 Ultrasound image of the terminal portion of the abdominal aorta from a dog with a right-to-left shunting patent ductus arteriosus (PDA). Agitated saline mixed with a small amount of blood was injected into a peripheral vein. The bubbles present in this mixture are visualized within the aorta, documenting a right-to-left shunt. No evidence of an intracardiac right-to-left shunt was found in this dog, confirming the presence of an extracardiac shunt, which is usually a PDA.

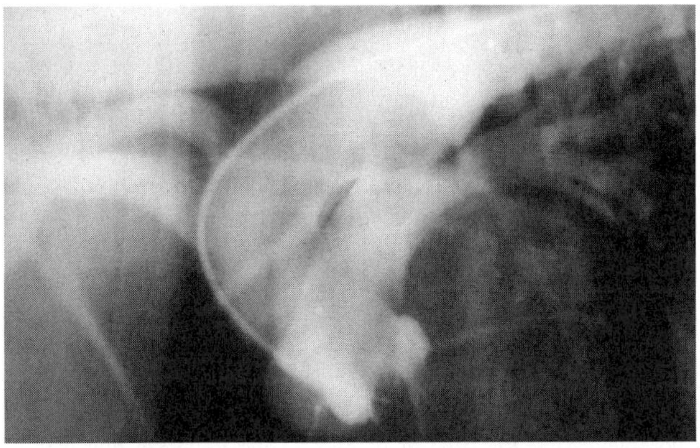

FIGURE 12-16 Angiogram of a left-to-right shunting patent ductus arteriosus (PDA). The catheter is placed in the aortic root. Contrast fills the aorta, PDA, and pulmonary artery. The anatomy is identical to that shown in Color Plate 38.

In the dogs with moderate-to–moderately large left-to-right shunting PDAs that present in heart failure in adulthood, the two-dimensional echocardiogram often resembles that of dilated cardiomyopathy. The end-systolic diameter is markedly increased because of severe myocardial failure. There is a severe, compensatory increase in the end-diastolic diameter. Shortening fraction is less than 20% and may be much lower.

CARDIAC CATHETERIZATION

Cardiac catheterization is rarely required to document the presence of a left-to-right shunting PDA. Radiopaque dye injection into the left ventricle or aorta confirms the presence of this type of PDA (Figure 12-16).

Cardiac catheterization may be required to document the presence of a right-to-left shunting PDA. Injection of radiopaque dye into the right ventricle outlines the right ventricle, the main pulmonary artery, the large PDA, and the descending aorta (Figure 12-17). Dye injection into the left heart may show some left-to-right flow through the PDA. Simultaneous right and left ventricular pressure measurement demonstrates identical systolic pressures in both ventricles. Simultaneous aortic and pulmonary artery pressure measurement also verifies equilibration of pressures.

DIFFERENTIAL DIAGNOSIS

Differential diagnoses at the time of physical examination include aorticopulmonary window, truncus arteriosus, ruptured sinus of Valsalva, systemic arteriovenous fistula in the chest, coronary artery fistula, pulmonary arteriovenous fistula, branch pulmonary artery stenosis, ventricular septal defect with aortic regurgitation, aortic stenosis with aortic regurgitation, and pulmonic stenosis with pulmonic regurgitation. The last three lesions produce to-and-fro murmurs rather than continuous murmurs. A to-and-fro murmur is a systolic murmur and diastolic murmur that occur together. These heart murmurs generally have a different character and are often

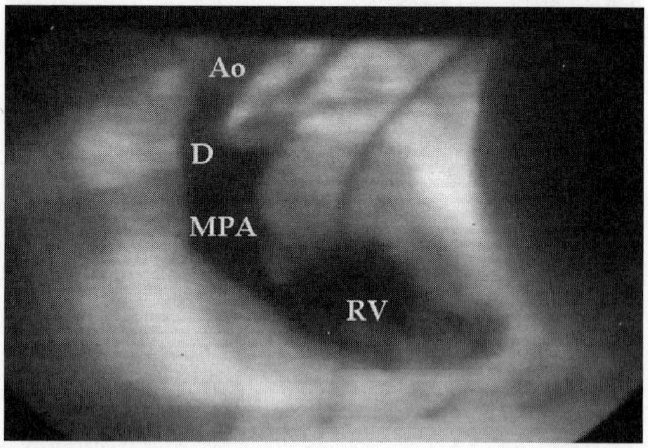

FIGURE 12-17 Computer-captured image from a videotape of an angiogram of a 2- year-old American cocker spaniel dog with a right-to-left shunting patent ductus arteriosus (PDA). A catheter has been advanced from a femoral vein into the right ventricle *(RV)*, where contrast material has been injected. The contrast material, along with blood, is ejected from the right ventricle into the aorta *(Ao)* dorsally and the pulmonary artery ventrally. The PDA *(D)* is the same size as the aorta and connects the dorsal portion of the main pulmonary artery *(MPA)* to the descending aorta.

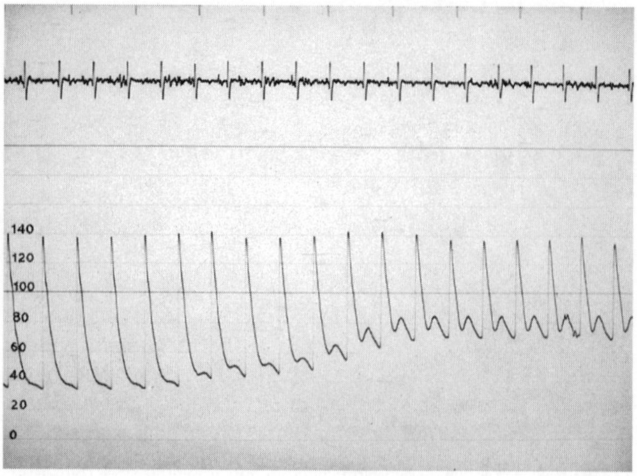

FIGURE 12-18 Recording of systemic arterial blood pressure during ligation of a patent ductus arteriosus in a 4-month-old Collie. Before ligation, the blood pressure is approximately 140 mm Hg in systole and 35 to 40 mm Hg in diastole in this anesthetized dog. The pulse pressure (systolic minus diastolic blood pressure) is increased to approximately 100 mm Hg. Following ligation, the systolic blood pressure remains at approximately 140 mm Hg, and the diastolic blood pressure increases to approximately 70 mm Hg. The aortic and carotid baroreceptors should sense this increase in blood pressure, resulting in a decrease in the heart rate in a patient that has not been administered atropine (Branham's sign).

heard in a different location than the typical PDA. All of the other defects are very rare in the dog and cat. Most, however, have been reported. If any doubt exists, a definitive echocardiographic diagnosis of a PDA should be made before surgery.

Treatment

SURGERY

Surgical ligation of a left-to-right shunting PDA is almost always recommended at the time of diagnosis. The youngest dog that we have sent to surgery was 2 weeks old. Many dogs with a large PDA will develop left heart failure if left untreated. Because surgical ligation is curative, surgery is always recommended in a patient with evidence of moderate-to-severe cardiac enlargement. In one study, of 14 dogs not treated surgically, nine died within 1 year of admission and the other five were lost to follow-up.[15] Some dogs have clinical or radiographic evidence of pulmonary edema at the time of diagnosis. Furosemide therapy for 24 to 48 hours before anesthetic induction should be carried out in these dogs. Elimination of pulmonary edema is the goal.

The surgery to ligate a PDA is described elsewhere.[20] Briefly, a thoracotomy is performed through the left fourth intercostal space. The PDA is visualized and palpated before dissection (Color Plate 42). Palpation reveals fremitus over the ductus and main pulmonary artery. Dissection is carefully performed straight down toward the opposite chest wall caudal to the PDA. Following this, dissection cranial to the ductus, between the aorta and pulmonary artery is carried out, again toward the opposite chest wall to a distance slightly greater than the width of the PDA. At this time, a curved forceps is used to dissect around the back side of the PDA, starting from the cranial dissection and carefully dissecting in a caudomedial direction, parallel to the long axis of the aorta. When the tips of the forceps are exposed, two 1-0 silk ligatures or strands of umbilical tape are drawn around the PDA, and tied down firmly (Color Plate 43). Diastolic systemic arterial blood pressure increases after ductal ligation. (Figure 12-18). Systolic pressure often remains the same. This results in a decrease in pulse pressure and normalization of the femoral pulse.

Operative mortality is low (less than 5%) for experienced surgeons, although mortality may approach 7% to 9%.[21] PDA surgery should not be performed by an inexperienced individual unless there is adequate supervision.

Postoperative complications are few. Most surgery is performed in young dogs that recover very quickly from thoracotomy. About 2% to 3% of dogs will have enough residual shunting to produce a continuous heart murmur. These dogs should be evaluated echocardiographically to determine if the residual shunt is hemodynamically significant. Most are not. If one is, the PDA may need to be religated. Many dogs will have a residual systolic heart murmur as a result of mitral regurgitation following surgery. Usually this murmur disappears over a week to several months following surgery. It is almost never hemodynamically significant in a young dog. "Silent" residual flow through the ligated ductus is more common. Residual flow can be identified in about 20% of patients using color flow Doppler.[22] A "silent" ductus does not produce any known significant clinical sequelae.

Following surgery, the end-diastolic diameter and volume of the left ventricle decrease while end-systolic diameter and volume tend to remain the same because myocardial function doesn't change. This results in a decrease in the amount of myocardial contraction, as evidenced by a decrease in shortening fraction. Shortening fraction can decrease to as low as 15% in some dogs. This is more common in dogs that are not young puppies. Although spectacular on an echocardiogram, left ventricular pump function is almost always adequate and the dogs show no evidence of heart failure. Myocardial function may improve over time.

Surgical ligation of right-to-left shunting PDAs is generally thought to be contraindicated. In these cases, pulmonary vascular disease is severe, resulting in a high and fixed pulmonary vascular resistance. In a right-to-left shunt, right heart output of blood is greater than left heart output, with much of the right heart output flowing through the PDA. When the PDA is ligated in this situation, the right heart continues to pump an increased quantity of flow into the fixed resistance, resulting in an even higher pulmonary artery pressure. Dogs with right-to-left shunting PDA that have had their PDA ligated, often die within the first 36 hours following surgery.[23] Partial ligation of a right-to-left shunting PDA may be theoretically sound. Our cardiovascular surgeon has tied off a right-to-left shunting PDA in two stages in one dog. He partially ligated the PDA and then completely closed it 2 weeks later. The dog lived but did not change clinically and still became cyanotic, presumably from chronic pulmonary disease. Any dog treated like this would be expected to have residual severe pulmonary hypertension. The prognosis for severe pulmonary hypertension resulting from pulmonary vascular disease is generally poor.

MEDICAL MANAGEMENT

Pharmacologic closure of the ductus with aspirin or indomethacin is effective in premature human infants whose ductus has adequate smooth muscle but lacks the stimulus to close.[3,4] Patent ductus arteriosus in the dog is due to lack of smooth muscle in the ductus arteriosus. Consequently, pharmacologic closure of the PDA in puppies examined by veterinarians at 5 weeks of age and beyond is not logical. Despite this fact, there is a report in the veterinary literature describing a 5-week-old Shi Tzu puppy with a continuous heart murmur that was administered indomethacin intravenously (0.15 mg/kg q12h for 48 hours).[24] This puppy clinically improved with an increase in body weight. The heart murmur changed in character but did not disappear. The puppy died 8 days later from congestive heart failure. The ductus arteriosus was patent.

Medical management of a left-to-right shunting PDA is aimed at treating heart failure. In young dogs with pulmonary edema as a result of a large PDA, furosemide administration before surgical ligation is all that is required. In the older dog with a moderate-to–moderately large ductus that has gone into heart failure because of the PDA and myocardial failure, furosemide, an ACE inhibitor, and digoxin should be administered and the PDA surgically ligated.

Medical management of the dog with a right-to-left shunting PDA is aimed at reducing the hematocrit. Most of the clinical signs noted in dogs with a right-to-left shunting PDA are a result of the hyperviscosity caused by the polycythemia. Consequently, successful management of the polycythemia can result in good long-term management of these patients. Phlebotomy is the procedure of choice. Mild decreases in hematocrit can produce significant clinical benefit. Overzealous phlebotomy decreases tissue oxygen delivery to the point that the patient becomes symptomatic (usually depressed). One method is to set a goal of restoring the hematocrit to 60% to 65%. To determine the amount of blood to remove one should use the following formula:

$$\text{Blood to be removed (mL)} = [\text{Body weight (kg)} \times 0.08] \times 1000\ \text{mL/kg} \times \frac{[\text{Actual hematocrit} - \text{Desired hematocrit}]}{\text{Actual hematocrit}}$$

Blood is removed through a large-bore catheter. The amount of blood removed is replaced with intravenous fluid (1 to 2 times the blood volume removed) while the blood is being withdrawn. It is common for the hematocrit to be greater than calculated once the phlebotomy is completed. This is probably due to release of stored red cells from extramedullary sites such as the spleen. Another method is to hospitalize the patient for the day and remove 10% of blood volume in the morning without replacing the blood volume with intravenous fluids. In the afternoon, another 2% to 10% of blood volume is removed and the patient sent home. This method has been used successfully in four dogs and for up to 8 years in one patient.[25] Hydroxyurea can be tried in cases that require frequent phlebotomies or that do not tolerate phlebotomy. Hydroxyurea is a myelosuppressive agent that produces reversible bone marrow suppression. It is administered initially as a loading dose of 30 mg/kg/day for 7 to 10 days followed by 15 mg/kg/day. Complete blood counts and platelet counts must be followed every 1 to 2 weeks. Leukopenia, thrombocytopenia, or anemia necessitate discontinuing the drug until the blood counts normalize. A lower dose may then be administered. Some dogs require higher doses to induce a decrease in hematocrit. The side effects of hydroxyurea in the dog include anorexia, vomiting, bone marrow hypoplasia, and sloughing of the nails.[26] As expected, some dogs do not tolerate hydroxyurea administration.

INTERVENTIONAL CLOSURE

Occlusion of a PDA with a percutaneous device is an alternative to surgical closure of a PDA. Closure of the PDA by an occlusion device has been described in dogs with naturally occurring PDAs.[27] Transcatheter occlusion involves placing a device in the PDA that stimulates clot formation or that itself occludes the ductus to completely interrupt blood flow. Several devices have been described, including discs, coils, and sacks. Gianturco helical coils (Cooke, Inc., Bloomington, Ind.) have been successfully placed in small dogs (5 to 20 lb) with naturally occurring PDAs.[27] Placement of these devices requires anesthesia, cardiac catheterization, and a skilled operator. Gianturco coils are made of wire coated with strands of wool to promote thrombosis. The coils are deployed through a cardiac catheter that is advanced from a femoral artery into the descending aorta and through the PDA into the pulmonary artery. One coil of the device is placed in the pulmonary artery and withdrawn to a point at which the end of the first coil hooks into the pulmonary artery end of the ductus. Subsequent coils are placed in the duct as the device is extruded. The device cannot be retrieved once it is deployed. The most common major complication is migration of the device immediately after it is deployed, resulting in embolization of a pulmonary artery. Pulmonary embolization, however, usually does not result in clinical sequelae, and the devices can be retrieved using a basket retrieval device (Med-Tech, Watertown, Mass.) or wire snare. The use of Gianturco coils to occlude PDAs is problematic and requires an experienced and skilled operator. The major advantage of this device is its price (approximately $30.00).

A newer device looks more promising for future use. The Gianturco-Grifka vascular occlusion device (Cooke, Inc., Bloomington, Ind.) consists of a nylon sack attached to an end-hole catheter. The catheter and sack are delivered to the ductus through a long delivery sheath. The sack is advanced into the ductus. It is then filled with modified guide wire (the stiff inner core has been removed) to distend it and fix it in place in the ductus. The filler wire is attached to a pusher wire. If the sack is not in proper position, the filler wire can be removed and the sack repositioned and filled again. Once placement is satisfactory, an angiogram is performed to confirm closure of the ductus. After confirmation, the sack is removed from the end of the catheter by pulling the catheter into the delivery sheath. Migration of this device is much less likely. An initial study performed in experimental dogs has confirmed that this device can occlude subclavian arteries and aortopulmonary shunts crafted from Gore-Tex.[28] The major drawback of this device is price ($650.00). The devices come in 3-, 6-, and 9-mm sizes, which make them useful only for small dogs, probably under 10 to 15 kg.

Although occlusion of PDAs by devices is feasible, it is doubtful that this procedure will find widespread utility in veterinary medicine within the near future. Coils, although inexpensive, are difficult to use and have potential complications. Very few individuals are currently trained to use them, and training of more individuals will require either trial-and-error learning or mentored-learning. Mentored-learning of individuals, other than residents training with experienced individuals, is unlikely. Use of the Gianturco-Grifka device may become popular in the future if the price for this device decreases. These devices have few advantages over surgery. The need for anesthesia and the time for anesthesia are similar. There is no postoperative pain or morbidity with occlusion devices, but most dogs that have surgery to ligate a PDA are young dogs. Young dogs are very resilient creatures that often are able to play the day following surgery. Older dogs with compromised cardiac function may be better candidates for this type of procedure. However, the lesser number of these dogs makes it difficult to gain and retain experience with these devices. Consequently, surgical ligation is still the procedure of choice in our hospital.

REFERENCES

1. Jones CL, Buchanan JW: Patent ductus arteriosus: anatomy and surgery in a cat, *J Am Vet Med Assoc* 179:364, 1981.
2. Heymann MA, Rudolph AM: Control of the ductus arteriosus, *Physiol Rev* 55:62, 1975.
3. Heymann MA, Rudolph AM, Silverman NH: Closure of the ductus arteriosus in premature infants by inhibition of prostaglandin synthesis, *N Engl J Med* 295:530, 1976.
4. Friedman WF, Hirschklau MJ, Printz MP et al: Pharmacologic closure of patent ductus arteriosus in the premature infant, *N Engl J Med* 295:526, 1976.
5. McCarthy JS, Zies LG, Gelband H: Age-dependent closure of the patent ductus arteriosus by indomethacin, *Pediatrics* 62:706, 1978.
6. Patterson DF: Genes and the heart: congenital heart disease, *Proc Acad Vet Cardiol,* 1991, p13.
7. Buchanan JW: Patent ductus arteriosus, ductal aneurysm, and pulmonary hypertension, *Proc Annu Vet Med Forum,* 1994, p 307.
8. Patterson DF: Congenital defects of the cardiovascular system of dogs: studies in comparative cardiology, *Adv Vet Sci Comp Med* 20:1, 1976.
9. Patterson DF, Pyle RL, Buchanan JW et al: Hereditary patent ductus arteriosus and its sequelae in the dog, *Circ Res* 29:1, 1971.
10. Pyle RL, Park RD, Alexander AF et al: Patent ductus arteriosus with pulmonary hypertension in the dog, *J Am Vet Med Assoc* 178:565, 1981.
11. Levin DL, Rudolph AM, Heymann MA et al: Morphological development of the pulmonary vascular bed in fetal lambs, *Circulation* 53:144, 1976.
12. Friedman WF. Congenital heart disease in infancy and childhood. In Braunwald E, ed: *Heart disease: a textbook of cardiovascular medicine,* ed 5, Philadelphia, 1997, WB Saunders.
13. Reddy VM, Meyrick B, Wong J et al: In utero placement of aortopulmonary shunts: a model of postnatal pulmonary hypertension with increased pulmonary blood flow in lambs, *Circulation* 2:606, 1995.
14. Espino-Vela J, Cardenas N, Cruz R: Patent ductus arteriosus: with special reference to patients with pulmonary hypertension, *Circulation* 38(suppl 5):V45, 1968.
15. Eyster GE, Eyster JT, Cords GB et al: Patent ductus arteriosus in the dog: characteristics of occurrence and results of surgery in one hundred consecutive cases, *J Am Vet Med Assoc* 168:435, 1976.
16. Perloff JK, Marelli AJ, Miner PD: Risk of stroke in adults with cyanotic congenital heart disease, *Circulation* 87:1954, 1993 (comments).
17. Oswald GP, Orton EC: Patent ductus arteriosus and pulmonary hypertension in related Pembroke Welsh corgis, *J Am Vet Med Assoc* 202:761, 1993.
18. Sidebottom RA, Williams PR, Kanarek KS: Glucose determinations in plasma and serum: potential error related to increased hematocrit, *Clin Chem* 28:190, 1982.
19. Chen K: Reevaluation and revision of electrocardiographic criteria for the diagnosis of left ventricular hypertrophy in dogs, *J Chin Vet Soc* 14:359, 1988.
20. Buchanan JW, Lawson DD: Cardiovascular surgery. In Archibald J: *Canine surgery,* ed 2, Santa Barbara, Calif, 1974, American Veterinary Publications.
21. Birchard SJ: Results of ligation of patent ductus arteriosus: 201 dogs (1969 to 1988), *J Am Vet Med Assoc* 196:2011, 1990.
22. Miller MW, Stepien RL, Meurs KM et al: Echocardiographic assessment of patent ductus arteriosus (PDA) after occlusion, *Proc Annu Vet Med Forum,* 1994, p 305.
23. Lombard CW, Knight DH, Buchanan JW et al: Clinico-pathologic conference: aorticopulmonary window, *J Am Vet Med Assoc* 172:75, 1978.
24. Atwell RB: Patent ductus arteriosus in a dog: attempted medical closure, *Vet Rec* 101:425, 1997.
25. Cote E, Ettinger SJ, Sisson DD: Long-term treatment of reversed patent ductus arteriosus (rPDA) in four dogs using phlebotomy alone, *J Vet Intern Med* 11:139, 1997 (abstract).
26. Campbell KL: Diagnosis and management of polycythemia in dogs, *Compend Cont Educ Pract Vet* 12:543, 1990.
27. Miller MW, Bonagura JD, Meurs KM et al: Percutaneous catheter occlusion of patent ductus arteriosus, *Proc Annu Vet Med Forum,* 1995, p 308.
28. Grifka RG, Mullins CE, Gianturco C et al: New Gianturco-Grifka vascular occlusion device: initial studies in a canine model, *Circulation* 91:1840, 1995.

CHAPTER 13

Septal Defects

Atrial Septal Defect

An atrial septal defect is a communication between the two atria that occurs because of a hole in the interatrial septum. In most situations, this results in shunting of blood from the left atrium into the right atrium and ventricle. When combined with right heart abnormalities, shunting may be right-to-left.

PREVALENCE

Atrial septal defects (ASD) are relatively common in humans, but they are relatively rare in dogs and cats. We have only definitively diagnosed ASD in 14 dogs over the past 10 years. Some of those were diagnosed as incidental defects, some as defects large enough to produce hemodynamic abnormalities, and some in conjunction with other defects. In the latter category, right-to-left shunting was commonly produced. Ostium secundum defects were the majority of the ASDs in these dogs. There was no predilection in this group of dogs, because 14 different breeds were represented. It is likely that many small ASDs go undetected in dogs, because they create no clinical signs and produce no heart murmur. There have been no clues that ASDs are hereditary in dogs. Within the same aforementioned period, we observed 15 cats with isolated ASD. Septum primum defects were more common in cats than in dogs. We also observed several cats that had no apparent interatrial septum.

Patent foramen ovale occurs when the septum primum and septum secundum fail to fuse and close the foramen ovale after birth. This results in a small communication between the left and right atria. A probe can be passed across the foramen ovale in approximately 30% of adult humans, but the defect is functionally closed.[1] In our experience, the presence of a probe patent foramen ovale is rare in dogs and cats. The only situation in which we think we commonly recognize a patent foramen ovale in dogs is in those with pulmonic stenosis. In these dogs, contrast echocardiography using agitated saline commonly identifies a small right-to-left shunt at the atrial level. This most likely occurs because the right atrial pressure in these dogs is probably always slightly higher than left atrial pressure, which prevents the foramen from closing.

EMBRYOLOGY

Two septa, the septum primum and the septum secundum, grow during fetal development to partition the two atria. The septum primum develops first. It starts as a ridge of crescent-shaped tissue along the roof of the primitive atria that grows apically toward the region of the atrioventricular valves. Extensions of the endocardial cushions grow along the edge of the septum primum. The defect that exists between these tissues and the floor of the atria is called the *ostium primum* of the septum primum. Proliferations of the septal tissue and fusion of the endocardial cushion tissue normally combine to close the ostium primum. Failure of this to occur results in a defect in the lower portion of the atrial septum and is termed an *ostium primum* atrial septal defect (ASD) (Figure 13-1). This most commonly occurs because of failure of the endocardial cushions to fuse in this region. Therefore an ostium primum defect is usually the result of an endocardial cushion defect. Before the ostium primum closes during fetal development, tissue resorption in the dorsal portion of the septum primum forms a second opening, creating the ostium secundum of the septum primum. Formation of this defect allows blood to continue to shunt from the right atrium to the left atrium in the fetus. At about the same time a second septum develops. This septum is positioned to the right of the septum primum and is termed the *septum secundum.* It also is a ridge of crescent-shaped tissue that originates from the roof of the atria. Its alignment and concave shape allow identification of two limbs of the septum secundum. The caudal limb fuses with the interatrial septum along the floor of the atria, and the cranial limb grows caudally to close the ostium secundum as the septum secundum grows to overlap the septum primum. The crescent shape of the septum secundum leaves a defect in its middle where it meets the septum primum. This opening is the foramen ovale, the last remaining communication between the left and right atria in the fetus. At birth, the change in hemodynamics pushes these two flaps of tissue into apposition and the foramen closes. Failure of the septum secundum to grow normally results in the ostium secundum remaining open and is termed an *ostium secundum* ASD (see Figure 13-1).

Besides ostium primum and ostium secundum types of ASDs, sinus venosus and coronary sinus defects are also described. Sinus venosus defects are thought to occur secondary to abnormal attachment of the right pulmonary veins to either the cranial or caudal vena cava. The defect occurs when the wall between these structures is resorbed (see Figure 13-1). Coronary sinus defects occur when the wall between the coronary sinus and the left atrium fails to develop.

PATHOPHYSIOLOGY

Small ASDs do not result in significant clinical abnormalities and are hemodynamically silent. In the absence of other cardiac abnormalities, moderate-to-large ASDs result in left-to-right shunting. The amount of shunting that occurs across the defect is related to the size of the defect and the relative compliances of the two ventricles in diastole. It is not directly related to the pressure gradient across the two atria, which is always small. Moderate-size defects provide resistance to blood flow and so help determine the amount of blood that flows from left-to-right. Large defects contribute no resistance to flow. In this situation, only the compliances of the two ventricles determine impedance to diastolic flow and so, in conjunction with

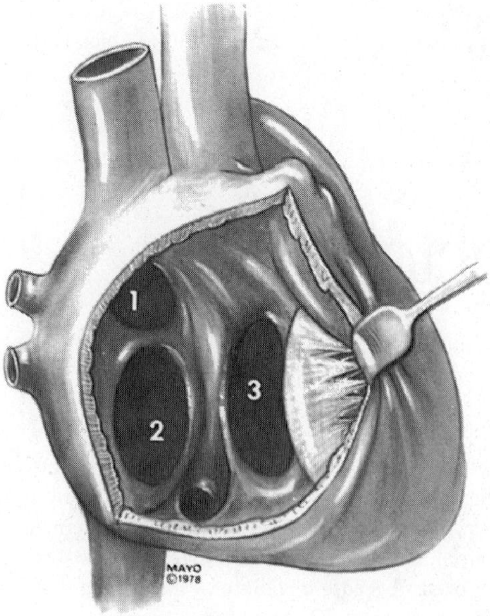

FIGURE 13-1 Drawing depicting three types of atrial septal defects. *(1),* Sinus venosus; *(2),* ostium secundum; and *(3),* ostium primum. (From Giuliani EM, Gersh BJ, McGoon MD et al, eds: *Mayo Clinic practice of cardiology,* St Louis, 1996, Mosby.)

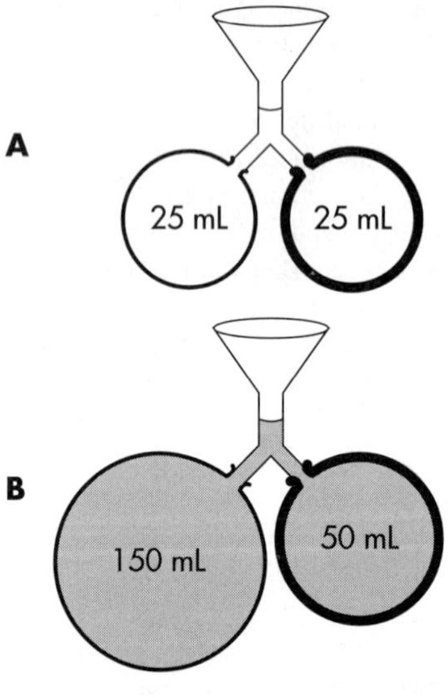

FIGURE 13-2 Schematic drawing demonstrating why blood flows from left-to-right through an atrial septal defect into the right ventricle. **A,** Two balloons are attached to either arm of a Y piece. The balloon on the right has a wall thickness 3 times greater than the one on the left. Both are filled with 25 mL of air. **B,** Two hundred milliliters of water have been poured into the top. The balloon with the thinner wall has filled to 3 times the capacity of the one with the thicker wall. This is similar to the way in which the thinner right ventricle fills in preference to the thicker-walled left ventricle during diastole in an atrial septal defect.

diastolic time, determine the amount of flow. To make this intuitively obvious, picture a Y piece with a funnel at the top, a thin-walled balloon connected to one arm of the Y, and a thick-walled balloon (3 times as thick as the thin-walled balloon) with the same initial volume connected to the other arm of the Y (Figure 13-2). Consider what would happen if water were poured into the funnel. The thin-walled balloon would fill to 3 times the volume of the

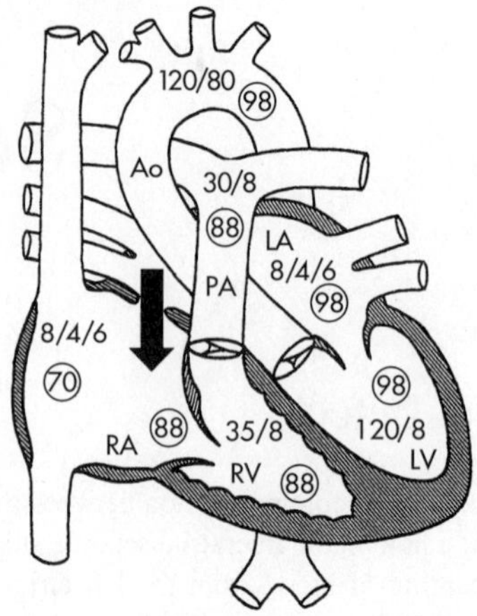

FIGURE 13-3 Schematic drawing of the circulation in a dog with a large left-to-right shunting atrial septal defect (ASD). The shunt results in right ventricular volume overload (not shown) and pulmonary overcirculation. There is mild systolic pulmonary hypertension. The oxygen saturation in the right ventricle is increased above the oxygen saturation in the proximal right atrium. Pulmonary blood flow (Q_p) is approximately 3 times systemic blood flow (Q_s). *RA,* Right atrium; *RV,* right ventricle; *LA,* left atrium; *LV,* left ventricle; *PA,* pulmonary artery; *Ao,* aorta. The arrow represents left-to-right flow through the ASD. Pressures are depicted as systolic/diastolic. Oxygen saturations are in circles.

thick-walled balloon. Because the right ventricle is approximately 2 to 3 times as compliant as the left ventricle (its walls are one half to one third as thick), the right ventricle can fill to 2 to 3 times the left ventricular quantity if there is no interatrial septum. In humans with a large ASD, pulmonary blood flow (right ventricular output) can exceed 3 times systemic blood flow (Figure 13-3).[1]

Atrial septal defects can occur in conjunction with other defects. When combined with pulmonic stenosis or pulmonary hypertension, significant right-to-left shunting and hypoxemia can occur. This occurs when the right ventricle concentrically hypertrophies, reducing its compliance. Tricuspid regurgitation also results in right-to-left shunting during systole as blood is ejected into the right atrium. We have seen mild-to-moderate but not severe polycythemia as a result of right-to-left shunting across an ASD in several cases. We have seen one case with pulmonic stenosis and an ASD in which balloon valvuloplasty resulted in tricuspid regurgitation. The acute tricuspid regurgitation resulted in marked right-to-left shunting and severe postoperative hypoxemia. The dog had to be taken to surgery, placed on cardiopulmonary bypass, and have its ASD closed.

CLINICAL FINDINGS

The classic auscultatory findings with a large left-to-right shunting ASD are a soft left basilar systolic heart murmur and a split second heart sound. The heart murmur is not due to flow across the ASD but rather to the increased flow of blood across the pulmonic valve. If 3 times the normal quantity of blood is ejected through the pulmonic valve in systole, blood flow velocity will increase to 3 times the normal value if ejection time remains the same. Usually ejection time is prolonged such that flow velocity does not increase quite to this degree. However, velocity can increase to the point that turbulence is created and a murmur generated (so-called relative pulmonic

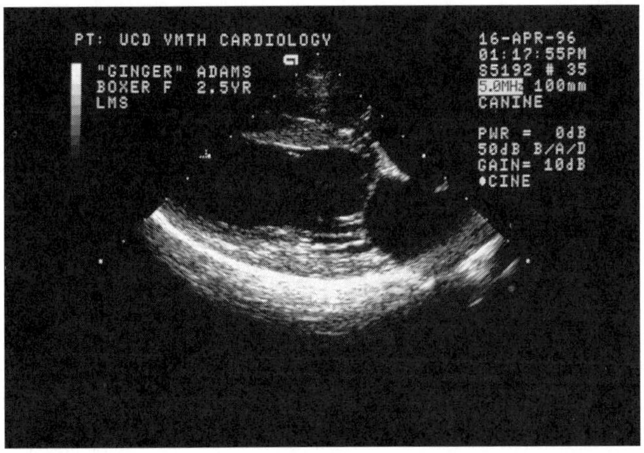

FIGURE 13-4 Two-dimensional echocardiogram from a 2-year-old male boxer with an atrial septal defect. This is a right parasternal long-axis view. The location of the defect in the atrial septum is consistent with an ostium secundum defect. It was identified as an incidental finding when the dog was screened for cardiomyopathy. The dog exhibited no clinical signs and did not have right heart enlargement. No treatment was recommended.

stenosis). The split second heart sound occurs because the right ventricular ejection time is longer than the left ventricular ejection time, delaying the closure of the pulmonic valve. Right ventricular ejection time is prolonged because of the marked increase in the amount of blood that the right ventricle must eject.

The left-to-right shunt at the atrial level results in right ventricular volume overload. The degree of right ventricular enlargement reflects the amount of blood that shunts left-to-right. In the absence of other cardiac abnormalities, a large defect will result in a large shunt, which will result in a large, eccentrically hypertrophied right ventricle. This is anatomically obvious on an echocardiogram and may be obvious on a thoracic radiograph.[2] An ECG may show evidence of right ventricular enlargement.[2-4] In addition, the pulmonary vasculature may be enlarged in proportion to the size of the defect and the shunt. The left ventricle may be smaller than normal in a large ASD.[2] The defect can be visualized using two-dimensional and color flow Doppler echocardiography (Figures 13-4 and Color Plate 44). When interrogating the interatrial septum, one should try to be as perpendicular to the septum as possible. Otherwise, "echo dropout" can occur, in which there appears to be an ASD when none exists (see Figure 6-7). This occurs when the ultrasound beam strikes a surface that is parallel with the beam, resulting in no ultrasound returning to the transducer. In general, a right-side parasternal long-axis view is used. ASDs, unless they are large and obvious, should be confirmed by identifying flow across the septum at the level of the defect with color flow Doppler. Pulsed-wave Doppler may also be used to interrogate this region.[2] In theory, the ratio of pulmonary blood flow to systemic blood flow (Q_p:Q_s) can be calculated by determining aortic and pulmonic velocity time integrals and multiplying them by their respective vessel diameters.[2] This has not been verified, however, by comparisons with other techniques in dogs or cats.

Patients that have concomitant right-side abnormalities that produce right-to-left shunting across an ASD may be presented because of exercise intolerance or cyanosis. These patients have complex cardiac disease and often have a poor prognosis. However, balloon valvuloplasty may benefit patients that have pulmonic stenosis and an ASD by reducing right ventricular hypertrophy and decreasing the amount of shunt.

TREATMENT

No treatment is necessary for small ASDs (Color Plate 45). Large ASDs can result in right heart failure and in syncope.[2,5] Standard medical therapy for heart failure is indicated when either of these occurs. Surgical repair of ASDs has been reported in two dogs. Both cases were performed using cardiopulmonary bypass. In the first case, a secundum type of defect was successfully closed and the dog lived for 4 years.[3] At that time, the dog developed right heart failure, and necropsy revealed a large granuloma in the right atrium that was caused by suture material. In the second case, an attempt was made to repair a sinus venosus type of defect with anomalous pulmonary venous return.[4] The dog died postoperatively from intrathoracic bleeding. The veterinary surgeons at the University of California, Davis, have successfully repaired several ASDs in dogs. Cardiopulmonary bypass has been used, and the defect has generally been repaired using a Dacron patch. Several of the dogs died during or soon after surgery. Consequently, surgery should only be attempted on dogs with large ASDs that have severe hemodynamic compromise in which the risk of the lesion outweighs the risk of the surgery.

Ventricular Septal Defect

LEFT-TO-RIGHT SHUNTING VENTRICULAR SEPTAL DEFECT

Ventricular septal defect (VSD) is an orifice in the interventricular septum that allows blood to flow from one ventricle to the other. It is the most common congenital cardiac abnormality identified in children.[6] The prevalence is much lower in dogs and cats. Whereas a busy pediatric cardiologist encounters a patient with a VSD on a weekly basis, a busy veterinary cardiologist encounters such a patient once a month or less. The etiology of VSDs is usually unknown. In most cases, dogs or cats with this defect present with no family history of the disease. Recently, a family of English springer spaniels has been reported in which the defect appears to be inherited as either an autosomal dominant trait with incomplete penetrance or as a polygenic trait.[7]

Prevalence. During the period between August 1, 1986 and August 1, 1996, we diagnosed an isolated VSD in 79 dogs. The English springer spaniel was the most common purebred dog represented in this population, with seven individuals. Thirteen dogs were mixed-breed dogs. The rest of the population consisted of numerous breeds with no more than two dogs of any breed represented. During that same period, 23 cats were diagnosed as having a VSD. Most of these had isolated VSDs. We did not include cats with a common atrioventricular canal or with tetralogy of Fallot in this population.

Anatomy. The ventricular septum is made up of the inlet septum; the outlet, or infundibular, septum; the trabecular septum; and the membranous septum (Figure 13-5).[8] The inlet septum is the smooth portion of the septum that starts at the tricuspid valve orifice and extends to the papillary muscles. The trabecular septum is the portion of the septum that is primarily apical and is heavily trabeculated. The outlet septum is the smooth region of the septum that is cranial to the crista supraventricularis and extends to the pulmonic valve. The membranous septum is small and lies immediately below the aortic valve on the left side and between the tricuspid valve and the pulmonic valve on the right side. Defects in the interventricular septum are defined by the region of the septum in which they reside. Most VSDs are perimembranous.[8] Defects that are situated high on the ventricular septum in the region of the membranous septum are currently termed *perimembranous trabecular defects.* These defects are immediately beneath the right and noncoronary cusps of the aortic valve on the left;

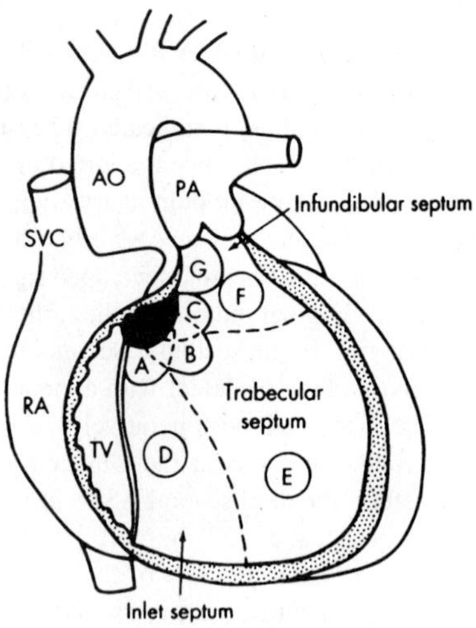

FIGURE 13-5 Schematic drawing of the right side of the interventricular septum. The anatomic regions of the interventricular septum and the anatomic locations of ventricular septal defects (VSD) are outlined. The black area is the membranous interventricular septum. *A,* Perimembranous inlet (atrioventricular canal type of defect) VSD; *B,* perimembranous trabecular (typical membranous) VSD; *C,* perimembranous infundibular (tetralogy type of defect) VSD; *D,* inlet muscular VSD; *E,* trabecular muscular VSD; *F,* infundibular or outlet muscular VSD; *G,* subarterial infundibular (supracristal) VSD; *SVC,* superior vena cava; *AO,* aorta; *PA,* pulmonary artery; *RA,* right atrium; *TV,* tricuspid valve. (From Park MK: *The pediatric cardiology handbook,* St Louis, 1997, Mosby.)

on the right they lie adjacent to the cranioseptal tricuspid valve commissure. Perimembranous inlet defects lie caudal to the septal leaflet of the tricuspid valve on the right side and beneath the aortic valve on the left. Perimembranous outlet septal defects also lie beneath the aortic valve on the left side but penetrate the septum from the outlet portion of the septum, beneath the pulmonic valve on the right side. Defects can also occur in the muscular portion of the septum. Muscular defects are rare in dogs and cats.

Pathophysiology. In an uncomplicated VSD, blood flows from the left ventricle to the right ventricle in systole and in diastole. Flow in either phase of the cardiac cycle may be trivial or substantial, depending on the size of the defect. With large defects, the relative impedances of flow through the systemic circulation vs. the pulmonary circulation is of major importance.

When the defect is small, it provides a high resistance to systolic flow and so produces a much higher impedance to flow than the pulmonary circulation. Consequently, the size of the defect and the aortic input impedance (primarily resistance and compliance) are the only variables that determine relative flow between the systemic and pulmonary circulations. Because flow through the pulmonary circulation is not greatly increased, right ventricular and pulmonary artery systolic pressures are normal. The small size of the defect also provides high resistance to diastolic flow. Moderate-size defects provide less resistance to systolic flow, but they still are the primary determinant of impedance to flow from the left ventricle to the pulmonary circulation in systole and possibly diastole. Therefore they are still "resistive" defects. Moderate-size and small VSDs are commonly termed *restrictive* VSDs in the human literature. This is commonly presented to mean that the size of the defect restricts the left ventricular pressure from being transmitted to the right ventricle. As one source states, "Moderate-size defects are those that offer resistance to pressure, but usually little resistance to flow."[8] Restriction is not a hemodynamic term, and resistance to pressure is a nonsensical term hemodynamically. Pressure is determined by flow and resistance (impedance). Pressure increases in the right heart with large, uncomplicated VSDs because of increased flow, not because pressure is transmitted from one chamber to another. Flow with a moderate-size VSD is greater than with a small VSD and may be great enough to increase pulmonary artery pressure and right ventricular systolic pressure.

Large VSDs have the same or greater surface area as the aortic valve region. Consequently, they provide no or very little resistance to systolic flow. Relative flows in this situation are purely determined by systemic and pulmonary vascular resistance or impedance. If pulmonary vascular resistance is normal at approximately one-fifth that of systemic vascular resistance, pulmonary blood flow increases to 5 times normal and left and right systolic pressures equalize. Consequently, pulmonary hypertension is always present with a large VSD. At this stage, the pulmonary hypertension is not due to pulmonary vascular disease but rather is due purely to the increased flow. With prolonged hypertension, however, pulmonary vascular disease is produced and pulmonary vascular resistance increases.

The blood that shunts in systole flows from the left ventricle into the right ventricle and out the pulmonary artery when the right ventricular myocardium is contracting. Consequently, the right ventricle only acts as a conduit for the shunt flow, and there is no stimulus for volume overload hypertrophy. Blood also shunts through VSDs in diastole. Shunt flow in diastole through a VSD occurs in much the same way as through an ASD and is determined by the size of the defect and the relative compliances of the two ventricles. Moderate-size and large defects have resistances that are low enough that substantial flow can occur in diastole. Large shunts result in a right ventricular pressure overload, which produces right ventricular hypertrophy and decreases right ventricular compliance. Consequently, in theory, a moderate-size VSD can have a greater right ventricular volume overload than a large VSD.

Moderate-size and large VSDs have a significant left heart volume overload. The blood shunted through the VSD flows through the pulmonary circulation and back to the left heart (recirculation). This extra quantity of blood must be accommodated and ejected. This is accomplished through volume overload hypertrophy. Large VSDs result in large shunts and markedly enhanced venous return to the left heart. The ability of the left ventricle to grow large enough to accommodate this increased volume can be overwhelmed if the shunt is large enough. This results in an increase in the left ventricular diastolic pressure. If it increases enough, pulmonary edema results. Pulmonary edema in a VSD is due to the increased left ventricular diastolic pressure backing up into the pulmonary capillaries, not to increased pulmonary blood flow per se.

Because VSDs are located immediately below the aortic valve, they can undermine the support for the valve cusps.[7] This results in aortic regurgitation. The aortic regurgitation can be mild or can be severe enough to contribute to the left ventricular volume overload. Significant aortic regurgitation creates a diastolic heart murmur. The combination of the systolic murmur resulting from the VSD and the diastolic murmur is termed a *to-and-fro murmur.* Although the murmur often lasts throughout systole and diastole, it sounds different from the continuous murmur created by a patent ductus arteriosus. However, this differentiation may not be obvious to someone who has not heard both types of murmurs previously.

Clinical findings. Patients with small defects often have a loud heart murmur with no clinical or radiographic evidence of disease

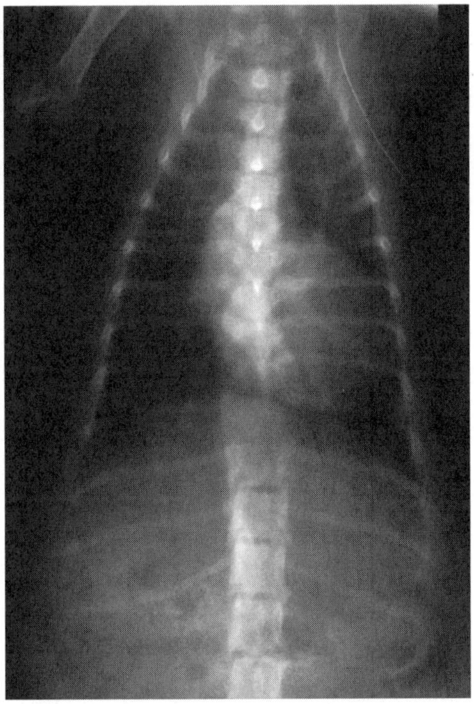

FIGURE 13-6 Dorsoventral radiograph from a 9-week-old female Maine coon kitten with a grade 5/6 systolic heart murmur. Echocardiography revealed a small ventricular septal defect with normal cardiac chamber sizes. The cardiac silhouette is rotated to the left, but otherwise the radiograph is normal.

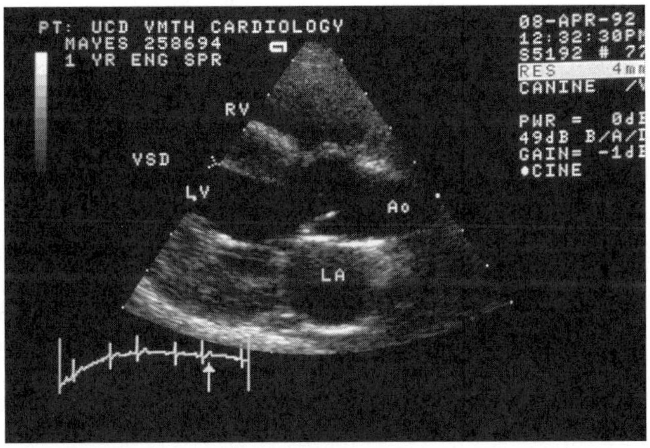

FIGURE 13-7 Two-dimensional echocardiogram from a 1-year-old female English springer spaniel with a small perimembranous ventricular septal defect. The view is a right parasternal long-axis view. The top of the interventricular septum and the root of the aorta *(Ao)* appear to be discontinuous. A membrane appears to overlie this region. Consequently, a defect cannot be definitively identified. *LA,* Left atrium; *LV,* left ventricular chamber; *RV,* right ventricular chamber, *VSD,* ventricular septal defect.

(Figure 13-6). The defect is often difficult to locate using two-dimensional echocardiography but can usually be identified using color flow Doppler echocardiography (Figure 13-7 and Color Plate 46). On color flow Doppler echocardiography, flow is laminar in the left ventricle and then accelerates toward the defect (Color Plate 46). At the defect, velocity increases dramatically to produce a turbulent jet that extends into the right ventricular cavity and strikes the right

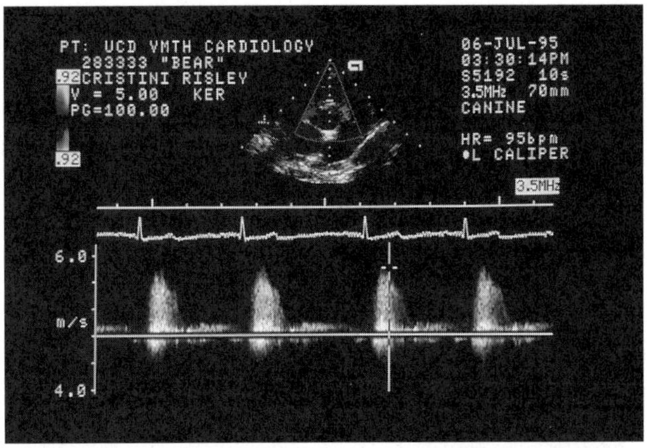

FIGURE 13-8 Continuous-wave Doppler ultrasound measurement of the velocity of the high-velocity jet of blood flow through the ventricular septal defect (VSD) during systole from a dog with a defect similar to the dog shown in Figure 13-6. The peak velocity is 5 m/sec, which translates into a pressure gradient of 100 mm Hg. This means the left ventricular systolic pressure is 100 mm Hg greater than the right ventricular systolic pressure and is characteristic of a small VSD in which resistance to flow is high (resistive VSD).

ventricular free wall. Because the resistance to flow is high and because the systolic pressures in the left ventricle and the right ventricle are normal, the velocity of the jet measured with continuous-wave Doppler is high. Normal left ventricular systolic pressure is 110 to 150 mm Hg, and normal right ventricular systolic pressure is 15 to 25 mm Hg. Using the modified Bernoulli equation ($4V^2$), one can quickly determine that jet velocity should be between 4.6 and 5.8 m/sec (Figure 13-8). Approximately 35% of small VSDs close spontaneously in children.[8] Occasionally a small defect may close spontaneously in a dog, although this is rare in our experience. Spontaneous closure has been reported in two dogs.[9] In one dog, the VSD was diagnosed at 8 weeks of age. The murmur disappeared, and the VSD was no longer evident on an angiocardiogram at 16 months of age. In the second dog, the VSD was diagnosed at 8 weeks of age and the murmur and angiocardiographic evidence of a VSD were gone at 1 year of age.

Patients with moderate-size defects have a loud heart murmur. They may show no clinical signs or may develop mild-to-moderate left heart failure early in life. Right heart failure may become evident later in life. Cardiomegaly and pulmonary overcirculation may be identified on thoracic radiographs. The VSD may be identified on two-dimensional echocardiography, usually from a right-side view. The defect can be seen immediately beneath the aortic valve on a long-axis view. On a short-axis view, the VSD may appear to be part of the aortic root. The location of the defect can be determined on the short-axis view, at approximately 11 o'clock to 12 o'clock (when the aortic root is viewed as a clock face) when the defect is a perimembranous inlet defect or a membranous defect and at 1 o'clock to 3 o'clock when it is a perimembranous outlet defect (Color Plates 47 and 48). The color flow jet may appear somewhat larger than with a small defect, although this should not be used as a distinguishing characteristic. Jet velocity is decreased from that seen with a small defect but is not laminar (Figure 13-9). The left ventricular and left atrial cavities are enlarged and left ventricular wall thickness is normal. Myocardial failure (a large end-systolic diameter and decreased shortening fraction) may be present. The right ventricular and right atrial cavities may also be enlarged.

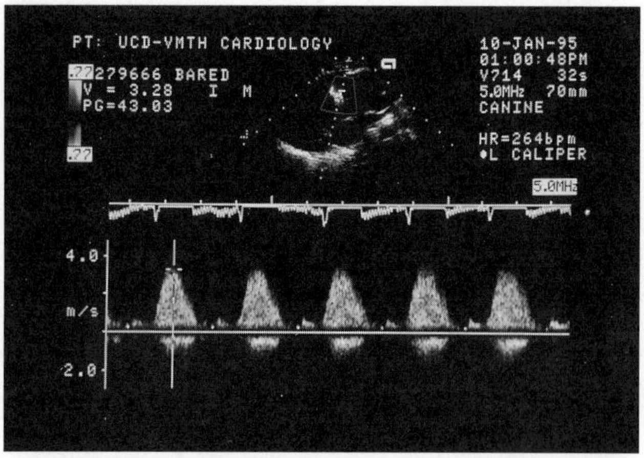

FIGURE 13-9 Continuous-wave Doppler ultrasound measurement of the blood flow velocity through the ventricular septal defect from a 4-month-old male Shar Pei puppy. The velocity is 3.3 m/sec (pressure gradient across the interventricular septum = 43 mm Hg). This low gradient suggests that the defect is large enough to allow enough blood to flow into the pulmonary circulation to increase the pulmonary artery and right ventricular systolic pressures. It also suggests that the defect is at least moderate in size. Pulmonary artery pressure at cardiac catheterization was normal under anesthesia. Oxygen saturation was measured in a systemic artery (87%), the cranial vena cava (65%), the caudal vena cava (40%), the body of the right atrium (55%), the body of the right ventricle (66%), and the right ventricular outflow tract (71%). The pulmonary to systemic flow ratio was determined to be approximately 2:1 ([87% − 55%]/[87% − 71%]). This was interpreted to be a moderate-size shunt. Because operative risk outweighed the risk of no therapy, surgery was not performed. The dog was well 2 years later.

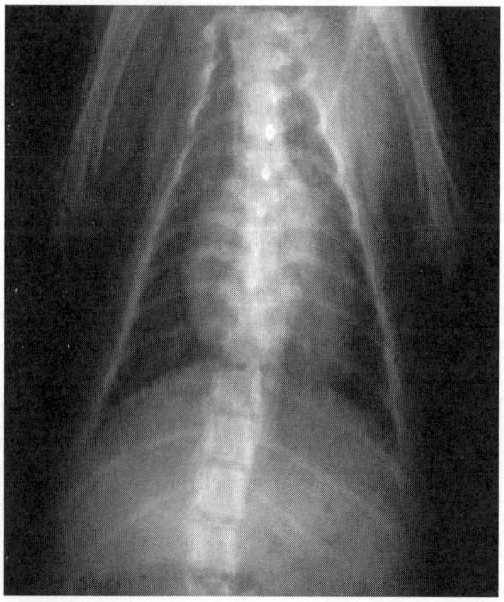

FIGURE 13-10 Dorsoventral radiograph from a sibling to the kitten shown in Figure 13-6. This kitten had a grade 4/6 systolic heart murmur. The left heart was enlarged on an echocardiogram in this kitten. The cardiac silhouette is enlarged. The caudal lobar pulmonary arteries and veins are enlarged compared with the vessels in the kitten in Figure 13-6. The pulmonary overcirculation (increased pulmonary blood flow) suggests that the kitten has a large ventricular septal defect. This was confirmed with echocardiography.

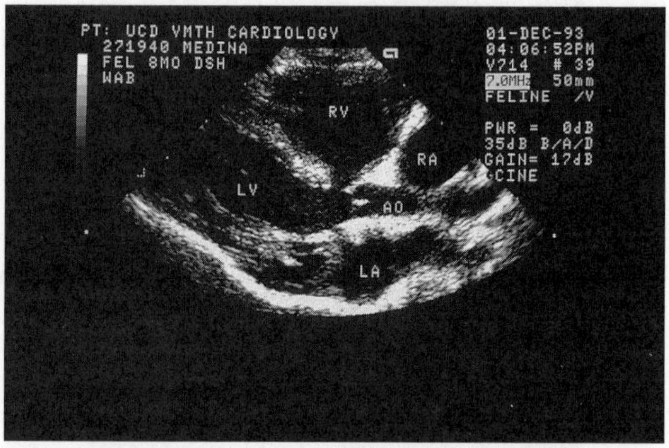

FIGURE 13-11 Two-dimensional echocardiogram from an 8-month-old domestic shorthaired cat. The view is a long-axis view taken from a right parasternal position. The owner noted that the cat had a distended abdomen. The referring veterinarian documented ascites. A defect in the interventricular septum between the right ventricular *(RV)* and the left ventricular *(LV)* chambers is clearly visible. The defect is immediately below the root of the aorta *(AO)*. The right ventricular chamber is clearly enlarged. The interventricular septum was flattened, suggesting that the right ventricular systolic pressure was increased. Pulmonary hypertension was verified by measuring the velocity of a pulmonic insufficiency jet to be 4.1 m/sec. *LA,* Left atrium; *RA,* right atrium.

Large VSDs are rare in clinical veterinary practice. It is likely that most puppies and kittens with large VSDs die within the first weeks of life from left heart failure, when pulmonary vascular resistance decreases into the normal range. Patients that do survive may present in left heart failure or they may present with Eisenmenger's complex and cyanosis (see below). Even in patients with left-to-right shunts, the heart murmur may be softer than with small- and moderate-size defects as flow velocity is decreased. The cardiac silhouette is usually enlarged on thoracic radiographs, and pulmonary overcirculation may be evident (Figure 13-10). Pulmonary edema may also be present. The large defect can be visualized and its location confirmed on two-dimensional echocardiography (Figure 13-11). The left ventricular and atrial cavities are enlarged. The right ventricular cavity may be enlarged because of diastolic flow through the VSD or because of pulmonary hypertension (see Figure 13-11). The right ventricular wall thickness may be increased, secondary to the right ventricular systolic hypertension (pressure overload). Because of the massive amount of flow through the defect, flow velocity is still usually increased in patients with a left-to-right shunt. Consequently, turbulent flow through the defect can be demonstrated with color flow Doppler echocardiography (Color Plate 49). Peak systolic flow velocity is decreased into the 1.0- to 2.5-m/sec range (Figure 13-12).

Although ventricular septal defects are usually identified using echocardiography, they can also be visualized using angiocardiography during cardiac catheterization (Figure 13-13). The right ventricle is opacified following the injection of a contrast agent into the left ventricle. The size of the VSD can also be evaluated during cardiac catheterization by measuring oxygen saturation in a chamber upstream from and a chamber downstream from the VSD (Figures 13-14 and 13-15).

Treatment. Treatment is not warranted in patients with small VSDs. Although a loud systolic heart murmur is present, the hemodynamic consequences are slight. Patients with moderate-size

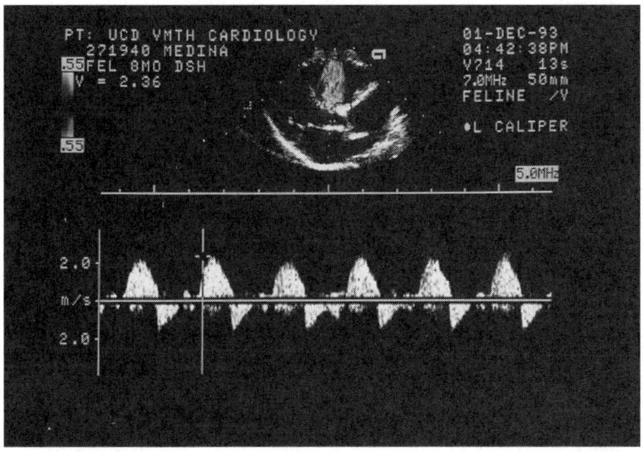

FIGURE 13-12 Continuous-wave Doppler tracings of the jet velocity from the cat in Figure 13-11. The velocity is low (2.4 m/sec), meaning the defect is large. The pulmonary hypertension in this young cat may be primarily flow-related or may be due to pulmonary vascular disease or both. The right heart enlargement and right heart failure is due to diastolic flow through the defect into the right ventricle and to the pulmonary hypertension.

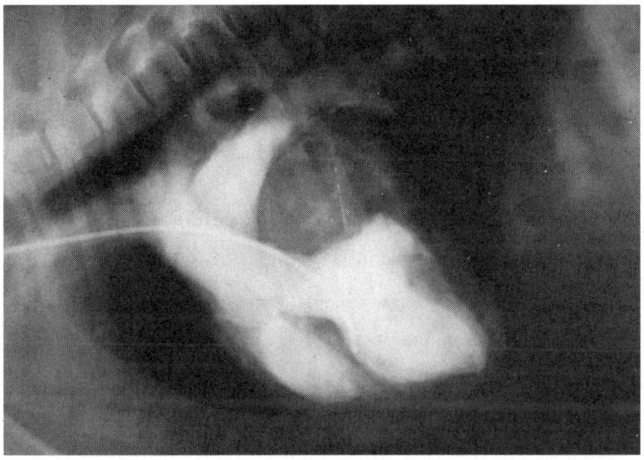

FIGURE 13-13 Angiocardiogram of a 1-year-old male collie with a ventricular septal defect (VSD). An iodinated contrast agent has been injected into the left ventricle. The left ventricular cavity, right ventricular cavity, aorta, and main pulmonary artery are densely opacified. Contrast material can be visualized passing through the VSD. The aorta overrides the interventricular septum. This likely makes this a form of tetralogy of Fallot.

defects may develop heart failure at a young age or as adults. Some may develop a right-to-left shunt because of pulmonary vascular disease. Others may tolerate the shunt and not develop clinically significant consequences. In other words, predicting the clinical course of a moderate-size VSD is difficult. Patients with large defects generally require therapy unless right-to-left shunting has occurred, in which surgical closure is contraindicated.

Patients that exhibit signs of congestive heart failure are treated with standard drugs, including furosemide, an angiotensin converting enzyme inhibitor, and, possibly, digoxin. Angiotensin converting enzyme inhibitors may have a small effect on the amount of left-to-right shunting by decreasing systemic vascular resistance.

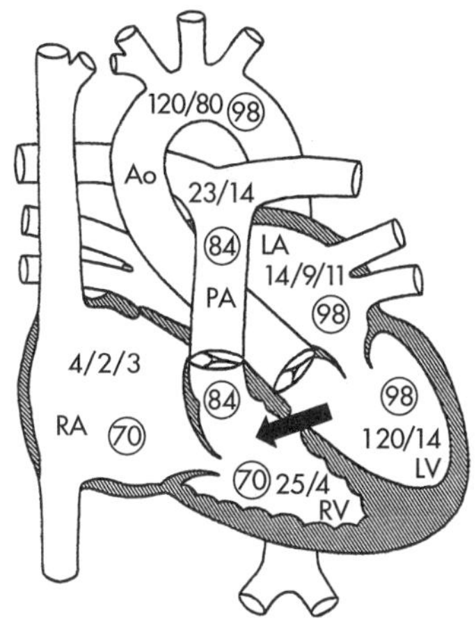

FIGURE 13-14 Schematic drawing of a medium-size ventricular septal defect. Oxygen saturation (O_2) is depicted as numbers in circles within chambers and vessels. The numbers beside the chambers and vessels are pressures in mm Hg. The diameter of the defect is less than the diameter of the aorta, so it imposes resistance to blood flow. Pulmonary vascular resistance is decreased. Pulmonary blood flow is 2 times systemic blood flow (SA O_2 – MV O_2/PV O_2 – PA O_2). *LA,* Left atrium; *RA,* right atrium; *LV,* left ventricle; *RV,* right ventricle; *Ao,* aorta; *PA,* pulmonary artery.

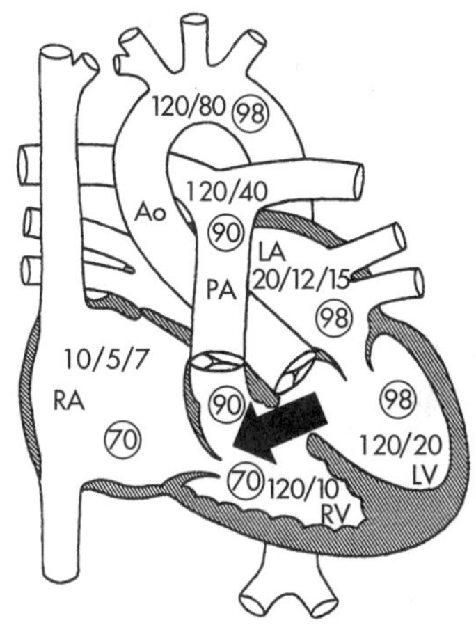

FIGURE 13-15 Schematic drawing of a large ventricular septal defect with left-to-right shunting. The diameter of the defect is the same as the diameter of the aortic root and so provides no-to-little resistance to blood flow. Pulmonary vascular resistance is mildly-to-moderately increased. Systolic pressure in the right ventricle and pulmonary artery is the same as in the left ventricle and aorta primarily because pulmonary blood flow is 3.5 times systemic blood flow. The left atrial pressure is increased, indicating mild-to-moderate left heart failure. Abbreviations are as in Figure 13-14.

Therapy aimed at reducing shunt flow is the most beneficial. Shunt flow can be reduced medically by administering a potent arteriolar dilator, such as hydralazine. It can also be reduced surgically by creating pulmonic stenosis. Of course, definitive surgery to close the defect is most effective.

In a patient with a large VSD, left-to-right flow through the VSD is determined by the relative resistances of the systemic and pulmonary circulations. Hydralazine administration decreases vascular resistance in the systemic circulation to a much greater degree than in the pulmonary circulation. Consequently, systemic flow through the aorta increases and shunt and pulmonary blood flow decrease. This decreases venous return to the left heart and decreases left ventricular diastolic pressure. The net result is improved hemodynamics and lessened heart failure. Prazosin produces an even better hemodynamic response in sheep.[10] We have found hydralazine administration to be particularly beneficial in cats and small dogs with large VSDs. Surgical risk is often greater in these patients, making medical management more attractive.

Pulmonary artery banding is another means of reducing shunt flow and improving hemodynamics in patients with VSDs large enough to cause clinical signs. In this situation, by creating pulmonic stenosis, pulmonary vascular resistance is increased, resulting in a decrease in pulmonary blood flow and shunt flow and a decrease in left ventricular venous return. This procedure has been reported in five dogs and two cats.[11,12] The procedure is carried out from a left-side surgical approach. The pericardium is opened and the pulmonary artery bluntly dissected away from the aorta. Umbilical tape is placed around the main pulmonary artery and then tightened using forceps until the pulmonary artery diameter is approximately one third of the pulmonary valve annulus diameter. The tape is sutured, the clamp removed, and the tape tied. The color of blood flowing through the pulmonary artery may change to a more blue color once the procedure is completed.[13] Excellent results have been reported with pulmonary artery banding, with some dogs reportedly living a normal life-span following the surgery.[8] Problems that can occur include right-to-left shunting if the band is tightened too far, no improvement in clinical signs if the band is not tightened enough, and hemorrhage.[11] Results are probably much better if the procedure is performed by an experienced cardiovascular surgeon. It has been recommended that pulmonary artery banding not be performed in dogs or cats less than 6 months of age because the supravalvular pulmonic stenosis that is created becomes worse as the animal grows and the stenotic region does not grow.[13] However, the procedure has been performed successfully in a 2-month-old dog.[11]

Closure of the VSD via open-heart surgery is the other potential means of treating a hemodynamically significant VSD. This can be performed using either deep hypothermic circulatory arrest or cardiopulmonary bypass.[13] In either case, the right ventricle is incised and the VSD repaired either by directly suturing the defect closed or by suturing a patch over the defect. Placing sutures in the caudal aspect of the defect must be avoided because the atrioventricular conduction system passes along this region. Damage to this area could result in complete atrioventricular block. There are few reports of surgical closure of VSDs in the veterinary literature.[14-16] In the only series of cases reported, the surgeon used aortic homografts to close the VSDs under deep hypothermia.[14] Potential problems with this procedure are many and include death as a result of hypothermia, hemorrhage, and failure of the myocardium to regain function following surgery. This procedure should only be performed by an accomplished cardiovascular surgeon.

RIGHT-TO-LEFT SHUNTING VENTRICULAR SEPTAL DEFECT (EISENMENGER'S COMPLEX)

Definition. Eisenmenger's *complex* is the combination of a ventricular septal defect with pulmonary vascular disease, leading to right-to-left shunting and cyanosis.[8] Eisenmenger's *syndrome* is the combination of other systemic-pulmonary communications, pulmonary vascular disease, and cyanosis. Eisenmenger's complex is rare in dogs and cats. Most ventricular septal defects are small and do not result in this type of significant hemodynamic abnormality.

Pathophysiology. Eisenmenger's complex occurs most readily in a patient with a large ventricular septal defect. When a VSD is large (same cross-sectional area of the aorta or more) and so produces no resistance to blood flow, blood flow distribution is based purely on the relative impedances (primarily resistances) of the systemic and pulmonary vascular beds. Systolic pressures are identical in both ventricles and the great arteries regardless of the amount of pulmonary vascular resistance. Because pulmonary vascular resistance is normally much lower than systemic vascular resistance, massive left-to-right shunting occurs if pulmonary vascular resistance decreases into the normal range in a neonatal person or animal. In infants, pulmonary vascular resistance decreases into the normal range in the third to fourth months of life. At this time, they present in severe left heart failure (as a result of the massive left-to-right shunting and volume overload and despite the fact that they have severe pulmonary hypertension). It is most likely that most puppies and kittens with large VSDs die of heart failure within the first several weeks of life. Consequently, they are never examined by a veterinarian. Rarely, the pulmonary vascular resistance does not decrease to the point of producing severe heart failure, and the dog or cat lives long enough to develop other problems. One potential problem is severe pulmonary vascular disease with shunt reversal and cyanosis.

In the situation of a large VSD, it is most likely that pulmonary vascular disease occurs primarily in response to the obligatory flow-related pulmonary hypertension. The pulmonary vasculature must thicken in response to the markedly increased pressure in an attempt to bring wall stress back toward normal and to prevent rupture. The damage to the pulmonary vasculature is progressive over time. When pulmonary vascular resistance increases to a value greater than systemic vascular resistance, right-to-left shunting occurs (Figure 13-16). In humans, pulmonary vascular disease can also occur, and can progress in children with moderate-size VSDs.[8] The reason for this is less clear. The only time we have observed this situation in dogs is when the dogs were born and raised in a

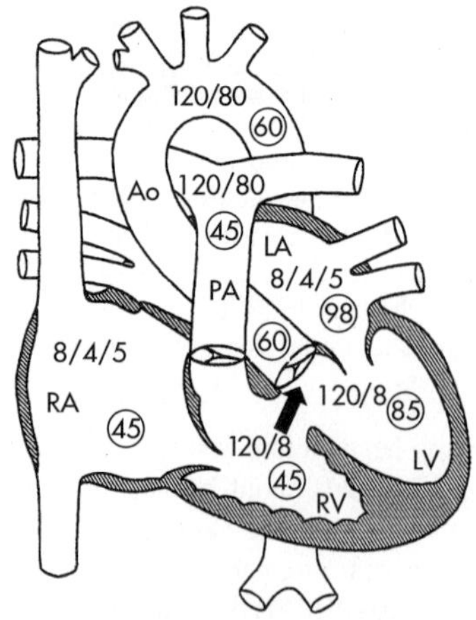

FIGURE 13-16 Schematic drawing of a large ventricular septal defect with right-to-left shunting (Eisenmenger's complex). The defect is large, as in Figure 13-15. Pulmonary vascular resistance has increased over time because of progressive pulmonary vascular disease. At this stage it is greater than systemic vascular resistance, resulting in the right-to-left shunt and consequent systemic hypoxemia. Pulmonary blood flow is 0.7 times systemic blood flow. Abbreviations are as in Figure 13-14.

high-altitude location or moved to a high-altitude location (Figure 13-17). Hypoxia is a known stimulant of pulmonary vasoconstriction and appears to be a modifying factor in dogs.

Clinical findings. Eisenmenger's complex has been described in three dogs in one series of case reports.[17,18] Unfortunately, the size of the VSDs in these dogs could not be well documented other than to note that the VSD was large in one dog. This dog also had a patent ductus arteriosus. All dogs presented with cyanosis, either at rest or with exercise, and polycythemia (PCV = 55% to 65%). Interestingly, each of these dogs still had a heart murmur, two in locations characteristic of a VSD. The primary owner complaints consisted of exercise intolerance, exercise-induced dyspnea, cyanosis, and seizure activity. Radiographs revealed a main pulmonary artery bulge in two dogs, enlarged proximal pulmonary arteries with normal distal arteries in one dog, decreased pulmonary artery size in one, and markedly enlarged caudal lobar pulmonary arteries in one (see Figure 13-17). The cardiac silhouette was enlarged in all dogs. The ECG suggested right ventricular enlargement in all three dogs. The arterial oxygen tension was 46 mm Hg in one dog that was not cyanotic at rest. In two dogs, cardiac catheterization confirmed the presence of a VSD and right-to-left or bidirectional shunting of blood. At necropsy, the VSDs were identified in each case, along with thickened right ventricular walls and dilated right ventricular chambers. The proximal main pulmonary artery was dilated in all of the dogs. The small pulmonary vasculature was abnormal but similar in each case. Dilation of the large elastic pulmonary arteries was present. The smaller elastic arteries had hypertrophied walls and large lumina. The muscular arteries had a marked increase in connective tissue and fibroblasts, focal subintimal proliferations that often obliterated the vessel lumen, medial muscular hypertrophy with severe disruption of the internal and external elastic laminae, and

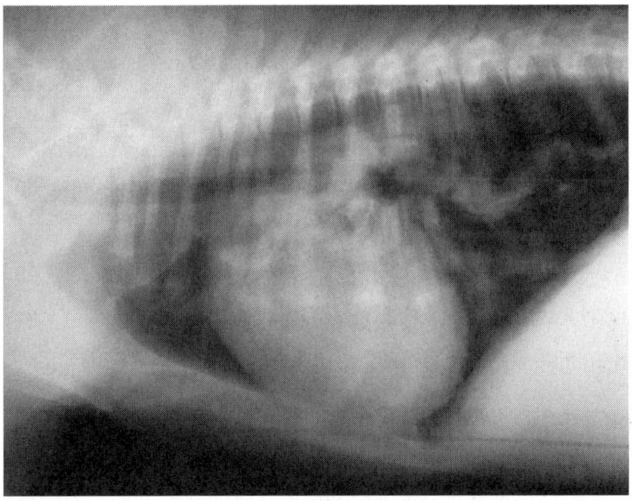

FIGURE 13-17 Thoracic radiograph from an 8-month-old female Siberian husky with Eisenmenger's complex. A large left-to-right shunting ventricular septal defect (VSD) had been diagnosed 3 months before presentation, when the dog lived in the Midwestern United States. She had been sold to owners who lived at approximately 5000 feet in the Sierra Nevada mountains. The owners noted dyspnea. She was cyanotic on presentation. The thoracic radiographs revealed large and tortuous pulmonary arteries as a result of the dog's severe pulmonary hypertension. The right ventricle was enlarged, as evidenced by the shifting of the apex off the sternum. The increased pulmonary blood flow as a result of the VSD coupled with the mild hypoxemia created by moving to a higher altitude probably caused this dog's severe increase in pulmonary vascular resistance and consequent right-to-left shunt.

plexiform lesions. Based on the Heath-Edwards classification the lesions in these dogs were grade 3 to grade 4.

A similar case has been reported of a 2-year-old, 25-kg Labrador retriever that presented with dyspnea at rest and exercise intolerance.[19] This dog had no cardiac murmur, a PCV of 55%, and an arterial oxygen tension of 39 mm Hg. The right ventricular systolic pressure was 60 mm Hg at cardiac catheterization, and a ventricular septal defect was identified using contrast radiography. At the postmortem examination, this dog had a 1.2-cm ventricular septal defect and concentric right ventricular hypertrophy. The diameter of this VSD was smaller than the normal aortic diameter of a 25-kg dog. The dog had medial hypertrophy and intimal fibrosis in the small muscular pulmonary arteries, along with some plexiform lesions.

Treatment. Surgical closure of a right-to-left shunting VSD is generally contraindicated.[8] Phlebotomy to relieve severe polycythemia or hydroxyurea administration may be tried to improve clinical signs. Long-term prognosis is poor.

REFERENCES

1. Vick GWI, Titus JL: Defects of the atrial septum including the atrioventricular canal. In Garson AJ, Bricker JT, McNamara DG, eds: *The science and practice of pediatric cardiology,* Philadelphia, 1990, Lea & Febiger.
2. Kirberger RM, Berry WL: Atrial septal defect in a dog: the value of Doppler echocardiography, *J S Afr Vet Assoc* 63:43, 1992.
3. Eyster GE, Anderson LK, Krehbeil JD et al: Surgical repair of atrial septal defect in a dog, *J Am Vet Med Assoc* 169:1081, 1976.
4. Jeraj K, Ogburn PN, Johnston GR et al: Atrial septal defect (sinus venosus type) in a dog, *J Am Vet Med Assoc* 177:342, 1980-346.
5. Chen KY: Persistent common atrioventricular canal and splenosis in a Persian cat, *J Chin Soc Vet Sci* 12:53, 1986.
6. Riopel DA: Pulmonary valve atresia with intact ventricular septum. In Garson AJ, Bricker JT, McNamara DG, eds: *The science and practice of pediatric cardiology,* Philadelphia, 1990, Lea & Febiger.
7. Brown WA: Ventricular septal defects in the English springer spaniel. In Bonagura JD, Kirk RW, eds: *Kirk's current veterinary therapy XII: small animal practice,* Philadelphia, 1995, WB Saunders.
8. Gumbiner CH, Takao A: Ventricular septal defect. In Garson AJ, Bricker JT, McNamara DG, eds: *The science and practice of pediatric cardiology,* Philadelphia, 1990, Lea & Febiger.
9. Breznock EM: Spontaneous closure of ventricular septal defects in the dog, *J Am Vet Med Assoc* 162:399, 1973.
10. Boucek MM, Chang R, Synhorst DP: Vasodilators and ventricular septal defect: comparison of prazosin, minoxidil, and hydralazine in a chronic lamb model, *Pediatr Res* 18:859, 1984.
11. Eyster GE, Whipple RD, Anderson LK et al: Pulmonary artery banding for ventricular septal defect in dogs and cats, *J Am Vet Med Assoc* 170:434, 1977.
12. Sheridan JP, Mann PG, Stock JE: Pulmonary artery banding in the cat: a case report, *J Small Anim Pract* 12:45, 1971.
13. Eyster GE: Atrial septal defect and ventricular septal defect, *Semin Vet Med Surg (Small Anim)* 9:227, 1994.
14. Northway RB: Aortic homograft for repair of septal defect in the heart, *Vet Med Small Anim Clin* 70:1303, 1975.
15. Zeiner FM: Two cases of coronary venous drainage by a persistent left superior vena cava in cats, *Anat Rec* 129:275, 1957.
16. Braden TD, Appleford MD, Hartsfield SM: Correction of a ventricular septal defect in a dog, *J Am Vet Med Assoc* 161:507, 1972.
17. Feldman EC, Nimmo-Wilkie JS, Pharr JW: Eisenmenger's syndrome in the dog: case reports, *J Am Anim Hosp Assoc* 17:477, 1981.
18. Nimmo-Wilkie JS, Feldman EC: Pulmonary vascular lesions associated with congenital heart defects in three dogs, *J Am Anim Hosp Assoc* 17:485, 1981.
19. Turk JR, Miller JB, Sande RD: Plexogenic pulmonary arteriopathy in a dog with ventricular septal defect and pulmonary hypertension, *J Am Anim Hosp Assoc* 18:608, 1982.

CHAPTER 14

Tetralogy of Fallot

Tetralogy of Fallot is a congenital cardiac abnormality characterized by the presence of a large ventricular septal defect, pulmonic stenosis, dextroposition of the aorta, and right ventricular hypertrophy (Color Plate 50). Blood shunts from the right ventricle to the left ventricle through the nonresistive ventricular septal defect. The blood usually flows from the right side of the heart to the left side because the pulmonic stenosis increases resistance to blood flow out of the right ventricle to a point that it is greater than systemic vascular resistance. The delivery of deoxygenated blood to the systemic circulation results in systemic hypoxemia. The hypoxemia is often severe enough to cause cyanosis, either at rest or with exercise.

Prevalence

Tetralogy of Fallot is an uncommon congenital cardiac defect in dogs and cats. Although the overall prevalence of congenital heart disease in dogs has been estimated to be approximately 27 per 4000, the prevalence of tetralogy of Fallot in dogs has been estimated to be 1 per 4000.[1] This is probably an underestimate because some severely affected dogs almost assuredly die at a young age, before a veterinarian examines them. However, tetralogy of Fallot is the most common of the cyanotic congenital cardiac defects in the dog.[2] We diagnosed tetralogy of Fallot in 19 dogs between August 1, 1986, and August 1, 1996. This is approximately two cases a year. The prevalence in our hospital patient population was also about 1 per 4000 (19 per 68,690). Tetralogy of Fallot comprised approximately 0.5% of our primary service caseload. Tetralogy of Fallot is an unusual, although reported, defect in the cat.[3-5] We diagnosed tetralogy of Fallot in four cats in the same period. We also diagnosed a ventricular septal defect with mild-to-moderate pulmonic stenosis with or without dextroposition of the aorta in three cats within that time.

Without palliative surgery the prognosis for this abnormality is poor, with most dogs dying within the first year of life from hypoxemia or complications from polycythemia.[1] Other congenital defects may be identified in dogs with tetralogy of Fallot. These include tracheal hypoplasia, peritoneal pericardial diaphragmatic hernia, ventral abdominal wall hernia and sternal deformity, retinal dysplasia, and persistent pupillary membranes.[2,6] Other congenital cardiac abnormalities may occasionally be noted in a patient with tetralogy of Fallot. They include but are not limited to patent ductus arteriosus (pentalogy of Fallot), atrial septal defect, and a persistent right aortic arch.

History

Nicholas Sten, a Danish scholar, provided the original description of this condition in children in 1673. Eduard Sandifort again described tetralogy of Fallot in 1777. In the mid-1800s, James Hope, Thomas Peacock, and Sir Thomas Watson provided descriptions of this abnormality. Etienne-Louis Arthur Fallot published his paper entitled "Contribution to the Pathologic Anatomy of Morbus Caeruleus" in 1888. In it he described what is now considered the classic description of the malady now known as tetralogy of Fallot. He described the following: (1) pulmonic stenosis, (2) large interventricular communication, (3) deviation of the origin of the aorta to the right, and (4) concentric right ventricular hypertrophy. The important features of this defect are the pulmonic stenosis and the large ventricular septal defect. The right ventricular hypertrophy is purely secondary to the right ventricular pressure overload. The overriding aorta is an important clue to the embryology of the defect and is an important consideration for surgical correction, but is not hemodynamically as important. With the large ventricular septal defect and pulmonic stenosis, blood shunts from the right ventricle through the ventricular septal defect and into the aorta and systemic circulation. This shunting of deoxygenated (venous) blood into the systemic circulation results in hypoxemia and, if the hypoxemia is severe enough, in cyanosis and polycythemia.

Embryology and Genetics

The name *tetralogy of Fallot* suggests that the patient has four separate congenital cardiac defects. It would be unusual for patients to have four primary cardiac abnormalities simultaneously. That tetralogy of Fallot is common suggests that the abnormalities observed stem from one abnormality. The embryology and heritability of tetralogy of Fallot and related defects have been studied in keeshond dogs.[7] The conotruncal (outlet or infundibular) septum is abnormal in keeshonds and presumably is also abnormal in other patients with the disease. This abnormality is inherited as a simple autosomal recessive trait. The conotruncal septum forms the upper portion of the interventricular septum.[8] In tetralogy of Fallot, this portion of the septum forms too far cranial. This results in malalignment with the lower portion of the interventricular septum and, consequently, a defect in the interventricular septum (a ventricular septal defect).[9] The formation of the conotruncal septum in this position also results in a narrowed right ventricular outflow tract and abnormal pulmonic valve formation (pulmonic stenosis) and in dextroposition of the origin of the aorta. The right ventricular hypertrophy occurs secondary to the pulmonic stenosis.

The trabecular septum forms the floor of the ventricular septal defect. The roof is formed by the aortic valve leaflets. The degree to which the aorta is shifted to the right is variable and has not been quantified in dogs. In humans, the amount of override ranges from 15% to 95%.[10]

Tetralogy of Fallot is not the only congenital cardiac abnormality identified when affected keeshonds are bred. Some dogs have subclinical defects in which the papillary muscle of the conus is absent and an aneurysm is present in the interventricular septum at the region of the membranous septum (Color Plate 13). Other dogs have just pulmonic stenosis or a ventricular septal defect. A few dogs have no formation of the conotruncal septum and so have truncus arteriosus where the aorta and pulmonary artery arise from the ventricles as one large great artery. A large ventricular septal defect is also present. These represent a spectrum of a genetic disease in which varying degrees of defective growth of the conotruncal cushions result in different degrees of embryologic abnormalities.[11]

Pathophysiology

Tetralogy of Fallot is a shunting defect in which there is usually no resistance to flow between the left and right ventricles. Consequently, blood flows to the right and left circulations proportional to systemic and pulmonary resistances (Figures 14-1 and 14-2). The pulmonic stenosis in symptomatic tetralogy of Fallot is severe such that resistance to flow through the pulmonic valve is greater than systemic vascular resistance. Consequently a significant amount of blood flows from the right ventricle, through the ventricular septal defect, and out the aorta (see Figure 14-1). The amount of blood that flows from the right heart into the aorta depends on the relative resistances between the two circulations. For example, if the pulmonic stenosis increases resistance to flow out the right ventricle to twice that of systemic vascular resistance and if we give pulmonary blood flow an arbitrary value of 100 mL, 200 mL will flow through the systemic circulation (pulmonary blood flow must be one-half of the systemic blood flow if pulmonary resistance is twice that of systemic vascular resistance). The Q_p/Q_s is 0.5. Because the ventricular septal defect provides no resistance to flow, blood will flow wherever it can in proportion to the resistances. Systolic intraventricular pressures will be equal on both sides. Because the amount of blood pumped into the pulmonary circulation equals left heart venous return, left ventricular output must also be 100 mL. Therefore 100 mL of blood must also flow through the ventricular septal defect and into the aorta (systemic flow = 200 mL; ventricular septal defect flow = systemic flow − pulmonary flow). In a patient with tetralogy of Fallot the amount of pulmonary blood flow is decreased from that seen in a normal animal because of the pulmonic stenosis and an apparent lack of response by the body to this decrease in pulmonary blood volume. The decrease in pulmonary blood flow results in a decrease in venous return to the left ventricle, with a resultant decrease in left ventricular size and stroke volume. The decrease in stroke volume results in a decrease in the amount of oxygenated blood that reaches the circulation.

The physiologic consequences of tetralogy of Fallot depend on two variables: the degree of pulmonic stenosis and systemic vascular

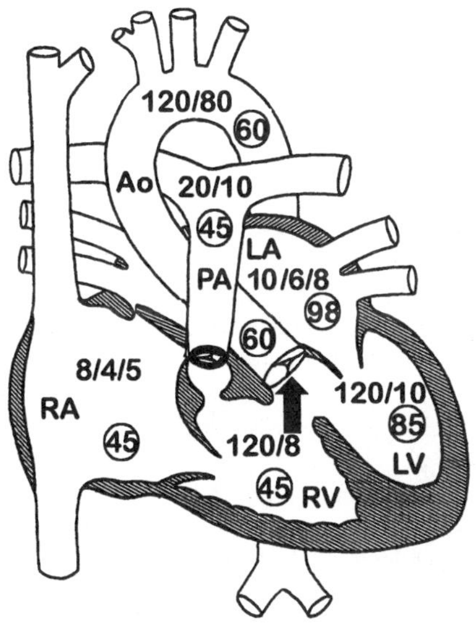

FIGURE 14-1 Drawing of the circulation in a patient with tetralogy of Fallot with severe right ventricular (RV) outflow obstruction. The course of the circulation, oxygen saturations *(circles),* and pressures are shown. Systolic pressures in the right ventricle, left ventricle (LV), and aorta (Ao) are identical (120 mm Hg). There is a pressure gradient of 100 mm Hg across the region of the pulmonic valve. Resistance to flow through the ventricular septal defect and systemic circulation are less than the resistance across the pulmonic valve region. Consequently, deoxygenated (oxygen saturation = 45%) blood from the right ventricle shunts into the left ventricle and systemic circulation. This results in systemic hypoxemia (oxygen saturation = 60%). Pulmonary blood flow is reduced to approximately 70% of systemic blood flow. Right atrial (RA) pressure is normal. *PA,* Pulmonary artery; *LA,* left atrium.

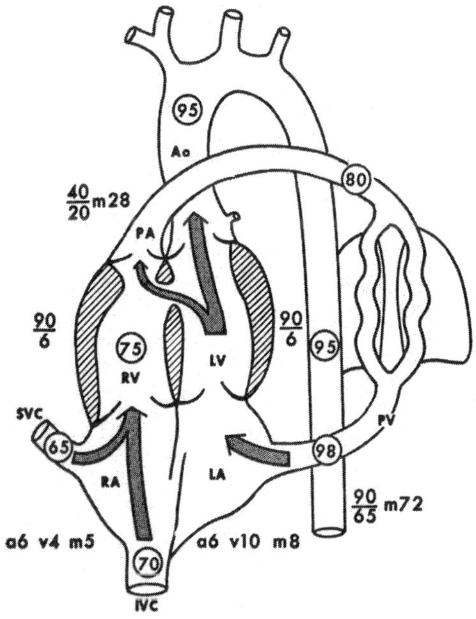

FIGURE 14-2 Drawing of the circulation in a patient with a large ventricular septal defect and moderate pulmonic stenosis. Systolic pressures in the right ventricle, left ventricle, and aorta are the same (90 mm Hg) because the large ventricular septal defect provides no resistance to blood flow. Resistance to blood flow through the pulmonic valve region is slightly less than systemic vascular resistance, resulting in a small left-to-right shunt. Abbreviations are as in Figure 14-1. (From Rudolph AM: *Congenital diseases of the heart,* St Louis, 1974, Mosby.)

resistance.[12] The degree of aortic override is not hemodynamically very important. The same amount of shunting will occur in an animal with a comparable-size ventricular septal defect and comparably severe pulmonic stenosis. Exercise exacerbates the right-to-left shunting as a result of vasodilation in skeletal muscle beds and a decrease in systemic vascular resistance. Because of the pulmonic stenosis, pulmonary resistance is fixed and right-to-left shunting increases, producing more severe systemic hypoxemia and cyanosis.

When the right ventricular output of blood contributes to aortic flow, venous blood is pumped into the systemic circulation. Blood that has a low partial pressure of oxygen (venous) then mixes with blood with a high partial pressure of oxygen (arterial). The net results are decreases in oxygen tension and oxygen content of the systemic blood that result in cyanosis. The severity of the hypoxemia directly reflects the degree of shunting. It is a sensitive and specific means of evaluating the severity of a right-to-left shunt. Symptomatic patients typically have an arterial oxygen tension less than 40 mm Hg at rest or with exercise.

Patients with tetralogy of Fallot do not necessarily have to be cyanotic, although the vast majority are, either at rest or with exercise. A patient with mild pulmonic stenosis (in which pulmonary resistance is still less than the systemic vascular resistance) and a large ventricular septal defect can have a predominantly left-to-right shunt and have the same hemodynamics as a patient with a small, isolated ventricular septal defect. A patient with equal pulmonary and systemic resistances as a result of moderate pulmonic stenosis can be "balanced" so that very little net shunting occurs, in either direction (see Figure 14-2). The latter type of patient would still be expected to develop more right-to-left shunting and arterial hypoxemia with exercise.

The pulmonic stenosis in tetralogy of Fallot does not necessarily have to be a fixed stenosis. Infundibular narrowing and hypertrophy can result in a stenosis that worsens when the contractility in this region increases (dynamic obstruction). This most commonly results in an increase in pulmonary resistance when the animal becomes excited or exercises. The fixed stenosis may be valvular, subvalvular, or infundibular (narrowing of the outflow tract).[4]

Because of the profound hypoxemia in patients with symptomatic tetralogy of Fallot, polycythemia is a common sequela. The polycythemia occurs when receptors in the kidney and, to a lesser extent, the liver are stimulated by hypoxemia to release erythropoietin.[13-15] Erythropoietin is a glycoprotein that has an oxygen-sensing site that probably contains heme.[13] Erythropoietin is produced in a subset of peritubular cells that lie along the capillary lumen and outside the tubular basement membrane in the inner renal cortex.[16] Serum erythropoietin concentration is increased in patients with chronic hypoxemia. For example, in one feline patient with tetralogy of Fallot that was reported in the literature, serum erythropoietin concentration was increased from the normal range of 5 to 22 mU/mL to 43 mU/mL.[17] Erythropoietin stimulates red cell production. It binds to receptors on erythroid cells in bone marrow and stimulates cell growth via a tyrosine protein kinase.[18] The protein kinases probably stimulate biologic activation of erythroid cells by phosphorylating nuclear proteins. The resultant increase in hematocrit increases the oxygen carrying capacity of the blood. This is beneficial to a hypoxemic patient if the hematocrit is in the 55% to 70% range. Blood viscosity increases exponentially with increases in hematocrit, and, at hematocrits exceeding 70%, blood viscosity increases dramatically. The increase in blood viscosity increases resistance to flow, decreasing cardiac output and so decreasing tissue oxygen delivery. Consequently, severe polycythemia is often detrimental. The hematocrit at which blood viscosity increases to the point of being detrimental varies tremendously from patient to patient. It should be noted that not all animals with tetralogy of Fallot have an increase in serum erythropoietin concentration. In one dog in one report a dog's serum erythropoietin concentration was within normal range despite an arterial oxygen tension of 28 mm Hg.[19]

Signalment and Medical History

Most dogs are presented to a veterinarian when they are young, most commonly between 2 and 8 months of age, and most are purebred dogs.[2] Many breeds have been identified with this defect. Tetralogy of Fallot has been diagnosed in 19 dogs at our hospital (University of California, Davis, Veterinary Medical Teaching Hospital) in the past 10 years. Seventeen of these were purebred dogs. Numerous breeds were represented, with three keeshonds and two wirehaired fox terriers identified. Other identified breeds at our hospital included an English bulldog, a rottweiler, a German shepherd, an American cocker spaniel, an English cocker spaniel, a Maltese, a Shar Pei, a miniature schnauzer, a Pomeranian, an Alaskan malamute, and a beagle.

The history obtained from the client can be quite varied. An animal may show no clinical signs, may be dyspneic, may have exercise intolerance, or may be less active than previously or less active than a litter mate.[2] The puppy or kitten may grow slower than litter mates. The owner may have noted cyanosis that may be continuous or occur in episodes, especially with exercise. The patient may be dyspneic or become dyspneic with stress or exercise.[3] Cyanotic episodes may culminate in syncope, especially with exercise.[20] There may be other central nervous system signs, including seizures, as a result of polycythemia. Right heart failure is rare.

Physical Examination

The patient may be smaller than normal. Cyanosis varies from absent to severe. When cyanosis is absent, exercise may produce cyanosis. When cyanosis is present at rest, exercise often makes it worse. The cyanosis is symmetrically distributed and is best appreciated by examining the mucous membranes (oral, penile, vulvar, anal) and the sclera (Color Plate 51). In animals with black oral mucous membrane color, cyanosis is difficult to impossible to appreciate in this region. The cyanotic color can range from a light scarlet to blue or purple. In one report, 12 of 13 dogs with tetralogy of Fallot were cyanotic at rest.[2]

A cardiac murmur is commonly, but not always, present.[5] The murmur is most commonly due to the pulmonic stenosis and is usually loudest at the left heart base. The ventricular septal defect in tetralogy of Fallot is large. Consequently, flow velocity is low and flow through the ventricular septal defect is laminar. The combination of pulmonic stenosis and a small-to-medium–size ventricular septal defect can occur but is uncommon. Here the ventricular septal defect does create a murmur. In dogs with right-to-left shunting, pulmonary blood flow decreases as the pulmonic stenosis increases in severity. Consequently, the murmur intensity varies inversely with the severity of the stenosis. This is opposed to the more usual situation of isolated pulmonic stenosis, in which the murmur may increase in intensity as the stenosis increases in severity. Occasionally a dog with tetralogy of Fallot does not have a murmur. With severe pulmonic stenosis and marked right-to-left shunting, flow through the pulmonic valve is markedly reduced. This decreases flow velocity across the stenotic region. In addition, such a case is commonly polycythemic.

Polycythemia increases blood viscosity. Producing turbulence in blood that is more viscous than normal is more difficult (e.g., producing flow disturbances in molasses is more difficult than in water). Consequently, turbulence and murmur intensity are decreased, occasionally to the point that there is no murmur. In one report, of 13 dogs examined, 11 had a heart murmur heard best at the left base, and in six of these dogs the murmur was a grade 5/6.[2]

Femoral artery pulse pressure is usually normal.[2] In dogs with decreased pulmonary blood flow, left heart venous return is decreased, resulting in a decreased left heart size. However, the combination of the decreased left ventricular stroke volume and shunt stroke volume combine to produce a normal amount of blood pumped into the aorta with each beat. The normal stroke volume combined with a normal aortic input impedance (resistance) result in a normal pulse pressure.

Diagnostic Tests

RADIOGRAPHY

The chest radiographic findings are variable, depending on the severity of the abnormalities, the chest configuration, and so on. The chest radiographs are almost always abnormal. The classic findings in tetralogy of Fallot include evidence of right ventricular enlargement and decreased pulmonary vascular markings. The right ventricular enlargement is due to concentric right ventricular hypertrophy. The enlargement may not be obvious. The decrease in pulmonary vascular markings is consistent in dogs with severe tetralogy of Fallot but may not be present in dogs with less severe disease. On a dorsoventral radiograph, the region of the main pulmonary artery may be normal, indented, or enlarged as a result of poststenotic dilatation (Figure 14-3).[2]

ELECTROCARDIOGRAPHY

The electrocardiogram is usually consistent with right ventricular enlargement.[2] Right axis deviation in the frontal plane, terminal orientation of the QRS complex toward the right ventricle, and a deep *S* wave in a left chest lead are all common in patients with severe right ventricular concentric hypertrophy. Arrhythmias can occur but are uncommon.

ECHOCARDIOGRAPHY

A definitive diagnosis of tetralogy of Fallot can usually be made using two-dimensional and color flow Doppler echocardiography. From a right parasternal long-axis view in which the aorta is seen, the large ventricular septal defect and overriding aorta can be visualized (Figures 14-4 and 14-5). Color flow Doppler imaging from this site may provide evidence for laminar blood flow from the right ventricle into the aorta (Color Plate 52). The right ventricular free wall is thickened, usually to the same degree as or to a greater degree than the left ventricular free wall. The right-to-left ventricular free wall thickness ratio was 1.0 to 2.3 in one study (normal = 0.4 to 0.8 in young dogs).[2] Contrast echocardiography is helpful and more reliable than color Doppler echocardiography in identifying the intracardiac right-to-left shunt. Injection of agitated saline into a peripheral vein results in microbubbles being visualized in the right ventricle (which is normal), the aorta, and, sometimes, in the left ventricle (both of which are abnormal).

From a right parasternal short-axis view of the heart base, the right ventricular outflow tract, pulmonic valve region, main pulmonary artery, and pulmonary artery branches can be visualized. The site of the pulmonic stenosis may be visualized by carefully examining for narrowed regions or immobile valve leaflets. Color flow Doppler may help in identifying the site of stenosis by delineating the site of origin of turbulent blood flow. Pulsed-wave Doppler can be used to

A

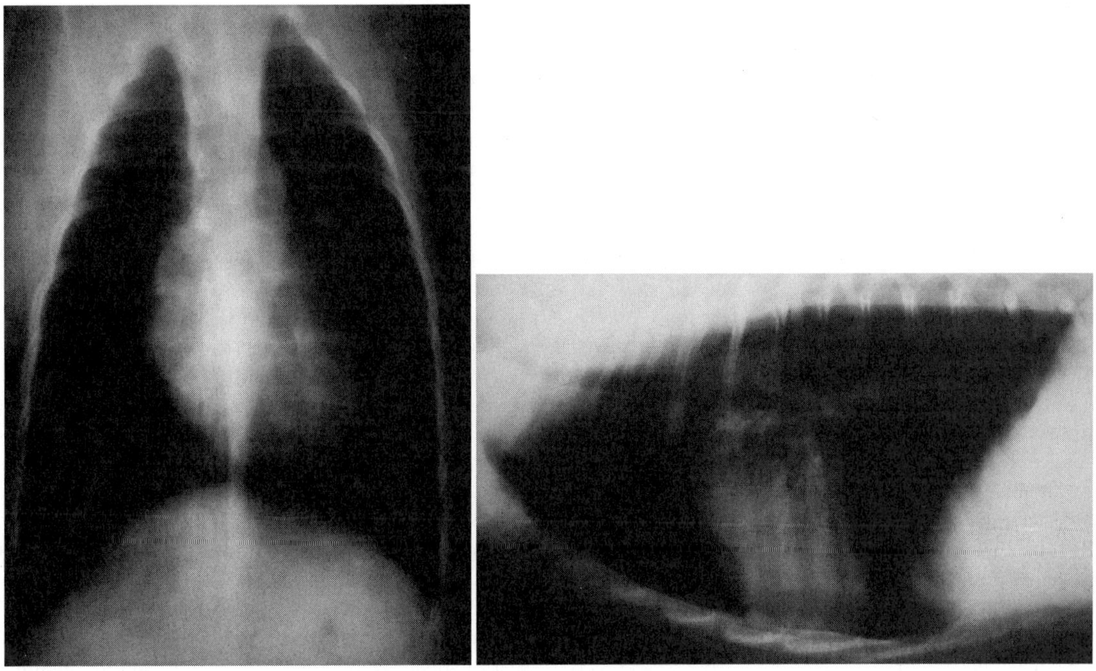

B

FIGURE 14-3 Dorsoventral (**A**) and lateral (**B**) thoracic radiographs from a 5-month-old male keeshond with tetralogy of Fallot. The cardiac silhouette does not appear to be enlarged. The lungs are hyperinflated, and the peripheral pulmonary vasculature is small. The main cranial and caudal lobar vessels are normal. The region of the main pulmonary artery on the dorsoventral radiograph is normal to slightly indented.

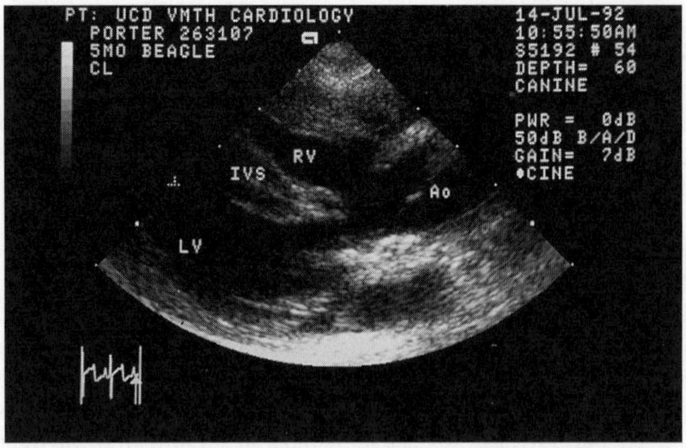

FIGURE 14-4 Long-axis two-dimensional echocardiogram taken from a right parasternal position from a 5-month-old beagle with tetralogy of Fallot. There is a large defect between the right ventricle *(RV)* and the left ventricle *(LV)*, at the top of the interventricular septum *(IVS)*. The root of the aorta *(AO)* is positioned to the right, such that more than 50% of it originates from the right ventricle. The right ventricular *(RV)* free wall is concentrically hypertrophied because of the pressure overload.

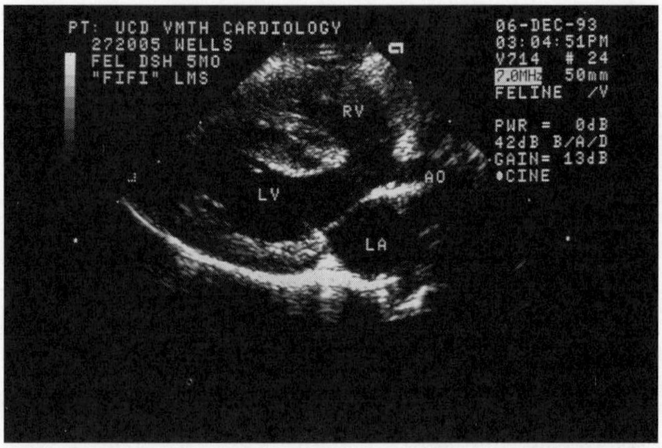

FIGURE 14-5 Long-axis two-dimensional echocardiogram from a 5-month-old cat with tetralogy of Fallot, taken from a right parasternal position. There is a large ventricular septal defect, and the aorta *(AO)* overrides the interventricular septum. *RV,* Right ventricular chamber; *LV,* left ventricular chamber; *LA,* left atrial chamber.

determine the site of stenosis in the same manner isolated pulmonic stenosis is evaluated. The ventricular septal defect can also be identified from the right parasternal short-axis view at the level of the aortic root. Color flow Doppler may aid in identifying the site of the ventricular septal defect. The ventricular septal defect is usually found in the perimembranous infundibular location (see Figure 13-5). The tricuspid valve and the aortic valve have fibrous continuity. Occasionally the defect will be supracristal, that is, below the pulmonic valve. A short-axis view at the level of the ventricles demonstrates the usually severe right ventricular concentric hypertrophy.

Continuous-wave Doppler is not a good measure of the severity of the stenosis in patients with tetralogy of Fallot and decreased pulmonary blood flow. The pressure gradient across a valve is related to the resistance to flow (determined by the size of the orifice) and blood flow (pressure gradient = flow × resistance). In the left heart, flow and resistance are maintained at a level to produce a pressure gradient of 100 to 150 mm Hg across the systemic circulation. In a circulation with a large ventricular septal defect imposed, the right ventricular pressure will also be maintained at 100 to 150 mm Hg, because maintenance of systemic pressure is highly regulated. Because this pressure is now regulated on both sides of the circulation, pulmonary flow and resistance will change in direct proportion to each other; that is, as resistance increases, flow always decreases in direct proportion and vice versa. Consequently, pressure gradient, and therefore flow velocity, are always the same (around 100 mm Hg and 5 m/sec, respectively).

From a left apical four-chamber view in which the aorta is visualized, the ventricular septal defect and the aortic override can be evaluated. Fibrous continuity between the aortic root and the tricuspid valve annulus will be present if the ventricular septal defect is perimembranous. From a left cranial view, the long-axis view of the right ventricular outflow tract can be viewed to examine the region of pulmonic stenosis.

LABORATORY EVALUATION

Many dogs and cats with tetralogy of Fallot have polycythemia. However, younger animals may be extremely hypoxemic and not have severe polycythemia. In one report, only five of 13 dogs had a packed cell volume (PCV) greater than 50% and only three had one greater than 60%.[2] All of the dogs that did not have a PCV greater than 50% in this report were either 4 months of age or less or not cyanotic at presentation. One must remember, however, that young dogs normally have a PCV that is much lower than an adult dog. The upper limit of normal for PCV in a 6-week-old dog is approximately 33% and in a 3- to 6-month–old dog is approximately 43%.[21] Using these values, 11 of 13 dogs in this report had a PCV that was at the upper limit of normal or greater than normal for its age range. The one dog that did not have an elevated PCV was the one dog in the report that was not cyanotic at rest. Consequently, it appears that PCV is increased in the vast majority of dogs with tetralogy of Fallot that are cyanotic at rest.

An arterial blood gas analysis is useful for determining the severity of the disease, especially in animals that are not polycythemic. Arterial oxygen tension has been reported to range between 39 and 64 mm Hg (normal is approximately 90 to 110 mm Hg, depending on elevation) in dogs with tetralogy of Fallot. However, some of these values were obtained from dogs that were being supplemented with oxygen.[2] Arterial oxygen tension was 28 mm Hg in one dog in another report.[19] In our experience, arterial oxygen tension is always less than 40 mm Hg and usually less than 35 mm Hg in an awake dog with tetralogy of Fallot that is cyanotic and not being administered supplemental oxygen.

CARDIAC CATHETERIZATION

In human medicine cardiac catheterization is important before performing open-heart surgery. It is used to assess the level of stenosis, the position of the ventricular septal defect, and the degree of aortic override and to identify complicating lesions, such as coronary artery anomalies. In veterinary medicine, in which open-heart surgery is almost never performed, cardiac catheterization is much less important, especially since the advent of echocardiography.

Cardiac catheterization is occasionally performed in veterinary patients with tetralogy of Fallot, and the findings are similar to those reported in human medicine.[2] When catheters are placed in the right and left ventricles so that simultaneous pressure recordings can be evaluated, right and left ventricular systolic pressures are identical. When radiopaque dye is injected into the

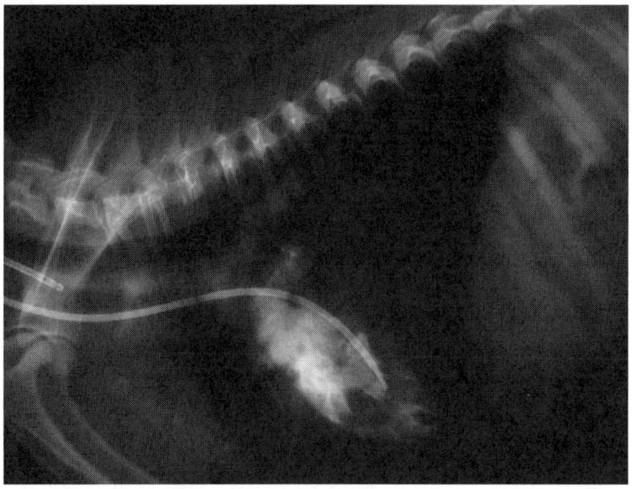

FIGURE 14-6 Angiocardiogram of the dog shown in Color Plate 51. The contrast agent was injected into the right ventricle, which is heavily trabeculated and clearly outlined. The contrast agent is ejected into both the pulmonary artery and the aorta. The proximal aorta is clearly outlined, as opposed to an angiogram from a dog with a right-to-left shunting patent ductus arteriosus.

right ventricle, the dye outlines the right ventricle, the pulmonary artery, and the aorta, confirming right-to-left shunting (Figure 14-6).[2-5] The region of stenosis may be visualized, but visualization may be difficult because of the aortic root overlying the stenotic region. The right heart catheter may pass into the left heart or aorta during catheterization, confirming the presence of the ventricular septal defect. An aortic root injection may be beneficial before performing palliative surgery. Identifying the side of the aortic arch and the anatomy of the brachiocephalic trunk and subclavian vessels may help a surgeon performing a systemic artery–to–pulmonary artery anastomosis.

Oximetry can be performed while the patient is inspiring 21% oxygen. With a pure right-to-left shunt, the oxygen tensions in the right atrium, right ventricle, and pulmonary artery are roughly equal and the oxygen tension in the aorta is less than in the left ventricular inflow tract and left atrium.[2] If bidirectional shunting is occurring, right ventricular and pulmonary artery oxygen tensions will be greater than right atrial oxygen tension. In one study, shunting appeared to be strictly right-to-left in seven dogs and bidirectional in the remaining six dogs.[2]

Bronchoesophageal arteries normally provide nutritional blood supply to the lungs. In dogs with tetralogy of Fallot, these vessels enlarge in an attempt to increase pulmonary blood flow.

Differential Diagnoses

Differential diagnoses include other congenital cardiac abnormalities that produce cyanosis. A right-to-left shunting patent ductus arteriosus most commonly results in differential cyanosis, with the caudal regions of the body being cyanotic and the cranial regions spared. However, generalized cyanosis can occur. Examples of other congenital cardiac abnormalities that produce cyanosis include Eisenmenger's complex, pulmonic stenosis with an atrial septal defect, double-outlet right ventricle with pulmonic stenosis, transposition of the great arteries, pulmonary atresia with intact ventricular septum, truncus arteriosus, and pseudotruncus arteriosus.

Treatment

MEDICAL MANAGEMENT

Phlebotomy. Medical management of tetralogy of Fallot is primarily aimed at alleviating clinical signs referable to polycythemia. Phlebotomy is the procedure of choice for the symptomatic patient with tetralogy of Fallot. Mild decreases in hematocrit can produce significant clinical benefit, whereas overzealous phlebotomy decreases tissue oxygen delivery to the point that the patient becomes more symptomatic (usually depressed). The goal should be to restore the hematocrit to between 60% and 65%. The following formula is used to determine how much blood to remove:

$$\text{Blood to be removed (mL)} = [\text{Body weight (kg)} \times 0.08] \times 1000\ \text{mL/kg} \times \frac{[\text{Actual hematocrit} - \text{Desired hematocrit}]}{\text{Actual hematocrit}}$$

Blood should be removed through a large-bore catheter. The blood removed must be replaced with intravenous fluid (1 to 2 times the blood volume removed) when the blood is withdrawn. It is common for the hematocrit to be greater than calculated once the phlebotomy is completed. This is probably due to release of stored red cells from extramedullary sites.

Hydroxyurea. Hydroxyurea can be tried in cases that require frequent phlebotomies. Hydroxyurea is a myelosuppressive agent that produces reversible bone marrow suppression. It is administered initially as a loading dose of 30 mg/kg/day for 7 to 10 days, followed by 15 mg/kg/day.[22] Complete blood counts and platelet counts must be determined every 1 to 2 weeks. Leukopenia, thrombocytopenia, or anemia necessitate stopping the drug until blood counts normalize. A lower dose may then be administered. Some dogs require higher doses to induce a decrease in hematocrit. The side effects of hydroxyurea in the dog include anorexia, vomiting, bone marrow hypoplasia, and sloughing of the nails.

β-Blockers. β-Adrenergic blocking drugs may be beneficial in relieving hypoxemic episodes. This strategy has been reported to be successful in a dog, and we have used it successfully in several cases.[20] It is also a commonly employed method in human patients.[23] Propranolol appears to be the β-blocker of choice. It can be used for acute termination of an hypoxemic episode or can be used chronically to prevent hypoxemic episodes. Presumably the patients that respond to β-blockade are having hypoxemic episodes because of adrenergic drive to hypertrophied myocardium in the right ventricular outflow tract causing dynamic infundibular narrowing. The β-blocker theoretically reduces the hypercontraction in this region, resulting in improved pulmonary blood flow. β-Blockers may also attenuate the β-adrenergic–mediated decrease in systemic vascular resistance during exercise. The dose used successfully in the aforementioned case report was 2.5 mg/kg q8-12 h. The dose reported in humans ranges between 1 and 1.25 mg/kg q8h.

Other drugs. Morphine is also used in human pediatric patients to relieve hypoxemic episodes. Its mechanism of action in this situation is unknown. It may decrease infundibular contraction or it may have a central effect or a peripheral vascular vagotonic effect. The use of morphine in veterinary patients with tetralogy of Fallot has not been reported.

In the same way that arteriolar dilators are useful for managing left-to-right shunts, arteriolar constrictors are beneficial in patients with right-to-left shunts that occur at the ventricular level or beyond. By increasing systemic vascular resistance, less blood is shunted right-to-left and more blood is ejected through the pulmonary vasculature. Unfortunately, no long-acting and orally available drugs have been formulated to constrict systemic arterioles. Consequently, this remains a theoretic modality for chronic management of right-to-left shunting lesions. Drugs such as phenylephrine can be used to manage an acute hypoxemic episode and are used in our hospital for managing hypoxemia during anesthesia. As an example, one of our patients with tetralogy of Fallot had an arterial oxygen tension of 33 mm Hg on room air. He was anesthetized for a procedure and placed on a ventilator with 100% inspired oxygen. His systemic arterial oxygen tension was 56 mm Hg, and his oxygen saturation was 84%. He was placed on a phenylephrine infusion, and his oxygen tension increased to 66 mm Hg and his oxygen saturation to 92%.

INTERVENTIONAL THERAPY

Balloon valvuloplasty of the pulmonic valve can be attempted in dogs with tetralogy of Fallot. Although results at the University of California, Davis, Veterinary Medical Teaching Hospital have been varied, successful outcomes have been identified. These patients have had apparent increases in pulmonary blood flow and decreases in right-to-left shunting, as evidenced by increased arterial oxygen tensions after valvuloplasty and improved clinical status. This improvement has been temporary in some cases and more long-lasting in others. Other canine patients have had no improvement. In one case the pulmonic stenosis was obliterated, resulting in acute, massive left-to-right shunting through the large ventricular septal defect, with resultant acute, massive pulmonary edema. This patient appeared to have a subarterial infundibular (supracristal) ventricular septal defect. A similar situation has been reported in a dog in which the pulmonic valve region was dilated at surgery, presumably using a valve dilator introduced through a small right ventriculotomy site within a purse-string suture.[2]

It should be noted that an improvement in the pulmonic stenosis cannot be verified using flow velocity or pressure gradient measurements. As explained in the echocardiography section, when balloon valvuloplasty successfully reduces pulmonary resistance by increasing the orifice size, flow increases proportionately. The net result is no change in pressure gradient or blood flow velocity.

SURGICAL MANAGEMENT

Palliative surgery can be performed in dogs with tetralogy of Fallot. The primary goal of any palliative treatment for this disease is to increase the oxygen tension in the systemic blood. Corrective surgery using cardiopulmonary bypass and open-heart surgery is commonplace in human medicine and is aimed at relieving the pulmonic stenosis and patching the ventricular septal defect. This has only been reported once in a dog, in 1983.[24] In this dog, cardiopulmonary bypass and mild hypothermia (32° C) were used and the heart was arrested with cold cardioplegia solution. The procedure consisted of resecting part of the hypertrophied pulmonary outflow tract (infundibulum), dilating the stenotic pulmonary valve until a 12-mm valve dilator could be passed freely through the orifice, and patching the ventricular septal defect with a Teflon patch through a right ventriculotomy. The patch was sutured with a continuous pattern, taking care not to disrupt the atrioventricular conduction system at the caudal-ventral portion of the ventricular septal defect. The apparent lack of success of this procedure, based on the paucity of reported cases, and the expense of cardiopulmonary bypass and open-heart surgery make this approach impractical in most situations in veterinary medicine.

Palliative surgery consists of producing systemic-to-pulmonary anastomoses (Figure 14-7). The most common is an anastomosis of the left subclavian artery to a pulmonary artery.[5,25] This type of

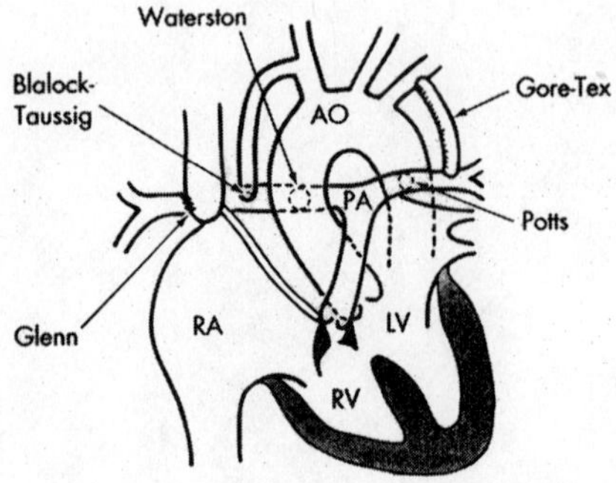

FIGURE 14-7 Schematic drawing of palliative surgical procedures for patients with cyanotic cardiac disease. The Blalock-Taussig, Potts, and modified Blalock-Taussig (Gore-Tex) shunts are used most commonly in patients with tetralogy of Fallot. Abbreviations are as in Figure 14-1. (From Park MK: *The pediatric cardiology handbook,* St Louis, 1997, Mosby.)

shunt was first described by Blalock and Taussig in 1945 and so carries their names.[26] A Blalock-Taussig shunt creates an artificial patent ductus arteriosus by connecting the left subclavian artery to a pulmonary artery using an end-to-side anastomosis. This "replumbing" takes some percentage of the blood that has shunted right-to-left through the ventricular septal defect and shunts it back into the pulmonary artery, increasing pulmonary blood flow and venous return to the left heart. Obviously, this is not ideal but it does take some of the less saturated blood that otherwise would be delivered to the systemic circulation and redistributes it to the pulmonary vasculature to be oxygenated. The net result is an increase in oxygenated blood returning to the left heart to be pumped into the systemic circulation. This type of shunt has been used successfully in veterinary medicine. In one case report, a 3.5-year-old wirehaired fox terrier with tetralogy of Fallot lived for 1.5 years after surgery.[25] However, the shunt closed after that time and the dog died.

Several other procedures have been described since Taussig and Blalock first described this technique. All these procedures create a communication between the systemic circulation and a pulmonary artery. They include a Potts shunt, a central graft shunt, a Waterston shunt, and a modified Blalock-Taussig shunt. The other procedure most commonly used in veterinary and human medicine is the modified Blalock-Taussig shunt, in which a synthetic graft made of Gore-Tex is interposed between a subclavian artery or the aorta and a pulmonary artery. Decision regarding technique is based on anatomy. A kink can form when the left subclavian artery is too short. The advantages that Blalock-Taussig or modified Blalock-Taussig shunts have are: (1) the surgery is performed outside the pericardial sac, (2) the subclavian artery or the graft is usually large enough to provide adequate flow, and (3) the subclavian artery or the graft is not so large that they result in too much flow, which could result in left heart failure or pulmonary hypertension. The Potts operation consists of directly creating a side-to-side anastomosis between the descending aorta and the left pulmonary artery. The potential problems with this shunt are the same as for a Blalock-Taussig shunt, plus the possibility of making the shunt too large and creating left heart failure. In one report of a series of four cases treated by this method, one dog developed left heart failure and one dog lived for 3 years and then became cyanotic again, although the shunt was still patent. One dog lived for 2 years and then developed exercise intolerance and died. The last dog developed cyanosis again 2 weeks after surgery and died with evidence of shunt closure at postmortem examination.[2] The second dog may have developed pulmonary vascular disease with subsequent recurrence of right-to-left shunting. End-to-end anastomosis of the left internal thoracic artery to the left middle lung lobe pulmonary artery has been performed successfully in one cat.[27] The lung lobe was removed after the anastomosis.

In any technique used, careful attention to surgical technique is mandatory. Poor surgical technique will result in thrombus formation in the shunt or stricture and may lead to shunt closure or a reduction in total shunt flow.[5] Patients being considered for palliative surgery should first be evaluated by a board-certified cardiologist, if possible, and then referred to a surgeon that has experience in placing Blalock-Taussig shunts or in vascular surgery. It remains uncertain whether balloon dilation should be routinely attempted before palliative surgery.

Successful palliative surgery increases systemic oxygen tension. This increase is not generally into the normal range. Instead, the PaO_2 usually increases into the 45- to 60-mm Hg range. This increase, however, usually results in clinical improvement. The improvement can be long-lasting.

REFERENCES

1. Patterson DF: Epidemiologic and genetic studies of congenital heart disease in the dog, *Circ Res* 23:171, 1968.
2. Ringwald RJ, Bonagura JD: Tetralogy of Fallot in the dog: clinical findings in 13 cases, *J Am Anim Hosp Assoc* 24:33, 1988.
3. Lombard CW, Twitchell MJ: Tetralogy of Fallot, persistent left cranial vena cava and retinal detachment in a cat, *J Am Anim Hosp Assoc* 14:624, 1978.
4. Bolton GR, Ettinger SJ, Liu SK: Tetralogy of Fallot in three cats, *J Am Vet Med Assoc* 160:1622, 1972.
5. Bush M, Pieroni DR, Goodman DG et al: Tetralogy of Fallot in a cat, *J Am Vet Med Assoc* 161:1679, 1972.
6. Stowater JL: Tetralogy of Fallot and peritoneopericardial diaphragmatic hernia in a dog, *Vet Med Small Anim Clin* 77:397, 1982.
7. Patterson DF, Pyle RL, Van Mierop L et al: Hereditary defects of the conotruncal septum in keeshond dogs: pathologic and genetic studies, *Am J Cardiol* 34:187, 1974.
8. Wenink ACG: Embryology of the heart. In Anderson RH, ed: *Paediatric cardiology,* Edinburgh, 1987, Churchill Livingstone.
9. Anderson RH, Lenox CC, Zuberbuhler JR: The morphology of ventricular septal defects, *Perspect Pediatr Pathol* 8:235, 1984.
10. Anderson RH, Allwork SP, Ho SY et al: Surgical anatomy of tetralogy of Fallot, *J Thorac Cardiovasc Surg* 81:887, 1981.
11. Patterson DF: Genes and the heart: congenital heart disease, *Proc Acad Vet Cardiol,* 1991, p 13.
12. Clark DR, Ross JN, Hamlin RL et al: Tetralogy of Fallot in the dog, *J Am Vet Med Assoc* 152:462, 1968.
13. Galson DL, Blanchard KL, Fandrey J et al: Cis elements that regulate the erythropoietin gene, *Ann N Y Acad Sci* 718:21, 1994.
14. Eckardt KU, Pugh CW, Meier M et al: Production of erythropoietin by liver cells in vivo and in vitro, *Ann N Y Acad Sci* 718:50, 1994 (discussion 61-3).
15. Epstein FH, Agmon Y, Brezis M: Physiology of renal hypoxia, *Ann N Y Acad Sci* 718:72, 1994 (discussion 81-2).
16. Liberato NL, Costa A, Barosi G: Erythropoietin: biological aspects and clinical usefulness, *Haematologica* 75:346, 1990.
17. Hasler AH, Giger U: Serum erythropoietin values in polycythemic cats, *J Am Anim Hosp Assoc* 32:294, 1996.
18. Sawyer ST: Introduction: the erythropoietin receptor and signal transduction, *Ann N Y Acad Sci* 718:185, 1994.
19. Cook SM, Lothrop CD: Serum erythropoietin concentrations measured by radioimmunoassay in normal, polycythemic, and anemic dogs and cats, *J Vet Intern Med* 8:18, 1994 (see comments).
20. Eyster GE, Anderson LK, Sawyer DC et al: Beta adrenergic blockade for management of tetralogy of Fallot in a dog, *J Am Vet Med Assoc* 169:637, 1976.
21. Reference intervals for canine blood values, Ralston Purina Company, 1986.
22. Peterson ME, Randolph JF: Diagnosis of canine primary polycythemia and management with hydroxyurea, *J Am Vet Med Assoc* 180:415, 1982.
23. Garson AJ, Gillette PC, McNamara DG: Propranolol: the preferred palliation for tetralogy of Fallot, *Am J Cardiol* 47:1098, 1981.
24. Herrtage ME, Hall LW, English TAH: Surgical correction of the tetralogy of Fallot in a dog, *J Small Anim Pract* 24:51, 1983.
25. Eyster GE, Braden TD, Appleford M et al: Surgical management of tetralogy of Fallot, *J Small Anim Pract* 18:387, 1977.
26. Blalock A, Taussig HB: The surgical treatment of malformation of the heart in which there is pulmonary stenosis or pulmonary atresia, *JAMA* 128:189, 1945.
27. Miller CW, Holmberg DL, Bowen V et al: Microsurgical management of tetralogy of Fallot in a cat, *J Am Vet Med Assoc* 186:708, 1985.

CHAPTER 15

Pulmonic Stenosis

Pulmonic stenosis is a narrowing anywhere from the right ventricular outflow tract to the main pulmonary artery. The lesion may be valvular, subvalvular, or supravalvular. Subvalvular lesions may be due to a fixed fibrous lesion or to thickened myocardium creating a dynamic narrowing of the outflow tract in systole. A combination of valvular and subvalvular stenosis is common.

Prevalence

Congenital obstruction to right ventricular outflow is a common lesion in dogs and is infrequently recognized in cats. In a survey of the records of North American veterinary schools for the years 1987 to 1989, isolated congenital pulmonic stenosis was the third most commonly diagnosed congenital cardiac defect in dogs (18%).[1] Only patent ductus arteriosus (32%) and subaortic stenosis (22%) were diagnosed with greater frequency.[1] In our clinic, pulmonic stenosis is also the third most commonly diagnosed congenital cardiac abnormality. From August 1, 1986, to August 1, 1996, we diagnosed isolated pulmonic stenosis in 181 dogs. The prevalence of the disease in our referral-based hospital population was two dogs per 1000 dogs examined. Pulmonic stenosis comprised approximately 5% of the primary cases we examined in our service during that period. Isolated pulmonic stenosis is rare in cats. We only diagnosed isolated pulmonic stenosis in eight cats within the same period. Pulmonic stenosis more often occurs in association with other defects in cats. Recently, dynamic obstruction of the right ventricular outflow tract, considered a form of pulmonic stenosis, has been identified in cats as an apparently incidental and benign finding (Chapter 3).[2,3] In dogs, pulmonic stenosis usually occurs as an isolated lesion, although it may occur along with other defects or in association with other defects in more complicated deformities (e.g., tetralogy of Fallot).[4,5]

Embryology and Genetics

During embryonic development, the pulmonic valve originates from three swellings (two truncus swellings and one intercalated swelling) within the developing truncus arteriosus, by a process of excavation in a proximal direction.[6] It has been postulated that a maldevelopment of the distal bulbous cordis, from which these swellings originate, may lead to pulmonary valve stenosis.[7] Infundibular or subvalvular stenosis probably results from an abnormal partitioning of the bulbous cordis during ventricular septal formation, whereas supravalvular stenosis may represent maldevelopment of the more distal portions of the truncus arteriosus.[8] However, little is known about the exact embryologic mechanisms responsible for each of the different types of pulmonic stenosis observed in dogs and cats. Even in man, the exact pathogenetic mechanism responsible for pulmonary valve stenosis is still speculative.[9]

A heritable basis for pulmonic stenosis has been proved in beagles and keeshonds and based on breeding studies of this and other defects is also suspected in other commonly affected breeds.[10-12] Other breeds at increased risk for pulmonic stenosis (based on calculated odds ratios) include the English bulldog, mastiff, Samoyed, miniature schnauzer, American cocker spaniel, and West Highland white terrier (Table 15-1).[1] Pulmonary valve dysplasia and stenosis have also been reported in the Boykin spaniel, bull mastiff, and beagle.[10,13,14] Both sexes may be affected, although in the English bulldog and bull mastiff, a male predominance has been reported.[1,14]

Anatomy

Congenital obstruction to right ventricular outflow can originate at the pulmonary valve or occur below (subvalvular) or above (supravalvular) the valve apparatus. Occasionally, multiple levels of obstruction are present in the same individual. The terms *valvular* and *valvar* imply "pertaining to the valve" and may be used interchangeably, although it is perhaps less confusing to simply use the word *valve* without modification (e.g., pulmonary valve stenosis). Deformation of the pulmonic valve or the adjacent regions generally results in stenosis, although isolated congenital pulmonic valve insufficiency has been reported in dogs.[15] Pulmonic insufficiency is more commonly associated with a stenotic valve and is generally mild and hemodynamically insignificant.

VALVULAR STENOSIS

Pulmonary valve stenosis resulting from commissural fusion is characterized by a thin-to-moderately thickened, pliant, conical or dome-shaped valve, with a narrowed outlet ("windsock").[9,10] Typically there are no discrete valve leaflets, although rudimentary raphe may extend from the orifice toward the wall of the pulmonary artery (Color Plate 53, *A*). Pulmonary valve stenosis resulting from pulmonary valve "dysplasia," on the other hand, usually consists of markedly thickened valve leaflets and annular hypoplasia without fusion of the commissures (Color Plate 53, *B*).[10,16,17] Commonly, the pathologic findings of both commissural fusion and valvular dysplasia coexist, and a more distinct subclassification cannot be made. Consequently, the term *pulmonary valve dysplasia* encompasses a variety of valvular abnormalities in dogs.[16] The leaflets of dysplastic valves are usually relatively immobile. This, in concert with the annular hypoplasia, leads to a reduction in effective orifice size. The most common form of pulmonic stenosis reported in dogs is valvular dysplasia (88%).[18]

SUPRAVALVULAR STENOSIS

Supravalvular pulmonic stenosis is rare in dogs (Color Plate 53, *C*). In humans, supravalvular pulmonic stenosis may result from narrowing of the main pulmonary artery or its main branches, or, less commonly, from a membranous obstruction immediately above the valve.[19] The anatomic features of supravalvular pulmonic stenosis have not been documented in dogs.

SUBVALVULAR STENOSIS

In dogs with subvalvular pulmonic stenosis, a fibrous ring is typically located at the base of the valve (usually accompanied by valvular deformity) or below the valve in a subvalvular ring (Color Plate 53, *B*). Occasionally, subvalvular obstruction consists of a fibromuscular narrowing of the infundibular region of the right ventricle, about 1 to 3 cm below the pulmonic valve.[4,18-20] In addition, excessive concentric infundibular or supraventricular crest hypertrophy may contribute to the outflow obstruction in some dogs, especially during exercise or stress provocation (i.e., dynamic obstruction).[4,13,18] The hemodynamic significance of infundibular hypertrophy is controversial. Dynamic outflow tract obstruction occurs in normal cats with heart murmurs. It tends to be mild, variable, and of little hemodynamic or clinical consequence.[2] There are no obvious anatomic deformities identified on echocardiographic examination in these cats; however, post mortem studies have not been evaluated.[2]

Subvalvular stenosis associated with a coronary artery anomaly. In the English bulldog and boxer breeds, subvalvular pulmonic stenosis may be associated with an R2A type of anomalous left coronary artery.[21-23] In this malformation, a single large coronary artery originates from the right coronary aortic sinus and quickly divides into right and left branches. The left main coronary artery encircles and apparently compresses the right ventricular outflow tract just below the pulmonary valve, before dividing into the left descending and left circumflex coronary arteries (Color Plate 53, *D*). The course of the right coronary artery is usually normal.

Commonly associated lesions. Mild, subclinical deformities of the tricuspid valve apparatus may accompany pulmonic stenosis in dogs. More severe tricuspid dysplasia with regurgitation may be a major complicating lesion.[5] We diagnosed pulmonary stenosis and tricuspid valve dysplasia in 15 dogs between August 1, 1986, and August 1, 1996, that were in right heart failure (ascites). Four of these dogs were boxers and three were English bulldogs. The foramen ovale may remain patent in dogs with pulmonic stenosis, and it may allow mild right-to-left shunting of blood because of the hypertrophied and therefore less compliant right ventricle.[24]

TABLE 15-1

Breed odds ratios[1]

Breed	*No.*	*Odds ratio*	*95% CL*	*P*
English bulldog	30	19.2	12.8-28.7	<0.0001
Mastiff	5	1.6	4.2-29.4	<0.0001
Samoyed	11	5.4	2.8-10.1	<0.0001
Miniature schnauzer	14	3.5	2.0-6.2	<0.0001
West highland white	5	3.3	1.2-8.3	0.020
Chow chow	5	2.2	0.8-5.5	NS
Cocker spaniel	18	1.7	1.0-2.8	0.026

Pathophysiology

PRESSURE OVERLOAD

Independent of the nature of the obstruction, the principle hemodynamic consequence of pulmonic stenosis is an increased resistance to the right ventricular systolic outflow, with a proportional elevation of right ventricular systolic pressure if flow remains constant (Figure 15-1). The pressure in the pulmonary artery is generally normal, but may be decreased if right ventricular stroke volume is significantly reduced. The magnitude of the resultant pressure gradient is directly related to both the quantity and rate of blood flow across the obstruction and to the cross-sectional area of the stenotic region. The pressure gradient is commonly used as an index of lesion severity. However, because it is affected by both lesion severity (resistance) and blood flow, it is less accurate than determinations of the lesion's cross-sectional area or resistance.

The increase in right ventricular systolic wall stress stimulates an increase in right ventricular muscle mass (concentric hypertrophy or hyperplasia), usually proportional to the severity of the obstruction.[20] In the fetus and neonate, the increase in mass occurs primarily from myocyte hyperplasia, with an associated increase in capillary growth, whereas in the mature animal, hypertrophy occurs with little or no associated hyperplasia.[9] The right ventricular hypertrophy normalizes right ventricular systolic function and usually allows right ventricular stroke volume to remain within the normal range. A massively hypertrophied right ventricle may reduce the right ventricular end-diastolic volume and may produce a relatively stiff ventricle, which may reduce the ability of the ventricle to fill properly and limit right ventricular stroke volume. Distal to the obstruction, blood flow velocity increases and flow becomes turbulent. The force

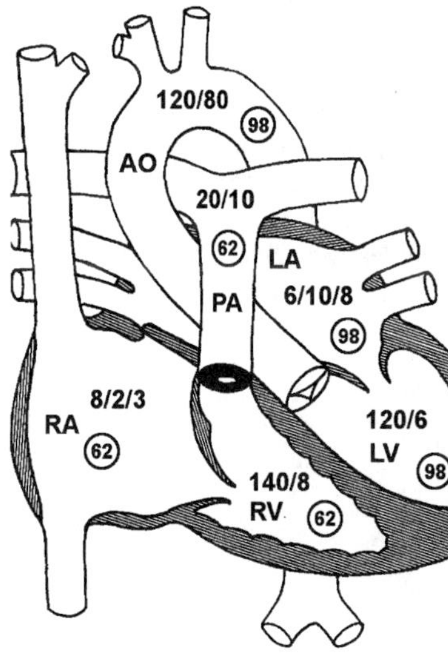

FIGURE 15-1 Schematic diagram depicting the hemodynamic alterations associated with severe valvular pulmonic stenosis. The resistance to flow at the pulmonary valve leads to an increase in right ventricular systolic pressure. The resultant concentric hypertrophy may lead to a mild increase in right ventricular diastolic pressure and right atrial pressure. Left-sided pressures remain normal. In the absence of an interatrial communication, both pulmonary and systemic hemoglobin saturation remain normal. *RA,* Right atrium; *RV,* right ventricle; *LA,* left atrium; *LV,* left ventricle; *PA,* pulmonary artery; *AO,* aorta. Intracardiac pressures are indicated in mm Hg as systolic/diastolic for LV, RV, PA, and AO and as *a* wave/*v* wave/mean for the LA and RA. Circled numbers indicate oxygen saturation.

of this turbulent jet results in main pulmonary artery enlargement (poststenotic dilation).

RIGHT HEART FAILURE

Congestive right heart failure is rare in patients with isolated pulmonic stenosis but is commonly observed in patients with concomitant tricuspid valve dysplasia. Between August 1, 1986, and August 1, 1996, we did not diagnose right heart failure in any dog with isolated pulmonic stenosis. Physiologic consequences of an elevated right ventricular systolic pressure may include reduced myocardial perfusion and ischemia. These may lead to ventricular arrhythmias and sudden death.

Diagnosis

MEDICAL HISTORY

Most dogs with pulmonic stenosis exhibit no clinical signs even with severe obstruction. Subtle decreases in exercise tolerance and activity may be noted by an observant owner or may be elucidated as having been present when the owner can evaluate these variables following successful treatment of pulmonic stenosis. The identification of a cardiac murmur during a routine physical examination is usually the first clue that pulmonic stenosis may be present. In severe cases, exertional fatigue, shortness of breath, or syncope may be reported. Although signs of right heart failure may occur, they are rare unless pulmonic stenosis is complicated by another anomaly, particularly by tricuspid valve dysplasia.

PHYSICAL EXAMINATION

On physical examination the most important finding is a systolic murmur of variable quality (usually harsh) heard best at the left heart base. The murmur may radiate to the right cranial thorax and is classically described as a systolic ejection murmur with a crescendo or crescendo-decrescendo quality (see Chapter 3).[4,20] Sometimes the murmur is heard lateral to the sternum on both sides of the cranial thorax.[4] Rarely, a soft diastolic murmur of pulmonic insufficiency may also be heard in the same location or may be heard radiating to the right side of the thorax. Dogs with pulmonic stenosis occasionally have a systolic ejection sound associated with the immobile valve leaflets snapping open (Figure 15-2). The jugular veins usually are not distended or pulsating, although a mildly exaggerated pulse may be noted in the lower third of the neck. In dogs with severe obstruction, mild pulsations (usually *a* waves) may be identified higher in the neck. If a marked jugular pulse is present or if jugular vein distension is observed, concurrent tricuspid valve dysplasia should be suspected. The arterial pulse is usually normal. In patients with an atrial or ventricular septal defect and right-to-left shunting, cyanosis of the mucous membranes may be observed.[24]

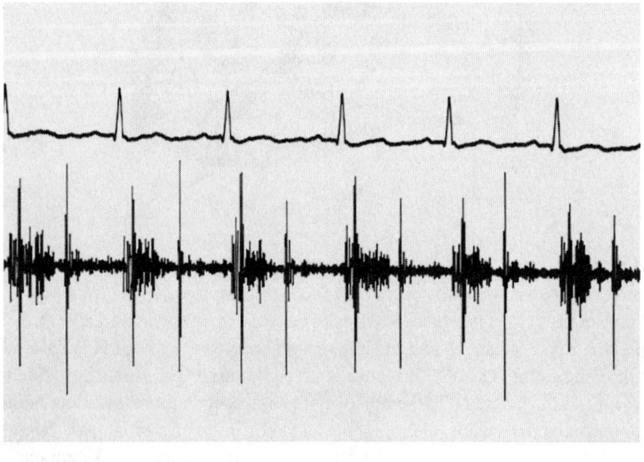

FIGURE 15-2 Phonocardiogram from a dog with pulmonic stenosis. The first heart sound occurs with the QRS complex of the ECG. Just after the first heart sound a loud ejection click can be seen, followed by a decrescendo systolic murmur and the second heart sound.

ELECTROCARDIOGRAPHY

In mild-to-moderate pulmonic stenosis, the electrocardiogram (ECG) is commonly normal. In dogs with severe right ventricular hypertrophy, evidence of right ventricular enlargement is commonly identified (see Chapter 5).[25-28] Right bundle branch block may be observed.[29] The *P* waves are usually normal. If the *P* waves are increased in amplitude, right atrial enlargement secondary to tricuspid dysplasia should be suspected.[29]

THORACIC RADIOGRAPHY

Thoracic radiographs are useful for supporting the diagnosis of pulmonic stenosis. However, radiographs often offer little specific information regarding the severity of the condition. In milder cases the radiographs may be normal. Radiographs are also helpful in identifying abnormalities that may suggest the presence of another defect.

Radiographs in dogs with moderate-to-severe pulmonic stenosis often demonstrate a prominent right ventricle and poststenotic dilatation of the main pulmonary artery (Figure 15-3).[26,30] The enlarged main pulmonic artery is most evident in the dorsoventral view. The pulmonary vasculature and parenchyma generally appear normal. If the heart appears markedly enlarged or if other segments appear significantly enlarged (e.g., the right atrium), an additional anomaly such as tricuspid dysplasia should be suspected.[29]

ECHOCARDIOGRAPHY

Echocardiography is the primary method of diagnosing pulmonic stenosis in animals. Invasive diagnostic techniques are usually unnecessary. The clinician can use two-dimensional echocardiography to accurately detect pulmonic stenosis. Doppler echocardiography provides an estimate of the severity of the obstruction (see Chapter 6). Right ventricular hypertrophy can be identified using M-mode echocardiography (Figure 15-4, *A*) but is identified just as well or better with two-dimensional echocardiography (Figure 15-4, *B* and 15-4, *C*). Paradoxical or flat systolic septal motion indicating elevated right ventricular systolic pressure, may also be recognized by M-mode examination (Figure 15-4, *C*). Otherwise, the M-mode echocardiogram provides little additional useful information toward the diagnosis of pulmonic stenosis, because the right atrium and pulmonic valve are not well visualized with this modality.[31]

Two-dimensional echocardiography can be used to identify most of the cardinal changes that occur in the heart in response to pulmonic stenosis. Moderate-to-severe right ventricular hypertrophy is usually readily identified; however, mild right ventricular hypertrophy may still be difficult to elucidate. The right ventricular papillary muscles may be notably enlarged. In severe cases, the septum may be flattened or may display paradoxical motion during ventricular systole because of the increased right ventricular systolic pressure.[32] The left ventricle may or may not assume its normal circular shape during diastole. In most cases, the poststenotic dilation of the main pulmonary artery, most apparent in the right parasternal short-axis view, can be visualized. However, the absence of this finding does not preclude the diagnosis. In the rare case, the pulmonary artery may be hypoplastic.

The pulmonary valve is difficult to image clearly using transthoracic echocardiography in most dogs because of interference with lung tissue. The valve can be visualized more clearly using transesophageal echocardiography. Multiple views from both sides of the chest are often necessary for complete evaluation when using transthoracic echocardiography. In dogs with pulmonary stenosis in which the valve is adequately visualized, several findings may be evident. With true pulmonary valve dysplasia the valve cusps are notably thickened and restricted in motion (Figure 15-4, *D*). A fused valve usually displays thin leaflets that "bow" into the main pulmonic artery during ventricular systole. Commonly, it is difficult to see enough detail of the pulmonary valve region to clearly define the exact location and anatomy of the deformity (i.e., whether there is valve thickening, valve fusion, fibrosis at the valve base, etc.). Subvalvular pulmonic stenosis usually produces an ill-defined and narrowed subvalvular area, and valvar anatomy is difficult to ascertain. In dogs with an anomalous left coronary artery, the obstructed region may be defined as subvalvular. The enlarged right coronary artery and the anomalous left coronary artery may be visualized in some cases in our experience. This is more easily seen with transesophageal echocardiography. In the mildest cases, the two-dimensional and M-mode examinations may be insensitive to the subtle changes that may be present.

In many cases of pulmonic stenosis, the right atrium is mildly enlarged. This probably occurs secondarily to an increase in the right atrial pressure that occurs because of decreased right ventricular compliance secondary to right ventricular hypertrophy. In some cases, mild tricuspid regurgitation may also exist.[33] Some dogs with pulmonic stenosis have an abnormal-appearing tricuspid valve, although they are functionally competent. If severe right atrial enlargement is present, severe tricuspid regurgitation as a result of concomitant tricuspid valve dysplasia should be suspected. The atrial septum should be evaluated from multiple views, because the foramen ovale may be patent in dogs with pulmonic stenosis and others may have an atrial septal defect.[24] Even in cases in which the atrial septum appears anatomically normal, contrast echocardiography should be performed to identify those patients with right-to-left shunting across a patent foramen ovale or atrial septal defect.[24] Although usually clinically insignificant, there are reports of right-to-left shunting atrial septal defects leading to cyanosis in dogs with pulmonic stenosis.[24]

Doppler echocardiography provides a means for estimating the severity of the stenosis and may be necessary for confirming the diagnosis in mild cases in which secondary findings on M-mode and two-dimensional examinations are equivocal.[34,35] Pulsed-wave Doppler can be used to identify the location of the stenosis.[36] Blood flow velocity proximal to the stenosis should be normal, and the flow pattern should be laminar (Figure 15-5, *A*). Blood flow velocity distal to the stenosis is increased, resulting in a turbulent flow pattern (Figure 15-5, *B*). To identify the narrowed region, the sample volume of the pulsed-wave Doppler should be placed proximal to the stenosis and then gradually advanced across the region of stenosis while recording. An increase in velocity and the development of turbulent flow as the sample volume crosses the narrowed region confirms the diagnosis and its location. Once the stenosis has been identified and localized using pulsed-wave Doppler, continuous-wave Doppler is used to determine peak blood flow velocity and semiquantify the severity of the stenosis (Figure 15-6). As in all stenoses, velocity increases as the cross-sectional area of the stenosis

A

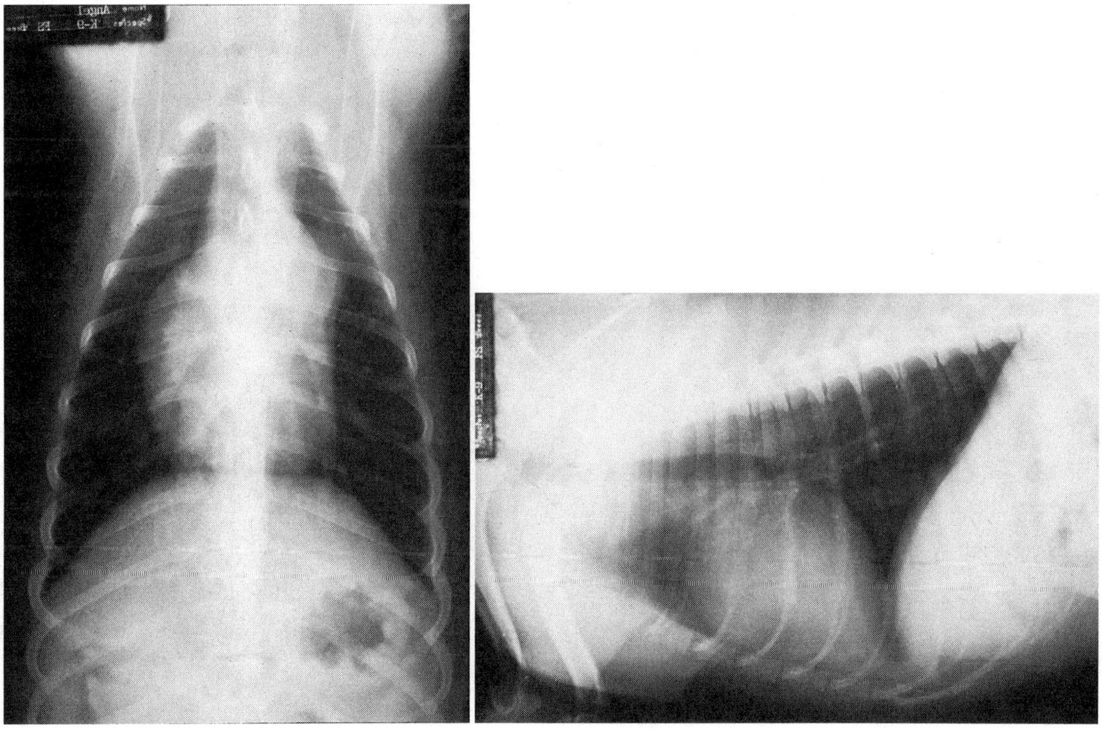

B

FIGURE 15-3 Thoracic radiographs from a dog with pulmonic stenosis. **A,** The dorsoventral projection shows right-sided cardiomegaly and an enlargement in the region of the main pulmonary artery. **B,** The lateral projection shows evidence of cardiomegaly, increased sternal contact, and a shift of the apex off the sternum due to right ventricular enlargement.

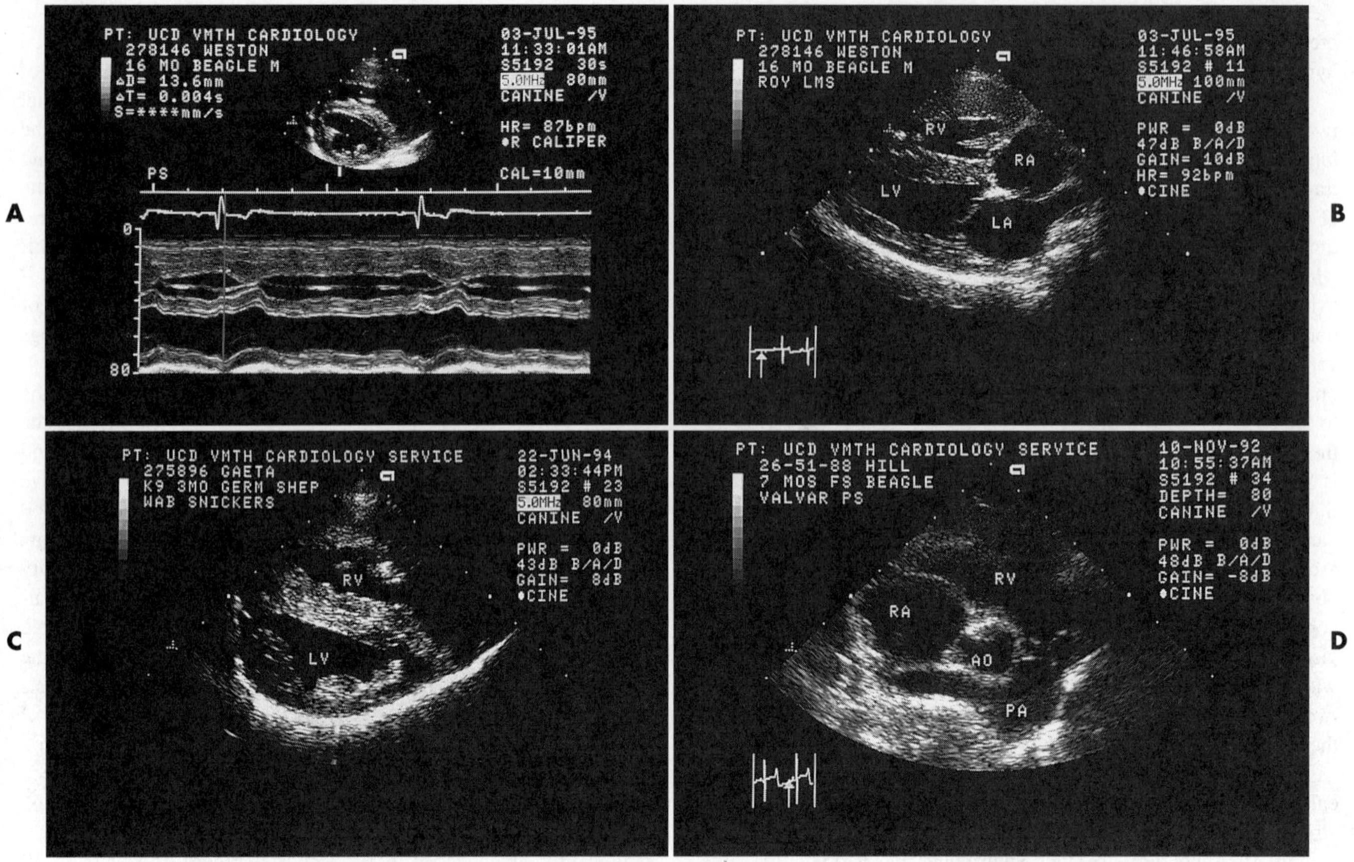

FIGURE 15-4 M-mode and two-dimensional echocardiographic images from dogs with pulmonic stenosis. **A,** This M-mode echocardiogram demonstrates right ventricular concentric hypertrophy and paradoxical motion of the interventricular septum toward the right ventricular free wall in systole. **B,** Two-dimensional echocardiogram taken from a right parasternal four-chamber view from the dog shown in **A.** Right ventricular concentric hypertrophy is evident as a thickened wall next to the transducer on top. The right ventricular free wall is thicker than the left ventricular free wall and interventricular septum. This echocardiogram was taken 10 months after successful balloon valvuloplasty and shows no regression of hypertrophy in this 16-month-old dog. **C,** Right parasternal short-axis view taken from another dog of the right and left ventricle in systole. Right ventricular concentric hypertrophy is evident and the interventricular septum is flattened, indicating an increase in right ventricular systolic pressure. Note that the left ventricular shape is ovoid rather than the normal spherical appearance. **D,** Right parasternal short-axis view of the aorta, pulmonary artery, and pulmonary valve. The pulmonary valve cusps are thickened, and there is a poststenotic dilation of the main pulmonary artery.

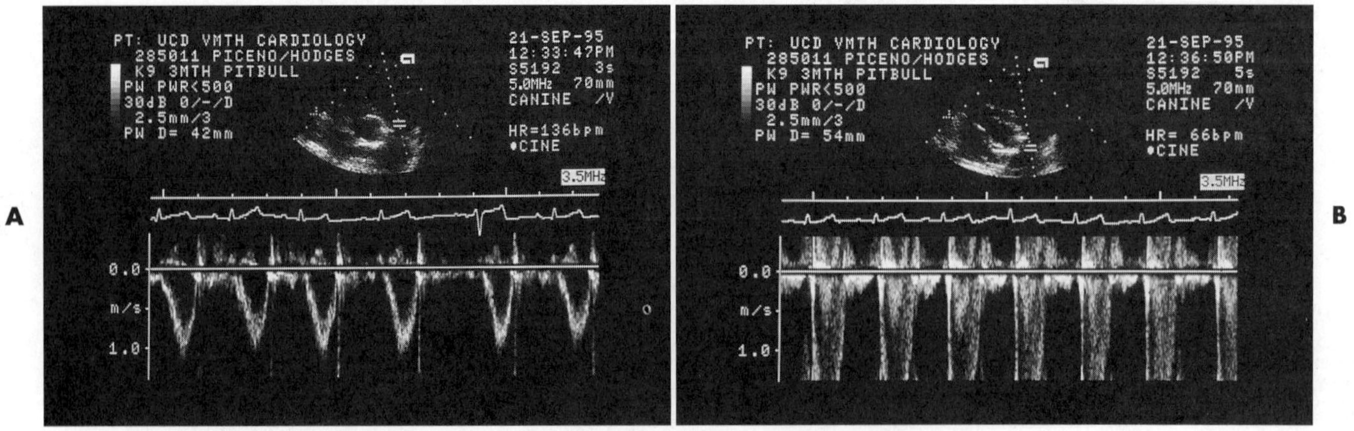

FIGURE 15-5 Doppler echocardiographic images from a dog with pulmonic stenosis. **A,** Pulsed-wave Doppler tracing taken proximal to the pulmonary valve. The tracing from this region displays normal laminar flow and velocity. **B,** Pulsed-wave Doppler tracing taken distal to the pulmonary valve. Note that the signal is aliased, indicating a step-up in velocity across the valve region. There is spectral broadening, indicating turbulent flow.

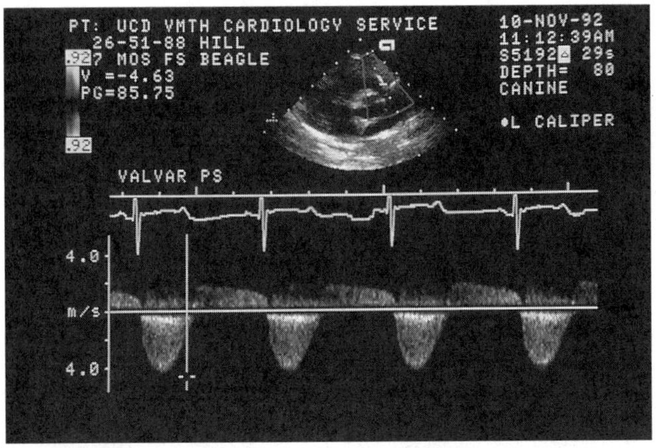

FIGURE 15-6 Continuous-wave Doppler tracing from a dog with pulmonic stenosis. The systolic velocity of pulmonary artery blood flow is increased to 4.6 m/sec (below the baseline), and there is a low-velocity (less than 2 m/sec) signal of pulmonary insufficiency in diastole (above the baseline).

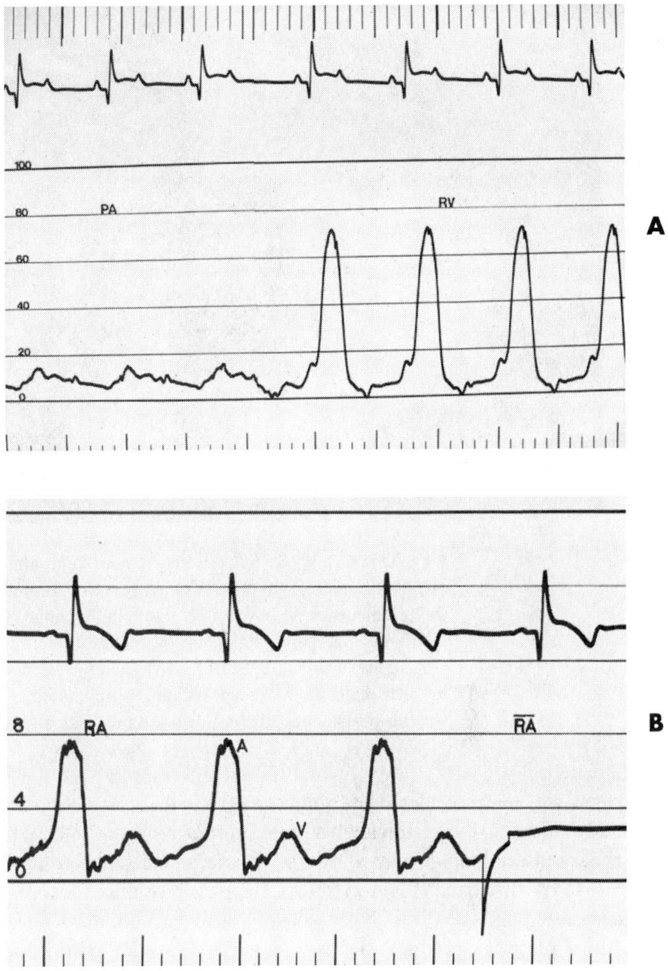

FIGURE 15-7 Intracardiac pressure tracings from a dog with pulmonic stenosis. **A,** Pressure tracing recorded while the catheter was pulled back from the pulmonary artery *(PA)* into the right ventricle *(RV)*. The right ventricular pressure is increased to approximately 70 mm Hg. The peak systolic pulmonary artery pressure is approximately 15 mm Hg. The pressure gradient is approximately 55 mm Hg (moderate pulmonic stenosis). **B,** Pressure tracing recorded from the right atrium (RA). The *a* wave pressure (A) is increased because of a reduction in compliance of the hypertrophied right ventricle. Mean right atrial pressure ($\overline{RA}$) is normal (no evidence of right heart failure).

decreases, assuming constant blood flow. As previously discussed, the Bernoulli equation ($\Delta P = 4V^2$) can be used to transform blood flow velocity into a pressure difference (pressure gradient) across the stenosis. Although exact numbers can be measured and calculated, only estimates of mild, moderate, and severe stenosis are clinically important. We arbitrarily consider peak blood flow velocities less than 3.5 m/sec (a pressure gradient less than 40 to 50 mm Hg) to indicate mild stenosis. Velocities between 3.5 and 4.5 m/sec (a pressure gradient between 50 and 80 mm Hg) indicate moderate stenosis, and flow velocities greater than 4.5 m/sec (a pressure gradient greater than 80 mm Hg) indicate severe stenosis. Doppler estimates of systolic pressure gradients in humans and dogs with pulmonic stenosis have shown very good correlation with invasive pressure measurements made under the same conditions.[34] Spectral Doppler confirmation and quantification of pulmonic stenosis are best accomplished using both the right parasternal short-axis and left parasternal long-axis views. Color flow Doppler echocardiography can be used to readily identify the turbulent systolic jet distal to the stenosis (Color Plate 54, *A*). It can also identify the mild and clinically insignificant pulmonic valve regurgitation that is present in many cases (Color Plate 54, *B*). It also may help to quickly identify the exact location of the obstruction by identifying the exact area where the turbulent flow begins. In patients with associated defects (e.g., tricuspid valve dysplasia), color flow Doppler evaluation may also allow accurate characterization of the other defect.

CARDIAC CATHETERIZATION

As with Doppler echocardiography, the pressure gradient across the obstruction can be measured invasively using cardiac catheterization (see Chapter 7). To assess severity, a catheter is introduced into the pulmonary artery via the jugular vein and pressure recorded from the distal end of the catheter. The pulmonic arterial pressure is usually normal. The catheter is withdrawn from the pulmonary artery, across the stenotic region, into the right ventricle. An increase in systolic pressure occurs as the catheter crosses the stenosis (Figure 15-7). As with Doppler-derived gradients in awake dogs, the magnitude of the pressure gradient reflects the severity of the obstruction, assuming blood flow across the obstruction remains constant. It may be helpful to measure cardiac output at the same time as the pressure gradient to facilitate comparisons between individuals and between subsequent measurements in the same patient (e.g., after balloon valvuloplasty). Anesthesia often decreases cardiac output. Consequently, pressure gradients measured under anesthesia may underestimate the true severity and therefore may not reflect the nature of the obstruction in the awake and active patient.[37] Despite these limitations, catheter-derived pressure gradients, with or without calculation of valve area, have been the method of choice for years in human medicine for determining prognosis and the need for intervention.[38] As with Doppler echocardiography, we arbitrarily consider gradients less than 40 mm Hg as mild, those between 40 and 80 mm Hg as moderate, and those greater than 80 mm Hg as severe. Right atrial pressure tracings usually demonstrate a normal or slightly elevated mean pressure with or without a relative increase in the *a* wave reflecting a loss of compliance in the hypertrophied right ventricle (Figure 15-7, *B*).

Following pressure measurement, a right ventricular dye injection is made. Right ventricular angiography readily demonstrates the region(s) of right ventricular outflow narrowing, poststenotic dilatation of the pulmonary artery, and right ventricular hypertrophy in most patients (Figure 15-8). In English bulldogs and

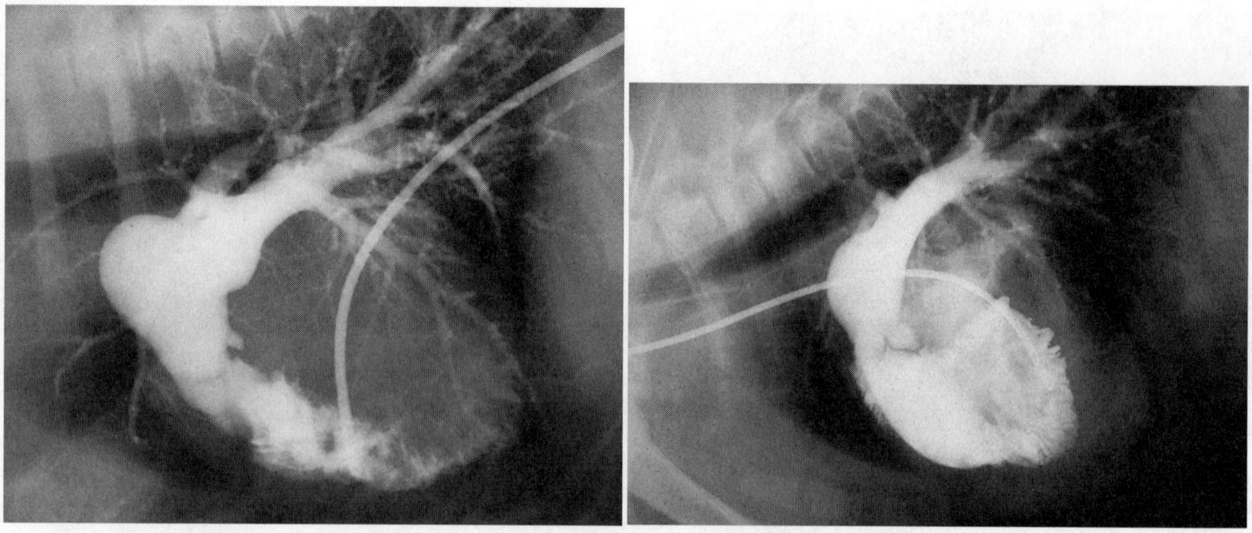

FIGURE 15-8 Selective right ventricular angiograms from dogs with pulmonic stenosis. **A,** The leaflets of the pulmonic valve are thickened (seen as filling defects in the angiogram), and the subvalvular region has filling defects caused by fibrous tissue in this dog with pulmonic valve dysplasia. There is marked poststenotic dilation of the main pulmonary artery. Right ventricular hypertrophy is evident as the space between the right ventricular chamber (edge of the dye) and the sternum is increased. **B,** This dog has pure valvular stenosis. The valve leaflets are thickened, creating filling defects. They bulge upward in this systolic frame. This dog has a smaller poststenotic dilation than the previous dog and has tricuspid regurgitation.

boxers with an anomalous left coronary artery, the obstruction is usually identified as subvalvular, and aortic root or selective coronary arteriography may allow the course of the left coronary artery to be visualized (Figure 15-9).[22] The poor resolution of some fluoroscopes and the difficulty in obtaining standard oblique views in dogs often make the exact nature of the valvular deformity difficult to detect.

Natural History and Prognosis

Standard guidelines for categorizing the severity of pulmonic stenosis in dogs and cats for purposes of prognosis and therapy have not been established. However, dogs with resting gradients in the severe category (greater than 80 mm Hg) may be at increased risk for sudden death. Balloon valvuloplasty is usually recommended for these dogs, whether or not they are symptomatic at the time of diagnosis. However, many of these dogs live many years without significant events. Consequently, any procedure that risks death should be avoided.[39] Although isolated pulmonic stenosis may produce symptoms in humans, the long-term survival rate without intervention is excellent.[17] Dogs with resting gradients in the mild category (less than 40 mm Hg) usually live normal lives and therapy is unnecessary.[18] In patients with concomitant tricuspid dysplasia, relief of the obstruction is often beneficial regardless of the resting pressure gradient. Dogs with intermediate resting gradients (40 to 80 mm Hg) often live normal lives, but the long-term prognosis is uncertain. In these dogs, therapeutic decisions are generally determined by the clinical presentation and the nature of progression.

Therapy

The options for treatment of pulmonic stenosis are all invasive techniques directed at reducing the right ventricular outflow obstruction. Medical therapy is of little benefit unless there are signs of congestion associated with the development of right heart failure. β-Blockers can be used in severe cases in an attempt to prevent sudden death. The general aim of therapy is to increase the size of the orifice. Generally one can only reduce the pressure gradient into the mild range, because complete relief of the obstruction is almost never achieved.

SURGERY

Surgical techniques used in dogs include (1) open valvulotomy by direct examination; (2) closed valvulotomy, using a valvulotome and dilating instruments inserted through a small incision in the right ventricular wall or pulmonary artery; (3) placement of a patch-graft over an arterioventriculotomy; and (4) implantation of a valved or nonvalved conduit from the right ventricle or proximal pulmonary artery to the distal pulmonary artery.[40-45] Each technique requires a left lateral thoracotomy and a detailed knowledge of cardiovascular surgery. All include significant surgical risk, depending on the skill of the surgeon. Variable success rates have been reported for each procedure; however, the limited availability, expense, and high associated risks have not allowed the systematic comparison of the techniques on a large number of animals. In a retrospective analysis of 129 treated and untreated dogs with pulmonic stenosis, Ewey et al[39] reported a significantly higher mortality in dogs undergoing patch-graft placement or valvulotomy compared with untreated dogs or those treated by balloon valvuloplasty at our institution. It is likely that risk and limited availability will continue to limit the number of animals subjected to these operative techniques, especially with the growing use and success of balloon valvuloplasty. However, in dogs with purely subvalvular pulmonic stenosis, in which the success of balloon valvuloplasty is limited, and in dogs with anomalous left coronary arteries, in which balloon valvuloplasty may be contraindicated, a surgical technique might still be considered.

Because of the variable nature of pulmonic stenosis in dogs, the diagnosis and differentiation of the types are important for choice of the most appropriate surgical correction. Differentiation is best

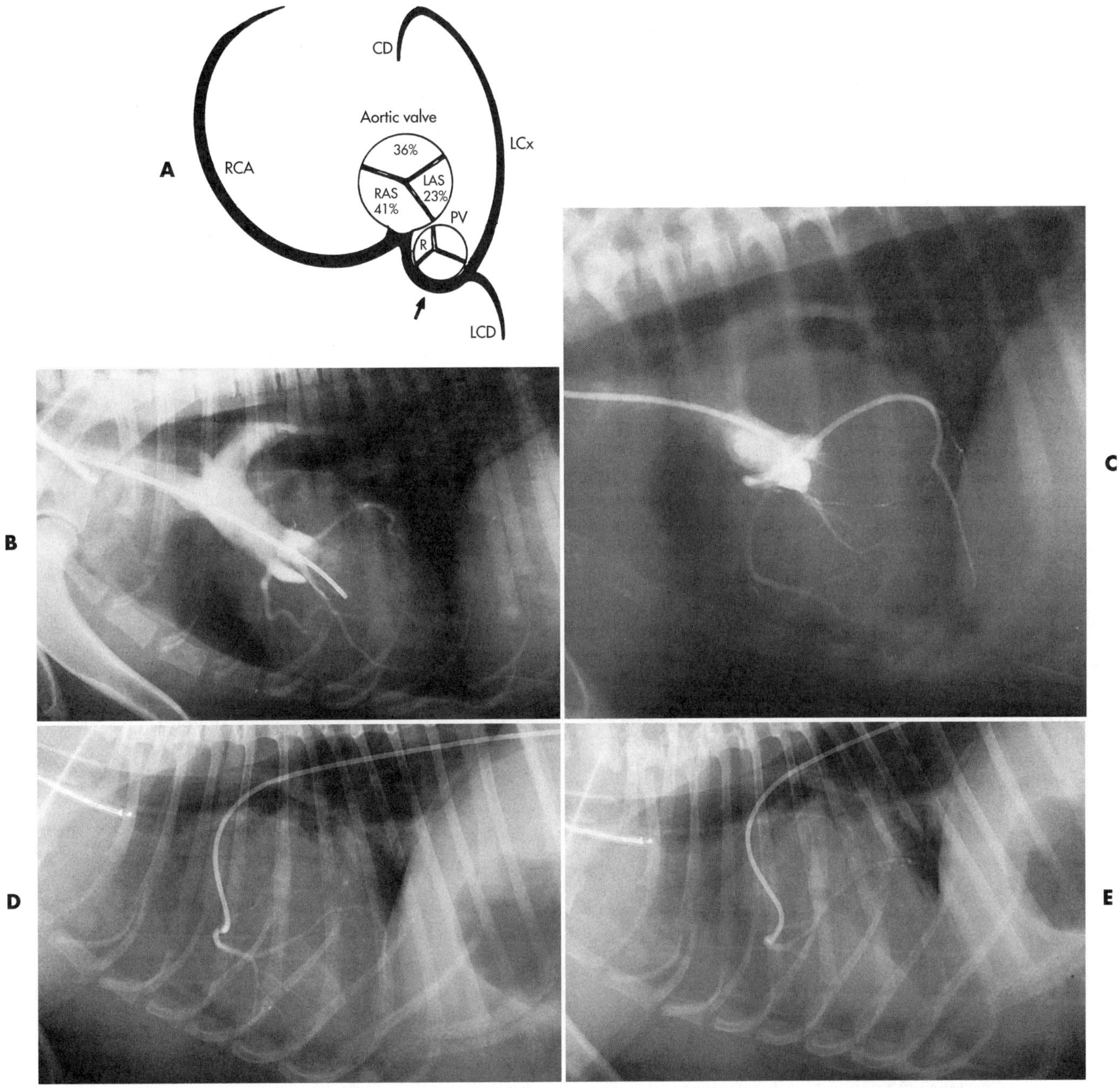

FIGURE 15-9 **A,** Schematic diagram of an R2A type of single right coronary artery *(RCA)* identified in some English bulldogs and boxers with pulmonic stenosis. The anomalous left main coronary artery *(arrow)* encircles and compresses the base of the pulmonary valve *(PV)*. The left aortic sinus of Valsalva *(LAS)* does not contain a coronary ostium and may be smaller than normal. *CD,* Caudal descending coronary artery; *LCx,* left circumflex coronary artery; *RAS,* right aortic sinus; *LCD,* left cranial descending coronary artery; *R,* right pulmonic valve leaflet. **B,** Aortic root angiogram from a normal dog showing normal coronary anatomy. The left circumflex coronary artery is to the right in the figure, the right coronary artery is to the left in the figure, and the left anterior descending coronary artery is in the middle, starting at the aortic root and projecting ventrally. **C,** Aortic root angiogram in an English bulldog with an R2A type of single right coronary artery. The right, left main, left descending, and left circumflex coronary arteries are evident. The left main coronary artery can be seen to originate from the region of the origin of the right coronary artery (on the left side of the picture) and curl back over the root of the aorta. **D,** Deep selective right coronary arteriogram in the dog with an R2A type of single right coronary artery shown in **C**. A normal right coronary artery is evident. **E,** Selective left coronary arteriogram in the dog shown in **D**. The catheter was first placed in the right coronary ostium and then directed into the anomalous left main coronary artery. The left main coronary artery originates from the right coronary artery, as evidenced by the catheter placement in the cranial aspect of the aortic root. The left anterior descending and left circumflex coronary arteries are evident.

achieved with a combination of echocardiography and cardiac catheterization. Brief descriptions of the more common procedures are provided. For more complete information, the reader is directed to the individual references provided.

Brock or modified Brock technique. The Brock or modified Brock technique is advocated for subvalvular forms of pulmonic stenosis.[45] It is performed via a left lateral thoracotomy. After the pericardium is opened parallel and ventral to the phrenic nerve, an infundibular rongeur is advanced into the right ventricular outflow tract through a purse-string stab incision in the right ventricle. The rongeur is used to grasp, cut, and remove the fibromuscular subvalvular lesion. The rongeur is then removed, and the purse-string suture is tightened and tied. The advantage of the Brock procedure is its simple nature and requirement of few additional instruments. The major disadvantage is the inability to directly observe the tissue being excised. The procedure is very risky in inexperienced hands.

Bistoury technique. The bistoury technique[45] is very similar to the Brock technique and is as simple. Instead of using an infundibular rongeur, a teat bistoury (a long, narrow-bladed knife) is inserted through the purse-string into the right ventricle and passed through the obstruction. Cuts are made in the fibromuscular subvalvular obstruction or in the pulmonary valve. The advantages of the bistoury technique include simplicity, ease of surgery, limited need for equipment, and the suitability for valvular and subvalvular pulmonic stenosis. The disadvantage, as with the Brock procedure, is the lack of direct visualization of the tissue being cut. The procedure is very risky in inexperienced hands. We have heard of anecdotal reports of aortic rupture and ventricular septal defect production with this technique even in experienced hands.

Valve dilator technique. In a procedure similar to the Brock or bistoury techniques, a valve dilator may be advanced via a right ventricular purse-string stab incision across a valvular obstruction.[45] Valve dilators act similarly to balloon valvuloplasty but have the added disadvantages of a thoracotomy and lack of fluoroscopic guidance. A combination instrument that both dilates and cuts is also available. The advantages and disadvantages are similar to the other "blind" techniques.

Pulmonary arteriotomy. The pulmonary ateriotomy[45] is also performed via a left lateral thoracotomy. Initially the cranial vena cava, caudal vena cava, and azygos vein are isolated, and Rommel tourniquets are placed around each. A double row of stay sutures may be placed in the pulmonic artery to manipulate the artery during the procedure and repose the vessel edges at the end of the procedure. The tourniquets are then tightened to provide inflow occlusion, stopping all venous return to the heart except coronary venous return. The heart is allowed to empty, and a pulmonary arteriotomy is made with a scalpel blade. The incision is extended with scissors, and suction is used to evacuate residual blood from the pulmonic artery. At this point the pulmonary valve may be repaired or excised, or a subvalvular or supravalvular obstruction may be surgically removed. The stay sutures are used to repair the arteriotomy site, along with vascular clamps or additional sutures. The inflow occlusion is released, and the thoracotomy site is closed in routine fashion. The period of inflow occlusion should not exceed 4 minutes at normal temperatures, but may be increased with hypothermia. The disadvantage of the procedure is its difficulty. The major advantage of the procedure is the ability to directly visualize the defect.

Patch-grafting. The patch-grafting technique[40,41,44,45] was developed to circumvent the problems associated with hypoplastic pulmonary valve annulus and infundibular obstruction (dynamic or fixed) that are commonly associated with pulmonic stenosis in the dog. The procedure may be performed with (open) or without (closed) pulmonary arteriotomy. A patch of either pericardium or woven Dacron is placed as a substitute for the right ventricular outflow tract. The graft is cut as a double ellipse to fit from the pulmonic artery across the obstruction to the right ventricle.

In the closed technique, a cutting suture or wire is inserted through the right ventricular wall, into the right ventricle, up the pulmonic artery, and out of the wall of the proximal main pulmonic artery. The patch is sutured from the pulmonic artery to the right ventricle over the outside portion of the cutting wire. The last two sutures in the ventral border of the graft are not completed, so that the two ends of the cutting wire emerge from the ventricular end of the graft. The wire is then withdrawn in a sawing motion, completely incising the pulmonic artery, the valve, and the right ventricular outflow tract. The graft suture is then completed.

The open patch-graft technique combines a pulmonary arteriotomy with the placement of a synthetic patch over the arteriotomy site and is performed using venous inflow occlusion and mild whole-body hypothermia. A partial-thickness incision is made in the right ventricular outflow tract parallel to the left descending coronary artery. The length and depth of the incision are generally guided by angiography. An elliptically shaped synthetic patch-graft (woven Dacron or polytetrafluoroethylene) is sutured to the margins of the partial ventriculotomy. Subsequently, the cranial margin of the patch-graft is sutured to the pulmonic artery, leaving the caudodorsal aspect of the patch over the pulmonic artery unattached. At this point the caval tourniquets are tightened to accomplish venous inflow occlusion, and the pulmonary arteriotomy is performed. In this case the pulmonary arteriotomy is extended dorsally to the tip of the patch and ventrally through the valve into the right ventricle, converting the partial-thickness ventriculotomy into a full-thickness incision. The valve is inspected and repaired or excised. The pulmonic artery is closed by suturing the caudal margin of the arteriotomy to the caudodorsal aspect of the patch.

The effect of patch-graft surgery is to widen the outflow tract by partially diverting blood into the patch. The advantages are that a right ventricular outflow tract of any size can be produced and the technique is effective for all forms of pulmonic stenosis. The open technique also offers the ability to directly visualize and repair or remove the defect. The disadvantages of the technique include placement of foreign material on the heart, operative difficulty, and, in the case of the open technique, increased risk because of inflow occlusion. This procedure is of questionable efficacy. No one has reported postoperative pressure gradients. In the few dogs that we have seen following this procedure, the pressure gradient was similar to the preoperative gradient.

Conduits. Vascular conduit repair[42,45] of pulmonic stenosis is relatively simple and inexpensive. It has the potential to be effective, especially for supravalvular pulmonic stenosis. However, this potential has not been realized in veterinary medicine. In this procedure the pericardium is opened dorsal to the phrenic nerve so that the pulmonary artery is more easily exposed. An appropriate Dacron conduit is chosen and preclotted with the patient's blood. A partially occluding vascular clamp is placed on the pulmonic artery distal to the obstruction, and the conduit is anastomosed end-to-side to the pulmonic artery with continuous sutures. The conduit is then clamped close to the anastomotic site, and the pulmonic artery clamp is moved proximal to the obstruction. For supravalvular pulmonic stenosis, the proximal end of the conduit is then anastomosed end-to-side to the pulmonic artery proximal to the obstruction. Valved or unvalved conduits have been successfully implanted between the right ventricle and pulmonic artery. Valved conduits are expensive, and the placement of the proximal (right ventricular) anastomosis is difficult. In general, conduits have been unsuccessful in veterinary medicine because of thrombotic complications and are usually considered only as a last resort.

BALLOON VALVULOPLASTY

Balloon valvuloplasty has rapidly become the initial treatment of choice for relieving cardiovascular obstructions in humans.[46] Balloon valvuloplasty has been particularly successful in humans with congenital valvular pulmonic stenosis, resulting in at least partial reduction of the obstruction in most patients.[47] The technique uses a catheter with a strong, cylindrical balloon at its end that is placed under fluoroscopic guidance via a vascular cut-down or percutaneous approach (Figure 15-10, *A*). The balloon is positioned across the obstruction and inflated with fluid under pressure. This fractures or stretches the obstructing tissue, increasing the effective size of the lumen. In general, balloon dilation techniques are simpler, less traumatic, less expensive, and less risky than open-chest surgical procedures.

The technique of transluminal angioplasty has been used for several decades in human patients for the treatment of obstructive vascular lesions. For more than 10 years balloon dilation techniques have been used for other congenital or acquired stenotic lesions in humans.[46] Balloon valvuloplasty can be performed safely in dogs with pulmonic stenosis, and the results parallel those seen in human medicine.[37,48,49] We have been performing balloon valvuloplasty for the treatment of pulmonic stenosis at our institution for over 10 years.

Technique. Standard techniques for vascular access and routine cardiac catheterization are described in Chapter 7. Following hemodynamic and angiographic studies, a stiff, long guide wire (longer than 200 cm in length, 0.03 to 0.038 inches in diameter) is introduced into either the left or right branch of the pulmonary artery through an end-hole catheter. An appropriate-size balloon dilation catheter is introduced over the guide wire and is positioned with fluoroscopic guidance across the obstruction. The balloon is rapidly inflated by hand using a 1:1 mixture of saline and contrast medium and a 20-mL syringe. The inflated balloon completely obstructs the systolic outflow from the right ventricle. Consequently, the balloon is kept fully inflated for only a few seconds and then is rapidly deflated. Full inflation is maintained for 5 to 10 seconds, and the average time from inflation to 90% deflation is generally less than 20 seconds. Multiple inflation-deflations are performed until a satisfactory degree of dilation is produced. Initially, when the balloon is inflated, an indentation of the balloon caused by the stenotic valve is visualized fluoroscopically (Figure 15-10, *B*). Upon successful balloon dilation, this indentation disappears (usually abruptly) during inflation of the balloon and is not evident on subsequent balloon inflations (Figure 15-10, *C*). Usually inward or outward traction on the guide wire by an assistant is necessary to maintain balloon position during inflation. Hemodynamic and angiographic studies are reevaluated after the dilation procedure.

Because of the variety of balloon catheters available it is necessary to choose an appropriate catheter for each individual patient. There are currently no standards available for balloon dilation catheter selection in veterinary medicine. Generally, the length of the balloon should extend from within the right ventricular outflow tract to several centimeters above the pulmonary valve. Balloon lengths between 4 and 10 cm are appropriate for most dogs. The balloon diameter is chosen based on pulmonary annulus size measured from the right ventricular angiogram or echocardiogram.

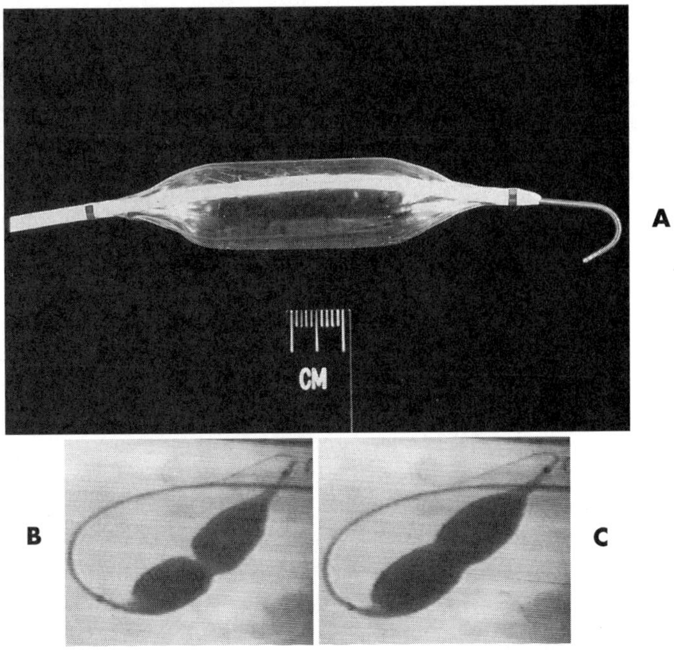

FIGURE 15-10 **A,** Illustration of the tip of a standard balloon valvuloplasty catheter with the balloon inflated with air. A J-tipped guide wire can be seen extending from the tip of the catheter. **B,** Fluoroscopic image of a valvuloplasty balloon partially inflated with a mixture of saline and angiographic dye. The balloon is placed across the stenotic pulmonary valve (indentation in the balloon). **C,** Further inflation of the balloon shows a decrease in the indentation in the balloon, indicating that the pulmonary valve has been torn open.

Balloon diameters 1.2 to 1.5 times the pulmonary annulus diameter are generally safe and effective.

Efficacy. Bright et al[49] first reported on the use of balloon dilation valvuloplasty in a dog in 1987. Since then it has become the preferred technique for the initial treatment of pulmonic stenosis in dogs.[37,48,50] Successful reduction of the obstructive pressure gradient by 50% or more has been reported in about 75% to 80% of dogs treated (Figure 15-11 and Color Plate 55). Complications are comparatively rare. Perforation of the heart with a catheter or guide wire may lead to cardiac tamponade, bleeding, and death. The most common complication is damage to the tricuspid valve. This may lead to right heart failure. We estimate that this complication occurs in about 5% of our patients. Minor complications are common and include hemorrhage at the access site, arrhythmias (ventricular premature contractions), and right bundle branch block.

Long-term follow-up studies in humans suggest excellent longevity and quality of life for patients following successful balloon dilation.[51] Although fewer studies are available for dogs, the results appear to be similar.[52,53] The initial reduction in the pressure gradient persists over succeeding months in most dogs, and the prognosis is probably improved, especially if the gradient can be reduced to less than 50 mm Hg.[37] In one report, untreated dogs had a 2.1 times greater risk of dying within the first 2 years compared with dogs following successful balloon dilation.[39] Aggressive selection of the balloon diameter relative to the pulmonary annular diameter and further experience with the technique may improve outcomes in the future. Additional work may also show that the technique can be applied to animals with pulmonic stenosis that is part of more complicated defects, such as tetralogy of Fallot.

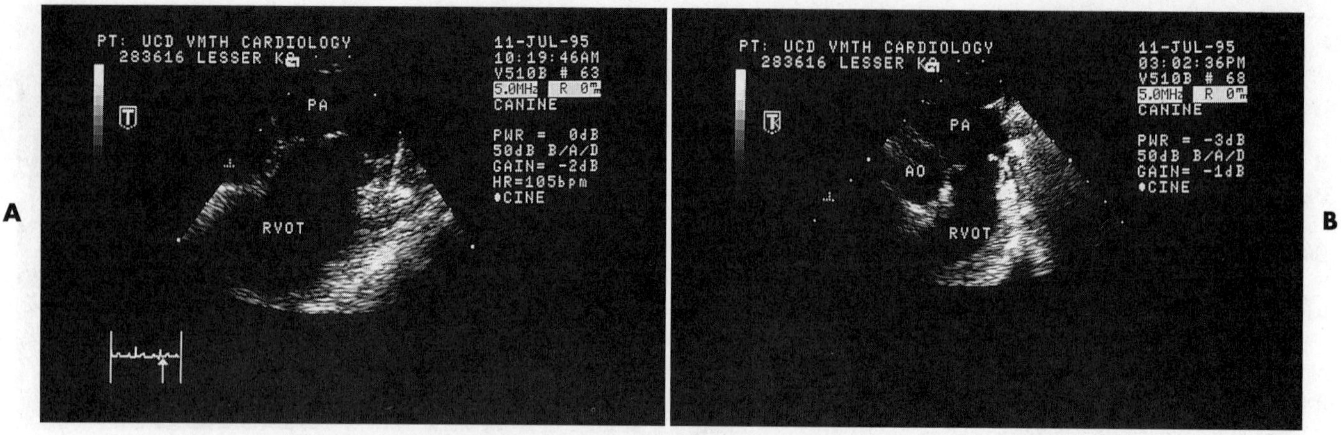

FIGURE 15-11 Transesophageal echocardiographic images from a dog with valvular pulmonic stenosis before **(A)** (see Color Plate 55, *A*) and after **(B)** (see Color Plate 55, *B*) balloon valvuloplasty. **A,** Cranial long-axis view of the pulmonary valve and main pulmonary artery in systole shows a thickened and domed pulmonary valve. The pulmonary valve orifice is small. **B,** Cranial long-axis view of the pulmonary valve and main pulmonary artery in systole at a lesser magnification than **A.** Although the valve is still thickened and domed, it now opens more completely.

TREATMENT OF DOGS WITH AN ANOMALOUS LEFT CORONARY ARTERY

The proper course of treatment in dogs with subvalvular stenosis associated with an anomalous left coronary artery is currently unresolved. Originally, death associated with transection of the anomalous vessel was reported resulting from patch-graft surgery.[22] Consequently, balloon dilation valvuloplasty was recommended in these patients. Two English bulldogs with this anomaly that died acutely during balloon dilation valvulotomy as a result of avulsion of the anomalous vessel from its origin at the right coronary have been reported.[21] Conduit implantation around the stenosis may be an option for these dogs. However, our experience with this procedure in this situation has been dismal. We currently opt not to treat these dogs, because we feel that the prognosis without therapy is better than with any type of intervention.

REFERENCES

1. Buchanan JW: Causes and prevalence of cardiovascular diseases. In Kirk RW, Bonagura JD, eds: *Current veterinary therapy XI,* Philadelphia, 1992, WB Saunders.
2. Rishniw M, Thomas WP, Kienle RD: Dynamic right mid-ventricular obstruction in 50 cats, *J Vet Intern Med* 10:159, 1996 (abstract).
3. Kienle RD, Rishniw M, Kittleson MD: Echocardiographic assessment of ventricular outflow tract dynamics during isoproterenol infusion in healthy sedated cats, *J Vet Intern Med* 10:162, 1996, (abstract).
4. Ettinger SJ, Sutter PF: Congenital heart disease. In Ettinger SJ, Sutter PF, eds: *Canine cardiology,* Philadelphia, 1970, WB Saunders.
5. Mulvihill JJ, Priester WA: Congenital heart disease in dogs: epidemiologic similarities to man, *Teratology* 7:73, 1973.
6. Netter FH: Embryology. In Yonkman FF, Netter FH, eds: *The Ciba collection of medical illustrations: the heart,* vol 5, Rochester, NY, 1974, Case-Hoyt Corp.
7. More GW, Hutchins GM, Brito JC et al: Congenital malformations of the semilunar valves, *Hum Pathol* 11:367, 1980.
8. Noden DM, DeLahunta A: Cardiovascular System. II. Heart. In Noden DM, DeLahunta A, eds: *The embryology of domestic animals: developmental mechanisms and malformations,* Baltimore, 1985, Williams & Wilkins.
9. Cheatham JP: Pulmonary stenosis. In Garson JA, Bicker JT, McNamara DE, eds: *The science and practice of pediatric cardiology,* vol II, Philadelphia, 1990, Lea & Febiger.
10. Patterson DF, Haskins ME, Schnarr WR: Hereditary dysplasia of the pulmonary valve in beagle dogs: pathologic and genetic studies, *Am J Cardiol* 47:631, 1981.
11. Patterson DF, Pyle RL, Van Mierop L et al: Hereditary defects of the conotruncal septum in keeshond dogs: pathologic and genetic studies, *Am J Cardiol* 34:187, 1974.
12. Van Mierop L, Patterson DF, Schnarr WR: Hereditary conotruncal septal defects in keeshond dogs, *Am J Cardiol* 40:936, 1977.
13. Jacobs GJ, Mahaffey M, Rawlings CA: Valvular pulmonic stenosis in four Boykin spaniels, *J Am Anim Hosp Assoc* 26:247, 1990.
14. Malik R, Church DB, Hunt GB: Valvular pulmonic stenosis in bull mastiffs, *J Small Anim Pract* 34:288, 1988.
15. Polzin DJ, Ogburn PN: Isolated pulmonary valvular insufficiency in a dog, *J Am Anim Hosp Assoc* 17:301, 1981.
16. Patterson DF: Two hereditary forms of ventricular outflow obstruction in the dog: pulmonary valve dysplasia, and discrete subaortic stenosis. In Nora JJ, Takao A, eds: *Congenital heart disease: causes and processes,* Mt. Kisko, NY, 1984, Futura.
17. Friedman WF: Congenital heart disease in infancy and childhood. In Braunwald E, ed: *Heart disease: a textbook of cardiovascular medicine,* ed 4, Philadelphia, 1992, WB Saunders.
18. Fingland RB, Bonagura JD, Myer CW: Pulmonic stenosis in the dog: 29 cases (1975-1984), *J Am Vet Med Assoc* 189:218, 1986.
19. Perloff JK: Congenital pulmonary stenosis. In Perloff JK, ed: *The clinical recognition of congenital heart disease,* ed 4, Philadelphia, 1994, WB Saunders.
20. Olivier NB: Congenital heart disease in dogs. In Fox PR, ed: *Canine and feline cardiology,* New York, 1988, Churchill Livingstone.
21. Kittleson MD, Thomas WP, Loyer C et al: Single coronary artery (type R2A), *J Vet Intern Med* 6:250, 1992 (letter).
22. Buchanan JW: Pulmonic stenosis caused by single coronary artery in dogs: four cases (1965-1984), *J Am Vet Med Assoc* 196:115, 1990.
23. Minami T, Wakao Y, Buchanan JW et al: A case of pulmonic stenosis with single coronary artery in a dog, *Nippon Juigaku Zasshi* 51:453, 1989.
24. Lombard CW, Ackerman N, Berry CR et al: Pulmonic stenosis and right-to-left atrial shunt in three dogs, *J Am Vet Med Assoc* 194:71, 1989.
25. Riepe RD, Gompf RE: ECG of the month, *J Am Vet Med Assoc* 202:374, 1993.
26. Anderson M: What is your diagnosis? Right-sided cardiomegaly associated with supravalvular pulmonic stenosis, *J Am Vet Med Assoc* 200:2013, 1992.

27. Trautvetter E, Detweiler DK, Bohn FK et al: Evolution of the electrocardiogram in young dogs with congenital heart disease leading to right ventricular hypertrophy, *J Electrocardiol* 14:275, 1981.
28. Hill JD: Electrocardiographic diagnosis of right ventricular enlargement in dogs, *J Electrocardiol* 4:347, 1971.
29. Liu SK, Tilley LP: Dysplasia of the tricuspid valve in the dog and cat, *J Am Vet Med Assoc* 169:623, 1976.
30. Farrow CS: Radiographic characterization of pulmonic stenosis in a dog, *Mod Vet Pract* 67:804, 1986.
31. Wingfield WE, Boon JA: Echocardiography for the diagnosis of congenital heart disease in the dog, *Vet Clin North Am Small Anim Pract* 17:735, 1987.
32. DeMadron E, Bonagura JD, O'Grady MR: Normal and paradoxical ventricular septal motion in the dog, *Am J Vet Res* 46:1832, 1985.
33. Bonagura JD, Herring DS: Echocardiography: congenital heart disease, *Vet Clin North Am Small Anim Pract* 15:1195, 1985.
34. Richards KL: Doppler echocardiographic quantification of stenotic valvular lesions, *Echocardiography* 4:289, 1994.
35. Richards KL: Assessment of aortic and pulmonic stenosis by echocardiography, *Circulation* 84(supp II):I-182, 1991.
36. Moise NS: Doppler echocardiographic evaluation of congenital heart disease, *J Vet Intern Med* 3:195, 1989.
37. Martin MWS, Godman M, Fuentes VL et al: Assessment of balloon pulmonary valvuloplasty in six dogs, *J Small Anim Pract* 33:443, 1992.
38. Carabello BA, Grossman W: Calculation of stenotic valve orifice area. In Grossman W, Baim DS, eds: *Cardiac catheterization, angiography and intervention,* ed 4, Philadelphia, 1991, Lea & Febiger.
39. Ewey DM, Pion PD, Hird DW: Survival in treated and untreated dogs with congenital pulmonic stenosis, *J Vet Intern Med* 6:114, 1992 (abstract).
40. Hunt GB, Pearson MR, Bellenger CR et al: Use of a modified open patch-graft technique and valvulectomy for correction of severe pulmonic stenosis in dogs: eight consecutive cases, *Aust Vet J* 70:244, 1993.
41. Orton EC, Bruecker KA, McCracken TO: An open patch-graft technique for correction of pulmonic stenosis in the dog, *Vet Surg* 19:148, 1990.
42. Ford RB, Spaulding GL, Eyster GE: Use of an extracardiac conduit in the repair of supravalvular pulmonic stenosis in a dog, *J Am Vet Med Assoc* 172:922, 1978.
43. Breznock EM: Surgical relief of pulmonic stenosis. In Bojrab M, ed: *Current techniques in small animal surgery,* ed 3, Philadelphia, 1990, Lea and Febiger.
44. Breznock EM, Wood GL: A patch-graft technique for correction of pulmonic stenosis in dogs, *J Am Vet Med Assoc* 169:1090, 1976.
45. Eyster GE: Basic cardiac surgical procedures. In Slatter D, ed: *Textbook of small animal surgery,* ed 2, Philadelphia, 1993, WB Saunders.
46. McKay RG, Grossman W: Balloon valvuloplasty for treatment of pulmonic, mitral, aortic, and prosthetic valve stenoses. In Braunwald E, ed: *Heart disease: a textbook of cardiovascular medicine,* ed 3, Philadelphia, 1988, WB Saunders.
47. Rao PS: Balloon dilation in infants and children with dysplastic pulmonary valves: short-term and intermediate-term results, *Am Heart J* 116:1168, 1988.
48. Sisson DD, MacCoy DM: Treatment of congenital pulmonic stenosis in two dogs by balloon valvuloplasty, *J Vet Intern Med* 2:92, 1988.
49. Bright JM, Jennings J, Toal R et al: Percutaneous balloon valvuloplasty for treatment of pulmonic stenosis in a dog, *J Am Vet Med Assoc* 191:995, 1987.
50. Brownlie SE, Cobb MA, Chambers J et al: Percutaneous balloon valvuloplasty in four dogs with pulmonic stenosis, *J Small Anim Pract* 32:165, 1991.
51. Masura J, Burch M, Deanfield JE et al: Five-year follow-up after balloon pulmonary valvuloplasty, *J Am Coll Cardiol* 21:132, 1993.
52. Thomas WP, Sisson DD, DeLellis LA: Technique and short term effects of balloon catheter dilation of congenital obstructive cardiac defects (pulmonic and subaortic stenosis) in dogs, *Proc Annu Vet Med Forum,* 1989, p 830.
53. Thomas WP, DeLellis LA, Sisson DD: Balloon dilation of congenital outflow obstruction in dogs: mid-term results, *Proc Annu Vet Med Forum,* 1990, p 907.

CHAPTER 16

Aortic Stenosis

Aortic stenosis is anatomically classified as valvular, supravalvular, or subvalvular. Further categorization is based on the functional characteristics of the obstruction, as either fixed or dynamic (labile). However, only subvalvular stenosis can be dynamic. The most common form of subvalvular stenosis is a fibrous ring of tissue that lies immediately below the aortic valve. It is termed *subaortic stenosis (SAS)* and is by far the most common type of aortic stenosis in dogs, constituting more than 95% of the lesions identified. Congenital fixed aortic stenosis is rare in cats, yet both subvalvular, valvular, and supravalvular forms have been recognized.[1,2] In congenital SAS, the dimensions of the restrictive orifice are static or "fixed" by the anatomic characteristics of the lesion. The severity of the obstruction is not altered from beat to beat and does not change as systole progresses. The dimensions of the lesion in dogs and cats with "dynamic" obstruction are labile. In this case, the severity of the obstruction is altered by changes in heart rate or inotropic state and usually varies as systole progresses.[3,4] In some cases, fixed and dynamic obstructions occur together.[5] Dynamic obstruction as a result of systolic anterior motion of the mitral valve is common in cats. It is usually associated with hypertrophic cardiomyopathy.

Prevalence

Subaortic stenosis is one of the most common forms of congenital heart disease recognized in the dog. Opinion varies as to the exact prevalence.[6-8] In a survey of the records of North American veterinary schools for the years 1987 to 1989, isolated congenital SAS was diagnosed in 22% of the canine cases, second only to patent ductus arteriosus (32%).[6] During the period October 1, 1986, to October 1, 1996, we diagnosed isolated SAS in 288 dogs; this was our most common diagnosis during that period. Golden retrievers and Newfoundland retrievers were the most commonly represented purebred dogs in this population. Many other breeds were represented, including large numbers of rottweilers, boxers, and German shepherds. Breeds at increased risk for developing SAS (based on calculated odds ratios) are presented in Table 16-1.

Embryology and Genetics

The embryologic basis for all forms of aortic stenosis is unclear and controversial. Valvular aortic stenosis is likely related to faulty development of the embryonic endocardial cushions in the truncoconal septum (truncus swellings), from which the semilunar valve leaflets originate.[9,10] Both subvalvular and supravalvular aortic stenosis occur in several anatomic forms, each of which likely has a unique embryologic basis. Supravalvular aortic stenosis is thought to be due to exaggerated development of the slight (normal) transverse infolding or plica of the aortic wall that is situated immediately above the sinuses of Valsalva.[9] Membranous, supravalvular stenosis is considered to be derived from aberrant tissue of the aortic cusps.[9] The left ventricular outflow tract is formed during the development of the conotruncal septum, the ventricular septum, and the anterior (septal) leaflet of the mitral valve.[10] Abnormal development of any of these structures may result in SAS. The common form of SAS seen in dogs is probably due to a primary developmental fault in the region of transition from the conus to the truncus, a site that favors inflammation in later stages of development in humans.[9] It has been suggested that in dogs the fibrocartilaginous ring of SAS is derived from persistent embryonal endocardial tissue that retains its proliferative capacity and has chondrogenic potential for some time after birth.[11]

Subaortic stenosis has been demonstrated to be an inherited trait in the Newfoundland retriever through selective breedings.[7,11,12] The initial results of breeding experiments were not consistent with any simple genetic hypothesis and indicated that SAS is inherited as a polygenic trait or as an autosomal dominant trait with gene modifiers.[11] However, in these test matings many of the offspring were sacrificed or died before 3 weeks of age. The same investigators have reported that lesions of SAS are not found in dogs before 3 weeks of age, and that only the mildest form of SAS is seen in dogs between 3 and 12 weeks of age.[11] The youngest dog with a detectable lesion in this report was 24 days old at the time of death. These findings suggest that SAS in the Newfoundland retriever is not a true congenital defect. Instead it develops in the postnatal period. If only dogs that survived beyond 3 weeks of age are considered in the genetic analysis, the results of all matings among Newfoundlands are consistent with an autosomal dominant pattern.[7] Also, recent reexamination of the breeding studies in SAS in the Newfoundland indicates that a single major gene abnormality underlies this defect.[13] Based on these studies, a heritable basis for SAS is also strongly suspected in other commonly affected breeds.[4]

Anatomy and Pathology

FIXED SUBAORTIC STENOSIS

The left ventricular outflow tract (LVOT) is defined by several structures: the craniolateral portion of the left ventricular free wall, the membranous and muscular portions of the basilar ventricular septum, and the anterior (cranial) mitral valve leaflet and associated structures. Abnormalities in any of these areas may produce subaortic obstruction to left ventricular outflow. The classic description of

TABLE 16-1

Estimated relative risks (odds ratios) by breed in dogs with SAS[37]

Breed	*Number*	*Odds ratio*	*95% CL*	p *Value*
Newfoundland	38	88.1	59.7-130	<0.001
Rottweiler	34	19.3	13.1-28.5	<0.001
Boxer	18	8.6	5.1-14.2	<0.001
Golden retriever	29	5.5	3.64-8.33	<0.001
German shepherd	20	1.3	0.79-2.1	0.28

SAS in the dog is that of a discrete fibrous ridge or collar that completely or partially encircles the LVOT immediately below the aortic valve (Color Plate 56).[7] Pathologic studies in breeding colonies have shown, however, that a range in severity of the lesion exists, the mildest form of which is clinically silent. Pyle et al[11] described three grades of SAS lesions based on postmortem studies in Newfoundland puppies. In the mildest form (grade 1), the lesions consisted of small, raised nodules of thickened endocardium on the interventricular septum below the aortic valve. Similar lesions were seen on the ventral surface of the aortic valve cusps in some animals. Grade 1 lesions were only identified in dogs between 3 and 12 weeks of age in this study. Grade 2 lesions formed a narrow ridge of whitish, thickened endocardium that partially encircled the LVOT below the aortic valve. In most cases this tissue originated at the base of the anterior mitral valve leaflet and traversed across the interventricular septum for a variable distance. In the most severe form (grade 3), a fibrous band, ridge, or collar completely encircled the LVOT immediately below the aortic valve. The ridge was raised, sometimes 1 to 2 mm, above the endocardial surface and extended around the entire LVOT, including the base of the anterior mitral valve leaflet (Color Plate 56). Grade 3 lesions were predominantly identified in dogs older than 6 months of age. In these dogs, the ventricular surfaces of the aortic valve leaflets were also thickened. Finding that the lesion severity was confined to specific age ranges documented that the lesion of SAS progressively worsens over at least the first 6 months of life.

The lesions of SAS are histologically characterized by large, uninucleated and multinucleated, rounded connective tissue cells that resemble chondrocytes.[14] Adjacent connective tissue is rich in acid mucopolysaccharides, small collagen fibrils, and poorly developed elastic and reticular fibers.[14,15] In advanced lesions, discrete bundles of collagen and cartilage may be found.[11,14] Dogs with pressure gradients across this region in excess of 35 mm Hg, demonstrate remodeling of the intramural coronary arteries and arterioles, characterized by luminal narrowing, intimal smooth muscle proliferation, medial hypertrophy, and medial smooth muscle disorganization.[11,16,17] Although the exact cause of the coronary lesions is not known, it is presumed that they may be precipitated by the increased left ventricular systolic pressure, increased systolic wall tension, and abnormal coronary blood flow associated with the subaortic lesion.[18,19] The coronary lesions are associated with focal areas of myocardial ischemia and fibrosis, which are most prevalent in the papillary muscles and subendocardial regions of the left ventricular wall.[16,17] The myocardial lesions are also influenced by a relative decrease in myocardial capillary density secondary to concentric hypertrophy.[17]

Associated findings on gross examination illustrate the pathologic consequences of SAS. Concentric hypertrophy of the left ventricle may be present, and its severity is thought to reflect the magnitude of left ventricular pressure increase in systole. However, a recent study demonstrated poor correlation between the Doppler pressure gradient and measurements of left ventricular wall thickness or mass.[20] In our experience, dogs with severe SAS always have echocardiographically demonstrable left ventricular concentric hypertrophy, whereas dogs with mild SAS do not. Dogs with pressure gradients in the moderate range are more variable but tend to have less concentric hypertrophy than expected. Mild left atrial enlargement may be present with severe SAS and is presumably due to a decrease in left ventricular compliance, myocardial failure, or concomitant mitral insufficiency. Dilatation of the ascending aorta and aortic arch occurs secondary to the turbulent flow forcefully striking the walls in those areas. Mild malformations of the mitral valve that are usually not functionally important are also common in dogs with SAS. However, some dogs do have concurrent moderate-to-severe mitral valve dysplasia. These dogs usually die at an early age from left congestive heart failure.

In colony-bred Newfoundland retrievers with grade 1 lesions, clinical examination and cardiac catheterization failed do identify the lesion.[11] Only soft, transient murmurs (1/6) were recognized in these puppies. Dogs with grade 2 lesions often had a soft systolic murmur (1 to 2/6) and a mild systolic pressure gradient across the subaortic region (less than 20 mm Hg). This means the peak systolic flow velocity in these dogs was less than 2.2 m/sec. Dogs with grade 3 lesions exhibited clear physical evidence of SAS (i.e., a readily detectable systolic heart murmur), and all had an abnormal pressure gradient across the subaortic lesion ranging from 36 to 95 mm Hg (this translates into a peak systolic flow velocity of 3 to 4.9 m/sec), and abnormal left ventricular angiography. Thus dogs with genetic coding for SAS may clearly remain unidentified using currently approved screening methods, especially when dogs less than 6 months of age are involved. This makes genetic counseling difficult in dogs of breeds known to be at increased risk for SAS when a soft systolic murmur of unknown or questionable origin is identified.

Pathologic studies of SAS in dogs clearly indicate that structural lesions either are not present or are not fully developed at birth.[11,21] They also indicate that the obstruction may, and often does, become progressively more severe during the developmental period. Further evidence suggests that any gradient, regardless of the age of the dog, may become progressively more severe over time.[21,22] However, this has only been documented in a few individuals and is not considered to be a common clinical course. It is uncertain at what age an obstruction becomes fully developed.

The progressive nature of SAS has clinical implications relative to the identification of affected puppies of breeds known to be at risk for SAS. Because the lesion may be clinically silent in dogs less than 3 months of age, dogs less than this age cannot be classified as free of the disease based on any type of clinical examination except for necropsy. The vast majority of dogs with SAS that are older than 3 months of age, and many younger dogs with the lesion will have a heart murmur. However, it may be difficult to definitively localize the origin of the murmur to SAS in some of these dogs because the lesion may not be fully developed and the pressure gradient and the peak flow velocity through the SAS region may be within normal limits. Dogs that are destined to develop only mild SAS may plateau at this stage and remain a clinical enigma. Only dogs that develop more severe SAS can be definitively recognized by current clinical examinations. Most dogs with SAS will have a heart murmur, and this diagnostic test is probably the most sensitive means of identifying an affected dog. Unfortunately, detection of a heart murmur does not specifically mean that a dog has SAS, because the murmur may be due to another cardiac malady or may be a "physiologic" or innocent murmur in a young dog. It is probably inappropriate to 'clear' dogs for SAS before they are full grown. It is inappropriate to judge a dog to be free of SAS if a soft systolic murmur of unknown origin is present. At best one can say the examination is 'equivocal,' indicating that the examiner cannot determine if the dog is affected or not. It is unlikely that any adult dog that does not demonstrate a cardiac murmur consistent with SAS has or will go on to develop SAS. Whenever mild-to-moderate SAS has been documented in a young dog, no prognosis should be given, because the obstruction may, and often does, ultimately become more severe.

The Congenital Heart Disease Committee of the Cardiology Specialty of the American College of Veterinary Internal Medicine has recently made recommendations for the standards for screening dogs for congenital heart disease. These recommendations were subsequently adopted by the Orthopedic Foundation for Animals for use in establishing a Congenital Heart Disease Registry. These recommendations were established largely to deal with the controversies surrounding congenital SAS, as discussed above, yet apply to all congenital defects. A careful clinical examination that emphasizes cardiac auscultation is cost-effective and expedient and is the preferred method for the initial identification of congenital heart disease in dogs. The noninvasive method of echocardiography with Doppler is the preferred method for establishing a definitive diagnosis in dogs when congenital heart disease is suspected from the clinical examination. Generally, echocardiography is an inappropriate screening tool. The recommendations stipulate that animals should be examined and classified by a veterinarian with expertise in the recognition of congenital heart disease. A *phenotypically* normal dog is defined as one without a cardiac murmur or as one with an innocent heart murmur that is found to be otherwise normal by virtue of an echocardiographic examination that included Doppler studies. Full certification is given to dogs examined at 12 months of age or older, whereas only provisional certification is given to dogs under 12 months of age. Dogs may be classified as equivocal when the findings do not clearly discriminate between normal and abnormal.

The mechanism by which SAS increases in severity is uncertain. Pyle et al[11] hypothesized that the fibrocartilaginous ring of SAS is derived from persistent embryonal endocardial tissue that retains its proliferative capacity and chondrogenic potential for some time after birth. It is unclear whether increases in body size and changes in the degree of left ventricular concentric hypertrophy may also contribute to the progression, although this is unlikely. Others have suggested that the real abnormality in SAS is a steepened angle between the LVOT and the proximal aorta producing abnormal blood flow patterns and increased septal shear stress in the region of the stenosis.[23] Although this could explain the abnormalities arising from the septal musculature, it seems unlikely that this type of abnormality would produce a complete ring.

DYNAMIC SUBAORTIC STENOSIS

Dynamic SAS is most commonly observed in veterinary medicine in cats with hypertrophic cardiomyopathy (see Chapter 21).[24,25] In this disease it is due to systolic anterior motion of the mitral valve. Hypertrophic cardiomyopathy is a primary myocardial disease that may or may not have a dynamic obstruction (dynamic SAS). The obstructive form of hypertrophic cardiomyopathy in humans is usually associated with both asymmetric septal hypertrophy and dynamic SAS. A similar obstructive form of hypertrophic cardiomyopathy is also recognized in cats; however, asymmetric septal hypertrophy is not a consistent feature.

Dynamic SAS associated with systolic anterior motion of the mitral valve is also seen in dogs, both as an isolated lesion and concurrently with fixed SAS.[3,26-29] Most dogs with dynamic SAS are members of breeds commonly affected by congenital fixed SAS and most reports of hypertrophic cardiomyopathy involve young dogs.[5,30] Dynamic subaortic stenosis has also been identified in dogs with pulmonic stenosis, tetralogy of Fallot, and idiopathic left ventricular concentric hypertrophy. Systolic anterior motion of the mitral valve is seen in humans with several congenital and acquired lesions.[30-32] Consequently, it is not yet clear in dogs whether dynamic SAS is the result of a primary myocardial disease (i.e., hypertrophic cardiomyopathy) or a congenital abnormality of the LVOT or mitral valve apparatus. It is also possible that both forms exist and that dynamic SAS is a nonspecific finding that does not represent one disease entity. Instead it may be a common result of altered LVOT hemodynamics from any cause.[33]

Left ventricular concentric hypertrophy without fixed obstruction to left ventricular obstruction, associated with abnormal LVOT hemodynamics is the hallmark of dynamic SAS. Global or septal left ventricular hypertrophy, a slightly narrowed LVOT, and a fibrous plaque on the intraventricular septum opposite the anterior leaflet of the mitral valve have been reported in dogs with dynamic SAS.[27,28] In conjunction, the mitral valve is often thickened and fibrotic, and secondary changes such as mild left atrial enlargement and left atrial endocardial jet lesions suggest the presence of mitral regurgitation. Mitral regurgitation may be secondary to either abnormal mitral leaflet coaptation related to the abnormal LVOT hemodynamics or coexisting mitral valve disease.[28,29]

Pathophysiology

Independent of the nature of the obstruction, the principle hemodynamic consequence of aortic stenosis is an increased resistance to the left ventricular systolic outflow. According to Ohm's Law (resistance = pressure gradient/blood flow), this increase in resistance results in one of three things—an increase in the pressure gradient across the stenotic region, a decrease in flow through the region, or a combination of both. In chronic SAS, the aortic pressure is usually normal and a pressure gradient across the subaortic lesion results in an increase in systolic left ventricular pressure (Figure 16-1). Concentric hypertrophy compensates for the increase in left ventricular systolic wall stress such that left ventricular function remains normal and flow through the subaortic narrowing usually remains within the normal range. Consequently, the pressure gradient across the narrowing usually increases in direct proportion to the increase in resistance (i.e., the decrease in the size of the narrowed opening). As long as flow is constant, the velocity of flow through the stenotic region also increases in direct proportion to the size of the stenotic ring (i.e., as the ring becomes smaller, blood flow velocity increases). This is similar to what happens when a wide, slowly flowing river suddenly narrows, producing rapids. Blood flow velocity (V) and pressure gradient have a constant relationship that is defined by the modified Bernoulli equation (pressure gradient = $4V^2$); either can be used to identify the abnormal hemodynamics associated with SAS, and both can be used to semiquantitatively determine the severity of the lesion. In summary, the primary physiologic abnormalities observed clinically in dogs with SAS are (1) an increase in the pressure gradient across the subaortic lesion, resulting in an increase in the systolic left ventricular pressure; (2) an increase

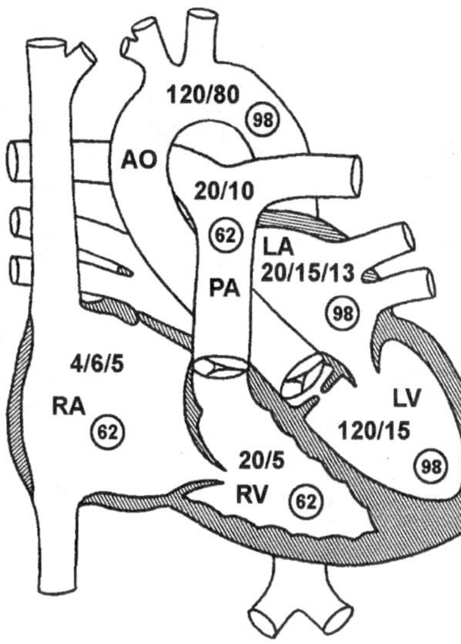

FIGURE 16-1 Schematic diagram depicting the hemodynamic alterations associated with subaortic stenosis. The resistance to flow at the subaortic narrowing leads to an increase in left ventricular systolic pressure, and the resultant concentric hypertrophy may lead to a mild increase in left ventricular diastolic pressure and left atrial pressure. Right-sided pressures remain normal. In the absence of other defects, both pulmonary and systemic oxygen saturation remain normal. *RA,* Right atrium; *RV,* right ventricle; *LA,* left atrium; *LV,* left ventricle; *PA,* pulmonary artery; *AO,* aorta. Intracardiac pressures are indicated in mm Hg as systolic/diastolic for the LV, RV, PA, and AO and as *a* wave/*v* wave/mean for the LA and RA. Circled numbers indicate oxygen saturation.

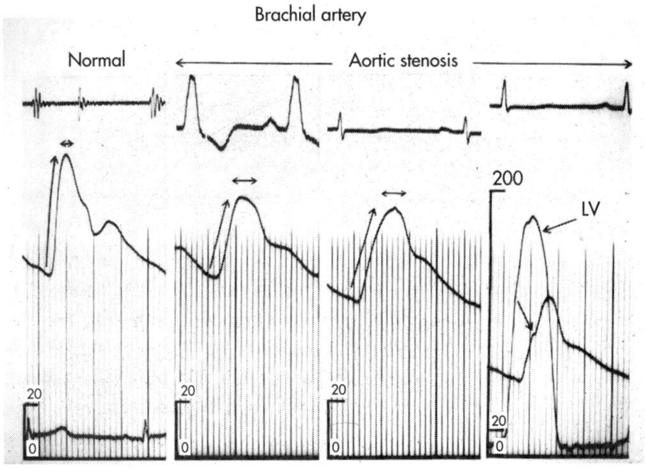

FIGURE 16-2 Systemic arterial pressure pulses from a normal human and three humans with aortic stenosis. The aortic stenosis pulse exhibits a relatively small pressure pulse, a slow rate of rise with a sustained peak, and a gentle decline. The last pane depicts an anacrotic notch in the ascending limb of the arterial pulse. *LV,* Left ventricle. (From Perloff JK: Congenital aortic stenosis: congenital aortic regurgitation. In Perloff JK, ed: *The clinical recognition of congenital heart disease,* ed 4, Philadelphia, 1994, WB Saunders.)

in blood flow velocity through the lesion; and (3) left ventricular concentric hypertrophy. The pressure gradient and blood flow velocity are commonly used as indexes of lesion severity. However, because they are affected by both lesion severity (resistance) and flow, they are less accurate than determinations of the lesion's cross-sectional area or resistance. For example, when a dog is anesthetized, cardiac function is usually compromised and cardiac output (i.e., flow) decreases. Consequently, the pressure gradient and the flow velocity through the lesion usually decrease even though the size of the narrowed region has not changed. Conversely, it is assumed that the pressure gradient, left ventricular pressure, and flow velocity increase dramatically during exercise when flow increases. Distal to the obstruction, flow becomes turbulent. The force of this turbulent jet striking the walls of the proximal aorta results in poststenotic dilation of the ascending aorta.

The increase in left ventricular systolic wall stress stimulates an increase in left ventricular muscle mass (concentric hypertrophy) usually proportional to the severity of the obstruction. The left ventricular hypertrophy normalizes ventricular systolic function and usually allows left ventricular stroke volume to remain within the normal range. However, because of the increased resistance, peak left ventricular ejection is delayed, resulting in a late-rising, variably diminished arterial pulse (Figure 16-2). A severely hypertrophied left ventricle may reduce the end-diastolic volume but usually not to the same degree as with hypertrophic cardiomyopathy. Severe hypertrophy produces an increase in ventricular stiffness. This in turn may reduce the ability of the ventricle to fill properly. An abnormal diastolic filling pattern may cause an increase in the *a* wave of the left atrial and pulmonary capillary wedge pressures and often leads to mild left atrial enlargement.

Mild degrees of aortic insufficiency are commonly observed in dogs with SAS and appear to be caused by thickening and impaired mobility of the aortic valve cusps. The thickening is secondary to the trauma created by the high-velocity jet striking the valve cusps during ejection.[34] Aortic insufficiency may be further aggravated by involvement of the leaflets within the fibrous ring, dilation of the ascending aorta, or infective endocarditis. All of these complications are rare. However, damage to the aortic valve cusps by the turbulent jet predisposes to the development of infective endocarditis in both dogs and humans with discrete subaortic stenosis.[16,35]

Exertional syncope and sudden death are the most common clinical signs related to SAS. The mechanisms behind these signs remain speculative. The most widely accepted explanation of exertional syncope is acute reflex peripheral arterial and venous dilation and bradycardia, possibly mediated by the exercise-induced effects of a sudden increase in left ventricular systolic pressure on ventricular baroreceptor activity.[36] However, some investigators contend that ventricular arrhythmias must also be considered as a causative factor. However, even though arrhythmias may be noted in some individuals that collapse, some studies indicate that syncope is the primary event, with malignant or fatal arrhythmias being secondary to the hemodynamic changes imposed by the collapse.[36] Malignant ventricular arrhythmias are probably responsible for sudden death. Whether they are associated with myocardial ischemia or induced by syncopal episodes is unknown.[19]

Although congestive left heart failure may ultimately result from severe SAS, the overall incidence is very low.[37] The left ventricle responds to sudden production of severe obstruction by dilation and reduction of stroke volume. However, in SAS the obstruction is either present at birth or gradually develops over time. Left ventricular output is maintained by concentric hypertrophy, and left ventricular end-diastolic volume usually remains relatively normal until late in the course of the disease.[38] The elevated left ventricular end-diastolic pressure resulting from decreased ventricular compliance is usually only mild and not generally high enough to produce pulmonary edema. If congestive heart failure does develop in a patient with SAS, it is likely due to slowly developing myocardial failure or complicating factors, such as moderate-to-severe mitral regurgitation or aortic insufficiency. We have observed only one dog with SAS and myocardial failure severe enough to cause heart failure. Consequently, this scenario appears to be rare.

PATHOPHYSIOLOGIC MECHANISM OF DYNAMIC SUBAORTIC STENOSIS

Dynamic subaortic obstruction is most commonly related to the development of systolic anterior motion (SAM) of the mitral valve. SAM of the mitral valve describes the pulling or pushing of the anterior mitral valve leaflet into the LVOT during ventricular contraction, with resultant mitral-septal contact. Several investigators have studied the pathophysiologic mechanism and anatomic structures responsible for the development of systolic anterior motion of the mitral valve; however, extensive controversy exists regarding the primary mechanism and the significance of SAM.[24] Early proposed mechanisms focused on hypertrophy of the interventricular septum causing narrowing of the LVOT.[39,40] It was believed that the narrow LVOT combined with rapid ejection created a negative pressure above the mitral valve (Venturi effect). The subsequent mitral-septal apposition resulted in the obstruction to LV outflow.[39,40] Others contend that the Venturi effect fails to explain several observed features of SAM, such as the location of mitral-septal contact point and how sufficient slack is produced in the mitral valve leaflets to permit SAM. Further, the Venturi hypothesis cannot explain the fact that the onset of SAM occurs before aortic valve opening, that the obstruction persists into late systole, or the fact that patients with primary mitral valve abnormalities (i.e., without septal hypertrophy) can also have SAM.[40,41] More recent investigations suggest that structural abnormalities or a malpositioning of the papillary-mitral apparatus play a fundamental role in altering the balance of forces acting upon the mitral valve leaflets, so that SAM is promoted by normal left ventricular ejection.[40-44] Anterior displacement of the papillary muscles and increased area and elongation of the anterior mitral valve leaflet appear to be important determinants of SAM.[40-44] This hypothesis would also explain the development of SAM in disorders other than hypertrophic cardiomyopathy, including congenital malformations of the mitral valve. Others have demonstrated that SAM can be produced in normal individuals by manipulating heart rate or contractility.[32] The induction and maintenance of SAM are probably multifactorial and are likely influenced by the anatomy of the mitral valve apparatus, the area of the LVOT, the contractile state of the ventricle, the heart rate, and other unidentified factors.[24,33]

The net result of SAM is the development of a pressure gradient across the LVOT and, in most instances, mitral regurgitation as the anterior mitral valve leaflet is forced away from its normal position into the outflow tract.[45,46] Doppler echocardiographic studies have shown that there is acceleration of flow in the LVOT just before the point of mitral-septal apposition, with turbulence and marked flow acceleration beyond the point of contact.[47] Continuous-wave Doppler flow tracings of dynamic gradients often demonstrate an increasing rate of acceleration (the velocity contour is concave to the left) and a peak systolic gradient in late systole, a phenomenon that has not been seen in patients with fixed obstructions (Figure 16-3). This increasing acceleration is due to progressive narrowing of the LVOT during systole.[43] Unlike a patient with a fixed obstruction, the estimated LVOT area also changes dramatically from beat to beat during perturbations that alter pressure and flow, such as exercise or infusions of vasoactive or inotropic agents.[46] Simultaneous recordings of phasic aortic flow and left heart pressure have shown that 80% to 90% of the left ventricular stroke volume is ejected in the first half of systole during the time when there is a relatively small pressure gradient followed by a concurrent increase in gradient and progressive reduction in flow during late systole.[46] As a result, patients with dynamic SAS tend to have a rapidly rising arterial pulse compared with the reduced amplitude and delayed systolic peak of fixed aortic stenosis.

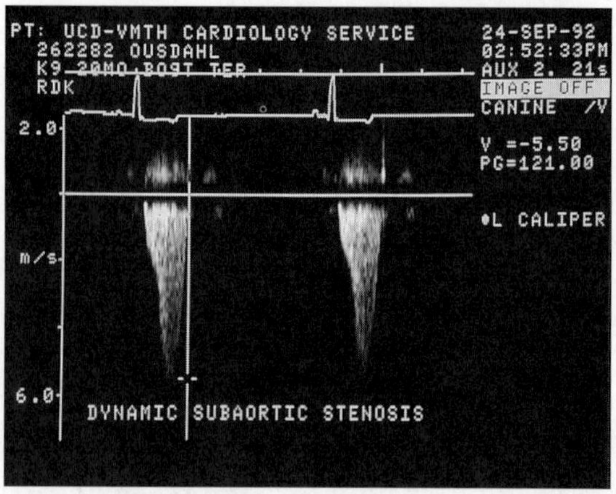

FIGURE 16-3 Continuous-wave Doppler tracing from the left ventricular outflow tract and aorta in a dog with dynamic subaortic stenosis. The peak systolic velocity is 5.5 m/sec, indicating a systolic pressure gradient between the left ventricle and aorta of 121 mm Hg. This finding is diagnostic of aortic stenosis. The concave appearance of the velocity tracing to the left and a delayed systolic peak indicate the gradient is dynamic in nature. This patient also had left ventricular concentric hypertrophy and systolic anterior motion of the mitral valve.

Diagnosis of Subaortic Stenosis

MEDICAL HISTORY

Clinical signs in puppies, almost all mildly-to-moderately affected individuals, and many severely affected individuals are absent. Most owners report a normal and apparently healthy individual when presenting the dog for routine examination. A heart murmur may have been previously identified in some dogs and may have been regarded as an innocent or functional murmur in a young puppy. More severely affected animals may be presented for exertional fatigue, syncope, or, rarely, for signs referable to congestive left heart failure. Sudden death without premonitory signs is common.

PHYSICAL EXAMINATION

The physical examination is often unremarkable except for the presence of a systolic ejection murmur, usually loudest in the left basilar region. The murmur intensity roughly correlates with lesion severity, with mildly affected dogs having a 1 to 3/6 murmur and more severely affected individuals having a 4 to 5/6 murmur. The radiation of the murmur, if present, is often characteristic. The murmur tends to radiate toward the left apex and the right cranial thorax. It might also be heard over the carotid arteries upon auscultation of the cervical region on either side of the trachea. In many dogs, the murmur is equally loud at the right cranial thorax and left basilar region, and, in some, it is loudest or only present at the right cranial

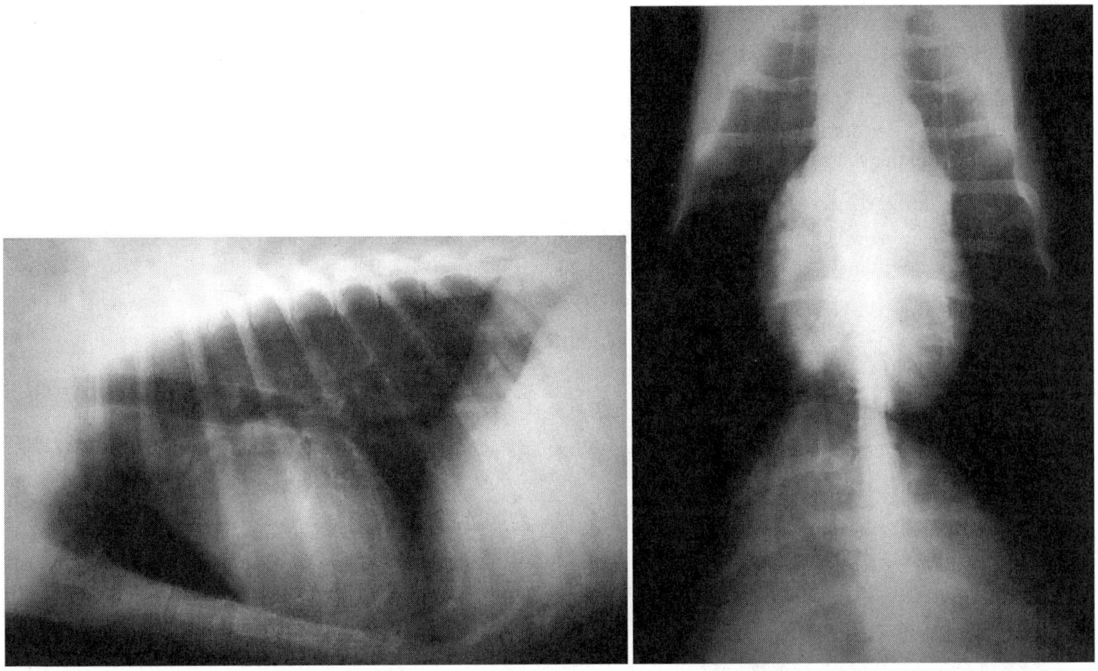

FIGURE 16-4 Thoracic radiographs from a dog with subaortic stenosis. **A,** Lateral projection exhibits mild generalized cardiomegaly, a loss of the cranial cardiac waste, and enlargement of the aortic root. **B,** The dorsoventral projection exhibits enlargement of the aortic root.

thorax. Because of the developmental nature of fixed subaortic stenosis, the murmur may increase in intensity during the first months of life. In dogs with a dynamic component, the murmur is similar but may vary in intensity from one examination to the next. In dogs with a severe obstruction, the arterial pulse may be hypokinetic (i.e., the pulse pressure is decreased) with a tardy or delayed peak (pulsus parvus et tardus) although pulse pressure may remain normal (see Figure 16-2). Occasionally, a diastolic murmur associated with mild-to-moderate aortic insufficiency is also audible in the left basilar region.

ELECTROCARDIOGRAPHY

The electrocardiogram is often normal in dogs with SAS, either fixed or dynamic. Left ventricular enlargement is suggested by the presence of an increased *R* wave amplitude in leads II and aV_F or the left chest leads in some dogs. The mean electrical axis is usually normal, although a left axis deviation may be rarely identified. The ST segment may be slurred, depressed, or elevated in some dogs with severe SAS. This is usually secondary to regional myocardial hypoxia. Ventricular premature contractions may also be identified in dogs with pressure gradients in the severe range. The latter findings may be induced or exaggerated by exercise.

Some veterinary cardiologists advocate long-term ambulatory ECGs (i.e., Holter monitor recordings) in patients with moderate-to-severe SAS to detect ventricular arrhythmias and ST segment changes that might suggest an increased probability of sudden death.[48] In a report of 14 dogs with SAS evaluated by Holter monitor, ventricular premature complexes were recorded in 10, which were multiform in 7.[49] Some dogs had ventricular tachycardia, triplets, or couplets. Although there was a tendency for the frequency of ventricular arrhythmias to increase in dogs with higher pressure gradients, considerable overlap occurred between the groups. Ventricular premature complexes were only identified on the resting electrocardiogram in 3 of 11 dogs in this study. When Holter recording was repeated 1 month after prescribing atenolol in 4 of the dogs, the frequency of ventricular premature contractions had decreased by 75%. ST segment deviation, probably related to regional myocardial ischemia, was identified in 50% of these dogs and developed more often in dogs with higher pressure gradients.

THORACIC RADIOGRAPHY

Thoracic radiographs are typically normal in mildly affected individuals and may show only apparent mild cardiomegaly as a result of left ventricular concentric hypertrophy in severely affected dogs. The most common finding in severely affected dogs is enlargement of the aortic root or widening of the mediastinum as a result of poststenotic dilation of the aorta (Figure 16-4).

ECHOCARDIOGRAPHY

Two-dimensional and M-mode echocardiographic findings are often normal in mildly-to-moderately affected individuals. Left ventricular hypertrophy is usually readily apparent only in moderately-to-severely affected dogs. In these cases, the M-mode echocardiogram demonstrates increased diastolic septal and left ventricular free wall thicknesses (left ventricular concentric hypertrophy) and a normal left ventricular shortening fraction. The narrowed subvalvular region can sometimes be identified while sweeping the M-mode transducer from the left ventricle to the level of the proximal aorta, but two dimensional evaluation is more accurate for this purpose.[50,51] Other findings may include poststenotic dilatation of the ascending aorta, secondary thickening of the aortic valve cusps, and midsystolic partial closure of the aortic valve cusps. In some cases of SAS, the mitral valve *E-F* slope decreases because of reduced compliance of the hypertrophied left ventricle.[52] This should not be misinterpreted as mitral stenosis. Overall, M-mode examination alone is not very reliable for identification or confirmation of congenital SAS except in severe cases.

In cases of moderate-to-severe SAS, the subvalvular lesion can usually be identified by an experienced echocardiographer. The secondary concentric hypertrophy is more readily identified. In mild cases, the obstruction may be difficult to distinguish except as minor irregularities in the left ventricular outflow tract. The obstruction appears as a narrowing between the ventricular septum and the base of the anterior mitral valve leaflet, just proximal to the aortic valve on the right parasternal or left cranial long-axis views. It usually appears as a discrete membranous or fibromuscular ridge (Figure 16-5). Rarely, it is as a longer, tunnel type of obstruction.[53] The subvalvular fibrous narrowing may also be identified in the right short-axis view as a circular or oval ring in the outflow tract, below

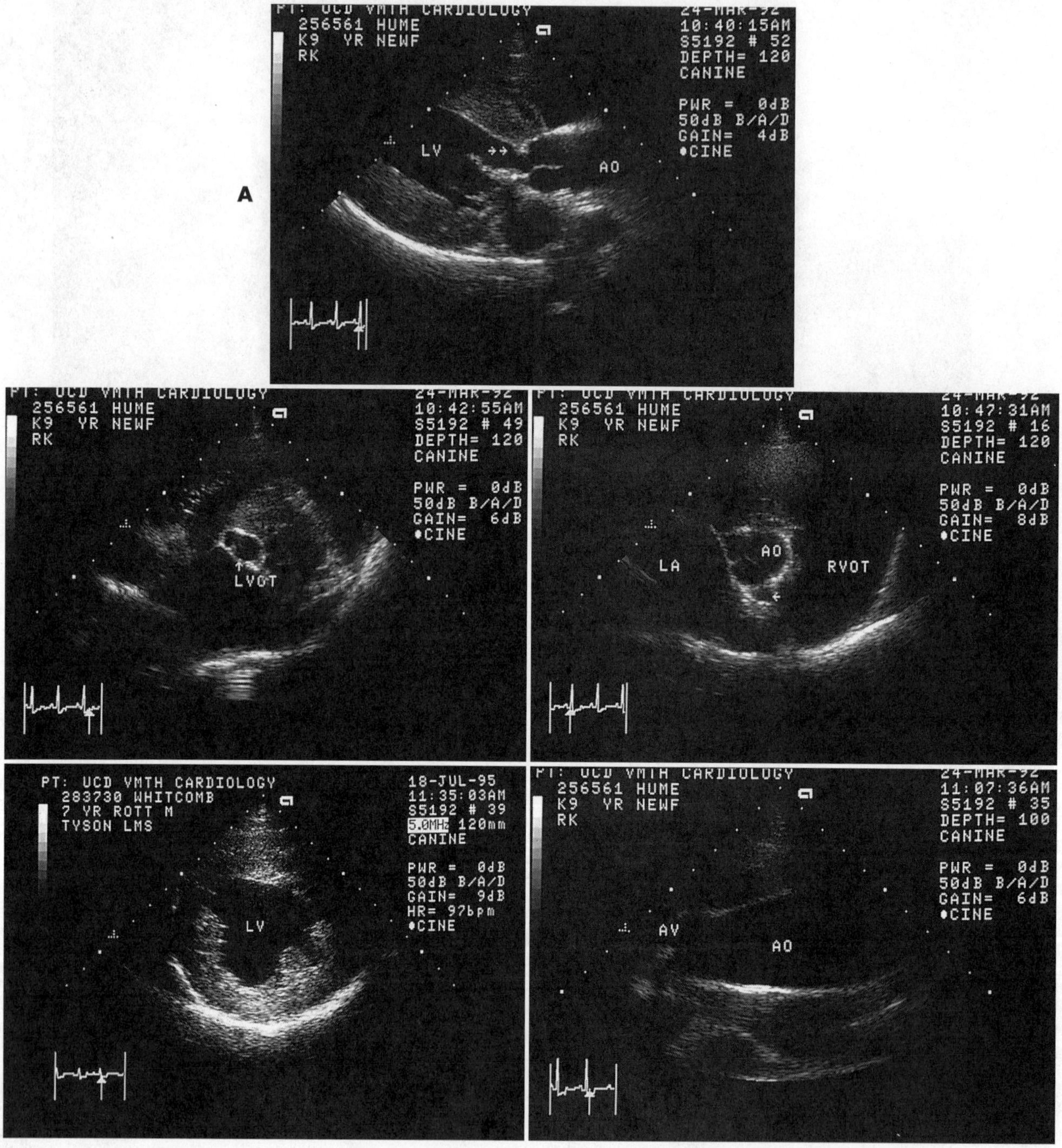

FIGURE 16-5 Two-dimensional echocardiograms from dogs with subaortic stenosis *AO,* Aorta. **A,** Right parasternal long-axis view exhibiting severe left ventricular *(LV)* concentric hypertrophy and a clearly identifiable, discrete narrowing of the left ventricular outflow tract *(LVOT)* below the aortic valve and thickening of the anterior mitral valve leaflet. **B,** Right parasternal short-axis view at the level of the LVOT, indicating that the fibrotic lesion identified in **A** completely encircles the LVOT. **C,** When the LVOT as seen in **B** is compared with the size of the aortic root just above, the degree of the stenosis can be appreciated. *Arrow,* Left coronary artery. *RVOT,* Right ventricular outflow tract. **D,** Right parasternal short-axis view at the level of the left ventricular papillary muscles exhibiting an increased echogenicity of the subendocardial region and papillary muscles suggestive of myocardial fibrosis. **E,** Left cranial long-axis view exhibiting poststenotic dilation of the aorta beyond the aortic valve *(AV).*

the aortic valve (see Figure 16-5, *B* and *C*). A recent study has demonstrated that the ratio of the cross-sectional area of the fibrous ring to the proximal aortic cross sectional-area from this view may be used to classify the severity of the lesion when Doppler echocardiography or cardiac catheterization are not available.[54] The areas of the fibrous ring and proximal aorta were determined planimetrically by tracing the outline of each structure from the right short-axis two-dimensional views. In this study, a logarithmic relationship between the fibrous ring/aorta ratio and the Doppler pressure gradient was obtained (r value = 0.88). When the ratio is divided into three ranges (greater than 0.5 = mild, 0.3 to 0.5 = moderate, and less than 0.3 = severe) it correctly predicts the severity of SAS (as determined by Doppler echocardiography) 84% of the time.

The aortic valve often appears mildly thickened from the continuous trauma associated with the stenotic jet. Areas of ischemic fibrosis appear as hyperechoic areas in the left ventricular papillary muscles or subendocardium (see Figure 16-5, *D*). In many cases, poststenotic dilation of the ascending aorta is recognized, but this can be slight in dogs less than 6 months of age. It may be identified in the right long-axis view, but is usually identified best in the left cranial long-axis view (see Figure 16-5, *E*). Mildly thickened mitral valve leaflets are commonly observed, but these valves are usually functionally competent. The left atrium is normal or mildly dilated in most dogs with SAS and normal mitral valve function. Cats with aortic stenosis display similar echocardiographic findings.[1,55]

An additional finding in a few dogs with SAS is systolic anterior motion (SAM) of the mitral valve, resulting in a dynamic left ventricular outflow obstruction between the anterior mitral valve leaflet and hypertrophied ventricular septum.[3,50,51,53,56] Mitral valve SAM is recognized by a movement of the anterior mitral valve leaflet toward the ventricular septum in midsystole, often approaching or contacting the septum either on the M-mode or two-dimensional echocardiogram (Figure 16-6, see Figure 21-4). Although reported in dogs with concurrent congenital fixed SAS, we have recognized SAM and dynamic SAS more often in young dogs and cats with hypertrophic cardiomyopathy.[28]

As with pulmonic stenosis, Doppler echocardiography is useful for determining the location of the stenosis and its severity, as well as accompanying complications. It is critical for the diagnosis of mild SAS in animals without clear abnormalities on the two-dimensional examination. Color flow Doppler examination demonstrates a broad

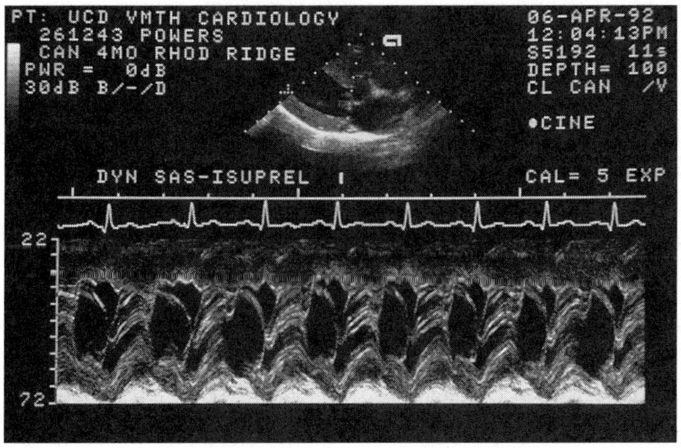

FIGURE 16-6 M-mode echocardiogram at the level of the mitral valve from a dog with dynamic subaortic stenosis resulting from systolic anterior motion of the mitral valve. Notice that the anterior mitral valve leaflet moves toward and comes in contact with the ventricular septum in midsystole.

systolic jet in the proximal aorta and diastolic aortic valve regurgitation in the left ventricular outflow tract (Color Plate 57). O'Grady found spectral Doppler evidence of mild aortic regurgitation in 87% of 53 dogs with SAS.[34] Our experience, using color Doppler imaging, is that mild aortic valve regurgitation is present in almost every dog with SAS, and that this may be one of the most sensitive indicators of SAS in dogs with the mildest defects (Color Plate 57). It is rare to find aortic regurgitation in normal dogs or dogs with other cardiac abnormalities, except for those with a ventricular septal defect or bacterial endocarditis of the aortic valve. Pulsed-wave Doppler studies in the left ventricle and aorta typically show a normal contour and velocity to the tracing in the left ventricular outflow tract (LVOT) below the lesion and spectral broadening and a step-up in velocity across the obstruction and in the ascending aorta (Figure 16-7). Continuous-wave Doppler examination of the LVOT and proximal aorta can be performed from the left apical position, a subcostal position, and a thoracic inlet (suprasternal) position. Lehmkuhl and Bonagura[57] recently studied 12 dogs with SAS and report that highest peak velocities were obtained from the subcostal position in 10 dogs (83%), the suprasternal position in one dog (8%), and the apical position in one dog (8%).The typical continuous wave tracing shows an increased systolic velocity toward the aorta and a high-velocity holodiastolic signal toward the left ventricle (aortic insufficiency) (see Figure 16-7). The modified Bernoulli equation is used to calculate the peak systolic pressure gradient. This is used, in combination with other clinical and echocardiographic findings, to estimate the severity of the lesion. Controversy exists as to what peak velocity measured in the LVOT and aorta is considered diagnostic for SAS. Most cardiologists agree that any velocity greater than 2 m/sec is supportive of the diagnosis. However, most normal dogs have peak velocities in this region less than 1.5 m/sec (usually less than 1.2 m/sec), such that there is a range of velocities between 1.5 and 2 m/sec that, in isolation, should not be used as diagnostic criteria for SAS. It is most appropriate to combine the peak velocity measurement with other echocardiographic findings, such as an increase in velocity between the LVOT and the aorta, the development of turbulence at the subaortic region, or the visual appearance of the lesion, and other clinical data to accept or refute the diagnosis. In general, dogs with a calculated pressure gradient less than 40 mm Hg are considered to have mild SAS, dogs with gradients greater than 80 to 90 mm Hg are considered to have severe stenosis, and those in between are regarded as moderately affected. These are arbitrary categorizations, however, that may not be appropriate in all cases. Doppler findings are similar in dogs with dynamic lesions, except the peak velocity may be quite variable and the continuous-wave Doppler tracing usually displays an increasing rate of acceleration (the velocity contour is concave to the left) and a peak systolic gradient in late systole, a pattern that is not seen in patients with a fixed obstruction (see Figure 16-3).

CARDIAC CATHETERIZATION

Left ventricular and aortic pressure measurements demonstrate a systolic pressure gradient across the obstruction and may also document an elevated end diastolic left ventricular pressure (Figure 16-8). This is usually accomplished by continuously recording the pressure while the catheter is withdrawn from the left ventricle, across the aortic valve and into the aorta. With good-quality tracings, the level of the obstruction may also be depicted from the pressure tracings using this technique (see Figure 16-8). The pressure gradient is invariably less than that recorded in the awake animal by Doppler echocardiography, often as much as 40% to 50%, because of decreased flow caused by the effects of general anesthesia.[58] Consequently, for purposes of prognosis and evaluating therapy,

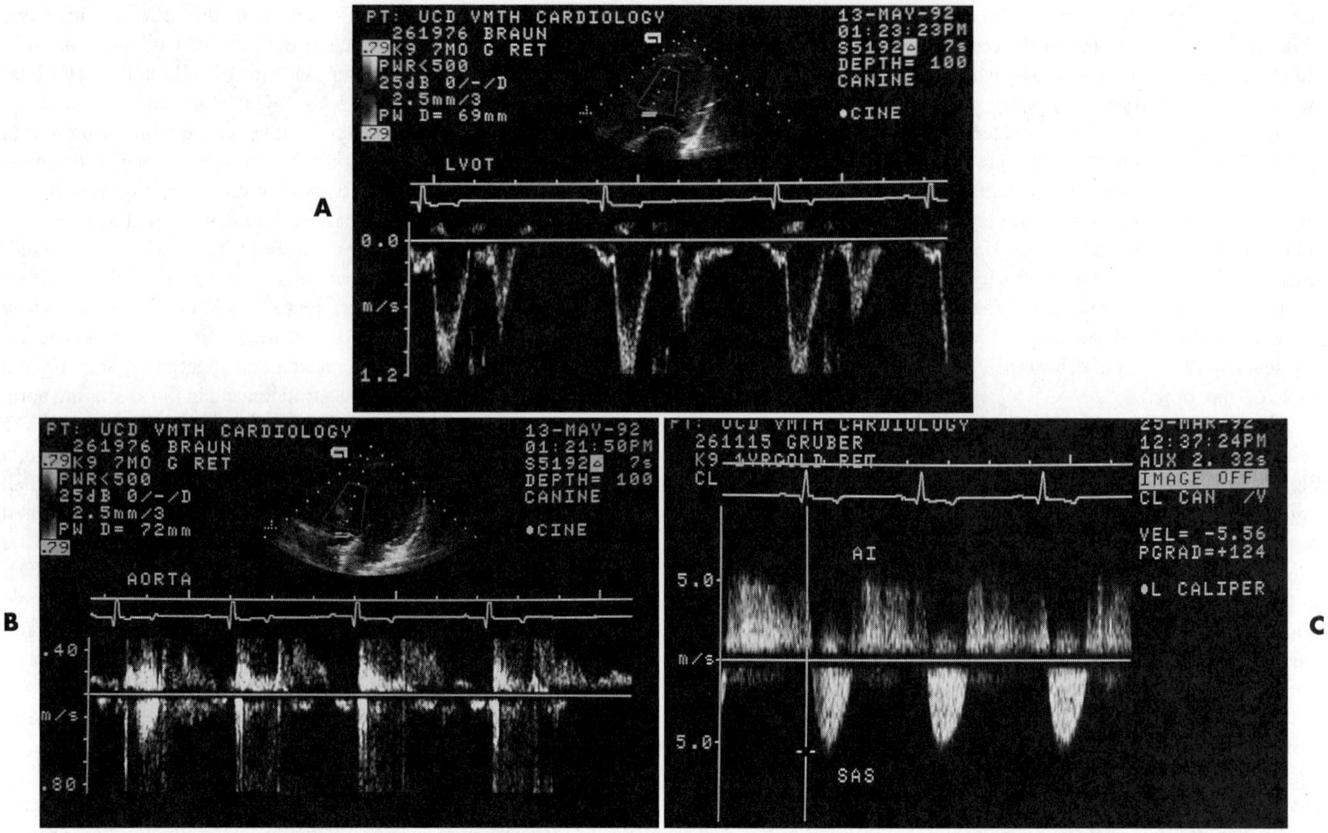

FIGURE 16-7 Spectral Doppler echocardiograms from dogs with subaortic stenosis. **A,** A normal LVOT pulsed-wave Doppler tracing (see Chapter 6 for details) **B,** As the pulsed-wave Doppler sample volume is moved across the LVOT, the signal becomes turbulent and increases in velocity. **C,** Continuous-wave Doppler tracing from the LVOT and aorta. The peak velocity of the systolic jet (directed toward the bottom of the figure) is increased (5.6 m/sec). Using the modified Bernoulli equation a LVOT-aortic pressure gradient of 125 mm Hg can be calculated. There is also a high-velocity diastolic signal directed toward the top of the figure, depicting aortic insufficiency. The velocity of this signal is not indicative of the severity of the insufficiency.

pressure gradients measured using Doppler echocardiography, in the awake patient, are more reliable. Recordings of left ventricular end-diastolic pressure, left atrial pressure, and pulmonary capillary wedge pressure often demonstrate an increased *a* wave amplitude and slightly increased mean diastolic pressures as a result of the decreased compliance of the hypertrophied left ventricle.

Left ventricular angiography outlines a normal to slightly smaller than normal left ventricular cavity and usually illustrates left ventricular concentric hypertrophy (Figure 16-9). In most cases, the actual obstruction and poststenotic dilation of the aorta are also readily identified. An aortic root angiogram may also be performed to assess the amount of secondary aortic insufficiency.

Natural History and Prognosis

Most dogs with severe SAS die suddenly or have symptoms that degrade their quality of life (Figure 16-10). Sudden death usually occurs in the first 3 years of life (the median age of sudden death is 14.4 months), mainly but not exclusively in dogs with severe obstructions (gradient greater than 80 mm Hg).[37] Up to 70% of severely affected dogs die suddenly during this time. Infective endocarditis and left heart failure are uncommon in dogs and tend to occur later in life. These complications usually occur in dogs with mild-to-moderate obstructions, probably because these dogs live long enough to develop secondary complications. Left heart failure is uncommon in the absence of additional congenital defects or infective endocarditis. Dogs born with moderate-to-severe mitral valve dysplasia that develop moderate-to-severe SAS usually develop severe left congestive heart failure between 3 and 6 months of age. Their prognosis is often poor. Dogs with a mild obstruction usually live a normal life expectancy and only rarely exhibit clinical signs.[37] The prognosis for long-term survival in dogs with untreated mild or moderate SAS is favorable; whereas the prognosis for dogs with severe SAS is usually poor (Figure 6-11).[37]

Therapy

Therapy is generally directed at preventing sudden death or reducing exercise intolerance or syncopal events. Therapy is usually unnecessary in mildly affected individuals, and the efficacy of treatment is unknown in patients with moderate-to-severe aortic stenosis.

MEDICAL

Although no scientific studies have documented efficacy, most veterinary cardiologists prescribe a β-adrenergic blocking agent for

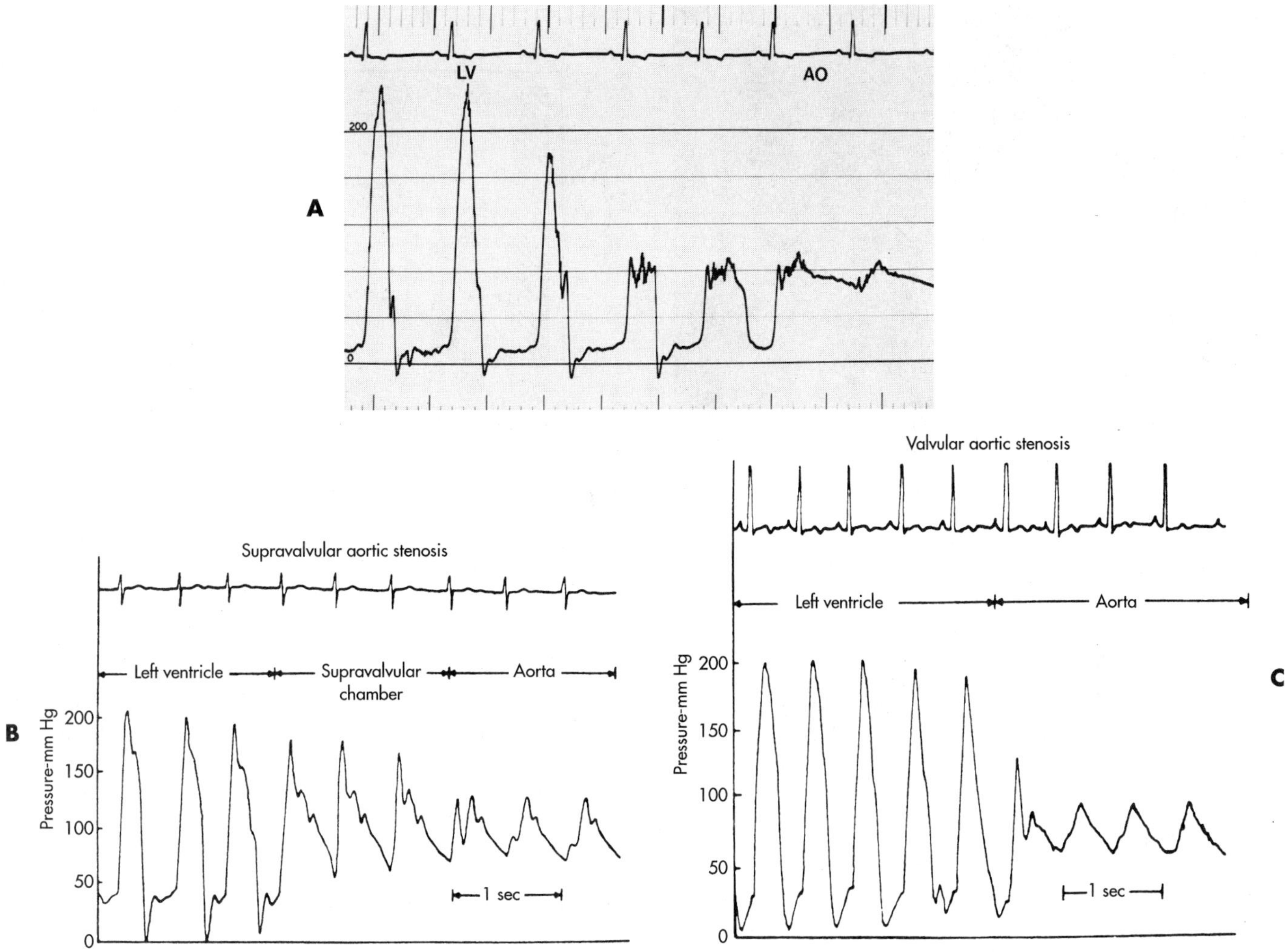

FIGURE 16-8 Pressure tracings from patients with various forms of aortic stenosis. **A,** Left ventricular (LV)-to-aortic pullback tracing in a dog with subaortic stenosis. The systolic left ventricular pressure is elevated (approximately 220 mm Hg), and the aortic systolic pressure is normal for a dog under general anesthesia (approximately 80 mm Hg). The peak-to-peak systolic pressure gradient in this dog is approximately 140 mm Hg, indicating a severe obstruction. LV end-diastolic pressure is also elevated (approximately 20 mm Hg) because of the LV concentric hypertrophy. The fourth and fifth pressure wave from the left displays systolic pressure the same as aortic and diastolic pressure the same as LV. This pressure was recorded from the space between the subaortic obstruction and the aortic valve and is diagnostic for subaortic stenosis. **B,** LV-to-aortic pullback tracing in a patient with supravalvular aortic stenosis. There is a peak-to-peak systolic pressure gradient of 80 mm Hg. The fourth, fifth, and sixth pressure waves depict LV systolic pressure with aortic diastolic pressure. These waves were recorded from the "chamber" between the aortic valve and the narrowing within the aorta (supravalvular). **C,** LV-to-aortic pullback tracing in a patient with valvular aortic stenosis. There is a peak-to-peak systolic pressure gradient of 80 mm Hg. There is no "transition" between LV and aortic pressure. (*B* and *C* from Perloff JK: In Perloff JK, ed: *The clinical recognition of congenital heart disease,* ed 4, Philadelphia, 1994, WB Saunders.)

dogs with a history of syncope or documented exercise intolerance, for dogs with frequent ventricular arrhythmias or ST segment depression, and for dogs with a pressure gradient in the moderate-to-severe range. β-Adrenergic blocking agents are used primarily in an attempt to prevent sudden death. β-Blockers prevent the arrhythmic effects of catecholamine surges on diseased myocardium. They also reduce myocardial oxygen demand and increase coronary perfusion by decreasing heart rate and contractility. The latter effects may prevent further myocardial ischemia associated with left ventricular hypertrophy, increased systolic wall stress, and abnormal coronary flow dynamics and therefore may reduce the incidence of lethal ventricular arrhythmias. Although probably beneficial in some patients, we have documented others that have died suddenly or have continued to have clinical signs while receiving β-adrenergic agents. Propranolol (1 to 2 mg/kg q8h) and atenolol (6.25 to 25 mg q12h) are the most commonly prescribed β adrenergic blocking drugs. The dose of both drugs must be increased as dogs grow. β-Receptor density in the myocardium increases during the administration of these drugs. Sudden cessation of β-blocker administration results in the sudden unmasking of an increased number of β-receptors. This can result in an exacerbation of a ventricular arrhythmia and can lead to sudden death.

Prophylactic antibiotics are advocated in humans with any degree of SAS during potential bacteremic episodes (dental procedures,

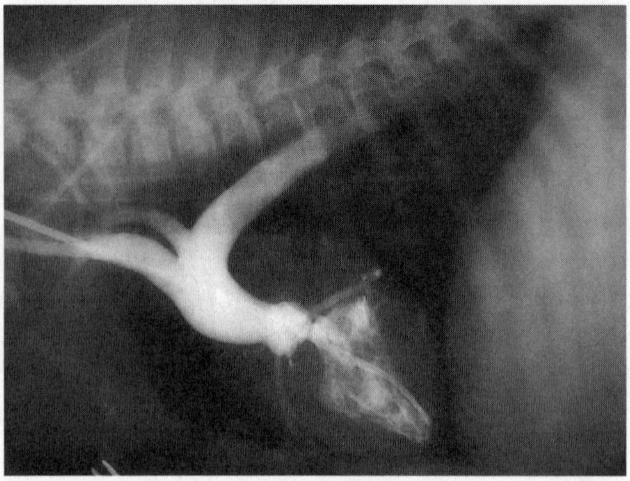

FIGURE 16-9 Left ventriculogram from a dog with subaortic stenosis. This diastolic frame shows LV concentric hypertrophy. The left ventricular outflow tract is narrowed, and there is a discrete band (filling defect) immediately beneath the aortic valve. The ascending aorta is dilated to the level of the brachiocephalic trunk.

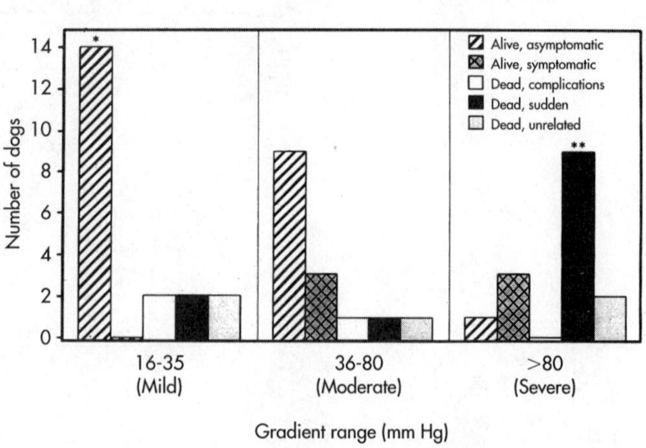

FIGURE 16-10 Distribution of outcomes for 50 dogs with SAS and different pressure gradients. In this study, dogs with mild SAS were 5.2 times more likely to be asymptomatic than other groups, and dogs with severe SAS were 16 times more likely to die suddenly than other groups. (From Kienle RD, Thomas WP, Pion PD: The natural clinical history of canine congenital subaortic stenosis, *J Vet Intern Med* 8:423, 1994.)

general surgery, severe skin disease) to reduce the risk of bacterial endocarditis. Therefore some veterinary cardiologists recommend the same precautions in dogs. The benefits of this approach are unproved.

BALLOON DILATION

Balloon dilation of SAS has been used to successfully relieve the obstruction of SAS in both children and dogs with discrete subaortic stenosis.[59-61] In humans, balloon dilation of discrete SAS only has long-term benefits in children with a thin membrane. In these patients there is usually dramatic and persistent relief of the obstruction because the procedure probably ruptures the membrane.[62] Thick and fibrous obstructing ridges, similar to the common form seen in dogs, generally only show a transient relief of the obstruction with rapid restenosis. In these cases, the lesion is probably only stretched rather than ruptured, allowing the lesion to remodel to its original form following the procedure. DeLellis et al[60] reported on balloon dilation of discrete fibrous SAS in nine dogs. Immediate follow-up showed that the peak-to-peak pressure gradient reduced by 60% or greater in 3 dogs and decreased by 25% to 49% in the remaining six dogs. Lehmkuhl and Bonagura[48] reported an average gradient reduction of 53% in 20 consecutive dogs. Long-term follow-up studies in these patients are less favorable, showing a significant return of the pressure gradient in most dogs.[63] Several dogs with very severe SAS (i.e., a pressure gradient of 200 mm Hg or greater) had a good long term outcome. Consequently, balloon valvuloplasty may be a viable option in dogs with very severe SAS but is usually not effective in dogs with lesser degrees of stenosis.

SURGERY

Surgical resection of the subaortic lesion with or without septal myectomy is the mainstay of therapy in children with discrete fibrous SAS.[64] Because of the lack of efficacy of medical therapy and balloon dilation, surgical correction has been investigated in dogs. However, the high cost, technical difficulty, lack of significant gradient reduction, and high operative mortality have made surgical options generally disappointing. Although closed valvotomy or valve dilation have been attempted, the most favorable results have been shown with direct resection of the lesion under cardiopulmonary bypass.[54,65-67] Recently Orton et al[54] and Komtebedde et al[67] have shown reasonable initial gradient reduction with open resection techniques combined with relatively low complication and mortality rates. In the study by Orton et al[54] the subvalvular ring and a portion of the interventricular septal musculature were resected. Fifteen of 17 dogs survived the procedure. Four died suddenly between 1 week and 30 months following the procedure, and the remaining eleven dogs were still alive at 1 to 48 months following surgery with no clinical signs or only minimal exercise intolerance. The mean Doppler derived pressure gradient reduced from 100 mm Hg to 29 mm Hg immediately following surgery and remained significantly decreased at 3 (37 mm Hg) and 6 months (43 mm Hg) following surgery. Komtebedde et al[67] reported successful surgical resection of the subaortic membrane only in seven dogs. No reports of pressure gradients obtained by Doppler echocardiography before or after surgery were reported in this study. All seven dogs were discharged alive and in stable condition. Six dogs were alive and in stable condition after a mean follow-up of 15.8 months. However, all but 1 of the dogs subsequently died of complications related to SAS. Most of these dogs died suddenly. One died of left congestive heart failure associated with progressive myocardial failure, and one died of congestive heart failure associated with mitral valve damage sustained during the surgery. Both of these dogs also had a persistent pressure gradient across the subaortic stenosis in the moderate-to-severe range. The one surviving dog suffers from chronic right congestive heart failure associated with constrictive pericarditis. Although open resection may be a viable treatment alternative for dogs with discrete SAS, demonstration of long-term survival in dogs undergoing this procedure will require further study. Although the results so far are impressive, most dogs that underwent this procedure were under a year of age. Even including follow-up time, most dogs were still younger than 3 years of age and many were still less than a year old at the last follow-up examination. The average age of sudden death in dogs with SAS is 14.4 months, and most dogs with severe SAS die suddenly within the first 3 years of life.[37] Therefore,

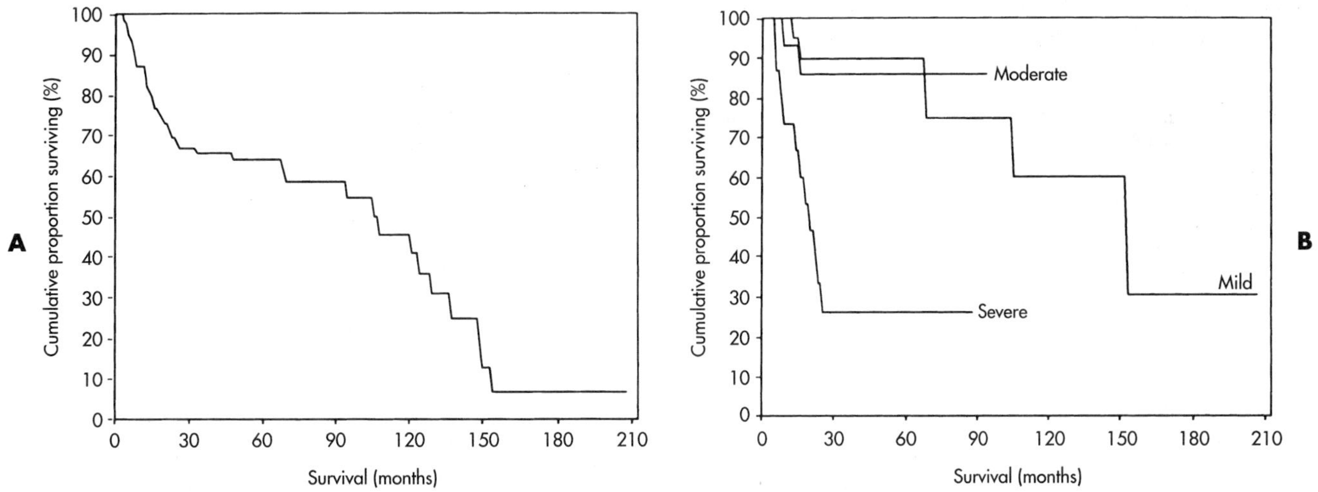

FIGURE 16-11 **A,** Survival curve of 86 dogs with untreated SAS is depicted as cumulative proportion surviving (%). Survival is from date of birth until date of death or end of study in those dogs still alive. **B,** Cumulative survival curves (%) for 50 dogs with SAS, divided into three severity groups based on left ventricular–aortic systolic pressure gradients. Mild = 15 to 35 mm Hg (*n*=20), moderate = 36 to 80 mm Hg (*n*=15), severe = greater than 80 mm Hg (*n*=15). (From Kienle RD, Thomas WP, Pion PD: The natural clinical history of canine congenital subaortic stenosis, *J Vet Intern Med* 8:423, 1994.)

based on these studies, the actual success of the open resection remains speculative. As with other surgical techniques, restenosis may limit the usefulness of this procedure and the costs are still relatively high.

REFERENCES

1. Stepien RL, Bonagura JD: Aortic stenosis: clinical findings in six cats, *J Small Anim Pract* 32:341, 1991.
2. Lui S: Supravalvular aortic stenosis with deformity of the aortic valve in a cat, *J Am Vet Med Assoc* 152:55, 1968.
3. Sisson DD, Thomas WP: Dynamic subaortic stenosis in a dog with congenital heart disease, *J Am Anim Hosp Assoc* 20:657, 1984.
4. Jones CL: Inheritable left ventricular outflow obstruction in the golden retriever, *Proc Annu ACVIM Forum,* 1989, p 851.
5. Buoscio DA, Sisson D, Zachary JF et al: Clinical and pathological characterization of an unusual form of subvalvular aortic stenosis in four golden retriever puppies, *J Am Anim Hosp Assoc* 30:100, 1994.
6. Buchanan JW: Causes and prevalence of cardiovascular diseases. In Kirk RW, Bonagura JD, eds: *Kirk's Current veterinary therapy XI,* Philadelphia, 1992, WB Saunders.
7. Patterson DF: Congenital defects of the cardiovascular system of dogs: studies in comparative cardiology, *Adv Vet Sci Comp Med* 20:1, 1976.
8. Bohn FK, Scabell G, Hanichen T: Supravalvulare Aortenstenose beim Hund, Zentralbl Vetarinarmed 14:85, 1967.
9. Bankl H: Aortic stenosis. In Bankl H, ed: *Congenital malformations of the heart and great vessels,* Baltimore, 1977, Urban & Schwartzenberg.
10. Titus JL, Edwards JE: The aortic root and valve: development, anatomy, and congenital abnormalities. In Emery RW, Arom KV, eds: *The aortic valve,* Philadelphia, 1991, Hanley & Belfus.
11. Pyle RL, Patterson DF, Chacko S: The genetics and pathology of discrete subaortic stenosis in the Newfoundland dog, *Am Heart J* 92:324, 1976.
12. Patterson DF: Two hereditary forms of ventricular outflow obstruction in the dog: pulmonary valve dysplasia, and discrete subaortic stenosis. In Nora JJ, Takao A, eds: *Congenital heart disease: causes and processes,* Mt. Kisko, NY, 1984, Futura.
13. Harpster NK, Jones CL, eds: Genes and the heart: congenital heart disease, *Proc Am Acad Vet Cardiol,* 1991 p 13.
14. Muna WF, Ferrans VJ, Pierce JE et al: Ultrastructure of the fibrous subaortic "ring" in dogs with discrete subaortic stenosis, *Lab Invest* 39:471, 1978.
15. Ferrans VJ, Muna WF, Jones M et al: Ultrastructure of the fibrous ring in patient with discrete subaortic stenosis, *Lab Invest* 39:30, 1978.
16. Muna WF, Ferrans VJ, Pierce JE et al: Discrete subaortic stenosis in Newfoundland dogs: association of infective endocarditis, *Am J Cardiol* 41:746, 1978.
17. Flickinger GL, Patterson DF: Coronary lesions associated with congenital subaortic stenosis in the dog, *J Pathol Bacteriol* 93:(1)133, 1967.
18. Pyle RL, Lowensohn HS, Khouri EM, et al: Left circumflex coronary artery hemodynamics in conscious dogs with congenital subaortic stenosis, *Circ Res* 33:34, 1973.
19. Bonagura JD, Darke PGG: Congenital heart disease. In Ettinger SJ, Feldman EC, eds: *Textbook of small animal internal medicine,* ed 4, Philadelphia, 1995, WB Saunders.
20. Oyama MA, Thomas WP: Echocardiographic predictors of congenital subaortic stenosis severity in dogs, *J Vet Intern Med* 11:140, 1997 (abstract).
21. Jones M, Picone AL, Ferrans VJ: Subaortic stenosis in Newfoundland dogs: an acquired congenital heart disease, *Circulation* 66(suppl 2):II, 1982 (abstract).
22. Nakayama T, Wakao Y, Ishikawa R et al: Progression of subaortic stenosis detected by continuous wave Doppler echocardiography in a dog, *J Vet Intern Med* 10:97, 1996.
23. Cape EG, Vanauker MD, Sigfusson G et al: Potential role of mechanical shear stress in the etiology of pediatric heart disease: septal shear stress in subaortic stenosis, *J Am Coll Cardiol* 30:247, 1997.
24. Wigle ED: Hypertrophic cardiomyopathy: a 1987 viewpoint, *Circulation* 75:311, 1987.
25. Kittleson MD, Kittleson JA, Mekhammer Y: Development and progression of inherited hypertrophic cardiomyopathy in Maine coon cats, *J Vet Intern Med* 10:165, 1996 (abstract).
26. Liu SK, Maron BJ, Tilley LP: Canine hypertrophic cardiomyopathy, *J Am Vet Med Assoc* 174:708, 1979.
27. Liu SK, Maron BJ, Tilley LP: Hypertrophic cardiomyopathy in the dog, *Am J Pathol* 94:497, 1979.
28. Thomas WP, Mathewson JW, Suter PF et al: Hypertrophic obstructive cardiomyopathy in a dog: clinical, hemodynamic, angiographic, and pathologic studies, *J Am Anim Hosp Assoc* 20:253, 1984.

29. Swindle MM, Huber AC, Kan JS et al: Mitral valve prolapse and hypertrophic cardiomyopathy in a pup, *J Am Vet Med Assoc* 184:1515, 1984.
30. Sisson D: Fixed and dynamic subvalvular aortic stenosis in dogs. In Kirk RW, Bonagura JD, eds: *Kirk's current veterinary therapy XI,* Philadelphia, 1992, WB Saunders.
31. Maron BJ, Gottdiener JS, Perry LW: Specificity of systolic anterior motion of anterior mitral leaflet for hypertrophic cardiomyopathy: prevalence in large population of patients with other cardiac diseases, *Br Heart J* 45:206, 1981.
32. Sakurai S, Tanaka H, Yoshimura H et al: Production of systolic anterior motion of the mitral valve in dogs, *Circulation* 71:805, 1985.
33. Moro E, ten Cate FJ, Leonard JJ et al: Genesis of systolic anterior motion of the mitral valve in hypertrophic cardiomyopathy: an anatomical or dynamic event? *Eur Heart J* 8:1312, 1987.
34. O'Grady MR: The incidence of aortic valve insufficiency in congenital canine aortic stenosis: a Doppler echocardiographic study, *J Vet Intern Med* 4:129, 1990 (abstract).
35. Roth L: Bacterial aortic valvular endocarditis associated with subaortic stenosis, *J Small Anim Pract* 35:169, 1994.
36. Jorgensen CR: The pathophysiology of aortic stenosis. In Emery RW, Arom KV, eds: *The aortic valve,* Philadelphia, 1991, Hanley & Belfus.
37. Kienle RD, Thomas WP, Pion PD: The natural clinical history of canine congenital subaortic stenosis, *J Vet Intern Med* 8:423, 1994.
38. Friedman WF: Congenital heart disease in infancy and childhood. In Braunwald E, ed: *Heart disease: a textbook of cardiovascular medicine,* ed 4, Philadelphia, 1992, WB Saunders.
39. Wigle ED, Adelman AG, Silver MD: Pathophysiologic considerations in muscular subaortic stenosis. In Wolstenholme GEW, O'Conner M, eds: *Hypertrophic obstructive cardiomyopathy,* London, 1971, Ciba Foundation Study Group.
40. Jiang L, Levine RA, King ME et al: An integrated mechanism for systolic anterior motion of the mitral valve in hypertrophic cardiomyopathy based on echocardiographic observations, *Am Heart J* 113:633, 1987.
41. Levine RA, Vlahakes GJ, Lefebvre X et al: Papillary muscle displacement causes systolic anterior motion of the mitral valve: experimental validation and insights into the mechanism of subaortic obstruction, *Circulation* 91:1189, 1995.
42. Klues HG, Roberts WC, Maron BJ: Anomalous insertion of papillary muscle directly into anterior mitral leaflet in hypertrophic cardiomyopathy: significance in producing left ventricular outflow obstruction, *Circulation* 84:1188, 1991.
43. Sherrid MV, Chu CK, Delia E et al: An echocardiographic study of the fluid mechanics of obstruction in hypertrophic cardiomyopathy, *J Am Coll Cardiol* 22:816, 1993.
44. Lefebvre X, Cagniot A, Yoganathan AP et al: Reproduction of systolic anterior motion of the mitral valve in a pulsatile flow model, *Circulation* 82(suppl III):III, 1990 (abstract).
45. Dinsmore RE, Sanders CA, Harthorne JW: Mitral regurgitation in idiopathic hypertrophic subaortic stenosis, *N Engl J Med* 275:1225, 1996.
46. Criley JM, Siegel RJ: Subaortic stenosis revisited: the importance of the dynamic pressure gradient, *Medicine (Baltimore)* 72:412, 1993 (comment).
47. Hoit BD, Penonen E, Dalton N et al: Doppler color flow mapping studies of jet formation and spatial orientation in obstructive hypertrophic cardiomyopathy, *Am Heart J* 117:1119, 1989.
48. Lehmkuhl LB, Bonagura JD: CVT update: canine subvalvular aortic stenosis. In Kirk RW, Bonagura JD, eds: *Kirk's current veterinary therapy XII,* Philadelphia, 1995, WB Saunders.
49. Lehmkuhl LB, Bonagura JD: Results of Holter monitoring in dogs with congenital subaortic stenosis, *Proc Annu Vet Med Forum* 1993, p 553.
50. Bonagura JD, Herring DS: Echocardiography: congenital heart disease, *Vet Clin North Am Small Anim Pract* 15:1195, 1985.
51. Wingfield WE, Boon JA, Miller CW: Echocardiographic assessment of congenital aortic stenosis in dogs, *J Am Vet Med Assoc* 183:673, 1983.
52. Feigenbaum H: *Echocardiography,* ed 4, Philadelphia, 1986, Lea and Febiger.
53. Kaplan PM: Congenital heart disease, *Prob Vet Med* 3:500, 1991.
54. Monnet E, Orton EC, Gaynor JS et al: Open resection for subvalvular aortic stenosis in dogs, *J Am Vet Med Assoc* 209:1255, 1996.
55. Moise NS: Doppler echocardiographic evaluation of congenital heart disease, *J Vet Intern Med* 3:195, 1989.
56. Moise NS: Echocardiography. In Fox PR, ed: *Canine and feline cardiology,* New York, 1988, Churchill Livingstone.
57. Lehmkuhl LB, Bonagura JD: Comparison of transducer placement sites for Doppler echocardiography in dogs with subaortic stenosis, *Am J Vet Res* 55:192, 1994.
58. Lehmkuhl LB, Bonagura JD, Stepien RL et al: Comparison of pressure gradients determined by doppler echocardiography and cardiac catheterization in dogs with subaortic stenosis, *J Vet Intern Med* 6:113, 1992 (abstract).
59. Thomas WP, Sisson DD, DeLellis LA: Technique and short term effects of balloon catheter dilation of congenital obstructive cardiac defects (pulmonic and subaortic stenosis) in dogs, *Proc Annu Vet Med Forum,* 1989, p 830.
60. DeLellis LA, Thomas WP, Pion PD: Balloon dilation of congenital subarotic stenosis in the dog, *J Vet Int Med* 7:153, 1993.
61. Lababidi Z, Weinhaus L, Stoeckle H et al: Transluminal balloon dilatation for discrete subaortic stenosis, *Am J Cardiol* 59:423, 1987.
62. Shrivastava S, Dev V, Kumar V et al: Echocardiographic determinants of outcome after percutaneous transluminal balloon dilatation of discrete subaortic stenosis, *Am Heart J* 122:1323, 1991.
63. Thomas WP, DeLellis LA, Sisson DD: Balloon dilation of congenital outflow obstruction in dogs: mid-term results, *Proc Annu Vet Med Forum,* 1990.
64. Coleman DM, Smallhorn JF, McCrindle BW et al: Postoperative follow-up of fibromuscular subaortic stenosis, *J Am Coll Cardiol* 24:1558, 1994.
65. Linn K, Orton EC: Closed transventricular dilation of discrete subvalvular aortic stenosis in dogs, *Vet Surg* 21:441, 1992.
66. Dhkarikar P, Caywood DD, Ogburn PN et al: Closed aortic valvotomy: a retrospective study in 15 dogs, *J Am Anim Hosp Assoc* 31:402, 1995.
67. Komtebedde J, Ilkiw JE, Follette DM et al: Resection of subvalvular aortic stenosis, surgical and perioperative management in seven dogs, *Vet Surg* 22:419, 1993.

CHAPTER 17

Congenital Abnormalities of the Atrioventricular Valves

Tricuspid Valve Dysplasia

Tricuspid valve dysplasia (TVD) is defined as congenital malformation of the tricuspid valve leaflets, chordae tendineae, or papillary muscles that usually results in tricuspid regurgitation. It is an uncommon congenital heart disease, seen in both dogs and cats. A specific type of congenital tricuspid valve malformation seen in humans, in which the basal attachments of the tricuspid valve are displaced ventrally into the right ventricle, is called *Ebstein's anomaly.* This anomaly is rare in dogs and not reported in cats.

PATHOLOGY

TVD is not just one type of lesion. Rather, numerous abnormalities can occur. These abnormalities almost always result in tricuspid valve regurgitation. Tricuspid stenosis occurs rarely. Described lesions in humans include focal or diffuse thickening of the valve leaflets, underdevelopment of chordae tendineae and papillary muscles, incomplete separation of valve components from the ventricular wall, and focal agenesis of valvular tissue.[1] In dogs and cats, chordae tendineae are commonly absent or very short.[2] Consequently, the papillary muscles often attach directly to the valve leaflets. The leaflets are often irregularly thickened and may contain fenestrations. Leaflets, especially the septal leaflet, may be directly adhered to the ventricular wall (Color Plate 58).

Other congenital heart defects may be present. These may include mitral valve dysplasia, septal defects, subaortic stenosis, and pulmonic stenosis.

PREVALENCE

TVD has been reported in numerous dog breeds, including old English sheepdogs, great Danes, German shepherds, and Irish setters.[2] We see a preponderance of Labrador retrievers in our clinic with this malformation. We identified 62 dogs with TVD between August 1, 1986, and August 1, 1996. Of these, 16 were Labrador retrievers. The majority of the dogs with this abnormality were purebred. Only eight mixed-breed dogs were identified. The vast majority of the dogs were large-breed dogs (greater than 20 kg). In the same period we diagnosed TVD in 23 cats. The majority of these were mixed-breed cats.[19]

CLINICAL FINDINGS

TVD in dogs and cats may initially be discovered because a heart murmur is identified. The heart murmur is systolic and generally loudest over the right apex. In many cases, however, the first clue that the patient has TVD is the discovery of ascites. At the time ascites is discovered, all dogs and most cats have a heart murmur. Some cats, however, apparently have a tricuspid orifice so large that regurgitant flow is laminar and no heart murmur is present. Most dogs and cats are young (less than 2 years of age) at presentation. We have identified TVD in cats as old as 12 years of age and dogs as old as 5 years of age.

PATHOPHYSIOLOGY

The malformed tricuspid valve in TVD allows blood to leak from the right ventricle into the right atrium during systole. The increase in systolic flow into the right atrium increases right atrial volume. The right atrium expands to accommodate this increased volume. The right ventricle grows larger (volume overload hypertrophy) to accommodate the increased venous return (normal venous return plus the return of the blood ejected into the right atrium in systole) in diastole. The increased right ventricular diastolic volume allows the right ventricle to eject a larger stroke volume, to compensate for the volume lost into the right atrium and maintain a normal forward (into the pulmonary artery) stroke volume. As the right heart grows larger, the tricuspid valve annulus increases in size. Because the tricuspid valve cannot grow to maintain coaptation, the orifice in the tricuspid valve becomes larger. The cycle of increasing right ventricular size leading to worsening tricuspid regurgitation leading to further increases in right ventricular size becomes a cycle of worsening hemodynamics that ultimately culminates in massive regurgitation that overwhelms the cardiovascular system's compensatory mechanisms. Congestive right heart failure is the end result. Right heart failure results from massive regurgitation into the right atrium resulting in increased right atrial pressure and decreased forward flow into the pulmonary vasculature. The decrease in pulmonary flow results in a decrease in venous return to the left heart. As a consequence, the left heart becomes underloaded and probably atrophies in response. The potential net result is a decrease in systemic blood flow.

Animals with severe TVD develop right heart failure. The most common manifestation of right heart failure is ascites. TVD is the most common cause of pure right heart failure leading to ascites in cats. Along with ascites, hepatomegaly and jugular vein distension may be identified. Pleural effusion may be identified on occasion but is rarely severe.

DIAGNOSTIC TESTS

Thoracic radiography. Thoracic radiographs of dogs and cats with severe TVD reveal severe cardiomegaly primarily as a result of massive right atrial enlargement (Figure 17-1). The enlarged right

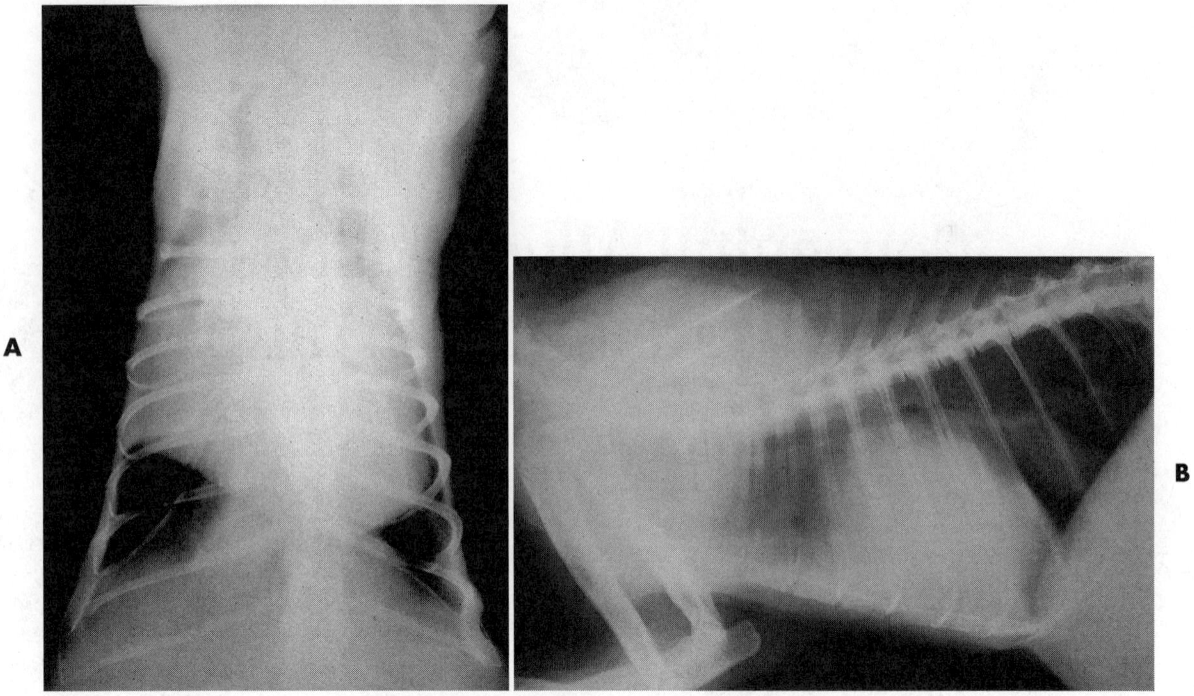

FIGURE 17-1 Thoracic radiographs from a 12-year-old neutered male cat with severe tricuspid valve dysplasia. **A,** The severe right atrial enlargement can be appreciated. The distended caudal vena cava can also be appreciated. **B,** The cardiac silhouette is grossly enlarged. The caudal vena cava is markedly distended.

atrium enlarges the entire right side of the cardiac silhouette, often pushing the left heart further to the left (Figure 17-2). The net result can be an impression of generalized cardiomegaly. More commonly, one can distinguish the markedly enlarged right atrium as a separate structure. Massive right atrial enlargement in a young animal with a right apical systolic heart murmur is pathognomonic for severe tricuspid regurgitation, usually as a result of TVD. Even in older animals, massive right atrial enlargement should suggest TVD, because acquired tricuspid regurgitation rarely produces such pronounced right atrial enlargement. Animals that present in right heart failure commonly have a massively enlarged caudal vena cava that can be identified on both views.

Electrocardiography. The electrocardiogram is commonly abnormal in dogs and cats with severe TVD. The most common finding is right axis-deviation as a result of deep *S* waves in leads I, II, III, and aV_F.[2] Tall *P* waves, indicative of right atrial enlargement, may also be present. However, this finding is not a sensitive means of detecting right atrial enlargement, and absence of this finding does not rule out right atrial enlargement in this or any other disease. Massive right atrial enlargement may lead to supraventricular tachyarrhythmias, most commonly atrial fibrillation.

Echocardiography. The most striking finding on the echocardiogram is the markedly enlarged right atrium (Figure 17-3). The right atrial size may be larger than the rest of the heart. A right ventricular volume overload is also present but never to the same degree as the right atrial volume overload. The left heart is often diminutive, with both the end-diastolic and end-systolic diameters smaller than normal. The left heart can be so small that it is difficult to identify during an examination. The valve leaflets are commonly abnormal. The septal leaflet may appear to be adhered to the interventricular septum and may have little movement. The mural leaflet may appear to be very large. The papillary muscles may be adherent to this leaflet or may be malpositioned. A large turbulent jet is always present during systole in the right atrium on color flow Doppler in dogs (Color Plate 59). In some cats, laminar regurgitant flow may be identified. Laminar regurgitant flow occurs when the tricuspid valve orifice is very large in systole, probably similar in size to the pulmonic valve orifice, resulting in very little resistance to blood flow. In dogs and cats with uncomplicated TVD, the velocity of the regurgitant jet, measured with continuous-wave Doppler, is in the 1.5- to 3-m/sec range.

Contrast echocardiography using microbubbles can be performed in dogs and cats with TVD. When the right heart is examined following injection of the saline, the bubbles remain in the right heart for a prolonged period. In severe tricuspid regurgitation, blood is pushed all the way back into the hepatic circulation in systole. Consequently, following a saline injection into a cephalic or jugular vein, bubbles can often be visualized in the hepatic veins. Retrograde hepatic vein flow can also be documented with spectral Doppler echocardiography.

TREATMENT

Medical therapy. Medical therapy is palliative and aimed at improving quality of life by reducing the amount of ascites. Standard therapy consists of administering furosemide and an angiotensin converting enzyme inhibitor. If the animal is uncomfortable at the first examination, the ascitic fluid is removed. Medical therapy is commonly effective at prolonging the time until the abdomen is severely distended again but is commonly ineffective at completely stopping fluid accumulation. Consequently, periodic abdominocentesis and fluid removal is often required. Periodic removal of ascitic fluid results in removal of large quantities of protein each time the procedure is repeated. However, in our experience this rarely results in clinically significant sequelae. Serum albumin concentration may decrease in these cases but rarely to less than 2 g/dL. Consequently, we never discourage an owner from returning for repeated

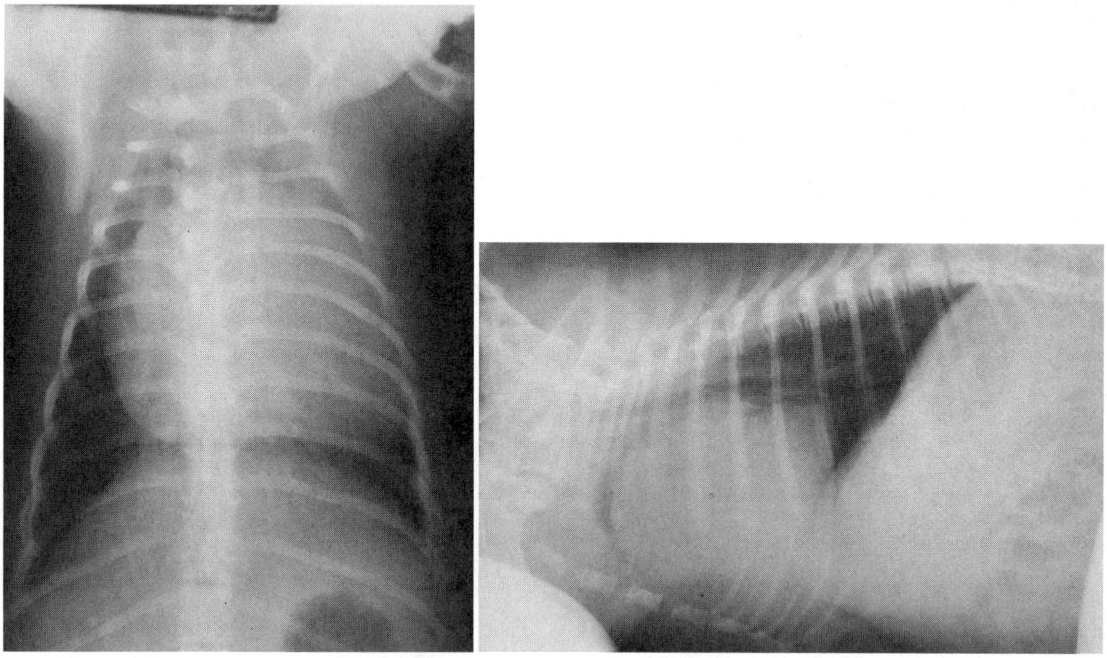

FIGURE 17-2 Thoracic radiographs from a 5-month-old female Shi Tzu with severe tricuspid valve dysplasia. **A,** The cardiac silhouette is grossly enlarged. The majority of this enlargement is due to right atrial enlargement. The border of the right atrium begins between 5 o'clock and 6 o'clock and extends around to 12 o'clock. The left heart is pushed to the left by the massively enlarged right heart. **B,** The heart is grossly enlarged. The cranial border of the heart bulges cranially because of the grossly enlarged right atrium.

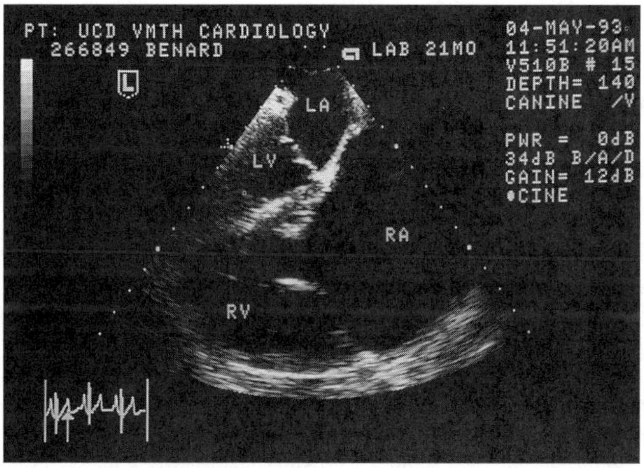

FIGURE 17-3 Two-dimensional transesophageal echocardiogram from a 21-month-old Labrador retriever with severe tricuspid valve dysplasia. A papillary muscle attaches directly to the tricuspid valve. The right atrium *(RA)* is massively enlarged. The right ventricular chamber *(RV)* is volume overloaded but not to the same degree as the right atrium. The left ventricular chamber *(LV)* and the left atrium *(LA)* are very small because of decreased right heart forward flow.

procedures. Some owners can even learn to do the procedure themselves. As opposed to dogs with left heart failure, dogs with right heart failure commonly feel good and so have a good quality of life between procedures. Ultimately, however, the interval becomes too short for most owners to tolerate, and euthanasia becomes a viable option.

Surgical therapy. Surgical therapy is usually a poor option, in our experience. We observed the clinical courses of three dogs following the replacement of the tricuspid valve with a bioprosthetic valve. In each case, the prosthetic valve was constructed from a stent and the dog's own pericardium. In each case, extensive thrombosis and fibrosis occurred shortly after surgery. One dog survived with moderate tricuspid stenosis, one dog died within 24 hours of surgery, and the last dog died 1 week following surgery, with severe tricuspid stenosis and possible pulmonary thromboembolism (Color Plate 60).

Mitral Valve Dysplasia

For this discussion, mitral valve dysplasia (MVD) is defined as an abnormally formed mitral valve that results in regurgitation. Abnormally formed valves usually result in mitral regurgitation, although mitral stenosis occasionally may be seen with the regurgitation. Mitral stenosis is considered as a separate entity below.

PATHOLOGY

Multiple abnormalities in the mitral valve apparatus have been described in dogs and cats with MVD. They include short and thick leaflets, cleft leaflets, short and stout chordae tendineae, long and thin chordae tendineae, upward malposition of atrophied (flat and small) or hypertrophied papillary muscles, leaflets adhered to the septum, and insertion of a papillary muscle directly onto one or both leaflets (Color Plate 61).[3-5] These lesions result in the valve leaflets leaking directly, the leaflets being tethered so that they cannot close properly, or the leaflets having inadequate support so that they do not coapt properly. The mitral valve annulus diameter and left atrial size are increased in size secondary to the primary mitral valve apparatus lesions. Diffuse endocardial fibrosis of the left atrium is a common finding in dogs.[3] Tricuspid valve dysplasia is occasionally identified in dogs with MVD.[3]

PREVALENCE

MVD occurred in nine of 325 dogs with congenital heart disease in one study.[6] In our hospital, we identified this abnormality in 58 dogs between August 1, 1986, and August 1, 1996. In dogs, MVD has been reported to occur most commonly in large dogs, such as great Danes and German shepherds.[3] In our population, many breeds were represented. Most of the abnormality was observed in purebred dogs, with only 15 mixed-breed dogs identified. The rottweiler was the most common breed.[7] We diagnosed MVD in only two German shepherds and no great Danes. The majority of our cases were large-breed dogs. MVD is reportedly one of the most common congenital cardiac abnormalities recognized in cats.[4,7] Within the same period, we diagnosed mitral valve dysplasia in only 11 cats—two Persians, one Burmese, and eight mixed-breed cats. MVD is rare in children.[8-10]

PATHOPHYSIOLOGY

The pathophysiology of mitral regurgitation is identical to the pathophysiology of mitral regurgitation secondary to myxomatous degeneration of the mitral valve (see Chapter 19). In our experience, one difference is that myocardial failure is a common sequel to severe mitral regurgitation in large dogs and in cats. At times, this can make the disease difficult to distinguish from dilated cardiomyopathy in dogs and from so-called intermediate cardiomyopathy in cats. We use three rules of thumb to make this distinction. First, having evidence of a large mitral regurgitant jet on color flow Doppler is unusual for a dog or cat with dilated cardiomyopathy. Instead, the jet is usually very small in dog breeds that typically develop dilated cardiomyopathy. Consequently, whenever a large jet is identified in a dog or cat with evidence of myocardial failure, the diagnosis of dilated cardiomyopathy should be strongly questioned. In the same vein, most dogs with dilated cardiomyopathy have a soft left apical heart murmur that occurs because of the small leak present in their mitral valve. If a dog has a moderate-to-loud murmur, the diagnosis of dilated cardiomyopathy should be questioned until other abnormalities have been ruled out. Second, developing heart failure with dilated cardiomyopathy is extremely unusual for a dog or cat until the shortening fraction is less than 15%. Consequently, if a dog or cat is presented in heart failure but has a shortening fraction greater than 15% the diagnosis of dilated cardiomyopathy should be questioned and the patient should be examined carefully for the presence of other lesions that can result in secondary myocardial failure. Severe mitral regurgitation in large dogs and in cats is the most common abnormality that can result in secondary myocardial failure. A left ventricle that has a larger-than-normal end-diastolic diameter and a shortening fraction greater than 15% usually has a larger-than-normal stroke volume. A dog with dilated cardiomyopathy has no reason for or no means of ejecting a larger-than-normal stroke volume. A dog with mitral regurgitation must generate a larger-than-normal stroke volume to compensate for the volume of blood that is pumped backward into the left atrium. As an example, it is not unusual for a large dog (25 to 30 kg) with dilated cardiomyopathy to present with a left ventricular end-diastolic diameter of 6 cm and an end-systolic diameter of 5.5 cm (shortening fraction = 8%). To calculate approximate end-diastolic and end-systolic volumes we can cube the end-diastolic diameter and end-systolic diameter and divide them by 1.5. This gives an end-diastolic volume of 144 mL and an end-systolic volume of 111 mL, meaning the total stroke volume of the left ventricle is 33 mL in this dog, which is a normal stroke volume. If this dog came in with an end-diastolic diameter of 6.0 cm and an end-systolic diameter of 4.8 cm, its shortening fraction would be 20%. The fact that the end-systolic diameter is greatly increased over normal is diagnostic of myocardial failure. This plus the lower-than-normal shortening fraction might suggest a diagnosis of dilated cardiomyopathy. However, if this dog's stroke volume is calculated in the same manner as before, it is approximately 70 mL. This is approximately twice normal and is diagnostic of a left ventricle that is compensating for a leak (regurgitation) or a shunt (e.g., a patent ductus arteriosus). Third, dogs and cats with myocardial failure secondary to primary mitral valve disease leading to severe regurgitation often develop severe myocardial failure of the left ventricular free wall; whereas the interventricular septal motion on an echocardiogram is usually normal or hyperdynamic. Although no or little free wall motion with normal to slightly reduced interventricular septal motion can be seen occasionally with primary myocardial failure (dilated cardiomyopathy), it is much more common to observe it in a patient with severe mitral regurgitation. In summary, a patient with heart failure that has a grade 3/6 left apical systolic heart murmur with a large jet of mitral regurgitation on color flow Doppler and a shortening fraction of 23% is much more likely to have primary mitral regurgitation than it is to have dilated cardiomyopathy. If the patient does have dilated cardiomyopathy in this situation it must have a combination of dilated cardiomyopathy (primary myocardial failure) and primary mitral regurgitation. Although this can occur, we believe that it is highly unusual. Cats with primary mitral regurgitation are commonly diagnosed as having intermediate or restrictive cardiomyopathy. These cats' left ventricles often are not markedly enlarged and do have evidence of myocardial failure. They may be somewhat misshapen. The left atrium is commonly larger than the left ventricle, and there may be right heart enlargement. Careful assessment of the mitral valve apparatus may identify the mitral valve abnormality.

DIAGNOSTIC TESTS

Radiography. The extent of the changes noted on thoracic radiographs and an echocardiogram depends on the severity of the mitral valve lesion. Cats with mild disease have only mild cardiac enlargement and may remain compensated for life.[11] Dogs and cats with severe disease usually present in the first year of life with clinical signs referable to heart failure.[3] However, heart failure may not develop until early adulthood in some dogs and cats. Animals with severe disease have severe left atrial enlargement and moderate-to-severe left ventricular enlargement on thoracic radiographs and an echocardiogram.

Electrocardiography. Prolonged *P* waves and a tall *R* wave in lead II may be seen on an ECG.[3] Cats are most commonly in sinus rhythm or have a sinus tachycardia. Supraventricular and ventricular premature beats may be observed. Sinus tachycardia, supraventricular premature contractions, supraventricular tachycardia, and atrial fibrillation are commonly observed in dogs with MVD. Ventricular premature contractions are less commonly observed.

Echocardiography

On echocardiography, the left ventricular enlargement is characterized by an increase in end-diastolic diameter and normal left ventricular wall thicknesses. The left atrium is larger than normal and is larger than the left ventricle (Figure 17-4). The left ventricular shortening fraction ranges from 15% to 45%, but in most large dogs is in the 20% to 40% range (Figure 17-5). As with acquired mitral valve disease, a shortening fraction in the normal range generally indicates that the end-sysolic diameter is increased and therefore myocardial failure is present. If the settings are correct and a careful and high-quality examination is performed, a large turbulent jet that reaches to the dorsal wall of the left atrium is identified using color flow Doppler in patients with severe regurgitation (Color Plate 62). Specific abnormalities in the mitral valve leaflets and chordae

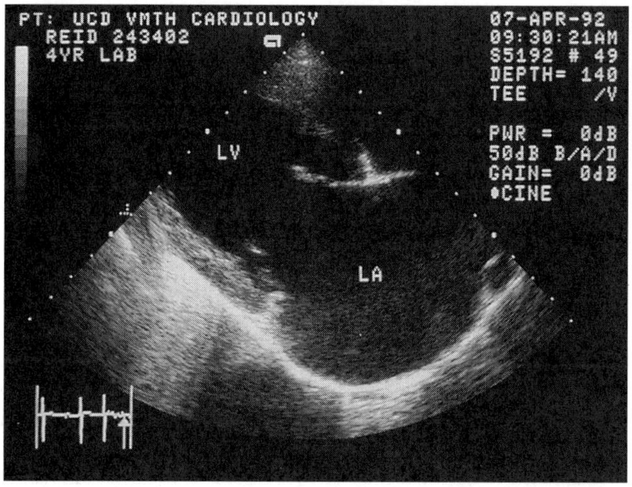

FIGURE 17-4 Two-dimensional echocardiogram from a 4-year-old Labrador retriever with severe mitral valve dysplasia. The left atrium *(LA)* is markedly enlarged. The left ventricular chamber *(LV)* is also enlarged but not to the same degree as the left atrium. This dog presented in atrial fibrillation and was in left heart failure.

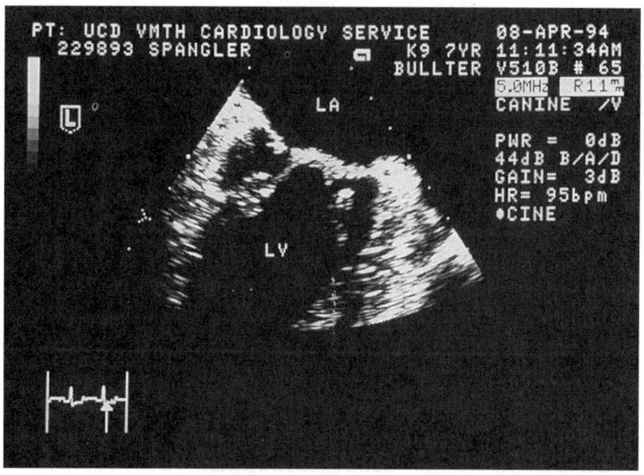

FIGURE 17-6 Transesophageal echocardiogram of the mitral valve from a 7-year-old bull terrier with mitral valve dysplasia. The papillary muscles are displaced dorsally. The chordae tendineae are short.

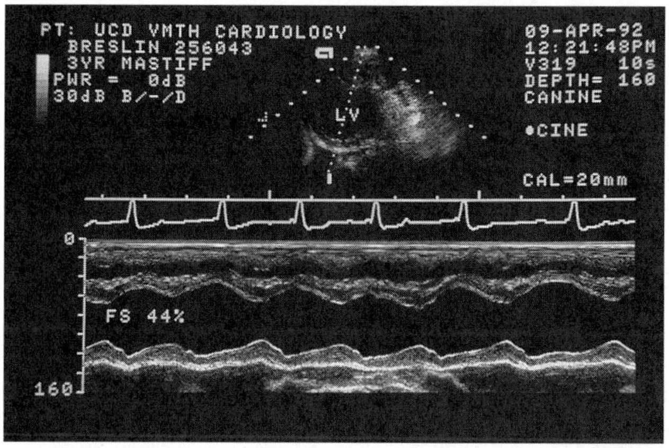

FIGURE 17-5 M-mode echocardiogram from a 3-year-old bull mastiff with severe mitral valve dysplasia and mild tricuspid valve dysplasia. The dog weighed 62 kg. The left ventricular chamber is markedly enlarged at 78 mm (normal = approximately 50 to 55 mm). The end-systolic diameter is approximately 44 mm (normal = 30 to 35 mm). The shortening fraction is 44%. The increased end-systolic diameter indicates that myocardial failure is present. This is consistent with the normal shortening fraction in the face of severe mitral regurgitation. This dog eventually developed right heart failure secondary to mild tricuspid dysplasia and moderate pulmonary hypertension.

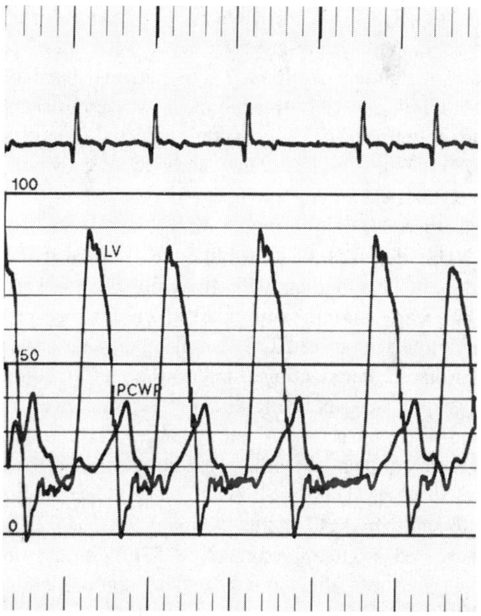

FIGURE 17-7 Simultaneously recorded pulmonary capillary wedge pressure (PCWP) and left ventricular *(LV)* pressure in a 4-year-old German shepherd with severe mitral valve dysplasia and atrial fibrillation. The diastolic pulmonary capillary and left ventricular pressures are identical and increased to approximately 17 mm Hg. In systole the *v* wave on the PCWP tracing increases severely to approximately 40 mm Hg. The resultant mean pulmonary capillary pressure in this dog was 28 mm Hg, which produced pulmonary edema.

tendineae may be identified in some dogs and cats, although this may be difficult (Figure 17-6). The right heart may also be enlarged. This is most commonly due to coexistent tricuspid valve dysplasia. Occasionally, it can be due to moderate-to-severe pulmonary hypertension that occurs secondary to increased pulmonary venous and capillary pressures. This is a rare occurrence in small dogs, is occasionally observed in large dogs, and appears to be more frequent in cats.

Cardiac catheterization. Cardiac catheterization is rarely performed in dogs or cats with MVD. If it is done, mitral regurgitation can be confirmed by injecting a radiopaque contrast agent into the left ventricle and noting its appearance in the left atrium.[12] In dogs in left heart failure, the left ventricular end-diastolic pressure is increased. If a catheter can be passed into the left atrium, the left atrial pressure will be increased, especially in systole, when an exaggerated *v* wave can be seen. If the left atrium cannot be catheterized, a Swan-Ganz catheter can be used to record the pulmonary capillary wedge pressure, to identify the same abnormalities seen in a left atrial pressure recording (Figure 17-7).

CLINICAL FINDINGS

Dogs and cats with MVD are most commonly presented for respiratory abnormalities that occur secondary to left heart failure. Right heart failure may also be present and is most common when tricuspid valve dysplasia is also present. The long-term prognosis is poor to grave in animals with severe disease. However, the short-term prognosis may be good with appropriate therapy. Some dogs with this disease die suddenly.[3]

TREATMENT

Medical therapy. Treatment for heart failure is standard and usually includes the administration of furosemide and an angiotensin converting enzyme (ACE) inhibitor. Digoxin is often indicated to control supraventricular arrhythmias. Digoxin may also be used in an attempt to improve myocardial function, normalize baroreceptor function, and produce additional diuresis. In dogs or cats that are refractory to standard therapy, hydralazine may be used in addition to the aforementioned drugs. If hydralazine is administered with an ACE inhibitor, it must be used cautiously and blood pressure must be monitored during titration (see Chapter 10). Alternatively, a thiazide diuretic can be administered with furosemide to promote further diuresis. Nitrates may also be beneficial.

Surgical therapy. Surgical treatment of MVD would be ideal in some canine patients. However, many dogs with severe MVD have myocardial failure that is too severe to tolerate mitral valve replacement or reconstruction. Humans with severe mitral regurgitation also develop moderate-to-severe myocardial failure secondary to a prolonged volume overload. Those patients that have severe myocardial failure generally tolerate mitral valve replacement very poorly and commonly die postoperatively.[13,14] Usually, an end-systolic volume index (end-systolic volume divided by body surface area) greater than 90 mL/m^2 predicts a poor outcome.[13]

Surgical therapy of presumed MVD has been reported in one dog.[15] This dog was a 3-year-old Saint Bernard that presented in left and right heart failure with atrial fibrillation. The dog had a grade 3/6 heart murmur with marked cardiomegaly and low-amplitude complexes on the ECG. Mitral regurgitation was demonstrated at cardiac catheterization. Surgery was performed in 1975, so echocardiography was not available. Attempts to convert the dog to sinus rhythm were unsuccessful before surgery. A mitral valve ball prosthesis was implanted during cardiopulmonary bypass and open-heart surgery. The dog recovered and was successfully converted to sinus rhythm 1 month after surgery. The forward stroke volume increased from approximately 25 mL before surgery to approximately 40 mL after surgery and to approximately 60 mL after cardioversion. The heart size decreased dramatically by 1 month after surgery. The dog did well for 15 months after surgery and was then euthanized because the owner no longer wanted to care for him. The prosthetic valve appeared to be functioning normally at postmortem examination. This dog was not treated with anticoagulants postoperatively and apparently did not develop thrombi associated with the prosthetic valve. In our experience this is unusual. Starr,[16] one of the original inventors of prosthetic valves, also considers this unusual. According to Starr, prototypes of prosthetic valves were developed by Edwards in the 1950s; Starr then placed the valves in dogs to test their feasibility. Each time the researchers tried a new type of valve, the dogs died of thromboembolic complications, despite anticoagulant therapy. This continued for several years. Finally, the researchers did identify one valve type that did not produce thrombi in several dogs. They immediately decided to try placing a prosthetic valve in a human, but for unknown reasons decided to use an earlier prototype. They had no problems with thrombosis in their human patients and never again attempted to place the valves in dogs.[17] They concluded that dogs produced thrombi much more avidly than did humans.

The preferable means of surgically treating diseased mitral valves is to repair them. Because of the thrombotic complications in dogs, this would seem to be the procedure of choice in this species. Besides this advantage, mitral valve repair with conservation of the chordal apparatus preserves left ventricular function in humans.[18] Unfortunately, mitral valve repair requires expertise that no veterinary surgeon currently possesses. The repair techniques used are unique for each patient, so the surgeon must have extensive experience to produce a successful outcome. Techniques used include chordal shortening, attachment of ruptured chordae to intact chordae, leaflet resection to exclude a leaflet unsupported by ruptured chordae, resection of redundant scallops of the mural leaflet, and translocation of chordae tendineae from the mural to the septal leaflet.[19] An incomplete or complete plastic ring is also sewn around the mitral valve annulus to decrease the size of the annulus in almost all cases. Mitral valve repair has been described in one dog from Japan, using deep whole-body hypothermia.[20] This dog had chronic myxomatous degeneration of the mitral valve rather than MVD. This dog only had mild mitral regurgitation but was subjected to surgery anyway. An annuloplasty ring was placed, and the septal leaflet of the mitral valve was plicated because the chordae tendineae to that leaflet were lengthened. The dog recovered and had no heart murmur postoperatively (see Chapter 19).

Mitral Valve Stenosis

Mitral valve stenosis is defined as a narrowed mitral valve orifice as a result of an abnormal mitral valve. The increased resistance to blood flow results in a pressure gradient across the mitral valve and an increase in left atrial pressure.

PREVALENCE

Mitral stenosis is a rare cardiac abnormality in dogs and cats. From others' and our experience, it appears that this abnormality is diagnosed in approximately 1 dog per year in a busy referral university hospital.[21] We diagnosed mitral stenosis in 12 dogs between August 1, 1986, and August 1, 1996. When mitral stenosis is identified in young dogs, it is often diagnosed in conjunction with another cardiac abnormality, most commonly subaortic stenosis in one series of cases.[21] Three (two Newfoundlands) of our 12 cases had subaortic stenosis in conjunction with mitral stenosis. We have also seen it in conjunction with pulmonic stenosis and with mitral dysplasia leading to mitral regurgitation. However, mitral stenosis can be diagnosed in younger and older dogs with no coexisting abnormalities. In older dogs, it is often impossible to determine if the abnormality is congenital or acquired. Acquired mitral stenosis in humans is almost always due to rheumatic fever.[22] Rheumatic fever does not exist in the dog or cat, and so postulating an etiology for acquired mitral stenosis in dogs and cats is diffficult. Of the 17 cases of dogs with mitral stenosis in the literature, five were diagnosed in bull terriers.[21,23] In four of these dogs, mitral stenosis was the only lesion present. The other dog also had subaortic stenosis. Postmortem examination of one of these dogs revealed MVD, with short, thickened, and fused chordae tendineae that inserted into the mitral valves behind the margins.[23] The papillary muscles were abnormal, being shifted upward and hypertrophied. This dog was 8 years old when it presented in atrial fibrillation. The one bull terrier that we have seen with mitral stenosis also had subaortic stenosis. Two of the cats reported with mitral stenosis also had evidence of MVD when examined echocardiographically.[24] These

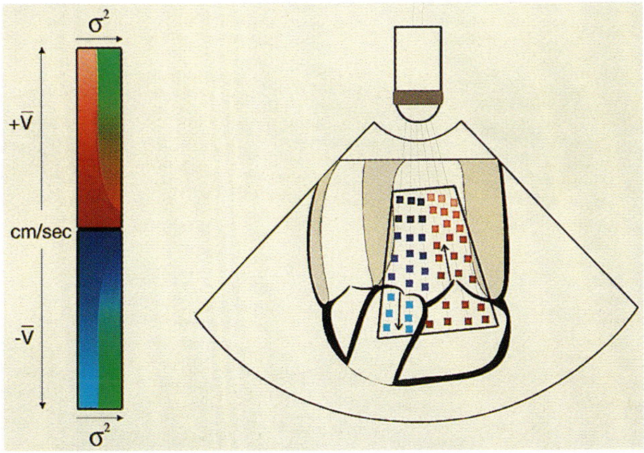

COLOR PLATE 29 Diagram of multiple Doppler sampling gates and color coding used to create a color display of blood flow velocity within a two-dimensional echocardiographic image. The color bar at the left indicates that increasingly lighter shades of red are applied to flow toward the transducer and increasingly lighter shades of blue are applied to flow away from the transducer. Variance is depicted by addition of green in this example. (See text for details.) (From Kienle RD, Thomas WP: Echocardiography. In Nyland T, Mattoon J, eds: *Textbook of veterinary ultrasound,* Philadelphia, 1995, WB Saunders.)

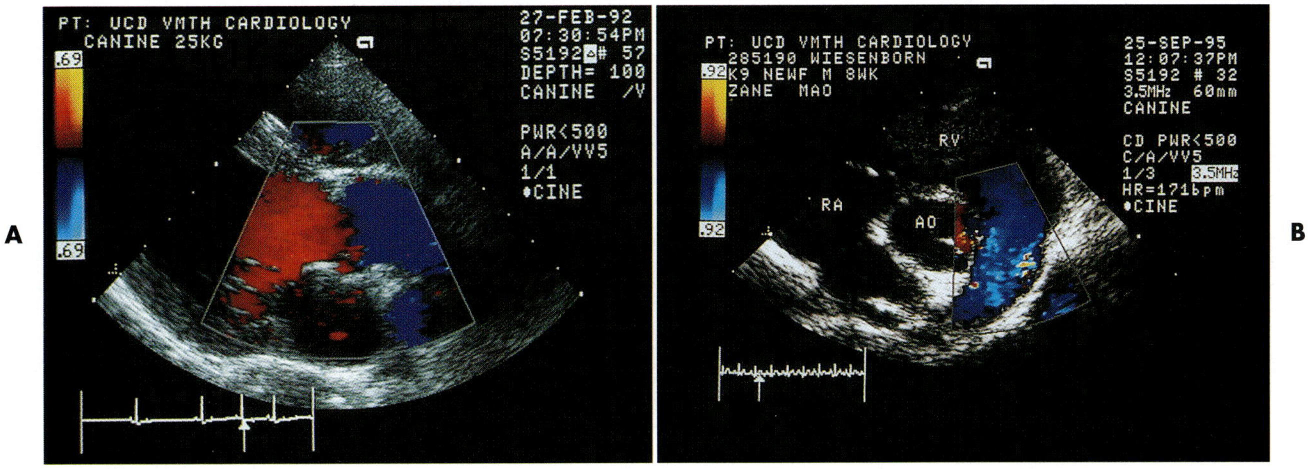

COLOR PLATE 30 Examples of two-dimensional color flow Doppler echocardiographic images in the dog. The color bar at the left codes flow toward the transducer from red to light orange, flow away from the transducer as darker to lighter shades of blue, and increased variance by addition of yellow or white, respectively. **A,** Normal left ventricular outflow from the right parasternal long-axis view. The blood flow is laminar, as indicated by the dark homogeneous colors. The dark red color in the left ventricle indicates flow coming slightly toward the transducer, and the dark blue flow in the aorta indicates flow slightly away from the transducer. **B,** Normal right ventricular outflow tract and main pulmonary artery flow. There are slightly higher velocities (indicated by lighter shades of blue) in the central portion of the stream. *RV,* Right ventricle; *RA,* right atrium; *AO,* aorta.

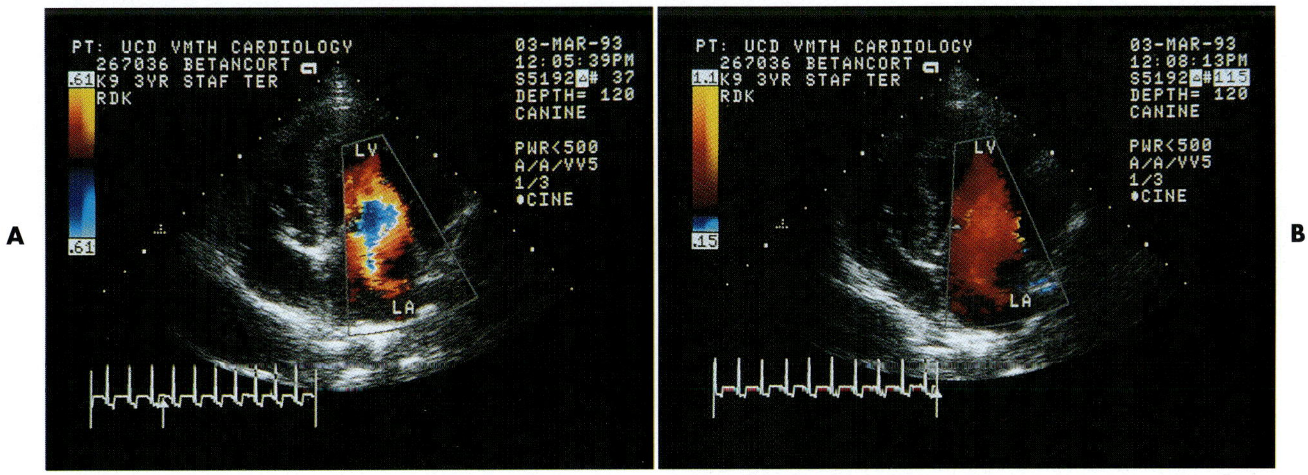

COLOR PLATE 31 Examples of color flow Doppler images depicting aliasing and turbulence. **A,** Normal left ventricular inflow with aliasing. The color Doppler appears as multiple layers of varying colors where flow velocity exceeds the Nyquist limit (see text for details). *LA,* Left atrium; *LV,* left ventricle. **B,** Same dog and view as in **A.** The velocity scale has been shifted to allow higher velocities to be measured toward the transducer (see color map to the left of the image); the color Doppler now displays a homogeneous red color indicating laminar flow toward the transducer. *LA,* Left atrium; *LV,* left ventricle.

Continued

C

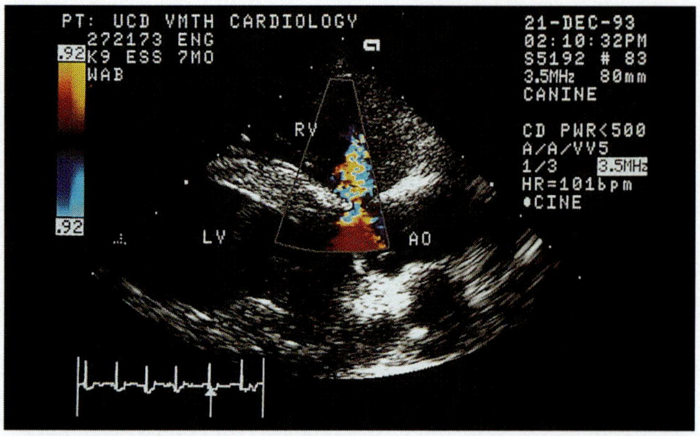

COLOR PLATE 31, cont'd **C,** Color flow Doppler image from a dog with a ventricular septal defect. The color jet in the right ventricle demonstrates turbulent flow, indicated by the random mixture (mosaic) of light yellow, orange, and blue colors. Note the laminar flow toward the defect beneath the aorta *(AO)*. *LV,* Left ventricle; *RV,* right ventricle.

A

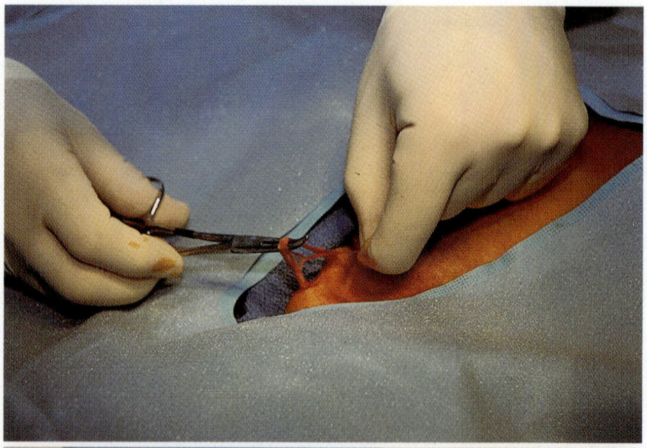

B

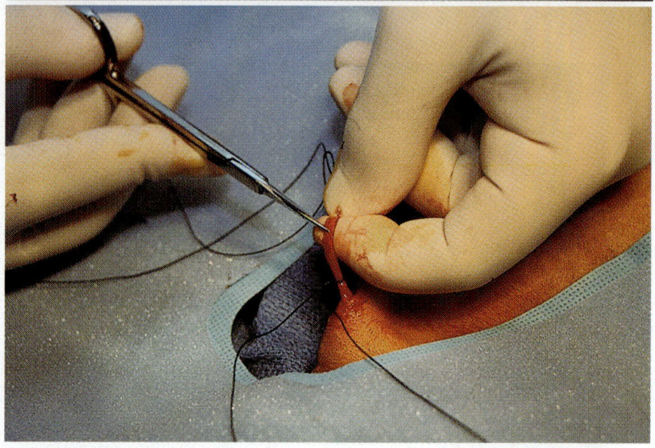

COLOR PLATE 32 Vascular cutdown of the jugular vein. The vessel is located by digital palpation. A ½- to 1-inch incision is made over the jugular vein, taking care to avoid laceration of the vein. **A,** The external jugular vein is easily exteriorized using blunt dissection. The fat and connective tissue adhered to the vein is carefully cleaned, and the vessel is brought out through the skin incision. **B,** The vein is maintained in an exterior position and hemostasis provided by securing it with a rubber band, umbilical tape, or nonabrasive suture material both proximal and distal to the intended venotomy site. A small venotomy is made using vascular scissors.

A

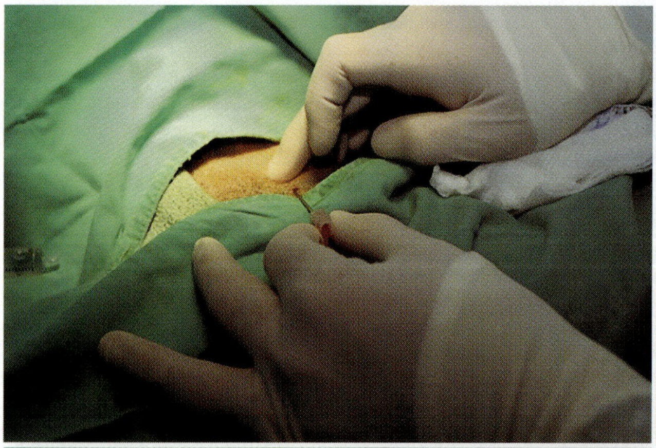

B

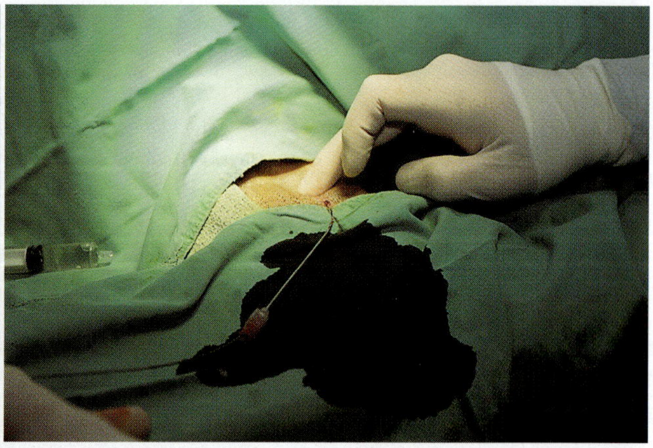

C

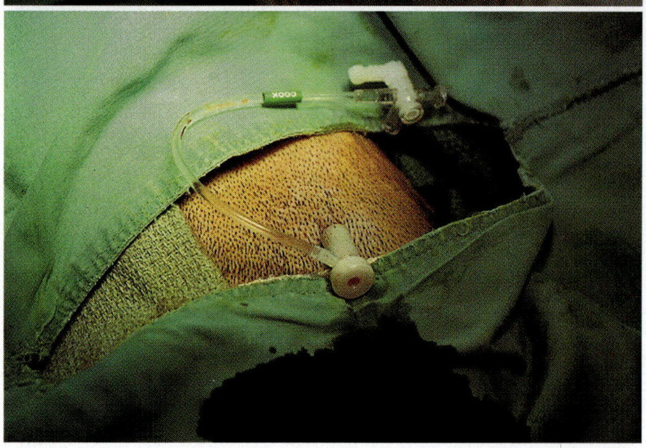

COLOR PLATE 33 Percutaneous access into the femoral artery. The area around the vessel to be accessed is clipped, scrubbed, and draped, and the vessel is located by means of digital palpation. A small puncture incision is made with a no. 11 scalpel to facilitate catheter or sheath passage through the skin. **A,** A vascular cannula (with stylet) or an 18- gauge vascular needle is inserted into the vessel using digital palpation as a guide. **B,** A flexible guidewire is inserted through the cannula or needle into the vessel. The needle or cannula is then removed, leaving the wire in place. An introducer sheath is inserted over the guidewire and gently guided into the vessel. **C,** The dilator and guidewire are removed, leaving the introducer sheath in the vessel.

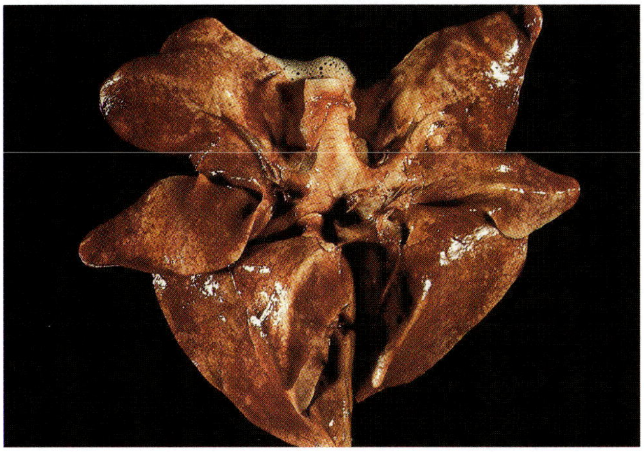

COLOR PLATE 34 Lungs from a beagle with left heart failure. There is marked pulmonary edema. Edema fluid is flowing from the trachea.

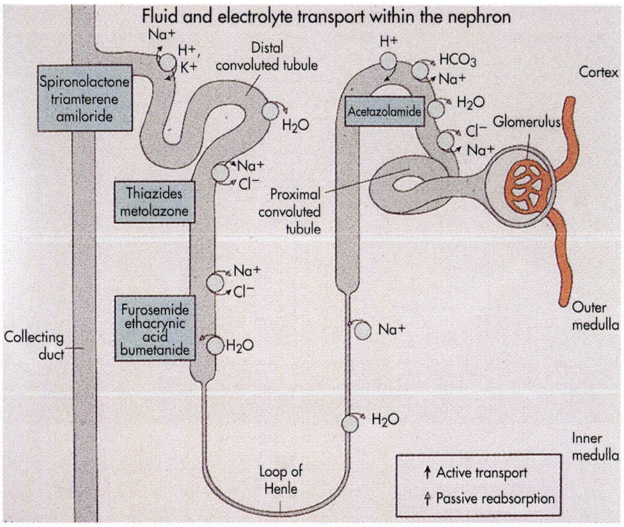

COLOR PLATE 35 Schematic drawing of a nephron, depicting fluid and electrolyte transport and the sites of action of diuretics. (From Willerson JT: *Treatment of heart diseases,* 1992, New York, Gower Medical.)

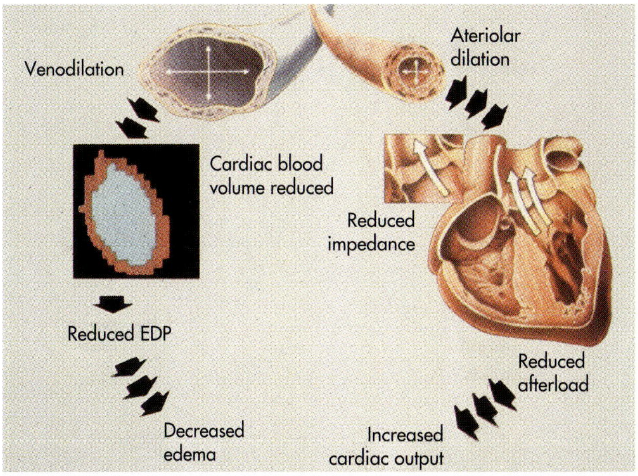

COLOR PLATE 36 Schematic drawing of the effects of venodilators and arteriolar dilators on the cardiovascular system.

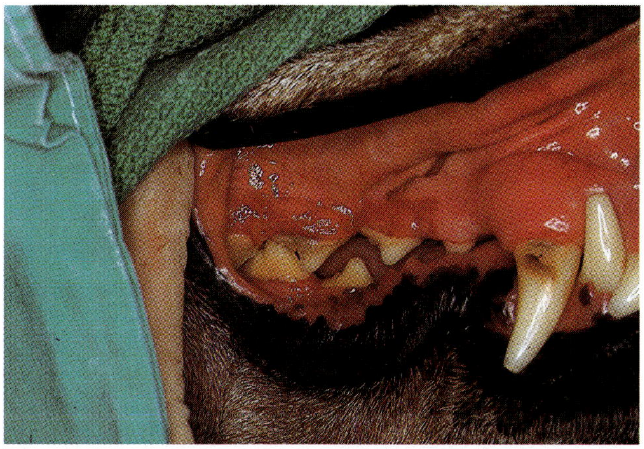

COLOR PLATE 37 The oral mucous membranes from a dog following hydralazine administration. The mucous membranes are hyperemic. Capillary refill time was approximately 0.25 seconds.

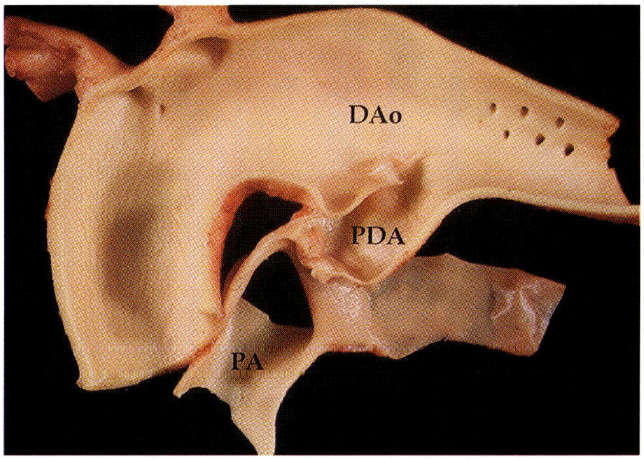

COLOR PLATE 38 Postmortem specimen from a young German shepherd dog of the transverse and proximal descending aorta *(DAo)* on top, the pulmonary artery *(PA)* branches ventrally, and a left-to-right shunting patent ductus arteriosus *(PDA)* between them. The aortic end of the PDA is wide open. The pulmonary artery end is partially constricted. This results in a funnel shape to the PDA. (Courtesy Dr. Mark Rishniw.)

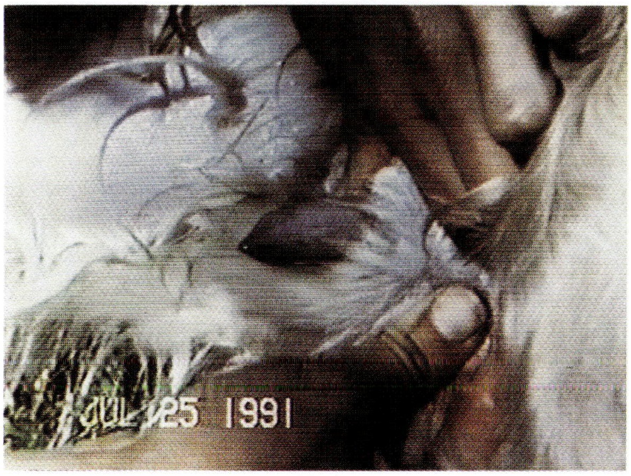

COLOR PLATE 39 Computer-captured image from a video tape of cyanotic penile mucous membranes from a 2-year-old American cocker spaniel with a right-to-left shunting patent ductus arteriosus. This image was taken immediately following exercise. The oral mucus membranes were not cyanotic (differential cyanosis).

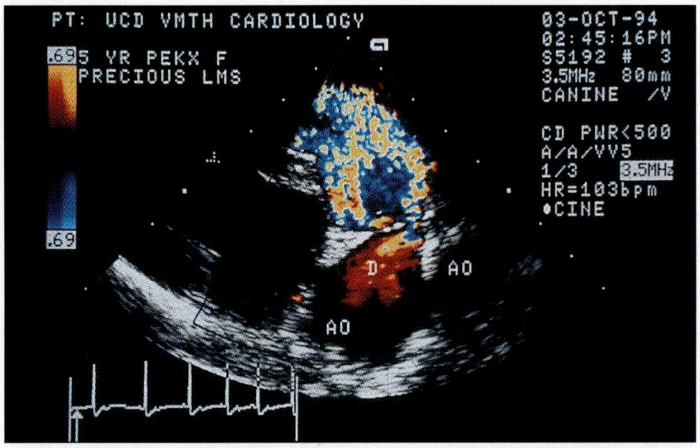

COLOR PLATE 40 Color flow Doppler echocardiogram from a dog with a left-to-right shunting patent ductus arteriosus (PDA). (See Figure 12-10.) Blood flow starts in the aorta *(AO)* as red, laminar flow then accelerates and aliases as it flows through the proximal region of the PDA *(D)*. At the pulmonary artery end of the PDA, blood flow becomes turbulent. The turbulent jet flows along the cranial border of the main pulmonary artery, strikes the pulmonic valve, and wraps back around within the main pulmonary artery.

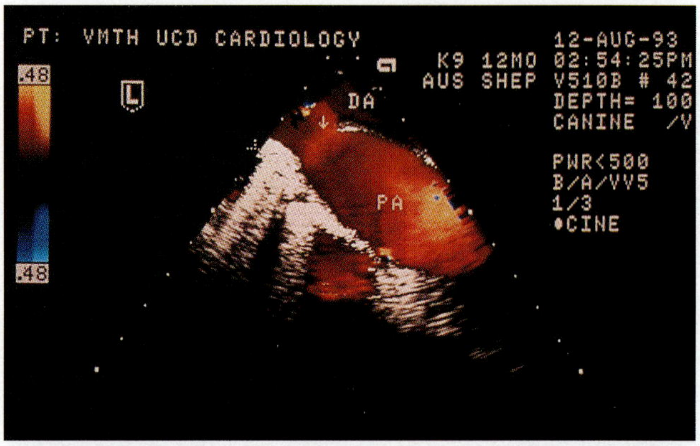

COLOR PLATE 41 Color flow Doppler transesophageal echocardiogram from the dog shown in Figure 12-13. Flow through the PDA *(arrow; DA)* is laminar and is directed toward the transducer *(red)*, flowing from the pulmonary artery *(PA)* into the aorta.

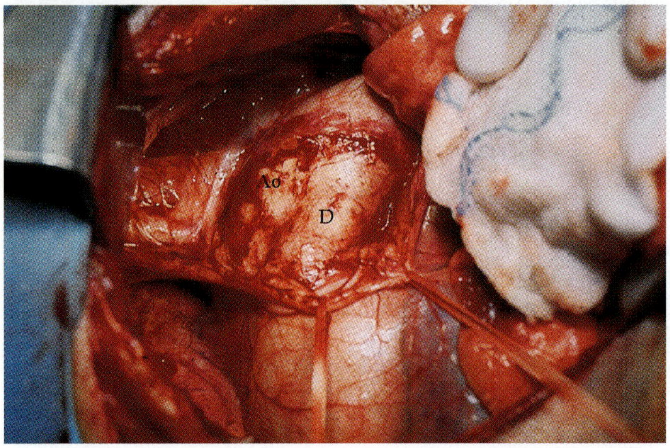

COLOR PLATE 42 Picture of the surgical site from a German shepherd cross with a left-to-right shunting patent ductus arteriosus (PDA). The region around the transverse and proximal portion of the descending aorta and the PDA have been dissected. The phrenic nerve has been isolated with umbilical tape and retracted ventrally. *Ao,* Aorta; *D,* patent ductus arteriosus.

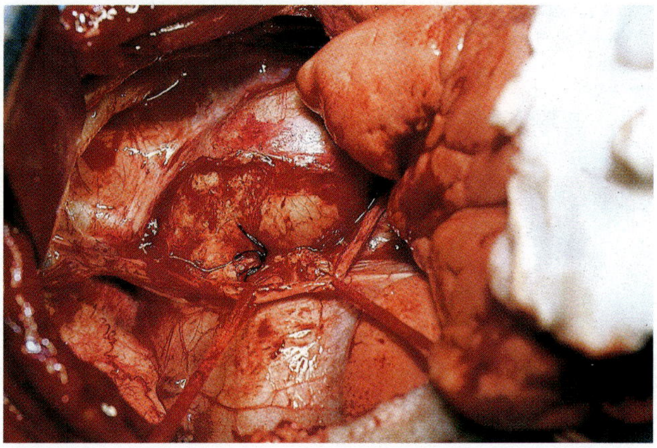

COLOR PLATE 43 Picture of the same surgical site shown in Color Plate 42. Silk sutures have been tied tightly, ligating the patent ductus arteriosus.

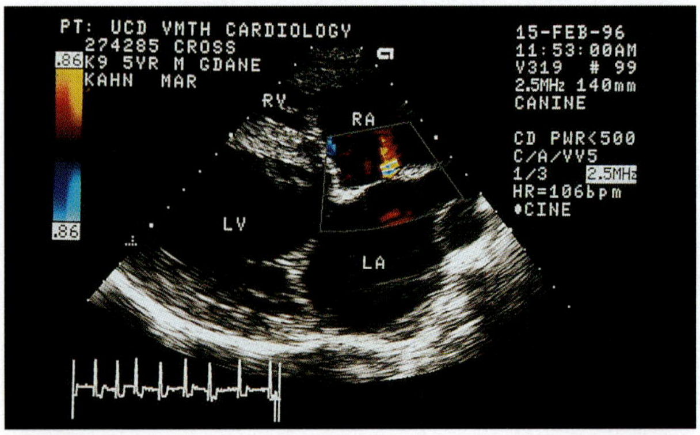

COLOR PLATE 44 Color flow Doppler echocardiogram from a 5-year-old male great Dane with a small atrial septal defect (ASD). The Doppler signal indicates that blood flows from the left atrium *(LA)* to the right atrium *(RA)* in ventricular systole. The signal is aliased. The dog had dilated cardiomyopathy. The ASD was an incidental finding. *LV,* Left ventricular chamber; *RV,* right ventricular chamber.

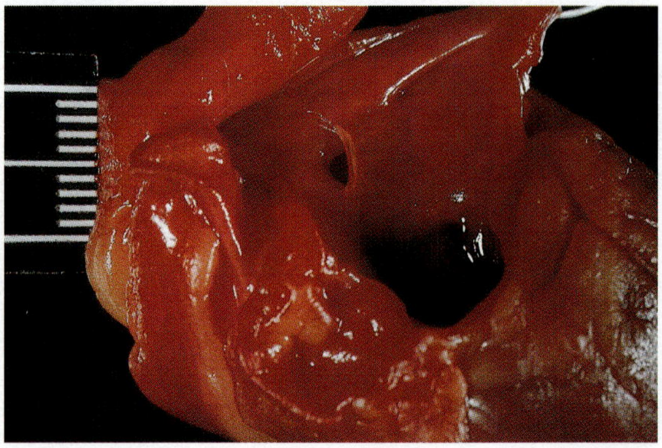

COLOR PLATE 45 Heart from a 1-year-old female American shorthair cat viewed at a postmortem examination. There is a small ostium secundum atrial septal defect (ASD). The cat died of heart failure secondary to hypertrophic cardiomyopathy. The ASD was an incidental finding.

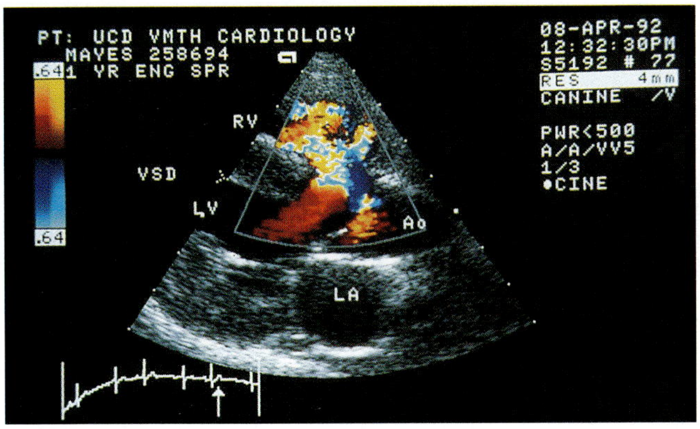

COLOR PLATE 46 Color flow Doppler echocardiogram from the dog shown in Figure 13-7, from the identical view. The color flow Doppler echocardiogram clearly demonstrates turbulent flow across the uppermost region of the interventricular septum and is diagnostic of a ventricular septal defect (VSD). Blood flow in the left ventricle *(LV)* is laminar and toward the VSD. At the defect, flow becomes turbulent. Turbulent flow projects into the right ventricular chamber *(RV)*. This dog had normal cardiac chamber sizes. *LA,* Left atrium; *Ao,* aorta.

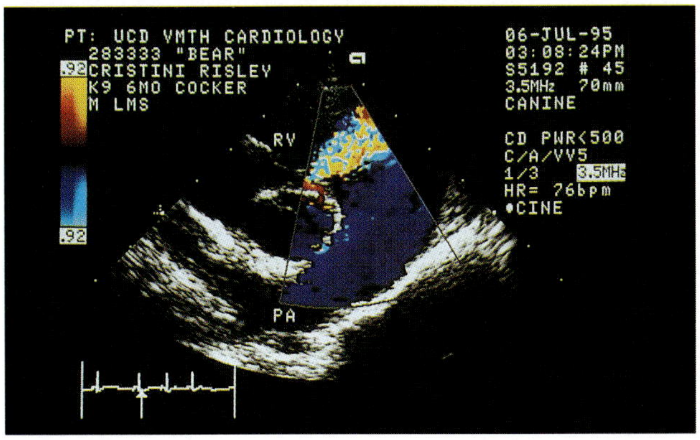

COLOR PLATE 47 Color flow Doppler echocardiogram from a 6-month-old male American cocker spaniel with a ventricular septal defect (VSD). The echocardiogram is taken from a right parasternal short-axis view at the base of the heart. Although the defect cannot be visualized, the color flow Doppler jet clearly originates immediately beneath the tricuspid valve (immediately to the left of the *RV* label). The jet strikes the right ventricular *(RV)* free wall. Flow in the right ventricular outflow tract is laminar and away from the transducer *(blue),* toward the pulmonary artery *(PA).*

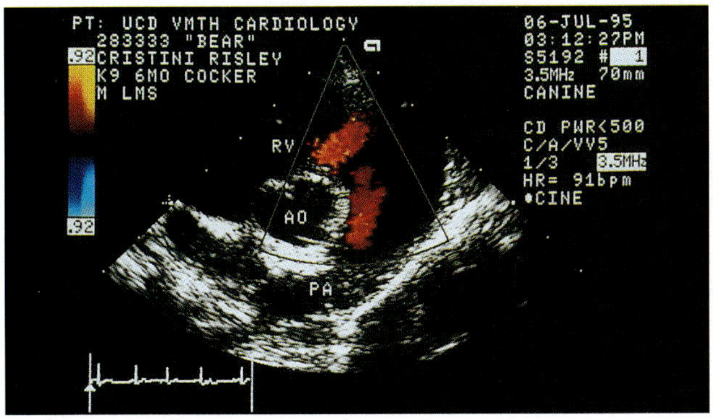

COLOR PLATE 48 Laminar diastolic flow through the ventricular septal defect (VSD) from the dog shown in Color Plate 46. Flow is into the right ventricular chamber *(RV)* and toward the transducer *(red).* There is also a laminar signal because of mild pulmonic insufficiency. The left ventricular end-diastolic diameter was 32 mm (normal = 25 to 30 mm), the end-systolic diameter was 18 mm (normal = 15 to 20 mm) in this 7-kg dog. The jet velocity was greater than 5 m/sec. The pulmonary to systemic blood flow ratio was calculated using pulsed-wave Doppler ultrasound to be 1.8:1.

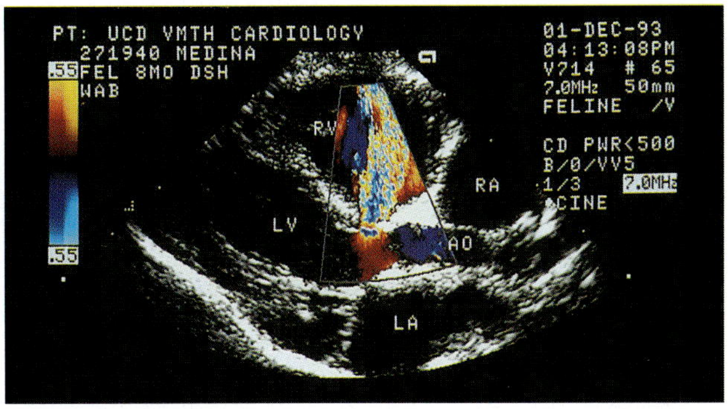

COLOR PLATE 49 Color flow Doppler recording of the turbulent jet caused by the ventricular septal defect in the cat shown in Figure 13-11. *RV,* Right ventricle; *LV,* left ventricle; *LA,* left atrium; *AO,* aorta; *RA,* right atrium.

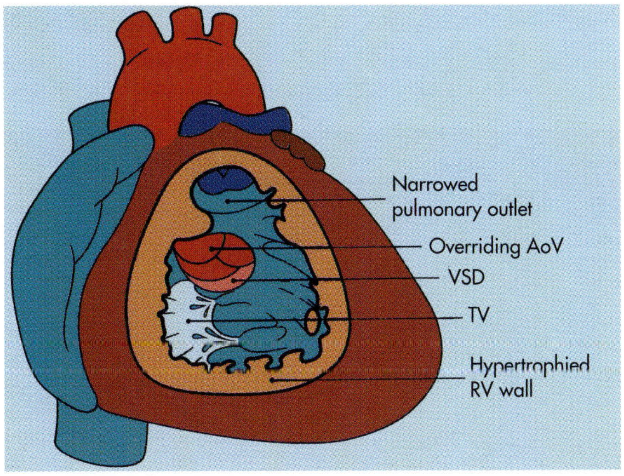

COLOR PLATE 50 Schematic drawing of the anatomy of tetralogy of Fallot. A portion of the hypertrophied right ventricular free wall has been cut away to reveal the inflow and outflow tracts of the right ventricle. A membranous ventricular septal defect (VSD) is present next to the cranioseptal commissures of the tricuspid valve (TV). The aorta is positioned rightward (dextroposition of the aorta), such that the aortic valve (AoV) lies over the top of the VSD. The outflow tract beneath the pulmonic valve is narrowed resulting in pulmonic stenosis.

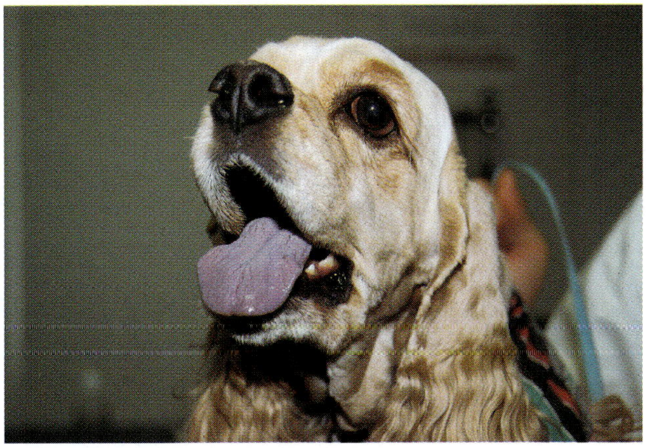

COLOR PLATE 51 Photograph of a 3-year-old male American cocker spaniel with tetralogy of Fallot. The dog is cyanotic, as evidenced by the blue color of his tongue. We had previously treated this dog surgically with a modified Blalock-Taussig shunt. The shunt had closed before this examination. The dog was successfully treated with propranolol.

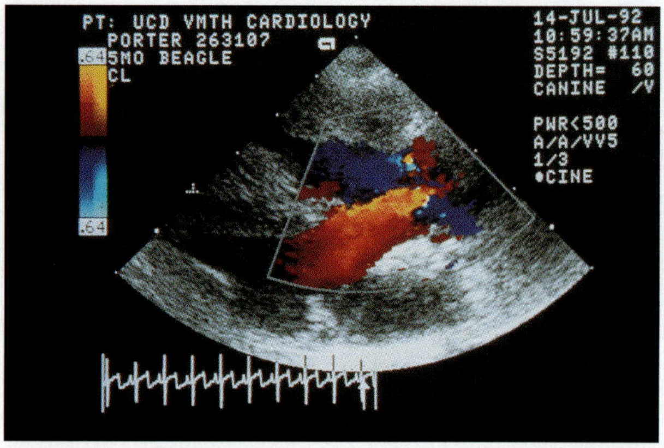

COLOR PLATE 52 Color flow Doppler echocardiography from a dog with tetralogy of Fallot. Laminar flow from the left *(red and gold)* and the right *(blue)* ventricles converge to enter the aorta. The flow through the ventricular septal defect is laminar because the defect is large such that velocity does not increase to the point of producing turbulence.

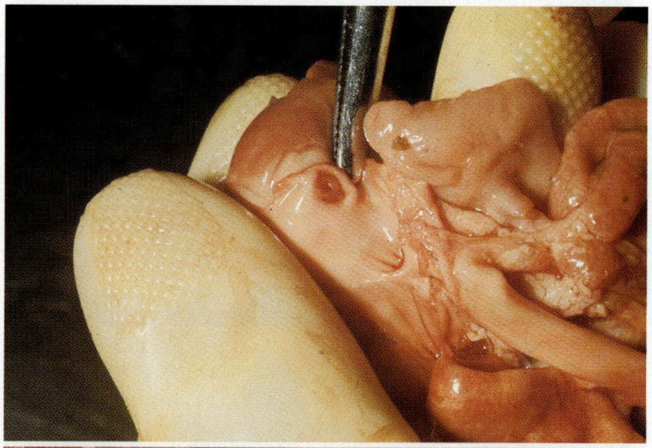

A

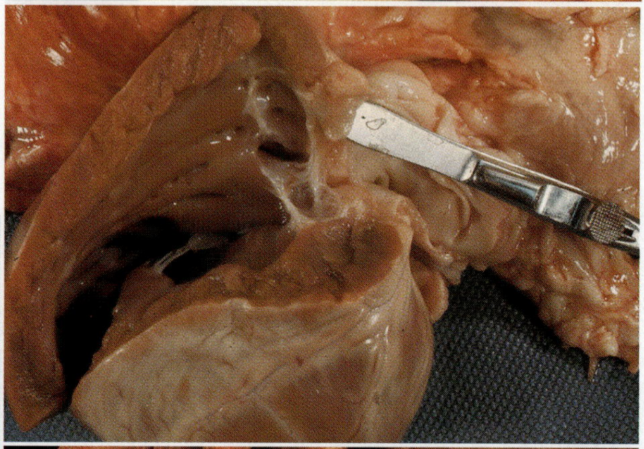

B

C

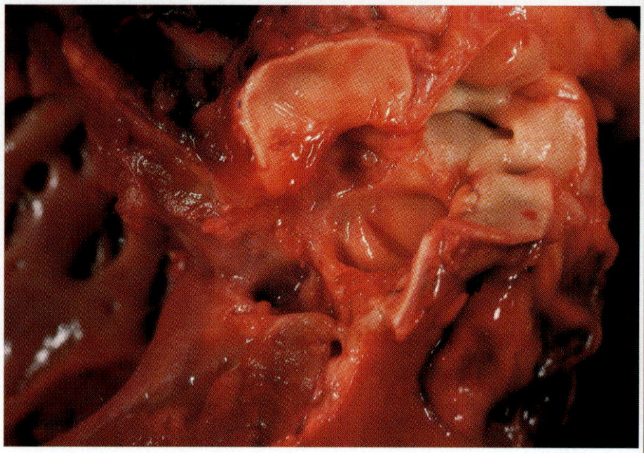

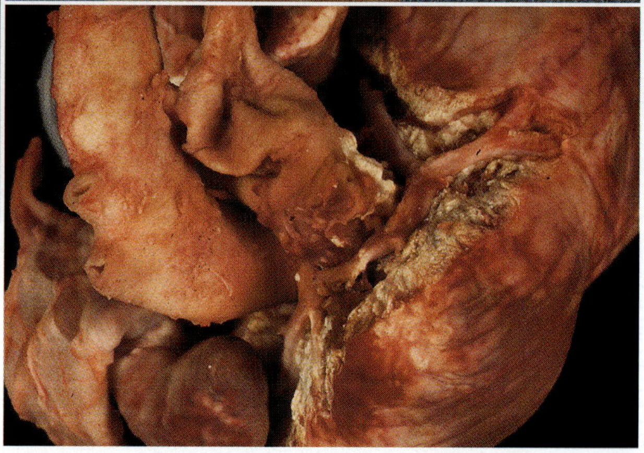

D

COLOR PLATE 53 Gross pathology specimens of pulmonic stenosis. **A,** Commissural fusion in a dog with pulmonic stenosis. The pulmonary valve (at the tip of the forceps) has a small orifice with no defined cusps. **B,** Pulmonary valve dysplasia in a dog. The valve cusps are thickened and deformed, and a discrete ring of fibrous tissue encircles the right ventricular outflow tract (subvalvular pulmonic stenosis) below the valve. **C,** A dysplastic pulmonary valve was surgically removed before death in this dog. A supravalvular narrowing of the main pulmonary artery, just above the sinuses and below the pulmonary artery bifurcation, is present. **D,** A dissected example of an R2A type of coronary anomaly in an English bulldog with subvalvular pulmonic stenosis. The left main coronary artery originates from the right coronary artery and encircles the origin of the the pulmonary artery (crosses to the right of the picture) before dividing into the left circumflex and left cranial descending coronary arteries. (Courtesy Dr. William Thomas.)

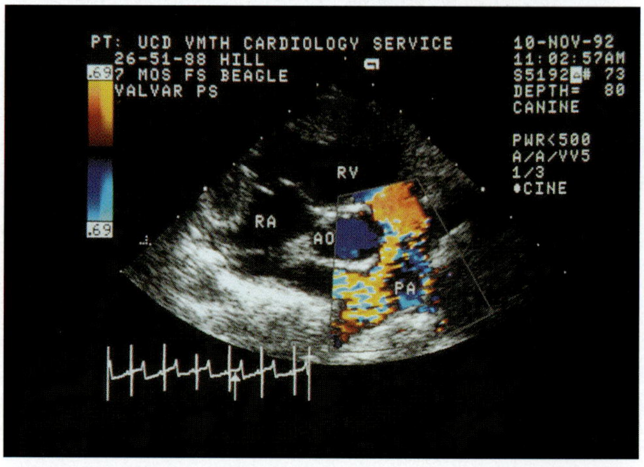

A

COLOR PLATE 54 **A,** Systolic color flow Doppler image taken from a right parasternal short-axis basilar view. The flow proximal to the pulmonic valve is laminar (single blue color that turns to a single gold color as blood flow velocity exceeds 0.69 m/sec, the Nyquist limit). There is a mosaic pattern in the main pulmonary artery *(PA),* indicating high-velocity, turbulent flow. *RA,* Right atrium; *RV,* right ventricle; *AO,* aorta.

B

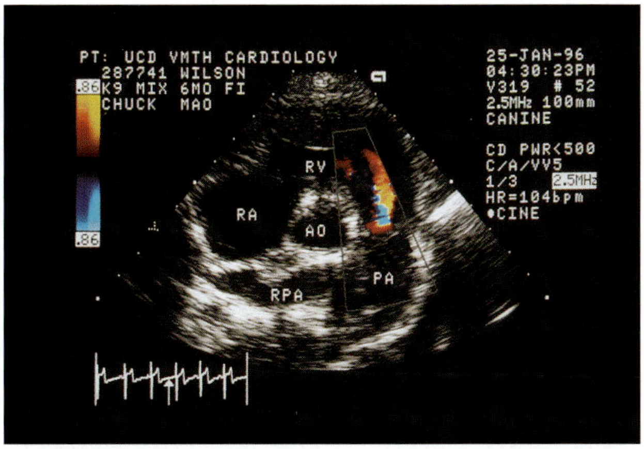

COLOR PLATE 54, cont'd **B,** Color flow Doppler image from the right ventricular outflow tract taken in diastole. There is a small turbulent jet from the pulmonary valve, indicating mild pulmonary insufficiency. There is poststenotic dilation of the main pulmonary artery as a result of pulmonic stenosis. *RPA,* Right pulmonary artery.

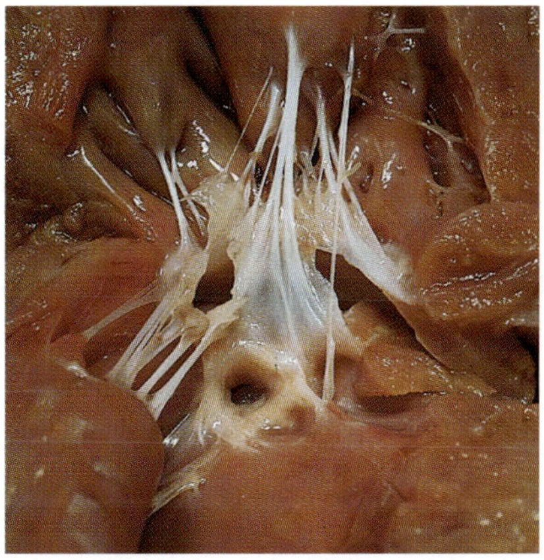

COLOR PLATE 56 Gross pathologic specimen from a dog with severe subaortic stenosis. The left ventricular free wall has been reflected. This photograph shows a close- up of the left ventricular outflow tract (LVOT). A fibrous ring completely encircles the LVOT below the aortic valve (not seen), including the base of the anterior mitral valve leaflet.

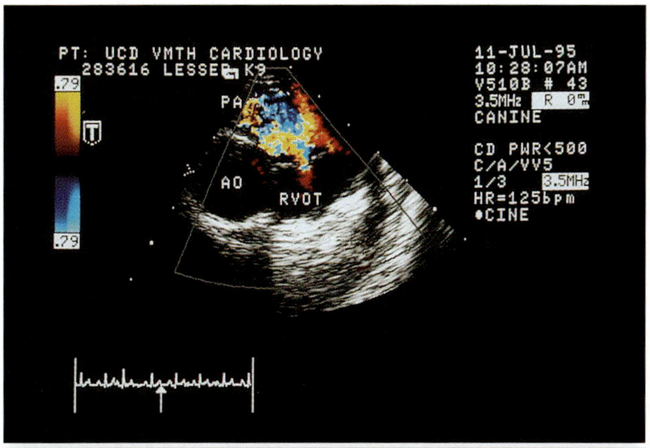

A

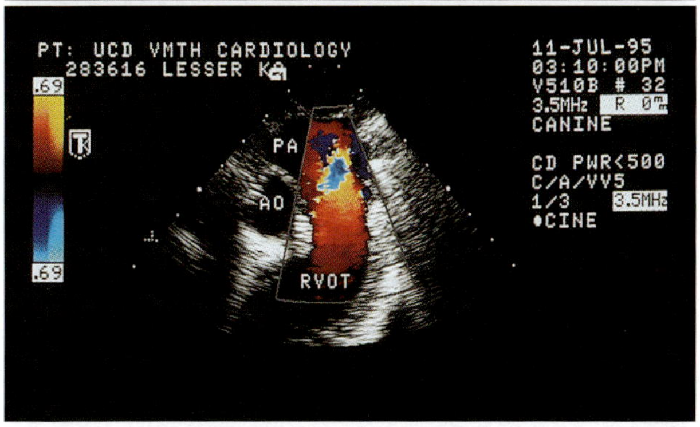

B

COLOR PLATE 55 **A,** Systolic color flow Doppler examination from the same view as in Figure 15-11, *A,* showing a mosaic, multicolored jet, indicating turbulence in the main pulmonary artery as a result of the valvular pulmonic stenosis. **B,** Systolic color flow Doppler frame from the same view as in Figure 15-11, *B.* Note that the flow is now laminar, as indicated by the homogenous red color. The peak velocity measured with continuous-wave Doppler decreased from 4.6 to 1.0 m/sec following balloon valvuloplasty (not shown).

A

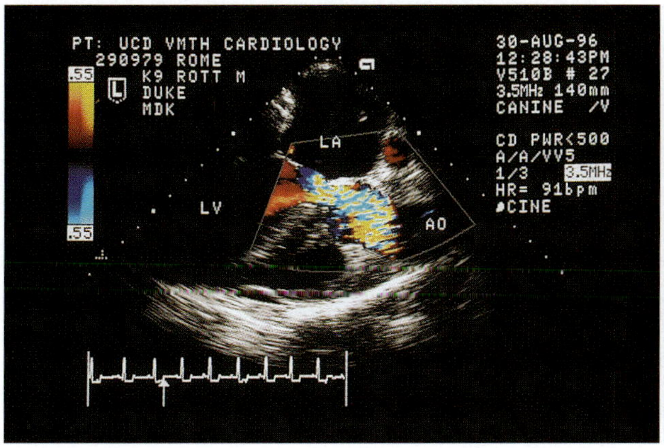

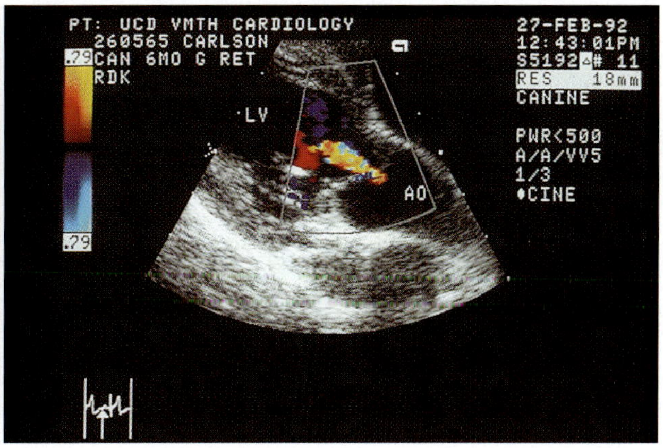

B

COLOR PLATE 57 Color flow Doppler echocardiograms from dogs with subaortic stenosis. **A,** Transesophageal view of the left ventricular outflow tract (LVOT), aortic valve, and ascending aorta. There is a broad, turbulent systolic jet originating in the narrowed region of the LVOT. *LA,* Left atrium; *LV,* left ventricle; *AO,* aorta. **B,** Left cranial long-axis view of the left ventricle *(LV)* and ascending aorta *(AO).* This is a diastolic frame depicting the turbulent jet of mild aortic insufficiency originating at the aortic valve and coursing through the left ventricular outflow tract.

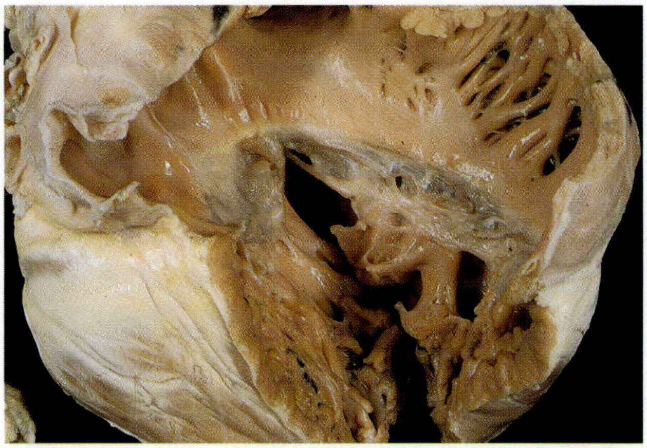

COLOR PLATE 58 Postmortem cardiac specimen from a dog with tricuspid valve dysplasia. The papillary muscles are attached directly to the valve leaflets. The leaflets have defects in them, and the septal leaflet is attached to the interventricular septum.

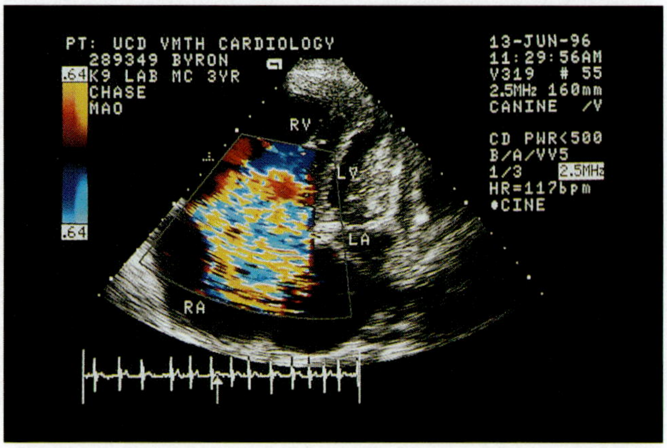

COLOR PLATE 59 Color flow Doppler echocardiogram (left apical four-chamber view) from a 3-year-old Labrador retriever with severe tricuspid valve dysplasia. A large jet of blood projects into the right atrium *(RA)* from the right ventricle *(RV)* in systole, characteristic of severe tricuspid regurgitation. The left ventricular chamber *(LV)* and the left atrium *(LA)* are small.

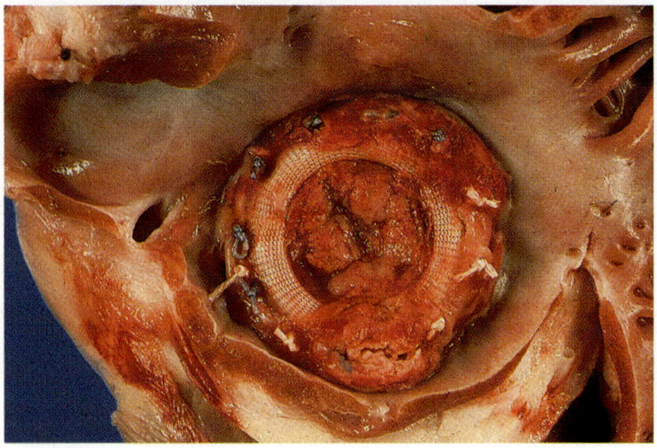

COLOR PLATE 60 Prosthetic valve viewed from the atrial side at the postmortem examination of a dog with severe tricuspid valve dysplasia. The prosthetic valve had been surgically placed 1 week before death. The dog died subacutely because of poor flow as a result of severe tricuspid stenosis. The prosthetic valve leaflets and valve ring have a large amount of organized thrombotic material adherent to their surfaces.

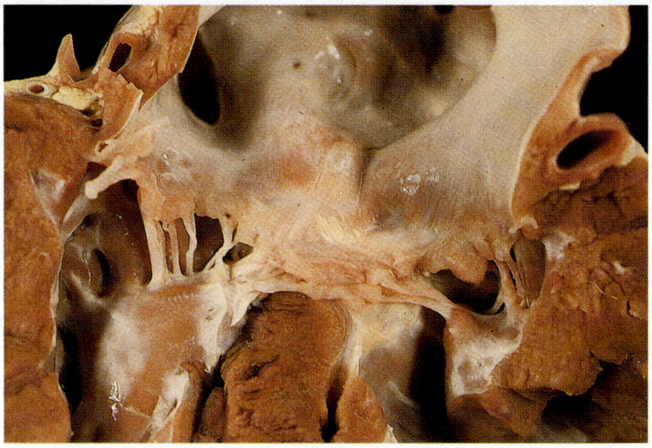

COLOR PLATE 61 Postmortem specimen of a heart from a 4-month-old golden retriever dog with mitral valve dysplasia. The chordae tendineae are short and thick. The edges of the valve leaflets are thickened. Echocardiography revealed moderately severe subaortic stenosis and severe mitral valve dysplasia. The dog was euthanized because of the poor prognosis.

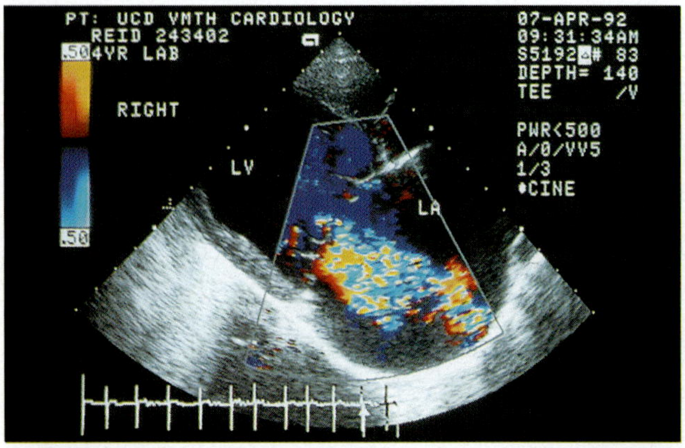

COLOR PLATE 62 Color flow Doppler echocardiogram from the dog shown in Figure 17-4. The blood flow is laminar in the left ventricular chamber *(LV)* and then accelerates to the mitral valve. At the valve, flow becomes turbulent. The turbulent jet extends from the valve to the dorsal wall of the severely enlarged left atrium *(LA)*.

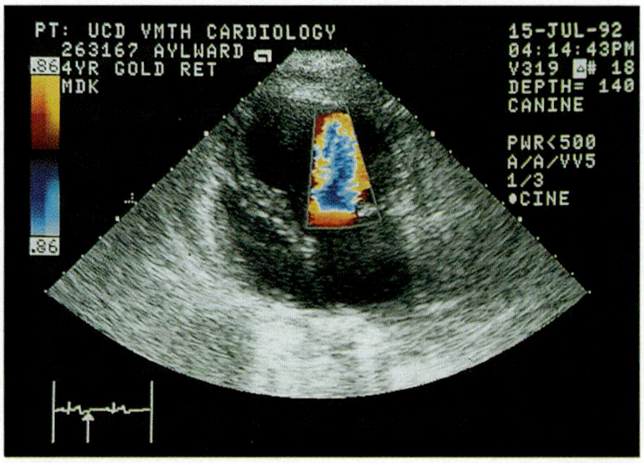

COLOR PLATE 63 Color flow Doppler echocardiogram from the dog shown in Figure 17-8. This diastolic frame shows flow into the left ventricle through the stenotic mitral valve orifice. The flow is laminar in the left atrium. Flow velocity exceeds the Nyquist limit at the mitral valve orifice and becomes aliased beyond that point.

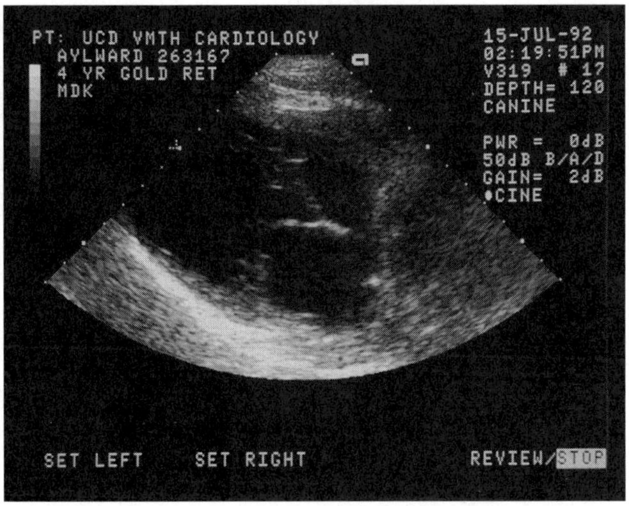

FIGURE 17-8 Two-dimensional echocardiogram from a 4-year-old golden retriever with moderate mitral stenosis. This frame is taken in diastole at the maximal mitral valve opening. The mural leaflet is immobile, maintaining a closed position throughout the cardiac cycle. The septal leaflet has decreased mobility. It never opened to within less than 6 mm of the interventricular septum, as would a normal valve leaflet.

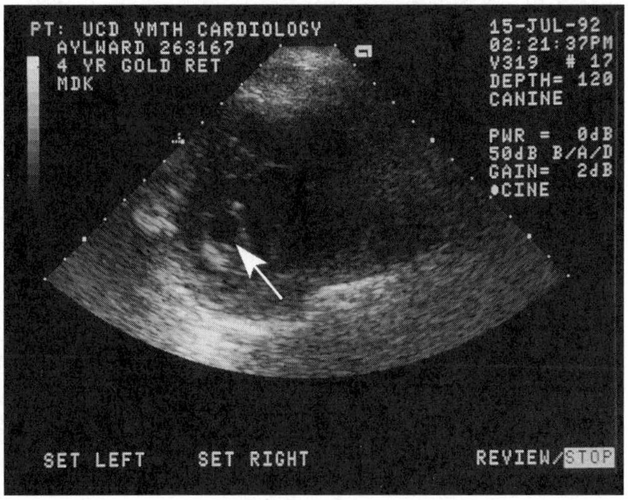

FIGURE 17-9 Two-dimensional echocardiogram taken to look at the mitral valve *(arrow)* from the dog shown in Figure 17-8 in cross-section. This is a diastolic frame. It shows that the mitral valve opens very poorly with an orifice that is only 1 to 1.5 cm in diameter. Normally it should open more than 4 cm. The mural leaflet is hyperechoic, either from fibrosis or calcification.

cats were 14 and 16 years old at presentation. Because of these data, we believe that most mitral stenosis in dogs and cats is probably the result of congenital MVD.

PATHOPHYSIOLOGY

Mitral stenosis produces obstruction to blood flow from the left atrium to the left ventricle in diastole. The increased resistance to blood flow results in an increase in left atrial pressure, with resultant increases in pulmonary vein and pulmonary capillary pressures. Consequently, severe mitral stenosis causes pulmonary edema. Exercise increases left atrial pressure even further, which may result in exercise-induced dyspnea. The obstruction to blood flow may also result in exercise-induced syncope in dogs.[21] Syncope may occur when flow cannot increase appropriately during exercise, resulting in inadequate flow to maintain systemic pressure during exercise-induced vasodilation, or it may be due to a tachyarrhythmia. Alternatively, syncope may occur when the inadequate left ventricular return during exercise results in a decrease in left ventricular chamber size, enhanced sympathetic response to the decrease in stroke volume, ventricular mechanoreceptor stimulation, and reflex vagally-mediated peripheral vasodilation and bradycardia.[25-27]

Reflex pulmonary vasoconstriction and pulmonary pathology leading to pulmonary hypertension, with or without right heart failure, is common in humans with mitral stenosis.[28] Although mild pulmonary hypertension has been reported in two dogs with isolated mitral stenosis, this amount of elevation is most likely due to the fact that pulmonary artery diastolic pressure must equal pulmonary capillary pressure, such that if pulmonary capillary pressure is increased, pulmonary artery pressure is also increased, albeit only mildly. No dog or cat with isolated mitral stenosis has been reported with severe pulmonary hypertension or right heart failure.

CLINICAL FINDINGS

Mitral stenosis is most commonly diagnosed in dogs and cats as an incidental finding or when the patient presents in left heart failure. The most common auscultatory abnormality in patients with isolated mitral valve disease is a systolic heart murmur characteristic of mitral regurgitation that occurs concomitantly with the mitral stenosis. The murmur ranges in intensity from grade 2/6 to grade 5/6. In dogs with concomitant disease, such as subaortic stenosis, the murmur caused by the predominant defect usually overshadows any other murmur. Mitral stenosis causes diastolic turbulence and routinely produces a diastolic heart murmur in humans.[22] In one report, only five of 15 dogs with mitral stenosis had a diastolic heart murmur recognized, and in one of these the murmur could only be heard after sedation.[21] The murmur in these dogs was characterized as a grade 1 to 2/6, low-frequency, diastolic murmur heard best at the left apex. Detecting a soft, low-frequency murmur in an uncooperative patient with a fast heart rate is extremely difficult, and it may easily be missed unless the examiner has a high index of suspicion. A diastolic murmur associated with mitral stenosis has not been reported in a cat, presumably because the fast heart rate taxes the skills of even the best examiner in this species.[24]

DIAGNOSTIC TESTS

Thoracic radiographs. The most striking and consistent feature identified on thoracic radiographs is left atrial enlargement.[21] Other congenital lesions and concomitant mitral regurgitation may result in enlargement of other chambers, particularly the left ventricle.

Electrocardiography. Prolongation of the *P* wave is the most common ECG abnormality, and was seen in seven out of 14 dogs in one study.[21] Interestingly, three dogs in this study had tall *P* waves in lead II in a disease that classically produces pure left atrial enlargement. Tall *R* waves in lead II were also observed in this study, but many dogs had concomitant subaortic stenosis. Supraventricular premature contractions, supraventricular tachycardia, and atrial fibrillation have all been reported in dogs with mitral stenosis.[21,23]

Echocardiography. The diagnosis of mitral stenosis in dogs and cats is generally made using echocardiography. The diastolic mitral valve excursion on two-dimensional echocardiography is subjectively decreased and is usually the abnormality that is first recognized (Figures 17-8 and 17-9). The leaflets, especially the septal leaflet, may dome toward the left ventricle as blood flow tries to force the valve open. The left atrium is enlarged, and often the valve leaflets

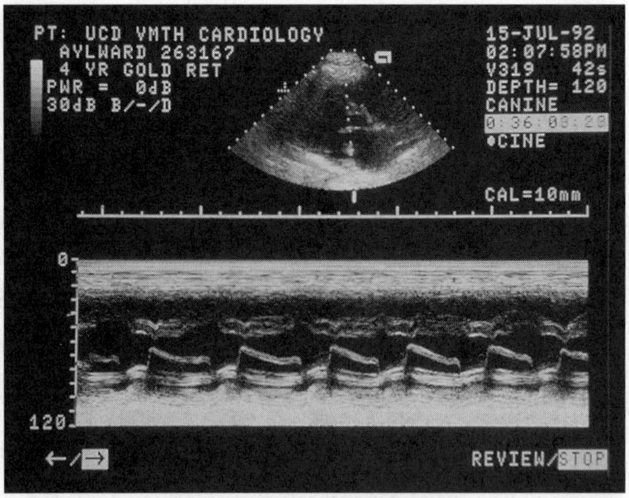

FIGURE 17-10 M-mode echocardiogram from the dog shown in Figure 17-8, taken at the mitral valve level. The mural mitral valve leaflet is thickened and immobile. The septal leaflet opens maximally in early diastole and then stays open throughout diastole in an attempt to allow a normal flow volume into the left ventricle. This results in a flat slope to the mitral valve opening throughout diastole (increased *E-F* slope).

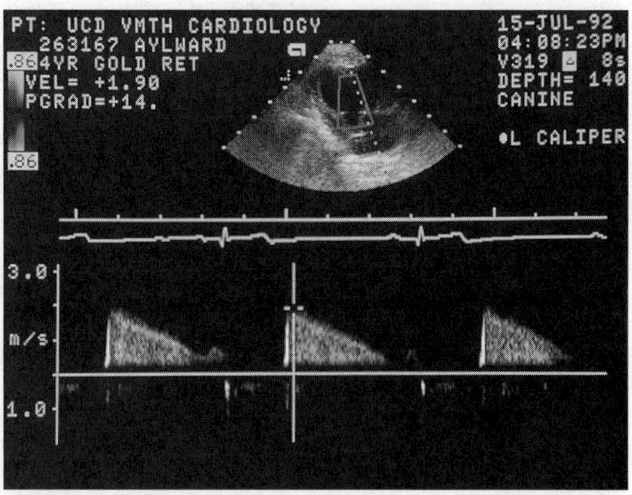

FIGURE 17-11 Continuous-wave Doppler tracing of mitral diastolic flow velocity from the dog shown in Figure 17-8. Peak diastolic flow velocity should not exceed 1.1 m/sec. Peak velocity in this dog is 1.9 m/sec. This translates into a pressure gradient of 14 mm Hg. This means the left atrial pressure is 14 mm Hg greater than the left ventricular diastolic pressure in early diastole. The time that it takes for the blood flow velocity to decelerate is prolonged. This results in a prolonged "ramp" that looks very similar to the motion of the septal leaflet of the mitral valve on the M-mode echocardiogram shown in Figure 17-10. The pressure half time is increased to approximately 80 ms.

are thickened. The left ventricle may be normal, increased, or decreased in size, depending on the amount of mitral regurgitation.[21] M-mode echocardiography is used to evaluate the diastolic mitral valve motion. The *E-F* slope of the septal leaflet (the slope of the leaflet echo between maximum opening in early diastole and maximum diastolic closure before the onset of systole) is flattened as a decreased amount of blood flows through the mitral valve orifice for a longer time (Figure 17-10). The motion of the mural leaflet is also flat, and the leaflet may move toward the septal leaflet during diastole. Color flow Doppler echocardiography is used to identify turbulent or aliased diastolic flow across the mitral valve (Color Plate 63). Aliased or turbulent flow occurs because of the increased flow velocity in this region. The jet begins at the mitral valve and projects into the left ventricle in diastole. Spectral Doppler is used to determine peak velocity and pressure half time (Figure 17-11). Maximum flow velocity occurs during early diastole and during atrial systole. Peak velocity is generally recorded during early diastole. Velocities greater than 1.1 m/sec are considered abnormally high in the dog.[29] However, other diseases, such as mitral regurgitation, can increase inflow velocity as a result of increased blood flow through a fixed orifice. Consequently, an increased flow velocity alone cannot be used to diagnose mitral stenosis. Peak flow velocities in one report ranged between 1.4 and 2.5 m/sec.[21] These translate into pressure gradients between 8 and 25 mm Hg. This means that the left atrial pressure was 8 to 25 mm Hg higher than left ventricular diastolic pressure in early diastole. Because left ventricular diastolic pressure is usually very low in early diastole (0 to 5 mm Hg), left atrial pressure was about 10 to 30 mm Hg in these dogs. The pressure difference between the left atrium and the left ventricle normally decreases very rapidly during diastole. The time for this pressure difference to drop in half has been reported to be less than 50 ms in dogs.[21] In dogs or cats with mitral stenosis, the time for this pressure gradient to decrease is prolonged because of the increased resistance to flow throughout diastole. Consequently, the time for the pressure difference to drop to one half of the starting pressure gradient (pressure half time) is prolonged in patients with mitral stenosis. This time can be measured at cardiac catheterization but is more easily determined with spectral Doppler by measuring the time that it takes for the velocity to decrease to 0.7 of the starting value. The value of 0.7 is used instead of 0.5 (one half) because pressure gradient is a square function of velocity ($\sqrt{0.5} = 0.7$). This value has been reported to be between 52 and 105 ms in dogs with mitral stenosis.[21] Pressure half time and pressure gradient do not necessarily provide the same information in a patient. In one study, the correlation coefficient *(r)* between these two variables was only 0.54.[21] Other more accurate measures of mitral stenosis severity have been devised in human medicine. Mitral valve area (MVA) is commonly calculated using the Gorlin equation in which:

$$MVA = F \div (C \times 44.5\sqrt{PG})$$

where *F* is the flow rate, *C* is a derived constant, and *PG* is the pressure gradient across the mitral valve. Because no normal values have been determined for dogs or cats of varying sizes, this method cannot be currently used in veterinary medicine.

TREATMENT

Medical therapy. Treatment of patients with mitral stenosis and with mild-to-moderate left heart failure is generally medical in dogs and cats. Furosemide administration and sodium restriction are reported to be effective in human patients, and this appears to be the case in dogs and cats.[21-24] Excessive diuresis or excessive preload reduction through diuresis and venodilation must be avoided, because transmitral flow depends on the pressure gradient across the mitral valve. An excessive reduction in left atrial pressure can decrease cardiac output precipitously. Digoxin is reported to be of no benefit in human patients with mitral stenosis unless it is used to slow the heart rate in patients with atrial fibrillation.

Surgical or interventional therapy. The treatment for moderate-to-severe mitral stenosis in humans that are in moderate-to-severe left heart failure is generally surgical or interventional.[22]

Surgical techniques in humans fall into the following three categories: (1) closed commissurotomy, (2) open commissurotomy, and (3) mitral valve replacement. The latter two require open-heart surgery and so cannot be used in cats, and, as mentioned previously, dogs tend not to tolerate prosthetic valves. Closed commissurotomy can be performed by placing a finger through a purse-string suture in the right atrial wall and digitally fracturing the stenotic material. The use of a transventricular dilator is preferred in this situation, however. Balloon valvuloplasty is also used in human medicine to relieve mitral stenosis. This requires passing a small balloon flotation catheter across the interatrial septum following transseptal puncture, enlarging the hole, passing a guide wire, and then advancing the larger balloon catheter over the guide wire and across the mitral valve. The primary danger of breaking down the stenotic tissue with a finger, a dilator, or a balloon, is exacerbation of mitral regurgitation. Because most dogs and cats with mitral stenosis have some degree of regurgitation and many have MVD, this danger appears to be very real. Consequently, these procedures should be performed only after serious consideration of alternatives. Surgical commissurotomy of the mitral valve has been reported in one dog, but this dog died in the early postoperative period.[21] Balloon valvuloplasty of an atrioventricular valve has only been reported once in a dog, and that was in a dog with tricuspid stenosis.[30] This was a dog with apparent tricuspid valve dysplasia that had tricuspid stenosis with no tricuspid regurgitation. Balloon valvuloplasty was successful at reducing the pressure gradient across the tricuspid valve, decreasing the right atrial pressure, and improving exercise tolerance in this dog. The valvuloplasty did not create tricuspid regurgitation in this dog.

REFERENCES

1. Becker AE, Becker MJ, Edwards JE: Pathologic spectrum of dysplasia of the tricuspid valve: features in common with Ebstein's malformation, *Arch Pathol* 91:167, 1971.
2. Liu SK, Tilley LP: Dysplasia of the tricuspid valve in the dog and cat, *J Am Vet Med Assoc* 169:623, 1976.
3. Liu S, K, Tilley LP: Malformation of the canine mitral valve complex, *J Am Vet Med Assoc* 167:465, 1975.
4. Liu SK, Brown B: Malformation of mitral valve complex associated with cardiac dysfunction in 120 cats, *Lab Invest* 58:56A, 1988.
5. Hamlin RL, Smetzer DL, Smith CR: Congenital mitral insufficiency in the dog, *J Am Vet Med Assoc* 146:1088, 1965.
6. Patterson DF: Epidemiologic and genetic studies of congenital heart disease in the dog, *Circ Res* 23:171, 1968.
7. Bolton GR, Liu SK: Congenital heart diseases of the cat, *Vet Clin North Am* 7:341, 1977.
8. LeBlanc JG, Sett SS, Vince DJ: Antiplatelet therapy in children with left-sided mechanical prostheses, *Eur J Cardiothorac Surg* 7:211, 1993.
9. Daliento L, Thiene G, Chirillo F et al: [Congenital malformations of the mitral valve: clinical and morphological aspects] Le alterazioni congenite della valvola mitrale: aspetti clinici e morfologici, *G Ital Cardiol* 21:1205, 1991.
10. Stellin G, Bortolotti U, Mazzucco A et al: Repair of congenitally malformed mitral valve in children, *J Thorac Cardiovasc Surg* 95:480, 1988.
11. Fox PR: Congenital feline heart disease. In Fox PR, ed: *Canine and feline cardiology,* New York, 1988, Churchill Livingstone.
12. Lord PF, Wood A, Liu S, K et al: Left ventricular angiocardiography in congenital mitral valve insufficiency of the dog, *J Am Vet Med Assoc* 166:1069, 1975.
13. Borow KM, Green LH, Mann T et al: End-systolic volume as a predictor of postoperative left ventricular performance in volume overload from valvular regurgitation, *Am J Med* 68:655, 1980.
14. Carabello BA, Nolan SP, McGuire LB: Assessment of preoperative left ventricular function in patients with mitral regurgitation: value of the end-systolic wall stress-end-systolic volume ratio, *Circulation* 64:1212, 1981.
15. Eyster GE, Weber W, Chi S et al: Mitral valve prosthesis for correction of mitral regurgitation in a dog, *J Am Vet Med Assoc* 168:1115, 1976.
16. Starr A: *History of cardiac surgery,* 1995, oral presentation, 68th Scientific Session of the American Heart Association Meeting.
17. Starr A, Edwards ML: Mitral replacement: clinical experience with ball-valve prosthesis, *Ann Surg* 154:726, 1961.
18. Rozich JD, Carabello BA, Usher BW et al: Mitral valve replacement with and without chordal preservation in patients with chronic mitral regurgitation: mechanisms for differences in postoperative ejection performance, *Circulation* 86:1718, 1992.
19. Carpentier A, Chauvaud S, Fabiani JN et al: Reconstructive surgery of mitral valve incompetence: ten-year appraisal, *J Thorac Cardiovasc Surg* 79:338, 1980.
20. Kanemoto I, Shibata S, Noguchi H et al: Successful mitral valvuloplasty for mitral regurgitation in a dog, *Jpn J Vet Sci* 52:411, 1990.
21. Lehmkuhl LB, Ware WA, Bonagura JD: Mitral stenosis in 15 dogs, *J Vet Intern Med* 8:2, 1994 [see comments].
22. Braunwald E: Valvular heart disease. In Braunwald E, ed: *Heart disease: a textbook of cardiovascular medicine,* ed 4, Philadelphia, 1992, WB Saunders.
23. Fox PR, Miller MW, Liu SK: Clinical, echocardiographic, and Doppler imaging characteristics of mitral valve stenosis in two dogs, *J Am Vet Med Assoc* 201:1575, 1992.
24. Stamoulis ME, Fox PR: Mitral valve stenosis in three cats, *J Small Anim Pract* 34:452, 1993.
25. Abboud FM: Ventricular syncope: is the heart a sensory organ? *N Engl J Med* 320:390, 1989 [editorial].
26. Grech ED, Ramsdale DR: Exertional syncope in aortic stenosis: evidence to support inappropriate left ventricular baroreceptor response, *Am Heart J* 121:603, 1991.
27. Shalev Y, Gal R, Tchou PJ et al: Echocardiographic demonstration of decreased left ventricular dimensions and vigorous myocardial contraction during syncope induced by head-up tilt, *J Am Coll Cardiol* 18:746, 1991.
28. Grossman W, Braunwald E: Pulmonary hypertension. In Braunwald E, ed: *Heart disease: a textbook of cardiovascular medicine,* ed 4, Philadelphia, 1992, WB Saunders.
29. Yuill CDM, O' Grady MR: Doppler-derived velocity of blood flow across the cardiac valves in the normal dog, *Can J Vet Res* 55:185, 1991.
30. Brown WA, Thomas WP: Balloon valvuloplasty of tricuspid stenosis in a Labrador retriever, *J Vet Intern Med* 9:419, 1995.

CHAPTER 18

Other Congenital Cardiovascular Abnormalities

Many types of congenital cardiac defects are observed much more frequently in human medicine than in veterinary medicine. Most children are examined within the first minutes to hours of life and are treated to maintain life. Presumably, most puppies and kittens with severe and complex congenital cardiac defects die early in life. Consequently, they are never examined by a veterinarian. Infants with abnormalities such as transposition of the great arteries with an intact ventricular septum, pulmonary atresia with an intact ventricular septum, and interrupted aortic arch develop clinical signs of disease within the first 3 days of life.[1] Others with abnormalities such as truncus arteriosus, tetralogy of Fallot with severe pulmonic stenosis, or pulmonary atresia present at 4 to 14 days of age, when the ductus arteriosus closes. Children with abnormalities such as a complete atrioventricular canal and a large ventricular septal defect develop clinical signs within the first 2 to 18 weeks of life, at the time that pulmonary vascular resistance falls. Not surprisingly, the abnormalities most commonly observed in small animal veterinary medicine, such as patent ductus arteriosus, noncritical aortic stenosis, noncritical pulmonic stenosis, and atrial and ventricular septal defects, are most commonly identified in children when they are 4 to 12 months old, very similar to when we diagnose these same abnormalities.

That many puppies and kittens die early from complex or severe congenital cardiac disease has been demonstrated in one study in which 368 kittens were examined at a postmortem. Thirteen kittens died of congenital heart disease, most between 1 day and 6 weeks of age.[2] Similar data have been reported in puppies.[3] Occasionally, a dog or cat will be born with a rare or complex defect that is not severe enough to cause death or that has a compensating defect (e.g., a patent ductus arteriosus). These animals may subsequently be presented for diagnostic work-up when they start to show clinical signs or when a heart murmur is discovered. These cases are often diagnostic challenges. This chapter is primarily a compilation of the veterinary literature on rare and complex congenital cardiac abnormalities. Abnormalities are listed in alphabetical order.

Anomalous Pulmonary Venous Connection

In anomalous pulmonary venous connection, a rare abnormality, pulmonary veins attach to the right atrium or a systemic vein (e.g., a vena cava, a coronary vein, or the portal vein), resulting in oxygenated blood flowing into the venous circulation (a left-to-right shunt). When one or more, but not all, pulmonary veins drain into the right atrium (directly or indirectly by venous connections), the lesion is termed a *partial anomalous venous connection.*[4] Total anomalous pulmonary venous connection occurs when all the pulmonary veins drain into the right heart or systemic veins. In total anomalous pulmonary venous connection, life is not possible without an associated communication between the left and right circulations, because all oxygenated blood recirculates into the pulmonary circulation. An associated atrial septal defect is the most common form of a communication present in these cases.

Very few reports of anomalous pulmonary venous connection in dogs are present in the veterinary literature.[5-8] In one case report, a 5-month-old great Dane presented in right heart failure.[6] The dog had a heart rate of 230 beats/min as a result of supraventricular tachycardia with a second-degree atrioventricular block. The right heart was grossly enlarged on the thoracic radiographs. The dog also had mild pulmonic stenosis and a poststenotic dilation of the main pulmonary artery. At cardiac catheterization, injection of a radiopaque contrast agent into the right ventricle resulted in the agent returning to the right atrium before it was present in the left atrium. An atrial septal defect was suspected. At postmortem examination, all of the pulmonary veins connected directly to the right atrium (total anomalous pulmonary venous connection). A moderate-size (1.5 cm) defect was present in the atrial septum in the region of the ostium secundum. There also was a fibrous ring at the base of the pulmonic valve.

The pathophysiology of this lesion is complex and differs depending on the size of the atrial septal defect (Figure 18-1).[4] When the defect is large, the amount of blood that flows into the right ventricle vs. the amount that flows into the left ventricle depends on the relative compliances of both chambers, just as in a large atrial septal defect. Because the right ventricle is more compliant, more blood flows into the right ventricle, resulting functionally in a large left-to-right shunt. In humans, pulmonary blood flow may be 5 times systemic blood flow. Consequently, much more oxygenated blood than deoxygenated blood returns to the right atrium. This results in right atrial blood that is only mildly-to-moderately desaturated. The blood mixes in the right atrium and flows right-to-left into the systemic circulation. Because this blood is not severely desaturated, these patients are usually not cyanotic. Human patients usually compensate for their disease into adulthood and then develop right heart failure.[4] When the atrial septal defect is small and presents resistance to blood flow, a massive functional left-to-right shunting exists. This shunting may be even worse

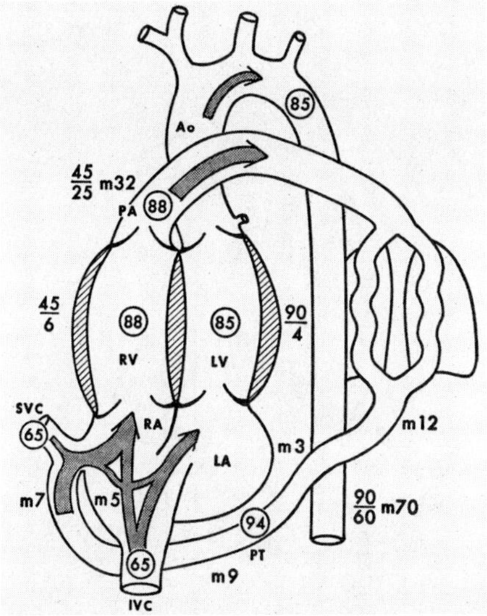

FIGURE 18-1 Schematic representation of the circulation in a patient with total anomalous pulmonary venous return. The pulmonary veins drain into the junction of the cranial or superior vena cava *(SVC)* and the right atrium. Here the oxygenated blood mixes with the deoxygenated blood and then shunts through an atrial septal defect into the left heart. The pulmonary blood flow is high, and the atrial septal defect is large in this patient, allowing for a reasonable arterial oxygen saturation of 85%. There is mild pulmonary hypertension because of the increase in pulmonary blood flow. *IVC,* Inferior (caudal) vena cava; *RV,* right ventricle; *LV,* left ventricle; *RA,* right atrium; *LA,* left atrium. Oxygen saturations are in circles. Pressures are represented as systolic pressure over diastolic pressure and mean *(m)* pressure.

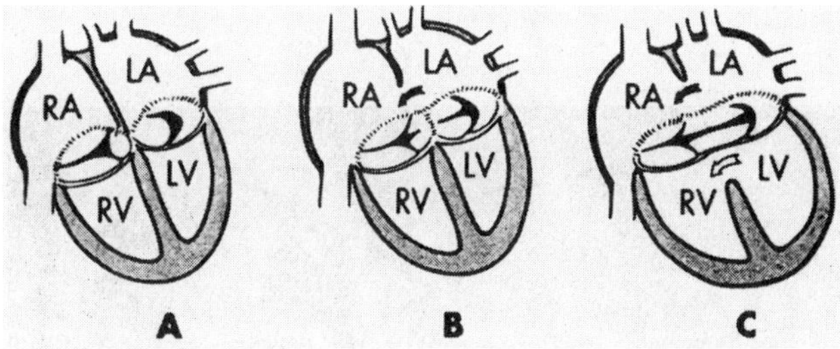

FIGURE 18-2 Schematic drawing of atrioventricular (AV) canal defects. **A,** Normal anatomic relationship of the AV valves and the cardiac septa. **B,** A partial AV canal defect with a septum primum atrial septal defect and abnormally formed AV valves, resulting in a left-to-right shunt at the atrial level and mitral regurgitation. **C,** Complete AV canal defect with a septum primum atrial septal defect, a ventricular septal defect, and one abnormally formed five-leaflet AV valve. (Abbreviations as in Figure 18-1.) (From Park MK: *The pediatric cardiology handbook,* ed 2, St Louis, 1997, Mosby.)

because the resistance to flow contributes even more to the impedance to blood flow going from the right side to the left side than does the compliance of the left ventricle. In addition, the resistance to blood flow increases the right atrial pressure even further than it would with massive left-to-right shunting. Consequently, human patients develop right heart failure within the first months of life. Because resistance to left heart venous return from the right atrium is increased, venous return to the left heart is decreased, the left heart is small on an echocardiogram, and systemic flow (cardiac output) is decreased. Systemic oxygen saturation is usually 85% to 90%.

Treatment of this abnormality is surgical.[4] In a patient with a small atrial septal defect and right heart failure, the defect can be enlarged via a balloon septostomy.

Atrioventricular Canal Defects

Atrioventricular (AV) canal defects are thought to occur because of abnormal development of the endocardial cushions, although this concept has been called into question.[9] AV canal defects have also been called *endocardial cushion defects, atrioventricular septal defects,* and *persistent atrioventricular ostium.*[10] The dorsal endocardial cushion fuses with the septum primum to close the ostium primum in the atrial septum. The dorsal and ventral endocardial cushions fuse to divide the common AV canal into the left and right AV canals. If they do not close, they cannot fuse with the septum primum to close the ostium primum. This failure to fuse also results in the AV valves being placed abnormally low in the ventricle and the aortic valve placed abnormally high. This results in a longer-than-normal left ventricular outflow tract. The long left ventricular outflow tract has been described in cats with this defect.[11] The normal partition between the left ventricular outflow tract and the right atrium is termed the *atrioventricular septum.* In AV canal defects, this septum is absent and a common AV orifice with a common fibrous ring and a five-leaflet valve are present.[12] Normal AV valves have two separate rings that lie at different levels in the heart. In AV canal defects, a five-leaflet valve is present and made up of a left mural leaflet, right mural leaflet, right cranial-ventral leaflet, and two bridging leaflets. The bridging leaflets have no counterpart in the normal heart. The papillary muscles are positioned abnormally, cranial and caudal rather than the normal cranial-medial and caudal-lateral positions. The defect recognized clinically depends on the relationship between the bridging leaflets and the cardiac septa (Figure 18-2). The common AV annulus can be divided into right and left AV orifices if the bridging leaflets connect to the ventricular or atrial septum. When the bridging leaflets are not connected to each other on the left side and are not connected to septa, the common AV annulus is wide open, with the large five-leaflet valve spanning the common orifice. This is termed a *complete atrioventricular canal,* and, in this condition, all four chambers communicate with each other through a septum primum atrial septal defect, a high ventricular septal defect, and AV valve regurgitation. If the bridging leaflets connect to each other on the left side at the septal region and connect with the interatrial septum, there is no atrial septal defect but there is a high ventricular septal defect. If they connect to each other and with the crest of the interventricular septum, an atrial septal defect lies between the floors of the two atria (a septum primum defect) (Figure 18-3). The bridging leaflets make the mitral valve look as if the anterior leaflet is cleft when the bridging leaflets connect on the left side. This cleft is really a commissure between the two bridging leaflets.

Patients with a complete AV canal defect have blood flow among all four chambers (Color Plate 64). Mitral regurgitation results in flow from the left ventricle into the left and right atria in systole (Figure 18-4). The atrial septal defect allows blood to flow from the left atrium to the right atrium. The ventricular septal defect allows blood to flow from the left ventricle to the right ventricle in systole. In diastole, atrial blood flow can enter either the left or the right ventricle. The massive left-to-right shunting and the regurgitation result in severe atrial and ventricular volume overload on both sides of the heart. Systolic pressures in the right and left ventricles are equal, with the pulmonary hypertension initially being due to

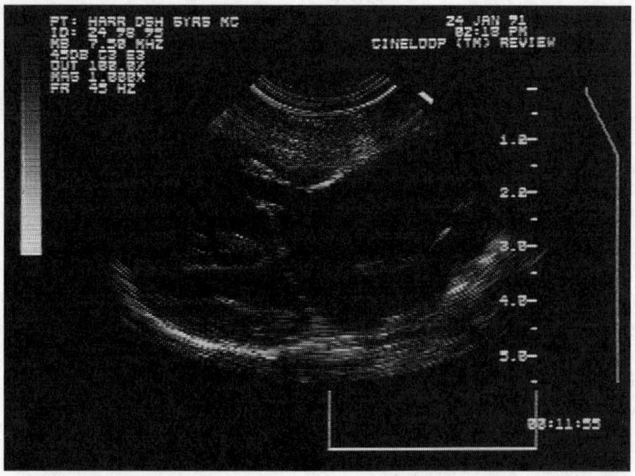

FIGURE 18-3 Two-dimensional echocardiogram from a 5-year-old cat with an atrioventricular (AV) canal defect. The cat originally presented with systolic heart murmurs and a history of dyspnea and collapse. He had been treated with furosemide. Radiographs revealed cardiomegaly and large pulmonary arteries. The echocardiogram shows a large defect between the atria, immediately above the AV valves (ostium primum atrial septal defect). The AV valves appear to bridge the interventricular septum and appear to attach to the top of the septum. The right atrium and right ventricular chamber are severely enlarged because of massive left-to-right shunting across the atrial septal defect. The tricuspid and mitral valves were malformed and leaking. A contrast echocardiogram using microbubbles demonstrated some right-to-left shunting across a small ventricular septal defect.

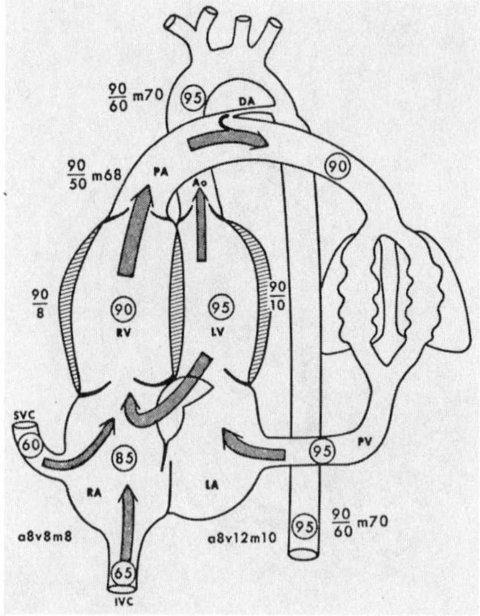

FIGURE 18-4 Schematic drawing of the hemodynamics in a patient with a partial atrioventricular canal defect. There is left-to-right shunting through a septum primum atrial septal defect. In addition, there is mitral regurgitation and regurgitant flow passes through the defect, exacerbating the shunt. (Abbreviations as in Figure 18-1.) (From Rudolph AM: *Congenital diseases of the heart,* Chicago, 1974, Mosby.)

massive pulmonary blood flow. Pulmonary artery pathology may develop over time if the animal survives, resulting in right-to-left shunting if pulmonary vascular resistance increases to the point that it exceeds systemic vascular resistance (Eisenmenger's syndrome).

Patients with primarily a ventricular septal defect have the same physiology as any patient with a large ventricular septal defect (see Chapter 13). Similarly, a patient with primarily an atrial septal defect will have the same physiology as a patient with a large atrial septal defect. Mitral regurgitation, however, commonly occurs with these lesions in patients with an AV canal defect. Moderate-to-severe regurgitation significantly adds to the volume overload.

Atrioventricular canal defects have been most commonly reported in cats.[11,13-15] However, they have also been reported in dogs.[13,16] This abnormality has been described as an apparently hereditary disease in one family of Persian cats in Japan.[11]

Cats with a complete AV canal defect or with an incomplete AV canal defect and severe mitral regurgitation are considered to have severe disease. They generally die at a very young age or present in heart failure when they are young.[17] In the reported Persian colony, kittens with severe disease were commonly in left heart failure at 3 to 6 weeks of age.[11] These cats all appear to have had incomplete forms of AV canal defects. In this colony, cats with less severe disease developed clinical signs at an older age or never developed clinical signs.[11] Pulmonary edema, or ascites, or both may be present in older kittens or cats.[15] Growth is often stunted. A loud heart murmur that is loudest over the left cranial ventral thorax is heard. The murmur is most likely primarily due to mitral regurgitation. The heart is markedly enlarged on the thoracic radiographs. Bundle branch blocks are common on the ECG, probably because the large defect interferes with normal bundle branch growth.[11]

Echocardiographic findings depend on the type of defect present. All four chambers may be enlarged because of volume overload, or variable degrees of enlargement may be present, depending on the exact physiology produced by the defects. A large atrial septal defect, low in the interatrial septum and immediately above the interventricular septum with or without mitral regurgitation, may be the most common finding (an incomplete AV canal defect). The AV valves appear to originate from the crest of the interventricular septum. In a complete AV canal defect, the bridging leaflets of the common AV valve cross the interventricular septum above the ventricular septal defect and below the atrial septal defect. From a short-axis right-sided view, two separate AV valves can be demonstrated in patients with incomplete AV canal defects. The left AV valve has three leaflets, with the commissure between the two leaflets that normally form the anterior leaflet pointing toward the right ventricle. In a complete AV canal defect, common leaflets are present that bridge the interventricular septum. These leaflets may attach to the interventricular septum or float over the septum. One cat has been described in which the cranial leaflet of the mitral valve was continuous with the tricuspid valve while the caudal leaflet was connected to the interventricular septum.[15] The valve leaflets may be thickened and gnarled or may attach directly to a papillary muscle.[18] Color flow Doppler echocardiography demonstrates the mitral regurgitation and the left-to-right shunting. The mitral regurgitant flow signal may course into the right atrium. Measurement of the tricuspid regurgitant jet velocity using continuous-wave Doppler echocardiography is helpful in determining right ventricular systolic pressure. In a patient with an atrial septal defect and mitral regurgitation, right ventricular systolic pressure is normal to slightly increased. Patients with a large ventricular septal defect will have right ventricular systolic hypertension.

Treatment of AV canal defects is usually aimed at treating the heart failure. Hydralazine administration has been effective in infants with AV canal defects at reducing the left-to-right shunting and the amount of mitral regurgitation.[10] Pulmonary artery banding is usually not effective in infants, because most symptomatic patients have significant mitral regurgitation. Attempted surgical

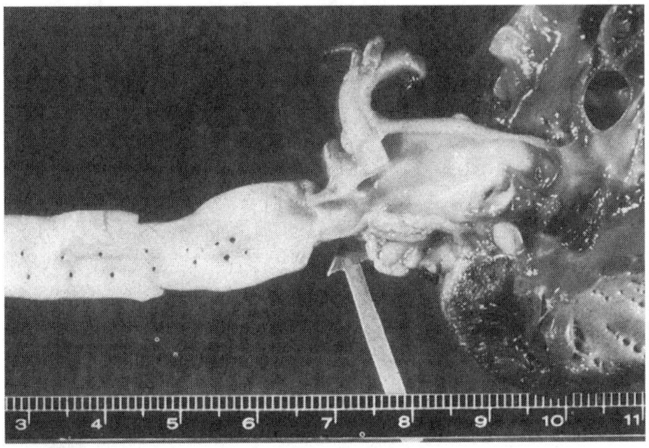

FIGURE 18-5 Postmortem specimen of an aorta from a dog with coarctation of the aorta. An arrow points to the narrowed region of the aorta, just beyond the left subclavian artery. (From Eyster GE, Carrig CB, Baker B, et al: Coarctation of the aorta in a dog, *J Am Vet Med Assoc* 169:426, 1976.)

correction of the atrial septal defect in a dog with an AV canal defect has been described.[13] However, the dog died postoperatively.

Coarctation of the Aorta

Coarctation of the aorta is a common congenital cardiac defect in humans but is extremely rare in the dog. It has not been reported in domestic cats. Coarctation is derived from the Latin verb *arctare* which means "to make tight." Coarctation of the aorta is a narrowing of the aorta. The narrowing usually occurs in the thoracic descending aorta, between the origin of the left subclavian artery and the insertion of the ligamentum arteriosum or ductus arteriosus (the "isthmus" of the aorta) (Figure 18-5). Aortic coarctation is caused by a ridgelike thickening of the media of the aortic wall that protrudes into the aortic lumen from the posterior and lateral wall in humans.[19]

Coarctation in essence produces a form of aortic stenosis. It results in increased aortic pressure proximal to the stenosis when the lumen has decreased to less than 45% to 55% of the normal cross-sectional area. This also results in an increase in systolic pressure within the left ventricle and left ventricular concentric hypertrophy. Systolic pressure increases more than diastolic pressure within the proximal aorta, resulting in an increase in pulse pressure. Distal to the coarctation, systolic pressure decreases more than diastolic pressure, resulting in a decrease in pulse pressure. The consequence is an inequality of pulse pressure in both the upper and lower extremities in humans.[19] The intercostal, internal mammary, and spinal arteries enlarge to provide collateral flow around the coarctation. Enlarged intercostal arteries may cause indentations ("notching") on the ribs, which are visible on radiographs in humans.

The heart murmur produced by aortic coarctation starts after the first heart sound and continues into diastole but is usually not continuous.[20] However, continuous murmurs may be produced in humans by the collateral vessels.[19]

Two reports of coarctation of the aorta in dogs are in the literature. In one case the dog showed no clinical signs.[21] The other dog was a 2-month-old female Boston terrier that presented in left heart failure.[20] The dog had a heart murmur that was loudest in systole but lasted into middiastole. The dog had marked left heart enlargement and what appeared to be a ductus diverticulum. It was initially thought to have a patent ductus arteriosus. Before surgery, a nonselective angiogram was performed and a narrowed region identified in the proximal descending aorta. The dog died of left heart failure following the procedure, and the diagnosis was confirmed at postmortem examination. The dog had a narrowed region of the aorta that started just distally to the subclavian artery and extended 7 mm distal from that point. In addition, the dog had a small ventricular septal defect and probably also had mitral valve dysplasia based on its radiographic findings. That the lesion contributed to the dog's left heart failure is of no doubt. However, it was not the primary cause of this dog's death.

Cor Triatriatum Sinister and Dexter

Cor triatriatum (three cardiac atria) occurs when a fibromuscular membrane divides either the left (sinister) or the right (dexter) atrium into two chambers. Cor triatriatum sinister has been reported in cats and cor triatriatum dexter in dogs.

COR TRIATRIATUM SINISTER

In cor triatriatum sinister it is thought that the common pulmonary vein fails to become incorporated into the left atrium.[22] A membrane divides the left atrium into upper/caudal and lower/cranial chambers. The left auricle is distal to the membrane. The membrane usually has one hole in it (a complete membrane would result in death), but can have multiple fenestrations in humans. The pulmonary veins drain into the upper, or caudal, chamber. The membrane with its small hole increases resistance to flow, resulting in increased pressure in this left atrial chamber and in the pulmonary veins and capillaries. Consequently, pulmonary edema develops or pulmonary hypertension occurs secondary to reactive pulmonary vasoconstriction.

One report of cor triatriatum sinister in a cat is in the veterinary literature.[23] We have seen this lesion in other cats in our clinic. Cats with this abnormality generally present at a young age because they are dyspneic. They may be small for their age. A heart murmur is not heard unless coexisting cardiac disease is present. Thoracic radiographs may reveal an enlarged left atrium and pulmonary edema. Echocardiographic examination reveals a membrane between a dorsal and a ventral left atrial chamber (Figure 18-6 and Color Plate 65). At postmortem examination, a fibromuscular membrane partitions the left atrium into cranial and caudal chambers. Heart weight is generally normal, although the right ventricle can be thickened, presumably because of pulmonary hypertension developing secondary to chronic pulmonary venous hypertension.[23] At postmortem examination, one of our patients had moderate medial hypertrophy of the pulmonary arteries.

Definitive treatment of this abnormality is surgical. Our surgeons have attempted to enlarge the opening in the abnormal septum in two cats during hypothermia and inflow occlusion of blood flow. Both cats have died, either during surgery or postoperatively. Palliative treatment of left heart failure with a diuretic and an angiotensin converting enzyme inhibitor may be beneficial.

COR TRIATRIATUM DEXTER

Cor triatriatum dexter is an uncommon congenital cardiac abnormality seen in dogs. It has been reported with surprising frequency in the veterinary literature.[24-30] Most cases have been reported since 1990. Persistence of the right sinus venosus valve is thought to produce the presence of the intraatrial partition in cor triatriatum dexter.[28,31] The partition is composed of fibromuscular tissue that divides the right atrium into cranial and caudal chambers. The cranial chamber communicates with the tricuspid valve, and the caudal vena

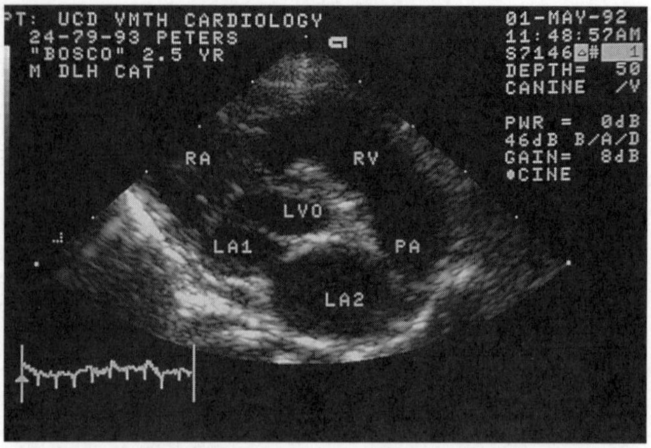

FIGURE 18-6 Two-dimensional echocardiogram from a 2-year-old cat with cor triatriatum sinister. This is a cross-sectional basilar view taken from a right parasternal position. The left atrium is divided into two chambers (*LA1* and *LA2*). The pulmonary veins drain into the upper chamber *(LA2)*. *LVO,* Left ventricular outflow; *RA,* right atrium; *RV,* right ventricular chamber; *PA,* main pulmonary artery. The cat also had an ostium primum atrial septal defect and moderate pulmonary hypertension. It lived until at least 4 years of age and was then lost to follow-up.

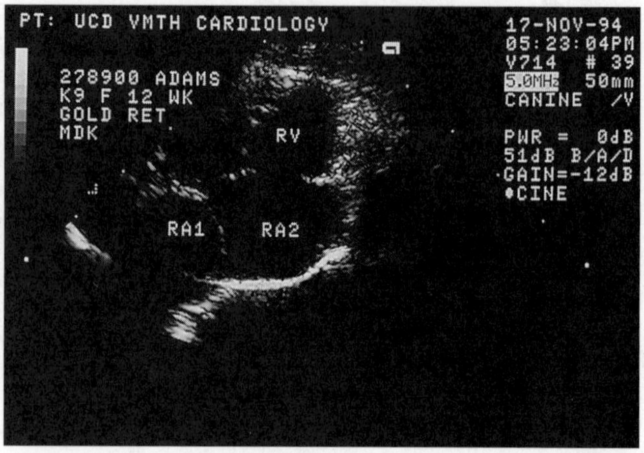

FIGURE 18-7 Two-dimensional echocardiogram from a 3-month-old golden retriever. The dog was referred because of ascites and a suspected portosystemic shunt. An abdominal ultrasound revealed enlarged hepatic veins. At consultation, no echocardiographic abnormalities were identified. A repeat echocardiogram revealed two right atrial chambers (*RA1* and *RA2*) separated by a membrane. This was diagnostic of cor triatriatum dexter. *RV,* Right ventricle.

cava and coronary sinus empty into the caudal chamber. The partition usually has one or more holes in it, although it may be imperforate. The increased resistance to caudal caval flow results in an increase in pressure in the caudal right atrial chamber, caudal vena cava, and hepatic veins. Hepatomegaly and ascites result. The ascites is the result of the increased capillary (sinusoidal) pressure in the liver, with resultant transudation of fluid from the liver into the peritoneal space. Because hepatic sinusoids are more porous than other capillary beds, protein leaks along with fluid, resulting in a high-protein modified transudate.

Obstruction of the caudal right atrium, caudal vena cava, or hepatic veins leading to ascites is often called *Budd-Chiari syndrome* or *Budd-Chiari–like syndrome.*[32] This syndrome includes many other lesions, including right atrial tumor, compression or invasion of the caudal vena cava by tumor, thrombosis of the caudal vena cava, kinking of the caudal vena cava following trauma, and venoocclusive disease of the hepatic veins.[33]

Clinical presentation. Dogs that present with cor triatriatum dexter are usually young. On physical examination, ascites is usually present. The fluid is usually a modified transudate with a protein content greater than 2 g/dL and few cells. The jugular veins are not distended, although the caudal superficial epigastric veins may be distended. No heart murmur is present. Some dogs may have diarrhea, presumably because of intestinal lymphangiectasia secondary to chronic intestinal venous hypertension.[30]

Diagnosis. The diagnosis is often first suspected when a markedly enlarged caudal vena cava is identified on a thoracic radiograph. The cardiac silhouette is normal in size and shape. The ECG is usually normal, although a tall *P* wave in lead II may be observed. Echocardiography usually provides the definitive diagnosis in our clinic. The membrane and the two right atrial chambers can be identified using either a right-sided long-axis view or a left-sided four-chamber view (Figure 18-7). Color flow Doppler can be used to identify flow through the perforation in the membrane (Color Plate 66). Flow velocity is low. Cardiac catheterization can be performed. Two catheters are usually used. One is passed from the femoral vein to the caudal chamber, and the other is passed from the jugular vein to the cranial chamber. Pressure in the cranial chamber is usually normal, whereas pressure in the caudal chamber is increased, usually to greater than 10 mm Hg. The pressure gradient can be calculated. Occasionally, the catheter can be passed through the orifice in the membrane, so that only one catheter is required to perform the catheterization. Injection of contrast medium into the cranial chamber reveals normal flow through the right heart. Injection into the caudal chamber usually reveals an enlarged caudal chamber and caudal vena cava with contrast medium jetting through the perforation in the membrane and into the cranial chamber. When the membrane is imperforate, collateral blood vessels must be present to route blood cranially to the right heart. In one such case that we treated, a vessel believed to be a remnant of a persistent left cranial vena cava originated from the coronary sinus. It carried blood dorsally to the vertebral venous circulation, probably using a hemiazygous vein.[28] Blood then flowed into the azygous vein and emptied into the cranial vena cava. This route was effective, because the dog did not show clinical signs until it was 7 years old.

Treatment of cor triatriatum dexter is surgical. Long-term medical management is generally unrewarding. Balloon dilation has been attempted but may be unsuccessful.[31] Presumably the membrane is commonly too fibrous to be amenable to rupture by a balloon. However, we have two anecdotal reports of successful balloon dilation of a cor triatriatum membrane, so it is feasible in some cases. Several surgical techniques have been described. In one, surgery is performed during occlusion of the venous return (inflow) to the heart, with or without total-body hypothermia.[28] After inflow is occluded, a side-biting vascular clamp is used to entrap part of the right atrial wall. An atriotomy is performed, the clamp removed, and the membrane visualized. The membrane is excised. The right heart is filled with saline to remove air, the vascular clamp is replaced, and inflow occlusion is released. Inflow occlusion should last no more than several minutes. The incision is then sutured closed. Another technique involves placing a purse-string suture around an incision in the right auricle and passing an instrument into the right atrium to tear the membrane.[25] This technique has the advantage of not requiring cessation of blood flow. However, the surgical site

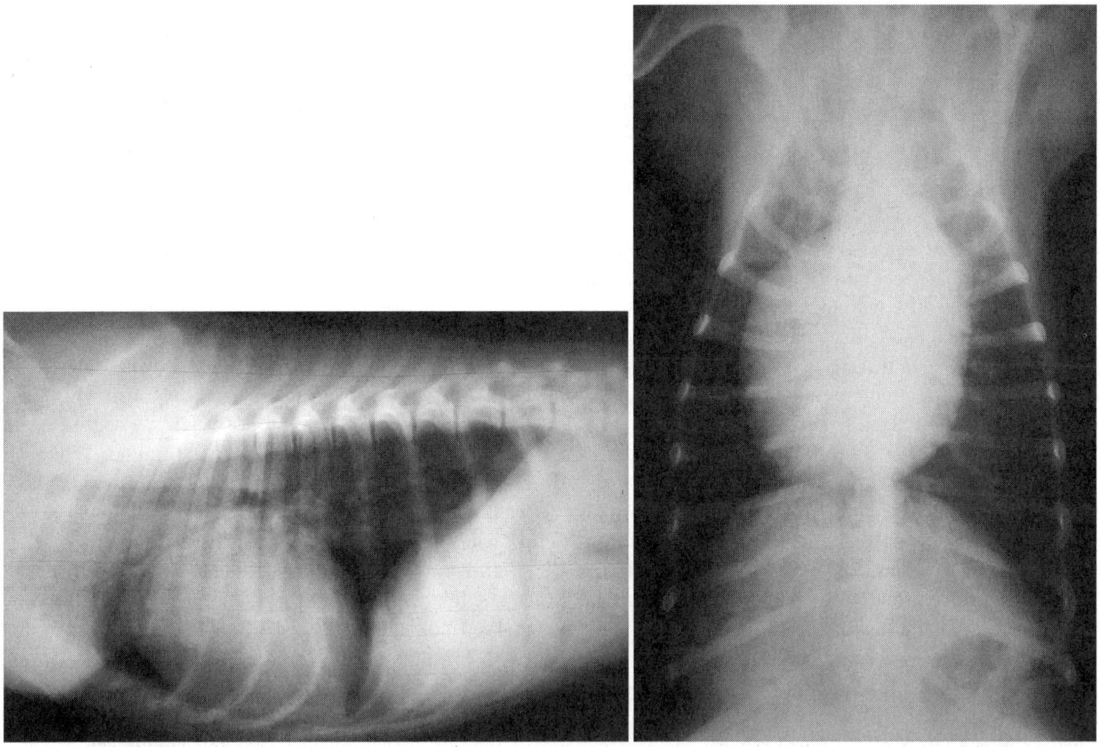

FIGURE 18-8 Thoracic radiographs from a young dog with a left-to-right shunting patent ductus arteriosus. On the dorsoventral view, the apex of the heart is in the right hemithorax. This is an example of dextrocardia.

within the heart cannot be visualized. Following surgery, recovery is usually uneventful and the ascites should reduce noticeably within several days.

A slight variation on the theme, in which a membrane is situated caudally to the coronary sinus, obstructing caudal caval flow, has also been reported in dogs.[30,34] One dog had a pleural effusion and ascites. Surgical resection was accomplished by occluding only the caudal vena cava.

A puppy with a three-chambered right atrium has been reported.[35] In this dog, the cranial vena cava and the caudal vena cava emptied into separate chambers, both of which communicated with a chamber ventral to these chambers. The third chamber communicated with the tricuspid valve. This puppy had ascites, pleural effusion, and subcutaneous edema, especially in the caudal limbs.

Dextrocardia and Situs Inversus

Dextrocardia means that the heart is positioned in the right hemithorax, with the apex pointing toward the right (Figure 18-8).[36] Dextrocardia can result from the heart being pushed to the right by fluid, air, or tissue, or it can be a primary congenital abnormality. When primary, it can be an isolated abnormality or associated with situs inversus, in which all organs in the body are formed as a mirror image of normal. Dextrocardia in the presence of situs solitus (normal organ orientation) is often associated with major intracardiac abnormalities in humans, including atrioventricular discordance and transposition of the great arteries.[37] In our experience, it is usually a benign abnormality in dogs and is usually noted as an incidental finding. The heart is normally situated in the right hemithorax in early gestation. Lack of normal leftward migration of the cardiac mass has been used to explain dextrocardia in situs solitus.[37]

Situs inversus usually is not associated with cardiac abnormalities other than dextrocardia in dogs, although abdominal vascular abnormalities may occur.[36,38-40] More commonly, situs inversus is associated with respiratory abnormalities such as sinusitis, bronchitis, and bronchiectasis. This syndrome was first described in humans in 1933 by Kartagener.[41] In 1976, it was shown that human patients with this syndrome lacked a portion of their respiratory cilia and sperm, called *dynein arms*.[42] The resultant lack of ciliary motility in this syndrome results in mucous accumulation in the upper and lower airways, leading to the clinical disease and clinical signs. It can also lead to decreased sperm motility. Similar abnormalities in ciliary ultrastructure have been reported in a dog.[38] However, another dog without the ciliary abnormalities has also been reported.[43]

Double-Outlet Right Ventricle

Double-outlet right ventricle (DORV) refers to a cardiac abnormality in which all of one great artery and most of the other great artery originate from the right ventricle. Associated congenital cardiac abnormalities are common. The resultant physiology and consequent clinical signs can simulate those of tetralogy of Fallot, a large ventricular septal defect, or transposition of the great arteries.[44] Anatomically, the great arteries can be related in three different ways. They can be normally related, with the aorta placed caudal and to the right of the pulmonary artery. The aorta can run parallel with the pulmonary artery but originate to the right and cranially to the pulmonic valve. Lastly, the aorta can lie cranially and the pulmonary artery caudally and to the right. Usually a large ventricular septal defect is present that is not resistive to blood flow. Consequently, the right and left ventricular systolic pressures are equal. The ventricular septal defect can lie beneath the aortic valve or pulmonic valve. Pulmonic stenosis is a common associated abnormality in humans.[44]

Patients with significant pulmonic stenosis can have either a subpulmonic or a subaortic ventricular septal defect. Because of the greater resistance to blood flow into the pulmonary circulation, right-to-left shunting and cyanosis occur. Blood flow streams from the left ventricle through the ventricular septal defect and out the aorta in patients with a subaortic ventricular septal defect without pulmonic stenosis. Consequently, the physiology mimics that of a large ventricular septal defect, and left heart failure is common early in life with pulmonary vascular disease and right-to-left shunting later in life. Patients with a subpulmonic ventricular septal defect and no pulmonic stenosis have clinical features similar to those of transposition of the great arteries. They have variable degrees of systemic desaturation and can develop heart failure.

Two dogs and six cats have been reported with this abnormality.[45-49] Three of the cats have been diagnosed at postmortem examination after they died between 1 and 6 days of age.[45] One kitten also had a complete atrioventricular canal. The second had no interventricular septum, and the aorta opened to the right of the pulmonic valve and the crista supraventricularis. The pulmonic valve opened to the left of the crista supraventricularis. The aortic opening was narrowed. The third kitten was identical, but the ventricular septal defect was smaller (2 to 3 m). Surgical repair of DORV has been reported in one cat.[48] The sibling of this kitten died of left heart failure. It had a DORV with a large subaortic ventricular septal defect and no pulmonic stenosis. A section of this kitten's aorta was harvested at the postmortem examination and used as a homograft to connect the ventricular septal defect with the aorta during open heart surgery of the first kitten. Surgery was performed under deep hypothermia. The kitten was alive at the time of the report, 2 years after surgery. The dog with DORV was a research dog diagnosed at 6 years of age.[49] It had a history of seizures and died unexpectedly. At postmortem examination, it had DORV, with the aorta to the right of the pulmonary artery. Pulmonic stenosis was present, and the circumference of the aortic valve was 4.5 cm and the pulmonic valve was 2.0 cm. The ventricular septal defect was 2 cm in diameter and subaortic. A kitten with DORV is presented in Figures 18-9 and Color Plates 67 and 68.

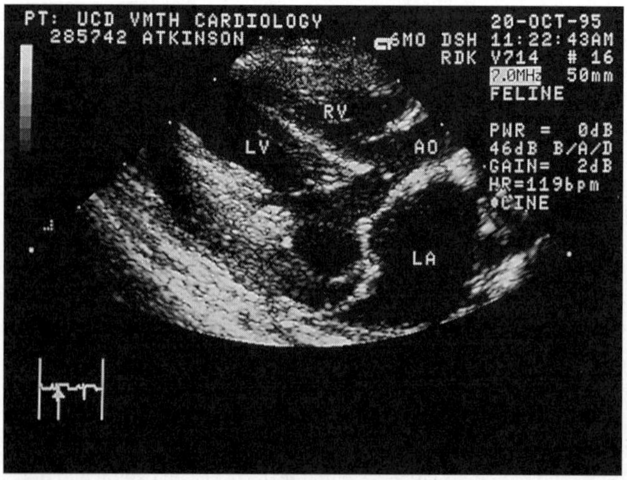

FIGURE 18-9 Two-dimensional echocardiogram from a 6-month-old cat with a double-outlet right ventricle. The aorta (AO) originates from the right ventricle. A ventricular septal defect is present. *LA,* Left atrium; *LV,* left ventricular chamber; *RV,* right ventricular chamber.

Interruption of the Aortic Arch

Interruption of the aortic arch is a rare congenital cardiac abnormality in which the ascending and descending aorta have no normal communication. This anomaly has been reported twice in dogs.[50,51] In humans the interruption occurs distally to the left subclavian artery (type A), between the left subclavian and the left carotid arteries (type B), or between the left and right carotid arteries (type C). Types A and B are the most common. A ventricular septal defect is commonly present. In infants, distal aortic flow is maintained through a patent ductus arteriosus. If the ductus arteriosus closes, infants become clinically ill and moribund. Without intervention they develop severe heart failure and die within the first days or weeks of life. Most puppies and kittens with this abnormality probably die before being seen by a veterinarian.

In the two cases in the veterinary literature, life was maintained in one by the presence of a patent ductus arteriosus and the other by marked collateral flow.[50,51] The first case was in a 3-month-old English bulldog that presented because of dyspnea and decreased vigor.[50] The dog had a left basilar ejection-quality heart murmur. A nonselective angiogram revealed subaortic stenosis and interruption of the aortic arch distal to the left subclavian artery. Flow to the descending aorta, however, was maintained by blood flowing through the costocervical trunk to the vertebral artery to the aorta. This abnormality was corrected surgically by placing a conduit between the ascending and descending aorta. The second case was a 4-month-old female Lakeland terrier. It was referred because of a heart murmur and exercise intolerance.[51] The dog had a crescendo-decrescendo heart murmur heard best over the left base and a plateau-quality murmur heard best at the right sternal border. Mild polycythemia (PCV = 55%) was present. It had evidence of right heart enlargement on its ECG and thoracic radiographs. Echocardiography revealed a right ventricle that was both eccentrically and concentrically hypertrophied and systolic anterior motion of the mitral valve. At cardiac catheterization, a left ventricular injection of a contrast medium identified complete interruption of the aortic arch between the brachiocephalic trunk and the left subclavian artery. Collateral vessels arose from the vertebral and right subclavian arteries that connected with the descending aorta but appeared to produce minimal flow. A right ventricular injection of contrast medium revealed a large (grade 6) patent ductus arteriosus with resultant shunting of blood from the pulmonary artery to the descending aorta, including the left subclavian artery. A small ventricular septal defect was also suspected. While the dog was breathing room air, the arterial oxygen tension in the carotid artery was 72 mm Hg and in the femoral artery was 46 mm Hg. The oxygen tension in the rear limbs apparently was not low enough to result in differential cyanosis, evidenced by the fact that this was not detected on physical examination. Life in this dog was maintained either because the ductus arteriosus remained physiologically patent after birth or because it was born with no smooth muscle in its ductus arteriosus so patency was maintained. At postmortem examination, the complete interruption of the aortic arch, the large patent ductus arteriosus, and the ventricular septal defect were verified. In addition, a discrete incomplete subaortic fibrous ring was present. Medial hypertrophy, sclerosis, and hyalinization of the pulmonary arterioles and small arteries, along with plexiform lesions in the arterioles were present. Duplication of elastic membranes in the large arteries was also present. These findings are all consistent with pulmonary hypertension that must have been present.

Persistent Left Cranial Vena Cava

During embryonic development, the cardinal venous system is paired. The left anterior (cranial) cardinal vein normally regresses, and the left common cardinal vein remains to drain the coronary circulation and form the coronary sinus. The right anterior (cranial) and right common cardinal veins remain to form the cranial vena cava. Occasionally the left cranial cardinal vein does not regress, resulting in a persistent left cranial vena cava. A persistent left cranial vena cava may occur in conjunction with a normal right cranial vena cava to form bilateral cranial vena cavae, or the left cranial vena cava may occur without a right cranial vena cava. Usually the persistent left cranial vena cava drains into the great cardiac vein and coronary sinus, resulting in enlargement of these structures. This abnormality has been reported in both dogs and cats.[52-56]

A persistent cranial vena cava can exist by itself or with other cardiac abnormalities. A persistent left cranial vena cava does not produce any clinically significant hemodynamic abnormality by itself. However, it can cause problems during cardiac catheterization, pacemaker implantation, and thoracic surgery. If a persistent left cranial vena cava is present and right heart catheterization or lead placement is attempted from the left jugular vein, the catheter or lead passes into the right atrium via the coronary sinus. From this direction passing the device into the right ventricle is usually impossible. For this reason, the right jugular vein is preferred for these procedures in dogs. Occasionally, during cardiac surgery the persistent left cranial vena cava will obstruct visualization of a cardiac structure, such as the ligamentum arteriosum in an animal with a persistent right aortic arch.[57,58]

The diagnosis of persistent left cranial vena cava can be made using either angiography or echocardiography.[54,55] On angiography, the persistent left cranial vena cava passes to the left of the heart in the atrioventricular groove and then behind the heart to empty via the coronary sinus (Figure 18-10). On echocardiography, a dilated coronary sinus may be seen in the right atrium or the persistent left cranial vena cava may be visualized passing behind the left atrium to the right atrium. (Figure 18-11)

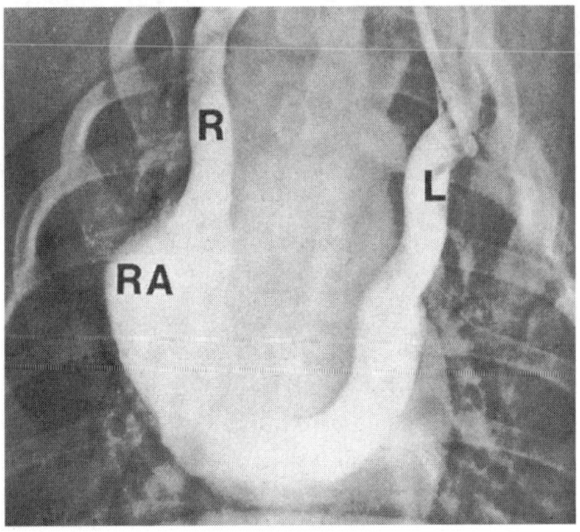

FIGURE 18-10 Angiogram from a dog with a persistent left cranial vena cava. A contrast agent has been injected simultaneously into right *(R)* and left *(L)* cranial vena cavae. *RA,* Right atrium. (From Ettinger SJ, Suter PF: *Canine cardiology,* Philadelphia, 1970, WB Saunders.)

Pulmonary Atresia with Intact Ventricular Septum

Pulmonary valve atresia with an intact ventricular septum can be viewed as the most severe form of pulmonic stenosis.[59] It is characterized by complete obstruction to forward flow from the right ventricle to the pulmonary artery because of an imperforate pulmonic valve. Usually this lesion is associated with varying degrees of hypoplasia of the right ventricle and tricuspid valve. An atrial septal defect and a source of pulmonary blood flow must be present to maintain life.

In infants, the ductus arteriosus is initially patent and is the only source of pulmonary blood flow. With this lesion, all the systemic blood returning to the right heart shunts across an atrial septal defect, mixes with the pulmonary venous blood returning to the left atrium, and then flows into the left heart and systemic circulation. The resultant desaturation of blood depends on the relative amounts of systemic flow and pulmonary flow. For example, if they are equal and pulmonary vein saturation is 90% and systemic vein saturation is 50%, systemic saturation will be 70%. Consequently, the amount of ductal flow determines the systemic arterial saturation. As the ductus arteriosus closes in early life, patients start to experience signs referable to hypoxia.[60] In infants, complete closure usually results in death. Ductal patency is maintained in these infants by infusing prostaglandin E_1. Infants change from blue and pale to pink within minutes of starting an infusion.[60]

A dog with pulmonary atresia with an intact ventricular septum has been reported.[61] This was a 7-week-old male wirehaired fox terrier that presented for stunted growth. The puppy was slightly cyanotic at presentation and had a heart murmur. The murmur was loudest at the left heart base and began with the first heart sound and continued past the second heart sound into diastole and at times sounded continuous. The ECG revealed sinus tachycardia, tall *P* waves, and terminal QRS forces directed toward the right. The radiographs suggested left ventricular enlargement, left atrial enlargement, and a decreased main pulmonary artery segment. Echocardiographic findings were not reported. At cardiac catheterization, injection of contrast medium into the right atrium revealed absence of flow into the right ventricle, retrograde flow into the vena cavae, and flow into the left atrium and left ventricle. A patent ductus arteriosus was not evident. Instead, a dilated bronchial artery originated at the level of T6 and coursed cranially and then caudally to the hilus. There it gave off branches to the lungs. At postmortem examination, the findings from cardiac catheterization were confirmed. A large fenestrated atrial septal defect was present. The tricuspid valve and right ventricle were markedly hypoplastic. The pulmonary valve was atretic and the pulmonary trunk had no lumen, although it was oriented normally. No evidence of a ligamentum arteriosum or a ductus arteriosus was found. Agenesis of the ductus arteriosus was diagnosed. The large bronchial artery that supplied the lungs was identified. Flow through this vessel was thought to cause the heart murmur in this dog. The agenesis of the ductus arteriosus may have facilitated collateral channels in utero and allowed life to continue in this pup after birth.

Transposition of the Great Arteries

Transposition of the great arteries is discordant ventriculoarterial connection of the great arteries in which the aorta originates from the morphologic right ventricle and the pulmonary artery originates from the morphologic left ventricle (Color Plate 69).[62] Consequently,

A

B

C

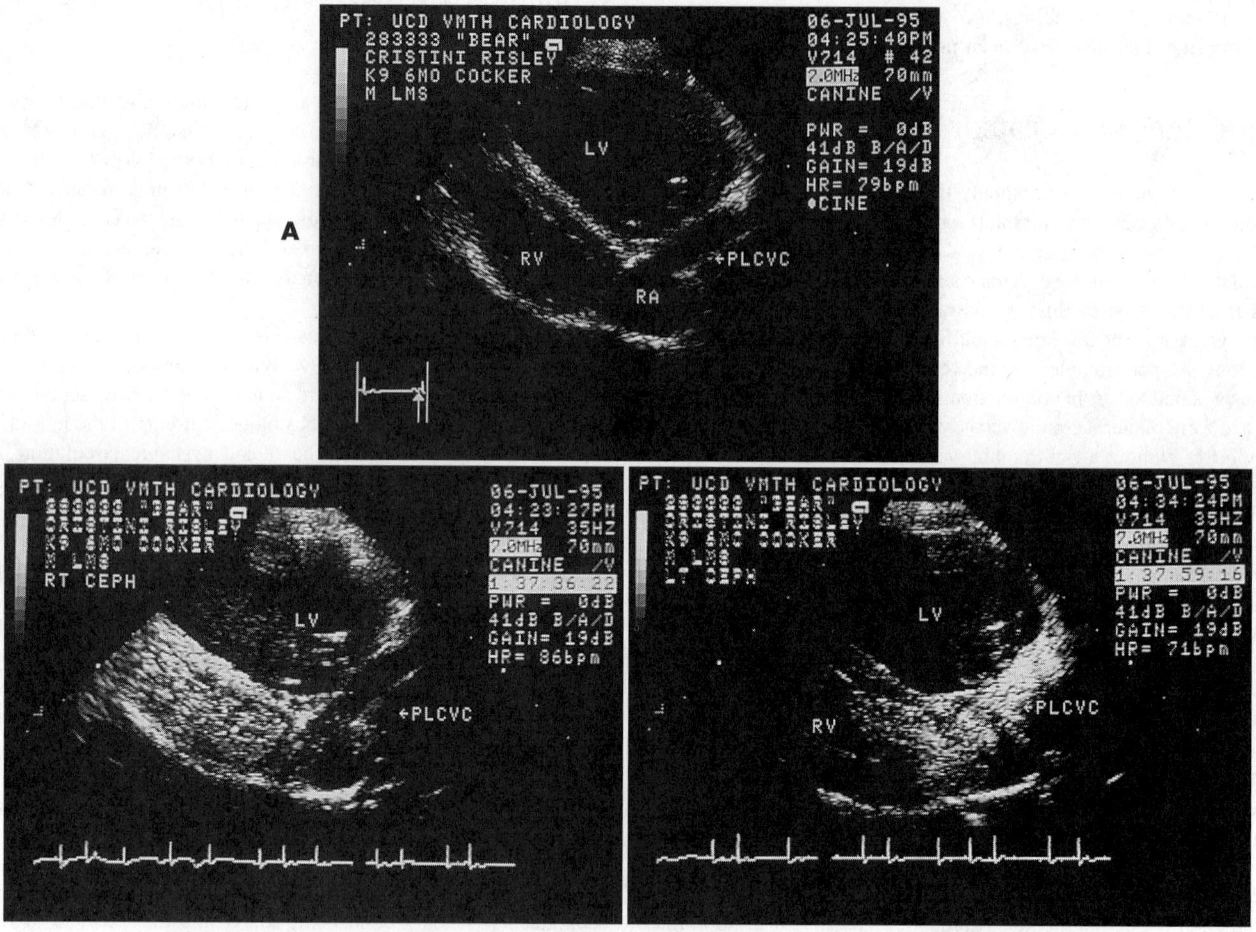

FIGURE 18-11 Two-dimensional echocardiograms from a 6-month-old cocker spaniel with a persistent cranial vena cava (PLCVC). **A,** The PLCVC is seen as it courses along the atrioventricular groove to the right atrium *(RA)*. **B,** To document that a right cranial vena cava was still present, microbubble-laden saline was injected into the right cephalic vein. The bubbles can be visualized in the right ventricle but not in the right atrium *(RA)* or PLCVC. **C,** Injection of saline into the left cephalic vein resulted in visualization of bubbles in the PLCVC, right atrium, and right ventricle. *LV,* Left ventricle.

instead of the circulation being in series, it is in parallel. For life to continue, a communication must exist between the systemic and pulmonary circulations. Before the advent of cardiac catheterization and surgery, 90% of infants with this abnormality died within the first year of life. Presumably, most puppies and kittens with this abnormality die before examination by a veterinarian. Only two kittens and one puppy have been reported with this abnormality.[63-65] The defect was produced in one kitten by the experimental administration of thalidomide.[65]

Physiologically, transposition of the great arteries is two circulations in parallel, with mixing of blood from the two circulations occurring via one or more communications between the two circulations. The communication may be a ventricular septal defect, an atrial septal defect, or either, along with a patent ductus arteriosus. Only left-to-right shunting occurs with a patent ductus arteriosus, so another communication must be present with a patent ductus arteriosus to maintain life. Left-to-right shunting and right-to-left shunting must occur, and the amount must be equal. Otherwise one circulation would become overloaded, and the other would become underloaded and empty. The larger the communication or the more communications there are, the more mixing that occurs. Most infants become dramatically worse when their ductus arteriosus closes a few days after birth.[62] Infusion of prostaglandin E_1 to open the ductus arteriosus often dramatically reduces the cyanosis. Infants with both a large ventricular septal defect and an atrial septal defect may not be cyanotic.

In one case report, a kitten was presented with this abnormality at 4 months of age for routine vaccination.[63] It had a loud continuous heart murmur on physical examination. Radiographs revealed a large heart with an enlarged main pulmonary artery and a hypervascular lung field with increased interstitial lung density (mild pulmonary edema). A nonselective injection of contrast medium entered the right heart and exited into the aorta. Subsequently, a selective injection of contrast material into the aortic arch demonstrated flow from the aorta to the pulmonary artery via a patent ductus arteriosus. In subsequent films, blood flowed from the left ventricle into the pulmonary artery. Oxygen tension in the right ventricle was 78 mm Hg and in the proximal aorta was 127 mm Hg, providing evidence of blood shunting from the left ventricle to the right ventricle through a ventricular septal defect. The kitten died after the procedure, and postmortem examination of the heart confirmed the presence of transposition of the great arteries with a ventricular septal defect and a patent ductus arteriosus. Apparently life was maintained in this kitten because of the predominant shunting of oxygenated blood from

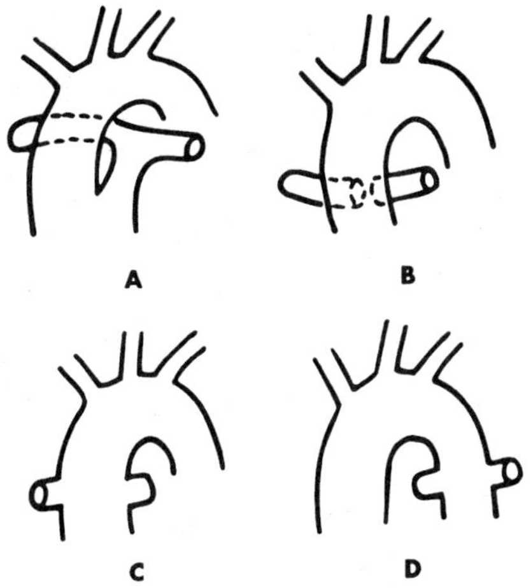

FIGURE 18-12 Anatomic types of persistent truncus arteriosus. **A,** Type I. **B,** Type II. **C,** Type III. **D,** Type IV. (From Park MK: *The pediatric cardiology handbook,* ed 2, St Louis, 1997, Mosby.)

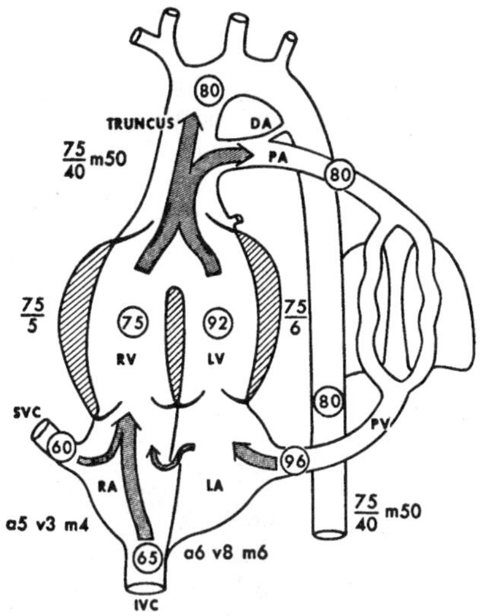

FIGURE 18-13 Schematic drawing of the hemodynamics in a patient with a truncus arteriosus. One large vessel originates from the heart. The pulmonary artery originates from this vessel, distal to its origin from the heart. In this example, both left-to-right shunting and right-to-left shunting of blood are shown. Shunting occurs in the ventricle through the ventricular septal defect and in the common trunk. (Abbreviations as in Figure 18-15.) (From Rudolph AM: *Congenital diseases of the heart,* St Louis, 1974, Mosby.)

the left ventricle to the right ventricle and aorta and the predominant flow of unoxygenated blood from the aorta to the pulmonary artery. Most likely the kitten would have died soon after birth if its ductus arteriosus had closed.

Truncus and Pseudotruncus Arteriosus

Truncus arteriosus is a rare congenital defect that has been described in dogs and cats.[45,66,67] It can be defined as a single great artery that arises from the base of the heart, giving origin to the systemic, pulmonary, and coronary arteries. This lesion appears in some keeshond dogs bred for conotruncal abnormalities and appears to be the most severe form of the phenotypic abnormalities associated with this genetic abnormality.[67] Consequently, the embryologic origin of this defect appears to be a complete failure of the conal septum and the truncal septum to septate (conotruncal hypoplasia) during fetal development. This makes persistent truncus arteriosus a "first cousin" of tetralogy of Fallot.

Several forms of truncus arteriosus have been described (Figure 18-12). In 1949 Collett and Edwards[68] devised the following classification of truncus arteriosus:

Type 1: A single pulmonary trunk and a single ascending aorta arise from the truncus arteriosus.

Type 2: The right and left pulmonary arteries arise close together from the dorsal wall of the truncus arteriosus.

Type 3: One or both pulmonary arteries come off independently from either side of the truncus arteriosus.

Type 4: No pulmonary arteries come off the truncus arteriosus. Pulmonary circulation is provided solely by bronchial arteries.

A ventricular septal defect is almost always present. In humans, the truncal root straddles the ventricular septal defect in about 60% of cases, and the truncus overrides either the right or left ventricle in the other 40%. The truncus arteriosus has one large valve. This valve is usually abnormal and may have 2 to 5 cusps in humans.[69] About 50% of humans with truncus arteriosus have aortic regurgitation, and in 50% of these it is moderate to severe.

Truncus arteriosus often results in a large left-to-right shunt as a result of the marked increase in pulmonary blood flow. In the early stages, pulmonary vascular resistance is much lower than systemic vascular resistance, so blood preferentially flows into the pulmonary circulation. This results in a left heart volume overload and may lead to left heart failure. Venous blood from the right ventricle is ejected into the systemic circulation (a right-to-left shunt), resulting in hypoxemia. In the early stages, pulmonary hypertension exists primarily because of increased flow, although pulmonary resistance is probably also physiologically increased. Over time, the increased pulmonary artery pressure and flow result in intimal and medial pulmonary artery hypertrophy, leading to progressive increases in pulmonary vascular resistance and greater and greater right-to-left shunting. In this way, the pathophysiology of truncus arteriosus is very similar to that of a large (right-to-left shunting) patent ductus arteriosus (Figure 18-13).

Truncus arteriosus is rarely observed in dogs and cats. Infants with truncus arteriosus usually develop left heart failure within the first few days of life. Presumably, puppies and kittens with truncus arteriosus die within this period and consequently are never observed by a veterinarian. A 5-week-old male mixed-breed terrier has been described in the literature.[66] This dog had a grade 4 systolic heart murmur and was euthanized at the time of presentation. It had primarily a type 4 truncus. It's main pulmonary artery originated from the truncus but was extremely hypoplastic. Most of the pulmonary blood flow came from a modified bronchial artery that originated in the descending aorta and delivered a branch to the right and left lungs. The opening to this artery was only 3 mm in diameter. Consequently, this dog probably did not have a large amount of pulmonary blood flow and so did not develop left heart failure. Histologically, the intrapulmonary pulmonary arteries had mild hypertrophy of the vascular muscle but no intimal hypertrophy. A kitten with truncus arteriosus is presented in Figure 18-14.

In pseudotruncus arteriosus, the pulmonary artery is present but is vestigial to hypoplastic (Figure 18-15). This represents an extreme form of tetralogy of Fallot. The aorta and aortic valve are large and lie over a ventricular septal defect. Consequently, on cardiac ultrasound the anatomy looks much like that of a truncus arteriosus. An 8-month-old Labrador retriever cross has been described in the literature with this lesion.[70] This dog presented after the owner noticed it collapse and turn grey. The dog was cyanotic on physical examination, and the cyanosis increased with exercise. The hematocrit was increased, at 61%. Thoracic radiographs revealed a markedly enlarged aorta and right heart enlargement. At cardiac catheterization, an injection of contrast medium into the right ventricle demonstrated right-to-left shunting of blood through a ventricular septal defect. The right and left ventricles pumped blood into a large aorta that straddled the ventricular septal defect. A small patent ductus ateriosus was present. The diagnosis was truncus arteriosus with a ventricular septal defect and a patent ductus arteriosus. At postmortem examination, the catheterization findings were verified, but a hypoplastic pulmonary artery was also identified adjacent to the aorta. The pulmonic valve was atretic, so no blood flowed from the right ventricle to the pulmonary artery. The patent ductus arteriosus was only 1 mm in diameter. Consequently, this dog had marked right-to-left shunting within the heart, with only a small amount of left-to-right shunting through the patent ductus arteriosus to the lungs. The dog also had numerous enlarged bronchial vessels present in an attempt to increase pulmonary blood flow, but based on his clinical presentation they were inadequate.

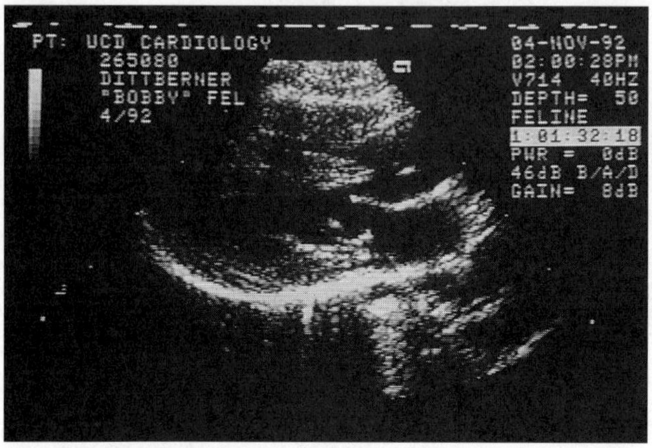

FIGURE 18-14 Two-dimensional echocardiogram from a 7-month-old cat with a presumed truncus arteriosus. One vessel lies over the top of the interventricular septum. The left and right ventricles clearly eject into this vessel. There was no evidence of a pulmonary artery originating from the heart. However, a very small vessel could not be ruled out completely. Consequently, this cat could have also had a pseudotruncus arteriosus. The cat presented with a heart murmur that was decreasing in intensity over time and exercise intolerance. It had mild polycythemia and had probably developed pulmonary hypertension by the time of the examination.

Vascular Ring Anomalies

Vascular rings occur when one or more aortic arch abnormalities, with or without a patent ductus arteriosus or ligamentum arteriosum, produce a ring that completely encircles the trachea and esophagus, leading to constriction of these structures (Figure 18-16).[71] Persistent right aortic arch with a left ductus arteriosus or ligamentum arteriosum is the most common type of vascular ring anomaly in dogs and cats.[57,72] It occurs with much greater frequency in the dog than in the cat. Vascular rings most commonly cause esophageal constriction and subsequent regurgitation.

During fetal development, the aortic arch exists as paired arteries that originate from the aortic sac on the ventral surface of the embryo and course cephalad (Color Plate 1).[71] They then turn and course dorsally and caudally to produce the paired dorsal aorta. Ventral and dorsal outgrowths from these structures come together in the middle to form the aortic arches. These arches develop and regress independently during fetal development.[58] Remnants persist and form parts of the adult circulation. In mammals, the first, second, and fifth aortic arches completely regress. The third aortic arches form the internal carotid arteries. The left fourth arch forms the roof of the aorta, and the right fourth arch forms the root of the subclavian artery. The sixth arches form the pulmonary arteries, and the left retains its

A

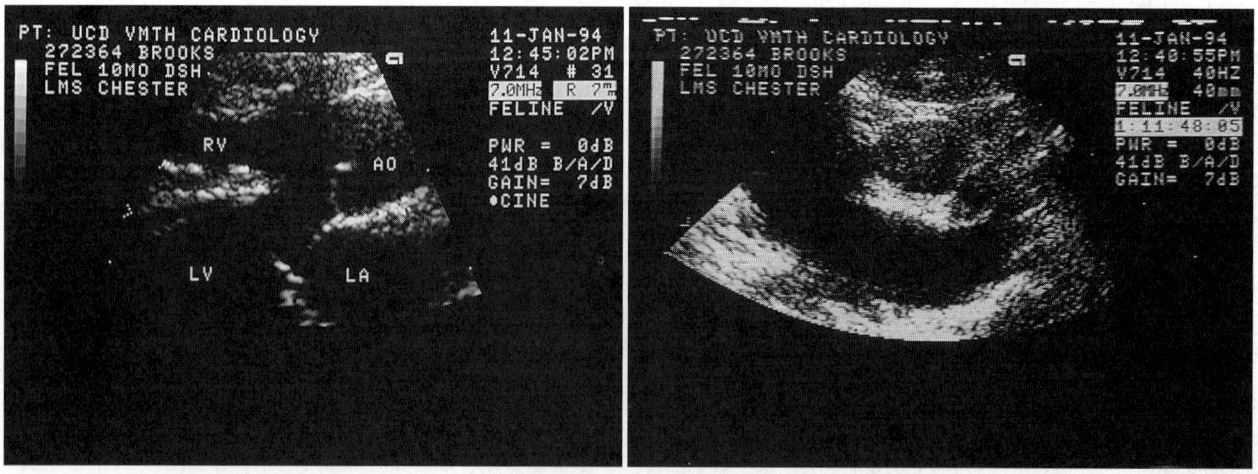

B

FIGURE 18-15 Two-dimensional echocardiograms from a cat with a pseudotruncus arteriosus. **A,** Similar to Figure 18-14, a large vessel originates above the interventricular septum. The left ventricle *(LV)* and the right ventricle *(RV)* eject into this vessel. **B,** In a cross-sectional view from the right side, the large vessel can be visualized. A smaller vessel at the 4-o'clock position (in relation to the large vessel) is also visualized. This is a small pulmonary artery. Identification of the pulmonary artery rules out truncus arteriosus. This means that the large vessel is an aorta *(AO)*. *LA,* Left atrium.

connection with the dorsal aorta to form the ductus arteriosus. The postbranchial period starts with the regression of the right sixth aortic arch.[73] The left and right subclavian arteries move cranially along the left and right dorsal aortas until they arise cranially to the sixth aortic arch. At this time, the right dorsal aorta, between the right subclavian artery and the junction of the dorsal aortas, disappears. The final vascular pattern is a left aortic arch with a brachiocephalic trunk that gives rise to the left and right common carotid arteries and the right subclavian artery, a left subclavian artery that originates just distally to the brachiocephalic trunk, and a left ductus arteriosus that courses from the left dorsal aorta to the origin of the left pulmonary artery.

Abnormalities of the aortic arch and its branches are more common than suggested by the occurrence of vascular rings. Most of these abnormalities do not result in vascular rings or esophageal compression. Nearly 20% of dogs dissected in one anatomy laboratory had an abnormality in the branching of the aortic arch.[74]

PERSISTENT RIGHT AORTIC ARCH

A right aortic arch may arise because of two mechanisms—one gives rise to a right aortic arch with mirror-image branching and the other without. The former results in the right aortic arch being connected to the pulmonary artery by a ductus arteriosus that originates from the right sixth aortic arch that lies to the right of the esophagus. The latter produces the type that forms a vascular ring. In this form, the part of the left dorsal aorta caudal to the fourth aortic arch disappears instead of the right and does so before the left subclavian has moved cranially along it. This results in a right, instead of a left, aortic arch that produces a bicarotid trunk that branches into the left and right common carotid arteries, a right subclavian artery, and a distal subclavian artery that originates just cranially to the left ductus arteriosus. The ductus arteriosus forms normally from the left sixth aortic arch that must lie on the left side and connect the aorta on the right to the pulmonary artery on the left. This leaves the right aortic arch to the right of the esophagus and trachea. The base of the heart, including the pulmonary artery, lies ventral and to the left of these structures. The ligamentum arteriosum or ductus arteriosus courses across the top of the esophagus, connecting the aorta to the pulmonary artery. The esophagus and trachea are trapped in the middle of these structures. Similar abnormalities, in which the left subclavian artery either is vestigial or arises from its normal position on the aorta, have also been described.[73]

Persistent right aortic arch appears to be a genetic disease. It has been reported to occur more frequently in German shepherds and Irish setters when these breeds were more popular.[75,76] In one large study of 191 dogs, 92% of affected dogs weighed more than 15 kg. In one study, mating of two affected dogs produced one affected dog, but this was out of 30 offspring produced.[76] Persistent left cranial vena cava and persistent right aortic arch may be linked in some manner, because 10 of 13 dogs with a persistent left cranial vena cava examined in one study had a persistent right aortic arch.[76]

Clinical signs referable to a vascular ring generally occur in puppies or kittens when they start to eat solid food at weaning. More than 80% are diagnosed within the first 6 months of life. However, the onset of clinical signs has been delayed in some dogs to as late

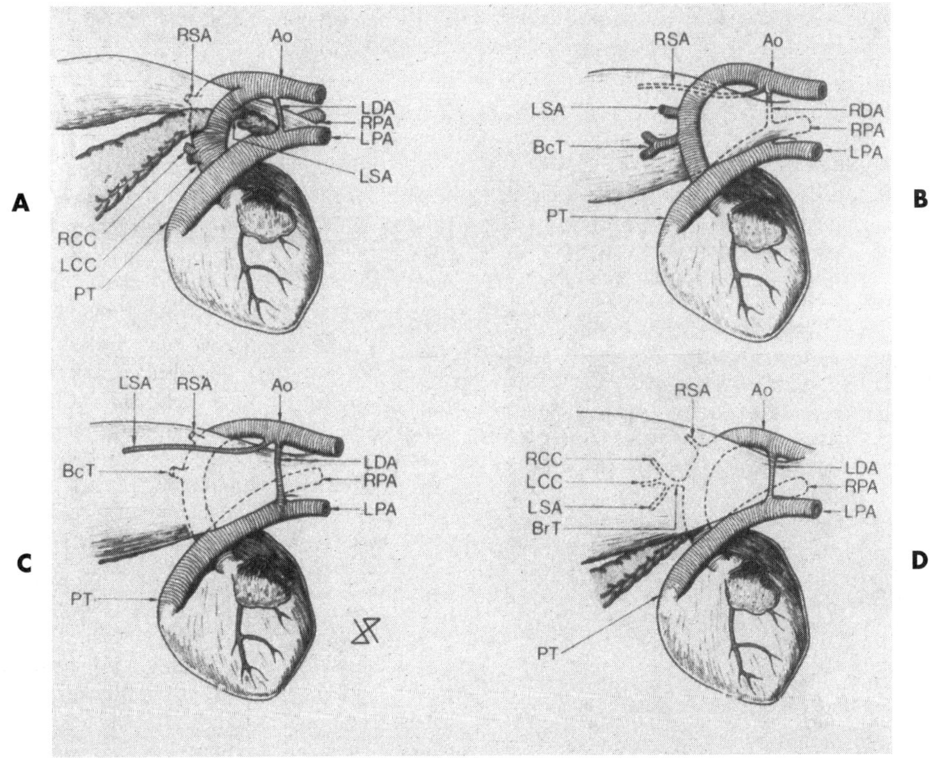

FIGURE 18-16 Anatomic drawings of the types of anomalous aortic arches. **A,** Double aortic arch. **B,** Left aortic arch with a right ductus arteriosus. **C,** Right aortic arch with a left ductus arteriosus and left subclavian artery. **D,** Right aortic arch with a left ductus arteriosus and left subclavian artery arising from the brachiocephalic trunk. *Ao,* Aorta; *PT,* pulmonary trunk; *LDA,* left ductus arteriosus; *RDA,* right ductus arteriosus; *LPA,* left pulmonary artery; *RPA,* right pulmonary artery; *BCT,* bicarotid trunk; *LSA,* left subclavian artery; *RSA,* right subclavian artery; *LCC,* left common carotid artery; *RCC,* right common carotid artery. (From van den Ingh TS, van der Linde-Sipman JS: Vascular rings in the dog, *J Am Vet Med Assoc* 164:939, 1974.

as 8 years of age and has been observed at postmortem examination in dogs that showed no clinical signs.[77,78] However, this is unusual with persistent right aortic arch. The clinical sign generally is regurgitation, although vomiting may occur. Dyspnea is rare and when present is more commonly due to aspiration pneumonia than to tracheal compression. Animals may have a ravenous appetite yet lose or fail to gain weight. Regurgitation most commonly occurs soon after eating, although it may be delayed for several hours.

On physical examination, the animals often are thin or emaciated. Auscultation of the heart and lungs is often normal. Occasionally the ductus arteriosus is patent, resulting in a continuous heart murmur. Animals with aspiration pneumonia may have respiratory crackles. In some animals, a bulge in the thoracic inlet may be felt or visualized. This bulge can be exacerbated by holding the mouth and nares and gently squeezing the abdomen.[58]

Radiographically, a vascular ring may be identified by observing an air or fluid-filled esophagus cranial to the heart. However, in most cases a barium contrast study of the esophagus is required to identify the cranial dilation of the esophagus (Figure 18-17). This dilation usually starts in the region of the thoracic inlet and ends abruptly at the base of the heart, around the fourth rib. Rarely, the dilation will extend into the cervical esophagus. The esophagus from the heart base to the diaphragm is rarely dilated. Persistent right aortic arch is so prevalent with this type of presentation that further studies to define the anatomy of the vascular ring before surgery are rarely performed. Instead, surgery is performed, and the vascular anatomy is defined at that time. Angiography can be performed if another form of a vascular ring is suspected. This is accomplished by injecting a radiographic contrast agent into the aortic root to outline the aortic arch and its branches. Both lateral and dorsoventral projections should be evaluated. Angiograms of a persistent right aortic arch have been previously published.[58]

Treatment of persistent right aortic arch is usually surgical. However, in one study of 191 dogs with persistent right aortic arch, 51 were treated medically.[75] In dogs and cats treated surgically, a ligamentum arteriosum is usually present and can be located, dissected, and severed following double ligation. More care must be taken if the ductus arteriosus is patent, because this structure is more friable and the ligation must be more secure. Overall survival of surgery and the postoperative phase (3 weeks) has been reported to be 80% for dogs treated at veterinary schools.[75]

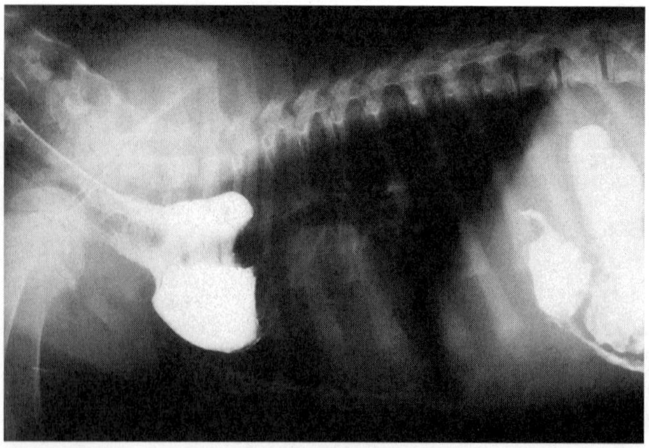

FIGURE 18-17 Lateral thoracic radiograph from a dog with chronic regurgitation of food. The radiograph was taken soon after the dog swallowed barium paste. Although the barium paste has passed into the stomach, a portion of it has accumulated in an esophageal dilation cranial to the heart. This appearance is typical for a vascular ring anomaly, most commonly a persistent right aortic arch.

Postoperative care is very important. Some dogs and cats can tolerate small frequent feedings following surgery. Other animals with severe esophageal dilation or esophagitis need to have small amounts of a watery high-protein food (gruel) fed frequently, with the dog supported in an upright position or standing with its legs on an elevated platform. This position should be maintained for 5 to 10 minutes after feeding.

One study has examined the long-term postoperative course of dogs with persistent right aortic arch.[75] Of 57 dogs, only five (9%) had an excellent outcome (i.e., no regurgitation even with solid food, weight gain, and no related problems). However, 67% of owners felt the response in their dog was good. These owners most frequently reported occasional regurgitation of any food and an intermittent inability to retain solid food. A poor response was reported by 24% of owners whose dogs continued to regurgitate frequently, lose weight, and have other problems, such as pneumonia. No factor or combination of factors could statistically predict a good or a poor outcome. In a more recent study of the long-term surgical outcome, 23 of 25 dogs no longer regurgitated on a solid food diet and the other two dogs regurgitated less than once a week.[79] Three dogs, however, were euthanized within 2 weeks after surgery because of continued regurgitation. One had aspiration pneumonia. Nineteen dogs were lost to follow-up.

DOUBLE AORTIC ARCH

In double aortic arch, a rare abnormality, both sides of the fourth aortic arch persist. This results in the ascending aorta branching into a right and left branch that ascend to either side of the esophagus and trachea and then reunite dorsally to form the descending aorta. The resultant esophageal and tracheal compression can result in regurgitation and dyspnea.[73,80,81] A patent ductus arteriosus may be present.[81]

Surgical treatment of this abnormality has been described in one dog.[80] This dog's littermate had a persistent right aortic arch. Surgery from the left side was performed in anticipation of finding a persistent right aortic arch. Dissection cranial and caudal to the aorta was required to identify the right aortic arch. Each arch was occluded and the femoral pulse evaluated. When the left arch was occluded, the femoral pulse was weak, and when the right arch was occluded it was normal. Consequently, the left arch was retracted, vascular clamps were placed on the right arch, and the right arch was transected between the clamps. The ends were then ligated and the stumps oversewn. Despite a good postoperative recovery, the dog died unexpectedly.

LEFT AORTIC ARCH WITH A RIGHT DUCTUS ARTERIOSUS

Left aortic arch with a right ductus arteriosus has only been reported once in a dog.[73] In this dog, the brachiocephalic trunk did not exist. Instead, a bicarotid trunk was present. The left subclavian artery emerged from its normal position, and the right subclavian originated from the descending aorta, just in front of the ductus arteriosus. The ductus arteriosus, instead of descending from the aorta to the left of the esophagus and attaching to the left pulmonary artery, descended to the right of the esophagus to the right pulmonary artery, entrapping the esophagus. This occurs when the distal right sixth aortic arch persists instead of the distal left sixth aortic arch.[71]

ANOMALOUS SUBCLAVIAN ARTERY

Anomalous subclavian arteries also rarely cause esophageal compression or deviation. An anomalous right subclavian artery can originate directly from the aorta, just distally to the left subclavian artery, or it can originate from the aorta, along with the left subclavian artery, as a short subclavian trunk. Instead of traversing from the brachiocephalic trunk on the left to the right front leg beneath the esophagus as normally occurs, the right subclavian courses dorsally from the aorta on the left, over the top of the esophagus to reach the right front leg. This compresses the esophagus downward.[58] Four English bulldogs have been reported with ventral deviation of the esophagus and regurgitation associated with anomalous left subclavian and brachiocephalic arteries.[82] In these dogs, instead of coursing from the aorta cranially as they normally do, the two arteries seemed to course dorsally toward the spine, trapping the esophagus between them.

REFERENCES

1. Danford DA, McNamara DG: Infants with congenital heart disease in the first year of life. In Garson AJ, Bricker JT, McNamara DG, eds: *The science and practice of pediatric cardiology,* Philadelphia, 1990, Lea & Febiger.
2. Hunt GB, Church DB, Malik R et al: A retrospective analysis of congenital cardiac anomalies (1977-1989), *Aust Vet Pract* 20:70, 1990.
3. van der Linde-Sipman JS, Wensing CJG. Pulmonary and aortic hypoplasia (pseudotruncus arteriosus) and persistence of the common arterial trunk (truncus arteriosus) in the dog and the pig, *Zentralbl Veterinarmed* 19A:15, 1972.
4. Ward KE, Mullins CE: Anomalous pulmonary venous connections; pulmonary vein stenosis; atresia of the common pulmonary vein. In Garson AJ, Bricker JT, McNamara DG, eds: *The science and practice of pediatric cardiology,* Philadelphia, 1990, Lea & Febiger.
5. Jeraj K, Ogburn PN, Johnston GR et al: Atrial septal defect (sinus venosus type) in a dog, *J Am Vet Med Assoc* 77:342, 1980.
6. Hilwig RW, Bishop SP: Anomalous pulmonary venous return in a great Dane, *Am J Vet Res* 36:229, 1975.
7. Bussadori C, Feretti A, Verona A: Anomalous pulmonary venous return with intact septa and stenosis of the conus arteriosus and pulmonary valve in a dog, *Boll Assoc Ital Vet Piccoli Anim* 23:83, 1984.
8. Ferencz C: Visceral heterotaxy with malformed heart: similar findings in a child and a puppy, *Anat Rec* 149:299, 1964.
9. Wenink AC, Zevallos JC: Developmental aspects of atrioventricular septal defects, *Int J Cardiol* 18:65, 1988.
10. Vick GWI, Titus JL: Defects of the atrial septum including the atrioventricular canal. In Garson AJ, Bricker JT, McNamara DG, eds: *The science and practice of pediatric cardiology,* Philadelphia, 1990, Lea & Febiger.
11. Kogure K, Miyagawa S, Ando M et al:AV canal defect in a feline species. In Nora JJ, Takao A, eds: *Congenital heart disease: causes and processes,* Mt. Kisco, NY, 1984, Futura.
12. Perloff JK: *The clinical recognition of congenital heart disease,* ed 4, Philadelphia 1994, WB Saunders Company.
13. Nakayama T, Wakao Y, Uechi M et al: A case report of surgical treatment of a dog with atrioventricular septal defect (incomplete form of endocardial cushion defect), *J Vet Med Sci* 56:981, 1994.
14. Chen KY: Persistent common atrioventricular canal and splenosis in a Persian cat, *J Chin Soc Vet Sci* 12:53, 1986.
15. Liu S, Ettinger S: Persistent common atrioventricular canal in two cats, *J Am Vet Med Assoc* 153:556, 1968.
16. Tanizawa K, Amano T, Kawai S et al: A case of canine atrioventricular canal malformation, *Adv Anim Electrocardiog* 13:34, 1980.
17. Bolton GR, Liu SK: Congenital heart diseases of the cat, *Vet Clin North Am* 7:341, 1977.
18. Liu SK, Hsu FS, Lee RCT: *An atlas of cardiovascular pathology,* Tainan, Taiwan, 1989, Pig Research Institute of Taiwan.
19. Morriss MJH, McNamara DG: Coarctation of the aorta and interrupted aortic arch. In Garson AJ, Bricker JT, McNamara DG, eds: *The science and practice of pediatric cardiology,* Philadelphia, 1990, Lea & Febiger.
20. Eyster GE, Carrig CB, Baker B et al: Coarctation of the aorta in a dog, *J Am Vet Med Assoc* 169:426, 1976.
21. Herrtage ME, Gorman NT, Jefferies AR: Coarctation of the aorta in a dog, *Vet Radiol Ultrasound* 33:25, 1992.
22. Strasburger JF: Cor triatriatum, pulmonary vein obstruction, supravalvular mitral stenosis, and congenital mitral valve disease. In Garson AJ, Bricker JT, McNamara DG, eds: *The science and practice of pediatric cardiology,* Philadelphia, 1990, Lea & Febiger.
23. Gordon B, Trautvetter E, Patterson DF: Pulmonary congestion associated with cor triatriatum in a cat, *J Am Vet Med Assoc* 180:75, 1982.
24. Stern A, Fallon RK, Aronson E et al: Cor triatriatum dexter in a dog, *Compen Contin Educ Pract Vet* 8:401, 1986.
25. Jevens DJ, Johnston SA, Jones CA et al: Cor triatriatum dexter in two dogs, *J Am Anim Hosp Assoc* 29:289, 1993.
26. Brayley KA, Lunney J, Ettinger SJ: Cor triatriatum dexter in a dog, *J Am Anim Hosp Assoc* 30:153, 1994.
27. Kaufman AC, Swalec KM, Mahaffey MB: Surgical correction of cor triatriatum dexter in a puppy, *J Am Anim Hosp Assoc* 30:157, 1994.
28. Tobias AH, Thomas WP, Kittleson MD et al: Cor triatriatum dexter in two dogs, *J Am Vet Med Assoc* 202:285, 1993.
29. van der Linde-Sipman JS, Stokhof AA: Triple atria in a pup, *J Am Vet Med Assoc* 165:539, 1974.
30. Miller MW, Bonagura JD, DiBartola SP: Budd-Chiari-like syndrome in two dogs, *J Am Anim Hosp Assoc* 25:277, 1989.
31. Fossum TW, Miller MW: Cor triatriatum and caval anomalies, *Semin Vet Med Surg Small Anim* 9:177, 1994.
32. Grooters AM, Smeak DD: Budd-Chiari-like syndromes in dogs. In Bonagura JD, ed: *Kirk's current veterinary therapy XII: small animal practice,* Philadelphia, 1995, WB Saunders.
33. Cohn LA, Spaulding KA, Cullen JM et al: Intrahepatic postsinusoidal venous obstruction in a dog, *J Vet Intern Med* 5:317, 1991.
34. Malik R, Hunt GB, Chard RB et al: Congenital obstruction of the caudal vena cava in a dog, *J Am Vet Med Assoc* 197:880, 1990.
35. Atwell RB, Sutton RH: Suspect three chambered right atrium in a pup, *Vet Rec* 113:86, 1983.
36. Carrig CB, Suter PF, Ewing GO et al: Primary dextrocardia with situs inversus, associated with sinusitis and bronchitis in a dog, *J Am Vet Med Assoc* 164:1127, 1974.
37. Gutgesell HP: Cardiac malposition and heterotaxy. In Garson AJ, Bricker JT, McNamara DG, eds: *The science and practice of pediatric cardiology,* Philadelphia, 1990, Lea & Febiger.
38. Afzelius BA, Carlsten J, Karlsson S: Clinical, pathologic, and ultrastructural features of situs inversus and immotile-cilia syndrome in a dog, *J Am Vet Med Assoc* 184:560, 1984.
39. Foodman MS, Giger U, Stebbins K et al: Kartagener's syndrome in an old miniature poodle, *J Small Anim Pract* 30:96, 1989.
40. Lohse CL, Selcer RR, Suter PF: Hepatoencephalopathy associated with situs inversus of abdominal organs and vascular anomalies in a dog, *J Am Vet Med Assoc* 168:681, 1976.
41. Kartagener M: Zur Pathogenese der Bronchiektasien bei Stius viscerum inversus, *Beitr Klin Tuberk* 83:489, 1933.
42. Afzelius BA: A human syndrome caused by immotile cilia, *Science* 193:317, 1976.
43. Edwards DF, Kennedy JR, Toal RL et al: Kartagener's syndrome in a chow chow dog with normal ciliary ultrastructure, *Vet Pathol* 26:338, 1989.
44. Silka MJ: Double-outlet ventricles. In Garson AJ, Bricker JT, McNamara DG, eds: *The science and practice of pediatric cardiology,* Philadelphia, 1990, Lea & Febiger.
45. van der Linde-Sipman JS, van den Ingh TS, Koeman JP: Congenital heart abnormalities in the cat: a description of sixteen cases, *Zentralbl Veterinarmed* 20A:419, 1973.
46. Wakao Y, Takahashi M, Suganuma T et al: A case of double outlet right ventricle of a dog with special reference to its clinical signs and hemodynamics, *Bull Azabu Vet Coll* 2:137, 1977.
47. Jeraj K, Ogburn PN, Jessen CA et al: Double outlet right ventricle in a cat, *J Am Vet Med Assoc* 173:1356, 1978.
48. Northway RB: Use of an aortic homograft for surgical correction of a double-outlet right ventricle in a kitten, *Vet Med Small Anim Clin* 74:191, 1979.

49. Turk JR, Miller LM, Hegreberg GA: Double outlet right ventricle in a dog, *J Am Anim Hosp Assoc* 17:789, 1981.
50. Nichols JB, Eyster GE, Dulisch ML et al: Aortic interruption in a dog, *J Am Vet Med Assoc* 174:1091, 1979.
51. Jacobs G, Patterson D, Knight D: Complete interruption of the aortic arch in a dog, *J Am Vet Med Assoc* 191:1585, 1987.
52. Hagio M: Persistent left cranial vena cava in a dog, *J Jpn Vet Med Assoc* 32:513, 1979.
53. Lombard CW, Twitchell MJ: Tetralogy of Fallot, persistent left cranial vena cava and retinal detachment in a cat, *J Am Anim Hosp Assoc* 14:624, 1978.
54. Jacobs G, Bolton GR, Watrous BJ: Echocardiographic features of dilated coronary sinus in a dog with persistent left cranial vena cava, *J Am Vet Med Assoc* 182:407, 1983.
55. Sales JP, Carvalho AP, Oliveira AL: Pulmonic stenosis and persistent left cranial vena cava in a dog, *Canine Pract* 20:24, 1995.
56. Zeiner FM: Two cases of coronary venous drainage by a persistent left superior vena cava in cats, *Anat Rec* 129:275, 1957.
57. Wheaton LG, Blevins WE, Weirich WE: Persistent right aortic arch associated with other vascular anomalies in two cats, *J Am Vet Med Assoc* 184:848, 1984.
58. Ettinger SJ, Suter PF: *Canine cardiology,* Philadelphia, 1970, WB Saunders.
59. Perloff JK: *The clinical recognition of congenital heart disease,* ed 4, Philadelphia, 1994, WB Saunders.
60. Riopel DA: Pulmonary valve atresia with intact ventricular septum. In Garson AJ, Bricker JT, McNamara DG, eds: *The science and practice of pediatric cardiology,* Philadelphia, 1990, Lea & Febiger.
61. Brown DJ, Patterson DF: Pulmonary atresia with intact ventricular septum and agenesis of the ductus arteriosus in a pup, *J Am Vet Med Assoc* 195:229, 1989.
62. Neches WH, Park SC, Ettedgui JA: Transposition of the great arteries. In Garson AJ, Bricker JT, McNamara DG, eds: *The science and practice of pediatric cardiology,* Philadelphia, 1990, Lea & Febiger.
63. Straw RC, Aronson EF, McCaw DL: Transposition of the great arteries in a cat, *J Am Vet Med Assoc* 187:634, 1985.
64. Ferency C: Visceral heterotaxy with malformed heart: similar findings in a child and a puppy, *Teratology* 11:65, 1996.
65. Khera KS: Fetal cardiovascular and other defects induced by thalidomide in cats, *Anat Rec* 149:299, 1964.
66. Chen HC, Bussian P, Whitehead JE: Persistent truncus arteriosus in a dog, *Vet Pathol* 9:379, 1972.
67. Temesy-Armos PN, Legenza M, Southworth SR et al: Effects of verapamil and lidocaine in a canine model of sudden coronary death, *J Am Coll Cardiol* 6:674, 1985.
68. Collett RW, Edwards JE: Persistent truncus arteriosus: a classification according to anatomic types, *Surg Clin North Am* 29:1245, 1949.
69. Williams RL, Sommerville RJ: Truncus arteriosus. In Garson AJ, Bricker JT, McNamara DG, eds: *The science and practice of pediatric cardiology,* Philadelphia, 1990, Lea & Febiger.
70. Fisher EW, Lee R, Pirie HM et al: Pseudo truncus arteriosus in a dog: a case report, *J Small Anim Pract* 15:627, 1974.
71. Morrow WR, Huhta JC: Aortic arch and pulmonary artery anomalies. In Garson AJ, Bricker JT, McNamara DG, eds: *The science and practice of pediatric cardiology,* Philadelphia, 1990, Lea & Febiger.
72. Buchanan JW: Thoracic surgery in the dog and cat. III. Patent ductus arteriosus and persistent right aortic arch surgery in dogs, *J Small Anim Pract* 9:409, 1968.
73. van den Ingh TS, van der Linde-Sipman JS: Vascular rings in the dog, *J Am Vet Med Assoc* 164:939, 1974.
74. Smollich A: Abweichungen im Bereich der Aste des Aortenbogens und ihre bedeutung, *Arch Exp Veterinarmed* 15:986, 1961.
75. Shires PK, Liu W: Persistent right aortic arch in dogs: a long term follow-up after surgical correction, *J Am Anim Hosp Assoc* 17:773, 1981.
76. Patterson DF: Epidemiologic and genetic studies of congenital heart disease in the dog, *Circ Res* 23:171, 1968.
77. Fingeroth JM, Fossum TW: Late-onset regurgitation associated with persistent right aortic arch in two dogs, *J Am Vet Med Assoc* 191:981, 1987.
78. Lawson D, Penhale B, Smith G: Persistent right aortic arch in the dog causing oesophageal obstruction, *Vet Rec* 69:326, 1957.
79. Muldoon MM, Birchard SJ, Ellison GW: Long-term results of surgical correction of persistent right aortic arch in dogs: 25 cases (1980-1995), *J Am Vet Med Assoc* 210:1761, 1997.
80. Aultman SH, Chambers JN, Vestre WA: Double aortic arch and persistent right aortic arch in two littermates: surgical treatment, *J Am Anim Hosp Assoc* 16:533, 1980.
81. Martin DG, Ferguson EW, Gunnels RD et al: Double aortic arch in a dog, *J Am Vet Med Assoc* 183:697, 1983.
82. Woods CB, Rawlings C, Barber D et al: Esophageal deviation in four English bulldogs, *J Am Vet Med Assoc* 172:934, 1978.

CHAPTER 19

Myxomatous Atrioventricular Valvular Degeneration

The mitral and tricuspid valves are the valves that separate the left and right atria from the left and right ventricles respectively. They are also termed the *atrioventricular valves.* Both act as one-way valves, allowing blood to flow into the ventricles during ventricular diastole and preventing blood from flowing backward into the atria during ventricular systole. The mitral valve apparatus is made up of the mitral valve leaflets, annulus of the mitral valve, chordae tendineae, and left ventricular papillary muscles. The tricuspid valve apparatus is composed of the tricuspid leaflets, chordae tendineae, and right ventricular papillary muscles. The function of the mitral valve can also be influenced by the left atrial wall and the left ventricle, and the tricuspid valve is likely similarly influenced by the right atrial wall and right ventricle.[1] Mitral regurgitation, also known as *mitral insufficiency,* is the leakage of blood through the mitral valve, from the left ventricle to the left atrium, during systole (Figure 19-1). Tricuspid regurgitation is the same situation on the right side of the heart. Greater force is generated in systole in the left ventricle than in the right ventricle. Consequently, greater regurgitation is produced for a given size of orifice in the valve in mitral regurgitation than in tricuspid regurgitation.

Atrioventricular regurgitation occurs secondary to numerous abnormalities. An abnormality in any component of the mitral or tricuspid valve apparatuses can result in valve leakage. Examples include (1) annular dilation and a displaced coaptation point secondary to increased ventricular chamber size (dilation), such as occurs with dilated cardiomyopathy, myxomatous valve degeneration, and so on; (2) abnormalities of the valve leaflets that include myxomatous degeneration and bacterial endocarditis; (3) abnormalities of the chordae tendineae that include lengthening and rupture in myxomatous degeneration; and (4) abnormalities of the papillary muscles that usually involves malorientation secondary to ventricular diseases, such as hypertrophic cardiomyopathy. The most common primary abnormality that causes atrioventricular regurgitation is myxomatous degeneration of a valve. Most of the abnormalities that result in secondary regurgitation are discussed in other sections of this book. Myxomatous degeneration of the atrioventricular valves and associated lesions are the primary abnormality discussed in this chapter.

Myxomatous valve degeneration (MVD) is also known in the veterinary literature as *endocardiosis, chronic degenerative valvular disease, chronic valvular disease, chronic valvular fibrosis,* and *acquired mitral* or *tricuspid regurgitation* or *insufficiency.* In human medicine this disease is commonly called *mitral valve prolapse* because this anatomic change in the valve (discussed below) is a common sequela. These are misnomers or incomplete definitions. Endocardiosis suggests degeneration of the endocardium. Although endocardium lines the valves, it does not appear that degeneration of this layer is the primary abnormality in this disease. *Chronic degenerative valvular disease* is a reasonable name for the disease but does not specifically address the type of degeneration. Chronic valvular disease is very nonspecific and theoretically could include numerous abnormalities, including chronic bacterial endocarditis. Chronic valvular fibrosis is an incomplete description because it only describes the pathologic changes seen in the atrialis layer and does not describe the more prominent, and most likely primary, changes in the spongiosa and fibrosa layers of the valve.[2] Acquired mitral or tricuspid insufficiency only distinguish the disease from congenital lesions of the atrioventricular valves. Mitral valve prolapse only describes one manifestation of the disease.

Anatomy

The mitral valve in the dog is made up of a large septal (anterior) leaflet, a medium-size mural (posterior) leaflet, and smaller commissural cusps placed between the two leaflets. Leaflets are defined as structures that have chordae tendineae from both papillary muscles. The commissural cusps only have chordae from one papillary muscle attached to them. Both leaflets are semicircular in shape. The septal leaflet has a larger radius of curvature than the mural leaflet. The edges of the leaflets, where the chordae tendineae attach to the ventricular surface, are rough to palpation and are opaque. This region is called the *rough zone.* The rough zone is where the leaflets come in contact during systole. The remaining portions of the leaflets are transparent. Leaflets and commissural cusps are attached to the mitral valve annulus, a fibrous ring that lies between the left atrium and the left ventricle. The base of the septal leaflet is contiguous with the root of the aorta, specifically with the regions of the aorta that form the left and noncoronary cusps. The mitral valve leaflets and cusps are attached to the two papillary muscles by first- and second-order chordae tendineae. Third-order chords are uncommon in dogs.

The *tricuspid valve* is a misnomer in the dog and cat because it consists of two, not three, primary leaflets and several unnamed commissural cusps. The largest leaflet is the mural leaflet, and the smaller leaflet is the septal leaflet. The chordae tendineae of the septal leaflet attach directly to small ridges on the interventricular septum. The chordae tendineae of the mural leaflet attach primarily to a

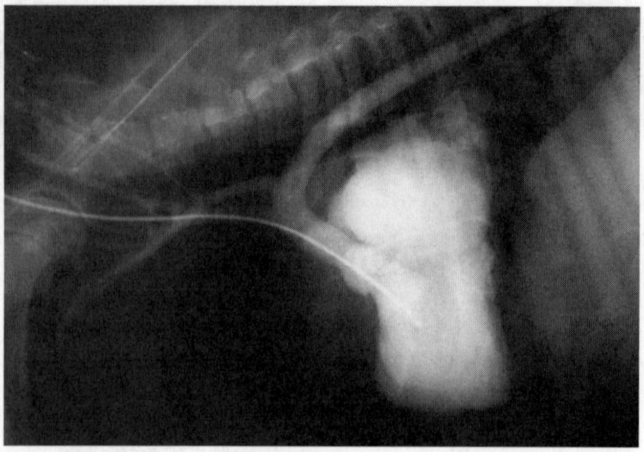

FIGURE 19-1 Angiocardiogram from a dog with severe mitral regurgitation. The contrast agent is ejected into both the aorta and left atrium. The left ventricle and the left atrium are enlarged. The intensity of the radiographic appearance of the contrast agent is at least the same or denser in the left atrium compared with the left ventricle (3+ to 4+). The intensity of the contrast material is greater in the left atrium than in the aorta, indicating that more blood is being ejected into the left atrium than into the aorta (the regurgitant fraction is greater than 50%). (Courtesy Dr. Bruce Madewell.)

variable number of papillary muscles (usually three) situated along the apical one third of the interventricular septum. The papillary muscle of the conus arises from the supraventricular crest and attaches to the portion of the mural leaflet closest to the pulmonic valve.

Histologically the atrioventricular valves have four layers. The atrial side and the ventricular side are endocardial layers and are called the atrialis and ventricularis. These layers consist of endothelial cells overlying a thin layer made up of collagen fibers, elastic fibers, and fibroblasts. The atrial side also has a thin layer of smooth muscle. Between these two layers are the spongiosa and the fibrosa layers. The fibrosa is the major structural portion of the valve and lies in apposition to the ventricularis. It is a dense, well-organized layer of collagen bundles. The spongiosa is between the fibrosa and the atrialis. It is a thin, loose collection of collagen fibers, fibroblasts, and elastic fibers in a bed of mucopolysaccharide ground substance, mostly made up of hyaluronic acid and chondroitin sulfate.

The chordae tendineae are chords of fibrous tissue that connect the valve leaflets and cusps to the papillary muscles. Histologically they are composed primarily of a collagenous central core that is continuous with the fibrosa layer of the valve.

Pathology

Myxomatous degeneration primarily affects the mitral and tricuspid valve leaflets and the chordae tendineae.[3] Mitral valve lesions are more common. In about 60% of cases the mitral valve alone is affected, whereas only the tricuspid valve is affected in about 10% of cases. The other 30% have both valves involved. The disease only rarely affects the aortic and pulmonic valves.

In myxomatous degeneration, the gross pathology of the valves is that of thickening and redundancy of the valve leaflets. The pathologic features of the disease are most pronounced at the free margins of the valves. This area is thickened, with prominent nodular thickenings in severely affected dogs. The affected regions of the valves are opaque, and the surface is smooth and glistening with no evidence of inflammation. Whitney has classified the progression of the lesions into four classes, and Kogure has modified it into three classes.[2,4] In class I, the lesions usually start as small, discrete nodules along the edge of the valve leaflets, The lesions increase in size and coalesce to form larger deformities toward the free edges of the leaflet. In class II, the free edges are thickened and the edges of the leaflets become irregular and more thickened as the disease progresses (Color Plate 70). Some rough zone chordae tendineae are thickened where they attach to the valve. In class III, the valve edges are grossly thickened and nodular (Color Plate 71). The thickening extends part way and sometimes all the way to the base of the valve leaflets. There appears to be redundant tissue.[2] This may result in some thickened tissue prolapsing into the left atrium. The rough zone chordae are thickened, and chordal rupture may be evident, resulting in mitral valve flail. Chordae tendineae to the septal leaflet also elongate in dogs with class III disease.[2]

On histopathology, the earliest changes occur along the atrial side of the atrioventricular valve. The endothelium proliferates, and there is an increase in the number of subendothelial fibroblasts. The elastic fibers between the atrialis and spongiosa split and separate. This is followed by the spongiosa increasing remarkably in size while the fibrosa layer of the valve degenerates. When it is thickened, the spongiosa has the appearance of embryonic mesenchymal tissue, therefore the name *myxomatous*. This is characterized by widely separated stellate and spindle-shaped cells and a marked increase in the extracellular matrix without a significant increase in mature collagen or elastic fibers. The extracellular matrix is comprised primarily of glycosaminoglycans (GAGs), mostly hyaluronic acid and chondroitin sulfate. Fibroblasts proliferate in the spongiosa, forming swirls and small nodules. In the fibrosa, the collagen bundles become swollen and hyalinized, fragment, and vanish. In severe cases, only scattered remnants of the fibrosa remain. Similar changes occur in the chordae tendineae.

Besides the valvular and chordal changes, the left atrium is dilated and the left ventricle is eccentrically hypertrophied. Jet lesions are commonly seen in the left atrium (Color Plate 72). They are fibrous plaques in the endocardium that occur in a region subjected to the impact of the high-velocity mitral regurgitant jet. Endomyocardial splits or tears may also be identified (Color Plate 71).[5] On occasion, a full-thickness left atrial tear occurs, resulting in hemopericardium, pericardial tamponade, and, usually, death (Color Plate 73). Rarely, a full-thickness endomyocardial tear will involve the interatrial septum, causing an acquired atrial septal defect.[5] Intramural coronary arteriosclerosis has been reported in dogs with chronic myxomatous mitral valve degeneration and has been used as an explanation for myocardial failure in this disease.[6] This type of lesion is also observed in older dogs without mitral valve disease, suggesting it is an incidental finding.[7]

Prevalence

Myxomatous degeneration of the atrioventricular valves is by far the most common cardiovascular disease identified in small animals. In past studies, it has accounted for approximately 75% of the cardiovascular disease seen in dogs.[8,9]

The prevalence of MVD in dogs is age- and breed-related. Older dogs and small breeds have the highest incidence of the disease. Males are slightly more prone to develop the disease than females and may be more prone to develop more severe disease.[3]

In past studies, small breeds most prone to developing MVD have been the poodle (miniature and toy), miniature schnauzer, cocker spaniel, Chihuahua, fox terrier, dachshund, and Boston terrier.[3] The Doberman pinscher has been the only large breed of dog identified as at increased risk for MVD. There is one cautionary note. These data were generated between 1973 and 1975, so demographics may have changed. The one breed that is obviously missing is the Cavalier King Charles spaniel, a breed frequently identified over the past decade. Numerous other breeds, such as the Lhasa apso, the Shi Tzu, and other terrier breeds frequently develop MVD. Prevalence data indicates an increase in expected frequency compared with the population. Just because a breed does not have an increased prevalence does not mean that the disease does not occur in that breed. Occasionally a large-breed dog, such as a great Dane or a German shepherd, presents with MVD.

MVD is unusual in most dogs less than 5 years of age. The exception to this rule is the Cavalier King Charles spaniel, in which the murmur of mitral regurgitation can be heard in 10% of dogs less than 1 year of age.[10] The incidence of heart murmurs in small breeds of dogs greater than 5 years of age is unknown. In one study, about 10% of all dogs had clinical evidence of MVD between 5 and 8 years of age, and about 25% had evidence when they were between 9 and 12 years of age.[3] The incidence increased to 35% in dogs greater than 12 years of age. These numbers increase when dogs are examined at necropsy. When all degrees of severity are included (Whitney grades I to IV), 93% of dogs between 9 and 12 years of age are affected, and all dogs 12 years of age or older are affected.[11] When only more severe lesions are included (Whitney grades III to IV), only 14% of dogs less than 9 years of age have MVD, whereas 58% of all dogs greater than 9 years of age have advanced disease.[11] Because these numbers include large dogs, the prevalence in small dogs must be higher.

Of more importance than the prevalence of heart murmurs in specific populations is the prevalence of severe disease that leads to heart failure. No data on this subject exist. All that we know is that not all dogs that have MVD of the mitral valve go on to develop heart failure.

Etiology

The etiology of MVD in dogs is unknown. Myxomatous degeneration is commonly confused with endocarditis. One reason for this may be that the disease has been termed *endocardiosis* in the past, which sounds like *endocarditis*. Endocarditis is inflammation and destruction of valvular tissue and is almost always due to an infectious agent. Myxomatous degeneration (endocardiosis) is a degenerative process not associated with inflammation or an infectious agent.

One popular theory of the etiology of MVD is that it occurs secondary to oral cavity and tooth disease. Many older small dogs have MVD, and many older small dogs have bad teeth. Consequently, an association has been made between the two. We are unaware of any scientific evidence to link these two entities. There is no evidence that bacteria that originate in the oral cavity either infect or somehow cause secondary changes in the atrioventricular valves.

In small breeds of dogs the disease is likely hereditary. This has been examined in Cavalier King Charles spaniels. In this breed, it has been suggested that myxomatous atrioventricular valve degeneration is inherited as a polygenic threshold trait.[12]

The same changes seen in the atrioventricular valves of dogs occur in the mitral valve of people with floppy valve syndrome (prolapsing mitral valve) and in people with collagen abnormalities, including Marfan syndrome, Ehlers-Danlos syndrome, and osteogenesis imperfecta.[13] The fact that these same histologic lesions are identified in people with collagen abnormalities suggests that a collagen abnormality may be the cause of MVD in dogs. The fact that these dogs frequently also have tracheobronchomalacia (collapsing large airways) and other potential maladies that could be due to abnormal collagen (intervertebral disc disease, ruptured anterior cruciate ligament), makes it attractive to speculate that these dogs could have a generalized collagen abnormality. The best means of identifying such an abnormality would be to identify an abnormal gene in these dogs. This may become feasible as more about the canine genome is discovered.

Pathophysiology

Myxomatous degeneration results in valve leaflet and chordae tendineae abnormalities. The initial changes appear to be lengthening of the chordae or redundancy and laxity of the valve leaflets. This results in mitral valve prolapse. Mitral valve prolapse is defined as some portion of the body of a valve leaflet protruding back toward the left atrium more than normal. Normally the mitral valve leaflets coapt in such a way that the coaptation point is on the left ventricular side of the plane of the mitral valve annulus. Mitral valve prolapse is diagnosed when the coaptation point or portions of the mitral valve leaflets are at or are on the left atrial side of the annular plane. Mitral valve prolapse is frequently identified in young Cavalier King Charles spaniels that have not yet developed mitral regurgitation and in older dogs with mitral regurgitation.[14] Mitral valve prolapse is common in humans with myxomatous degeneration of the mitral valve. The prolapsing valve commonly produces a systolic click in humans. The incidence of systolic clicks appears to be much less in dogs with prolapse. Following the period in which isolated prolapse occurs, the leaflets thicken along the edges and curl on themselves. This results in the valve leaking (mitral regurgitation). At this time the heart must compensate for the disease.

A clear understanding of the pathophysiology of mitral regurgitation is required to understand the changes noted on radiographic, electrocardiographic, and echocardiographic examinations and to formulate logical therapeutic plans for patients with this abnormality. A good way to gain understanding of pathophysiology is to examine the changes that occur in left ventricular mechanics and hemodynamics over the course of the disease.

MILD MITRAL REGURGITATION IN SMALL DOGS

Figure 19-2 depicts schematic drawings of a left ventricle from a dog with acute mild mitral regurgitation before any compensation has taken place. Normal left ventricular function using such a schematic was described in Chapter 2. All variables in this figure are normal except for the presence of a small regurgitant leak leading to a small decrease in forward stroke volume. This drawing mimics a right parasternal cross-sectional echocardiographic view of the left ventricle at three phases during the cardiac cycle: end-diastole, immediately before the onset of ejection, and end-systole. Springs are placed in the left ventricle to represent left ventricular pressure. Muscles are placed in parallel and in series in the left ventricular wall to represent sarcomeres (contractile elements). Each muscle represents thousands of sarcomeres. Values for different echocardiographic and hemodynamic variables are depicted below the drawings. All values are normal for a dog that weighs 25 to 30 kg (1 m^2 of body surface area). Please note that there are nine "muscles" in series around the outside row in this figure. Left ventricular weight is approximately 120 g/m^2.

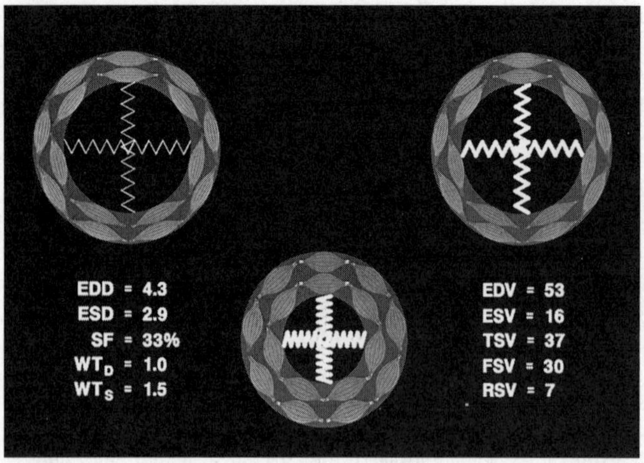

FIGURE 19-2 Schematic drawing of the left ventricle from a dog with acute, mild mitral regurgitation. The schematics are drawn in cross-section at different stages in the cardiac cycle. The end of diastole is depicted in the upper left corner of the picture. The ventricle is drawn immediately before ejection in the upper right corner, and the ventricle is pictured at the end of systole on the bottom. Sarcomeres are depicted as "muscles" within the myocardium. The sarcomeres are arranged in parallel and in series with each other. The intraventricular pressure is depicted as springs within the ventricular chamber, pushing out against the myocardium. Higher pressure in systole is depicted as thicker springs. The end-diastolic diameter *(EDD)*, end-systolic diameter *(ESD)*, and shortening fraction *(SF)* are normal. The wall thicknesses in diastole *(WT_D)* and in systole *(WT_S)* are also normal. The end-diastolic volume *(EDV)*, end-systolic volume *(ESV)*, and the total stroke volume *(TSV)* ejected by the ventricle are normal. The presence of a regurgitant stroke volume *(RSV)* confirms that mitral regurgitation is present. The forward stroke volume *(FSV)* is decreased because some blood is ejected back into the left atrium.

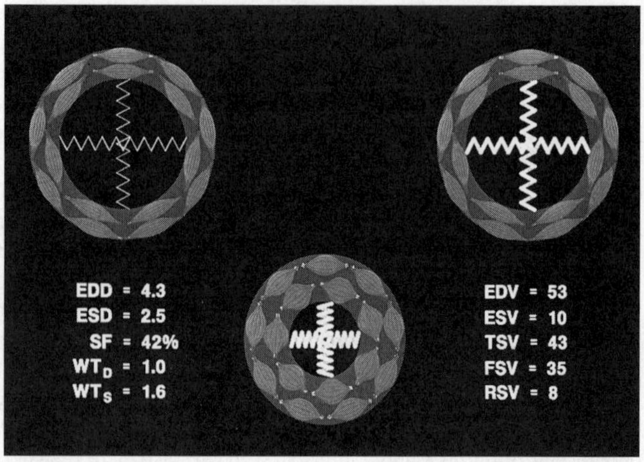

FIGURE 19-3 Cross-sections of a left ventricle from a dog with mild mitral regurgitation and β-receptor stimulation. Myocardial contractility is increased, which decreases end-systolic diameter and volume. The decrease in end-systolic volume increases total stroke volume ejected from the chamber. This compensates for the volume of blood pumped into the left atrium and brings forward stroke volume back to normal. Abbreviations are as in Figure 19-2.

To depict the changes that occur from the onset of mitral regurgitation to the end-stage of the disease, imagine a 7-year-old Lhasa apso with MVD of the mitral valve that suddenly develops mild mitral regurgitation. In actuality, a dog like this would start with a very small leak that would gradually worsen. For illustration purposes it is easier to imagine an acute insult, as described. From recent studies we know that dogs with clinically mild mitral regurgitation have a regurgitant fraction less than 50%.[15] Regurgitant fraction is regurgitant stroke volume divided by total stroke volume (end-diastolic volume − end-systolic volume) and is the percentage of the total stroke volume of the ventricle ejected into the left atrium. In this case we will choose the regurgitant fraction to be 20%. Figure 19-2 schematically represents this situation before any compensatory changes have occurred. Note that the left ventricular chamber size at end-diastole and end-systole is normal, so total stroke volume is normal. However, some (7 mL) blood leaks back into the left ventricle so that the blood volume ejected into the aorta (forward stroke volume) is decreased to 30 mL. Thus the consequences of the development of peracute mild mitral regurgitation in this dog are a decrease in flow through the systemic circulation (hypoperfusion) and an increase in left atrial volume and therefore pressure. The increased left atrial pressure backs up into the pulmonary veins and capillaries and, if severe enough, could produce pulmonary edema. Before any compensation occurs, the decrease in blood flow into the systemic circulation results in a decrease in systemic arterial blood pressure and a decrease in renal blood flow. Compensation stems from these two abnormalities. The baroreceptors immediately sense the decrease in pressure, and the kidneys sense the decrease in flow. Baroreceptor stimulation results in activation of the sympathetic nervous system. Sympathetic nervous system activation results in an increase in the sinus node rate, an increase in contractility (through β_1-receptor stimulation in myocardium), and systemic arteriolar constriction. The increase in the heart rate and the increase in contractility increase cardiac output (blood flow per minute), which helps increase blood pressure and improves perfusion. The arteriolar constriction also helps increase blood pressure. The expected net result is normalization of hemodynamics, with an increase in contractility, as seen in Figure 19-3. This rapid compensation takes place before the kidneys have a chance to produce a significant hemodynamic response.

The sympathetic response results in complete compensation. However, β_1-receptors down-regulate quite rapidly. It is known that enough are still present that if a β-blocker is administered, contractility becomes significantly decreased in mitral regurgitation.[16] In chronic heart failure it appears that about 50% of the β_1-receptors are no longer able to be stimulated. We will assume that a similar number are down-regulated within 3 days of the increase in stimulation. At this stage, contractility is increased but not to the same degree as before. Consequently flow is still decreased. Because increasing contractility further is no longer an option, the cardiovascular system must find another means of increasing stroke volume back to normal.

Volume overload hypertrophy is the major mechanism by which the cardiovascular system compensates for this disease chronically (see Chapter 9). The decreases in blood flow and blood pressure stimulate the kidney to elaborate hormones and increase sodium and water retention. The resultant increase in blood volume increases venous return to the heart, and, in mitral regurgitation, the left ventricle grows larger. The major difference between dilated cardiomyopathy and mitral regurgitation is that myocardial contractility and end-systolic volume stay normal in mitral regurgitation. Figure 19-4 depicts the changes expected to occur with chronic mild mitral regurgitation. The ventricle has grown larger (volume overload or eccentric hypertrophy), so that for any given degree of contraction,

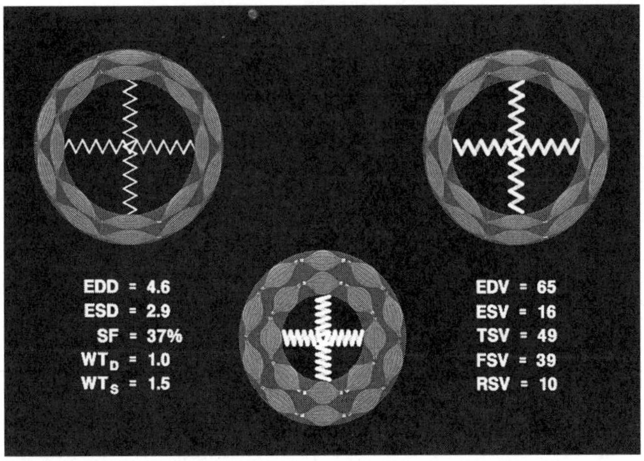

FIGURE 19-4 Cross-sections of a left ventricle from a dog with mild mitral regurgitation and mild volume overload (eccentric) hypertrophy. Contractile elements (muscles) in the outer row have increased from 9 to 10. Myocardial contractility has returned to normal, so end-systolic volume is again normal. The volume overload hypertrophy has resulted in an increase in end-diastolic volume and a resultant increase in total stroke volume to compensate for the regurgitant flow. Abbreviations are as in Figure 19-2.

the stroke volume will be larger than normal. The increase in total stroke volume allows the ventricle to compensate for the blood "lost" through the leak in the mitral valve. When compensation is complete at this early stage, end-diastolic volume is increased to 65 mL/m^2 (EDD = 4.6 cm/m^2), end-systolic volume is normal at 16 mL/m^2 (ESD = 2.9 cm/m^2), shortening fraction is increased to 37%, total stroke volume is increased to 49 mL/m^2, forward stroke volume is normal (39 mL/m^2), and regurgitant stroke volume is 10 mL/m^2. The left atrium enlarges (eccentrically hypertrophies) to accommodate the increased amount of blood flowing into it.[17] Consequently, left atrial pressure does not increase and pulmonary edema does not form. Compensation is complete. Note that contractile element numbers around the outside row have increased from nine to ten (an increased number linked in series). Left ventricular weight is now 137 g/m^2. This dog has a soft systolic heart murmur heard best at the left apex. Otherwise, he is clinically normal.

MODERATE MITRAL REGURGITATION IN SMALL DOGS

Myxomatous mitral valve degeneration insidiously progresses as time passes. At 9 years of age, our patient now has clinically moderate mitral regurgitation (regurgitant fraction = 45% to 75%) (Figure 19-5). The regurgitant stroke volume is now 47 mL/m^2, and the regurgitant fraction is 55% (47 mL/85 mL = 0.55). The end-systolic volume (16 mL/m^2) is normal. This is due either to normal innate myocardial contractile function or mildly reduced innate myocardial contractile function coupled with increased adrenergic stimulation. The end-diastolic volume has increased to 99 mL/m^2 (EDD = 5.3 cm/m^2), therefore total stroke volume has increased to 83 mL/m^2, greater than twice normal. The increase in end-diastolic volume caused by the volume overload hypertrophy has allowed the forward stroke volume to remain normal, at 38 mL/m^2. Shortening fraction is increased to 46%. Note that this variable, which is commonly equated with "contractility," is increased in this disease. However, contractility is actually normal, as evidenced by the normal end-systolic diameter. The increase in shortening fraction is due to the increase in the end-diastolic diameter and so is increased by the presence of volume overload hypertrophy, not contractility. Left ventricular weight is increased to 160 g/m^2.

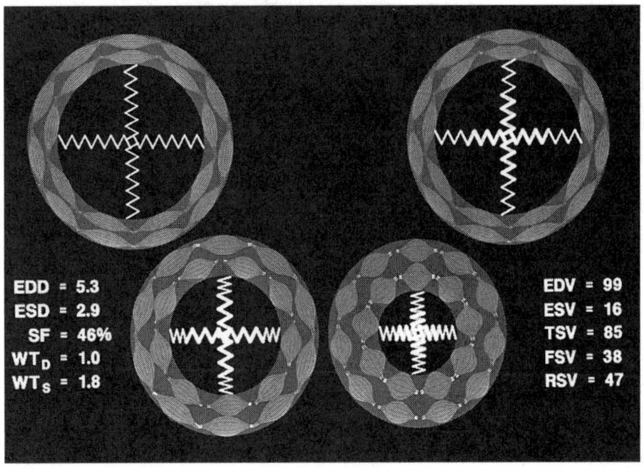

FIGURE 19-5 Cross-sections of a left ventricle from a dog with moderate mitral regurgitation and moderate eccentric hypertrophy. The regurgitant fraction (regurgitant stroke volume ÷ total stroke volume) is 55%. Notice that the springs in systole now have two components. The thinner, outer component represents the lower pressure in early systole, during which contraction can occur in mitral regurgitation (ventricular unloading). The thicker, inner portion represents the normal pressure in later systole. An additional cross-section is presented to show the end of the early part of systole. Eccentric hypertrophy has compensated perfectly for the amount of mitral regurgitant flow so that forward stroke volume is normal. Abbreviations are as in Figure 19-2.

At this stage, the dog has a moderate-intensity systolic heart murmur but is otherwise clinically normal. Thoracic radiographs would show moderate cardiomegaly with a moderately enlarged left atrium.

The plasma concentration of immunoreactive atrial natriuretic peptide (ANP) has been measured in Cavalier King Charles spaniels at this phase of the disease. The concentration was not increased.[18]

SEVERE MITRAL REGURGITATION IN SMALL DOGS

In MVD, only dogs with severe mitral regurgitation develop heart failure. Dogs with chronic MVD that are in heart failure have a moderately-to-severely enlarged left atrium. The left atrium can be normal in size with acute mitral regurgitation resulting from chordal rupture.

At 11 years of age, the Lhasa apso in Figure 19-6 has severe mitral regurgitation (regurgitant fraction greater than 75%). In this example, the regurgitant fraction is 76% and is now severe enough to produce clinical signs of heart failure at rest. Forward stroke volume is mildly decreased. The heart rate would be expected to increase to compensate for this, so the dog would be unlikely to have clinical evidence of hypoperfusion.[19] Note that end-systolic diameter and end-systolic volume are still normal because myocardial contractility either is normal or is reduced with adrenergic support.[19,20] Left ventricular wall motion is hyperdynamic, as evidenced by the increased shortening fraction, and is due to the increase in end-diastolic diameter. In mitral regurgitation at this stage the diastolic intraventricular pressure is increased because the body continues to retain sodium and water to compensate for the leak but the ventricle is reaching the end-stage of its ability to increase in size. Consequently, blood is being forced into a chamber that can no longer distend or grow larger. Because the left ventricular diastolic pressure is increased, the left atrial diastolic pressure increased. The systolic leak of blood into the left atrium produces an even higher systolic left atrial pressure, which would be seen as an increased *v* wave on a left

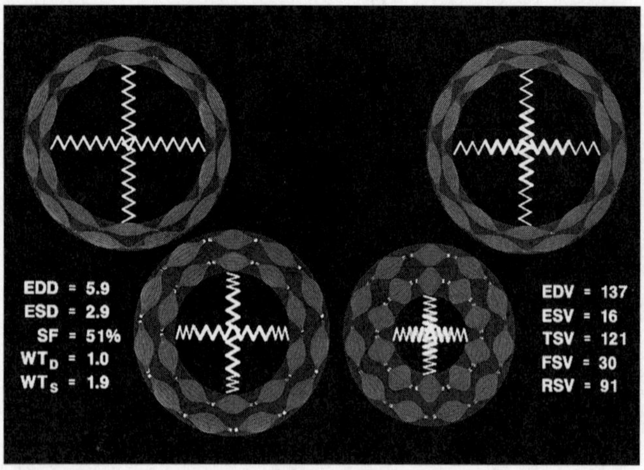

FIGURE 19-6 Cross-sections of a ventricle from a dog with severe mitral regurgitation and normal myocardial function. Note that the springs in systole are the same as in Figure 19-5. The regurgitant fraction is 76%. There is marked volume overload hypertrophy, with the end-diastolic volume approximately 2.5 times normal. The end-systolic diameter and volume are normal. Consequently, the left ventricle is pumping a total stroke volume of 121 mL with each beat, approximately 3.3 times normal. The shortening fraction has increased to 51%. because of the volume overload hypertrophy (the increase in end-diastolic diameter). Note the marked wall thickening that takes place at the end of systole. Abbreviations are as in Figure 19-2.

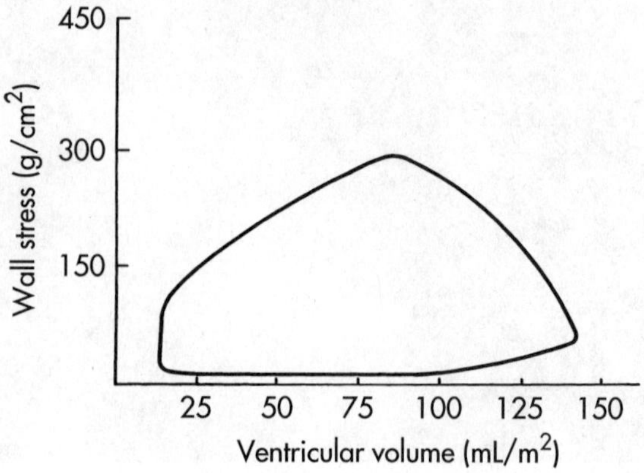

FIGURE 19-7 Schematic drawing of a wall stress–volume loop from a dog with severe mitral regurgitation and normal myocardial function, as seen in Figure 19-6. Wall stress starts to decrease as soon as the ventricle starts to develop force. This is the result of the ventricle's ability to eject blood into the low-pressure left atrium in early systole. When ejection takes place, the chamber size decreases and the wall thickens, resulting in a decrease in wall stress. Consequently, peak systolic wall stress does not increase. Rather, it stays within the normal range. Consequently, one would not expect myocardial oxygen consumption to increase.

atrial pressure tracing (see Figure 17-7). Increased left atrial pressure results in increased pulmonary capillary pressure that results in the transudation of fluid from the capillary spaces into the lung tissue (pulmonary edema). The increased left ventricular diastolic pressure in Figure 19-6 is depicted as a thicker spring in diastole. Left ventricular weight is now 200 g/m^2.

At this phase of the disease, the plasma concentration of ANP is increased.[18] The plasma concentration of aldosterone is generally also increased.[21] Heart rate variability is decreased, providing evidence for increased sympathetic and decreased vagal tone.[22]

This dog has mild-to-moderate respiratory signs, usually coughing. He has a loud systolic heart murmur and a markedly enlarged left atrium on thoracic radiographs and on an echocardiogram. This dog needs drug administration to treat congestive heart failure.

Ventricular unloading in mitral regurgitation. Note in Figures 19-5 and 19-6 why the left ventricle moves so well in systole in this disease. In a normal heart, the left ventricle does not eject blood in early systole. Instead it only develops pressure while volume remains the same (isovolumic systole). In mitral regurgitation the left ventricle is allowed to eject blood into the left atrium during early systole. In fact, it can eject up to 50% of the total left ventricular stroke volume into the left atrium before the aortic valve opens.[23] Consequently, the ventricular walls move immediately during early systole as the ventricle ejects blood into the left atrium. As a result, the left ventricle decreases in size as soon as systole begins. This unloading of the left ventricle gives it a hemodynamic advantage. The initial motion is very easy because the pressure in the ventricle is low and therefore systolic wall stress (afterload) is low. This is depicted as a thinner spring toward the outside of the spring in Figures 19-5 and 19-6. In the lower left portions of these figures, the initial easy contraction during early systole is complete. Later in systole, pressure is normal, the chamber radius is smaller, and the wall is thicker than at the onset of systole because some contraction has already occurred. Consequently the afterload (systolic wall stress) is never increased. Because contractility is normal, the left ventricle can go through its normal motion later in systole as normal systolic pressure is achieved and the aortic valve opens. In summary, the left ventricle goes through two phases of contraction: an initial easy contraction (low pressure and wall stress) and, later, more normal contraction (because of the normal systolic pressure, the smaller radius, and the increased wall thickness at this time). Obviously in real life this abrupt change from low to normal wall stress does not occur. Instead, there is a progressive change throughout systole.

A wall stress–volume loop from a dog with severe mitral regurgitation and normal myocardial function, similar to the dog in Figure 19-6, is presented in Figure 19-7. This figure shows the lack of an isovolumic phase to systole, the resultant decrease in chamber volume and size before the aortic valve opens, the normal peak systolic wall stress, the markedly increased total stroke volume, and the normal end-systolic volume.

VERY SEVERE (REFRACTORY) MITRAL REGURGITATION IN SMALL DOGS

In small dogs with mitral regurgitation, myocardial contractility may become depressed in the late stages of the disease. Commonly, when this stage is reached, the dog is refractory to conventional drug therapy. Our imaginary case at 12 years of age is depicted in Figure 19-8. This patient is now on maximum doses of furosemide and on an angiotensin converting enzyme inhibitor. When myocardial contractility decreases, the end-systolic volume increases. In Figure 19-8 it has increased from 16 to 40 mL/m^2 (ESD = 3.9 cm/m^2). End-diastolic volume has increased even further to 159 mL/m^2 to compensate. Forward stroke volume is decreased to 20 mL/m^2, and the total stroke volume of the left ventricle is still markedly increased at 119 mL/m^2. The regurgitant stroke volume is now massive (99 mL/m^2), as is the regurgitant fraction at 83% (for every 10 mL/m^2 of blood ejected, approximately 8 mL/m^2 goes into the left atrium and 2 mL/m^2 goes into the aorta). Shortening fraction is 37%. Notice

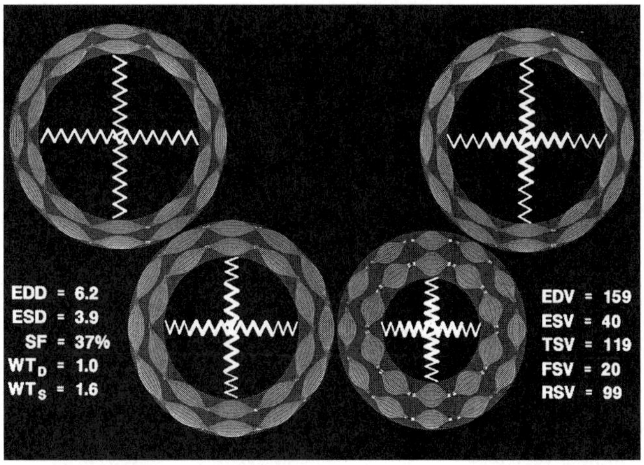

FIGURE 19-8 Cross-sections of a ventricle from a dog with end-stage mitral regurgitation and mild-to-moderate myocardial failure. Note the increase in end-systolic diameter and volume and the normal shortening fraction. The forward stroke volume is decreased. Abbreviations are as in Figure 19-2.

that shortening fraction is within the normal range when myocardial failure is present in this disease. Left ventricular wall thickness remains 1 cm/m^2. Left ventricular weight, however, has increased to 219 g/m^2, almost double that of a normal dog. Left ventricular diastolic chamber volume has tripled, and the number of muscles around the outside row has increased from nine to 12. The left ventricular weight is similar to that attained in one study in which aorto-caval fistulas were produced in dogs to cause chronic heart failure.[24] This appears to be the maximum size attainable by the left ventricle. This figure would also be appropriate for depicting the changes seen in a large dog with severe mitral regurgitation, because large dogs commonly develop myocardial failure earlier than small dogs, in our experience. Dogs at this stage have severe cardiomegaly. The left atrium is especially enlarged. They have a poor long-term prognosis and are at risk for developing atrial fibrillation because of the markedly enlarged left atrium. The plasma aldosterone and ANP concentrations are markedly increased at this stage when the patient is in heart failure.[21]

In summary, small dogs with primary mitral regurgitation as a result of mitral valve degeneration compensate for mild-to-moderate disease very well, primarily through volume overload (eccentric) hypertrophy. This compensation usually lasts for years as the leak in the mitral valve gradually worsens. Myocardial function during this stage in small dogs stays normal. When heart failure begins it is due to massive regurgitation of blood and not to myocardial failure. By the time the patient has become refractory to furosemide administration, myocardial failure may be evident but is still mild compared with that of a patient with dilated cardiomyopathy, while massive regurgitation is present.

LARGE DOGS WITH MYXOMATOUS MITRAL VALVE DEGENERATION

As opposed to small dogs with primary mitral valve disease, myocardial failure is more severe and develops earlier in larger dogs with mitral regurgitation. Experimental studies of mitral regurgitation routinely use large (20 to 25 kg) dogs as the model of the disease, and myocardial contractility is routinely decreased in these studies.[25-27] In clinical cases, the end-systolic diameter and end-systolic volume are moderately increased, along with a moderate increase in end-diastolic diameter and end-diastolic volume. Consequently, shortening fraction is usually within the normal range, although it may be mildly decreased. Large dogs should have the same hemodynamic advantage as small dogs, yet more problems with myocardial function develop. Because humans with mitral regurgitation also develop myocardial failure, there is something obviously different between small patients and large patients, but the origin of that difference is unknown. Few studies have addressed the issue of why myocardial failure develops in myocardium subjected to an increased workload. One recent study examined the role of oxidative stress on production of myocardial failure in guinea pigs with supravalvular aortic stenosis.[28] It was found that vitamin E prevented the development of ultrastructural myocardial damage and heart failure in this species. Although the same amount of hypertrophy was present in guinea pigs with aortic stenosis with and without vitamin E administration, there was less oxidative stress and less lipid peroxidation in the hearts from the animals that were administered vitamin E.

MITRAL REGURGITATION COMPLICATED BY ATRIAL FIBRILLATION

Dogs with severe mitral regurgitation can develop atrial fibrillation. The onset of atrial fibrillation in a small dog with mitral regurgitation is often related to the onset of worsening clinical signs and a poor prognosis. Atrial fibrillation significantly worsens hemodynamics in large dogs with mitral regurgitation and presumably in small dogs with mitral regurgitation. In one study of dogs with experimentally produced mitral regurgitation, six dogs went into atrial fibrillation at the time of cardiac catheterization.[29] They were studied at that time and again later when they were not in atrial fibrillation. When in atrial fibrillation the cardiac index was approximately 25% less, stroke volume index was approximately 50% less, and pulmonary capillary pressure was approximately 6 mm Hg higher than when the dogs were not in atrial fibrillation. The heart rate was only 150 beats/min on average when these dogs were in atrial fibrillation vs. 110 beats/min when they were not in atrial fibrillation. Consequently, blaming inadequate ventricular filling time for these marked changes is difficult. Apparently the loss of atrial systolic left ventricular filling can be catastrophic to dogs with atrial fibrillation and mitral regurgitation.

TRICUSPID REGURGITATION

The pathophysiology of tricuspid regurgitation is very similar to that of mitral regurgitation. The major differences are as follows. First, when tricuspid regurgitation becomes severe and the right heart fails, ascites is most commonly produced. Second, because the right heart generates much less pressure than the left side, a similar size orifice in the tricuspid valve results in a smaller leak than on the left side. Consequently, the orifice size must be much larger on the right side to produce heart failure. As a consequence, right heart failure usually develops later than left heart failure in dogs with myxomatous atrioventricular valve disease, if it develops at all. In our experience, right heart failure in dogs with primary tricuspid regurgitation as a result of MVD is most commonly identified in dogs with preexisting pulmonary disease and moderate-to-severe pulmonary hypertension caused by pulmonary vascular disease. Pulmonary vascular disease increases pulmonary vascular resistance, which decreases forward flow and increases regurgitant flow.

PULMONARY HYPERTENSION IN MITRAL REGURGITATION

When dogs with chronic myxomatous atrioventricular valve degeneration develop right heart failure it is often thought to be a result of their preexisting left heart failure. In people, horses, and some cats, left heart failure can produce right heart failure even when right heart disease is not present.[30] In these species, a reflex pulmonary arteriolar vasoconstriction occurs secondary to pulmonary venous hypertension, which can result in severe pulmonary hypertension. The pulmonary vasoconstriction may be due to enhanced endothelin-I release in these species.[31] It has been reported that left heart failure can also produce severe pulmonary hypertension and resultant right heart failure in dogs.[32] In our experience this can occur but is unusual in dogs. Although left heart failure can certainly exacerbate existing right heart disease in dogs, in our experience it is very unusual for it to result in right heart failure when right heart disease is not already present. This is because reflex pulmonary vasoconstriction appears to be unusual in dogs.

In most of the dogs that we see with left heart failure, pulmonary artery pressure is increased, but only mildly. This mild increase is to be expected. In dogs with severe left heart failure, the left ventricular end-diastolic pressure can be expected to be in the 30- to 40-mm Hg range. For illustration purposes, assume that the left ventricular end-diastolic pressure is 35 mm Hg. During diastole the mitral valve is open and left ventricular pressure and left atrial pressure are similar, so we can assume that left atrial, pulmonary vein, and pulmonary capillary pressures are 35 mm Hg. If we assume a reasonable diastolic interval, diastolic pressure in the pulmonary artery should equalize with pulmonary capillary pressure. This makes pulmonary artery diastolic pressure 35 mm Hg, also. The normal pulmonary artery diastolic pressure is approximately 10 mm Hg. The pulmonary artery diastolic pressure is now increased by 25 mm Hg. Normal pulmonary artery systolic pressure is approximately 25 mm Hg. If we assume a normal pulse pressure, pulmonary artery systolic pressure would be 50 mm Hg in this case. This means that in severe left heart failure, right ventricular systolic pressure (which is the same as pulmonary artery systolic pressure in this case) would be 50 mm Hg instead of 25 mm Hg. This is comparable to mild pulmonic stenosis. Because dogs with isolated mild pulmonic stenosis are normal clinically and never go into right heart failure, it is difficult to rationalize how this mild increase in right ventricular systolic pressure could result in right heart failure. On the other hand, if such a dog also had moderate tricuspid regurgitation, mild systolic hypertension could exacerbate moderate regurgitation into severe regurgitation and produce right heart failure.

Natural History

Clinical evidence of valvular regurgitation (presence of a typical heart murmur) in dogs is commonly initially present between 6 and 9 years of age. The exception to this rule is the Cavalier King Charles spaniel, in which the heart murmur commonly is present at an earlier age. From the point of murmur identification, the disease may progress relatively rapidly such that the dog is in heart failure within 1 to 2 years (most common in Cavalier King Charles spaniels), but it more commonly progresses gradually. Acute progression to heart failure occurs in some dogs with chordal rupture. Gradual progression is best followed on radiographs. Here the left heart progressively enlarges over several years. Heart failure ultimately ensues in some dogs. In other dogs the progression may be so slow that heart failure is never produced within the dog's lifetime. Consequently, the long-term prognosis for a dog diagnosed with a heart murmur typical of atrioventricular valve regurgitation is unknown in the early stages of the disease. In our experience, most dogs with moderate-to-severe heart enlargement will progress to heart failure.

Once a dog is in heart failure, the survival time is variable, and therefore long-term prognosis is guarded in an individual patient. However, there are some facts that can be related to a client. Data derived from clinical trials of the use of milrinone in dogs encompass the largest number of dogs with valvular disease studied.[33] The addition of milrinone to the therapeutic regimen could have altered survival and so these data may not be truly representative of dogs treated with conventional drugs. However, the data do not appear to be grossly skewed in one direction or the other. Of the 93 dogs in this study, 40 were in mild-to-moderate heart failure at presentation and 53 were in severe heart failure. In the dogs with severe failure, 25% died within the first 3 months, 50% within the first 7 months, and 75% within the first year after diagnosis. In the dogs with mild-to-moderate heart failure, 25% died within the first 6 months, 50% within the first year, and 75% within 1 year and 9 months.

Myxomatous valve degeneration in Cavalier King Charles spaniels. Cavalier King Charles spaniels represent a unique breed of dog with MVD. The prevalence of the disease is high in this breed, and the disease appears in some dogs at a very early age. In one study, 10% of very young Cavalier King Charles spaniels (less than 1 year of age) had a murmur characteristic of mitral regurgitation.[10] In another study, 13% of these dogs 3.0 ± 2.7 years had a characteristic heart murmur.[34] In another group aged 6.4 ± 2.8 years, 52% had a heart murmur.[34] Similarly, in dogs greater than 4 years of age, 56% had a heart murmur.[10] Almost all Cavalier King Charles spaniels have MVD by the time they are 10 years of age.[10] Apparently, heart failure also occurs earlier in this breed. One study in the United States has documented that the first visit to a referral veterinary hospital for Cavalier King Charles spaniels occurred at an average age of 6.25 years.[10] For other breeds of dogs, this value was 12 years. In Sweden, Cavalier King Charles spaniels may live somewhat longer with their heart disease. In one study, the average age when heart failure occurred was 9.6 years.[19]

Diagnosis

The diagnosis of mitral regurgitation resulting from MVD is commonly based on signalment, history, physical examination findings, and thoracic radiographs. Electrocardiography is usually not helpful in making the diagnosis, although it may be helpful in identifying chamber enlargement. Echocardiography identifies the abnormal valve anatomy and the chamber enlargements, and Doppler echocardiography can be used to definitively identify the regurgitant jet and its peak velocity.

HISTORY AND CLINICAL SIGNS

Dogs with chronic atrioventricular valve regurgitation secondary to MVD commonly present to the veterinarian in two ways. The most common presentation is a dog with mild-to-moderate disease and no history of clinical abnormalities. This type of patient is commonly presented for vaccination or for another problem, and a heart murmur is ausculted during a routine physical examination. The owner should be counseled about the dog's disease at this time and told that this is a progressive disease that can culminate in heart failure. They can be told that the progression to heart failure can be relatively rapid (especially if a chordal structure ruptures) or it can take years. They should be reassured that most dogs have mitral regurgitation for many years before heart failure becomes evident and that some dogs never develop heart failure. Radiographs should be taken to stage the disease and establish a baseline.

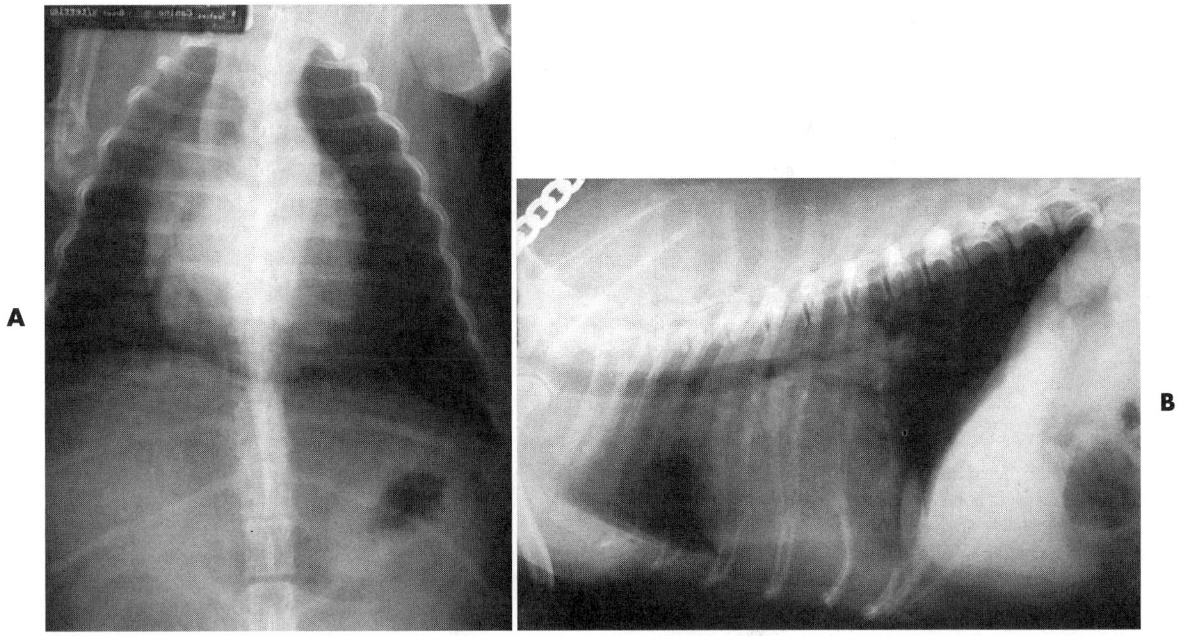

FIGURE 19-9 Dorsoventral (**A**) and lateral (**B**) radiographs from a 14-year-old terrier cross with a severe cough and a heart murmur characteristic of mitral regurgitation. The referring veterinarian noted a heavy interstitial pattern in the right caudodorsal lung field. He treated the dog with an antibiotic and furosemide, but the dog continued to cough. Physical examination revealed the heart murmur and inspiratory crackles and pops. On the thoracic radiographs, the left atrium was severely enlarged and the infiltrate was no longer present. The mainstem bronchi appeared compressed on the lateral view. **A,** The left mainstem bronchus is compressed from the seventh to the tenth ribs. The accessory lobe bronchus is also compressed between the seventh and ninth ribs. The dog was treated with aminophylline and improved but did not completely stop coughing. A cough suppressant was then administered with good results.

Dogs that are in heart failure secondary to mitral regurgitation usually present because the owner has noted abnormal respiratory signs. These signs include cough, tachypnea, and dyspnea and are secondary to the presence of pulmonary edema. Clinical signs may develop gradually in dogs as the disease progresses or signs may appear to develop suddenly. In the latter situation, either the dog hides its clinical signs successfully until heart failure is moderate to severe or the owner is not attentive and so misses the early clinical signs. In these cases a disease that is actually chronic appears to be an acute disease to the owner. This occurs most frequently in sedentary dogs. In some dogs clinical signs actually do develop acutely. In these cases, an acute rupture of a chorda tendineae, an acute onset of an arrhythmia (usually atrial fibrillation), or an acute salt load can produce acute heart failure. Dogs that present acutely, for whatever reason, are often presented with severe-to-fulminant pulmonary edema and require immediate attention.

Cough. Coughing is a common presenting complaint in dogs with a murmur of mitral regurgitation. The cough secondary to pulmonary edema in small dogs may be soft or may be harsh. In large dogs it is more commonly soft. The cough is often exacerbated by excitement or exercise. Occasionally it is present more often at night. However, this aspect is often overplayed in the veterinary literature, probably because paroxysmal nocturnal dyspnea is common in humans with heart failure. The clinician must be aware that coughing is a common sequela to respiratory disease, and older small dogs with mitral regurgitation commonly have concomitant respiratory disease. Consequently, the combination of a cough and a typical heart murmur do not necessarily indicate heart failure. Further diagnostic tests, primarily radiography and echocardiography, must be performed to make the diagnosis of heart failure secondary to mitral regurgitation. Dogs that are in heart failure have evidence of pulmonary edema and a large left atrium on a thoracic radiograph, unless heart failure is secondary to a ruptured chord. On echocardiography, the left atrium must at least be moderately enlarged to be compatible with left heart failure, except in the instance of a ruptured chorda tendineae, in which case the left atrial size may be normal.

Dogs with mitral regurgitation not only develop a cough secondary to pulmonary edema. Left atrial enlargement often compresses the left mainstem bronchus or the accessory lobe bronchus (Figure 19-9). Normal airways probably do not collapse with this compression. However, bronchomalacia is a common malady in older, small-breed dogs in which mitral regurgitation commonly occurs. The combination of bronchomalacia and severe left atrial enlargement commonly results in airway compression and collapse. The airway collapse produces a cough that is often severe and refractory to therapy.

Other clinical signs. Dogs with heart failure may also lose weight and, if they exercise, have exercise intolerance. Syncope may also accompany the signs of heart failure or be present by itself. Syncope may be due to an arrhythmia or acute vasodilation or may be secondary to severe coughing (see Chapter 28). It is the result of the dog's heart disease but is not a sign of heart failure. It is not due to a low cardiac output as a result of heart failure. Ascites as a result of concomitant tricuspid regurgitation and right heart failure occurs occasionally either without evidence of left heart failure or as a very late finding in a dog with severe mitral regurgitation.

Dogs with severe myxomatous mitral valve degeneration may die suddenly. The most common cause is a left atrial tear with resultant

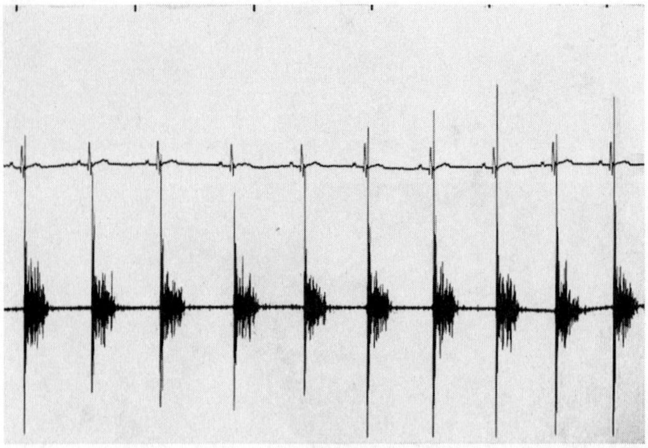

FIGURE 19-10 Phonocardiogram recorded at the left apex from a dog with severe mitral regurgitation. The first heart sound is very loud. The heart murmur starts immediately after the first heart sound. The murmur has the same intensity throughout systole on most of the recordings. In some the murmur decreases in intensity. The second heart sound cannot be seen because the heart murmur continues through it (pansystolic heart murmur).

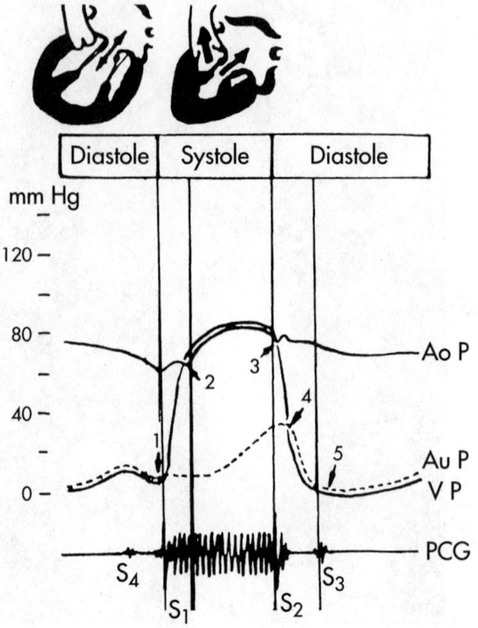

FIGURE 19-11 Schematic drawing presented to explain the reason that the heart murmur lasts through the second heart sound in patients with severe mitral regurgitation. Aortic *(Ao)*, left ventricular *(V)*, and left auricular *(Au)* pressures *(P)* are drawn simultaneously with a phonocardiogram *(PCG)*. The mitral valve closes when left ventricular pressure exceeds left atrial pressure *(1)*, coincident with the first heart sound *(S_1)*. The heart murmur starts immediately after mitral valve closure and extends through systole. Regurgitation occurs as long as left ventricular pressure exceeds left atrial pressure. The second heart sound *(S_2)* is generated when left ventricular pressure drops below aortic pressure and the aortic valve closes. Note that left ventricular pressure continues to exceed left atrial pressure for a short time after aortic valve closure, during isovolumic relaxation. Consequently, the regurgitation and the heart murmur continue after the second heart sound. Note the third heart sound *(S_3)*, which occurs at the end of rapid ventricular filling, and the fourth heart sound *(S_4)*, which occurs with atrial systole.

acute pericardial tamponade (Color Plate 73). Occasionally a dog with a left atrial tear will survive for a short time and present to a veterinarian in acute collapse or collapse in the veterinarian's office. The cardiac silhouette may or may not appear enlarged on thoracic radiographs. The heart sounds may or may not be muffled. Pulsus paradoxus may or may not be present. Echocardiography is the best diagnostic test and usually reveals a small amount of pericardial effusion and a linear thrombus in the pericardial space. Acute rupture of a primary chord can also produce sudden or acute death.

PHYSICAL EXAMINATION

Heart murmur. A heart murmur is almost always identified in a dog with MVD of an atrioventricular valve severe enough to cause a clinically significant leak. The murmur secondary to mitral valve regurgitation is heard best over the left apex. The intensity of the murmur is usually constant (plateau) and blowing (Figure 19-10). This type of murmur occurs secondary to the vibrations created by turbulent blood flow that occurs secondary to the high-velocity jet of blood that shoots into the left atrium in systole. Because the jet is directed dorsally into the left atrium, one might expect to hear the murmur over the mid-to-upper chest. This does not occur because of a large acoustic mismatch between the soft tissue of the heart and the lung tissue that surrounds it. This mismatch prevents the sound from transmitting well through the lung to the thoracic wall. Where the heart touches the chest wall (at the apex beat), there is a much smaller acoustic mismatch, and sound travels more readily from soft tissue to soft tissue and so to the surface of the chest. When loud, the murmur commonly radiates widely to other regions of the chest, especially to the right apex, dorsally, and caudally. The murmur is usually either holosystolic (lasting throughout systole) or pansystolic (lasting through the second heart sound). Regurgitation starts as soon as the left ventricle begins to tense and left ventricular pressure exceeds left atrial pressure. Consequently, the murmur starts immediately after the first heart sound. The murmur then continues until left ventricular pressure decreases below left atrial pressure. This occurs after left ventricular pressure decreases below aortic pressure, the time that the second heart sound occurs (Figure 19-11). Consequently, the murmur of mitral regurgitation commonly lasts through, and so obliterates, the second heart sound.

Occasionally, a single-frequency murmur that is commonly high-pitched (whooping) can be heard (Figure 19-12). This type of heart murmur is usually created by a portion of a valve leaflet vibrating. On occasion, this can be seen as high-frequency vibrations of a valve leaflet on an M-mode echocardiogram and may be the result of at least second-order chordal rupture.

The intensity of the heart murmur roughly corresponds to the severity of the disease. In one study, all dogs with a grade 2 or less heart murmur had mild disease and most dogs with a grade 5 or 6 heart murmur had severe disease. None had mild disease.[35] Those dogs with grade 3 and 4 murmurs, the most common grades, had mild-to-severe disease. In this study, the murmur intensity increased in individual dogs as the disease progressed in severity. These data exclude the "honking" or musical type of murmur in which the murmur is very loud and the disease is usually mild.

That murmur intensity has some relationship with disease severity in mitral regurgitation might be expected. The force generated by turbulent blood flow and therefore the intensity of the murmur at its origin is determined by blood flow velocity (cm/s) and the flow rate (cm^3/s or g/s) where velocity × flow = force [dynes or grams cm/sec^2]. In mitral regurgitation, the velocity of blood flow across the mitral valve is determined by the pressure gradient across the valve in systole, according to the modified Bernoulli equation, where velocity = ($\sqrt{\text{pressure gradient}} \div 4$). Systolic pressure in the left

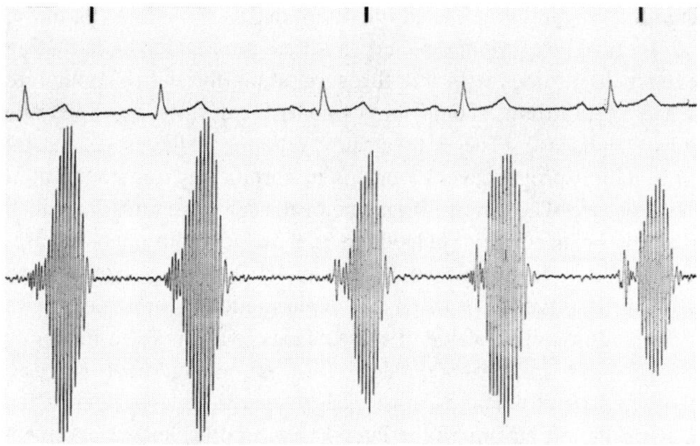

FIGURE 19-12 Phonocardiogram from a dog with mitral regurgitation and a single-frequency, or musical, heart murmur. The murmur is of low frequency and sounded like a "honk."

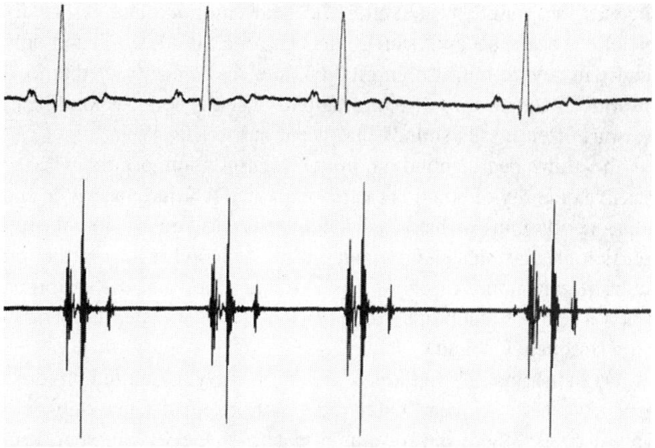

FIGURE 19-13 Phonocardiogram and an electrocardiogram from a dog with a systolic click. The click is a high-frequency sound that occurs between the first heart sound *(S_1)* and the second heart sound *(S_2)*. In this dog the click was louder than the first and second heart sounds.

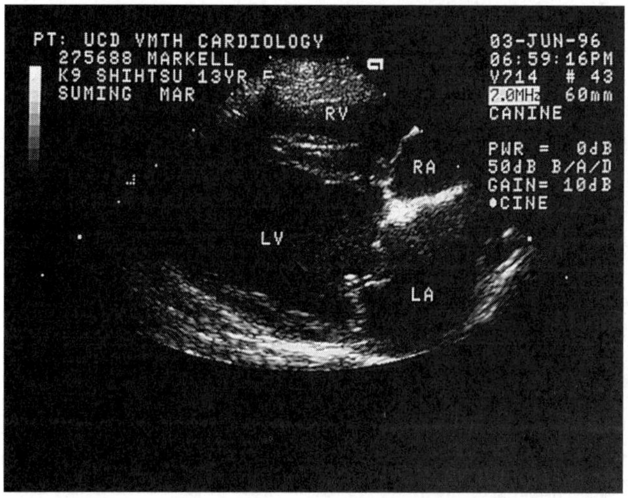

FIGURE 19-14 Two-dimensional echocardiogram from a dog with severe mitral valve prolapse. The mid-portion of the septal leaflet bulges back into the left atrium in systole.

ventricle is maintained at 120 to 150 mm Hg until the very late stages of the disease. Left atrial pressure gradually increases from less than 10 mm Hg to greater than 30 mm Hg as heart failure worsens. This means the pressure gradient can range from 90 mm Hg to 140 mm Hg. Consequently, velocity ranges from approximately 4.7 to 5.9 m/sec; therefore it has the potential of changing within the range of about 20%. Conversely, we have documented flow rates through the mitral valve as low as 40 mL/sec in dogs with mild mitral regurgitation and as high as 800 mL/sec in dogs with severe regurgitation.[15] Obviously, the flow rate experiences a much greater change than does flow velocity and therefore must be the major factor that determines murmur intensity at the origin of the murmur (the intensity you might hear if you were able to place your stethoscope in the turbulent jet). The flow rate and the size of a color flow Doppler jet correlate to each other. Consequently, the size of the jet on ultrasound and the intensity of the heart murmur should also correlate. The intensity of the heart murmur at the surface, however, is determined by many variables. These include the intensity of the heart murmur at its origin, the direction of the turbulent jet in relation to the region ausculted, the character of the tissues between the turbulent jet and the area being ausculted, the frequency of the murmur, the quality of the stethoscope, and the ability of the examiner to hear. Because of this it is expected that murmur intensity would have a rough correlation with disease severity but that there would be variability from dog to dog and examiner to examiner. It is also expected that the relationship between disease severity and murmur intensity would improve dramatically if the same examiner listened to the same dog with the same stethoscope over time.

First heart sound. The intensity of the first heart sound is increased in dogs with mitral regurgitation (see Figure 19-10).[35] The mitral valve opens very wide in dogs with mitral regurgitation, and the velocity of force generation is increased. Both variables, alone or in combination, increase the intensity of the first heart sound.

Systolic click. Occasionally a systolic click is ausculted in dogs with early mitral valve disease (Figure 19-13). A systolic click is a high-frequency sound that occurs between the first and second heart sounds. It is commonly mistaken for a gallop sound. There are three ways to rule out a gallop sound in this situation. First, if one has heard a systolic click before, making the same mistake again is unusual because the sound is unique. It has a higher pitch than a gallop sound and sounds like a click rather than a thud. Second, a phonocardiogram can be recorded. The phonocardiogram allows one to distinguish between a third diastolic sound (gallop sound) and a third systolic sound (systolic click). Third, one can use logic. If one hears three heart sounds in a middle-age, small-breed dog that has no or only mild cardiovascular pathology (which can be verified by taking a thoracic radiograph) then logic dictates that it is most likely a systolic click. Gallop sounds do not occur in dogs without significant cardiac disease and there are no other common types of extra heart sounds in otherwise normal dogs.

Systolic clicks are produced by mitral valve prolapse in humans. Although prolapse does occur in myxomatous mitral valve degeneration in dogs and can be identified using echocardiography, we have not documented this in all cases in which systolic clicks were heard (Figure 19-14). Most likely a small region of the valve prolapses and is not readily discerned on echocardiography.

Third heart sound. A third heart sound is common in dogs with severe mitral regurgitation.[35] However, the third heart sound in this disease is not readily discerned by most veterinarians. This occurs for three reasons. First, the sound is of low frequency, and most veterinarians are not trained to listen to low-frequency sounds.

Second, the sound occurs after the heart murmur and is usually mistaken for the second heart sound. Third, a third heart sound only occurs in severe mitral regurgitation, and the intensity of the heart murmur in severe mitral regurgitation is usually loud. A loud heart murmur often masks sounds that occur subsequent to it.

The third heart sound in mitral regurgitation occurs when a massive quantity of blood is ejected into the left atrium in systole and subsequently joins with normal venous return to "dump" into the left ventricle in diastole. The massive inflow of blood results in the left ventricle distending rapidly to its maximum point of distensibility. When it reaches this point, the walls shudder or vibrate, resulting in a low-frequency sound.

Arrhythmias. Arrhythmias are commonly ausculted in dogs with advanced atrioventricular regurgitation, most commonly premature beats. There is no reliable means of identifying supraventricular vs. ventricular premature depolarizations on auscultation. Consequently, an electrocardiogram must be evaluated to determine the origin. Atrial fibrillation sounds like "tennis shoes in a dryer," with an admixture of variable-intensity first heart sounds, present or absent second heart sounds, and third heart sounds. Ventricular tachyarrhythmias may sound like atrial fibrillation, therefore an electrocardiogram must be evaluated. Respiratory sinus arrhythmia is common in breeds predisposed to MVD. In dogs with mild MVD, respiratory sinus arrhythmia may be mistaken for a more serious arrhythmia by auscultation alone and lead one to believe the valvular insufficiency is more severe.

Lung sounds. Lung sounds in dogs with MVD of the mitral valve are variable. In dogs that have no clinical signs, the lung sounds are usually normal. In dogs presented for coughing, lung sounds may be normal or snaps, crackles, and wheezes may be present. Although abnormal lung sounds may occur in dogs with pulmonary edema, loud abnormal sounds are much more common in dogs that have chronic airway disease (collapsing airways, chronic bronchitis, etc.). Dogs that are hyperpneic because of moderate pulmonary edema, commonly have only increased bronchovesicular sounds as a result of an increased amount of air moving through the airways. Some dogs with pulmonary edema, however, will have fine crackles to coarse pops. This is more common with severe edema in which edema fluid actually fills the airways. Even with severe edema, some dogs do not have abnormal lung sounds. In one study only 68% of dogs with severe edema had crackles.[36]

Femoral pulse quality. The femoral pulse in dogs with mild-to-moderate mitral regurgitation is usually normal. In dogs with severe regurgitation the pulse is commonly "brisk." A brisk pulse has a steep rise and a steep descent with a normal-to-mild increase in pulse pressure that occurs over a shorter-than-normal interval. In mitral regurgitation the left ventricle must develop force rapidly and eject its contents rapidly. If a slow contraction occurred, more blood would flow into the left atrium than would with a fast contraction. Consequently, the left ventricle contracts rapidly and blood is ejected into the aorta rapidly. Ejection time is commonly decreased in mitral regurgitation.[36]

Right heart disease. Tricuspid regurgitation is difficult to diagnose based on auscultation in dogs with concomitant mitral regurgitation. The mitral murmur commonly radiates to the right side, which makes it difficult to discern if the right-sided murmur is a radiation or a primary murmur. The jugular veins may be distended or have a systolic pulsation with severe tricuspid regurgitation. Severe regurgitation may, however, be present with no discernible jugular vein abnormality. Dogs that are in right heart failure secondary to tricuspid regurgitation usually have ascites. Pleural effusion and subcutaneous edema can also occur but are unusual.

RADIOGRAPHY

The thoracic radiograph is an important means of diagnosing mitral and tricuspid regurgitation and is often crucial for determining severity. In all dogs with mitral regurgitation, the radiographic size of the left atrium should be evaluated carefully to stage the patient's disease. The left atrium reliably enlarges as mitral regurgitation progressively worsens in chronic myxomatous mitral valve disease. The left atrium is one of the few structures for which size can be accurately judged on a thoracic radiograph. Consequently, the radiographic impression of left atrial size can be used to judge the severity of the mitral regurgitation in most dogs with myxomatous mitral valve disease. Dogs with mild-to-moderate disease have mild-to-moderate left atrial enlargement (Figures 19-15 and 19-16). This is most clearly seen as enlargement of the body of the left atrium on the lateral view in dogs and enlargement of the left auricle on the dorsoventral view. Dogs with severe, chronic mitral regurgitation almost always have radiographic evidence of severe left atrial enlargement (Figure 19-17). Dogs with severe left atrial enlargement often have pulmonary edema. The radiographic impression of left ventricular enlargement is usually more difficult to evaluate and depends on the size of the left ventricle, the size of the right ventricle, the chest conformation of the dog, the phase of respiration, and the position of the heart in the thorax.

The lungs should be evaluated for the presence of pulmonary edema. By definition, dogs with mitral regurgitation that are in heart failure have pulmonary edema. Severe and moderate pulmonary edema are readily diagnosed. Mild pulmonary edema, however, is often difficult to diagnose. Mild-to-moderate pulmonary edema is usually perihilar and is centrally located. Consequently, it is best evaluated on a lateral thoracic radiograph (Figure 19-18). In many cases, pulmonary edema as a result of MVD of the mitral valve occurs in older dogs that already have chronic pulmonary parenchymal changes. In most dogs, obtaining an adequate inspiratory radiograph is impossible. Consequently, when one is trying to evaluate the caudodorsal lung fields for mild pulmonary edema, one is also looking at lung fields that have increased interstitial density because of the age-related changes and the expiratory phase. In this situation examining the size of the pulmonary veins may be helpful. However, these veins are not always readily discernible, and, when they are, the increase in size is often subtle. Consequently, if mild pulmonary edema is suspected but cannot be proved, a trial regimen of diuretic therapy may be required to see if clinical signs improve.

Most dogs with severe mitral regurgitation and pulmonary edema have an enlarged left atrium. Dogs with severe regurgitation secondary to acute chordal rupture, however, may not have left atrial enlargement. Conversely, some dogs with chronic, severe mitral regurgitation have a remarkably large and compliant left atrium that can accommodate the massive flow into it without an increase in pressure. The net result is massive left atrial enlargement without pulmonary edema.

ELECTROCARDIOGRAPHY

The electrocardiogram provides critical information in dogs that have an arrhythmia secondary to mitral regurgitation. Atrial premature depolarizations and atrial fibrillation are the most common arrhythmias identified in these dogs.

The ECG may provide useful information about chamber enlargement but it is often normal, even with demonstrable chamber enlargements. Left atrial enlargement may result in a wide and sometimes notched *P* wave. However, this abnormality may be detected in as few as 40% of patients with moderate-to-severe

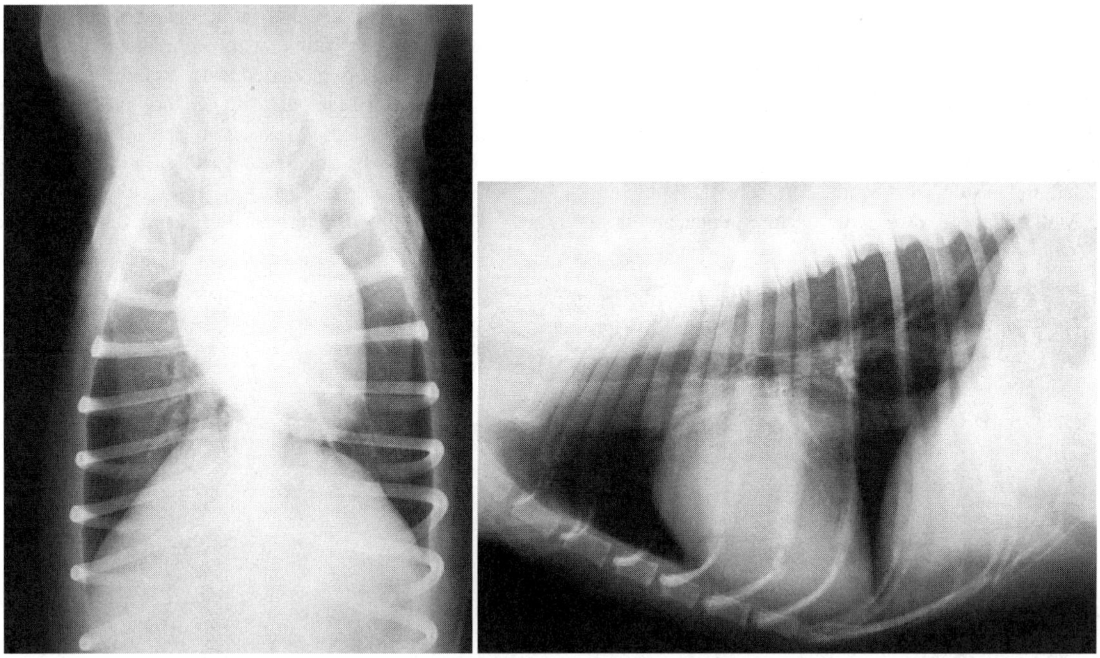

A B

FIGURE 19-15 Dorsoventral **(A)** and lateral **(B)** thoracic radiographs from a 7-year-old dog with mild mitral regurgitation as a result of myxomatous mitral valve degeneration. The left atrium is mildly enlarged on the lateral radiograph. **A,** The left auricle is mildly enlarged.

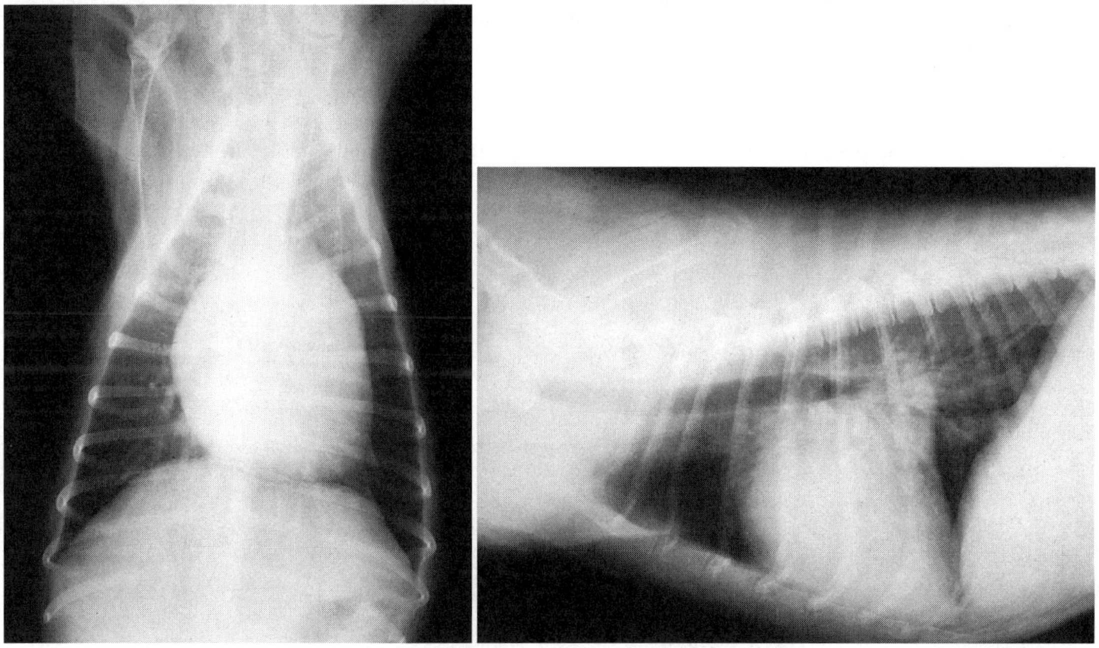

A B

FIGURE 19-16 Dorsoventral **(A)** and lateral **(B)** thoracic radiographs from the dog shown in Figure 19-15, taken 2 years later. The dog now has moderate mitral regurgitation. **A,** The left auricle and the left ventricle are enlarged. **B,** The left atrium is moderately enlarged. Because the two chambers are similarly enlarged, the left auricular bulge is not clearly visible in **A.**

enlargement and is usually normal in patients with mild left atrial enlargement.[37] Detection of left ventricular enlargement is also poor. The electrocardiogram probably detects less than 50% of cases with significant left ventricular enlargement secondary to mitral regurgitation.[37] If one does not have access to echocardiography, the thoracic radiographs and the electrocardiogram should be combined in an attempt to identify left ventricular enlargement. If echocardiography is available, left ventricular enlargement is much more accurately identified using this tool.

ECHOCARDIOGRAPHY

The echocardiogram is useful but not critical for the diagnosis and management of myxomatous atrioventricular valve degeneration. Two-dimensional echocardiography allows the clinician to examine the anatomy of the affected valve and to identify the nodular thickening of the tips of the valve leaflets (Figure 19-19). The valve lesions of bacterial endocarditis can look identical to those of MVD. Consequently, the distinction between the two often cannot be based on the echocardiographic examination. However, lesions of endocarditis may be solitary and more echodense. Usually the signalment and the history make the distinction between endocarditis and MVD possible. Dogs with bacterial endocarditis may have a history of fever, systemic illness, a new heart murmur, and clinical signs compatible with thromboembolic disease. Bacterial endocarditis occurs most frequently in large dogs. Dogs with MVD tend to be older, are afebrile, do not have systemic signs, and commonly have a long history of a heart murmur typical of mitral regurgitation. Myxomatous valve degeneration occurs most commonly in small dogs.

The two-dimensional echocardiogram can also be used to identify

A

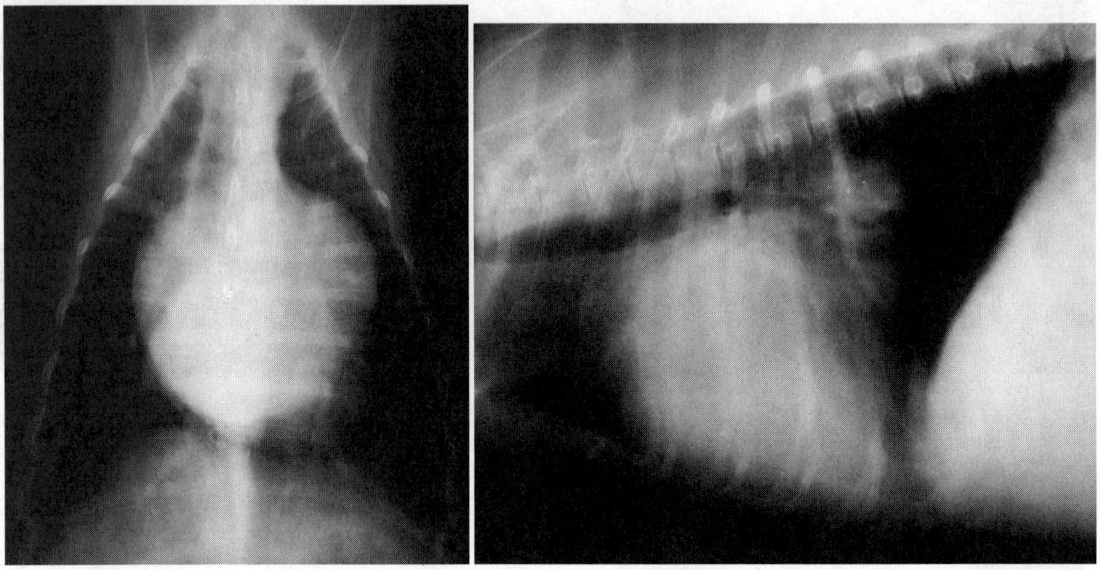

B

FIGURE 19-17 Dorsoventral **(A)** and lateral **(B)** thoracic radiographs from the dog shown in Figures 19-15 and 19-16, 1 year later than Figure 19-16. The dog now has severe mitral regurgitation, as evidenced by severe left atrial enlargement. **B,** The left atrial shadow contacts the spine on the lateral view. The left mainstem bronchus is compressed by the enlarged left atrium. **A,** The left atrium can be seen caudally as a more dense portion of the cardiac silhouette. The left auricular bulge is very large.

A

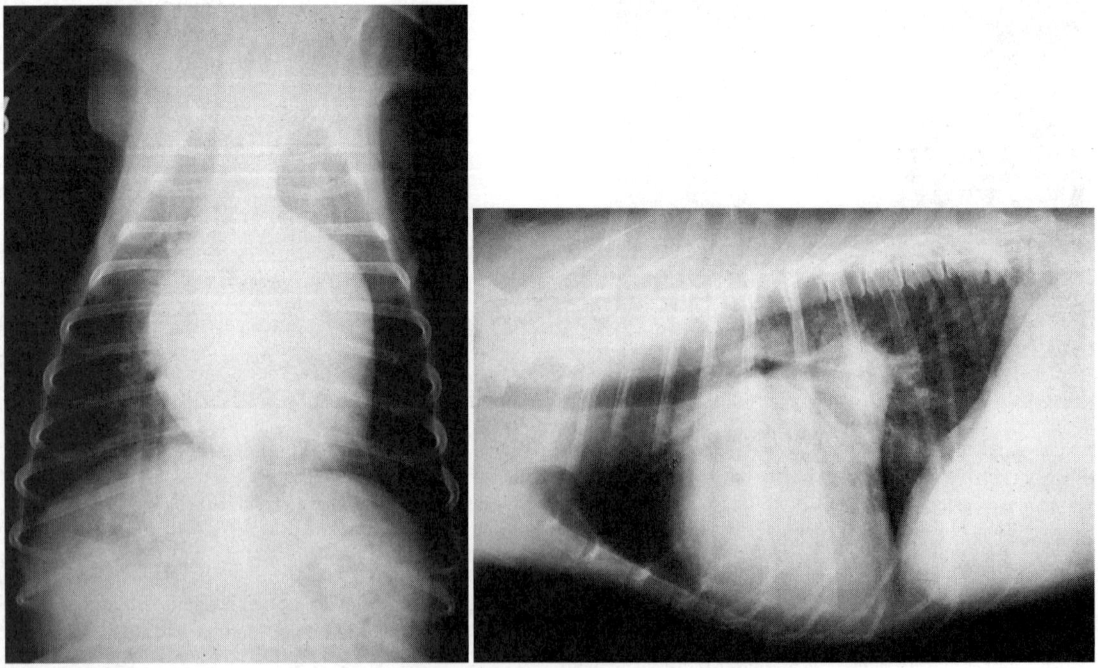

B

FIGURE 19-18 Dorsoventral **(A)** and lateral **(B)** thoracic radiographs from a dog with severe mitral regurgitation and left heart failure. The left atrium and left ventricle are very large. **A,** Most of the pulmonary edema is centrally located and cannot be seen. A small amount of edema can be visualized in the right caudal and accessory lung lobes. **B,** Moderate pulmonary edema is present.

regions of valve prolapse and to identify valve flail. Valve prolapse is defined as a portion of the body of the leaflet buckling into the left atrium in systole. It occurs in association with the MVD (see Figure 19-14). Valve flail is the edge of a leaflet moving into the left atrium in systole. It occurs secondary to chordae tendineae rupture. Occasionally, one can visualize the ruptured chord in the left atrium or in the left ventricle (Figure 19-20).

Left atrial size. The left atrium should be viewed from the right parasternal position in a cross-sectional view with the left auricle and body of the left atrium in view. In dogs with chronic mitral regurgitation as a result of MVD, the most useful information garnered from the two-dimensional echocardiogram is the size of the left atrium. Dogs with acute severe mitral regurgitation secondary to ruptured chordae tendineae may have pulmonary edema with a normal to mildly enlarged left atrium. Some dogs that have had moderate mitral regurgitation and then experience an acute chordal rupture have a moderately enlarged left atrium but severe mitral regurgitation. In all other cases the size of the left atrium corresponds to the severity of the disease. Dogs with pulmonary edema as a result of chronic mitral regurgitation always have a moderately-to-severely enlarged left atrium. Dogs with mild mitral regurgitation always have a small or normal-size left atrium. Left atrial size can be examined from a right parasternal long-axis view, a right parasternal short-axis view, and a left apical four-chamber view on a two-dimensional echocardiogram. When viewed from a right parasternal short-axis view, the size of the left atrium can be readily compared with the size of the aortic root. The size of the aortic root is relatively constant in a given-size dog. No absolute criteria for left atrial size from this view have been firmly established in the dog or cat. Consequently, we use a subjective grading scale of normal, mildly enlarged, moderately enlarged, and severely enlarged (see Figure 6-12). Normal values for a ratio of a left atrial dimension divided by the aortic root dimension on an M-mode echocardiogram have been reported to be 0.8 to 1.2 (mean ± 2 SD).[38] However, in dogs and some cats, the left atrial dimension recorded from this view is not the largest dimension. If one uses this criterion when examining a two-dimensional echocardiogram, one must be sure to use the same orientation as that recorded on an M-mode echocardiogram to measure the dimension. When measured at its greatest width on a two-dimensional echocardiogram, our impression is that the diameter of the left atrium divided by the aortic root diameter should be less than 1.5 to 1.7. Dogs that are in heart failure generally have a ratio greater than 2.0.[18]

Left ventricular function in small dogs. Assessment of left ventricular size and function is also important in mitral regurgitation.

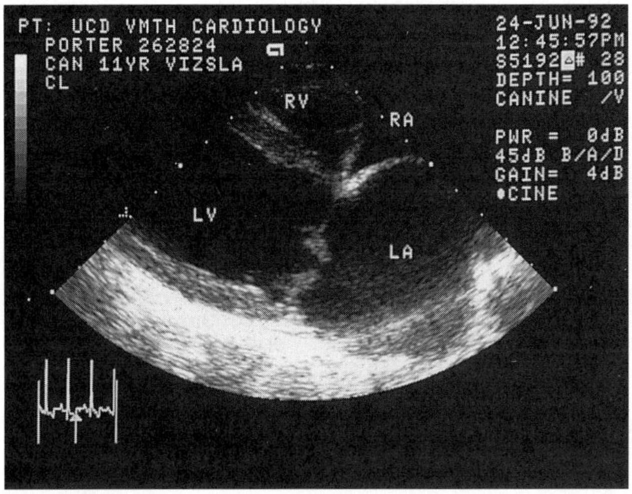

FIGURE 19-19 Two-dimensional echocardiogram from an 11-year-old Vizsla dog with severe myxomatous mitral valve disease and severe mitral regurgitation. The edges of the mitral valve leaflets are markedly thickened. Both leaflets bend backward into the left atrium, most likely because of small chordal ruptures. The left atrium *(LA)* is markedly enlarged and is larger than the left ventricular *(LV)* chamber. The right ventricle *(RV)* and the right atrium *(RA)* are normal.

A

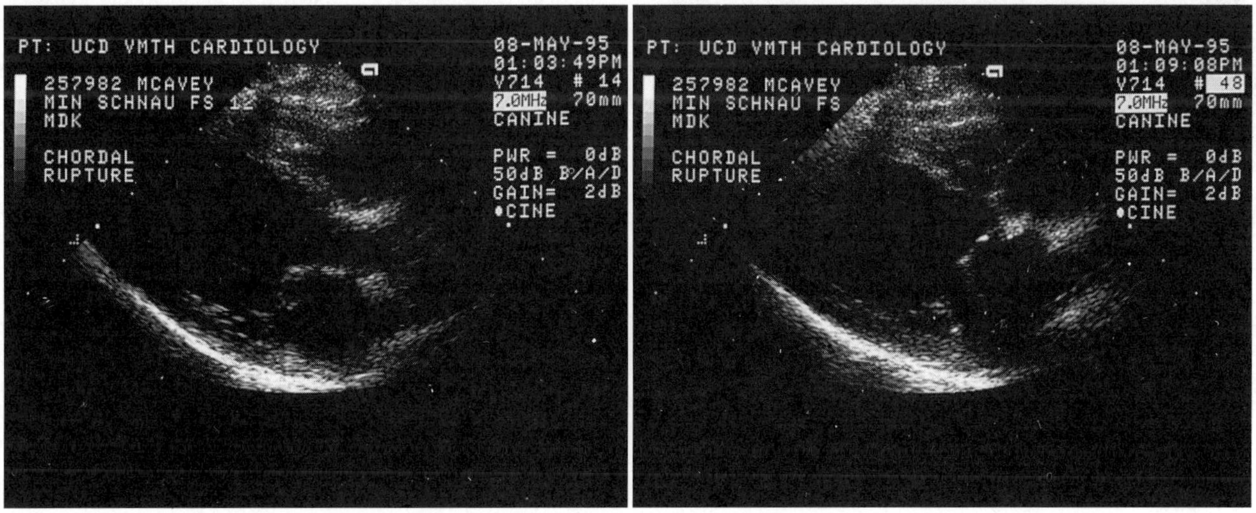

B

FIGURE 19-20 A, Two-dimensional echocardiogram from a 12-kg, 12-year-old miniature schnauzer with a loud heart murmur. This dog was hospitalized to control its diabetes mellitus. During the hospitalization period, the dog developed tachypnea and mild-to-moderate dyspnea. Thoracic radiographs revealed pulmonary edema without a marked increase in left atrial size. **A,** The echocardiogram shows mitral valve flail, with the edge of the septal leaflet of the mitral valve buckling into the left atrium in systole. This is highly suggestive of a ruptured chorda tendineae. Note that the left atrium and left ventricle are not markedly enlarged. **B,** Another view showing a long piece of a chorda tendineae in the left atrium in systole. This is diagnostic of a ruptured chorda tendineae.

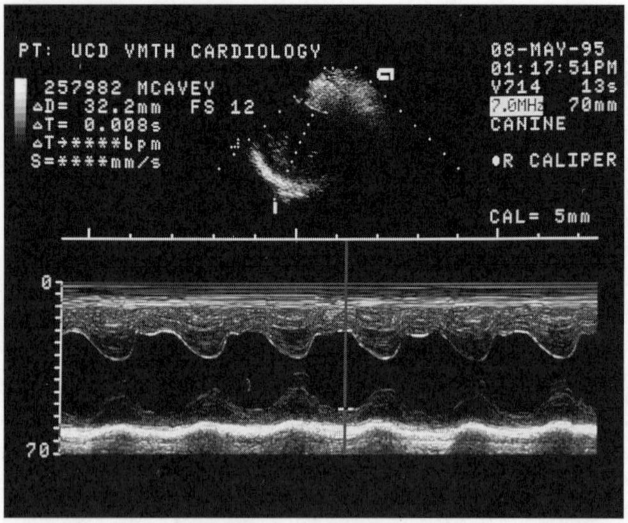

FIGURE 19-21 M-mode echocardiogram from the dog shown in Figure 19-20. The end-diastolic diameter of the left ventricle is 32 mm, which is mildly increased. The end-systolic diameter is 13 mm, which is moderately decreased. The decrease in end-systolic diameter is most likely due to a catecholamine-induced increase in myocardial contractility.

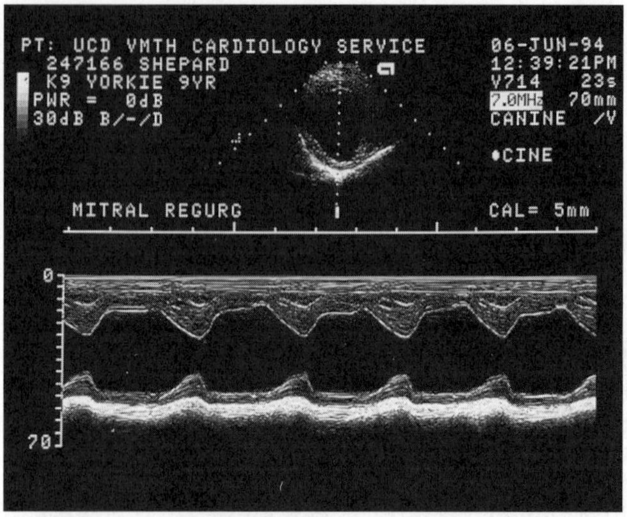

FIGURE 19-22 M-mode echocardiogram from a 3-kg, 9-year-old Yorkshire terrier with severe mitral regurgitation. The normal end-diastolic diameter (EDD) for a dog this weight is approximately 25 mm, and the normal end-systolic diameter (ESD) is 15 mm. This dog's EDD is approximately 38 mm and the ESD is approximately 17 mm. The shortening fraction is approximately 55%. The dog was not in heart failure at the time of presentation but had an intractable cough caused by compression of the left mainstem bronchus by the severely enlarged left atrium.

In dogs with acute mitral regurgitation secondary to chordal rupture with no preexisting mitral regurgitation and in dogs with mild mitral regurgitation, the left ventricle is commonly not enlarged (normal end-diastolic diameter) and the end-systolic diameter is decreased from normal in response to enhanced sympathetic tone (Figure 19-21). In chronic mitral regurgitation, left ventricular diastolic size increases in concert with left atrial size and severity of mitral regurgitation.[18] However, the degree of enlargement is usually

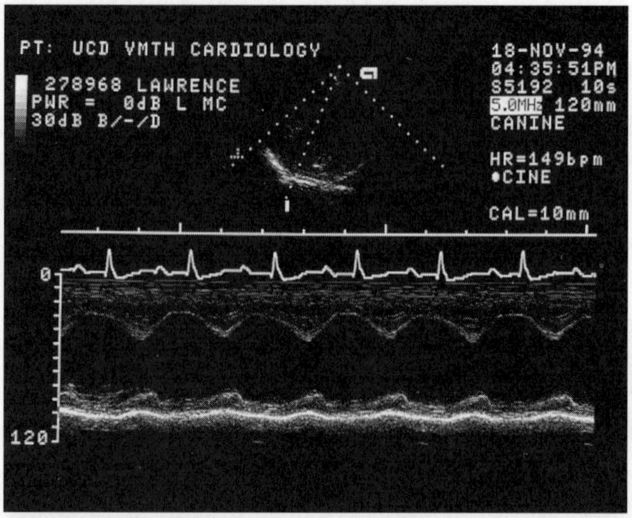

FIGURE 19-23 M-mode echocardiogram from a 24-kg Australian cattle dog with severe mitral regurgitation reveals that the end-diastolic diameter is markedly increased to 60 mm (normal is 40 mm) and the end-systolic diameter is increased to 40 mm (normal is 25 mm). The shortening fraction is 33%. Note that the shortening fraction is normal and some motion of the LV free wall occurs after the end of systole as the entire LV moves rightward, toward the transducer.

greater for the left atrium. Left ventricular wall thickness is usually within normal limits. The increase in chamber size combined with the normal wall thickness provides proof that volume overload (eccentric) hypertrophy is present. In small dogs, the end-systolic diameter of the left ventricle commonly remains within normal limits until the very late stages of the disease.[18,39] This is evidence that myocardial function remains normal. The left ventricular diastolic diameter increases with increasing disease severity. Consequently, shortening fraction increases as the disease severity worsens. Small dogs with severe mitral regurgitation commonly have a shortening fraction greater than 50% (Figure 19-22). In the end-stage of the disease, the end-systolic diameter increases, causing the shortening fraction to decrease more toward normal.[36]

Large dogs with mitral regurgitation. As opposed to small dogs that have supranormal shortening fractions when mitral regurgitation is severe and the dogs are in heart failure, large dogs commonly have a shortening fraction in the 25% to 40% range when they present in heart failure (Figure 19-23). The mitral valve leaflets may or may not look as severely affected in large dogs as they do in small dogs. The exact reason for the more prominent myocardial failure and the reason that the valves do not appear to be as severely affected yet leak so badly in some dogs is a mystery. One possibility is that some large-breed dogs with mitral regurgitation actually have mitral valve dysplasia rather than degenerative disease. We have also seen one dog at postmortem examination that had only mild-to-moderate MVD of the mitral valve but had severe mitral regurgitation. It had a split in one of the commissural cusps at postmortem examination. There was a jet lesion above this region and a partial-thickness tear in the left atrial wall. In this dog, it appeared that the degenerative lesion had weakened this cusp, allowing it to split and subsequently to leak.

Mitral regurgitation and a lower-than-normal shortening fraction in large dogs is often mistaken for dilated cardiomyopathy. Usually these dogs are presented for signs of heart failure and have the

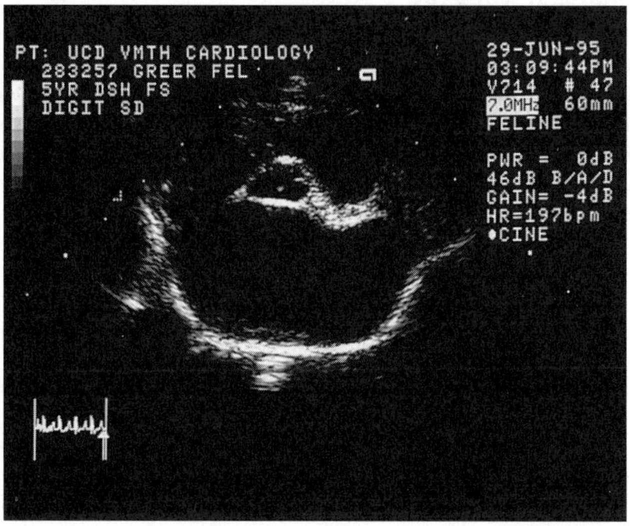

FIGURE 19-24 Echocardiographic recording from a cat with mitral regurgitation and left heart failure. The cat was examined by a referring veterinarian, who removed 270 mL of fluid from the cat's pleural space 2 days before our examination. Approximately 100 mL of a modified transudate had been removed the day before presentation, and furosemide was administered. The cat presented to us severely dehydrated and moribund. A two-dimensional echocardiogram of the left atrium showed it to be markedly enlarged. (See text for details.)

aforementioned shortening fractions. Dogs with dilated cardiomyopathy do not develop heart failure until the shortening fraction is less than 15%. Consequently, the diagnosis of dilated cardiomyopathy should always be questioned in a dog in heart failure with a shortening fraction greater than 15%. In large dogs with mitral regurgitation, one of the characteristic findings is normal-to-hyperdynamic septal wall motion and decreased free wall motion. Whenever normal-to-enhanced septal motion is identified in a dog in heart failure, a careful examination to identify the mitral regurgitation should be carried out.

Doppler echocardiography. Spectral and color flow Doppler evaluation is useful in dogs with primary mitral regurgitation. Color flow Doppler echocardiography confirms the presence of mitral regurgitation (Color Plate 74). The size of the color flow jet can be compared with the size of the left atrium. This comparison is semiquantitative in dogs and cats with mitral regurgitation. A small jet almost certainly rules out the presence of moderate-to-severe regurgitation. The presence of a large jet, however, can sometimes be visualized in a dog with only moderate regurgitation, so one must be careful when making this type of interpretation. The severity of mitral regurgitation in dogs with chronic primary mitral regurgitation is best assessed by determining left atrial size. Spectral Doppler can be used to identify the mitral regurgitatant jet and map its size when color flow Doppler is not available. The velocity of the mitral regurgitant jet is usually in the 5 to 6 m/sec range using continuous-wave Doppler.

The velocity of the mitral and tricuspid regurgitant jets may be clinically useful. Systemic hypertension increases the jet velocity, and the clinician should suspect its presence whenever the velocity exceeds about 6 m/sec. Jet velocity is decreased in systemic hypotension, when the orifice is large, or with dramatic increases in left atrial pressure.

An example of the clinical utility of measuring jet velocity is provided in Color Plate 75 and Figure 19-24. This cat presented in left heart failure with pulmonary edema, pleural effusion, cold extremities, and a low rectal temperature (98° F). The echocardiogram revealed a left ventricular end-diastolic chamber diameter of 19 mm (normal is less than 17 mm), indicating left ventricular volume overload. The end-systolic diameter was 11 mm (normal is less than 10 mm), indicating mild myocardial failure. The left atrium was markedly enlarged. The wall thicknesses of the ventricles were normal. The right heart was moderately enlarged. A large mitral regurgitant jet and a smaller tricuspid regurgitant jet were identified. The tricuspid regurgitation jet velocity was 3.2 m/sec, which translates into a pressure gradient of approximately 40 mm Hg across the tricuspid valve in systole. We assumed that the right atrial pressure was normal, because there was no evidence of right heart failure in this cat. Because the right heart was mildly enlarged, we assumed that the right atrial pressure was at the upper end of normal (5 mm Hg). This means that systolic right ventricular pressure had to be approximately 45 mm Hg. Because there was no evidence of pulmonic stenosis in this cat we also assumed that pulmonary artery systolic pressure was 45 mm Hg. The upper limit of normal for systolic pulmonary artery pressure is approximately 30 mm Hg, so the velocity of the tricuspid jet indicated that this cat had mild pulmonary hypertension. Next, the velocity of the mitral regurgitant jet was measured and it was 3.5 m/sec, which translates into a pressure gradient of approximately 50 mm Hg, which is very low. The ruled out items for a low-pressure gradient across the mitral valve are systemic hypotension, left atrial hypertension, or both. This cat's systolic systemic blood pressure was measured to be 80 mm Hg using a Doppler unit. This means the cat had systemic hypotension, probably because of its severe heart failure. The cat's hypothermia and hypotension are evidence of cardiogenic shock. Because there was no evidence of aortic stenosis in this cat, the left ventricular systolic pressure also had to be 80 mm Hg. Because the pressure gradient was approximately 50 mm Hg, the left atrial pressure had to be approximately 30 mm Hg. This figure was compatible with the cat's signs of left heart failure. The left atrial pressure and the pulmonary artery diastolic pressure should be about equal, which means the cat's pulmonary artery diastolic pressure was approximately 30 mm Hg. Because normal pulse pressure (systolic − diastolic blood pressure) in the pulmonary artery is approximately 15 mm Hg, the previous calculation of a systolic pulmonary artery pressure of 45 mm Hg and the current calculation of a diastolic pulmonary artery pressure of 30 mm Hg are compatible with each other. Myxomatous mitral valve degeneration was confirmed at postmortem examination in this cat (Color Plate 76).

CARDIAC CATHETERIZATION AND HEMODYNAMICS

Cardiac catheterization is rarely performed on dogs or cats with mitral regurgitation. The diagnosis of mitral regurgitation can be confirmed and the severity assessed by injecting a contrast agent into the left ventricle through a catheter (see Figure 19-1). Severity can be graded on a 1+ to 4+ scale. Following the injection of contrast agent, the left atrium does not fully opacify in very mild, or 1+, regurgitation. When the agent fills the left atrium but the density of the agent does not achieve the density of the agent in the left ventricle, the patient has mild, or 2+, regurgitation. When the density in the left atrium and the left ventricle are equal, the patient has moderate, or 3+, regurgitation. When the density in the left atrium exceeds the density in the left ventricle, severe, or 4+, regurgitation is present. A Swan-Ganz catheter can be wedged in a distal pulmonary artery to estimate left atrial pressure. This catheter can be placed in either awake or anesthetized dogs. In patients in left heart failure, the pulmonary capillary wedge pressure (PCWP) is increased. In patients with mild pulmonary edema, the PCWP is usually in the 20- to 25-mm Hg range. Patients with moderate edema have a PCWP in the 25- to 30-mm Hg range, and patients with severe pulmonary edema have a PCWP in the 30- to 45-mm Hg range.[40] A large *V* wave secondary to systolic flow into the left atrium may be recorded on the PCWP. Cardiac output can be measured by the thermodilution technique using the Swan-Ganz catheter. Cardiac index is variable in dogs with severe heart failure secondary to primary mitral regurgitation, ranging from low to normal (1.93 to 3.82 L/min/m^2 in one study).[40] Stroke volume index, however, is uniformly low in these patients, ranging from 10 to 23 mL/m^2 in one study (normal is approximately 30 to 40 mL/m^2). The average heart rate for dogs with severe heart failure secondary to mitral regurgitation is increased at 161 beats/min. Mean arterial blood pressure is normal (average of 104 mm Hg in one study).[40]

Treatment

MEDICAL THERAPY

Based on the pathophysiology of the disease, small dogs with mitral regurgitation should be given medication to decrease blood volume, to venodilate, and to decrease regurgitation through dilation of systemic arterioles. Positive inotropes should be administered to small dogs late in the course of their disease and to large dogs with moderate-to-severe mitral regurgitation. Mitral valve repair or replacement would be the ideal treatment but is not technically feasible at this time.

As seen above, at the end stages of the disease, renal retention of sodium and water into the vascular space is no longer beneficial and, in fact, becomes detrimental. Its major detriment is the production of an increased left ventricular diastolic pressure causing pulmonary edema. Measures to decrease blood volume or to counteract the continuous attempt by the kidneys to retain sodium and water are indicated at this stage and are beneficial. Diuretic administration, especially furosemide administration, is the most efficient means of decreasing blood volume and the most efficacious means of treating heart failure. Angiotensin converting enzyme inhibitor administration and salt intake restriction are good adjunct means of reducing blood volume.

Venodilation is a means of redistributing the central blood volume and in theory should be beneficial. Unfortunately there are no venodilators known to produce consistent benefits in veterinary medicine. Angiotensin converting enzyme inhibitors have some venodilating properties but they seem relatively mild. Nitroglycerin cream and isosorbide dinitrate are other potentially useful venodilators.

The amount of blood ejected from the left ventricle into the aorta vs. the amount ejected into the left atrium depends on the relative impedances of the two circulations. If the impedance of the systemic circulation is decreased, more blood flows forward into the systemic arteries, resulting in a decrease in blood flow into the left atrium (see Figure 10-10). The most efficient means of decreasing aortic input impedance is to decrease systemic vascular resistance via systemic arteriolar dilation. Several arteriolar dilators are currently available. The angiotensin converting enzyme inhibitors act as arteriolar dilators but are mild. Hydralazine, a more potent arteriolar dilator, is more effective but also more difficult to use with more side effects. Certain types of calcium channel blockers, such as amlodipine, may also be beneficial but have not been studied in dogs or cats.

SURGICAL THERAPY

The treatment of choice for treating mitral regurgitation in humans is surgical intervention. Mitral valve repair is the current method of choice.[41,42] Replacement of the mitral valve with a prosthetic valve is also commonly performed. Four variables combine to make surgical intervention in dogs with primary mitral regurgitation uncommon. First, most dogs with primary mitral regurgitation are small, making cardiopulmonary bypass more difficult. Second, there are very few trained veterinary cardiovascular surgeons with the skills necessary to perform either valve replacement or valve repair. Third, cardiopulmonary bypass and open-heart surgery are very expensive ($5000.00 to $6000.00 in our hospital, just to recoup costs). Lastly, in the case of mitral valve replacement, dogs avidly thrombose and fibrose foreign material in the heart, resulting in systemic thromboembolism and dysfunction of the prosthetic valve.

A few case reports of successful mitral valve surgery have been reported. Bioprosthetic valves have been placed successfully in two dogs with mitral valve dysplasia.[43,44] One dog was a Saint Bernard and the other a bull terrier. Successful mitral valve repair has been reported in one 10-year-old Maltese with severe myxomatous mitral valve degeneration.[45] The surgery was performed by an experienced surgeon in human medicine in this case. Sections of mitral valve leaflets that were severely affected or were unsupported because of chordal rupture were excised. The annulus size was decreased by imbricating the annulus with pledgetted sutures. This dog improved dramatically after surgery and its heart decreased remarkably in size on radiographs. Other surgeries performed by this same team have not been as successful, however.

Therapeutic Strategies for Treating Mitral Regurgitation

Medical therapy for mitral regurgitation must be tailored for each patient based on the stage of the disease and the response of the patient to the medication (Table 19-1).

ASYMPTOMATIC DISEASE

There are no clinical studies in veterinary medicine to suggest that anything slows the progression of mitral valve degeneration or slows the progression of the altered hemodynamics. Even in humans, as stated in a 1996 review article, "There are no long-term studies that support the use of vasodilator therapy in asymptomatic patients with chronic mitral regurgitation."[46] Despite this, many veterinarians place dogs with mitral regurgitation as a result of MVD on angiotensin converting enzyme (ACE) inhibitors before the onset of heart failure. This is commonly done based on theory and data generated in human clinical trials.

Studies have been performed in humans to determine if early administration of ACE inhibitors to patients with dilated cardiomyopathy decreases the progression of myocardial failure and so reduces mortality. In the SAVE study, captopril was found to decrease mortality and morbidity in patients with left ventricular dysfunction following acute myocardial infarction.[47] In a similar study (CONSENSUS II), enalapril did not improve survival in patients after acute myocardial infarction.[48] Regardless, acute myocardial infarction is a disease that is very dissimilar to chronic mitral regurgitation, and data from these studies cannot be extrapolated to dogs with chronic myxomatous degenerative mitral valve disease. Another study (the prevention limb of the SOLVD trial) also examined the issue of early intervention with an ACE inhibitor in patients with left ventricular dysfunction.[49] Patients enrolled in this

TABLE 19-1

Drugs used in various stages of heart failure secondary to mitral regurgitation

Drugs	*None*	*Mild to moderate*	*Severe*	*Fulminant*	*Refractory*
Furosemide	No	1-3 mg/kg q8-12h PO	2-4 mg/kg q8-12h PO	4-8 mg/kg q1-2h IV	4 mg/kg q8h PO
ACEI	?	Yes	Yes	No*	Yes
Digoxin	No	?	?	No*	Yes
Nitroglycerin	No	No	?	OK	OK
Hydralazine	No	No	No	Yes	Yes
Nitroprusside	No	No	No	Yes	No
Low-salt diet	No	?	OK	No*	Yes
Thiazide diuretic	No	No	No	No	Yes

No, Do not use; *No**, do not use at this time, although the drug may be beneficial once the patient is stabilized; *Yes,* indicated for use, although the drug doesn't necessarily have to be used; *?,* efficacy has not been established; *OK,* the drug may be beneficial.

study had to have moderate-to-severe myocardial failure (ejection fraction less than 35%, which corresponds to a shortening fraction less than 15%) and could not have hemodynamically serious valvular disease. Consequently, the data from this study may have some bearing on dogs with dilated cardiomyopathy but, again, cannot be extrapolated in any form to dogs with chronic mitral regurgitation. This study found that enalapril administration delayed the onset of heart failure symptoms but did not influence mortality. A conclusion from this study was that there was a trend toward reduced mortality but the trend was not statistically significant. This trial enrolled 4228 patients. Investigators examine data for trends when pilot studies are performed. A trial of this size looks for definitive answers, not trends. Consequently, the conclusion of this study should be that there is no reduction in mortality when ACE inhibitors are administered to patients with left ventricular myocardial failure that are not yet in heart failure.

The results of the prevention limb of the SOLVD trial are not surprising. That administering an agent to treat heart failure would result in a delay in the onset of heart failure signs seems expected. Most likely this could also be accomplished with the early administration of a diuretic. In humans, in whom the economics of medicine is quite different from the economics of veterinary practice, it makes sense to spend several hundred dollars a year to delay hospitalization, because each hospitalization costs thousands of dollars. In veterinary medicine it may make more sense to wait until the onset of heart failure signs before initiating therapy with expensive agents like ACE inhibitors. Cost for enalapril in a 5- to 10-kg dog at the our hospital for 1 year is approximately $400.00 to $500.00. This is roughly twice the cost of a hospital visit to initiate heart failure therapy in a patient with mild-to-moderate heart failure. Obviously, this is a personal decision that must be made by the veterinarian and the client.

MILD-TO-MODERATE HEART FAILURE

Patients with mild-to-moderate heart failure generally present to a veterinarian because of respiratory signs, most commonly cough, tachypnea, or mild-to-moderate dyspnea. Pulmonary edema is usually present on thoracic radiographs, although appreciating it in dogs with small chest cavities may be difficult (because of obesity, chest configuration, lack of full inspiration, or all these) when the edema is mild. These patients have apparent normal myocardial contractility and moderate-to-severe regurgitation. The left ventricle and left atrium at this stage are consistently enlarged. Usually this enlargement is severe.

Treatment at this stage is always indicated. Primary therapy is diuretic and ACE inhibitor administration. The ACE inhibitor dose is relatively fixed at 0.5 mg/kg (frequency of administration depends on the particular ACE inhibitor used). The dose of diuretic should be tailored to eliminate the edema at the lowest dose possible. This dose may be as low as 1 mg/kg every other day or as high as 3 mg/kg q8h.

SEVERE HEART FAILURE

Patients with severe heart failure have evidence of heavy interstitial-to-alveolar pulmonary edema. They need to be treated more aggressively than patients with mild-to-moderate heart failure. In patients that present for the first time with severe heart failure, hospitalization is usually required. Patients with dyspnea benefit from oxygen administration and moderate-to-high dose intravenous or intramuscular furosemide administration (4 to 6 mg/kg q2h-q6h). Topical nitroglycerin cream may also be administered but is of questionable efficacy. Once stabilized, patients that presented with moderate-to-severe dyspnea benefit from oral furosemide administration and ACE inhibitor administration. Patients that are clinically stable on presentation may also be treated with oral administration of furosemide and an ACE inhibitor. The dose of furosemide should be kept as low as possible, but doses usually range between 2 to 4 mg/kg q8-12h. A low-salt diet may also be beneficial.

FULMINANT HEART FAILURE

Patients that present with severe, life-threatening (fulminant) pulmonary edema should be treated as emergency patients. These patients are markedly dyspneic as a result of severe hypoxemia caused by severe pulmonary edema. They may cough up white or pink-tinged froth (pulmonary edema fluid). They are easily stressed to the point of death, and therefore must be handled gently, if at all. Patients present in this condition either because they have chronic heart failure that the owner has not noticed or has ignored or because they have acute rupture of a major chorda tendineae. On admission, a cursory physical examination should be performed, if possible. Commonly, these are small geriatric dogs with a history of a heart murmur compatible with mitral regurgitation. On physical examination they have a loud left apical murmur that may radiate widely. Auscultation of the lungs may reveal abnormal lung sounds or may only reveal increased bronchovesicular sounds. *Absence of abnormal lung sounds does not rule out pulmonary edema.* These dogs are very dyspneic and tachypneic, with respiratory rates in the 60- to 90-breaths/min range. A thoracic radiograph may be obtained if the patient is reasonably stable and the radiograph can be obtained quickly and with little stress. Severe, alveolar infiltrates confirm pulmonary edema. If the patient is not stable or struggles during radiographic examination, radiographs should be delayed. The patient should then receive intravenous furosemide at doses ranging from 4 to 8 mg/kg. If the patient will not tolerate catheter placement, furosemide should be administered intramuscularly.

Following the administration of furosemide, supplemental oxygen should be administered using an oxygen cage, nasal insufflation, or a tight-fitting mask. A mask should not be used if the patient fights its use. If an oxygen cage is used, FIO_2 should be 40% to 50%. Administration of a potent arteriolar dilator may also be contemplated at this time. The choice is either to administer hydralazine per os or to administer nitroprusside intravenously. Hydralazine is effective within 30 minutes of oral administration, and administration of an intravenous form is generally not required. If the patient is not currently on an ACE inhibitor, titration of hydralazine is generally abandoned because of the emergency situation, and 2 mg/kg is administered per os. This dose should be effective in 80% to 90% of patients. This dose does have the potential of making the dog clinically hypotensive. Clinical hypotension is defined as a mean systemic arterial blood pressure less than 50 to 60 mm Hg or a systolic blood pressure less than 90 mm Hg resulting in signs of weakness. Clinical hypotension in this case is of some concern but almost never results in clinical sequelae. In humans, for whom data are routinely gathered on cause of death, there has never been a recorded death resulting from hydralazine administration. The largest recorded dose is 10 g (1000 10-mg tablets). If the patient is already on an ACE inhibitor, titration must be carried out carefully, starting at a dose of 0.5 mg/kg and using blood pressure monitoring. Overdose of hydralazine in the presence of an ACE inhibitor can produce lethal complications, such as renal failure. The alternative to hydralazine administration is nitroprusside administration. Nitroprusside is a very potent arteriolar dilator and a potent venodilator and is very effective in this situation. The drawbacks are that it must be administered intravenously and blood pressure must be monitored to avoid overdosing and to confirm efficacy. Intravenous catheter placement is not always possible or advisable when dealing with a patient that is severely dyspneic and easily stressed. Monitoring blood pressure in such a case is even more problematic. Intraarterial catheter placement generally requires time and rigid restraint. Noninvasive blood pressure measurement is often unreliable or difficult to repeat frequently. However, the primary drawback to blood pressure monitoring is the lack of equipment in many private veterinary practices. Consequently, nitroprusside is not a commonly used therapeutic agent.

Once the patient has received initial drug therapy, it should be handled or disturbed as little as possible. The respiratory rate and effort should be monitored every 15 to 30 minutes. If the respiratory rate has not decreased by at least 10 breaths/min within the first hour, another dose of furosemide (4 to 8 mg/kg) should be administered intravenously, and, if the rate has not decreased by another 10 breaths/min in the next 2 hours, the dosage should be repeated. Once the respiratory rate starts to decrease, the furosemide dose should be curtailed sharply using clinical judgment. For example, if the dog received 8 mg/kg twice and the respiratory rate decreased from 80 to 65 breaths/min after the second dose and remained at that level for 2 hours, a 4-mg/kg dose of furosemide might then be administered intravenously. If the respiratory rate then decreased to 50 breaths/min, the furosemide dose might be decreased to 4 mg/kg per os every 6 hours until the respiratory rate was normal (less than 40 breaths/min). Many other scenarios exist, and medical management must be based on clinical judgment.

High-dose intravenous furosemide therapy commonly results in hyponatremia, hypochloremia, hypokalemia, and dehydration. If the dehydration is severe, fluids should be replaced cautiously. Usually the dehydration is not severe and is corrected when the animal starts to feel better and eat and drink on its own. The same is true of electrolyte abnormalities. Usually these are only laboratory abnormalities that do not result in clinical problems. These abnormalities usually correct themselves when the patient starts to eat and drink. Aggressive fluid and electrolyte replacement is usually not indicated, because the fluid therapy can easily reproduce heart failure.

REFRACTORY HEART FAILURE

Patients with refractory heart failure are those that are on maximum chronic oral doses of furosemide (4 mg/kg q8h), an appropriate dose of an ACE inhibitor, and a low-salt diet but are still showing signs of mild-to-severe heart failure. In patients with mild-to-moderate heart failure, choices for additional drug therapy at this time include the addition of a thiazide diuretic, digoxin, hydralazine, or all three. Patients that are refractory to furosemide and an ACE inhibitor usually improve following the addition of a thiazide diuretic. Some patients respond to the addition of digoxin. Most will respond to the addition of hydralazine. However, hydralazine administration to a patient already receiving an ACE inhibitor must be done with utmost caution by someone that can monitor systemic arterial blood pressure. Alternatively, furosemide can be administered intravenously to increase its delivery to the nephron. However, this can only be done periodically, which limits its usefulness.

When hydralazine is administered to a patient that is already receiving an ACE inhibitor, a baseline measurement of systemic arterial blood pressure must be obtained. The most accurate means of obtaining blood pressure is direct femoral artery puncture with a 20- to 22-gauge needle connected directly to a pressure transducer. This method is also the most difficult. Measurement of systolic blood pressure using a Doppler flow detecting device and an appropriate-size cuff is a reasonable substitute. The major disadvantage is that only systolic blood pressure is obtained. However, in almost all cases both systolic and diastolic blood pressures decrease after hydralazine administration; therefore systolic blood pressure can be used for monitoring the response to hydralazine. Alternatively, an oscillometric device can be used to obtain systolic and diastolic blood pressures. The disadvantage of these devices is inaccuracy in small dogs.

Once a blood pressure measurement is obtained, 0.5 mg/kg hydralazine should be administered per os and the blood pressure measurement repeated 1 hour later. If blood pressure (mean, diastolic, or mean) has decreased by at least 15 mm Hg, a response is identified and that dose is administered q12h after that. If the blood pressure has not decreased by at least 15 mm Hg, another 0.5 mg/kg should be administered. The total dose administered is now 1.0 mg/kg. Blood pressure is checked 1 hour later, looking for a response to the hydralazine. This procedure is repeated until the required decrease in blood pressure is identified. A total dose greater than 2.0 mg/kg is unusual, although the rare case may require up to 3.0 mg/kg. The duration of hydralazine's effect is 12 hours, so the total dose administered during titration (less than 6 hours) is the cumulative dose. This is the dose that should be administered every 12 hours.

Comments on Selected Drugs Commonly Used to Treat Heart Failure Secondary to Mitral Regurgitation

FUROSEMIDE

With the arrival of some of the newer agents for treatment of heart failure, some older agents may be inadvertently overlooked. Consequently it is important to remember that furosemide is still the most efficacious drug for treating any type of heart failure in the dog. It is efficacious in treating acute or chronic heart failure. It can be administered by several different routes, therefore onset of action and duration of effect can be tailored to the situation. Its dosage can be adjusted over a wide range to treat mild-to-severe heart failure. In the dog, it has very few side effects. For these reasons, it is almost the ideal drug for treating heart failure in the dog.

In dogs with mild-to-moderate heart failure as a result of mitral regurgitation, furosemide generally is administered at dosages ranging from 1 to 3 mg/kg PO q8-12h. At these dosages, complications with furosemide are almost nonexistent. As opposed to human patients, electrolyte abnormalities at these dosages are rare. Similarly, dehydration and prerenal azotemia are rare as long as the patient continues to eat and drink. Any patient that becomes anorexic while on furosemide may rapidly become dehydrated, and owners must be cautioned about this situation.

In dogs with severe chronic heart failure, furosemide should be administered at dosages ranging up to 4 mg/kg PO q8h. Even at this dose, electrolyte abnormalities are uncommon if the patient is eating and drinking, although electrolytes should be monitored on occasion. Clinical dehydration is also uncommon at this dose as long as the patient is not anorexic. Subclinical dehydration is probably common and beneficial. Mild prerenal azotemia may be present at this dose, but if this dose is required to alleviate the edema and the patient is eating, mild, and sometimes even moderate, azotemia can be ignored.

ANGIOTENSIN CONVERTING ENZYME (ACE) INHIBITORS

By blocking the conversion of angiotensin I to angiotensin II, ACE inhibitors decrease plasma concentrations of aldosterone and angiotensin II. This results in less sodium and water retention (diuretic effect), mild arteriolar dilation, and mild venodilation. These effects become evident at different times following the onset of administration. Arteriolar dilation is observed after the first dose is administered; whereas the lessening of sodium and water retention takes days to become clinically significant. Because most dogs presenting for severe heart failure are dying from pulmonary edema, the ACE inhibitors are poor emergency heart failure drugs.

ACE inhibitors act acutely and chronically as arteriolar dilators. In most canine patients, however, this effect is relatively mild compared with the more potent arteriolar dilators, such as hydralazine and nitroprusside. This explains the reduced number of hypotensive events observed with this drug. This probably also explains why the effect of the drug on edema formation and cardiac output in dogs with mitral regurgitation is usually not as profound as with hydralazine.

Studies of enalapril use in dogs with dilated cardiomyopathy and in dogs with primary mitral regurgitation have been completed and reported. Enalapril is beneficial in dogs with mitral regurgitation but of less benefit for the group as a whole than possibly expected. In our clinical experience, some dogs with mitral regurgitation have dramatic responses to an ACE inhibitor, many improve clinically, and a significant number have little response.

In the IMPROVE study, which included 22 dogs with mitral regurgitation, enalapril did not significantly improve any clinical variable.[50] Almost no echocardiographic variable was significantly altered. Hemodynamic variables were statistically significantly altered, with mean systemic arterial blood pressure decreasing an average of approximately 5 mm Hg and pulmonary capillary wedge pressure (the pressure that determines the amount of pulmonary edema) decreasing approximately 3 to 5 mm Hg. The decrease in systemic blood pressure is clinically insignificant because cardiac output did not increase significantly. The decrease in pulmonary capillary wedge pressure is very small and probably clinically insignificant for the group. Almost assuredly some dogs within this group did experience a more clinically significant decrease in pulmonary capillary pressure, however. In the LIVE study, dogs with mitral regurgitation (n = 88) were treated with either placebo (n = 41) or enalapril (n = 47).[51] Treatment was continued until the investigator thought the dog's heart failure was not adequately responding to treatment (at which time the investigator was unblinded about whether the dog was receiving placebo or enalapril and switched to enalapril if on the placebo), the patient died, the patient was dropped from the study for other reasons, or the study was terminated. Time until treatment failure was not significantly different between these two groups that had mitral regurgitation. A survival study using clinical patients with mitral regurgitation has not been conducted. In the COVE study, dogs with mitral regurgitation were enrolled but the exact number has not been published. One hundred and ninety dogs were enrolled, the vast majority with either mitral regurgitation or dilated cardiomyopathy. In this study, more dogs with mitral regurgitation receiving enalapril experienced improvement in class of heart failure than dogs on placebo.[52] The overall evaluation also improved in more dogs on enalapril than in dogs on placebo. These data underscore the clinical impression that the clinical response to ACE inhibitors can be quite varied (some dogs have dramatic responses, some have no response, and most have mild-to-moderate improvement). They also underscore the fact that clinical improvement with these drugs is commonly more dramatic than the hemodynamic or echocardiographic response.

REFERENCES

1. Perloff JK, Roberts WC: The mitral valve apparatus: functional anatomy of mitral regurgitation, *Circulation* 46:227, 1972.
2. Kogure K: Pathology of chronic mitral valvular disease in the dog, *Nippon Juigaku Zasshi* 42:323, 1980.
3. Buchanan JW: Chronic valvular disease (endocardiosis) in dogs, *Adv Vet Sci Comp Med* 21:75, 1977.
4. Whitney JC: Cardiovascular pathology, *J Small Anim Pract* 8:459, 1967.
5. Buchanan JW, Kelly AM: Endocardial splitting of the left atrium in the dog with hemorrhage and hemopericardium, *J Am Vet Radiol Soc* 5:28, 1964.
6. Luginbuhl H, Detweiler DK: Cardiovascular lesions in dogs, *Ann NY Acad Sci* 127:5, 1965.
7. Jonnson L: Coronary arterial lesions and myocardial infarcts in the dog, *Acta Vet Scand* 38:5, 1972.
8. Detweiler DK, Patterson DF: The prevalence and types of cardiovascular disease in dogs, *Ann NY Acad Sci* 127:481, 1965.
9. Das KM, Tashjian RJ: Chronic mitral valve disease in the dog, *Vet Med Small Anim Clin* 60:1209, 1965.
10. Beardow AW, Buchanan JW: Chronic mitral valve disease in Cavalier King Charles spaniels: 95 cases (1987-1991), *J Am Vet Med Assoc* 203:1023, 1993.
11. Whitney JC: Observations on the effect of age on the severity of heart valve lesions in the dog, *J Small Anim Pract* 15:511, 1974.
12. Swenson L, Haggstrom J, Kvart C et al: Relationship between parental cardiac status in Cavalier King Charles spaniels and prevalence and severity of chronic valvular disease in offspring, *J Am Vet Med Assoc* 208:2009, 1996.
13. Braunwald E: Valvular heart disease. In Braunwald E, ed: *Heart disease: a textbook of cardiovascular medicine,* ed 4, Philadelphia, 1992, WB Saunders.
14. Pedersen HD, Kristensen BO, Lorentzen KA et al: Mitral valve prolapse in 3-year-old healthy Cavalier King Charles spaniels: an echocardiographic study, *Can J Vet Res* 59:294, 1995.
15. Brown WA, Kittleson MD: Color flow Doppler estimation of mitral regurgitation using the proximal flow convergence method in dogs with chronic degenerative mitral valve disease, *J Vet Int Med* 8:143, 1994.

16. Nagatsu M, Zile MR, Tsutsui H et al: Native beta-adrenergic support for left ventricular dysfunction in experimental mitral regurgitation normalizes indexes of pump and contractile function, *Circulation* 89:818, 1994.
17. Kihara Y, Sasayama S, Miyazaki S et al: Role of the left atrium in adaptation of the heart to chronic mitral regurgitation in conscious dogs, *Circ Res* 62:543, 1988.
18. Haggstrom J, Hansson K, Karlberg BE et al: Plasma concentration of atrial natriuretic peptide in relation to severity of mitral regurgitation in Cavalier King Charles spaniels, *Am J Vet Res* 55:698, 1994.
19. Haggstrom J, Hansson K, Karlberg BE et al: Effects of long-term treatment with enalapril or hydralazine on the renin-angiotensin-aldosterone system and fluid balance in dogs with naturally acquired mitral valve degeneration, *Am J Vet Res* 57:1645, 1996.
20. Assey ME, Zile MR, Usher BW et al: Effect of catheter positioning on the variability of measured gradient in aortic stenosis, *Cathet Cardiovasc Diagn* 30:287, 1993.
21. Knowlen GG, Kittleson MD, Nachreiner RF et al: Comparison of plasma aldosterone concentration among clinical status groups of dogs with chronic heart failure, *J Am Vet Med Assoc* 183:991, 1983.
22. Haggstrom J, Hamlin RL, Hansson K et al: Heart rate variability in relation to severity of mitral regurgitation in Cavalier King Charles spaniels, *J Small Anim Pract* 37:69, 1996.
23. Eckberg DL, Gault JH, Bouchard RL et al, Mechanics of left ventricular contraction in chronic severe mitral regurgitation, *Circulation* 47:1252, 1973.
24. Legault F, Rouleau JL, Juneau C et al: Functional and morphological characteristics of compensated and decompensated cardiac hypertrophy in dogs with chronic infrarenal aorto-caval fistulas, *Circ Res* 66:846, 1990.
25. Tsutsui H, Spinale FG, Nagatsu M et al: Effects of chronic beta-adrenergic blockade on the left ventricular and cardiocyte abnormalities of chronic canine mitral regurgitation, *J Clin Invest* 93:2639, 1994.
26. Nagatsu M, Ishihara K, Zile MR et al: The effects of complete versus incomplete mitral valve repair in experimental mitral regurgitation, *J Thorac Cardiovasc Surg* 107:416, 1994.
27. Tsutsui H, Urabe Y, Mann DL et al: Effects of chronic mitral regurgitation on diastolic function in isolated cardiocytes, *Circ Res* 72:1110, 1993.
28. Dhalla AK, Hill MF, Singal PK: Role of oxidative stress in transition of hypertrophy to heart failure, *J Am Coll Cardiol* 28:506, 1996.
29. Sisson D, Brown W, Riepe R: Hemodynamic effects of atrial fibrillation in dogs with experimentally induced mitral regurgitation, *J Vet Intern Med* 9:200, 1995 (abstract).
30. Grossman W, Braunwald E: Pulmonary hypertension. In Braunwald E, ed: *Heart disease: a textbook of cardiovascular medicine,* ed 4, Philadelphia, 1992, WB Saunders.
31. Sakai S, Miyauchi T, Sakurai T et al: Pulmonary hypertension caused by congestive heart failure is ameliorated by long-term application of an endothelin receptor antagonist: increased expression of endothelin-1 messenger ribonucleic acid and endothelin-1-like immunoreactivity in the lung in congestive heart failure in rats, *J Am Coll Cardiol* 28:1580, 1996.
32. O'Grady MR: Pulmonary hypertension in dogs with mitral regurgitation, *Proc Annu Vet Med Forum,* 1994, p 343.
33. Keister DM: *A summary of phase IV clinical data on milrinone (Wincardin): a canine cardiotonic—protocol H,* New York, 1988, Sterling Winthrop.
34. Haggstrom J, Hansson K, Kvart C et al: Chronic valvular disease in the Cavalier King Charles spaniel in Sweden, *Vet Rec* 131:549, 1992.
35. Haggstrom J, Kvart C, Hansson K: Heart sounds and murmurs: changes related to severity of chronic valvular disease in the Cavalier King Charles spaniel, *J Vet Intern Med* 9:75, 1995.
36. Amberger C, Glardon O, Lombard CW: Validite des examens complementaires dans l'evaluation de l'insuffisance cardiaque par endocardiose mitrale: etude a partir de 106 cas, *Prat Med Chir Anim Comp* 30:659, 1995.
37. Lombard CW, Spencer CP: Correlation of radiographic, echocardiographic, and electrocardiographic signs of left heart enlargement in dogs with mitral regurgitation, *Vet Radiol* 26:89, 1985.
38. Lombard CW: Normal values of the canine M-mode echocardiogram, *Am J Vet Res* 45:2015, 1984.
39. Kittleson MD, Eyster GE, Knowlen GG et al: Myocardial function in small dogs with chronic mitral regurgitation and severe congestive heart failure, *J Am Vet Med Assoc* 184:455, 1994.
40. Kittleson MD, Johnson LE, Oliver NB: Acute hemodynamic effects of hydralazine in dogs with chronic mitral regurgitation, *J Am Vet Med Assoc* 187:258, 1985.
41. Tischler MD, Cooper KA, Rowen M et al: Mitral valve replacement versus mitral valve repair: a Doppler and quantitative stress echocardiographic study, *Circulation* 89:132, 1994.
42. Carpentier A, Chauvaud S, Fabiani JN et al: Reconstructive surgery of mitral valve incompetence: ten-year appraisal, *J Thorac Cardiovasc Surg* 79:338, 1980.
43. Eyster GE, Weber W, Chi S et al: Mitral valve prosthesis for correction of mitral regurgitation in a dog, *J Am Vet Med Assoc* 168: 1115, 1976.
44. White RN, Stepien RL, Hammond RA et al: Mitral valve replacement for the treatment of congenital mitral dysplasia in a bull terrier, *J Small Anim Pract* 36:407, 1995.
45. Boggs L: *Heart surgery in dogs,* Veterinary Information Network, August 11, 1996.
46. Levine HJ, Gaasch WH: Vasoactive drugs in chronic regurgitant lesions of the mitral and aortic valves, *J Am Coll Cardiol* 28:1083, 1996.
47. Pfeffer MA, Braunwald E, Moye LA et al: Effect of captopril on mortality and morbidity in patients with left ventricular dysfunction after myocardial infarction: results of the survival and ventricular enlargement trial: The SAVE Investigators, *N Engl J Med* 327:669, 1992 (comments).
48. Swedberg K, Held P, Kjekshus J et al: Effects of the early administration of enalapril on mortality in patients with acute myocardial infarction: results of the Cooperative New Scandinavian Enalapril Survival Study II (CONSENSUS II), *N Engl J Med* 327:678, 1992 (comments).
49. The SOLVD Investigators: Effect of enalapril on mortality and the development of heart failure in asymptomatic patients with reduced left ventricular ejection fractions, *N Engl J Med* 327:685, 1992.
50. Sisson DD: Hemodynamic, echocardiographic, and clinical effects of enalapril in dogs with chronic heart failure: The IMPROVE Study Group, *ProcVet Med Forum,* 1992.
51. Ettinger SJ, Benitz AM, Ericsson GF: Relationships of enalapril with other CHF treatment modalities, *Proc Vet Med Forum,* 1994.
52. Ettinger SJ, Lusk R, Brayley K: Evaluation of enalapril in dogs with heart failure in a large multicenter study: Cooperative Veterinary Enalapril (COVE) Study Group, *Proc Vet Med Forum,* 1992.

CHAPTER 20

Primary Myocardial Disease Leading to Chronic Myocardial Failure (Dilated Cardiomyopathy and Related Diseases)

Dilated Cardiomyopathy

Myocardial contractility is the inherent capability of the myocardium to contract without any forces acting on it. It is the sum of numerous variables that determine the inherent ability of the myocardium to contract. *Myocardial contraction* is the amount that the myocardium contracts from end-diastole to end-systole (the amount of wall motion on an echocardiogram) and is determined by myocardial contractility, preload, afterload, and other variables. It is commonly measured by calculating shortening fraction. *Myocardial failure* is defined as a decrease in myocardial contractility. *Dilated cardiomyopathy (DCM)* is the term given to diseases in which myocardial failure is present for unknown reasons (idiopathic). The disease cannot be secondary to a valvular abnormality or to a congenital shunt (i.e., it must be primary). If the cause of the myocardial failure is known, then a different name is given to the disease, which describes the inciting feature of the disease (e.g., adriamycin cardiotoxicity or cardiomyopathy). Because there are other causes of myocardial failure, the diagnosis of DCM is a diagnosis of exclusion.

DCM is characterized on echocardiography by a primary increase in left ventricular end-systolic diameter and volume (because of the decrease in myocardial contractility) and usually (but not always) by a compensatory increase in left ventricular end-diastolic diameter and volume. Because end-diastolic diameter does not have to increase as much as the end-systolic diameter increases to maintain a normal stroke volume, shortening fraction (the amount of wall motion) decreases. The increase in chamber size is a compensatory, not a primary, mechanism and does not define the disease. Left ventricular wall thickness is normal to decreased (Figure 20-1).

Dilated cardiomyopathy, literally translated, means "a heart muscle disease in which the heart is dilated." Although the ventricular chambers are increased in size in this disease, the ventricles themselves have undergone volume overload (eccentric) hypertrophy, therefore the term *dilated* may be a misnomer. In addition, the term *dilated* describes a secondary feature of the disease, the chamber dilation, rather than the primary abnormality, the myocardial disease leading to the decrease in myocardial contractility. Consequently, we would prefer the name "idiopathic primary myocardial failure" for this disease. This term adequately describes the disease but is cumbersome, is not popular, and is not accepted nomenclature by the World Health Organization (WHO).[1] Consequently, the term dilated cardiomyopathy will be used in this chapter. Although it may not be grammatically correct, dilated cardiomyopathy is the term accepted by the WHO. Other terms in the literature, such as *congestive cardiomyopathy, dilative cardiomyopathy,* and *dilatative cardiomyopathy* are generally not used. The term *idiopathic* is sometimes placed in front of the accepted name (i.e., idiopathic dilated cardiomyopathy); however, this is redundant.

There are numerous known (not idiopathic) causes of myocardial failure in the dog and cat, as shown in Box 20-1. Most of these rarely cause clinically significant myocardial failure. Instead, the vast majority of the cases of myocardial failure observed are idiopathic. That is, no known etiology can be identified in most of the cases of primary myocardial failure seen in a veterinary clinic, and, consequently, most are called *DCM.* Therefore, although the diagnosis is one of exclusion, if myocardial failure is identified in a typical dog breed and there is no obvious inciting cause, DCM is usually diagnosed without a further extensive diagnostic workup.

Most cases of DCM diagnosed by veterinarians have clinical signs; however, evidence of heart failure, syncope, arrhythmia, or sudden death are not necessarily present in a dog with DCM. The disease has a long subclinical phase during which myocardial function, along with cardiac compensatory mechanisms, are adequate to maintain normal hemodynamics.[2] This phase of the disease during which echocardiographic or electrocardiographic evidence of the disease is present but clinical signs of the disease are not present has been termed *occult* in the literature. Occult denotes the phase of a disease during which it cannot be identified. Because the disease can often be readily identified with echocardiography (currently the most sensitive means of identifying the disease) or with a 24-hour ECG recording (Holter monitor) during this phase, the disease is not occult. The true occult phase of the disease is the stage in which echocardiographic evidence of myocardial failure and electrocardiographic evidence of ventricular arrhythmia are absent, yet the disease is present. A patient with DCM spends most of its life in a subclinical phase and only has clinical signs for a short time. Because veterinarians usually only see the patient during the time that it has clinical signs, we often think of the disease only in this context. We hope this will change as veterinarians become more aware of the natural history of this disease.

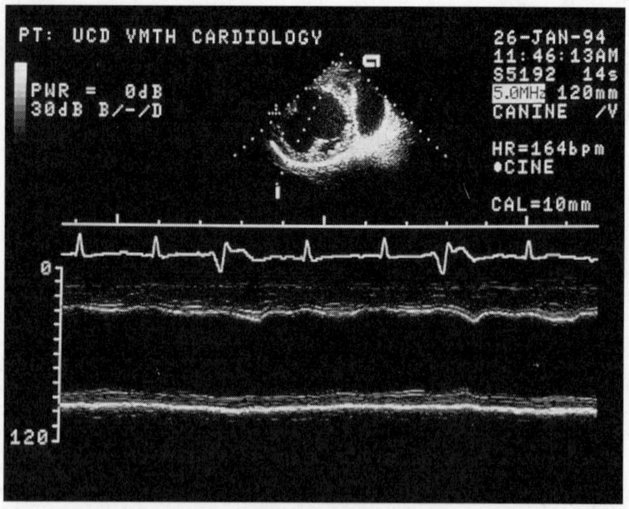

FIGURE 20-1 M-mode echocardiogram from a Doberman pinscher with dilated cardiomyopathy and ventricular premature depolarizations. The left ventricular end-systolic diameter is markedly increased, indicating severe myocardial failure. The end-diastolic diameter is increased to compensate for the decreased myocardial contractility. Shortening fraction is less than 10%. The left ventricular free wall thickness is normal. The interventricular septal thickness is decreased. The premature depolarizations produce better contractions than the sinus beat, which is unusual. The contractions appear to be delayed.

BOX 20-1

Causes of myocardial disease that might lead to chronic myocardial failure in dogs and cats**

Infectious agents

Viral

Parvovirus*
Distemper virus
Canine herpes virus

Fungal

Rickettsial

Ehrlichia canis
Rickettsia rickettsii
Bartonella elizabethae

Spirochetal

*Borrelia burgdorferi**

Parasitic

*Trypanosoma cruzi**
Toxoplasma gondii
Toxocara canis

Endocrinologic

Severe hypothyroidism
Hyperthyroidism*
Pheochromocytoma

Drugs and toxins

Adriamycin*
Cobalt
Gossypol

Physical injury

Electric shock
Trauma
Heat stroke

Nutritional deficiencies

Taurine*
Carnitine*

Ischemia/Infarction

Septic coronary artery embolus*
Atherosclerosis*

Muscular dystrophy

Duchenne's muscular dystrophy*

*Clinically documented causes of myocardial failure in veterinary medicine.
**These causes constitute less than 10% of the clinical cases of severe myocardial failure seen clinically. The remainder are idiopathic.

PREVALENCE

The prevalence of DCM is relatively low compared with other acquired cardiovascular diseases, such as myxomatous mitral valve disease. In the Veterinary Medical Data Base from Purdue University, between January, 1985, and December, 1991, DCM was listed as a diagnosis in 0.5% of the cases.[3] The prevalence in our hospital between August 1, 1986, and August 1, 1996, was 0.35% (245 ÷ 68,690 = 0.35%). These data are compiled from University veterinary hospitals and so represent primarily referral populations. The prevalence of DCM in private practice must be much lower. A prevalence of 0.5% translates into seeing one dog with DCM for every 200 dogs examined. In a busy practice, 200 dogs can be examined within a 2-week period. Even if one half of these were recheck examinations, a 0.5% prevalence could translate into every busy practice seeing a dog with DCM every month. It is more likely that a busy practice examines a dog with DCM once or twice a year.

Most of the time, DCM is identified in particular breeds of dogs. In the listings from the Veterinary Medical Data Base at Purdue University from January, 1986, to December, 1991, only 0.16% (131 out of 83,417 dogs) of mixed-breed dogs have had a diagnosis of dilated cardiomyopathy compared with a prevalence of 0.65% for purebred dogs.[3] Out of 1314 dogs listed with the diagnosis of DCM, 1183 (90%) were purebred dogs. Breeds in this database listed in descending order of number of cases in the United States were: Doberman pinscher (603), boxer (131), great Dane (122), Labrador retriever (73), American cocker spaniel (53), golden retriever (42), Irish wolfhound (38), Saint Bernard (29), springer spaniel (25), Newfoundland retriever (22), English sheepdog (18), Afghan hound (15), Scottish deerhound (7), and English cocker spaniel (5). At the University of California, Davis, Veterinary Medical Teaching Hospital, only 16 of the 260 cases (6%) diagnosed with DCM between August 1, 1986, and August 1, 1996, were mixed-breed dogs. Doberman pinschers accounted for 33% of the cases and boxers for 15%. Great Danes and American cocker spaniels each accounted for 10% of the cases. Golden and Labrador retrievers each represented 4% of the population. We only observed 7 (3%) Irish wolfhounds with DCM during that period. Obviously the Doberman pinscher dominated the DCM world in the late 1980s and early 1990s. Almost 6% of Doberman pinschers examined at University referral hospitals had severe DCM.[3] Other breeds, such as the German shepherd, English cocker spaniel, and Newfoundland are frequently identified in other regions of the world.[4-6] We only identified three German shepherds, three Newfoundlands, and no English cocker spaniels in our population. Although the disease is reported to be prevalent in the Scottish deerhound population, the population of these dogs is so small that we identified only two of these dogs with DCM.[3]

ETIOLOGY

By definition the etiology of DCM is unknown. What, in theory, could result in decrease in myocardial contractility without an obvious cause? There are numerous potential causes. Abnormalities in sarcomere structure or function may be one potential cause. However, we know that sarcomere abnormalities are compensated for by sarcomere hyperplasia, which results in primary concentric hypertrophy (hypertrophic cardiomyopathy; see Chapter 21). Decreased cellular energy production is another possible cause. Mitochondrial abnormalities would be the most likely cause of this type of dysfunction. Reduced sarcomere contraction would be the net result. Such abnormalities have been identified in skeletal muscular dystrophies.[7,8] Abnormal sarcoplasmic reticulum function could also result in reduced sarcomere contraction. Although these types of abnormalities have been identified on occasion in types of cardiomyopathy, they appear to be secondary abnormalities.[9] No primary abnormality in sarcoplasmic reticulum function has been identified. The aforementioned abnormalities would result in reduced sarcomere contraction and, consequently, reduced myocardial function. Abnormal cytoskeletal function could also result in reduced myocardial function without altering sarcomere function. The cytoskeleton of the myocardium is made up of numerous intracellular and extracellular proteins that hold myosin and actin in place, link sarcomere to sarcomere, link sarcomeres to the cell membrane, and attach cell to cell. Alterations in cytoskeletal structure or function could result in reduced linkage between sarcomere contraction and myocyte contraction or between myocyte contraction and global myocardial contraction. This could result in decreased global contraction. These abnormalities could also result in cell damage and death. Dystrophin abnormalities result in myocyte death. Abnormalities in cytoskeletal proteins are just now being recognized as causes of DCM in humans and hamsters.[10-12]

Ischemic myocardial disease is a common cause of myocardial failure in humans. This is a rare cause of myocardial failure in dogs and cats but can occur. In cats, ischemic disease most commonly results in a region of myocardium that is hypokinetic or akinetic and is usually thin.[13]

Taurine. From 1986 to 1987, taurine deficiency was discovered to be the primary cause of DCM in cats.[14] Since this discovery, the proper name for this disease should be taurine deficiency–induced myocardial failure. Because this name is cumbersome, the disease is still commonly called *feline DCM,* although not all cases of feline DCM are due to taurine deficiency.

Taurine is a sulfur-containing amino acid first isolated from ox bile.[15] One of its functions is to conjugate bile acids, along with glycine in some species. Although it is an amino acid, it is not a constituent of proteins. Its definitive role in cellular function is not known, but it is concentrated in the cytoplasm up to 250 times that in plasma.[16] This concentration is maintained by active transport and is modulated by β-adrenergic receptors. The highest cellular concentration is found in excitable tissue, such as myocardium, retina, central nervous system, and skeletal muscle.[17] It is also present in a high concentration in leukocytes and platelets.[18] In the heart, taurine has been postulated to help modulate intracellular osmolality, calcium concentration, and transmembrane ion fluxes.[19]

In a study reported in 1987, all cases of DCM in cats presented to our hospital (University of California, Davis, Veterinary Medical Teaching Hospital) were taurine-deficient.[14] In addition, echocardiographic measures of cardiac function returned either to normal or close to normal following 2 to 3 months of taurine supplementation (Figure 20-2). Following this discovery, it was quickly discovered that the source of the taurine deficiency was nutritional. Dry cat foods contained too little taurine, and the taurine in canned foods was not biologically available in adequate amounts. This was quickly remedied by the cat food manufacturing industry adding more taurine to their dietary formulations. Subsequently the prevalence of feline DCM decreased to less than 10% of pre-1987 levels.[20] All these facts are compatible with the theory that taurine is the only factor responsible for feline DCM. However, when experimental cats are fed taurine-deficient diets and are made systemically deficient, only about 30% develop echocardiographic evidence of myocardial failure.[21] This suggests some other factor or factors may also be involved. It is interesting that cats that develop myocardial failure on a taurine-deficient diet will redevelop myocardial failure if they are first treated with taurine to restore myocardial function and then redepleted of taurine. Cats that do not develop myocardial failure the first time do not subsequently develop it. This suggests something unique about individual cats and their sensitivity to taurine deficiency. One study has suggested that a genetic factor may be involved.[22] Because the disease has all but disappeared, interest in additional research has decreased markedly. Consequently, the other factor or factors involved may never be identified.

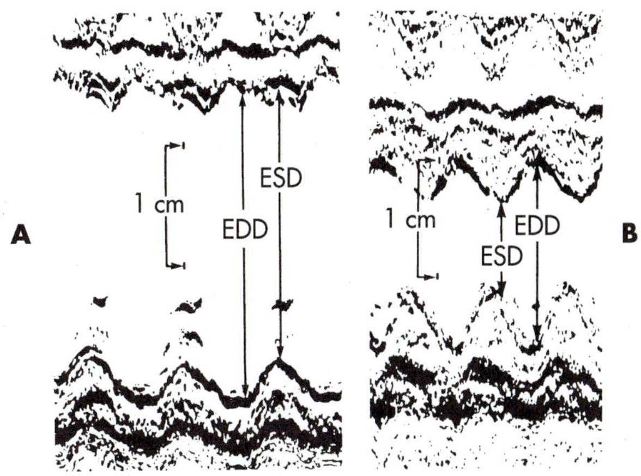

FIGURE 20-2 M-mode echocardiograms from a cat before and 3 months after taurine supplementation (250 mg q12h). **A,** Before supplementation, the echocardiogram shows a markedly increased left ventricular end-systolic diameter (ESD) of 23 mm, markedly increased end-diastolic diameter (EDD) of 26 mm, and a shortening fraction of 12%. **B,** After taurine supplementation, the ESD has decreased to 8 mm, the EDD has decreased to 15 mm, and the shortening fraction has increased to 47%. (From Pion PD, Kittleson MD, Rogers QR et al: Myocardial failure in cats associated with low plasma taurine: a reversible cardiomyopathy, *Science* 237:764, 1987.)

Cats are obligate carnivores with an absolute dietary requirement of taurine. Taurine is not an essential amino acid in dogs (i.e., they can maintain a normal plasma concentration without dietary intake). However, taurine deficiency is occasionally associated with DCM in dogs. In one report, plasma taurine concentration was low in 17% of the 75 dogs with DCM studied.[23] Plasma taurine concentration was not decreased in the breeds that are more commonly afflicted with DCM. Instead, all of the American cocker spaniels, three of the five golden retrievers, and four of the seven atypical or mixed breeds with DCM in this study had a low plasma taurine concentration. The first two American cocker spaniels treated with taurine supplementation, however, did not respond. L-carnitine was given as a supplement, along with taurine, in the next two American cocker spaniels with DCM, and both dogs responded, although plasma carnitine concentration was not decreased in these dogs. Following this, a clinical trial examining exclusively American cocker spaniels was completed. This study found all 11 American cocker spaniels to be systemically taurine-deficient. Echocardiographic measures of myocardial performance improved, the dogs clinically improved, and cardiovascular drug support could be removed 3 to 4 months after starting supplementation with taurine and carnitine. Consequently, it is now known that American cocker spaniels with DCM are taurine-deficient, and it is assumed that the taurine deficiency is at least a part of the etiology of the disease in this breed. Exactly how L-carnitine is related to the disease in this breed is unknown. We have documented echocardiographic improvement in some dogs with only taurine supplementation, so carnitine may not be involved at all. Exactly why American cocker spaniels are systemically taurine-deficient is unknown. We have examined renal clearance of taurine in one American cocker spaniel with DCM and a very low plasma taurine concentration. The urine concentration was also extremely low, suggesting that excess renal excretion of taurine is not the underlying abnormality in this breed. However, the fractional excretion of taurine in this dog was modestly increased.

Although taurine is not an essential amino acid in dogs, we have noted systemic taurine deficiency occasionally in dogs fed vegetarian diets. One situation involved a household in which two dogs were fed tofu and brown rice exclusively. Both dogs had DCM and a low plasma taurine concentration. One dog died before supplementation could improve its myocardial function. The other dog improved.

Carnitine. Carnitine deficiency appears to cause myocardial failure occasionally in dogs. Carnitine is a quaternary amine synthesized by the body from the amino acids lysine and methionine. It transports long-chain fatty acids across the inner mitochondrial membrane and modulates the intramitochondrial coenzyme A/acyl-coenzyme A ratio.[24] Consequently, carnitine deficiency results in poor mitochondrial function, reduced cellular energy production, and accumulation of triglycerides in the tissues. The net result is reduced myocardial performance. Carnitine deficiency has been diagnosed in a family of boxers.[25] This family was composed of the sire, the dam, and two littermates. All four had DCM at some stage. Of these, only one had a low plasma L-carnitine concentration. This dog also had a low myocardial L-carnitine concentration and was treated with high-dose L-carnitine (220 mg/kg/day) per os. His shortening fraction increased from 18% to 28%. This dog's littermate had a normal-to-high plasma L-carnitine concentration with a low myocardial concentration and responded to high-dose L-carnitine administration (shortening fraction increased from 2% to 24%). This dog also experienced a decline in myocardial function after L-carnitine therapy was withdrawn. The sire and dam both had a normal plasma L-carnitine concentration and a low myocardial concentration. They were treated with L-carnitine but died too soon for the L-carnitine to have much effect. Unfortunately these data are somewhat difficult to interpret. A low myocardial L-carnitine concentration has been identified in other dogs with DCM that have no apparent response to L-carnitine supplementation. This indicates that the myocardium can become carnitine-deficient secondary to other disease processes. Consequently, the finding of a low myocardial concentration in these dogs may or may not be significant for identifying a primary deficiency. Finding a low plasma L-carnitine concentration suggests a systemic deficiency, which occurs with much less frequency and is more difficult to blame on other causes. Consequently, the finding of a low concentration in the one dog in this report is intriguing. The response to supplementation is also intriguing and possibly even exciting. Because endomyocardial biopsies are not routinely done in veterinary medicine, myocardial concentration can be decreased in other myocardial diseases not associated with a primary carnitine deficiency, and plasma concentration did not identify which dogs would respond to L-carnitine in this report, it appears that the only method of identifying boxers that might be responsive to L-carnitine supplementation is to supplement them and observe their response. Consequently, it seems prudent to supplement boxers identified with DCM with 110 mg/kg L-carnitine per os q12h for 3 to 6 months and note their clinical and echocardiographic response. If no response is noted in that time and the dog is still alive, we recommend that supplementation be discontinued because L-carnitine is expensive. If an echocardiographic response is identified, the dose could be decreased and left ventricular function watched closely to determine if any deterioration was occurring. Any deterioration, of course, would require that the dose be increased again.

Cystinuria has been identified as a possible risk-factor for L-carnitine deficiency in dogs. Cystinuric dogs have impaired renal tubular reabsorption of cystine and other amino acids.[26] Some may also have excessive urinary loss of L-carnitine. A dachshund with this problem has been described.[27] It had cystinuria, a very low plasma L-carnitine concentration, and DCM that was responsive to L-carnitine supplementation.

Coenzyme Q_{10}. It has been suggested that coenzyme Q_{10} administration might be beneficial for veterinary patients with DCM.[28] Coenzyme Q_{10} (ubiquinone) is an essential component of the mitochondrial respiratory chain providing a redox link between flavoproteins and cytochromes in the inner mitochondrial membrane.[29,30] It is present in meats, fishes, nuts, dairy products, various vegetables, rapeseed oil, and soybean oil.[31] Primary genetic deficiencies of this and related compounds have been described in humans.[32,33] These deficiencies result in mitochondrial encephalomyopathies. Syndromes described include the MELAS (mitochondrial myopathy, encephalopathy, lactic acidosis, and stroke-like episodes) syndrome and Leigh syndrome.[7,34,35] The myopathies primarily involve skeletal muscle but can also affect cardiac muscle to produce DCM.[34,36] Carnitine deficiency may result from these abnormalities.[37] Abnormalities involving coenzyme Q_{10} are rare in human medicine, and mitochondrial defects such as this produce multisystem disease, as one might expect. Consequently, it is unlikely that a deficiency of coenzyme Q_{10} produces DCM in dogs.

Apparently, plasma and myocardial concentrations of coenzyme Q_{10} are decreased in human patients with DCM.[38,39] One group of researchers has been examining the administration of coenzyme Q_{10} to human patients with DCM since 1982.[40-43] They claim remarkable success, increasing ejection fraction from about 40% to about 60% and improving survival compared with historical controls. The major problems with their studies is the lack of a large placebo controlled clinical trial to document efficacy and the lack of corroboration by another group. Although they have reported similar findings several times, this mode of therapy apparently has not been accepted, because it is not mentioned in the standard human cardiology textbooks. It did, however, produce a review published in 1990.[44] Interested individuals are referred to this review. No studies have looked at this issue in veterinary medicine.

Breed predilection and genetics. Because of the breed predilection, DCM is almost certainly genetic in origin and almost certainly heritable. This, however, has not been proved. Some form of heritable biochemical or structural abnormality in the myocardium is suspected. The disease is predominantly diagnosed in male dogs. In one study, 79% of the dogs were male.[45] Because most of the diagnoses are made in symptomatic dogs, this male predilection may be for the disease or may be for developing severe disease. In Doberman pinschers, the disease appears to be more evenly distributed between males and females.[46] Male Doberman pinschers generally present with heart failure at a younger age than do the females.[47]

The prevalence of DCM increases with age.[3] In Doberman pinschers, the disease is most commonly identified between 7 and 10 years of age. A significant number, however, are diagnosed with the disease between 4 and 7 years of age and after 10 years of age. In great Danes, most of the disease is identified in 4-to-10-year-old dogs. Because the natural life span of great Danes is commonly less than 10 years, few cases are seen in dogs more than 10 years of age.

In boxers, the disease has been reported to be more prevalent in certain breeding lines, and multiple affected dogs in litters have been observed.[48] A small pedigree has been reported that suggests the disease may be inherited as an autosomal dominant trait.[49] Similarly, in Doberman pinschers, the disease has been reported to be more prevalent in certain breeding lines.[50]

The inheritance pattern of DCM in Doberman pinschers has not been determined. However, it appears that the prevalence of the disease is very high when these dogs are screened for the disease using echocardiography or are followed over time. One small study (n = 46) has estimated the prevalence to be 50% using left ventricular wall thickening on echocardiography and ejection fraction using angiocardiography as the distinguishing characteristics.[51] Another larger study suggested that 45% of the Doberman pinschers examined (n = 103) had evidence of DCM.[52] The high prevalence suggests a dominant trait. One study in which pedigrees were analyzed also suggests that DCM is inherited as an autosomal dominant trait with reduced penetrance.[53]

Myocardial abnormalities have been identified in Doberman pinschers with DCM. Most Doberman pinschers with DCM have a decreased myocardial carnitine concentration.[54] Response to supplementation is generally poor, and plasma L-carnitine concentration is usually normal. Consequently, the myocardial L-carnitine deficiency is probably secondary to another abnormality rather than a primary abnormality. Myocardial myoglobin concentration is decreased in Doberman pinschers with DCM.[55] It is also decreased in experimental dogs with myocardial failure induced by rapid ventricular pacing. The reduction, however, is greater in Doberman pinschers that are in heart failure. The reduction in asymptomatic Doberman pinschers with DCM is similar to paced dogs. The fact that myoglobin is decreased in another form of myocardial disease makes it most likely that this observation is also a secondary abnormality. Myoglobin function can be obliterated chemically with no change in myocardial oxygen consumption.[56] Consequently, it is unlikely that a reduction in myoglobin concentration would have a significant effect on myocardial function. The mitochondria of Doberman pinschers with DCM do not function normally.[57] Electron transport is decreased, energy (ATP) production is decreased, and lactate concentration is increased. Total creatine kinase concentration is decreased, and the isoenzyme CK-MB is decreased to less than 50% of normal.[58] Because enzyme systems normally must be decreased to a level less than 10% of normal to result in clinically significant derangement, this level of alteration suggests that this abnormality is not a primary abnormality. It is known that in experimental preparations, decreasing total creatine kinase concentration to less than 2% of normal only results in a decrease in myocardial reserve, not in resting myocardial function.[59] Sarcoplasmic reticulum calcium transport is also decreased.[60,61] These types of abnormalities are described in other myocardial diseases and almost certainly represent secondary, not primary (causal) abnormalities.

In humans, genetic causes of DCM are now being identified. An abnormality of myocardial dystrophin causes X-linked dilated cardiomyopathy in a few human families.[62] Families with X-linked DCM do not have a clinically apparent skeletal muscular dystrophy (Duchenne's muscular dystrophy). Males develop DCM in their 20s to 40s and die or are transplanted within several years. Heterozygote females present later in life with atypical chest pain and don't develop heart failure for more than a decade. Gene mutations have been identified in several families.[63] In one family, a point mutation in the 5′ splice site of the first intron of the muscle dystrophin gene has been identified. In this family, it was shown that skeletal muscle could express brain dystrophin to compensate for the loss of muscle dystrophin, whereas myocardium could not. A missense mutation in exon 9 of the gene that encodes for dystrophin has also been reported in three human families.[64] In another family there is a mutation that affects the muscle promoter region of the dystrophin gene.[65] One individual has been identified with a deficiency of another cytoskeletal protein, metavinculin.[66] Linkage analysis has also identified an abnormal gene on the long arm of chromosome 9 in one family and on chromosome 1q32, 1p1-1q1, 9q13-q22, and 3p22-25 in others.[67-69] To date all that can be concluded is that abnormalities in structural proteins are one cause of heritable DCM in humans. It is possible that similar abnormalities will be identified in dogs.

Dalmations are also at risk for developing DCM. In one study of nine cases, all affected Dalmations were male and eight were eating Hill's Prescription Diet u/d.[70] Four dogs were tested for taurine deficiency in this study, and values ranged from 41 to 144 nmol/mL. We consider any value less than 50 nmol/mL to be deficient, which means that at least one of these dogs appeared to be taurine-deficient. Two dogs were supplemented with taurine but apparently for only a short time. The diet was switched in six dogs, but only one had a documented improvement in left ventricular function following a change. We have observed only one case of DCM in a Dalmatian. This dog presented in heart failure with a shortening fraction between 5% and 10%. He was being fed a home-cooked vegetarian diet, and his plasma taurine concentration was 16 nmol/mL (normal is greater than 50 nmol/mL). He continued to have clinical signs referable to heart failure for several months while on digoxin, captopril, and furosemide. Within 3 months of starting taurine supplementation his shortening fraction improved to 20%, his cardiac silhouette decreased remarkably in size, and his EPSS decreased. This dog went on to live for at least another 3 years. Hill's supplemented u/d with additional taurine after a possible association between their diet and DCM in Dalmations was made. The instances of DCM in Dalmations reported to Hill's since that time have reportedly decreased.

PATHOLOGY

In dogs and cats with severe DCM, the most striking gross finding is moderate-to-marked dilation of all four cardiac chambers (Color Plate 77). Often the left heart appears more affected than the right heart. The myocardium of fresh specimens often appears flabby. The heart commonly collapses when placed on a table, rather than retaining its shape (Color Plate 78). The walls of the ventricles may appear thin, but this judgement is usually made by comparing wall thickness to chamber size. When measured, the wall thicknesses may be normal or they may, in fact, be thin. The papillary muscles appear flattened. When the heart or specific chambers are weighed, the weight is greater than normal, indicating the presence of hypertrophy.[71] On cut-section, the left ventricular myocardium appears remarkably normal in many cases, although pale regions may be noted.

Histologic findings may primarily indicate hypertrophy rather than marked tissue destruction. This is especially true in cats with taurine deficiency in which other histologic findings are commonly absent (Color Plate 79). In dogs, there commonly is evidence of myocardial disease, but it is often not severe enough to cause the marked degree of myocardial failure observed clinically. Histologically, there is evidence of myocytolysis, myofibril fragmentation, abnormal mitochondria, and vacuolization, but these changes may be only mild to moderate and are often identified in other cardiac diseases.[71] Similar findings are reported in humans with DCM.[72] Doberman pinschers most frequently have focal cardiac muscle atrophy, some foci of fibrosis, occasional sarcoplasmic vacuoles, and lipofuscin in the cytoplasm of myocardial cells.[73] There may also be regions of more severe replacement fibrosis and fatty replacement (Color Plate 80). The most severe lesions are commonly in the left ventricular papillary muscles.[47] There are no differences in histologic lesions or lesion severity in dogs with mild or severe disease.[47] This may mean that the histologic changes are not the primary abnormality responsible for the depressed myocardial function.

Boxers may be unique in that they commonly have more diffuse and severe myocardial changes.[48] Active and chronic myocardial changes are present. Active changes are less frequent and consist of focal areas of myocytolysis, myofiber necrosis, hemorrhage, and mild mononuclear cellular infiltration. Chronic changes consist of myofiber atrophy, marked variation in the size and shape of myofibers, extensive fatty infiltration, and fatty change. Myxomatous change in the atrioventricular valves is also common.

The finding that many dogs do not have extensive myocyte loss or damage suggests that the myocardial disease process in dogs may also be due to some form of biochemical or structural abnormality. Such abnormalities could result in poor contractile function but not cellular destruction. The lack of extensive myocyte damage suggests that if the specific cause of the disease in dogs could be identified, the disease might be reversible, as it is in cats, or at least partially reversible, as it is in American cocker spaniels.

PATHOPHYSIOLOGY

The pathophysiology of DCM is outlined in Chapter 9. Briefly, a myocardial disease of unknown etiology results in a progressive decrease in myocardial contractility. This starts as a mild decrease and may progress over months to years to a severe decrease in contractility.[2] The decrease in contractility results in an increase in end-systolic diameter and end-systolic volume, which results in a decrease in stroke volume. Chronically the heart compensates for this decreased function by growing larger ventricular chambers through eccentric (volume overload) hypertrophy. This growth occurs secondary to many factors. One primary factor is renal sodium and water retention, leading to an increase in blood volume that leads to an increase in intracardiac volumes. This places stretch on the myocardium that stimulates the myocytes to grow longer and the chambers to grow larger. This results in an increase in end-diastolic diameter and end-diastolic volume. The increased chamber size allows the stroke volume to return to normal when the disease is mild to moderate. At some stage the myocardial failure becomes so severe that the ability of the cardiovascular system to compensate for the disease is overwhelmed and the ventricular chambers can grow no larger. At this stage, left ventricular end-diastolic pressure increases, which results in pulmonary edema (congestive heart failure). If the right heart is also severely involved, right ventricular end-diastolic pressure increases, which most commonly results in ascites in dogs. Stroke volume is reduced at this stage. Increased sympathetic tone increases the heart rate, which helps compensate for the decrease in stroke volume. However, cardiac output ultimately decreases also (low-output heart failure). In the terminal stages of the disease, cardiac output may decrease to the point that, even with a marked increase in peripheral vascular resistance, systemic arterial blood pressure decreases to a clinically significant level (cardiogenic shock).

Other abnormalities may also contribute to the production of heart failure. Myocardial diseases not only result in systolic dysfunction but also in diastolic dysfunction. The primary abnormality that results in clinically significant impairment of diastolic function is altered ventricular compliance. A stiffer or less compliant left ventricle results in a higher diastolic pressure for any given diastolic volume, and therefore more pulmonary edema for any degree of volume overload. A decrease in left ventricular compliance has been documented in dogs with DCM.[74] Mitral regurgitation is also commonly present in dogs with DCM. Diseases in which the left ventricle becomes volume overloaded commonly have secondary changes that cause an atrioventricular valve to leak. In DCM, two changes can occur that result in atrioventricular valve regurgitation. First, the atrioventricular annulus dilates as the left ventricle enlarges.[75] Second, the papillary muscles are displaced laterally and apically as the ventricular chamber enlarges.[76,77] Both result in the leaflets failing to close completely during systole (incomplete valve closure). This manifests as the coaptation point (the point where the valve leaflets come together) being displaced apically. This may be observed on an echocardiogram. Functional valvular regurgitation results. This type of regurgitation is usually mild on the left side of the heart, however; therefore its contribution to the production of heart failure is probably minimal in most cases (Color Plate 81). The fact that hydralazine usually does not result in a decrease in pulmonary capillary wedge pressure or pulmonary edema in dogs with DCM suggests that the mitral regurgitation in DCM is not usually an important component of the disease.

Arrhythmias can also contribute to the genesis of heart failure. Atrial fibrillation is probably the most important. The acute production of atrial fibrillation usually results in an increase in heart rate. In normal dogs, a marked increase in heart rate in association with atrial fibrillation results in a decrease in cardiac output. Whether or not this also occurs in dogs with severe myocardial failure is unknown. We have noted that venous oxygen tension commonly decreases when the heart rate is pharmacologically decreased in dogs with atrial fibrillation and DCM. This suggests that the high heart rate in this situation may aid in maintaining cardiac output. However, it is well known that rapid ventricular pacing at a rate as low as 180 beats/min produces myocardial failure.[78,79] Because further myocardial failure in a patient that already has severe myocardial failure must be detrimental, reducing the heart rate in dogs with atrial fibrillation to a heart rate less than 170 beats/min is necessary for long-term function, even if cardiac output may be compromised further. Besides atrial fibrillation, fast ventricular arrhythmias may also compromise ventricular function if they are sustained.

Oxygen delivery to myocardium appears to be inadequate for myocardial oxygen consumption in dogs with severe DCM. We have verified this by measuring coronary sinus oxygen tension in five dogs with DCM.[80] Venous oxygen tension is a measure of the adequacy of oxygen delivery for a given amount of oxygen consumption. When it decreases below about 21 mm Hg, oxygen diffusion into cells is compromised. Normal coronary sinus oxygen tension in dogs ranges from 24 to 29 mm Hg. In these five dogs, the coronary sinus oxygen tension was 13, 15, 17, 18, and 23 mm Hg. The dog with the highest value was not in heart failure and had a shortening fraction between 15% and 20%. All of the other dogs were less than 15% and were in or had been in heart failure. The blood that is obtained from the coronary sinus of dogs with severe DCM is black. This finding indicates that the myocardium in dogs with severe DCM is severely hypoxic. This severe hypoxia is almost certainly secondary to the abnormalities present in a heart with severe DCM (e.g., a marked increase in systolic myocardial wall stress) and is not a primary abnormality. However, severe myocardial hypoxia almost certainly contributes to a further degradation in myocardial function which shortens survival time.

Dogs with DCM die suddenly from their disease. Some of these dogs may faint or have episodes of weakness that are probably aborted instances of sudden death. Ventricular tachyarrhythmias are most likely responsible for most of these cases although severe bradyarrhythmias may also occur.[81]

NATURAL HISTORY

The natural history of DCM in most breeds of dogs has not been studied in detail. It has been better studied in Doberman pinschers and cats. The studies in cats have been done on cats experimentally fed a diet low in taurine content.

Cats. Only about 30% of taurine-deficient cats develop echocardiographic evidence of myocardial failure.[82] Of the cats with myocardial failure, about 30% develop severe myocardial failure (shortening fraction less than 15%). Cats with severe myocardial failure are often stable for months to years. Some of these cats appear to develop heart failure suddenly. More likely they develop heart failure more slowly and then reach a critical point. Consequently, they only appear to have an acute onset of heart failure.

Before the discovery that taurine was the cause of DCM in cats, the prognosis for survival in these cats was poor to grave. They usually presented with severe congestive heart failure and severe low-output heart failure. Survival time was hours to a few months. Taurine supplementation to a cat with DCM caused by taurine deficiency does not change the short-term prognosis. Cats that live longer than 2 to 3 weeks, however, almost all survive, and their myocardial function normalizes over 3 to 5 months. Consequently, their long-term prognosis is excellent. In cats with DCM that is not due to taurine deficiency, the prognosis is usually grave. The median survival time on one study was only 2 weeks.[13]

Doberman pinschers. Like cats, Doberman pinschers have a long period during which they have myocardial failure but no clinical signs. Affected dogs develop echocardiographic evidence of myocardial failure at some stage, and then their myocardial function usually deteriorates over months to years.[2] However, in some dogs the disease stabilizes for several years.[52] Female Doberman pinschers tend to be older (median age = 9.5 years) than male dogs (median age = 7.5 years) at the time their myocardial failure becomes severe enough for them to go into heart failure.[83] Although it appears that males and females are equally affected, more males develop heart failure and die of their disease than do females.[83] In one study, of 66 Doberman pinschers that either died from heart failure or died suddenly, 55 (83%) were males. Doberman pinschers, like cats, often appear to develop heart failure acutely. The presentation is often so acute that an owner thinks that someone has poisoned the dog. Instead, dogs hide their clinical signs well until heart failure is severe and only show obvious clinical signs when heart failure is severe. Doberman pinschers may be diagnosed with DCM at almost any age, but they present in heart failure between 2 and 14 years of age.[83] The time course of the disease appears to be accelerated in Doberman pinschers that develop echocardiographic evidence of the disease at less than 2 years of age and more prolonged when it develops after 6 to 7 years of age.[50] Approximately 75% are between 5 and 10 years of age at the time they die.[50]

Ventricular arrhythmias are a consistent finding in affected Doberman pinschers. The number and the complexity of the ventricular arrhythmias increase as the disease progresses. One investigator reported a study of 129 Doberman pinschers with no clinical signs of disease.[84] Of these, 87 (57%) had a shortening fraction between 30% and 34% and had no or fewer than 50 ventricular premature depolarizations on a 24-hour ECG recording (Holter monitor). All of these dogs were alive and healthy 3 years later. Thirty-four dogs had a shortening fraction less than 25% and had more than 100 ventricular premature depolarizations per 24 hours. Eight had a shortening fraction between 25% and 29% and 50 to 100 ventricular premature depolarizations per 24 hours. Of these 42 dogs, 21% died suddenly ($n = 9$) and 62% died of heart failure ($n = 26$) within 3 years. From these data a shortening fraction less than 25% in a Doberman pinscher clearly indicates the presence of DCM. A shortening fraction between 25% and 30% is suspicious of the disease. In addition, the presence of more than 50 ventricular premature depolarizations within a 24-hour period on a Holter monitor recording is indicative of DCM in Doberman pinschers. The type of arrhythmia appears to be important. All of the dogs with complex ventricular arrhythmias (pairs of ventricular premature depolarizations, runs of ventricular premature depolarizations, and periods of nonsustained ventricular tachycardia) in the above study died suddenly, presumably from the ventricular tachyarrhythmia degenerating into ventricular fibrillation.[85] Large numbers of single ventricular premature depolarizations did not appear to predict sudden death. However, in a more recent report by the same author, even complexity of a ventricular arrhythmia did not predict sudden death, because many dogs that died suddenly and many dogs that went on to develop heart failure had complex ventricular arrhythmias.[47] Only the presence of sustained (greater than 30 seconds) ventricular tachycardia predicted which dogs would die suddenly in this report. Approximately 30% of Doberman pinschers are in atrial fibrillation at the time they are diagnosed with heart failure.[83]

When the shortening fraction decreases to less than 15%, dogs can go into heart failure.[47] It is extremely unusual for a dog with DCM in heart failure to have a shortening fraction greater than 15%, and they are commonly less than 10%. Consequently, the diagnosis of DCM should always be questioned in a dog that is in heart failure and has an accurately measured shortening fraction greater than 15%. Although dogs can theoretically have both DCM and primary mitral regurgitation (usually myxomatous mitral valve disease), this appears to be uncommon. More often, large-breed dogs with primary mitral regurgitation develop secondary myocardial failure and present in heart failure with a shortening fraction between 20% and 40%. Most of the Doberman pinschers we see with primary mitral valve disease and myocardial failure do not have ventricular arrhythmias present on a Holter monitor.

Once they are in heart failure, dogs with DCM have both a poor short-term and long-term prognosis despite adequate medical therapy. They commonly present in fulminant heart failure that can be difficult to manage. Consequently, they may die shortly after presentation. These dogs are also commonly euthanized once the owners are made aware of the poor long-term prognosis. Most symptomatic Doberman pinschers die within the first 3 months after diagnosis. About 20% die suddenly during this stage.[83] The median and mean survival times have been reported to be 10 and 6 weeks.[83,86] Approximately 25% are dead within 2 weeks of presenting in heart failure, 40% are dead within 4 weeks, and 65% are dead within 8 weeks. Survival of Doberman pinschers with DCM has been reported to correlate inversely with the degree of myocardial failure, as measured by end-systolic diameter.[87] Doberman pinschers that present in both left and right heart failure have a worse prognosis (median survival time = 3 weeks) than those that have left heart failure alone (median survival time = 7.5 weeks).[83] Doberman pinschers in atrial fibrillation have a median survival time of 3 weeks. Occasionally (about 10% of the time) a Doberman pinscher with DCM will stabilize and do well clinically for a longer time, sometimes up to a year.

Other breeds. Other breeds with DCM do slightly better but not to a clinically significant degree. In one clinical trial of the use of milrinone in dogs with heart failure, 117 dogs with DCM were enrolled.[45] Milrinone had no apparent clinically significant effect on survival. Consequently, the data from these dogs are probably representative of a normally treated population of dogs with symptomatic DCM. In this study, 50% of the dogs with heart failure resulting from DCM died within the first 3 months and 75% were dead within the first 6 months after diagnosis (Figure 20-3). About 10% of the dogs lived for 1 year and 5% for 2 years. Dogs with

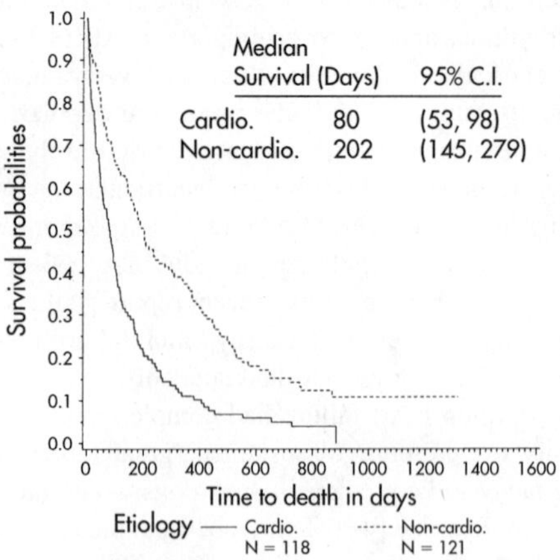

FIGURE 20-3 Kaplan-Meier survival curves for dogs with dilated cardiomyopathy (DCM) (cardio.) and dogs with heart failure from other causes (non-cardio). All were treated with furosemide and milrinone and most were administered digoxin. Most of the dogs with other cardiac disease had myxomatous degeneration of the mitral valve producing severe mitral regurgitation. The median survival time for the dogs with DCM was 80 days and for the other dogs was 202 days.

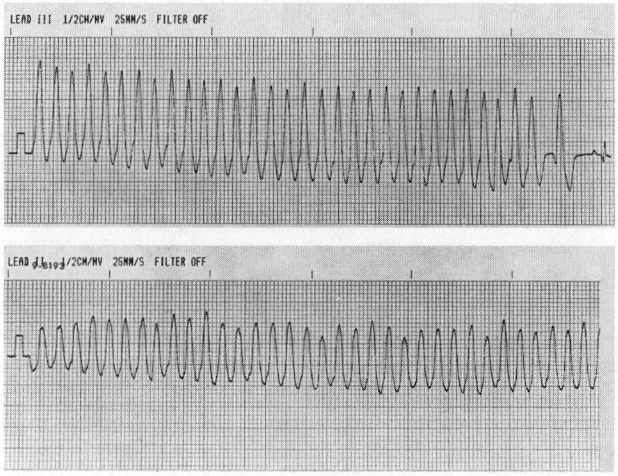

FIGURE 20-4 Lead III electrocardiographic tracings from a boxer with category 2 boxer cardiomyopathy taken at a time during which the dog was having syncopal events. The primary rhythm is a fast (rate = 375 beats/min) ventricular tachycardia that is bordering on ventricular flutter. The rhythm spontaneously slows and then reverts to sinus rhythm at the end of the first trace. (Paper speed = 25 mm/sec.)

severe heart failure faired somewhat worse than dogs with mild-to-moderate heart failure. Approximately 50% of the dogs with severe heart failure were dead within 2 months and 75% were dead within 4 months, whereas 50% of the dogs with mild-to-moderate heart failure died within 4 months and 75% died within 7.5 months. About 20% of the dogs with mild-to-moderate heart failure lived for 1 year, and 10% lived for 2 years. Another study has examined survival time in 37 symptomatic and asymptomatic dogs with DCM.[88] Approximately 50% of these dogs also died within the first 3 months after diagnosis. This can be compared to survival in humans with DCM, of which approximately 50% die within 36 months and 75% die within 72 months.[89] Box 20-2 presents a case example of a Doberman pinscher with dilated cardiomyopathy.

Boxers. Boxers have different forms of the disease. Consequently, they may present differently and may have a different natural history. Harpster[48] has divided so-called boxer cardiomyopathy into three categories. Boxers with mild ventricular arrhythmias are placed in category 1. These dogs have ventricular arrhythmias most commonly identified on a Holter monitor recording. They commonly have a small number of ventricular premature depolarizations. The natural history of this group of dogs is unknown with or without therapy, although Harpster has reported that many of these dogs do well for more than 2 years.[48] Dogs in category 2 have severe ventricular arrhythmias and commonly are presented because of syncope (Figure 20-4). The rate of the ventricular tachyarrhythmia commonly exceeds 300 beats/min. Dogs in this category are prone to sudden death. The syncopal events seen in these dogs are in reality more likely instances of aborted sudden death. The events are most likely due to episodes of fast ventricular tachycardia or ventricular flutter that spontaneously revert to sinus rhythm. The prognosis is guarded. Some of these dogs go on to die suddenly (Figure 20-5). Others do well with antiarrhythmic therapy. At presentation, some of these dogs have myocardial failure, and an approximate equal number have normal myocardial function. Most dogs without myocardial dysfunction at presentation go on to develop myocardial failure. Some, however, never seem to develop myocardial failure, although it is possible that these dogs have not been followed for an adequate time and would ultimately develop it. Dogs in category 3 have severe myocardial failure, heart failure, and, usually, ventricular tachyarrhythmias. Some, however, may have supraventricular tachyarrhythmias, most commonly atrial fibrillation. The prognosis for these dogs is poor. These dogs either die of heart failure or die suddenly. The majority (approximately 85%) of these dogs are

BOX 20-2

Case example of a Doberman pinscher with dilated cardiomyopathy

"Rascal" was an 8 year-old male Doberman pinscher that was presented for a urinary tract infection. His turned out to be a "typical" case of dilated cardiomyopathy in the Doberman pinscher. The owner was a breeder who knew that several of Rascal's relatives had died of DCM and so wanted to have him examined echocardiographically. Rascal was completely normal clinically and on physical examination. Echocardiography revealed a left ventricular end-diastolic diameter of 67 mm (normal = 50 mm), an end-systolic diameter of 53 mm (normal = 35 mm), a left ventricular wall thickness of 9 mm (normal), an *E*-point–septal separation of 12 mm (normal is less than 6 mm), and a shortening fraction of 22% (normal is approximately 25% to 40%). On a resting ECG he had no premature ventricular depolarizations. On a Holter monitor recording, he had approximately 280 premature ventricular depolarizations in 24 hours. The owner donated the dog to the University of California, Davis, Veterinary Medicine Teaching Hospital. He was examined periodically over the next 2.5 years. During that time his myocardial function gradually deteriorated. Nine months after presentation his shortening fraction was 16%, end-systolic diameter was 57 mm, and end-diastolic diameter was 68 mm. On the Holter recording he had approximately 830 premature ventricular depolarizations in 24 hours. All of these were single. He was still clinically normal. At this time he was adopted by a secretary from the hospital. He was presented for periodic reexaminations, and his left ventricular function was stable for approximately 1 year. One and one-half years after he was adopted, he was presented in acute respiratory distress. At this time his shortening fraction was 12% and his left ventricular end-systolic and end-diastolic diameters were markedly increased (64 and 73 mm, respectively). He was managed medically with furosemide, an ACE inhibitor, and digoxin. Over the next 4 months, his diuretic dose was gradually increased to control his clinical signs. At the end of this time, he was euthanized because of clinical deterioration.

A

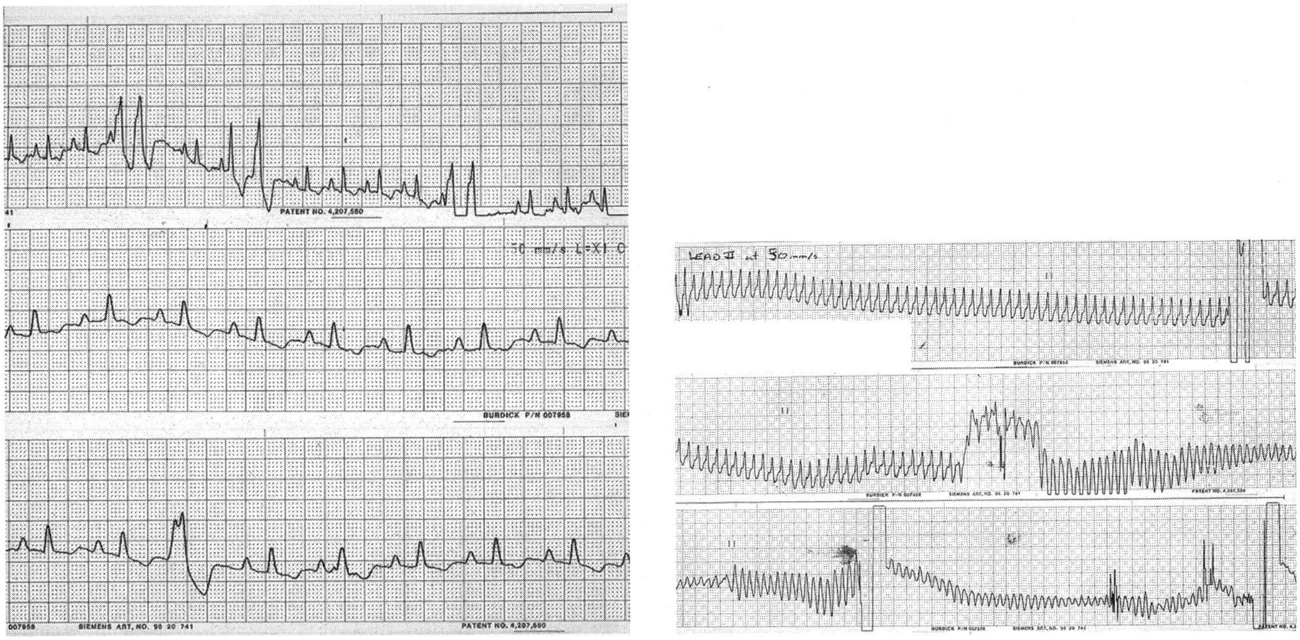

B

FIGURE 20-5 **A,** Three lead II ECG tracings from a 7-year-old boxer with dilated cardiomyopathy and a history of syncopal events. The top tracing is taken at 25 mm/sec and shows pairs of ventricular premature depolarizations (VPDs). The first VPD in the pair occurs late, coming in immediately before the sinus depolarization reaches the ventricles. The second VPD occurs at a variable interval after the first, achieving a rate as fast as approximately 300 beats/min. The first VPD of the second pair is a fusion beat. The second and third tracings are recorded at 50 mm/sec. The second tracing shows sinus rhythm. The third tracing has one VPD (third complex). The VPDs are upright and appear to originate from the right ventricle. **B,** Semicontinuous monitoring lead ECG tracings from the dog shown in **A,** taken several hours later when the dog collapsed in the hospital. The ECG was recorded while the dog died suddenly. Although the paper speed is labeled at the time of recording as being 50 mm/sec, tracings are actually recorded at 25 mm/sec. The top tracing shows fast ventricular tachycardia with the ventricular focus firing at a rate of approximately 400 beats/min. Artifact occurs at the end of this tracing. The second tracing shows the same ventricular tachycardia in the first half of the tracing. There is artifact in the middle of the tracing. After the artifact, the dog's rhythm has degenerated into ventricular flutter at a rate of approximately 500 beats/min. In the bottom tracing, the ventricular flutter degenerates into coarse ventricular fibrillation. Resuscitation attempts were unsuccessful. (Courtesy Dr. Dean Beyerinck.)

between 6 and 12 years of age at the time of diagnosis, with only 10% being less than 6 years of age. Median and mean ages are 8 to 8.5 years. Males are slightly more represented than females (58% vs. 42%).

CLINICAL SIGNS

Dogs with mild-to-moderate myocardial failure usually show no clinical signs. Syncope is occasionally observed, more commonly in boxers and Doberman pinschers. Most of the dogs and cats diagnosed with DCM have severe myocardial failure and are in heart failure at the time of presentation. Most of these dogs have had a short history of problems. Many are presented for acute clinical signs, prompting the owner to suspect trauma or toxins as the cause. Respiratory signs secondary to pulmonary edema predominate and include tachypnea, dyspnea, and a soft cough. Dogs with fulminant pulmonary edema are severely dyspneic, have respiratory rates that usually exceed 70 breaths/min, and may cough up pink-tinged pulmonary edema fluid from their airways (Color Plate 82). Some dogs may also exhibit signs of right heart failure (i.e., ascites). A few dogs will have pleural effusion, most likely as a result of a combination of left and right heart failure. Weight loss may also be present and can be profound. Other dogs present with no evidence of weight loss. Some dogs also present with evidence of poor perfusion, including cold extremities, cold ears, and weakness. When the hypoperfusion is profound, total body hypothermia (rectal temperature less than 100° C) may also be present. Dogs with DCM that become dehydrated more commonly have clinical signs referable to poor perfusion.

Some dogs with DCM present with a history of syncopal episodes or episodes of weakness. These signs are more common in Doberman pinschers and boxers, in which ventricular arrhythmias are common.[48] These episodes are most commonly due to short periods of severe ventricular tachyarrhythmias and are probably aborted instances of sudden death. Approximately 20% of Doberman pinschers will die suddenly from their disease.[90] Syncope is a clinical sign in about 35% of boxers with myocardial disease.[48] Whereas Doberman pinschers that present because of syncope usually have evidence of myocardial failure, many boxers have apparently normal ventricular function on echocardiography and normal thoracic radiographs. Boxers with ventricular arrhythmias are at risk for sudden death regardless of whether or not myocardial function is depressed (see Figure 20-5).

PHYSICAL EXAMINATION

Dogs with early DCM that are not in heart failure are usually normal on physical examination. An arrhythmia, most commonly ventricular premature depolarizations, may be identified. Dogs that present with severe DCM that are in heart failure have many abnormal findings on physical examination. The most obvious signs are those of left and, sometimes, right congestive heart failure. Pulmonary edema produces tachypnea and dyspnea. A soft cough may be present in the examination room or may be elicited by tracheal palpation. If the rear quarters are elevated, blood-tinged fluid may run out of the mouth or nose in dogs with fulminant pulmonary edema. Auscultation of the lungs most commonly reveals increased bronchovesicular sounds as a result of the hyperpnea (increased air moving through the airways). Some dogs have soft crackles, and some will have more coarse crackles. These are more commonly ausculted in dogs with severe edema. In dogs with right heart failure, ascites is usually present. Hepatomegaly and sometimes splenomegaly may be palpated. Jugular vein distension may be present.

Auscultation of the heart often reveals a soft systolic heart murmur, a gallop sound, or an arrhythmia. The murmur is most commonly due to mild mitral regurgitation and is usually grade 3 or softer. The gallop sound is usually a third heart sound. This sound is heard best in dogs that are in sinus rhythm and is impossible to distinguish from the other heart sounds in dogs in atrial fibrillation. The gallop sound is often subtle, and to hear it one must listen carefully and know what one is listening for. In some dogs the sound is very loud and on occasion can be felt by placing one's fingers over the left apex beat.

Arrhythmias are common in dogs with DCM. Atrial fibrillation is very common in dogs with symptomatic DCM and especially common in giant breeds with DCM. The heart rate is rapid in these dogs when they are in heart failure. This is due to high circulating catecholamine concentrations enhancing the conduction patterns of the atrioventricular node. The heart rate commonly exceeds 200 beats/min. The fast rate, the variability of the rate, and the admixture of heart sounds often make it impossible to count the heart rate on auscultation. Ventricular arrhythmias are common in Doberman pinschers and boxers with DCM. These range from isolated premature beats to salvos of rapid ventricular tachycardia to sustained ventricular tachycardia. Occasionally, ventricular arrhythmias will be mistaken for atrial fibrillation on auscultation. Femoral pulse quality can range from normal to severely decreased. Pulse deficits and alternating pulse strength are common in dogs with atrial fibrillation and ventricular arrhythmia.

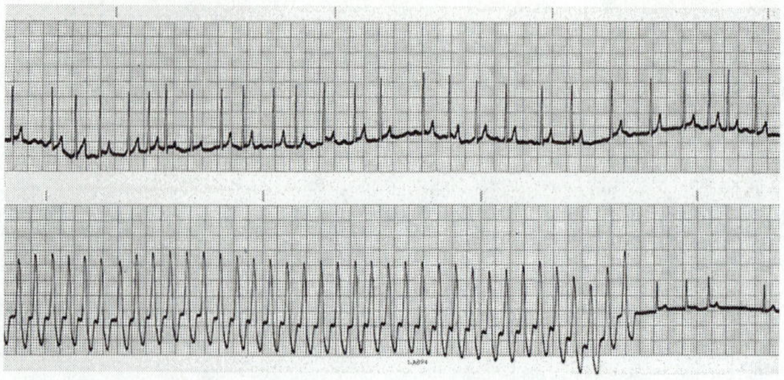

FIGURE 20-6 Lead II ECG tracings from a boxer presented for syncope. On an echocardiogram the dog had moderate-to-severe myocardial failure and an enlarged left atrium. The top ECG tracing shows atrial fibrillation. On the bottom tracing the dog is having a bout of nonsustained ventricular tachycardia at a rate of 260 beats/min. The dog did not faint during this episode. Most likely the episodes of ventricular tachycardia that precipitated syncope were longer, faster, or both. (Paper speed = 25 mm/sec; 1 cm = 1 mV.)

DIAGNOSTIC STUDIES

Electrocardiography. The electrocardiogram is used primarily to identify the type of arrhythmia present in a patient with DCM. Although QRS and *P* wave abnormalities are commonly present, they are nonspecific and rarely contribute to the diagnosis. Abnormalities include increased *R* wave height in leads II and aV_F, prolonged QRS complexes and *P* waves, QRS complex notching and slurring, and ST segment and *T* wave abnormalities.

Atrial fibrillation is present in 75% to 80% of giant-breed dogs at the time of presentation.[91] In Doberman pinschers and boxers, ventricular tachyarrhythmias are common, although atrial fibrillation is also often present (Figure 20-6). An examination room ECG usually only encompasses about 30 seconds of information and may not typify the ventricular arrhythmias that occur during the rest of the day. In one report of three boxers, ventricular ectopy constituted more than 20% of the depolarizations during the morning hours and only 2% at night.[49] This can be reversed, however, such that most of the premature depolarizations occur while the dog is sleeping.[92] The office ECG may show single, unifocal ventricular premature depolarizations on one end of the extreme or can show sustained, fast ventricular tachycardia at the other end (see Figure 20-5). We have observed dogs that had severe ventricular arrhythmias in an examination room have less than 100 single premature beats during a 24-hour recording. We have also seen dogs with a single premature ventricular complex during an ECG recording that had thousands of premature ventricular complexes on a 24-hour recording.

The ventricular premature complexes in boxers are often upright in leads II, III, and aV_F and so most likely originate from the right ventricle. Cats often only have sinus tachycardia, although atrial fibrillation, premature depolarizations, isorhythmic atrioventricular dissociation, and sinus bradycardia may also occur.

In Doberman pinschers with DCM, ventricular arrhythmias are a consistent finding on 24-hour ECG (Holter) recordings. Doberman pinschers with echocardiographic evidence of the disease almost always have more than 50 premature ventricular depolarizations on a Holter recording. The number of premature depolarizations and the complexity of the premature depolarizations increases as the disease progresses.[84] Doberman pinschers with ventricular tachyarrhythmias are at increased risk of sudden death.

Thoracic radiography. Dogs with severe myocardial failure as a result of DCM consistently have cardiomegaly on thoracic radiographs. Dogs with lesser stages of the disease may or may not have cardiomegaly. Cardiomegaly ranges from mild to severe and depends on the severity of the disease and, to some degree, on the breed involved. Giant-breed dogs and American cocker spaniels usually have severe cardiomegaly present (Figures 20-7 and 20-8). Doberman pinschers may only have apparent mild-to-moderate cardiomegaly, although on echocardiography their cardiac enlargement is often severe. The severe cardiomegaly may not be readily detected on thoracic radiographs in this breed, presumably because of their chest configuration and possibly because they do not have as much right heart enlargement as giant breeds (Figure 20-9).[93] The same may be true for boxers.

Evidence of heart failure is commonly present on thoracic radiographs. Dogs in left heart failure have pulmonary edema that can range from mild to severe. Enlarged pulmonary veins (pulmonary congestion) may also be evident. Dogs with both left and right heart failure may have pleural effusion.

Cats with DCM commonly have evidence of pleural effusion that obscures their cardiac silhouette. In cats without pleural effusion, cardiomegaly is present. Figure 20-10 shows thoracic radiographs from a cat with DCM after pleurocentesis and diuretic therapy and the same cat after supplementation with taurine.

Echocardiography. The echocardiographic changes with DCM are the same in dogs and cats. The primary abnormality is an increase

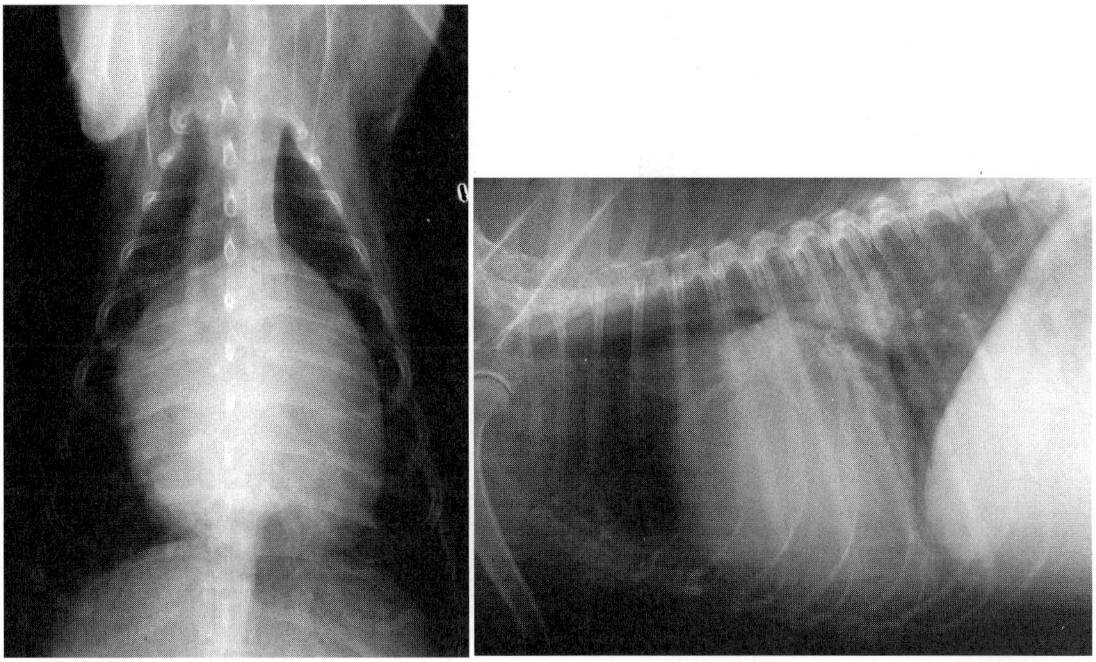

FIGURE 20-7 Dorsoventral (**A**) and lateral (**B**) thoracic radiographs from an American cocker spaniel with dilated cardiomyopathy. Marked generalized cardiomegaly is present. The lateral radiograph is taken during expiration. Consequently, it is impossible to determine if the interstitial infiltrate in the caudodorsal lung fields is due to pulmonary edema or not. The dog did not have an increased respiratory rate while at rest at home the evening before these radiographs were taken. Therefore it is unlikely that pulmonary edema is present.

in the left ventricular end-systolic diameter (Figure 20-11). This increase can range from mild to severe depending on the severity of the disease. A compensatory increase in the left ventricular end-diastolic diameter also is usually present when the disease is moderate to severe (see Figure 20-11). It often is not present in a patient with mild myocardial failure (mild increase in the end-systolic diameter) and may, on occasion, not be present in a patient with severe myocardial failure. The increase in the end-systolic diameter decreases the shortening fraction. The compensatory increase in the end-diastolic diameter increases the shortening fraction. Consequently, even in DCM shortening fraction is not a very accurate estimate of myocardial function. However, in most patients with DCM the shortening fraction is decreased, although in patients with mild disease the decrease may be subtle. For classification purposes, using shortening fraction is easier than using end-systolic diameter as a measure of left ventricular function because it does not change between different-size dogs. Consequently, a shortening fraction between 20% and 25% is considered evidence of mild disease, between 15% and 20% is moderate disease, and less than 15% is considered severe disease.

Controversy exists as to the lower limit of normal for shortening fraction, especially in large-breed dogs. Studies have been performed to determine normal values for shortening fraction and other echocardiographic variables in specific large breeds.[5,52] Because DCM is prevalent in these populations, these studies probably have not established values for normal. Instead they have established values for a mixture of normal dogs and dogs with DCM. Consequently, shortening fractions as low as 13% have been reported as normal. This is almost assuredly incorrect. It is known that sarcomeres normally contract about 30% (end-diastolic length of 2.2 μm to an end- systolic length of 1.5 μm). With normal coupling of sarcomeres together, this should translate into a 30% change in circumference of the left ventricle from end-diastole to end-systole and so also a 30% change in chamber diameter. The aforementioned studies have based assessment of normal on the fact that the investigators saw no progression of disease within a 2- to 3-year period. Unfortunately, this measure of normalcy is probably incorrect, that is, dogs with DCM can most likely stabilize for long periods. We have observed cats with taurine deficiency stabilize for several years, which sets a precedence for this type of behavior. Studies that have correlated other characteristics of DCM in certain breeds, such as ventricular arrhythmias, with shortening fraction are probably more accurate in predicting which dogs are normal and which have DCM.[47,84] In these studies, dogs with shortening fractions less than 25% have been identified as being abnormal.

Dogs with heart failure secondary to DCM always have severe disease and so have a shortening fraction less than 15% (see Figure 20-1).[47] If a patient that is in heart failure is shown to have a shortening fraction greater than 15%, the diagnosis of DCM should be reconsidered. It may be possible that DCM can be present along with another disease, such as primary mitral regurgitation, such that the patient does have DCM and is in heart failure and has a shortening fraction greater than 15%. However, in our experience this is very unusual. Secondary myocardial failure (i.e., an increase in end-systolic diameter) is common in large dogs with primary mitral regurgitation. These dogs usually have a shortening fraction in the 20% to 40% range when they present for heart failure. The increase in the end-systolic diameter in these cases is secondary to myocardial failure caused by the mitral regurgitation and so is not DCM (primary idiopathic myocardial failure).

The left ventricular wall (free wall and interventricular septum) thickness is normal or thinner than normal. Wall thinning usually does not occur until the end-stages of the disease. It probably represents slippage of myofilaments that occurs secondary to a

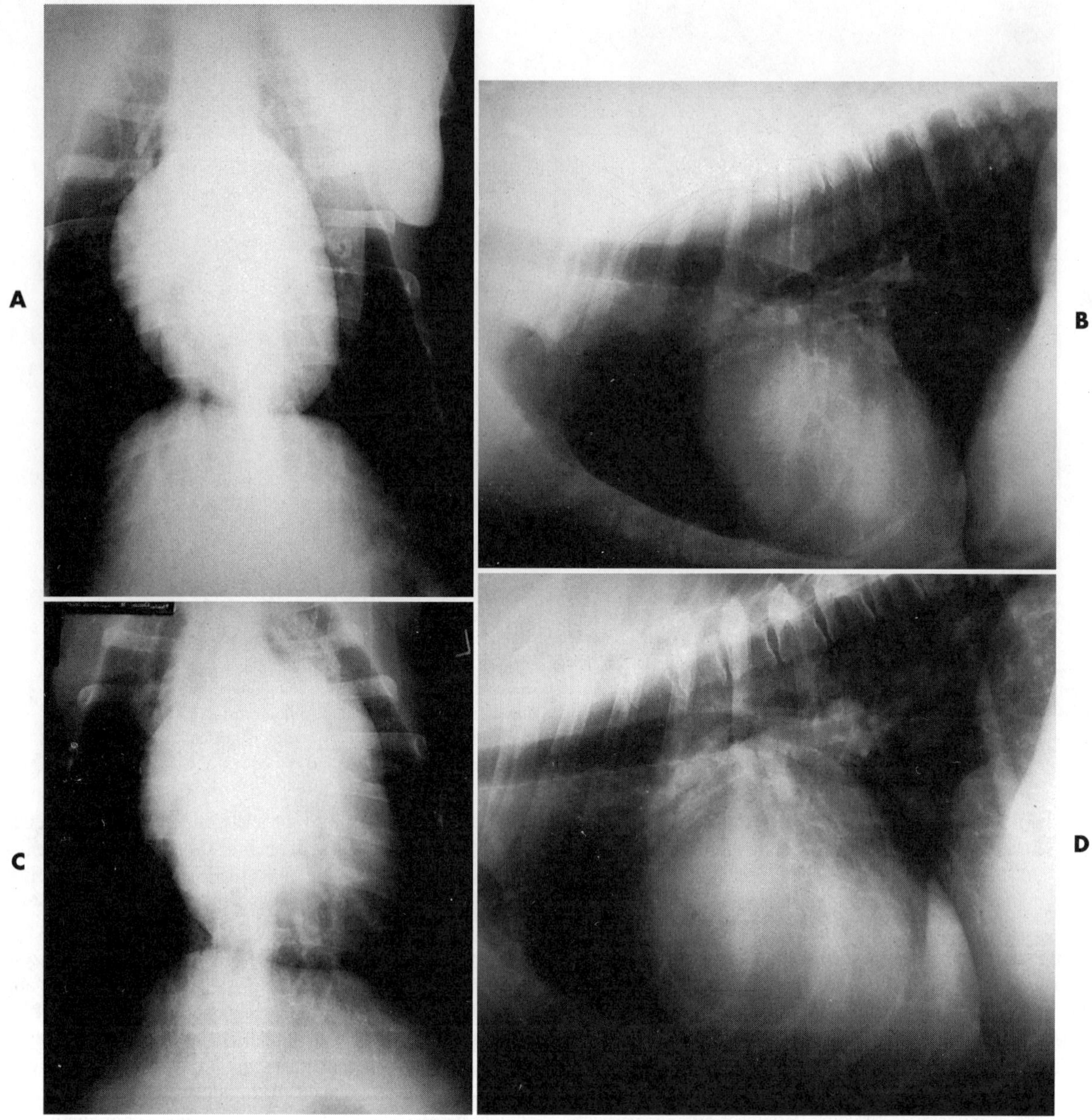

FIGURE 20-8 Dorsoventral (**A** and **C**) and lateral (**B** and **D**) thoracic radiographs from a great Dane taken before (**A** and **B**) and after (**C** and **D**) the dog developed dilated cardiomyopathy (DCM). There is generalized cardiomegaly following the development of DCM.

prolonged and marked increase in diastolic intraventricular pressure. Systolic wall thickening (thickening fraction) is decreased. Myocardial function is often reduced similarly throughout the left ventricle (i.e., myocardial contractility is decreased similarly in the free wall and septum). However, there can be regional heterogeneity of myocardial function. Most commonly the free wall moves and thickens less than the interventricular septum, although sometimes the septum may be more affected. Occasionally, more discrete regions of heterogeneity exist within the free wall and septum. In the latter type of case, obtaining an accurate estimate of left ventricular function is more difficult because the shortening fraction differs depending on the site of measurement.

The left ventricular and left atrial chambers are increased in size on a two-dimensional echocardiogram in severe DCM (Figure 20-12). Usually the increase in atrial size is comparable to the increase in left ventricular size. This is compared with the patient with primary mitral regurgitation, in which the increase in left atrial size is commonly greater than the increase in left ventricular size. The right heart may also be enlarged.

Mitral valve diastolic excursion during rapid ventricular filling is decreased in patients with moderate-to-severe DCM. This results in an increase in the separation between the mitral valve E-point and the interventricular septum (EPSS) (Figure 20-13). The decreased early diastolic excursion of the mitral valve is due to decreased blood flow and flow velocity through the mitral valve orifice. Increased chamber size may also contribute to the increase in EPSS. In severe DCM, forward stroke volume is commonly decreased. Hemodynamically, whatever is pumped into the aorta in systole is replaced through the mitral valve in diastole. If systolic forward flow is decreased, diastolic mitral flow must also be decreased. Hence, the decrease in

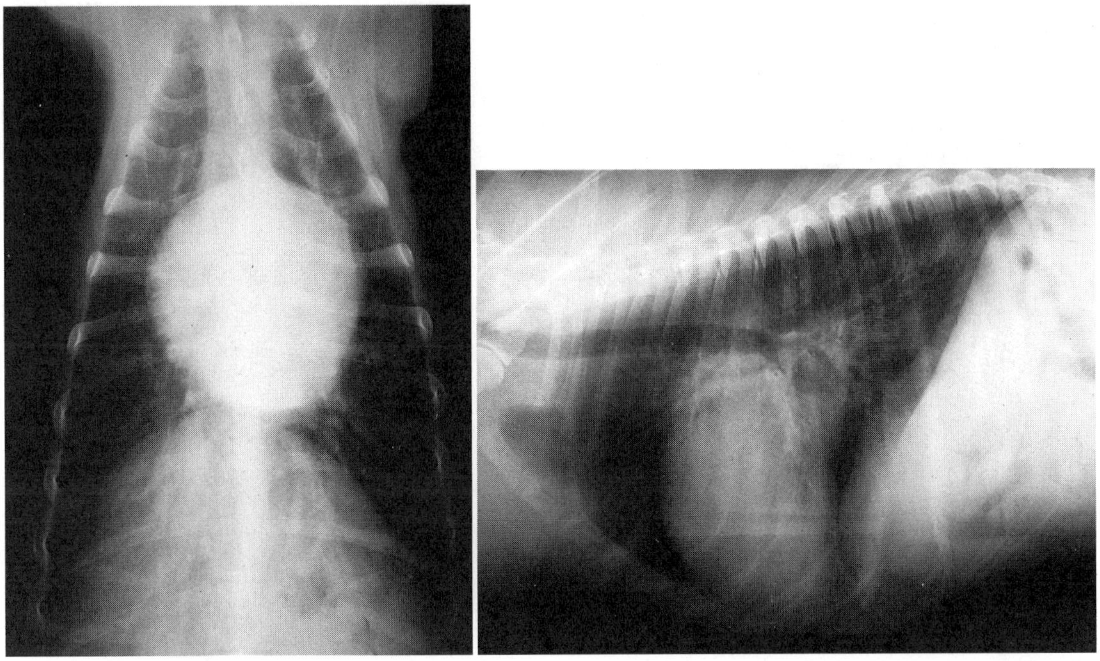

FIGURE 20-9 Dorsoventral **(A)** and lateral **(B)** thoracic radiographs from a Doberman pinscher with dilated cardiomyopathy (DCM). The cardiac silhouette does not appear markedly enlarged. However, on an echocardiogram all four chambers were severely enlarged. The left atrium is enlarged on the lateral view.

mitral valve diastolic excursion. In moderate DCM, forward stroke volume may be normal. Flow velocity, however, is commonly decreased, and mitral inflow velocity during early diastole may also be decreased, resulting in a lesser mitral valve excursion.

Aortic motion may be reduced on an M-mode echocardiogram. Effects of arrhythmias on hemodynamics may also be noted (Figure 20-14).

Hemodynamic studies. A Swan-Ganz thermodilution catheter can be placed to measure hemodynamic abnormalities in dogs with DCM. In dogs that are in left heart failure, the mean pulmonary capillary wedge pressure, which is a measure of left atrial pressure, is increased, usually to a value greater than 20 mm Hg (normal is less than 12 mm Hg) in dogs with mild-to-moderate pulmonary edema and to a value greater than 30 mm Hg in dogs with severe pulmonary edema. Cardiac output is routinely decreased in dogs with severe disease. In dogs that are also in right heart failure, the mean right atrial pressure is increased to a value greater than 5 mm Hg and to greater than 10 mm Hg in dogs that have ascites. Systemic arterial blood pressure is normal to moderately decreased.

Plasma concentrations of amino acids. Plasma taurine concentration should be measured in any cat or American cocker spaniel diagnosed to have DCM. This may also be true for golden retrievers. The blood should be drawn into a heparinized syringe or placed in a heparinized tube and placed on ice. Red cells and platelets concentrate taurine. Consequently, hemolysis and clot formation will markedly increase the concentration of taurine in plasma and must be avoided. Red cells will slowly leak taurine into plasma if the plasma is not separated from the red cells soon after collection. Consequently, the blood sample should be centrifuged within 1 hour of collection and the plasma harvested and placed in a separate tube. The plasma sample should be frozen until it is assayed. Some heparinized blood may also be saved to measure whole blood taurine concentration. A plasma taurine concentration less than 50 nmole/mL in dogs or cats is considered low. Most cats with DCM resulting from taurine deficiency have a plasma concentration less than 20 nmole/mL. Dilated cardiomyopathy is rare in cats since the discovery that taurine deficiency causes DCM. In addition, of the cats identified with DCM, very few are taurine-deficient. However, because taurine-induced feline DCM is reversible with supplementation, it must be ruled out in each case.

Plasma L-carnitine concentration may be measured in selected cases. Occasionally a giant-breed dog has been identified as carnitine-deficient. Most, however, are not. To our knowledge no Doberman pinscher with DCM has been diagnosed as systemically deficient and responsive to L-carnitine supplementation. Boxers may or may not have a low plasma L-carnitine concentration, and it appears that response to supplementation may be the only method of identifying affected dogs. Consequently, measuring plasma L-carnitine concentration is up to the discretion of the veterinarian and owners of this breed.

There currently is no evidence that dogs with DCM are deficient in coenzyme Q_{10} nor that they are responsive to its supplementation.

Laboratory abnormalities. Prerenal azotemia is common in dogs and cats with severe DCM. This may be due to a low cardiac output because of severe disease or to dehydration added to a low cardiac output as a result of severe disease. Subclinical dehydration is common with diuretic administration and commonly contributes to the azotemia. Mild-to-moderate prerenal azotemia should be noted because it is usually a sign of a marked reduction in cardiac output. The dose of the diuretic should be reduced if it can be. However, if severe heart failure is present and any reduction in diuretic results in recrudescence or exacerbation of clinical signs, the dose of the diuretic should be maintained and the azotemia ignored, as long as the patient continues to eat and drink normally. Mild-to-moderate prerenal azotemia does not cause death and often produces no clinical signs. Heart failure does.

Patients that present in heart failure may have electrolyte abnormalities, with hyponatremia and hypokalemia more commonly

A

B

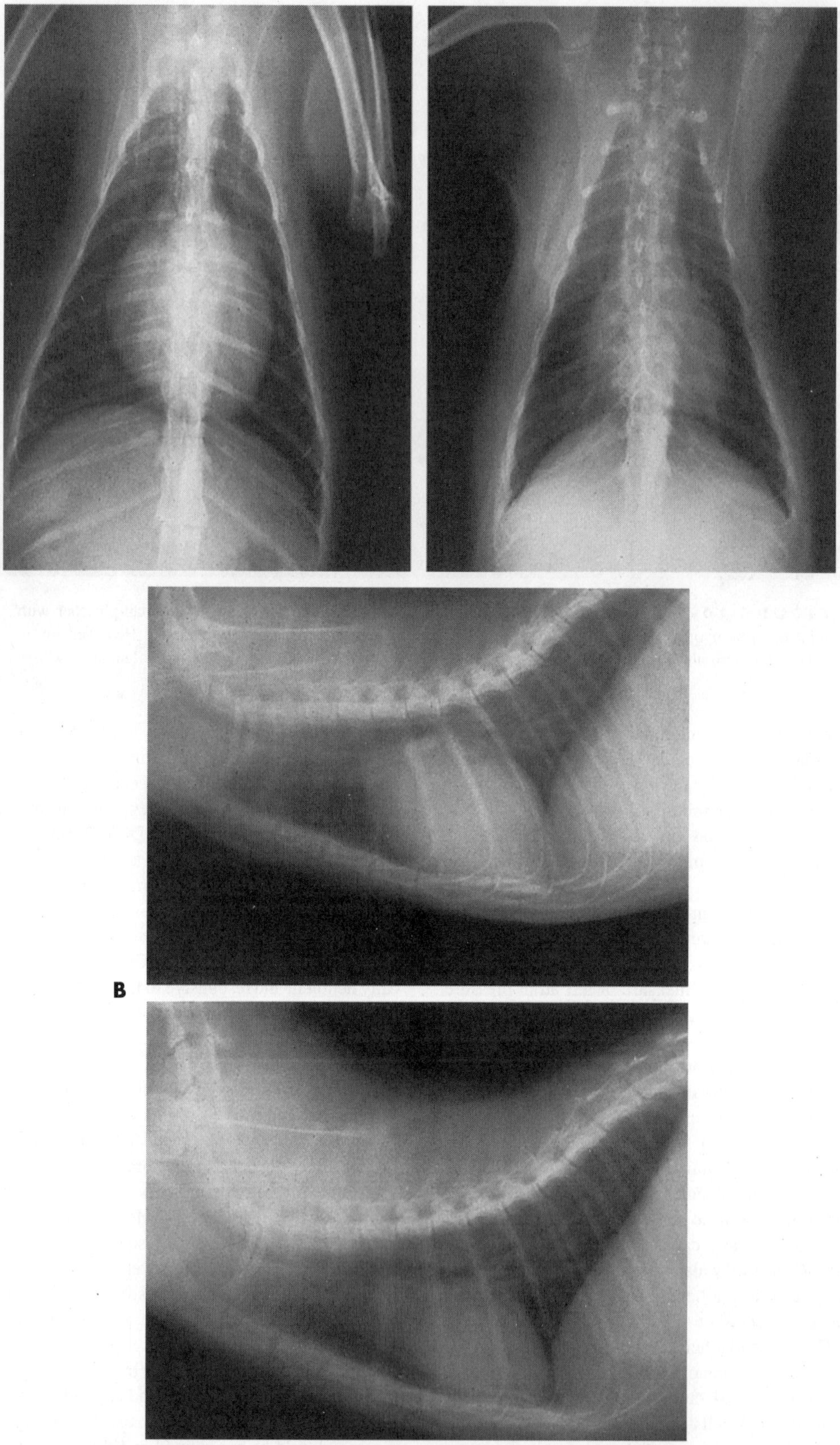

FIGURE 20-10 Dorsoventral **(A)** and lateral **(B)** thoracic radiographs from a 4-year-old cat with dilated cardiomyopathy before (*left* and *top*) and 6 months after (*right* and *bottom*) beginning taurine supplementation. Note the marked reduction in cardiac size after supplementation.

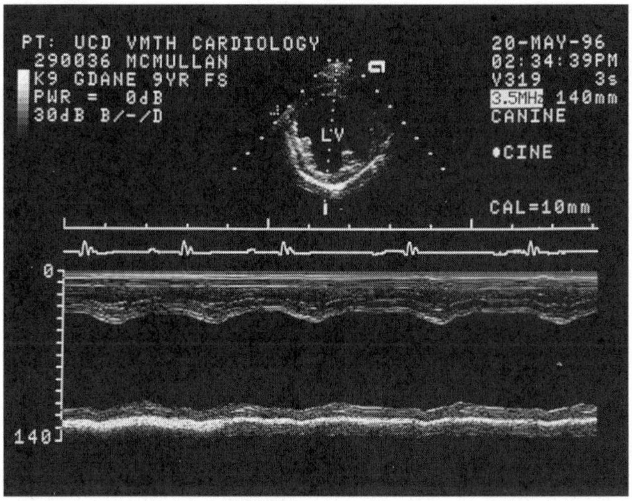

FIGURE 20-11 M-mode echocardiogram from a 9-year-old great Dane with dilated cardiomyopathy. This dog presented with a gastric dilation/volvulus. Following surgery a Swan-Ganz catheter was placed to measure pulmonary capillary wedge pressure (PCWP) and cardiac output. Following a whole blood transfusion, the PCWP increased from 11 to 30 mm Hg (normal is less than 12 mm Hg). One dose of furosemide decreased the PCWP back to normal. This prompted the ultrasound examination of the heart. The echocardiogram shows marked increases in the end-systolic diameter (73 mm) and the end-diastolic diameter (83 mm), with a reduced shortening fraction (12%). Although the left ventricular free wall appears to contract, its motion occurs very late and after the interventricular septum contracts. This motion is most likely due to the entire heart moving toward the transducer in early diastole rather than to myocardial contraction. The left ventricular wall thicknesses are normal at approximately 10 mm.

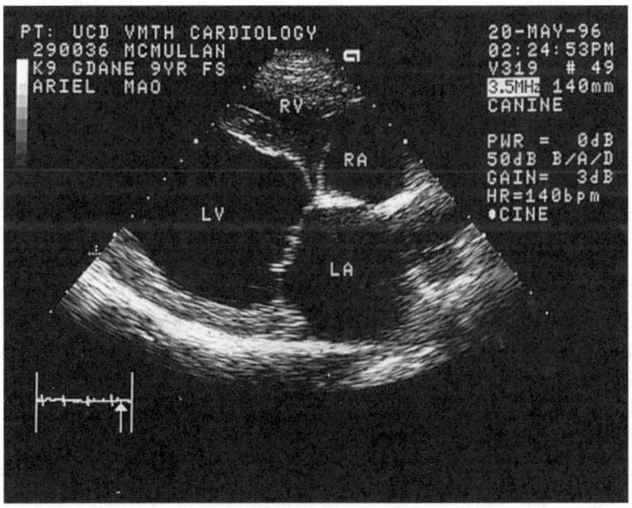

FIGURE 20-12 Two-dimensional echocardiogram from the dog shown in Figure 20-10 shows similarly enlarged left ventricular *(LV)* and left atrial *(LA)* chambers. The right atrium *(RA)* and right ventricle *(RV)* may also be mildly enlarged.

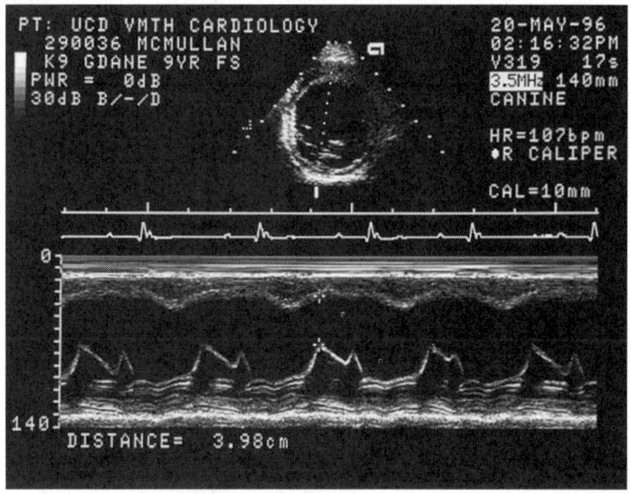

FIGURE 20-13 M-mode echocardiogram from the dog shown in Figure 20-10, taken at the mitral valve level. It demonstrates a marked increase in the *E*-point–to–septal separation (EPSS) to 40 mm (normal is less than 6 mm).

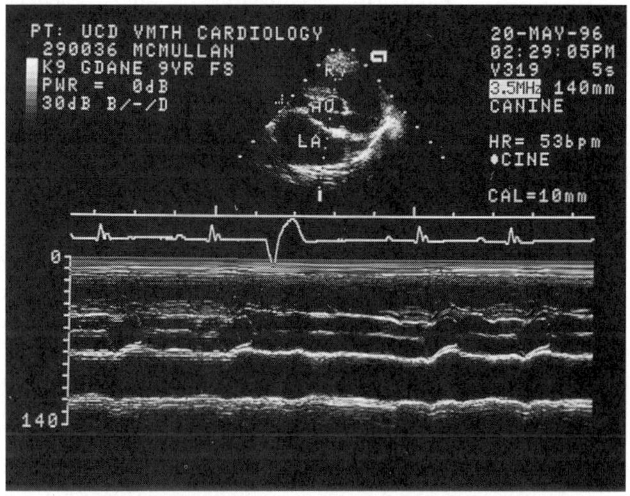

FIGURE 20-14 M-mode echocardiogram from the dog shown in Figure 20-10, taken at the heart base, across the aorta and left atrium. Although the left atrium is moderately enlarged, it appears to be normal-to-mildly enlarged on the M-mode echocardiogram because the ultrasound beam transects a portion of the left auricle rather than the body of the left atrium in this view. For this reason, subjective evaluation of left atrial size is preferred. The aortic valve cusps appear as boxes during ejection and as a line in the center of the aorta when not open. A pulse deficit associated with a ventricular premature depolarization is demonstrated. Following the premature depolarization on the electrocardiogram, the aortic valve fails to open.

seen. Hyponatremia in a patient not receiving diuretic therapy is most often dilutional (i.e., the sodium concentration is low because of excess water retention, not decreased total body sodium content). This is most commonly because of excessive ADH secretion resulting in excessive renal water retention.[94] Hyponatremia in a patient not receiving diuretic therapy is almost always seen in patients with severe heart failure. It is a poor prognostic sign in humans and may also be in dogs and cats.[95] Hypokalemia is uncommon in dogs that are eating normally.

The blood lactate concentration may be increased in dogs with a severe decrease in cardiac output. The venous oxygen tension may also be decreased in these patients.

TREATMENT

Treatment of DCM is aimed at reducing the clinical signs that result in heart failure, improving survival time, and delaying or abolishing sudden death. Success at achieving any of these goals is generally poor in most dogs with DCM. Taurine supplementation (250 mg q12h) cures DCM in cats. Taurine and L-carnitine supplementation improves ventricular function in most American cocker spaniels to the point that they can be removed from drug therapy and are clinically normal.

Acute medical therapy

Dogs. Dogs with DCM that initially present to a veterinarian commonly present with moderate-to-fulminant pulmonary edema. Clinical evidence of poor perfusion may also be present but usually does not predominate at this stage. Consequently, treatment is aimed at reducing pulmonary edema formation and improving oxygenation. These dogs are tachypneic, hyperpneic, and dyspneic on presentation. They are hypoxemic and must be handled gently to avoid acute exacerbation of clinical signs and to prevent provoking an acute agonal crisis. Thoracic radiographs may be obtained if they can be obtained with a minimum of stress. Only one view may be necessary to document the presence and the severity of the pulmonary edema. A lateral view is usually the most helpful. The dog should receive supplemental oxygen as soon as possible. Placing an oxygen source close to the dog's nose is of little benefit. Administering oxygen via a face mask can be beneficial if the face mask fits snugly and the dog does not resist its placement. If the dog struggles with a face mask, the stress may be more detrimental than the oxygen is beneficial. Nasal insufflation of oxygen or placing the dog in an oxygen cage is preferred for any type of long-term oxygen administration.

Drug therapy known to be effective at reducing edema formation in this type of situation is limited to furosemide or nitroprusside administration. Dobutamine and dopamine may be effective supplemental agents. Dogs with severe-to-fulminant pulmonary edema as a result of DCM are emergency cases that will die within a short period without aggressive medical management. Before starting aggressive therapy, clients must be made aware of the poor long-term prognosis so that they can decide whether to continue. Once the decision to proceed is made, a baseline respiratory rate should be obtained and a decision made regarding the type of drug therapy to use. Nitroprusside can be a very effective agent in this situation. However, it is not an easy drug to use. The dosage must be titrated, starting at a low dose and titrating up. Titration should be performed by measuring systemic arterial blood pressure at baseline, administering a low dose, and titrating the dose until the mean blood pressure decreases by at least 15 mm Hg. If the drug is administered without blood pressure monitoring, the most common mistake is to not achieve an adequate infusion rate. If an adequate infusion rate is not attained, no benefit is obtained and the patient will die. Consequently, we do not recommend using nitroprusside unless a veterinarian has a means of monitoring blood pressure. If nitroprusside is used successfully, weaning the patient off it and onto another drug may be difficult.

Dobutamine has been used successfully in combination with nitroprusside in dogs with severe pulmonary edema secondary to DCM. We have done echocardiograms on several dogs with DCM before and after dobutamine administration. Usually the contractile response has been surprisingly poor. Consequently, we believe that the nitroprusside is the more effective agent in this combination. Dobutamine administration has been shown to have long-lasting beneficial effects in humans.[96] This benefit is marginal at best, with an average increase in shortening fraction of 2 percentage points.

High-dose furosemide administration is also very effective in this situation and is the method we prefer. We initially administer 6 to 8 mg/kg IV every 1 to 2 hours. Generally this dosing is continued until the respiratory rate decreases significantly. Most patients with severe pulmonary edema present with a respiratory rate greater than 70 breaths/min at baseline. In this situation it is recommended that high-dose furosemide be administered until the respiratory rate decreases by at least 20 breaths/min (the respiratory rate is usually 50 to 60 breaths/min). When this occurs, the furosemide dose should be curtailed, usually to approximately 4 mg/kg every 4 to 6 hours. When the respiratory rate decreases to less than 50 breaths/min, a high-end maintenance dose of 4 mg/kg every 8 hours can be used. Dobutamine may be used in conjunction with this regimen, although we have successfully treated many dogs with fulminant pulmonary edema without it.

Complications routinely occur with high-dose furosemide therapy. However, our success rate approaches 80% with this method, and the complications are usually not clinically significant. Complications include dehydration, hyponatremia, hypochloremia, and hypokalemia. If this protocol is used and the dose curtailed appropriately when the respiratory rate starts to decrease, the dehydration produced is usually mild. Mild dehydration does not require therapy in this situation and is corrected when the dog feels good enough to start eating and drinking again. Severe dehydration can result in a further and significant decrease in cardiac output. Intravenous fluid therapy can be used if more severe dehydration occurs, but fluid administration should be cautious and not aimed at producing full rehydration. The hyponatremia produced is usually moderate (130 to 140 mEq/L), produces no clinical sequelae, and should not be treated. It usually normalizes once the dog starts to eat again. Serum potassium concentration most commonly is in the 3.0- to 3.5-mEq/L range after high-dose furosemide administration. This is not clinically significant in the short term and does not require treatment. It usually normalizes once the patient is eating again. More severe hypokalemia may require supplementation.

Other drugs can be administered to the patient that presents with acute fulminant pulmonary edema but should not be relied on to produce significant clinical benefit. Digoxin and an ACE inhibitor can be started soon after admission. However, both take days to a week to produce any significant benefit, and the benefits of these drugs usually are much fewer than those of furosemide or nitroprusside. Topical nitroglycerin cream can be administered but should only be used as an adjunctive agent. Its benefits are too mild and too variable to be relied on without administering other agents.

In dogs with severe tachyarrhythmias, antiarrhythmic therapy is also required. For ventricular tachyarrhythmias, lidocaine is usually the drug of choice. Lidocaine is effective at suppressing ventricular tachyarrhythmias and is also probably effective at preventing sudden death resulting from ventricular fibrillation. An initial loading dose of 2 to 4 mg/kg should be administered over 2 to 5 minutes followed by a constant-rate infusion of 30 to 100 μg/kg/min. Other class I agents and sotalol may also be effective. Atrial fibrillation is often the primary rhythm in dogs with DCM. Commonly the heart rate is greater than 200 beats/min. Although it is important to reduce the heart rate over time in these dogs, it is not imperative to reduce the heart rate immediately. In dogs with ventricular rates greater than 260 beats/min, subacute heart rate reduction is more important. This may be accomplished by administering digoxin at twice the maintenance dose orally for 1 day or by administering low doses of either a β-blocker or diltiazem orally.

Cats. Cats with DCM also commonly present with acute respiratory distress. Their distress may be due to pulmonary edema, pleural effusion, or both. Thoracocentesis should be performed as soon as possible to determine if pleural effusion is present and to remove as much fluid as possible. Severe pulmonary edema in cats should be treated as it is in dogs, except the furosemide dose should be cut in half (3 to 4 mg/kg IV or IM). Dehydration in cats can produce anorexia. Consequently, judicious fluid replacement may be necessary.

Chronic medical therapy. Treatment of chronic heart failure is generally attempted using a combination of a diuretic, an ACE inhibitor, and a digitalis glycoside. The primary clinical signs in dogs with DCM are usually referable to pulmonary edema. Consequently, drug therapy aimed at reducing pulmonary edema usually results in the most clinical benefit. All three drug types mentioned have the potential of reducing edema formation. They differ markedly in their ability to achieve this endpoint, however. Diuretics reduce blood volume, ventricular diastolic volumes, and therefore ventricular diastolic pressures. Diuretics are by far the most efficacious of the three drug classes, with furosemide being very efficacious and the most commonly used diuretic.

ACE inhibitors produce venodilation and reduce renal sodium and water retention by decreasing aldosterone secretion. In so doing, they reduce ventricular diastolic volumes, and therefore ventricular diastolic pressures. They are also efficacious drugs in this disease and should be used routinely to treat DCM. Their efficacy is less than that of furosemide, however. The fact that moderate-to-severe pulmonary edema can usually be controlled with just furosemide and almost never controlled with just an ACE inhibitor is a primary reason for this judgement. ACE inhibitors also produce arteriolar dilation, which helps increase cardiac output.

Digoxin increases myocardial contractility, increases cardiac output and renal blood flow, and so reduces renal sodium and water retention in some dogs and cats. Digoxin is efficacious at reducing pulmonary edema in some dogs and not in others. We estimate that 20% to 30% of dogs with DCM have a clinically significant response to digoxin. Digoxin also increases vagal tone, which helps decrease heart rate. It may also have a diuretic effect.

In some dogs, clinical signs of low-output heart failure predominate. These dogs may be weak and usually have cold extremities and ears. Often these dogs are clinically dehydrated. The dehydration, coupled with the decreased myocardial contractility, is often the primary cause of the severe decrease in cardiac output in these patients. The dehydration is most commonly due to anorexia, with or without concomitant diuretic administration. If dehydration is severe, cautious intravenous fluid administration is warranted. Complete rehydration will commonly result in edema formation. Diuretic administration must be discontinued in this type of case. Prerenal azotemia is commonly present in these dogs. Consequently, drugs that are cleared by the kidneys, such as digoxin, should also be discontinued or the dose reduced drastically. Inotropic support with a sympathomimetic such as dobutamine may be beneficial.

Supplemental therapy. Cats with DCM should be administered 250 mg taurine PO q12h until the results of the plasma analysis for taurine can be assessed or until a response to therapy can be assessed if plasma concentration is not measured. Echocardiographic response to therapy generally takes 2 to 4 months, although clinical signs often start to improve within 3 weeks. If a cat is not taurine-deficient or does not respond to supplementation, further taurine administration is not warranted.

Taurine (500 mg q12h) should also be administered to American cocker spaniels with DCM because these dogs are usually taurine-deficient. Taurine in combination with L-carnitine supplementation (1 g q12h) usually results in a clinically significant improvement in myocardial function within 3 to 4 months of starting supplementation (Figure 20-15). Plasma L-carnitine concentration is not decreased in these dogs, and some or most may respond to taurine supplementation alone. However, we have documented no response to taurine alone in some American cocker spaniels and have documented a uniform response to taurine and L-carnitine (1 g q12h) supplementation. Consequently, we recommend that both amino acids be administered to these dogs unless a specific contraindication to the L-carnitine supplementation exists. L-carnitine may be expensive. Consequently, the most common contraindication to its administration is an inability of the client to afford supplementation. Most American cocker spaniels that present with severe DCM and heart failure have a shortening fraction in the 10% to 15% range, a left ventricular end-diastolic diameter in the 45- to 50-mm range (normal is approximately 30 mm), and a left ventricular end-systolic diameter in the 40- to 45-mm range. After 4 to 6 months of supplementation the end-diastolic diameter commonly decreases into the 40- to 45-mm range, end-systolic diameter decreases into the 30- to 35-mm range, and the shortening fraction increases into the 20% to 25% range. The EPSS usually decreases about 5 mm. Once echocardiographic improvement has been documented, the dog should be weaned off cardiovascular drugs. Digoxin can be withdrawn first. The owners should count the dog's respiratory rate at rest to document that pulmonary edema is not recurring during the time that therapy is being withdrawn. If no untoward effects are observed over 4 to 7 days, the ACE inhibitor therapy can be stopped. If this is tolerated, the furosemide dose can be halved for 3 days, then halved again, and then stopped. All of the American cocker spaniels that we have treated have been weaned off drug therapy. Only one has had a subsequent worsening of cardiomyopathy. All of the others have remained clinically normal until they developed other diseases.

Some golden retrievers, some mixed-breed dogs, some breeds in which DCM is unusual, and some dogs on vegetarian diets may also be taurine-deficient. Plasma taurine concentration should be measured in all these dogs, and taurine supplementation should be attempted to reverse the myocardial failure partially. We have successfully treated or witnessed successful treatment with taurine of two golden retrievers, a Welsh corgi, a Tibetan terrier, and a Dalmatian.

Taurine and carnitine can be purchased at health food stores. However, it is less expensive to purchase these products wholesale (Ajinomoto U.S.A., Inc., 19675 Mariner Ave., Torrance, CA 90503). By this route, carnitine costs approximately $0.25/g and taurine costs about $0.025/g.

Antiarrhythmic therapy. Atrial fibrillation is a common arrhythmia that requires therapy in dogs with DCM. The goal of therapy is to decrease the ventricular rate, usually into the 140- to 160-beats/min range. Faster ventricular rates are known to produce myocardial failure in the dog.[78] The goal of therapy is not to convert the rhythm to a sinus rhythm, because this goal is almost never attainable. Instead, the ventricular rate is reduced in atrial fibrillation by administering pharmacologic agents that prolong the refractory period and the conduction time of the AV node. At presentation, dogs commonly have ventricular rates in the 200- to 240-beats/min range. The atrial rate in atrial fibrillation is probably greater than 500 beats/min in dogs. Consequently, only every 2 to 3 atrial depolarizations traverse the AV node. Drugs that prolong the AV nodal refractory period and AV nodal conduction time decrease the number of atrial depolarizations that reach the ventricles and so slow the ventricular rate. The AV node in a dog with atrial fibrillation and no underlying cardiac disease usually keeps the ventricular rate in the 90- to 120-beats/min range. The reason the ventricular rate is faster in patients that are in heart failure is that sympathetic tone and circulating catecholamine concentrations are increased and parasympathetic tone is decreased in heart failure. Parasympathetic tone to the AV node can be chronically increased by administering digoxin.

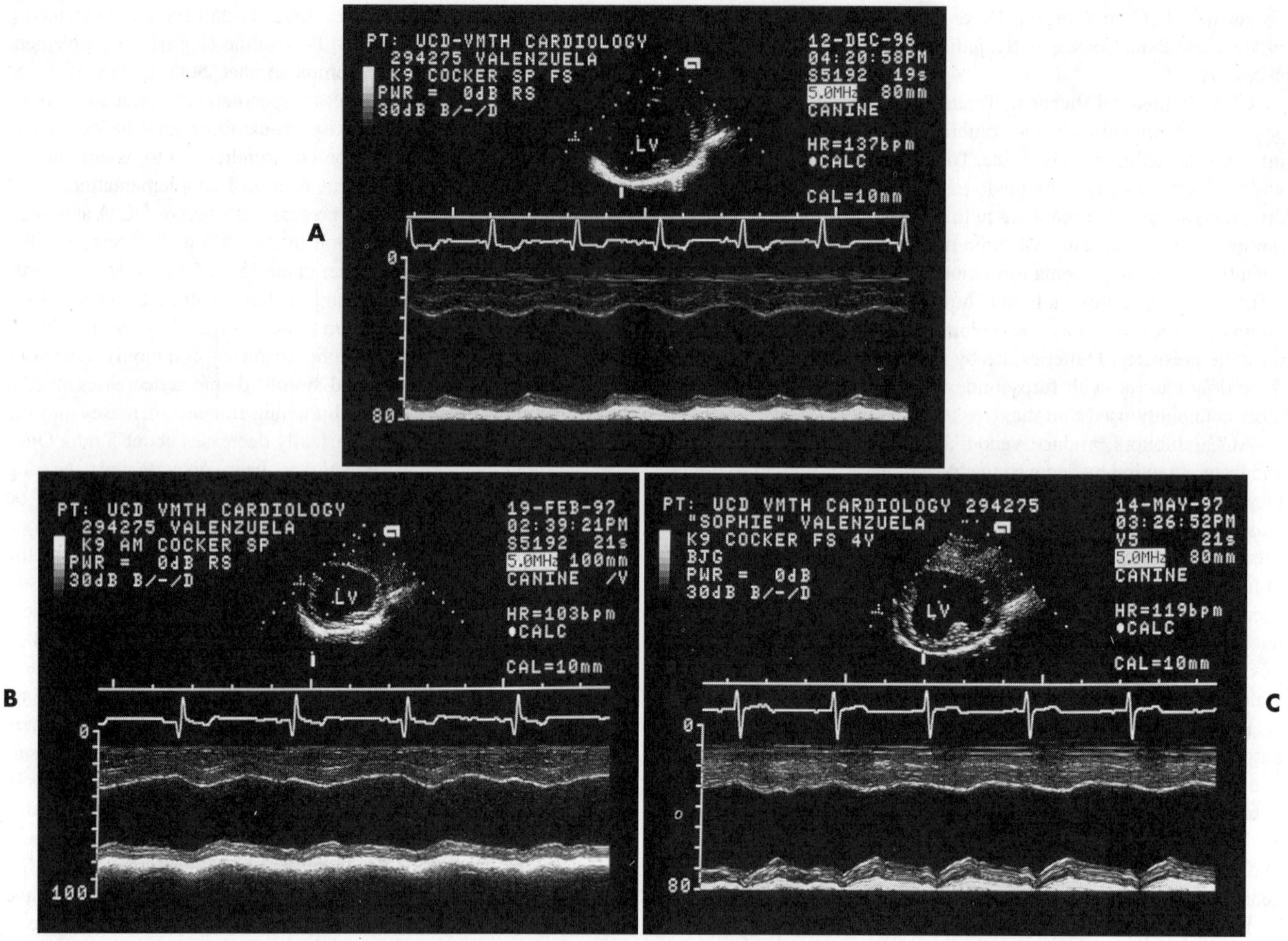

FIGURE 20-15 M-mode echocardiograms from a 4-year-old American cocker spaniel with dilated cardiomyopathy, taken before **(A)** starting taurine supplementation and 2 months **(B)** and 5 months **(C)** after starting supplementation. Myocardial function improved following supplementation. The shortening fraction increased from the 10% to 15%. range to the 20% to 25% range. The end-diastolic and end-systolic diameters decreased, and the left ventricular walls increased in thickness (ventricular remodeling).

Digoxin is moderately effective at reducing the ventricular rate in patients with atrial fibrillation for this reason. The other drugs used to treat atrial fibrillation have potential negative inotropic effects. Because digoxin has no negative inotropic effects, it is commonly the first drug administered to a patient with DCM. It is administered at a dose of 0.25 mg/m^2 of body surface area. Frequently the ventricular rate does not decrease or only decreases mildly. Consequently, other drugs are often required to help reduce the ventricular rate. The logical way to counteract the effects of catecholamines on the AV node is to administer a β-adrenergic blocking drug, such as propranolol or atenolol. Catecholamines also help maintain whatever myocardial contractility remains in patients with DCM. Consequently, a potential complication of administering a β-adrenergic blocking drug to a patient with DCM is a decrease in contractility, resulting in a further reduction in cardiac output and more edema formation. Fortunately, low doses of β-adrenergic blockers often decrease heart rate without significantly affecting contractility. Because of this fact, the dose of propranolol that is initially administered to a dog with atrial fibrillation is in the 0.1- to 0.2-mg/kg range. This dose is then gradually increased to 0.3 to 0.5 mg/kg if the initial response is suboptimal. Alternatively, a calcium channel blocker can be administered. The AV node depolarizes via slow calcium channels. Consequently, calcium channel–blocking drugs slow conduction and prolong the refractory period of the AV node. Diltiazem is commonly administered to dogs with atrial fibrillation to slow their ventricular rate. The dose of diltiazem is titrated, starting at 0.5 mg/kg q8h. If an adequate response is not produced, the dose is gradually increased to an endpoint of 1.5 mg/kg q8h. A β-adrenergic blocking drug and a calcium channel–blocking drug should not be administered together because of the enhanced adverse effects that can be produced on heart rate and myocardial contractility.

Dogs with DCM, especially Doberman pinschers and boxers, can die suddenly. Sudden death definitely occurs secondary to ventricular tachyarrhythmias that terminate in ventricular fibrillation. Sudden death or syncope may also occur as a result of severe bradyarrhythmias.[81] Dogs with DCM that present with severe ventricular arrhythmias (nonsustained ventricular tachycardia with a ventricular rate greater than 200 beats/min; sustained ventricular tachycardia) should be treated with lidocaine. An initial bolus of 2 to 4 mg/kg over 1 to 3 minutes should be administered, followed by a constant-rate infusion of 40 to 100 μg/kg/min. Chronic suppression of ventricular arrhythmias is controversial in dogs with DCM. This subject is also controversial in human medicine. One author has stated in a human cardiology text, "Efficacy of antiarrhythmic therapy for both suppression of chronic PVCs and prevention of VT (ventricular tachycardia) and VF (ventricular fibrillation) in patients with DCM is unclear. Nonetheless, treatment remains customary. The selection of a drug or drug combination for high-risk patients with chronic PVCs is complex."[97] Commonly perceived goals are reduction of the number of ventricular premature depolarizations, decrease of the periods of ventricular tachycardia, and decrease of the rate of the ventricular focus. Because the number of ventricular premature depolarizations does not predict sudden death in Doberman pinschers, simply reducing the number is probably not a worthwhile goal. Because complex ventricular arrhythmias may predict sudden death, abolishing these may be a worthwhile goal. Whether or not this can be achieved is unknown. Whether or not the rapidity at which the ventricular focus fires predicts sudden death is unknown because it has not been studied. The fact that a normal left ventricle can be fibrillated when stimulated at rates greater than 300 beats/min suggests that a ventricular focus firing at this rate or, possibly, less in a diseased heart, has the potential for producing ventricular fibrillation. Class IA antiarrhythmic agents, (e.g., procainamide and quinidine) are commonly prescribed for the purposes of reducing the number of premature depolarizations, abolishing complex ventricular arrhythmias, and reducing the rate at which the ventricular focus fires.[50] We believe that these agents commonly reduce the number of premature beats and reduce the rate of firing but that dogs still die suddenly while on these drugs. Other authors have noted that dogs often become refractory to these drugs within 3 to 6 months and that many dogs have died suddenly while on these agents.[50] Class IC antiarrhythmic agents (flecainide, encainide) are not used in veterinary medicine. Class IB agents are lidocaine and its derivatives. We have been disappointed with the results of tocainide at a dosage range of 10 to 15 mg/kg. Calvert[50] notes efficacy at a dose of 15 to 20 mg/kg q8h. However, the incidence of severe side effects, including a high incidence of corneal endothelial dystrophy and renal failure, has been unacceptable.[98] Mexiletine (5 to 10 mg/kg q8h) does not have the toxicity of tocainide and has been reported to have good efficacy.[50] Growing evidence in human medicine suggests that class I agents are ineffective at preventing sudden death in patients with DCM, and that occasionally their proarrhythmic properties may promote sudden death. Consequently, we do not routinely use class I antiarrhythmic agents in patients with DCM. We use them to control sustained ventricular tachycardia or frequent runs of nonsustained ventricular tachycardia, but we do not rely on these agents to prevent sudden death. Unfortunately there are no drugs proved to prevent sudden death in dogs with DCM.

In humans, β-adrenergic blocking drugs and class III antiarrhythmic agents are moderately effective at preventing sudden death. Veterinarians and veterinary cardiologists have more experience with β-adrenergic blocking drugs. However, the dose required to prevent sudden death is not known. It is known that high doses (1 to 2 mg/kg) of propranolol and atenolol produce negative inotropic effects. Consequently, high-dose β-adrenergic blocking therapy is either contraindicated in patients with severe DCM or at least must be used very cautiously in these patients. Lower doses may be effective, but this is unproved. Amiodarone, a class III drug, has gained popularity in human medicine since 1990 and may be an effective agent at preventing sudden death resulting from ventricular tachyarrhythmias. There is very little experience with this drug in veterinary medicine, however. Amiodarone has a very long half-life (greater than 3 days) in the dog.[99] Therefore it takes a long time to reach a therapeutic serum concentration and a long time for the drug to clear from the body after it is discontinued. Consequently, an initial loading dose must be administered. A dose of 10 to 15 mg/kg q12h for 7 days, followed by a dose of 7.5 mg/kg q12h, followed by 7.5 mg/kg q24h has been used in Doberman pinschers with reported success.[50] Beneficial effects may not be seen for 1 to 3 weeks. Numerous toxic effects of amiodarone have been reported in humans, including interstitial pneumonitis and alveolitis, increased liver enzymes, exacerbation of the existing arrhythmia, and symptomatic bradycardia. Amiodarone administration increases the serum digoxin concentration. The digoxin dose should be halved when amiodarone administration begins.

Sotalol is a β-blocking drug and a class III antiarrhythmic drug that may also be promising for preventing sudden death in patients with DCM (see Chapter 29). Preliminary experience in boxers with DCM, ventricular arrhythmias, and syncope has been positive. The dose in boxers is 40 to 80 mg q12h. Because of its β-blocking properties, sotalol must be used cautiously in patients with moderate-to-severe myocardial dysfunction (shortening fraction less than 20%). Weakness because of low cardiac output or exacerbation of edema can occur. If either occurs, the dose should be decreased or the drug discontinued.

Surgical therapy. The treatment of choice for humans with severe DCM is cardiac transplantation. Cardiac transplantation is commonly performed on experimental dogs, and the surgical procedure is not difficult. Rejection of the organ is one primary obstacle to this procedure in dogs. Newer, promising antirejection agents may become available that may surmount this problem. The other major problem is availability of donor organs. Although thousands of donor organs are disposed of daily, the political influence of the animal rights lobby is sure to have an impact on the availability of donor organs.

Dynamic cardiomyoplasty is a surgical technique by which the right latissimus dorsi muscle is isolated on its nervous pedicle, transposed into the thoracic cavity, and wrapped around the ventricles. The muscle is electrically stimulated progressively to induce it to change from a fast-twitch to a slow-twitch type of muscle so that it acts more like cardiac muscle. The technique is experimental in human medicine (400 cases worldwide as of 1994) and barely tried in veterinary medicine.[100,101] In one report, of five dogs treated in this manner, two died shortly after surgery, one died 8 weeks later of progressive heart failure, one dog died suddenly 8 months later, and one dog lived at least 2 years after surgery.[102] In the dog that lived 2 years, shortening fraction initially increased from the 5% to 10% range to the 25% to 30% range and then decreased into the 15% to 20% range. Contraindications to the procedure are said to be advanced systolic dysfunction, refractory ventricular arrhythmia, and severe right heart failure. Unfortunately most dogs have severe systolic dysfunction at the time of diagnosis. The one long-term survivor described above had severe systolic dysfunction, however.

Recently, left ventriculectomy has been described as a possible procedure to reduce left ventricular wall stress and improve left ventricular function in humans.[103,104] In this controversial procedure, a large section of left ventricular myocardium is surgically removed to reduce left ventricular size in patients with DCM. The reduction in size results in reduction in systolic wall stress via the decrease in chamber radius. This reportedly has resulted in a greater decrease in end-systolic volume than in end-diastolic volume and therefore an increase in wall motion (i.e., shortening fraction and ejection fraction). It also has reportedly resulted in clinical improvement in some human patients with heart failure. Hopefully future studies will delineate the types of patients that benefit from this procedure.

Myocarditis

Myocarditis is a rare cause of myocardial failure in dogs and cats. A list of infectious agents that can cause myocarditis is presented in Box 20-1. Of these, only parvovirus and *Trypanosoma cruzi* are agents identified with any degree of frequency in dogs presented for evidence of DCM. The lack of identifiable lesions in most dogs with DCM makes myocarditis an unlikely, but not impossible, cause of most cases of DCM.

CHAGAS' MYOCARDITIS

Chagas' disease is caused by *Trypanosoma cruzi*, a hemoflagellate protozoan parasite. The disease is named after Carlos Chagas, who first described the disease in 1909.[105] Chagas' disease is the leading cause of DCM in humans in Latin America. It is a rare cause in North America. In veterinary medicine, Chagas' disease occurs most commonly in dogs in Texas and Louisiana.[106-108] However, the incidence appears to be very low in dogs. In one report, of 315 canine serum samples submitted to the Texas Veterinary Diagnostic Laboratory over a 6-year span, 25 were positive for Chagas' disease.[109] Dogs infected with *T. cruzi* have also been reported from Oklahoma, South Carolina, and Virginia.[110] There have been no reports of feline trypanosomiasis in North America, although it does occur in South America.[111]

The vectors for *T. cruzi* are insects in the family Reduviidae (e.g., the Mexican kissing beetle). These insects inhabit bedding, where they feed at night. Hosts for the *T. cruzi* include raccoons, armadillos, opossums, dogs, cats, and guinea pigs. In blood, the organism exists as a trypomastigote. The organism enters the insect as the trypomastigote form, presumably when the insect ingests the blood of an infected animal. In the insect it transforms to the epimastigote form and multiplies by binary fission. It then transforms in the hindgut back to the trypomastigote form. This form is excreted in the feces of the reduviid vector and deposited into a fresh bite wound during a feeding. Vectors in the United States do not defecate during feeding and so transmit the infection less efficiently (20%) than do their counterparts in South America (up to 100%). The parasite is spread hematogenously within the host as trypomastigotes. They enter the cytoplasm of macrophages and striated myocytes (including myocardium), where they transform to the amastigote form and multiply, rupturing the cells.[111] Before cell rupture, the parasite transforms back to the trypomastigote form to be carried in the bloodstream. The vector then ingests this form to complete the life cycle.

Raccoons, armadillos, and opossums are the principal reservoir hosts for *T. cruzi* in the southern United States. Infected raccoons have been found in Maryland and Oklahoma. Mice, rats, and squirrels have been found to be infected in New Mexico and California, and antibodies to *T. cruzi* have been identified in dogs in northern California.[112] A small number of dogs from Virginia have also been reported to have either *T. cruzi* infection or antibodies.[110]

The acute form of the disease produces no echocardiographic changes. However, electrocardiographic changes are often noted. These changes are variable and include conduction abnormalities (first- and second-degree atrioventricular block, complete atrioventricular block, right bundle branch block), sinus tachycardia, and depressed *R* wave amplitude.[111,113] Sudden death can occur, and presence of the conduction disturbances predicts sudden death.[114] Dogs may also have evidence of generalized lymphadenopathy, splenomegaly, hepatomegaly, pale mucous membranes, slowed capillary refill time, anorexia, diarrhea, and multifocal neurologic signs.[111] There may be a small amount of ascites. Following the acute phase of the disease, a latent phase occurs, in which dogs show no clinical signs, although sudden death may still occur. This phase lasts for 27 to 120 days in dogs. The electrocardiogram may be normal or have residual changes from the acute phase of the disease. The echocardiogram is still normal during this phase. The chronic stage of Chagas' myocarditis is indistinguishable from DCM on clinical examination. It is characterized by myocardial failure, heart failure, and ventricular arrhythmias.[113] Right heart failure may occur first or predominate the clinical picture, but left heart failure usually follows. Evidence of primarily right ventricular systolic dysfunction should warrant further investigation of Chagas' myocarditis. On the left side, myocardial depression is commonly worse in the left ventricular free wall than in the interventricular septum.[113] The reason for the slow progression to myocardial failure is unknown, but the cause may be microvascular vasospasm.[115]

The diagnosis of chronic Chagas myocarditis is based on a high index of suspicion; typical clinical, electrocardiographic, and echocardiographic findings; and identifying circulating antibodies to *T. cruzi*. Indirect fluorescent antibody, direct hemagglutination, and complement fixation tests on serum are used to identify the circulating antibodies. An ELISA test for detecting antibodies to North American isolates of *T. cruzi* has also been described.[111] Antibody tests are sensitive and specific for *T. cruzi* in North America.[111] The acute form of Chagas' myocarditis can be diagnosed by identifying trypomastigotes in peripheral blood.[109] However, the number of circulating organisms is low, which makes finding these organisms difficult. This, coupled with the fact that the clinical signs of Chagas' disease are nonspecific, makes diagnosis at this stage rare. At a postmortem examination, hearts that have been chronically infected with *T. cruzi* have multifocal regions of interstitial lymphoplasmacytic and histiocytic infiltrates. Marked fibrosis is also present.[111]

Treatment for the chronic phase of this disease is unrewarding and is primarily the symptomatic treatment of the heart failure and arrhythmias. Therapy directed at killing the organism does not alter the course of the disease at this stage. Treatment of experimentally infected mice with verapamil, starting in the acute phase of the disease, decreased mortality from 60% to 6% and decreased the amount of myocardial pathology in one study.[116] This may be due to a beneficial effect on the microvasculature, decreasing microvascular spasm.[115]

PARVOVIRUS

Parvovirus is an infectious agent that invades numerous cell types, including myocardial cells. Parvovirus myocarditis was an extensive problem in young puppies in the late 1970s and early 1980s, when this virus first appeared. At this time, bitches had no maternal antibody to pass on to their puppies. Very young puppies (3 to 8 weeks of age) exposed to the virus developed a fulminant infection resulting in acute death secondary to pulmonary edema.[117] Two-to-four-month-old puppies also often died subacutely (within 24 hours) as a result of heart failure.[118] Apparently, some dogs that were acutely exposed to parvovirus developed a more subtle myocarditis that allowed them to survive the neonatal period. Some of these dogs may have gone on to develop a disease clinically indistinguishable from DCM, usually at less than 1 year of age.[119]

Gross examination of the heart at necropsy of acutely affected puppies reveals cardiac enlargement and pale myocardium or pale streaks in the myocardium.[118] Histopathologic features of the disease are myofiber loss, myocytolysis, and mononuclear cell infiltrate of variable intensity. Large, basophilic intranuclear inclusion bodies are found in the myocardium of acutely infected younger puppies. Intranuclear inclusions are absent in older puppies.[120] Older dogs have gross myocardial scarring with multiple pale streaks throughout the myocardium and myocardial thinning.[119]

This disease is primarily of historical interest. No cases of parvovirus-induced myocarditis, including those of older dogs, have been identified in the literature since the early 1980s. The incidence of intranuclear inclusions in hearts at necropsy is very low.[121] Although pale, fibrous streaks in the myocardium may be observed occasionally in a dog with DCM, the lesions are almost never extensive enough to explain the degree of myocardial failure and are unlikely to be due to parvovirus.

LYME CARDITIS

Lyme carditis is a rare cause of myocardial disease in dogs. In humans, the spirochete *Borrelia burgdorferi* can cause a transient cardiac disease in about 10% of patients infected with the organism. The most common manifestation is a transient third-degree atrioventricular block, although first- and second-degree atrioventricular blocks may also occur. Ventricular arrhythmias and myocardial failure occasionally occur. There is one report of one dog that developed third-degree atrioventricular block that possibly had organisms in the myocardium at necropsy.[122] This dog also had a very high antibody titer to *B. burgdorferi*. It did not receive a pacemaker and died 1 month after diagnosis because of extreme bradycardia and long periods (up to 30 seconds) of ventricular asystole. We have treated one dog with severe myocardial failure that also had a high antibody titer. Whether or not this dog's cardiomyopathy was due to Lyme disease or not is unknown. If Lyme carditis is suspected, diagnosis can be confirmed by antibody titers, endomyocardial biopsy, and necropsy. Third-degree atrioventricular blocks may require temporary cardiac pacing. Permanent pacemaker therapy is rarely required in humans. The efficacy of antibiotic therapy in Lyme carditis associated with atrioventricular block in humans is not established.[123] However, intravenous penicillin G and tetracycline are commonly used. The benefit of antiinflammatory agents is also unclear.

TRANSMISSIBLE MYOCARDITIS AND DIAPHRAGMITIS

In 1993, Pedersen et al[124] described a group of cats with transient fever (103 to 107° F) and depression. Whole blood from naturally infected cats was injected into experimental cats, and the disease was reproduced. The fever in these cats was usually biphasic, occurring 9 to 16 days and 17 to 27 days after inoculation. The fever lasted 1 to 3 days the first time and about 5 days the second time. Affected cats had normal hemograms, blood chemistries, thoracic and abdominal radiographs, and urinalyses. They were negative for feline leukemia virus, feline immunodeficiency virus, and feline infectious peritonitis. Blood cultures for aerobic and anaerobic bacteria were negative. Some (3 of 7) cats had an increase in creatine phosphokinase during the febrile stage. Postmortem examination of cats euthanized during the second febrile episode revealed 1- to 3-mm pale foci within the myocardium and the diaphragm. The foci were discrete and numbered five to 25 per organ. Microscopically, the lesions consisted of myonecrosis with an inflammatory cell infiltrate. The inflammatory cells were predominantly neutrophils with scattered macrophages. One cat had primarily macrophages. Mesenteric lymphadenopathy and splenomegaly were common. Although a viral etiology was suspected, no organism was identified.

Myocardial Infarction

Myocardial infarction as a result of major coronary artery occlusion is a rare cause of regional left ventricular hypokinesis or akinesis in dogs and cats. The most common cause of myocardial infarction in dogs is septic embolism of a coronary artery secondary to bacterial endocarditis, especially endocarditis of the aortic valve. Coronary atherosclerosis, the primary cause of myocardial infarction in humans, is rare in the dog. It can, however, be recreated in the canine species by producing hypothyroidism and feeding a high-cholesterol diet. This scenario could occur in a client-owned dog. Consequently, atherosclerosis leading to myocardial infarction is not an impossible scenario in a dog. In one report, 21 dogs were diagnosed at necropsy with atherosclerosis over a 14-year period at the Animal Medical Center in New York City.[125] Some of these dogs did have evidence of myocardial infarction. Hypercholesterolemia, hyperlipidemia, and hypothyroidism were common in affected dogs.[125]

The clinical diagnosis of myocardial infarction is most commonly entertained when regional hypokinesis is observed on an echocardiogram. Regional hypokinesis is not pathognomonic for myocardial infarction. The left ventricular free wall commonly is more hypokinetic than the interventricular septum in large dogs with severe mitral regurgitation. This phenomenon also occurs in tachycardia-induced myocardial failure in dogs. Regional akinesis with wall thinning is more likely to be due to myocardial infarction and has been identified in cats with myocardial failure.[13] However, other causes, such as myocarditis and DCM, exist. The only practical way to definitively diagnose myocardial infarction antemortem is to perform a coronary angiogram.

Tachycardia-Induced Myocardial Failure

It has been well established that when an experimental dog's heart is electrically paced at a rate greater than 200 beats/min, myocardial failure, severe enough to produce heart failure, is produced within 2 to 6 weeks.[78,79] All four chambers become enlarged. Hypertrophy commonly is not present. Instead, true dilation of the heart occurs as the chambers enlarge and the walls thin.[126] Ascites is usually present, and pulmonary edema may be present. At the cellular level, myocytes are elongated as in volume overload hypertrophy, but these elongated cells have a decreased number of sarcomeres instead of an increased number.[127] Glycogen stores appear depleted. Mitochondria are swollen and the cristae are disorganized. The mechanism by which this failure occurs is unknown. It is not due to myocardial hypoxia, although myocardial blood flow reserve is reduced.[128] In addition to reduced glycogen stores, there are decreased stores of creatine, phosphocreatine, and ATP.[126] Mitochondrial function appears abnormal, with reduced cytochrome oxidase staining and creatine kinase activity. Abnormal calcium handling is present and may be a primary or a secondary abnormality.[126] Myocardial failure rapidly reverses once the tachycardia is terminated. Cardiac output and ventricular filling pressures are almost normal within 48 hours after pacing is stopped. Shortening fraction recovers dramatically within the same time frame and is normal within 1 to 2 weeks.[126] During this time, sarcomeres are added to the cells and the heart weight increases. End-diastolic and end-systolic volumes remain increased for at least 12 weeks, documenting that myocardial function is not fully recovered.

A sustained tachycardia can result in severe myocardial failure and heart failure in canine patients. An old English sheepdog with a sustained supraventricular tachycardia (rate = 320 beats/min) whose myocardial failure completely resolved following successful treatment of the supraventricular tachycardia is presented in Figure 20-16. More commonly a dog with a tachycardia and myocardial failure becomes a chicken and egg story in which it is difficult to tell if the myocardial failure is due to the tachycardia or the tachycardia is the result of myocardial disease. Generally the tachycardia must be sustained to produce myocardial failure. If the tachycardia is controlled and myocardial function improves, one can usually assume one is dealing with tachycardia-induced myocardial failure.

Doxorubicin-Induced Myocardial Failure

Doxorubicin is a widely used cancer chemotherapeutic agent used to treat a variety of tumor types in human and veterinary medicine. It is also a known cardiotoxic agent. Cardiotoxicity is manifested as arrhythmias, myocardial failure, or both. Cardiotoxicity is dose-dependant and irreversible. At doses of 80 mg/m^2/day for 2 days or 25 mg/m^2/week for 4 to 11 weeks, approximately 80% of experimental dogs will develop ventricular arrhythmias. About 30% will develop periods of fast (180 to 300 beats/min) nonsustained ventricular tachycardia.[129] Slower ventricular rhythms, atrial arrhythmias, and conduction blocks can also be produced at these high doses (Figure 20-17). When doxorubicin is administered at approximately 25 mg/m^2/week for 20 weeks, all experimental dogs develop myocardial failure. In one study, approximately 65% of the dogs died of heart failure or died suddenly, usually after 17 weeks of drug administration.[130] In this study, the dogs that died had more severe histopathologic myocardial lesions than those dogs that survived. The worst lesions were in the subendocardium of the left ventricular free wall and interventricular septum. Lesions were primarily vacuolar degeneration of myocytes. Ultrastructurally, these vacuoles were caused by distension of the sarcoplasmic reticulum. This is consistent with the current theory that doxorubicin permanently alters the calcium release channels on the sarcoplasmic reticulum. Studies have shown that when doxorubicin is initially administered it sensitizes the calcium release channel to activation by calcium.[131] Continued exposure and continued sensitization result chronically in a progressive and irreversible reduction in the number of functional calcium release channels.[132]

In humans, usually doses higher than 400 to 550 mg/m^2 must be administered to produce cardiotoxicity. Dogs and cats are much more sensitive to the cardiotoxic effects. Consequently, smaller doses are used to treat neoplasia in small animal veterinary medicine. Even so, in one study in which only two doses of 30 mg/m^2 were administered, 3% of the dogs studied developed cardiomyopathy.[133] Cardiotoxicity is more common at cumulative doses exceeding 250 mg/m^2 in dogs.[133] Consequently, the dose is generally maintained lower than this threshold.

The true prevalence of clinically significant doxorubicin cardiotoxicity is unknown. In one study that examined 175 canine patients that were administered adriamycin, cardiac abnormalities were identified in 32 (18%).[134] Of these, 31 (18%) developed ECG abnormalities and 7 (4%) developed heart failure. In another set of studies, 52 dogs were administered either doxorubicin (30 mg/m^2 every 3 weeks; cumulative dose = 180 mg/m^2) alone or doxorubicin in combination with hyperthermia.[135,136] These dogs were studied prospectively with ECGs and echocardiograms. The hyperthermia did not appear to increase the prevalence of clinical cardiotoxicity. Eleven of the 52 dogs (21%) developed cardiotoxicity. Four dogs (8%) developed heart failure either during therapy or within 8 weeks of treatment completion. Seven dogs (13%) developed echocardiographic evidence of myocardial failure without heart failure. One of these dogs developed myocardial failure after the second dose.[135] Three of these dogs developed ECG abnormalities that included ventricular premature beats (n = 2) and right bundle branch block (n = 1). The ECG abnormalities did not occur before the onset of myocardial failure.

A

B

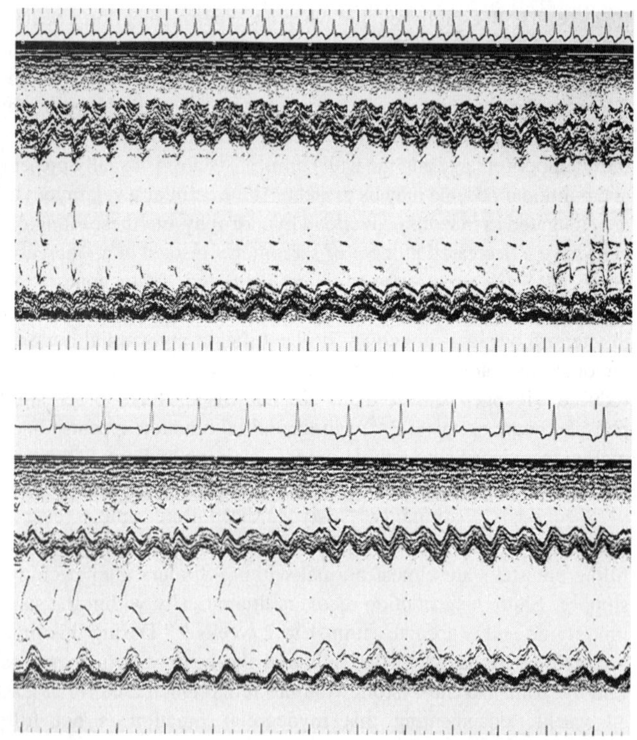

FIGURE 20-16 **A,** M-mode echocardiogram and an ECG from an Old English sheepdog with sustained supraventricular tachycardia and subsequent severe myocardial failure. The shortening fraction was in the 10% to 15% range. The dog was in heart failure at presentation. **B,** M-mode echocardiogram and an ECG taken a week after the arrhythmia was abolished with drug therapy. Myocardial function has improved (shortening fraction is approximately 30%). Signs of heart failure had abated.

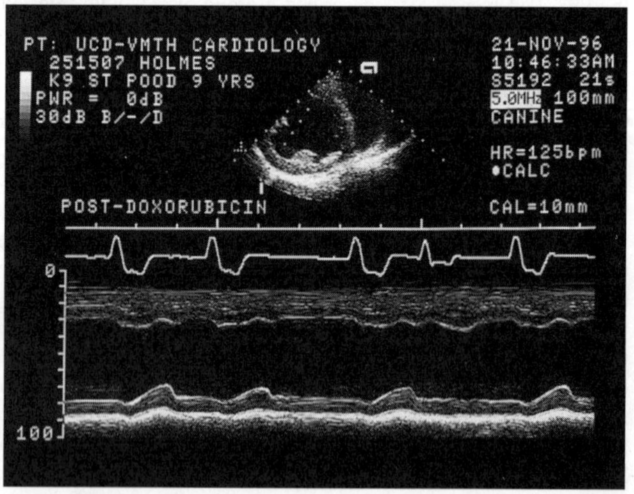

FIGURE 20-17 M-mode echocardiogram from a dog with adriamycin cardiotoxicity. This 26-kg dog had a mild increase in end-systolic diameter with no increase in end-diastolic diameter and a shortening fraction between 20% and 25%. The interventricular septum contracts poorly but at the appropriate time. It can also be seen to move away from the transducer when the left ventricular free wall relaxes. The free wall contracts normally but very late. The dog was in atrial fibrillation with a left bundle branch block and occasional ventricular premature beats.

Atrial Standstill Resulting from Cardiomyopathy or Myocarditis

A particular form of cardiomyopathy that destroys the atrial and, sometimes, ventricular myocardium is seen in dogs, most commonly in English springer spaniels.[137] The disease has also been reported in other breeds, including the Old English sheepdog, a Shi-Tzu, a German shorthaired pointer, and mixed-breed dogs.[138] We have also diagnosed this condition in a boxer, a Chesapeake Bay retriever, a Labrador retriever, and a pit bull terrier. It has been reported in cats, although the cats reported have also had DCM.[137] It is unclear whether or not these cats were taurine-deficient, because the report was published in 1983, before the discovery of taurine deficiency as the cause of most DCM in cats.

This cardiomyopathy appears to first effect the atria, destroying most of the atrial tissue. The destruction of the atrial myocardium (and the sinus node (SA) and internodal tracts) results in loss of SA pacing or conduction from the sinus node to the atrioventricular node (AV), forcing the AV node to take over the pacing function of the heart.[139] Consequently, the cardiac rhythm observed in these dogs is a nodal escape rhythm with a heart rate usually between 40 and 60 beats/min. No *P* waves or, occasionally, very small *P* waves are observed on the ECG. The heart rate does not increase following atropine administration, as expected. The atria do not contract, as evidenced by lack of fluoroscopic atrial motion and lack of echocardiographic mitral valve opening during late diastole. The atrial cardiomyopathy may be followed by ventricular myocardial failure.

Clinically, these dogs commonly present with signs referable to their bradycardia. Clinical signs include exercise intolerance, weakness, episodic weakness, and syncope. They may also have signs of heart failure. Right or left heart failure may predominate. On echocardiography the atria are markedly enlarged and ventricular function is normal to moderately depressed (Figures 20-18 and 20-19). Atrioventricular valvular regurgitation is commonly present, and the appropriate ventricle may be volume overloaded (Color Plate 83). Over time, ventricular myocardial function often deteriorates.

Histopathologically, at the end stage, this disease is characterized by almost complete loss of atrial myocardium with replacement by fibrous tissue. Steatosis may also be a histologic feature.[140] Grossly this results in the atria being markedly enlarged and translucent (Color Plate 84). In one report, three dogs with atrial standstill also had marked muscle wasting that involved the muscles of the upper foreleg and scapula.[137] Histopathology of these muscles was compatible with a muscular dystrophy. Features included hyalinized, degenerated muscle fibers and mild-to-moderate steatosis.[140] This was termed a *facioscapulohumeral* type of muscular dystrophy after that seen in humans. Because there was no facial involvement in these dogs, it has been speculated more recently that this might more likely be an Emery-Dreifus muscular dystrophy.[141] We stress that in most dogs there is no evidence of muscular involvement, and the relationship to any form of human muscular dystrophy is unknown and purely speculative. Interestingly, there is one published report of an English springer spaniel with atrial standstill that did not have atrial fibrosis but rather had evidence of myocarditis in the atria and ventricles and atrial standstill.[139] The heart from this dog had an active myocarditis with large numbers of lymphocytes. In another report, a German shorthaired pointer died soon after presenting with atrial standstill. This dog also had mild-to-extensive focal accumulations of lymphocytes along with severe fibrosis and hemorrhage in both atria.[138] The AV node and bundle of His were also infiltrated with lymphocytes. The left ventricular free wall had focal areas of hemorrhage. In one case of an English springer spaniel reported to us, marked infiltration of the atrial myocardium by mononuclear cells was identified.[142] We have also observed a boxer with a severe lymphocytic, plasmacytic, eosinophilic polymyositis that also had a myocarditis, in which the atrial myocardium was destroyed producing atrial standstill. These four patients may represent cases in which the disease was identified before its end stage. We have looked extensively for evidence of a muscular dystrophy in one case of atrial standstill in an English springer spaniel and found no evidence of skeletal muscle pathology. Consequently, we believe that this disease is most likely the result of a myocarditis of unknown etiology in many cases.

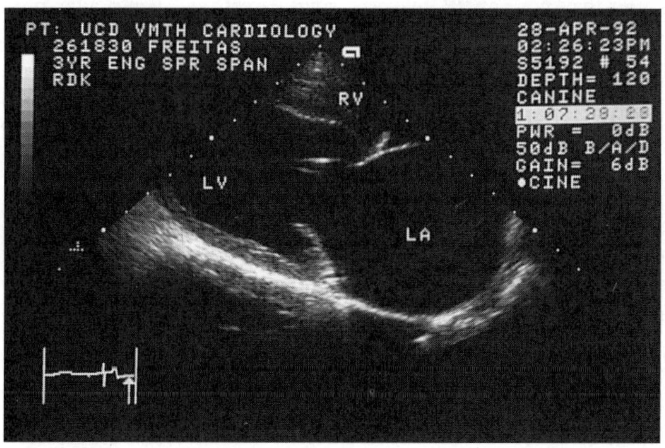

FIGURE 20-18 Two-dimensional echocardiogram taken from a right parasternal long-axis view in diastole from an English springer spaniel with atrial standstill. The left ventricular chamber is enlarged, and the left ventricular free wall thickness is normal, indicating volume overload hypertrophy. The left atrium is dilated.

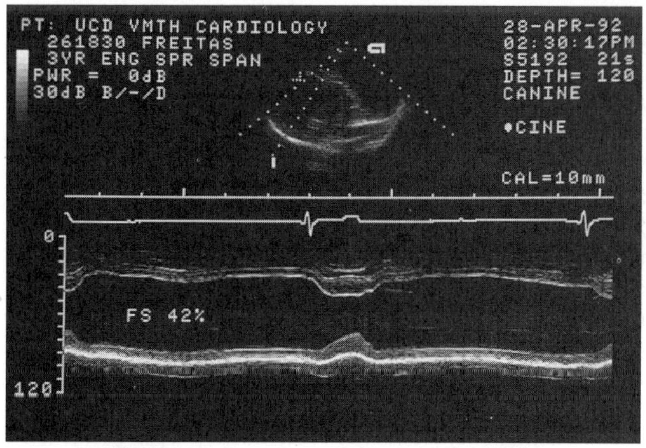

FIGURE 20-19 M-mode echocardiogram and an ECG from the dog shown in Figure 20-18. The heart rate is approximately 45 beats/min. There are no *P* waves. The left ventricular end-diastolic diameter is approximately 60 mm (normal = 45 mm), indicating volume overload hypertrophy. The end-systolic diameter is approximately 35 mm (normal = 30 mm), indicating mild myocardial failure. The shortening fraction is 42%, indicating a mild hyperdynamic contraction.

Treatment for this condition is often unrewarding. A pacemaker may be implanted to improve the clinical signs that occur secondary to the bradycardia. Clinical signs secondary to heart failure may also improve because of the increase in heart rate and therefore cardiac output. Catecholamines may be administered acutely to increase the rate of the AV node pacemaker in dogs that are showing clinical signs referable to poor perfusion while waiting to implant an external pacemaker.[139] The improvement in clinical signs following pacemaker implantation is usually temporary. Dogs ultimately succumb to heart failure or die suddenly. Heart failure is usually treated with furosemide and an ACE inhibitor. The boxer described previously was treated with corticosteroids with little response.

Endocardial Fibroelastosis

Endocardial fibroelastosis is a rare cause of myocardial failure in young dogs and cats. It is characterized by focal thickening of the endocardium of the left atrium, left ventricle, and mitral valve.[143] Grossly, the thickened endocardium imparts a diffuse white appearance to the normally translucent endocardial surface. Histologically, there is proliferation of collagenous and elastic tissue within the endocardium. Elastic fibrils may extend into the myocardium.[143,144]

Endocardial fibroelastosis has been reported in various dog breeds, including the Labrador retriever, great Dane, English bulldog, boxer, springer spaniel, and pit bull.[144,145] It has also been reported in Burmese and Siamese cats.[146,147] Whether or not the lesion was primary in many reported cases is questionable. Many reported cases have had subaortic stenosis and apparent mitral valve dysplasia, along with the endocardial thickening. Experimental endocardial fibroelastosis has been produced in dogs by ligating the cardiac lymphatics.[145] The abnormality is reportedly an inherited abnormality in Burmese cats.[148] In Burmese cats with the disease, there are no lesions in kittens that are less than 2 days of age.[148] Kittens between 5 and 19 days of age have endocardial edema and fibroblast proliferation. Left ventricular chamber enlargement and endocardial thickening are seen in kittens greater than 19 days of age. Postmortem examination has revealed dilated lymphatic capillaries at the endomyocardial junction plus collagen and elastic fibers that were 3 to 5 times as thick as normal. The facts that cardiac lymphatic ligation can produce endomyocardial fibroelastosis, that the earliest lesion is edema, and that dilated lymphatics were seen in these hearts suggests that the disease in Burmese cats may be caused by obstruction to cardiac lymphatic drainage.

Dogs, cats, and humans with this disease develop heart failure. That the lesion in this disease is not confined to the endocardium is obvious because diffuse myocardial failure is a hallmark of this disease and is the primary cause of the heart failure. If endocardial thickening produced all of the abnormalities in this disease, the pathophysiologic principle underlying the heart failure would be diastolic dysfunction caused by ventricular restriction. If the lesion truly is due to the blockage of lymphatics, it would make sense that the entire myocardium would be involved.

Affected animals present when they are young, often less than 6 months of age. They are usually in heart failure at presentation. On echocardiography, the left chambers are dilated and myocardial failure is evident as an increased end-systolic diameter and a decreased shortening fraction. Diffuse endocardial thickening on the echocardiogram has been reported in humans but apparently is not a consistent feature.[143] This feature has not been examined in dogs or cats. Mitral or tricuspid regurgitation are usually present. Otherwise, the clinical presentation, treatment, and prognosis are the same as for DCM.

Duchenne's Cardiomyopathy

Duchenne's muscular dystrophy is a common inherited neuromuscular disorder in humans. It is inherited as an X-linked trait (only males are severely affected) and is due to mutations of the gene that encodes for dystrophin.[149] Dystrophin is a cytoskeletal protein that is present in skeletal and cardiac muscle.[150] Human patients with the disease experience continual skeletal muscle necrosis, regeneration, and fibrosis. Patients lose their ability to ambulate in their early teens and usually die in their early twenties. Patients not only develop skeletal abnormalities but also myocardial abnormalities that can lead to severe myocardial failure and heart failure.[151] Rarely, dogs can be affected with Duchenne's muscular dystrophy. It has been best characterized in the golden retriever breed.[152] A similar condition, however, has been reported in Irish terriers, Samoyeds, and rottweilers.[152] The disease is known as *canine X-linked muscular dystrophy* in dogs. Myocardial disease can also be a component of the canine disorder. The myocardial disease is characterized by hyperechoic lesions on the echocardiogram.[153] These lesions are present in almost all affected dogs (males) and about one half of carrier dogs (females). They are often present by 6 to 7 months of age. The lesions are most prominent in the left ventricular free wall and papillary muscles. These hyperechoic areas decrease in size after 2 years of age. The hyperechoic regions correspond to regions of calcified and fibrotic myocardium at postmortem examination. In one study, of six dogs examined that were more than 2 years of age, three had myocardial failure.[153] Two of these had severe myocardial failure (left ventricular end-systolic diameters of 52 mm each, shortening fractions of 7% and 13%, and *E*-point septal separations of 18 and 29 mm). One of these dogs died of heart failure. The interventricular septum in both dogs was 1 to 2 mm thinner than normal, and the left ventricular free wall was thinner than normal in one of these dogs.

Dogs with canine X-linked muscular dystrophy also have electrocardiographic abnormalities. All affected golden retrievers have deep and narrow *Q* waves in leads II, III, aV_F, CV_6LL, and CV_6LU. All carrier dogs with hyperechoic lesions have deep and narrow *Q* waves in leads II, III, and aV_F. A reduced electromotive force in affected regions of the myocardium and increased forces in the nonaffected regions accounts for the deep *Q* waves. A shorter-than-normal PR interval, sinus arrest, and ventricular premature depolarizations have also been reported.

Arrhythmogenic Right Ventricular Cardiomyopathy

Cardiomyopathy restricted to the right heart is rare in dogs and cats, having only been reported twice.[154,155] These cases resembled a condition in humans termed *right ventricular dysplasia, Uhl's disease, parchment heart,* or *arrhythmic right ventricular cardiomyopathy.*[156] Human patients have severe and complex arrhythmias, may die suddenly, and may develop right heart failure. The myocardium in this abnormality is partially or totally replaced by adipose or fibrous tissue. The loss of myocardium seems progressive and the result of inflammation, degeneration, and necrosis of right ventricular myocardium.[157] Whether the inflammation that is present is primary or secondary to cell death is unknown. The cause of right ventricular cardiomyopathy is unknown, although recent investigations have localized gene loci to specific chromosome regions in human families with the disease.[69,158] The dog presented in the veterinary literature was a 3.5-year-old dachshund in right heart failure.[155] On echocardiography, there was a marked volume overload of the right heart, a markedly enlarged tricuspid valve annulus, and severe tricuspid regurgitation with no evidence of tricuspid valve dysplasia. The postmortem examination confirmed the absence of any valvular abnormality. Gross pathology revealed an enlarged right ventricular chamber with a wall that was very thin, to the point of being translucent in some areas. Histopathologic examination of the right ventricular myocardium revealed widespread loss of myocardium with replacement by fibrous and adipose tissue. There were moderate numbers of mononuclear cells surrounding the fibrotic areas. Smaller numbers of mononuclear infiltrates were present in the interventricular septum and left ventricular free wall. The cat in the literature was 4 years old when it presented in right heart failure.[154] At postmortem examination it had a large translucent region of its right ventricular free wall. Histopathology of this region revealed endocardium and epicardium separated by adipose and fibrous tissue.

REFERENCES

1. Report of the WHO/ISFC task force on the definition and classification of cardiomyopathies, *Br Heart J* 44:672, 1980.
2. Calvert CA, Brown J: Use of M-mode echocardiography in the diagnosis of congestive cardiomyopathy in Doberman pinschers, *J Am Vet Med Assoc* 189:293, 1986.
3. Sisson DD, Thomas WP: Myocardial diseases. In Ettinger SJ, Feldman EC, eds: *Textbook of veterinary internal medicine,* ed 4, Philadelphia, 1995, WB Saunders.
4. Gooding JP, Robinson WF, Wyburn RS et al: A cardiomyopathy in the English springer spaniel: a clinico-pathological investigation, *J Small Anim Pract* 23:133, 1982.
5. Koch J, Pedersen HD, Jensen AL et al: M-mode echocardiographic diagnosis of dilated cardiomyopathy in giant breed dogs, *Zentralbl Veterinarmed (A)* 43:297, 1996.
6. Tidholm A, Jonsson L: Dilated cardiomyopathy in the Newfoundland: a study of 37 cases (1983-1994), *J Am Anim Hosp Assoc* 32:465, 1996.
7. Fujii T, Ito M, Okuno T et al: Complex I (reduced nicotinamide-adenine dinucleotide-coenzyme Q reductase) deficiency in two patients with probable Leigh syndrome, *J Pediatr* 116:84, 1990.
8. Ogasahara S, Engel AG, Frens D et al: Muscle coenzyme Q deficiency in familial mitochondrial encephalomyopathy, *Proc Natl Acad Sci U S A* 86:2379, 1989.
9. O'Brien PJ, Gwathmey JK: Myocardial Ca(2+)- and ATP-cycling imbalances in end-stage dilated and ischemic cardiomyopathies, *Cardiovasc Res* 30:394, 1995.
10. Towbin JA, Hejtmancik JF, Brink P et al: X-linked dilated cardiomyopathy: molecular genetic evidence of linkage to the Duchenne muscular dystrophy (dystrophin) gene at the Xp21 locus, *Circulation* 87:1854, 1993.
11. Kawaguchi N, Fujitani N, Schaper J et al: Pathological changes of myocardial cytoskeleton in cardiomyopathic hamster, *Mol Cell Biochem,* 144:75, 1995.
12. Schaper J, Mollnau H, Hein S et al: [Interactions between cardiomyocytes and extracellular matrix in the failing human heart] Wechselwirkungen zwischen Kardiomyozyten und der extrazellularen Matrix im insuffizienten menschlichen Herzen, *Z Kardiol* 84(suppl) 4:33, 1995.
13. Fox PR, Petrie JP, Liu SK et al: Clinical and pathological features of cardiomyopathy characterized by myocardial failure in 49 cats, 1990-1995, *J Vet Intern Med* 11:139, 1997 (abstract).
14. Pion PD, Kittleson MD, Rogers QR et al: Myocardial failure in cats associated with low plasma taurine: a reversible cardiomyopathy, *Science* 237:764, 1987.
15. Tiedemann F, Gmelin L: Einige neue Bestandtheile der Galle des Ochsen, *Physik Chem* 9:326, 1827.
16. Azari J, Huxtable RJ: The mechanism of the adrenergic stimulation of taurine influx in the heart, *Eur J Pharmacol* 61:217, 1980.
17. Huxtable RJ: Taurine in the central nervous system and the mammalian actions of taurine, *Prog Neurobiol* 32:471, 1989.
18. Laidlaw SA, Sturman JA, Kopple JD: Effect of dietary taurine on plasma and blood cell taurine concentrations in cats, *J Nutr* 117:1945, 1987.
19. Chesney RW: Taurine: its biological role and clinical implications, *Adv Pediatr* 32:1, 1985.
20. Pion PD, Kittleson MD, Thomas WP et al: Clinical findings in cats with dilated cardiomyopathy and relationship of findings to taurine deficiency, *J Am Vet Med Assoc* 201:267, 1992.
21. Pion PD, Kittleson MD, Rogers QR et al: Taurine deficiency myocardial failure in the domestic cat, *Prog Clin Biol Res* 351:423, 1990.
22. Lawler DF, Templeton AJ, Monti KL: Evidence for genetic involvement in feline dilated cardiomyopathy, *J Vet Intern Med* 7:383, 1993.
23. Kramer GA, Kittleson MD, Fox PR et al: Plasma taurine concentrations in normal dogs and in dogs with heart disease, *J Vet Intern Med* 9:253, 1995.
24. Breningstall GN: Carnitine deficiency syndromes, *Pediatr Neurol* 6:75, 1990.
25. Keene BW, Panciera DP, Atkins CE et al: Myocardial L-carnitine deficiency in a family of dogs with dilated cardiomyopathy, *J Am Vet Med Assoc* 198:647, 1991.
26. Bovee KC, Thier SO, Rea C et al: Renal clearance of amino acids in canine cystinuria, *Metabolism* 23:51, 1974.
27. Sanderson S, Osborne C, Ogburn P et al: Canine cystinuria associated with carnitinuria and carnitine deficiency, *Proc Annu Vet Med Forum,* 1995, p 1027 (abstract).
28. Bucci LR: Coenzyme Q10 and heart disease, *Vet Forum,* March 1994, p 78.
29. Urban PF, Klingenberg M: On the redox potentials of ubiquinone and cytochrome b in the respiratory chain, *Eur J Biochem* 9:519, 1969.
30. Kroger A, Klingenberg M: On the role of ubiquinone in mitochondria. II. Redox reactions of ubiquinone under the control of oxidative phosphorylation, *Biochem Z* 344:317, 1966.
31. Kamei M, Fujita T, Kanbe T et al: The distribution and content of ubiquinone in foods, *Int J Vitam Nutr Res* 56:57, 1986.
32. Koga Y, Nonaka I, Kobayashi M et al: Findings in muscle in complex I (NADH coenzyme Q reductase) deficiency, *Ann Neurol* 24:749, 1988.
33. Fischer JC, Ruitenbeek W, Gabreels FJ et al: A mitochondrial encephalomyopathy: the first case with an established defect at the level of coenzyme Q, *Eur J Pediatr* 144:441, 1986.
34. Cristofari M, Bertocchi P, Vigano M: [The MELAS syndrome and dilated-hypertrophic cardiomyopathy: a case report] Sindrome MELAS e cardiomiopatia dilatativa-ipertrofica: descrizione di un caso, *G Ital Cardiol* 25:69, 1995.
35. Kobayashi M, Morishita H, Sugiyama N et al: Two cases of NADH-coenzyme Q reductase deficiency: relationship to MELAS syndrome, *J Pediatr* 110:223, 1987.
36. Nishizawa M, Tanaka K, Shinozawa K et al: A mitochondrial encephalomyopathy with cardiomyopathy: a case revealing a defect of complex I in the respiratory chain, *J Neurol Sci* 78:189, 1987.
37. Di Donato S, Frerman FE, Rimoldi M et al: Systemic carnitine deficiency due to lack of electron transfer flavoprotein:ubiquinone oxidoreductase, *Neurology* 36:957, 1986.
38. Littarru GP, Ho L, Folkers K: Deficiency of coenzyme Q 10 in human heart disease. II. *Int J Vitam Nutr Res* 42:413, 1972.
39. Folkers K, Littarru GP, Ho L et al: Evidence for a deficiency of coenzyme Q10 in human heart disease, *Int Z Vitaminforsch* 40:380, 1970.
40. Folkers K, Langsjoen P, Langsjoen PH: Therapy with coenzyme Q10 of patients in heart failure who are eligible or ineligible for a transplant, *Biochem Biophys Res Commun* 182:247, 1992.
41. Langsjoen PH, Folkers K: Long-term efficacy and safety of coenzyme Q10 therapy for idiopathic dilated cardiomyopathy, *Am J Cardiol* 65:521, 1990.
42. Langsjoen PH, Folkers K, Lyson K et al: Pronounced increase of survival of patients with cardiomyopathy when treated with coenzyme Q10 and conventional therapy, *Int J Tissue React* 2:163, 1990.

43. Langsjoen PH, Folkers K: A six-year clinical study of therapy of cardiomyopathy with coenzyme Q10, *Int J Tissue React* 12:169, 1990.
44. Greenberg S, Frishman WH: Co-enzyme Q10: a new drug for cardiovascular disease, *J Clin Pharmacol* 30:596, 1990.
45. Keister DM: A summary of phase IV clinical data on milrinone (Wincardin), a canine cardiotonic: protocol H, New York, 1988, Sterling-Winthrop.
46. O'Grady MR: Occult dilated cardiomyopathy in the Doberman pinscher, *Proc Annu Vet Med Forum,* 1995, p 298.
47. Calvert CA, Hall G, Jacobs G et al: Clinical and pathologic findings in Doberman pinschers with occult cardiomyopathy that died suddenly or developed congestive heart failure: 54 cases (1984-1991), *J Am Vet Med Assoc* 210:505, 1997.
48. Harpster NK: Boxer cardiomyopathy. In Kirk RW, ed: *Kirk's current veterinary therapy VIII: small animal practice,* Philadelphia, 1983, WB Saunders.
49. Goodwin JK, Cattiny G: Further characterization of boxer cardiomyopathy, *Proc Annu Vet Med Forum,* 1995, p 300.
50. Calvert CA: Diagnosis and management of ventricular arrhythmias in Doberman pinschers with cardiomyopathy. In Bonagura JD, ed: *Kirk's current veterinrary therapy, XII: small animal practice,* Philadelphia, 1995, WB Saunders.
51. Smucker ML, Kaul S, Woodfield JA et al: Naturally occurring cardiomyopathy in the Doberman pinscher: a possible large animal model of human cardiomyopathy*?* *J Am Coll Cardiol* 16:200, 1990.
52. O'Grady MR: Outcomes of 103 asymptomatic Doberman pinschers: incidence of dilated cardiomyopathy in a longitudinal study, *J Vet Intern Med* 9:199, 1995 (abstract).
53. Hammer TA, Venta PJ, Eyster GE: The genetic basis of dilated cardiomyopathy in Doberman pinschers, *Anim Genet* 27:109, 1996 (abstract).
54. Keene BW: L-carnitine supplementation in the therapy of canine dilated cardiomyopathy, *Vet Clin North Am Small Anim Pract* 21:1005, 1991.
55. O'Brien PJ, O'Grady M, McCutcheon LJ et al: Myocardial myoglobin deficiency in various animal models of congestive heart failure, *J Mol Cell Cardiol* 24:721, 1992.
56. Chung Y, Xu D, Jue T: Nitrite oxidation of myoglobin in perfused myocardium: implications for energy coupling in respiration, *Am J Physiol* 271:H1166, 1996.
57. McCutcheon LJ, Cory CR, Nowack L et al: Respiratory chain defect of myocardial mitochondria in idiopathic dilated cardiomyopathy of Doberman pinscher dogs, *Can J Physiol Pharmacol* 70:1529, 1992.
58. O'Brien PJ: Deficiencies of myocardial troponin-T and creatine kinase MB isoenzyme in dogs with idiopathic dilated cardiomyopathy, *Am J Vet Res* 58:11, 1997.
59. Hamman BL, Bittl JA, Jacobus WE et al: Inhibition of the creatine kinase reaction decreases the contractile reserve of isolated rat hearts, *Am J Physiol* 269:H1030, 1995.
60. Cory CR, Shen H, O'Brien PJ: Compensatory asymmetry in downregulation and inhibition of the myocardial $Ca2^{++}$ cycle in congestive heart failure produced in dogs by idiopathic dilated cardiomyopathy and rapid ventricular pacing, *J Mol Cell Cardiol* 26:173, 1994.
61. Cory CR, McCutcheon LJ, O'Grady M et al: Compensatory downregulation of myocardial Ca channel in SR from dogs with heart failure, *Am J Physiol* 264:H926, 1993.
62. Beggs AH: Dystrophinopathy, the expanding phenotype: dystrophin abnormalities in X-linked dilated cardiomyopathy, *Circulation* 95:2344, 1997.
63. Milasin J, Muntoni F, Severini GM et al: A point mutation in the 5' splice site of the first intron of the dystrophin gene responsible for X-linked dilated cardiomyopathy, *J Am Coll Cardiol* 27:226A, 1996 (abstract).
64. Ortiz-Lopez R, Li H, Su J et al: Evidence for a dystrophin missense mutation as a cause of X-linked dilated cardiomyopathy, *Circulation* 95:2434, 1997.
65. Muntoni F, Cau M, Ganau A et al: Brief report: deletion of the dystrophin muscle-promoter region associated with X-linked dilated cardiomyopathy, *N Engl J Med* 329:921, 1993 (comments).
66. Maeda M, Holder E, Lowes B et al: Dilated cardiomyopathy associated with deficiency of the cytoskeletal protein metavinculin, *J Am Coll Cardiol* 27:51A, 1996 (abstract).
67. Krajinovic M, Pinamonti B, Sinagra G et al: Linkage of autosomal dominant familial dilated cardiomyopathy to chromosome 9, *J Am Coll Cardiol* 27:226A, 1996 (abstract).
68. Durand JB, Bachinski L, Beiling L et al: Localization of the gene for familial idiopathic dilated cardiomyopathy to chromosome 1q32, *J Am Coll Cardiol* 27:2A, 1996 (abstract).
69. Coonar AS, McKenna WJ: Molecular genetics of familial cardiomyopathies, *Adv Genet* 35:285, 1997.
70. Freeman LM, Michel KE, Brown DJ et al: Idiopathic dilated cardiomyopathy in Dalmations: nine cases (1990-1995), *J Am Vet Med Assoc* 209:1592, 1996.
71. Van Vleet JF, Ferrans VJ, Weirich WE: Pathologic alterations in congestive cardiomyopathy of dogs, *Am J Vet Res* 42:416, 1981.
72. Rose AG, Beck W: Dilated (congestive) cardiomyopathy: a syndrome of severe cardiac dysfunction with remarkably few morphological features of myocardial damage, *Histopathology* 9:367, 1985.
73. Calvert CA, Chapman WLJ, Toal RL: Congestive cardiomyopathy in Doberman pinscher dogs, *J Am Vet Med Assoc* 181:598, 1982.
74. Lord PF: Left ventricular diastolic stiffness in dogs with congestive cardiomyopathy and volume overload, *Am J Vet Res* 37:953, 1976.
75. Sagie A, Schwammenthal E, Padial LR et al: Determinants of functional tricuspid regurgitation in incomplete tricuspid valve closure: Doppler olor flow study of 109 patients, *J Am Coll Cardiol* 24:446, 1994.
76. Kono T, Sabbah HN, Rosman H et al: Left ventricular shape is the primary determinant of functional mitral regurgitation in heart failure, *J Am Coll Cardiol* 20:1594, 1992.
77. Kono T, Sabbah HN, Stein PD et al: Left ventricular shape as a determinant of functional mitral regurgitation in patients with severe heart failure secondary to either coronary artery disease or idiopathic dilated cardiomyopathy, *Am J Cardiol* 68:355, 1991.
78. Wilson JR, Douglas P, Hickey WF et al: Experimental congestive heart failure produced by rapid ventricular pacing in the dog: cardiac effects, *Circulation* 75:857, 1987.
79. Riegger AJ, Liebau G: The renin-angiotensin-aldosterone system, antidiuretic hormone and sympathetic nerve activity in an experimental model of congestive heart failure in the dog, *Clin Sci* 62:465, 1982.
80. Kittleson MD: Coronary sinus oxygen tension in dogs with heart disease, *Proc AnnuVet Med Forum,* 1992, p 594.
81. Calvert CA, Jacobs GJ: Bradycardia resulting in syncope during exercise in Doberman pinscher dogs with cardiomyopathy, *J Vet Intern Med* 9:202, 1995.
82. Pion PD, Kittleson MD, Skiles ML: Dilated cardiomyopathy associated with taurine deficiency in the domestic cat: relationship to diet and myocardial taurine content, *Adv Exp Med Biol* 315:63, 1992.
83. Calvert CA, Pickus C, Jacobs GJ et al: Signalment, survival, and prognostic factors in Doberman pinschers with end-stage cardiomyopathy, *J Vet Int Med* 11:323, 1997.
84. Calvert C: Long-term ambulatory electrocardiographic (Holter) monitoring as an aid in the diagnosis of occult cardiomyopathy in Doberman pinschers, *Proc Annu Vet Med Forum,* 1991, p 691.
85. Calvert CA: Arrhythmias and sudden death in Doberman pinschers with dilated cardiomyopathy, personal communication, 1990.
86. Jacobs GJ, Calvert CA: Survival and prognostic factors in Doberman pinschers with congestive heart failure, *J Vet Intern Med* 9:203, 1995.
87. Calvert CA: Canine dilated cardiomyopathy. In Kirk RW, Bonagura JD, eds: *Kirk's current veterinary therapy, XI: small animal practice,* Philadelphia, 1992, WB Saunders.
88. Monnet E, Orton EC, Salman M et al: Idiopathic dilated cardiomyopathy in dogs: survival and prognostic indicators, *J Vet Intern Med* 9:12, 1995.
89. Roberts WC, Siegel RJ, McManus BM: Idiopathic dilated cardiomyopathy: analysis of 152 necropsy patients, *Am J Cardiol* 60:1340, 1987.
90. Kittleson MD: The efficacy and safety of milrinone for treating heart failure in dogs, *Vet Clin North Am Small Anim Pract* 21:905, 1991.

91. Liu SK, Tilley LP: Animal models of primary myocardial diseases, *Yale J Biol Med* 53:191, 1980.
92. Moise NS, Gilmour RFJ, Riccio ML et al: Diagnosis of inherited ventricular tachycardia in German shepherd dogs, *J Am Vet Med Assoc* 210:403, 1997.
93. Thomas WP: Myocardial diseases of the dog. In Bonagura JD, ed: *Contemporary issues in small animal practice: cardiology,* New York, 1997, Churchill Livingstone.
94. Szatalowicz VL, Arnold PE, Chaimovitz C et al: Radioimmunoassay of plasma arginine vasopressin in hyponatremic patients with congestive heart failure, *N Engl J Med* 305:263, 1981.
95. Saxon LA, Stevenson WG, Middlekauff HR et al: Predicting death from progressive heart failure secondary to ischemic or idiopathic dilated cardiomyopathy, *Am J Cardiol* 72:62, 1993.
96. Unverferth DV, Magorien RD, Lewis RP et al: Long-term benefit of dobutamine in patients with congestive cardiomyopathy, *Am Heart J* 100:622, 1980.
97. Myerburg RJ, Kessler KM: Clinical assessment and management of arrhythmias and conduction disturbances. In Hurst JW, Schlant RC, eds: *The heart,* ed 7, 1995, New York, McGraw-Hill.
98. Calvert CA, Jacobs GJ: Use of tocainide for ventricular tachyarrhythmias in Doberman pinscher dogs with cardiomyopathy, *J Vet Intern Med* 9:199, 1995 (abstract).
99. Brien JF, Jimmo S, Brennan FJ et al: Disposition of amiodarone and its proximate metabolite, desethylamiodarone, in the dog for oral administration of single-dose and short-term drug regimens, *Drug Metab Dispos* 18:846, 1990.
100. el Oakley RM, Jarvis JC: Cardiomyoplasty: a critical review of experimental and clinical results, *Circulation* 90:2085, 1994.
101. Orton EC, Monnet E, Brevard SM et al: Dynamic cardiomyoplasty for treatment of idiopathic dilatative cardiomyopathy in a dog, *J Am Vet Med Assoc* 205:1415, 1994.
102. Orton EC: Dynamic cardiomyoplasty: an update, *Proc Annu Vet Med Forum,* 1995, p 303.
103. Batista JVR, Santos JLV, Takeshita N et al: Partial left ventriculectomy to improve left ventricular function in end-stage heart disease, *J Cardiol Surg* 11:96, 1996.
104. Takeshita N, Kawaguchi AT, Lima PRN et al: Hemodynamic changes in patients undergoing left ventricular diameter reduction (Batista operation), *J Am Coll Cardiol* 29:64A, 1997 (abstract).
105. Chagas C: Nova tripanosomiase humana. Estudos sobre a morfologia e o ciclo evolutivo do *Schizotrypanum cruzi* n. gen., n. sp., agente etioloico de novo entradade morbiba do homen, *Mem Inst Oswaldo Cruz* 1:1, 1909.
106. Barr SC, Simpson RM, Schmidt SP et al: Chronic dilatative myocarditis caused by *Trypanosoma cruzi* in two dogs, *J Am Vet Med Assoc* 195:1237, 1989.
107. Barr S, Baker D, Markovits J: Trypanosomiasis and laryngeal paralysis in a dog, *J Am Vet Med Assoc* 188:1307, 1986.
108. Snider TG, Yaeger RG, Dellucky J: Myocarditis caused by *Trypanosoma cruzi* in a native Louisiana dog, *J Am Vet Med Assoc* 177:247, 1980.
109. Meurs KM, Miller MW, Helman RG: Canine Chagas' myocarditis. In Bonagura JD, ed: *Kirk's current veterinary therapy, XII: small animal practice,* Philadelphia, 1995, WB Saunders.
110. Barr SC, Van Beek O, Carlisle-Nowak MS et al: *Trypanosoma cruzi* infection in Walker hounds from Virginia, *Am J Vet Res* 56:1037, 1995.
111. Barr SC: American trypanosomiasis in dogs, *Compend Cont Educ Pract* 13:745, 1991.
112. Navin TR, Roberto RR, Juranek DD et al: Human and sylvatic *Trypanosoma cruzi* infection in California, *Am J Public Health* 75:366, 1985.
113. Barr SC, Holmes RA, Klei TR: Electrocardiographic and echocardiographic features of trypanosomiasis in dogs inoculated with North American *Trypanosoma cruzi* isolates, *Am J Vet Res* 53:521, 1992.
114. Barr SC, Holmes RA, Klei TR: Electrocardiographic features of trypanosomiasis in dogs inoculated with North American *Trypanosoma cruzi* isolates, *Am J Vet Res* 53:521, 1992.
115. Sole MJ, Liu P: Viral myocarditis: a paradigm for understanding the pathogenesis and treatment of dilated cardiomyopathy, *J Am Coll Cardiol* 22:99A, 1993.
116. Morris SA, Weiss LM, Factor S et al: Verapamil ameliorates clinical, pathologic and biochemical manifestations of experimental chagasic cardiomyopathy in mice, *J Am Coll Cardiol* 14:782, 1989.
117. Hayes MA, Russell RG, Babiuk LA: Sudden death in young dogs with myocarditis caused by parvovirus, *J Am Vet Med Assoc* 174:1197, 1979.
118. Meunier PC, Cooper BJ, Appel MJ et al: Experimental viral myocarditis: parvoviral infection of neonatal pups, *Vet Pathol* 21:509, 1984.
119. Cimprich RE, Robertson JL, Kutz SA et al: Degenerative cardiomyopathy in experimental beagles following parvovirus exposure, *Toxicol Pathol* 9:19, 1981.
120. Robinson WF, Huxtable CR, Pass DA: Canine parvoviral myocarditis: a morphologic description of the natural disease, *Vet Pathol* 17:282, 1980.
121. Liu SK, Keene BW, Fox PR: Myocarditis in the dog and cat. In Bonagura JD, ed: *Kirk's current veterinary therapy, XII: small animal practice,* Philadelphia, 1995, WB Saunders.
122. Levy SA, Duray PH: Complete heart block in a dog seropositive for *Borrelia burgdorferi:* similarity to human Lyme carditis, *J Vet Intern Med* 2:138, 1988.
123. Wynne J, Braunwald E: The cardiomyopathies and myocarditides: toxic, chemical, and physical damage to the heart. In Braunwald E, ed: *Heart disease: a textbook of cardiovascular medicine,* ed 4, Philadelphia, 1992, WB Saunders.
124. Pedersen NC, Griffey SM, Grahn R et al: A transmissible myocarditis/diaphragmitis of cats manifested by transient fever and depression, *Feline Pract* 21:13, 1993.
125. Liu SK, Tilley LP, Tappe JP et al: Clinical and pathologic findings in dogs with atherosclerosis: 21 cases (1970-1983), *J Am Vet Med Assoc* 189:227, 1986.
126. Shinbane JS, Wood MA, Jensen DN et al: Tachycardia-induced cardiomyopathy: a review of animal models and clinical studies, *J Am Coll Cardiol* 29:709, 1997.
127. Spinale FG, Fulbright BM, Mukherjee R et al: Relation between ventricular and myocyte function with tachycardia-induced cardiomyopathy, *Circ Res* 71:174, 1992.
128. Spinale FG, Tanaka R, Crawford FA et al: Changes in myocardial blood flow during development of and recovery from tachycardia-induced cardiomyopathy, *Circulation* 85:717, 1992.
129. Kehoe R, Singer DH, Trapani A et al: Adriamycin-induced cardiac dysrhythmias in an experimental dog model, *Cancer Treat Rep* 62:963, 1978.
130. Van Vleet JF, Ferrans VJ, Weirich WE: Cardiac disease induced by chronic adriamycin administration in dogs and an evaluation of vitamin E and selenium as cardioprotectants, *Am J Pathol* 99:13, 1980.
131. Pessah IN, Schiedt MJ, Shalaby MA et al: Etiology of sarcoplasmic reticulum calcium release channel lesions in doxorubicin-induced cardiomyopathy, *Toxicology* 72:189, 1992.
132. Pessah IN: Calcium release channel of sarcoplasmic reticulum: an important target for doxorubicin-mediated cardiotoxicity, *Adv Exp Med Biol* 311:409, 1992.
133. Ogilvie GK, Richardson RC, Curtis CR et al: Acute and short-term toxicoses associated with the administration of doxorubicin to dogs with malignant tumors, *J Am Vet Med Assoc* 195:1584, 1989.
134. Mauldin-Smith GE, Matus RE, Bond BR: Doxorubicin cardiotoxicity in thirty-two dogs, *Proc AnnuVet Cancer Soc Conf,* 1987, p 41 (abstract).
135. Novotney CA, Page RL, Macy DW et al: Phase I evaluation of doxorubicin and whole-body hyperthermia in dogs with lymphoma, *J Vet Intern Med* 6:245, 1992.
136. Page RL, Macy DW, Ogilvie GK et al: Phase III evaluation of doxorubicin and whole-body hyperthermia in dogs with lymphoma, *Int J Hyperthermia* 8:187, 1992.
137. Tilley LP, Liu SK: Persistent atrial standstill in the dog and cat, *Proc Am Coll Vet Int Med,* 1983, p 43 (abstract).

138. Robinson WF, Thompson RR, Clark WT: Sinoatrial arrest associated with primary atrial myocarditis in a dog, *J Small Anim Pract* 22:99, 1981.
139. Jeraj K, Ogburn PN, Edwards WD et al: Atrial standstill, myocarditis and destruction of cardiac conduction system: clinicopathologic correlation in a dog, *Am Heart J* 99:185, 1980.
140. Liu SK, Hsu FS, Lee RCT: *An atlas of cardiovascular pathology,* Tainan, Taiwan, 1989, Pig Research Institute of Taiwan.
141. Miller MS, Tilley LP, Atkins CE: Persistent atrial standstill (atrioventricular) muscular dystrophy. In Kirk RW, Bonagura JD, eds: *Kirk's current veterinary therapy, XI: small animal practice,* Philadelphia, 1992, WB Saunders.
142. Shelton D: Personal communication, Dr. Diane Shelton, 1996.
143. Paquet M, Hanna BD: Cardiomyopathy. In Garson A, Bricker JT, McNamara DG, eds: *The science and practice of pediatric cardiology,* Philadelphia, 1990, Lea & Febiger.
144. Lombard CW, Buergelt CD: Endocardial fibroelastosis in four dogs, *J Am Anim Hosp Assoc* 20:271, 1984.
145. Wegelius O, von Essen R: Endocardial fibroelastosis in dogs, *Acta Path Microbiol Scand* 77:66, 1969.
146. Zook BC: Some spontaneous cardiovascular lesions in dogs and cats, *Adv Cardiol* 13:148, 1974.
147. Paasch LH, Zook BC: The pathogenesis of endocardial fibroelastosis in Burmese cats, *Lab Invest* 42:197, 1980.
148. Zook BC, Paasch LH, Chandra RS et al: The comparative pathology of primary endocardial fibroelastosis in Burmese cats, *Virchows Arch* 390:211, 1981.
149. Hoffman EP, Brown RHJ, Kunkel LM: Dystrophin: the protein product of the Duchenne muscular dystrophy locus, *Cell* 51:919, 1987.
150. Bonilla E, Samitt CE, Miranda AF et al: Duchenne muscular dystrophy: deficiency of dystrophin at the muscle cell surface, *Cell* 54:447, 1988.
151. Farah MG, Evans EB, Vignos PJJ: Echocardiographic evaluation of left ventricular function in Duchenne's muscular dystrophy, *Am J Med* 69:248, 1980.
152. Valentine BA, Winand NJ, Pradhan D et al: Canine X-linked muscular dystrophy as an animal model of Duchenne muscular dystrophy: a review, *Am J Med Genet* 42:352, 1992.
153. Moise NS, Valentine BA, Brown CA et al: Duchenne's cardiomyopathy in a canine model: electrocardiographic and echocardiographic studies, *J Am Coll Cardiol* 17:812, 1991.
154. Atwell RB: Uhl's anomaly in a cat associated with severe right-sided cardiac decompensation, *J Small Anim Pract* 21:121, 1980.
155. Simpson KW, Bonagura JD, Eaton KA: Right ventricular cardiomyopathy in a dog, *J Vet Intern Med* 8:306, 1994.
156. Marcus FI, Fontaine GH, Guiraudon G et al: Right ventricular dysplasia: a report of 24 adult cases, *Circulation* 65:384, 1982.
157. Thiene G, Nava A, Corrado D et al: Right ventricular cardiomyopathy and sudden death in young people, *N Engl J Med* 318:129, 1988.
158. Coonar AS, Protonotarios N, Tsatsopoulou A et al: A gene locus for arrythmogenic right ventricular cardiomyopathy maps to chromosome 17p1-q3, *J Am Coll Cardiol* 29:4A, 1997 (abstract).

CHAPTER 21

Hypertrophic Cardiomyopathy

Definition

Hypertrophic cardiomyopathy (HCM) is a disease of the ventricular (primarily left ventricular) myocardium characterized by mild-to-severe primary concentric hypertrophy. The word *primary* in this context means that the hypertrophy is due to an inherent problem in the myocardium and is not secondary to a pressure overload or hormonal stimulation. Concentric hypertrophy (a thickened wall with a normal-to-small chamber size) of the left ventricle has numerous secondary causes, including aortic stenosis, systemic arterial hypertension, hyperthyroidism, and acromegaly. When any of these diseases are present, the diagnosis of HCM is excluded and the cardiac abnormality should not be called *HCM.* Instead the abnormality should be called *concentric hypertrophy secondary to the primary abnormality* (e.g., concentric hypertrophy secondary to hyperthyroidism). These disorders typically produce symmetric concentric hypertrophy and a maximum increase in wall thickness of 50% or less, even with severe disease. If severe or asymmetric concentric hypertrophy is present in a patient with one of these disorders, concomitant HCM should be considered. Besides concentric hypertrophy, the myocardium can also thicken as a result of infiltration (e.g., with lymphoma).[1]

Prevalence

HCM is the most commonly diagnosed cardiac disease in cats. From August 1, 1986, to August 1, 1996, we diagnosed moderate-to-severe HCM in 249 cats. This was more than twice the number of congenital cardiac defects diagnosed in cats in this same period. This is a similar incidence to another report, in which 46 cats were diagnosed with HCM during a 2-year period at the Animal Medical Center in New York.[2] HCM is a reported but rare disease in dogs.[3,4] In the dog it has been reported as an isolated lesion, like it is in the cat, and in association with pulmonic stenosis.[5] We diagnosed HCM in 11 dogs in the same 10-year period. Eleven breeds were represented.

Etiology

SARCOMERIC GENE MUTATIONS IN HUMANS WITH HCM

The etiology of HCM in most cats is unknown. It has been known since 1958 that HCM is often familial in humans.[6] It has been demonstrated that approximately 50% of the human cases of HCM are inherited in an autosomal dominant pattern, with the other cases being sporadic (although often still genetic in origin). Since 1989, several specific gene abnormalities associated with HCM have been identified in human families. The first abnormality was a point mutation identified on the β-myosin heavy-chain gene.[7-10] Since then more than 50 point mutations associated with HCM have been identified on this gene.[11] Most commonly these mutations have been identified in families as inherited abnormalities, but de novo (spontaneous) mutations in individuals with no family history have also been identified.[12] Mutations in the α-tropomyosin gene, the cardiac troponin T and I genes, and the myosin-binding protein C gene have also been identified as causes of familial HCM in humans.[11,13-15] Most recently, mutations in the genes that encode for essential and regulatory light chains have been associated with a rare form of HCM in humans, in which midventricular obstruction occurs.[16] Because mutations in genes that encode for myosin, troponin, tropomyosin, myosin-binding protein C, and light chains have now been identified, it appears that familial HCM in humans is most commonly or perhaps exclusively a disease of the sarcomere (contractile element). Approximately 35% to 40% of familial human HCM appears to be due to β-myosin heavy-chain gene mutations.[11] The percentage resulting from troponin and tropomyosin gene mutations are about 15% and 5%, respectively.[17] Consequently, it appears that many other mutations remain to be identified. Another locus in humans has been mapped to chromosome 11q11, but the gene has not been identified.[18]

It has been demonstrated that myosin gene mutations are not just associated with but cause HCM.[19] One laboratory first reported producing a transgenic mouse model in which a specific myosin gene mutation was introduced into developing mice.[20] Another laboratory successfully reproduced this model and documented severe HCM in these mice, thus fulfilling Koch's postulates.[19] Interestingly, although all of the mice have the same genotype, the phenotype varies in that male mice are more severely affected than female mice, similar to the occurrence in cats and humans. This laboratory also demonstrated that more sudden death occurs in exercised mice than in sedentary mice.

Hypertrophy secondary to sarcomeric gene mutations. Why does hypertrophy occur with β-myosin heavy chain gene mutations? DNA comes in pairs of alleles, one inherited from the father and one from the mother. If your father, for example, has HCM because of a mutation in one of his alleles that codes for myosin, then you have a 50-50 chance of inheriting a gene that codes for abnormal myosin (half his myosin genes are normal and half are abnormal). We're assuming that your mother does not have the disease. If you inherit your father's abnormal gene, half your genes that make myosin are abnormal (father) and half are normal (mother). This means that half your myosin is abnormal. The contractility of mutated β-myosin is decreased, so the sarcomere involved does not function correctly.[21,22] Presumably this increases the stress on the normal sarcomeres. Consequently, the heart tries to replace the abnormal sarcomeres by producing new sarcomeres.[11,23,24] When the heart turns on its DNA, it has a 50-50 chance of replacing the defective sarcomere with a sarcomere that has normal myosin and a 50-50 chance of replacing it with another sarcomere with defective myosin. If it replaces it with a defective sarcomere, it must try again and has the same chance again. The net result is that the heart ends up having twice as much myosin and twice as many sarcomeres as it should have. Because sarcomeres make up a large part of the heart muscle, the heart muscle ultimately almost doubles in thickness. Consequently, instead of producing dilated cardiomyopathy, as one might expect if contractile proteins are abnormal, HCM is produced instead.

FAMILIAL FELINE HCM

Recently we identified the first family of cats (Maine coon cats) with HCM, 35 years after the first identification of a human family.[25] We reproduced the disease by mating affected to unaffected and affected to affected Maine coon cats. We demonstrated that the course of the disease is accelerated in affected cats produced by mating affected to affected cats. These data strongly suggest that the disease is inherited in this breed. The pattern of inheritance produced by selected matings suggests that the disease is inherited in a simple autosomal dominant pattern, as it is in humans. In Maine coon cats there appears to be complete penetrance, which means that all cats with a mutation have HCM. The disease is progressive. In most affected Maine coon cats HCM has not been apparent at 3 months of age but has become apparent by 6 months to 2.5 years of age (Figure 21-1).[26] Some cats that have evidence of the disease early in life have only mild thickening and systolic anterior motion of the mitral valve. Offspring from mating affected to affected cats can have severe disease by 6 months of age. Studies are currently in progress to determine if specific sarcomeric gene abnormalities exist in this family of cats.

We also identified a family of American shorthair cats with primarily systolic anterior motion of the mitral valve, but with evidence of HCM also. The disease in this breed also appears to be inherited as an autosomal dominant trait.[27]

Some mutations in humans produce malignant disease in which survival time is short, whereas other mutations produce benign

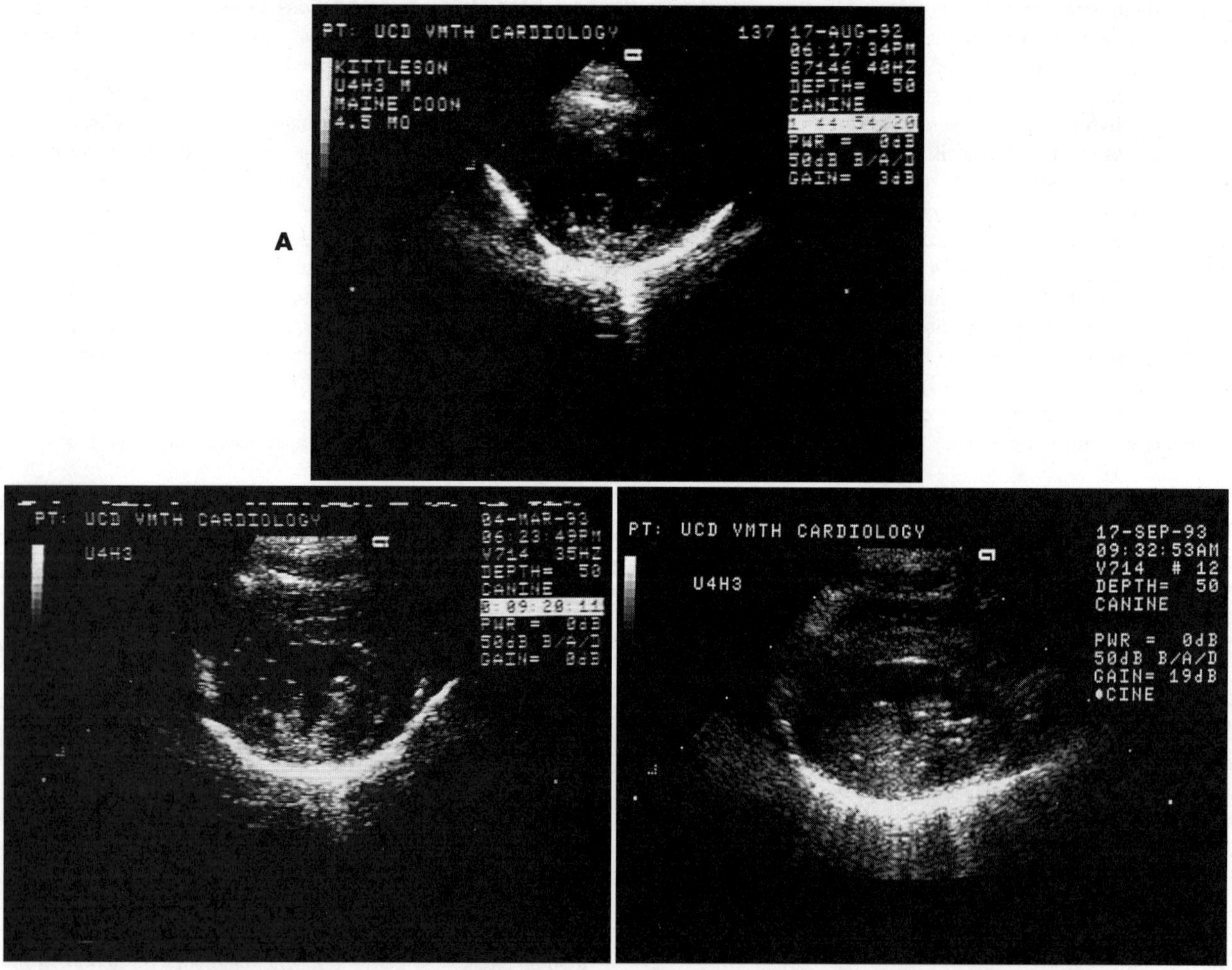

FIGURE 21-1 Two-dimensional echocardiograms taken from an intact male Maine coon cat that developed hypertrophic cardiomyopathy over the first 1 to 1.5 years of life and died of heart failure at 2.5 years of age. **A,** Cross-sectional view of the heart taken at 4.5 months of age. No evidence of hypertrophic cardiomyopathy was present at this time. **B,** The same view, taken at 11 months of age. The papillary muscles appear prominent. **C,** The same view, taken at 17 months of age. The left ventricular free wall and papillary muscles are grossly thickened. The interventricular septum is not thickened. The appearance of the left ventricle remained stable until the cat died at 2.5 years of age from heart failure.

disease with little change in survival.[28,29] Whereas the Maine coon breed appears to have a very malignant disease, the American shorthair appears to have a more benign disease.

GROWTH HORMONE

An increase in serum growth hormone concentration was identified in about 60% of the cats with HCM studied in our clinic.[30] Growth hormone is a known inducer of myocardial hypertrophy. Cats with acromegaly can have quite severe concentric hypertrophy of the left ventricular myocardium.[31] In humans, serum growth hormone concentration is increased in patients with heart failure. In cats with HCM, elevations were identified in cats both with and without heart failure. Whether the increase in serum growth hormone concentration is the cause, is the result, or is unrelated to feline HCM is unknown.

Pathology

GROSS PATHOLOGY

Cats with severe HCM have severe thickening of the left ventricular myocardium (the interventricular septum and free wall), with the entire wall commonly being 8 to 11 mm thick (Color Plate 85). As in many pathologic specimens, hearts from cats with HCM may undergo contraction following death, resulting in a wall thickness that is closer to the end-systolic wall thickness in life rather than the end-diastolic thickness. Papillary muscle hypertrophy is often very prominent. The left ventricular chamber is often smaller than normal because of the myocardial thickening encroaching on the left ventricular cavity. The volume may again be closer to an end-systolic volume because of rigor. In most cats, the left ventricular free wall and the interventricular septum are equally thickened (symmetric hypertrophy).[2,32] In some cats the interventricular septum is significantly thicker than the free wall, whereas in a few others the free wall is thicker (asymmetric hypertrophy).[2,33] The left atrium is usually enlarged, often markedly so. However, with early, severe disease we have identified normal left atrial size in some Maine coon cats. Occasionally a thrombus is present in the body of the left atrium or within the left auricle.

Cats with milder forms of the disease (mild-to-moderate HCM) have lesser wall thickening and a more normal-size left ventricular chamber. The left atrium may be normal in size or mildly-to-severely enlarged. Papillary muscle hypertrophy may be the predominant lesion.

Heart weight is a useful indicator of disease severity and is useful to identify hearts with hypertrophy. For this procedure, the pericardium should be removed from the heart and the aorta and pulmonary artery transected so that no more than 2 to 4 cm are left. Normal heart-weight–to–body-weight ratio has been reported to be 4.8 ± 1.8 g/kg with cats, with HCM having a ratio of 6.0 ± 1.4 g/kg.[2] This results in a large overlap between the two groups. In our experience, most normal-size cats (4 to 6 kg) have a heart that weighs less than 20 g, and most cats in this size range with HCM have a heart that weighs more than 20 g. Cats with severe HCM almost always have a heart that weighs more than 25 g, and it can weigh as much as 35 g.

HISTOPATHOLOGY

Histopathologically, there is a wide range of abnormalities. In some hearts, only myocyte hypertrophy is evident. On the other end of the spectrum, some cats have severe interstitial and interfibril fibrosis and dystrophic mineralization.[32] Moderate-to-severe interstitial or replacement fibrosis is present in about 20% to 40% of cases.[32] Intramural coronary arteriosclerosis is present in approximately 75% of cats with HCM.[2,32] This appears to result from proliferation of smooth muscle cells and connective tissue elements in the media and the intima. The lumenae of these small arteries are often obliterated. In humans, intramyocardial small artery disease is not specific for HCM, because it is also identified in patients with systemic hypertension.[34] The myocardial fibrosis seen in some cats may be secondary to the small intramural coronary artery obstructions, as speculated to be the case in humans.[35,36] However, this association is controversial.[37] Maine coon cats consistently have both moderate-to-severe intramural coronary artery disease and fibrosis.

In humans, myocardial fiber disarray that involves at least 5% of the myocardium in the interventricular septum is found in 90% of patients.[38,39] This finding is also quite specific for HCM in humans. Other diseases that produce concentric hypertrophy can also cause myocardial fiber disarray, but this almost always involves less than 1% of the myocardium. In cats with HCM, myocardial fiber disarray in the interventricular septum of the same magnitude observed in humans is only identified in approximately 30% of cases (Color Plate 86).[32,40] However, myocardial fiber disarray is a consistent feature of HCM in Maine coon cats. Sarcomeres also have disarray in human patients with HCM. Interestingly, investigators in one study have examined whether or not myosin mutations cause myofiber disarray in cats by infecting isolated feline cardiocytes with an adenoviral vector containing a full-length mutated human β-myosin heavy-chain gene.[41] Within 5 days, 50% of the cardiocytes had evidence of severe sarcomere disruption.

Pathophysiology

HYPERTROPHY

Severe HCM is characterized by a thick left ventricular myocardium with a normal-to-small left ventricular chamber. The concentric hypertrophy results in a stiff chamber and also results in a decrease in afterload because of the increase in wall thickness. The stiff chamber causes an increase in diastolic intraventricular pressure, left atrial enlargement, and congestive heart failure. The decreased afterload results in a decrease in end-systolic volume, often to zero (cavity obliteration). Abnormal papillary muscle orientation and other unexplained factors commonly also produce systolic anterior motion of the mitral valve and therefore mitral regurgitation in this disease.

The increased chamber stiffness results in an increased left ventricular diastolic pressure, as seen in Figure 21-2. Stiffness is Δpressure/Δvolume. This means there is a greater increase in pressure for any given increase in volume when the ventricle fills in diastole. The myocardium from cats with HCM also takes a longer time to relax in early diastole.[42] This can cause an increase in diastolic pressure if the heart rate is very fast (if diastole is so short that the ventricle cannot relax to a normal point in the time allotted). Incomplete relaxation of the myocardium may also occur. Increased chamber stiffness can be demonstrated by blowing up a normal balloon and then blowing up a thick-walled balloon and noting the pressure in your mouth "chamber" necessary to distend the two balloons. It takes a larger pressure to distend the thick-walled balloon than it does to distend a thin-walled ventricle. The increased stiffness results in elevated left atrial and pulmonary venous pressures, which can cause pulmonary edema or pleural effusion in cats and humans.[43] Myocardial fibrosis exacerbates the abnormal diastolic function in most cats and probably worsens with age.

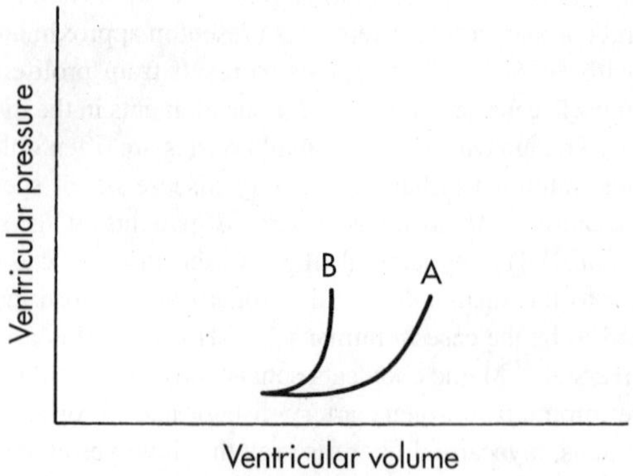

FIGURE 21-2 Theoretical pressure-volume diagram of two diastolic curves. The curve labeled *A* is normal, and the curve labeled *B* is from a patient with HCM. Curve *B* is steeper and shifted to the left. The shift to the left occurs because the chamber is smaller than normal. The steepness reflects an increase in left ventricular wall stiffness (decreased compliance) that occurs because of the increase in wall thickness and possibly increased fibrosis.

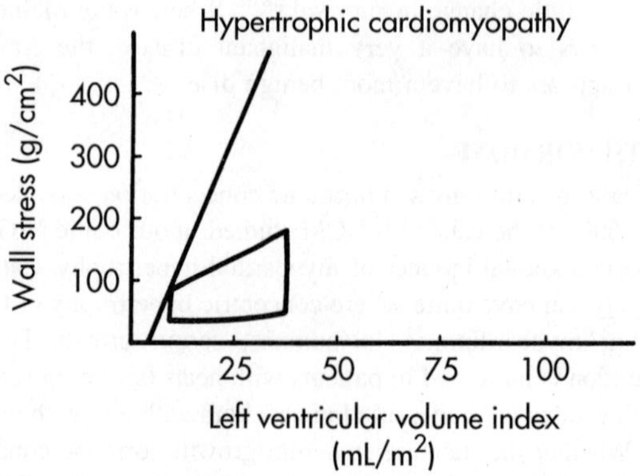

FIGURE 21-3 Theoretical wall stress–volume loop from a patient with HCM. Contractility is normal, as evidenced by the normal relationship between end-systolic volume and end-systolic wall stress (E_{max}). Peak systolic wall stress (afterload) is decreased because of the increase in wall thickness. Consequently, end-systolic volume is decreased. End-diastolic volume is decreased because the thickened wall has encroached on the chamber space.

The schematic in Color Plate 87 demonstrates the changes in left ventricular volumes and mass. This figure is a schematic drawing of the left ventricle similar to those in Chapters 2 and 9. Because HCM occurs most frequently in cats, it seems appropriate to make the left ventricular volumes cat-size. To be consistent, however, the same size (25 to 30 kg) of animal as used in the previous chapters has been used.

When left ventricular hypertrophy is severe, it is common for the left ventricular wall thickness to be twice normal thickness. Consequently, left ventricular wall thickness is 2 cm/m^2 in Color Plate 87. This severe concentric hypertrophy encroaches on the left ventricular cavity so that it decreases in size (the left ventricular end-diastolic volume has decreased from 53 to 37 mL/m^2). Anyone who has seen an angiogram from a cat with HCM is aware that the end-systolic volume is also greatly reduced. The chamber often appears to almost completely empty, and the walls may actually touch (cavity obliteration). End-systolic volume could be decreased from an increase in contractility or a decrease in afterload. Studies in humans have shown that global myocardial contractility is normal; that is, the properties of the myocardial cells themselves have not changed at all.[44] Instead the increased thickness of the walls and the reduced chamber size result in a decrease in systolic wall stress or afterload (wall stress = [pressure × radius] ÷ [2 × wall thickness]) and consequently end-systolic volume decreases (Color Plate 87). In this theoretical case, end-systolic volume has decreased from a normal value of 16 mL/m^2 to 2 mL/m^2. Total stroke volume is preserved at 35 mL/m^2. Mitral regurgitation may be present, however; therefore, instead of all of the stroke volume going into the aorta, 10 mL/m^2 might go into the left atrium and 25 mL/m^2 into the aorta. Heart rate would have to increase to compensate for the decrease in forward (aortic) stroke volume. Note that shortening fraction is greater in this situation than in the normal animal presented in Chapter 2 (60% vs. 33%), yet the stroke volume is the same because of the decreases in end-diastolic and end-systolic volumes. The left ventricular weight has increased to 294 g, the largest increase illustrated. The weight increase is due to the increased number of contractile elements laid down in parallel to each other (concentric hypertrophy) and possibly is also due to myocardial cell hyperplasia.[45]

In addition to hypertrophy producing a stiff chamber, it encroaches on the diastolic volume of the chamber, making it smaller. If the end-diastolic volume becomes small enough, stroke volume must also decrease. Stroke volume could decrease to the point that total body perfusion (cardiac output) decreases. Reduction in renal blood flow would result in renin release with subsequent aldosterone secretion. We have measured plasma aldosterone concentration in six cats with heart failure secondary to HCM and found it to be elevated. An increase in plasma aldosterone concentration leads to an increase in blood volume, which further increases the left ventricular filling pressure and left atrial pressure.

In Figure 21-3, a wall stress–volume loop from a cat with HCM is depicted. Contractility is normal, as evidenced by the normal end-systolic wall stress–volume relationship but end-systolic volume is markedly decreased because of the decrease in systolic wall stress. Wall stress is decreased because of the increase in wall thickness, the decrease in chamber radius, and the normal systolic intraventricular pressure.

SYSTOLIC ANTERIOR MOTION OF THE MITRAL VALVE

A phenomenon called *systolic anterior motion (SAM)* of the mitral valve is a common abnormality identified in cats with HCM. In one survey of 46 cats, SAM was present in 67%.[2] SAM of the mitral valve is the process of the septal (anterior) mitral valve leaflet being pulled into the left ventricular outflow tract during systole. It is then caught in the blood flow and pushed toward or against the interventricular septum (Figures 21-4 and 21-5). The mechanism by which SAM occurs is controversial. The most popular theory is that the Venturi effect creates SAM (much like blowing between two sheets of paper that are close together results in the papers being drawn toward one another instead of being blown apart). For the Venturi effect to occur, the anterior leaflet of the mitral valve must already be close to the interventricular septum for the high-velocity flow to draw it toward the septum. This theory does not explain how the leaflet gets to the initial position. Normally the septal leaflet is far from the septum in systole and is closed, with its coaptation point in the center of the chamber. Consequently, we do not believe that the Venturi effect is the major contributor to the production of SAM. The initial pulling of the mitral valve leaflet toward the left ventricular outflow tract in systole is probably due to the malorientation of the papillary muscles in the grossly hypertrophied left ventricle in patients with HCM. This

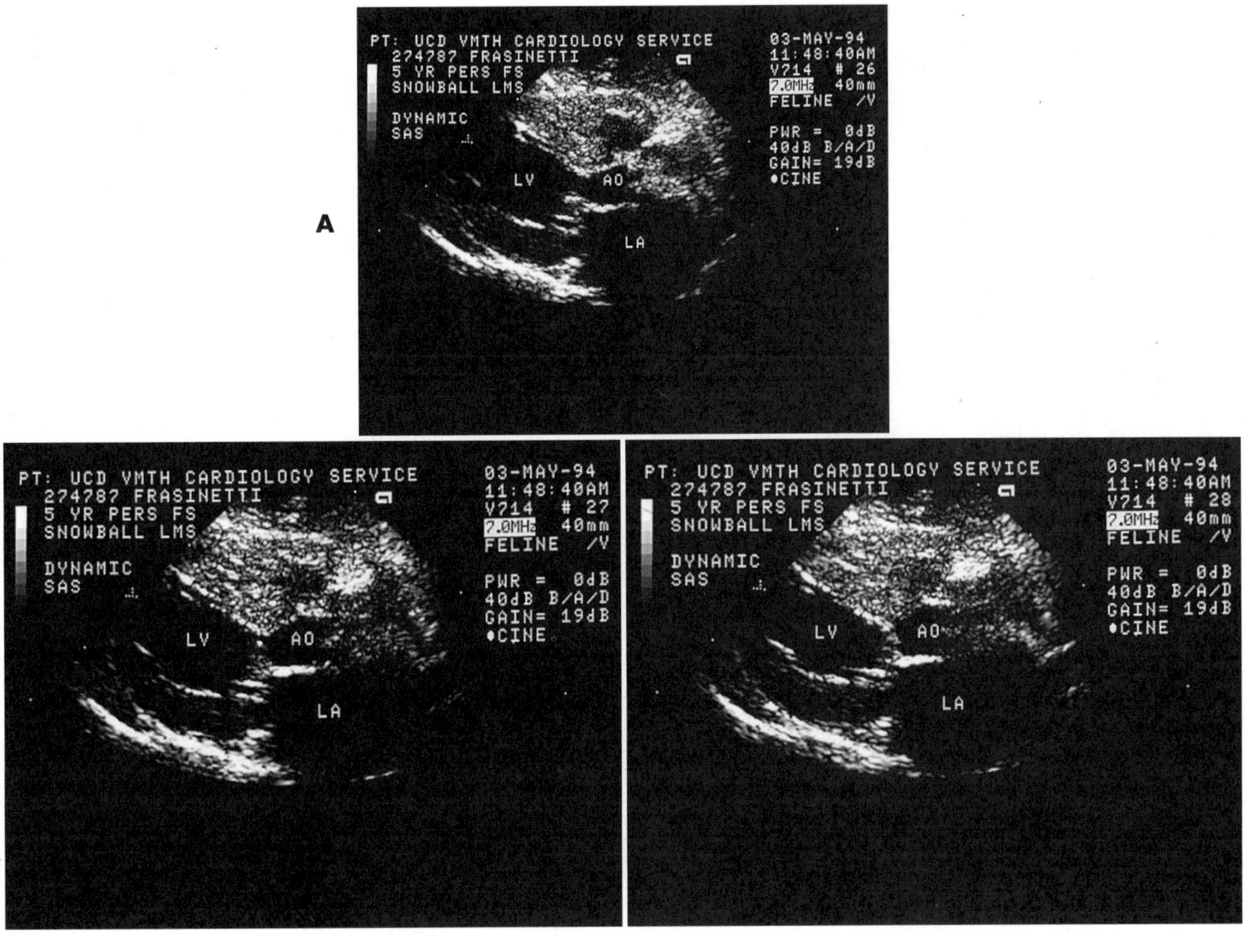

FIGURE 21-4 Sequential two-dimensional echocardiographic frames (*26, 27,* and *28*) showing systolic anterior motion of the mitral valve in a cat with hypertrophic cardiomyopathy. **A,** Long-axis view of the left ventricle *(LV),* left atrium *(LA),* and aorta *(AO)* taken in early systole. The mitral valve leaflets are closed. **B,** One frame later, a small portion of the septal mitral valve leaflet is present in the subaortic region. **C,** One more frame later, a portion of the septal mitral valve leaflet almost touches the interventricular septum.

situation has been reproduced experimentally in dogs by surgically displacing their papillary muscles cranially.[46] We believe that the septal leaflet of the mitral valve is pulled toward the left ventricular outflow tract by the abnormally positioned papillary muscles. The tip of the leaflet then gets caught in the blood flow. Blood flow slams the leaflet tip up against the interventricular septum once it is pulled into the outflow tract. When the septal leaflet is pulled toward the interventricular septum, this leaves a gap in the mitral valve, creating a leak (mitral regurgitation). Simultaneously, a dynamic subaortic stenosis is created that increases systolic intraventricular pressure in mid-to-late systole. Consequently, SAM produces two abnormalities. First, it obstructs flow out of the left ventricle in systole (dynamic subaortic stenosis). This increases the velocity of blood flow through the subaortic region and may produce turbulence (Color Plate 88 and Figure 21-6). Second, by drawing the septal leaflet out of its normal position, SAM creates mitral regurgitation (Color Plate 88). Mitral regurgitation may be the abnormality of primary significance caused by SAM in cats if the mitral regurgitation is severe enough to contribute to the development of heart failure in feline HCM. The argument against this happening is that the color flow Doppler jet that is present in the left atrium is commonly small compared with patients that have primary mitral regurgitation and heart failure. However, color flow Doppler may underestimate the amount of

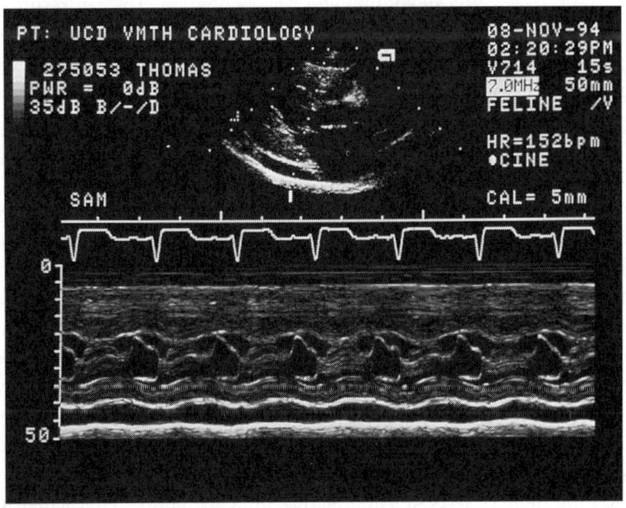

FIGURE 21-5 M-mode echocardiogram from a cat with severe hypertrophic cardiomyopathy showing systolic anterior motion of the mitral valve. The systolic anterior motion occurs between the diastolic openings of the mitral valve leaflets. The septal leaflet moves toward the interventricular septum in systole.

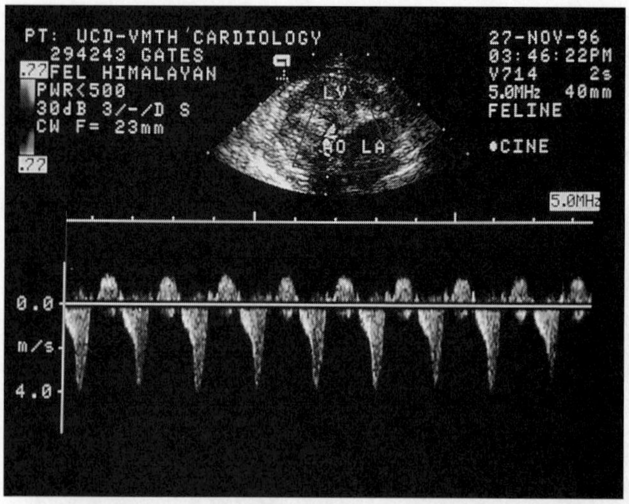

FIGURE 21-6 Continuous-wave Doppler tracing from a Himalayan cat with hypertrophic cardiomyopathy. The transducer has been placed at the left ventricular apex and the beam directed across the obstructed left ventricular outflow tract and aorta. Blood flow velocity is markedly increased to 4.0 m/sec. This translates into a pressure gradient of 64 mm Hg. The shape of the tracing is typical for a dynamic subaortic stenosis showing the marked increase in velocity that starts in midsystole.

regurgitation in cats because of the fast heart rate compared with the slow frame rate in current machines. Even if the amount of regurgitation is less than that seen in primary mitral regurgitation, it may contribute to the generation of heart failure.

SUMMATION OF PROBLEMS THAT LEAD TO HEART FAILURE

We now have four interrelated problems. (1) The increased wall thickness encroaches on the end-diastolic volume, making it smaller. (2) The increased wall thickness and possibly fibrosis causes an increase in left ventricular chamber stiffness. (3) The mitral regurgitation secondary to SAM may increase left atrial pressure further. (4) Decreased perfusion may increase renin and aldosterone secretion, resulting in sodium and water retention. The net result is increased left ventricular diastolic, left atrial, and pulmonary vein pressures that increase pulmonary capillary pressure and capillary pressure in the visceral pleura. Pulmonary edema and sometimes pleural effusion result.

PLEURAL EFFUSION

Cats with severe HCM that present in heart failure most commonly have pulmonary edema secondary to the left heart abnormalities. However, some cats with HCM have pleural effusion. Usually this is only a small amount of an effusion, but in a few cases the effusion can be considerable (Figure 21-7). Pleural effusion in cats with heart failure can be a modified transudate or can be pseudochylous or true chylous in nature. It is unknown exactly why pleural effusion develops in these cats. There are two likely possibilities. The first is that the elevation in pulmonary vein and pulmonary capillary pressures results in pulmonary vasoconstriction, pulmonary hypertension, and right heart failure. This scenario commonly occurs in humans and horses with left heart failure but does not usually occur in dogs. It may occur in cats, but in our experience identifying evidence of right heart enlargement on an echocardiogram in these cases is unusual. It is also unusual to identify other evidence of right heart failure, such as an increase in central venous pressure, jugular vein distension, hepatic vein distension on ultrasound, or ascites. The second possibility is that feline visceral pleural veins drain into the pulmonary veins such that elevated pulmonary vein pressure (congestive left heart failure) causes the formation of pleural effusion. It has been known since 1907 that the visceral pleura in the dog is supplied by pulmonary arteries and drained by pulmonary veins.[47] In 1961, McLaughlin et al[48] described comparative lung types and grouped the dog, cat, and monkey together as having type II lungs. One characteristic of type II lungs is that the visceral pleura is thin (as opposed to thick, as in the cow, pig, sheep, and horse) and is supplied not by bronchial arteries but by pulmonary arteries. Presumably this means that cat visceral pleura is also drained by pulmonary veins, and therefore pulmonary venous hypertension secondary to left heart failure could cause pleural effusion in cats. A right atrial pressure tracing from a cat with HCM and pleural effusion is presented in Figure 21-8. This cat had no right heart enlargement on an echocardiogram, no jugular vein distension when he was standing, and no hepatic vein distension on an ultrasound examination. He did, however, have distended jugular veins when in sternal recumbency and when steady pressure was applied to his abdomen (a positive hepatojugular reflux test). His mean right atrial pressure was normal, proving that he did not have right congestive heart failure. Consequently, it was presumed that pleural effusion formed secondary to left heart failure.

THROMBOEMBOLISM

Thrombi in cats with HCM may develop in the left atrium or left auricle (Figure 21-9). Left atrial thrombi commonly break loose (become emboli) and are carried by blood flow, most commonly to the terminal aorta, where they lodge. These thromboemboli occlude aortic blood flow and elaborate substances that constrict collateral vessels. The net result is cessation of blood flow to the caudal legs, resulting in acute paresis/paralysis and pain. In humans, the presence of echocardiographic "smoke" (an amorphous, swirling, light gray haze also known as *spontaneous echo contrast*) in the left atrium is associated with increased risk of thromboembolic disease.[49] Echocardiographic "smoke" is probably the result of red cell aggregation that occurs when blood flow velocity is low.[50] We and others have noted echocardiographic "smoke" in some cats with HCM and an enlarged left atrium, in some cats with HCM and left atrial thrombi, and in some cats with HCM and thromboembolic disease. Believing that blood flow velocity would be decreased in an enlarged atrium is rational, especially in the auricle. Consequently, the presence of moderate-to-severe left atrial enlargement in a cat with HCM should probably be considered a risk factor for development of thromboembolic disease. Identification of echocardiographic "smoke" should probably be considered an additional risk factor. For additional discussion regarding systemic thromboembolism see Chapter 31.

Clinical Presentation

DEVELOPMENT

In humans, familial HCM develops in most individuals over the first 2 decades of life.[51] The disease has been observed in cats as young as 6 months of age and as old as 16 years of age. We have documented one Maine coon cat without evidence of HCM at 3 months of age that died of the disease at 1 year of age, another in which the disease progressed from 6 months to 18 months of age, another in which the disease was fully progressed by 15 months of age, and yet another in which the disease was not fully developed until 2.5 years of age. Consequently, the HCM

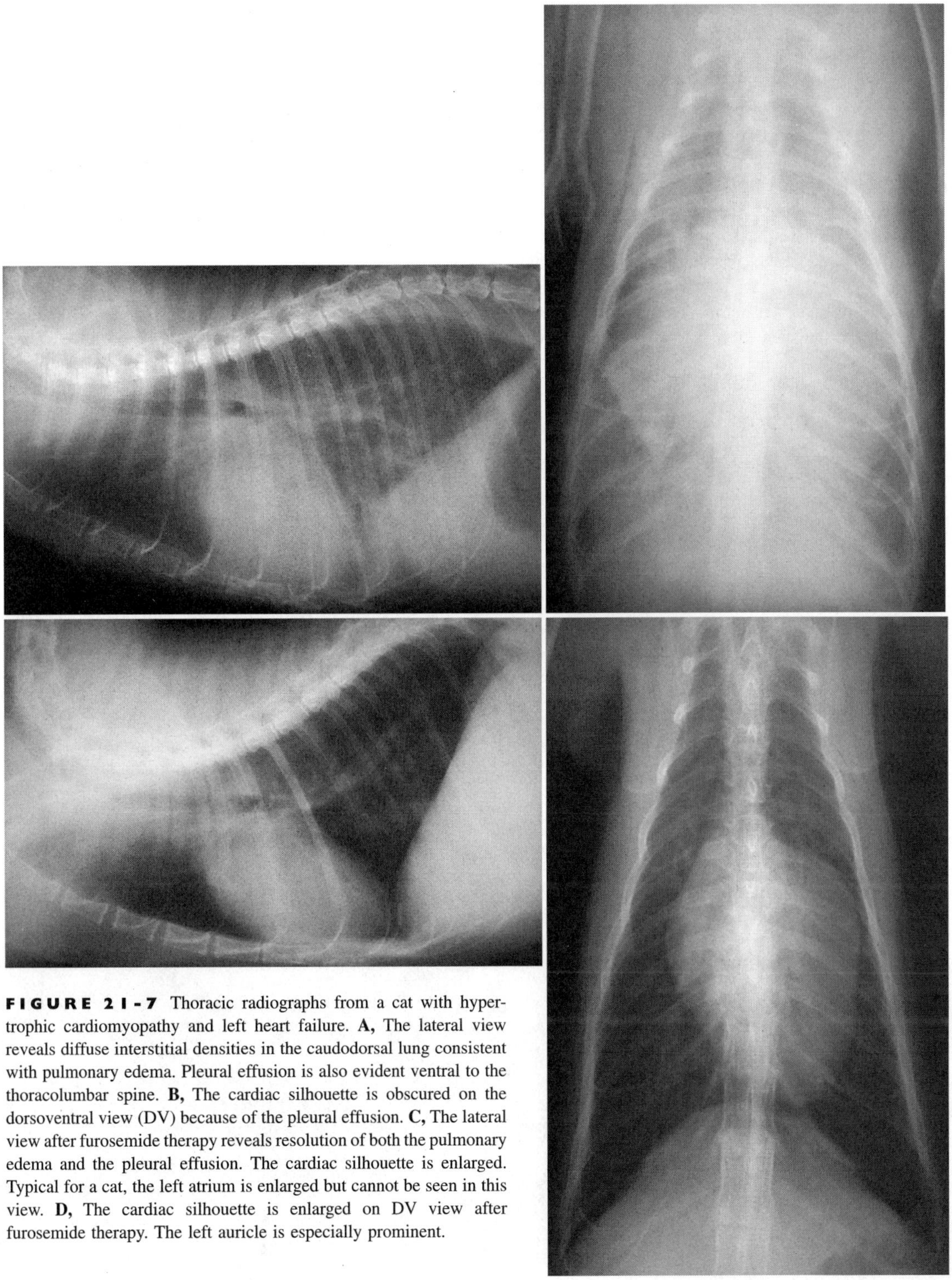

A B C D

FIGURE 21-7 Thoracic radiographs from a cat with hypertrophic cardiomyopathy and left heart failure. **A,** The lateral view reveals diffuse interstitial densities in the caudodorsal lung consistent with pulmonary edema. Pleural effusion is also evident ventral to the thoracolumbar spine. **B,** The cardiac silhouette is obscured on the dorsoventral view (DV) because of the pleural effusion. **C,** The lateral view after furosemide therapy reveals resolution of both the pulmonary edema and the pleural effusion. The cardiac silhouette is enlarged. Typical for a cat, the left atrium is enlarged but cannot be seen in this view. **D,** The cardiac silhouette is enlarged on DV view after furosemide therapy. The left auricle is especially prominent.

in this breed appears to develop over the first 1 to 3 years of life. We have also seen Maine coon cats that have had moderate-to-severe hypertrophy all of their life die suddenly or from heart failure between 7 and 10 years of age. This means that it is possible that when a veterinarian examines an older cat with HCM, the disease has been present for all of the cat's life.

PRESENTATION

Cats with HCM may be completely asymptomatic, may be presented to a veterinarian with subtle signs of heart failure, may have moderate-to-severe heart failure, or may be presented because of thromboembolic disease. They may also die suddenly. Asymptomatic cats can have mild-to-severe left ventricular thickening. However, those with severe thickening usually go on to develop heart failure. Cats with severe disease that appear to be asymptomatic often show subtle signs of heart failure that can be detected by an observant owner. The respiratory rate is often increased in these cats at rest, and they may become more tachypneic or even dyspneic if stressed, although they usually recover quickly following stress. Cats with mild-to-moderate thickening may never develop clinical signs referable to their disease and may live normal lives. In others, the left ventricular wall may thicken further and complications (heart failure, thromboembolism) may develop.

Cats with severe HCM and moderate-to-severe heart failure are usually presented to a veterinarian because of respiratory abnormalities, usually tachypnea or dyspnea. Coughing is less common in cats than in dogs. However, coughing in cats is commonly mistaken for vomiting. Consequently, the owner's chief complaint at presentation can be vomiting. The respiratory abnormalities observed in cats with HCM are due to pulmonary edema, pleural effusion, or both. Because household cats are generally sedentary, owners usually do not notice that they are having respiratory difficulty until the dyspnea is advanced. At that time, the onset of the disease commonly appears to be acute or peracute to the owner, whereas in reality the disease has been present for years, and the heart failure has probably been gradually worsening over months to years.

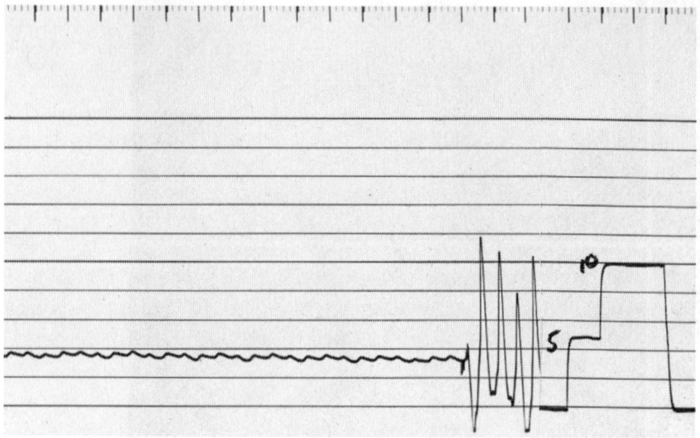

FIGURE 21-8 Right atrial pressure tracing from a cat with hypertrophic cardiomyopathy and pleural effusion. The mean right atrial pressure is normal (approximately 4 mm Hg). The tip of the catheter appears to be close to the tricuspid valve, resulting in large variations in the pulsatile pressure. This probably artifactually increased the mean pressure.

THROMBOEMBOLISM

Cats with thromboembolic disease present most commonly because of the peracute onset of posterior paresis or paralysis and pain resulting from a large thromboembolus lodging at the aortic trifurcation. These cats do not have palpable femoral artery pulses, have pale–to–blue-tinged pads or nail beds, and have turgid gastrocnemius muscles. Lack of flow to the rear limbs can be documented by Doppler examination or by cutting a nail back to the "quick" and observing for lack of blood flow. Smaller thromboemboli may exit the aorta, causing a variety of signs. One of the more common signs resulting from a smaller thromboembolus is right front leg lameness. This occurs when a small thromboembolus takes the first major exit off the aorta (the brachiocephalic trunk) and then the next exit (the right subclavian artery) to the right front leg. Smaller thromboemboli may also lodge in one femoral artery, resulting in loss of blood flow to only one rear leg. (See Chapter 31 for the discussion of thromboembolism.)

SUDDEN DEATH

Cats with severe HCM may die suddenly, often with no prior clinical signs referable to heart failure. To our knowledge, an electrocardiogram has not been recorded during sudden death of any cat that had HCM. Consequently, we do not know what causes the sudden death. In humans, sudden death appears to be due to either arrhythmic or hemodynamic causes.[52] The hemodynamic cause is usually an acutely worsening outflow tract obstruction associated with strenuous exercise (which probably ultimately leads to a terminal arrhythmia). Because cats are not usually subjected to strenuous exercise, this is a less likely cause in cats, although it could occur with extreme excitement. In our experience, sudden death in Maine coon cats is usually not associated with any type of physical stress. It is more likely that these cats die of an acute

A

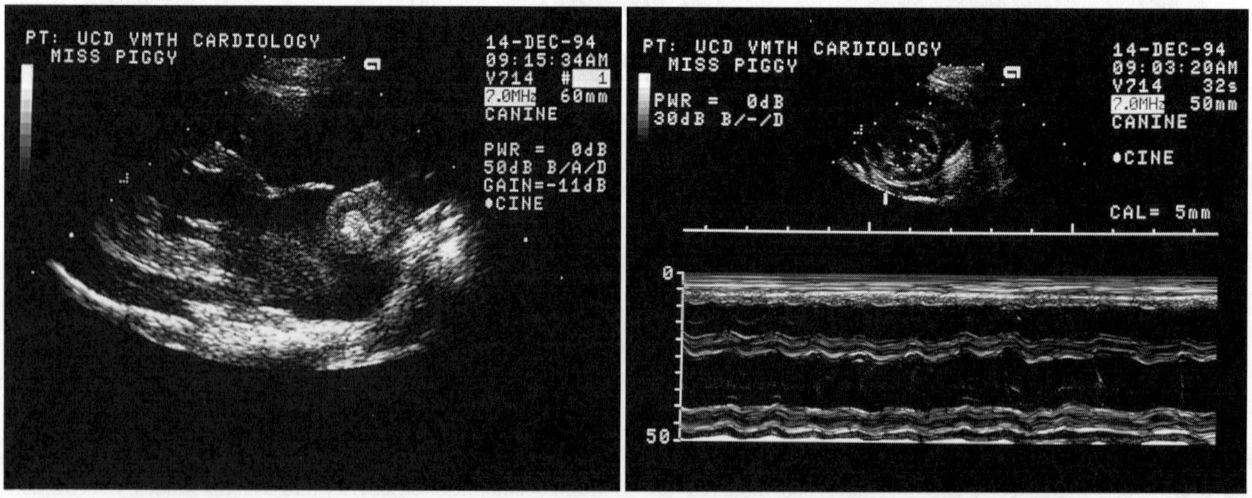

B

FIGURE 21-9 Two-dimensional (**A**) (right parasternal long-axis view) and an M-mode echocardiogram (**B**) from a Maine coon cat with terminal hypertrophic cardiomyopathy. A large thrombus is present in the left atrium, which was mobile. It is surrounded by spontaneous echo contrast ("smoke"). This cat's left ventricular walls are thinner, and the left ventricular cavity is larger than they had been previously. Left ventricular wall motion is poor on the M-mode echocardiogram, indicating that myocardial failure has developed. The cat died 4 hours later from global hypoperfusion. At postmortem examination, the thrombus had increased in size and occluded the left ventricular cavity.

ventricular tachyarrhythmia that degenerates into ventricular fibrillation. The incidence of sudden death in feline HCM is probably underrepresented in the veterinary literature because cats that die suddenly are not presented to veterinarians. Owners commonly do not report their cat's death to a veterinarian, especially if the event is not witnessed and the cat is just found dead. We have also documented one cat in which a large and mobile left atrial thrombus was noted 4 hours before death (see Figure 21-9). The cat died subacutely from severe hypoperfusion. At postmortem examination, the thrombus had increased in size and completely occluded the left ventricular cavity.

AUSCULTATION

Cats with severe HCM usually have auscultatory abnormalities. A systolic murmur, heard best over the cranial sternum or left apex is common and is probably due either to outflow tract obstruction or mitral regurgitation or both (SAM). The murmur is often dynamic, increasing in intensity when the cat becomes excited, with heart rate and contractility increasing and decreasing in intensity or disappearing when the cat is calm. A gallop sound is also common, especially in cats in heart failure. In cats with fast heart rates, rapid ventricular filling and atrial systole (the two times at which gallop sounds are generated) occur very close together, so that on an M-mode echocardiogram the mitral valve only opens once. Consequently it is often impossible to tell in a cat with tachycardia whether the gallop sound is an audible third, fourth, or summated heart sound. It is only of academic interest because differentiation of the third heart sound from the fourth heart sound does not distinguish the type of heart disease present. Interestingly, even if the gallop sound is present after the *P* wave on an electrocardiogram, it may still be a third heart sound if the heart rate is fast, as illustrated in Figure 21-10.

DOGS

Dogs with HCM may present in heart failure, may die suddenly, or may die during anesthetic procedures.[3] A systolic heart murmur is often present. Heart failure can be severe.

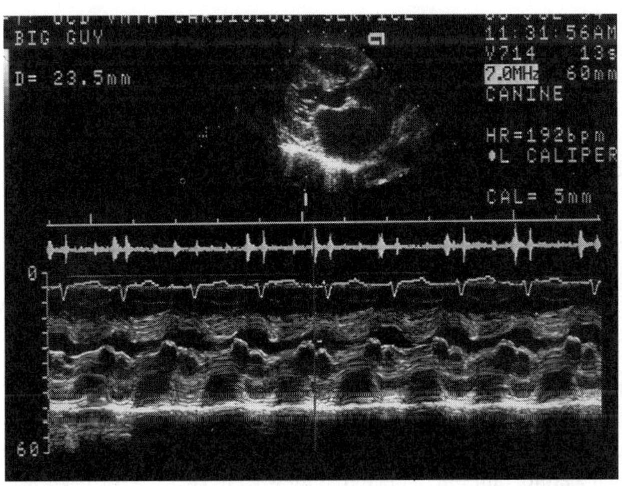

FIGURE 21-10 Simultaneous recordings of a phonocardiogram, an electrocardiogram, and an M-mode echocardiogram. During the fourth cardiac cycle, a vertical line has been placed to show the relationship between the gallop sound, the *P* wave on the electrocardiogram, and the mitral valve. The gallop sound occurs after the *P* wave but before the *A* point on the mitral valve on the echocardiogram, documenting that it is a third heart sound.

Diagnosis

ECHOCARDIOGRAPHY

The diagnosis of HCM is most commonly and preferably made using echocardiography. Angiocardiography can be used to make the diagnosis but is invasive and associated with a much higher complication rate (Figures 21-11 and 21-12). On echocardiography, cats with severe HCM usually have markedly thickened left ventricular walls (8 to 10 mm), papillary muscle hypertrophy, and an enlarged left atrium (Figure 21-13). The hypertrophy can be global, affecting all areas of the left ventricular wall or can be more regional or segmental (see Figure 21-1).[2] In segmental forms the entire interventricular septum or free wall or a region of them may be primarily affected, the apex primarily affected, or the papillary muscles (and often the adjacent free wall) primarily affected. Because of these forms, HCM is a diagnosis that should be made by examining several two-dimensional echocardiographic views and measuring wall thicknesses in diastole from the region or regions of thickening on the two-dimensional images. M-mode echocardiography may miss regional thickening unless it is guided by the two-dimensional view. An M-mode echocardiogram taken from immediately below the mitral valve leaflets (the standard view for measuring left ventricular wall thicknesses and chamber diameters) may miss regional wall thickening. Dogs with HCM have similar echocardiographic findings and usually also have SAM (Figure 21-14).

Systolic anterior motion of the mitral valve. Color flow Doppler echocardiography can be used to demonstrate the hemodynamic abnormalities associated with SAM. With this modality two turbulent jets can be observed originating from the same region, one regurgitating back into the left atrium and the other projecting into the aorta (Color Plate 88). Mitral valve SAM can be identified definitively on an M-mode echocardiogram or on a two-dimensional

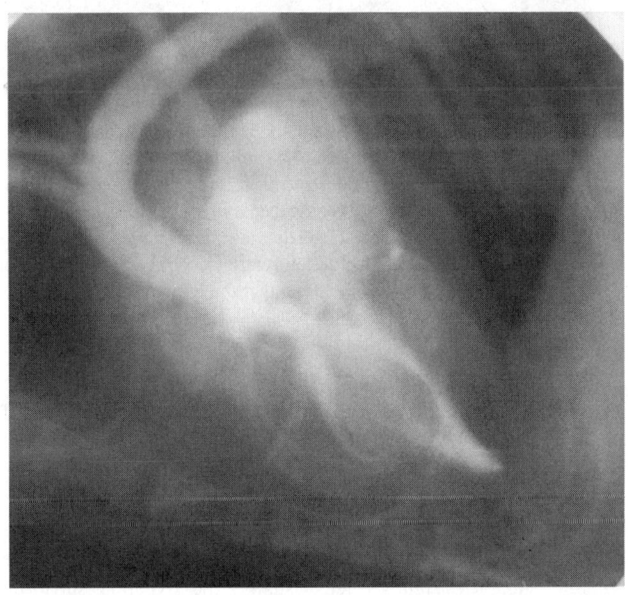

FIGURE 21-11 Angiocardiogram taken during systole from a cat with hypertrophic cardiomyopathy. The catheter was placed in the left ventricle from the carotid artery. The left ventricular cavity is smaller than normal and has filling defects from the hypertrophied papillary muscles. Contrast medium is present in the left atrium, indicating mitral regurgitation that appears to be moderately severe (3+).

A 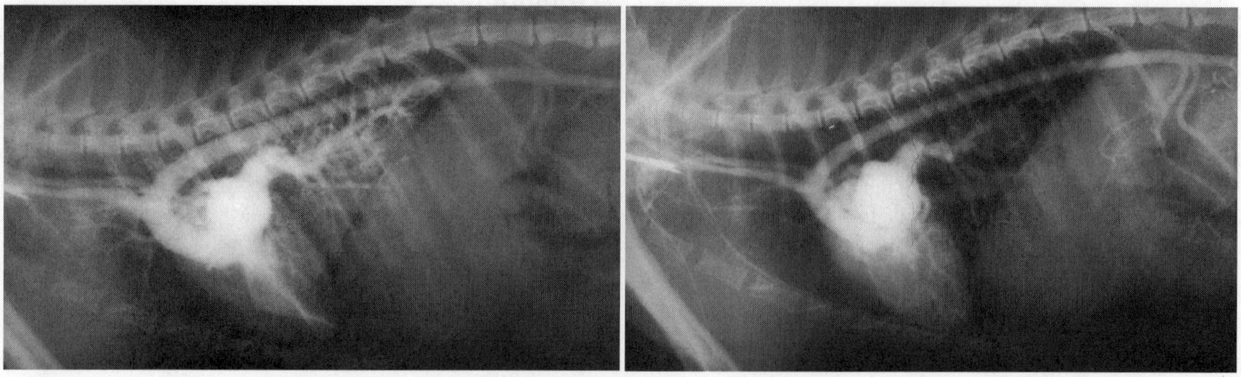 B

FIGURE 21-12 Nonselective angiocardiograms from a cat with hypertrophic cardiomyopathy. **A,** The contrast medium is in the pulmonary circulation, the pulmonary veins, the left heart and the aorta. The pulmonary veins are enlarged and tortuous, indicating pulmonary venous hypertension. The left atrium is enlarged. The left ventricular cavity is small and has filling defects. **B,** This frame was taken at end-systole. No to very little contrast agent remains in the left ventricular cavity (the end-systolic volume is negligible). This is known as *cavity obliteration* and is characteristically seen in HCM.

A 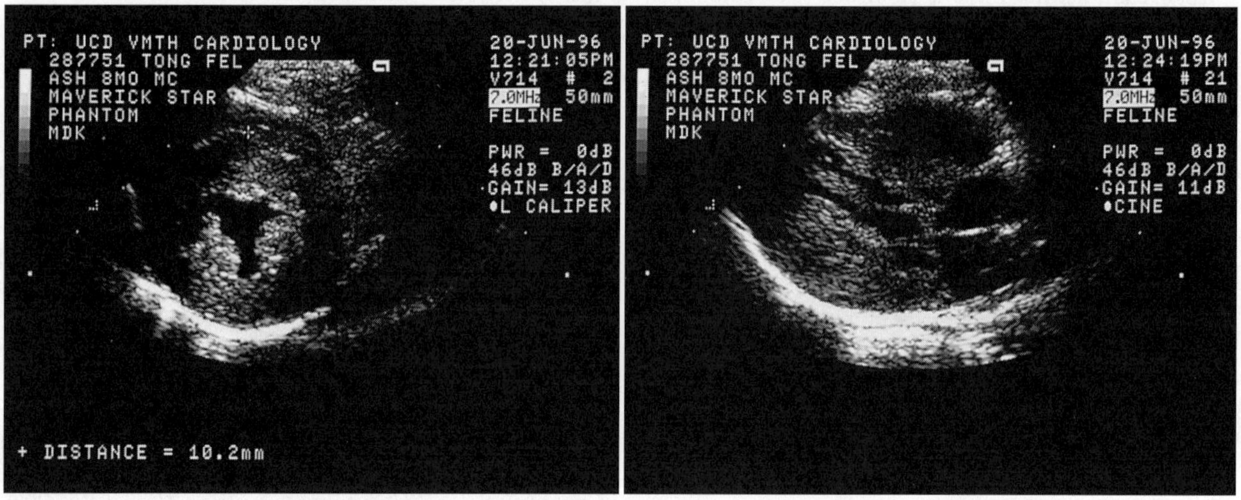 B

FIGURE 21-13 Two-dimensional echocardiograms from an 8-month-old American shorthair cat with severe hypertrophic cardiomyopathy. **A,** In the cross-sectional view taken in diastole, the interventricular septum is 10 mm thick and the left ventricular free wall is 8 mm thick. The papillary muscles are prominent and encroach on the left ventricular cavity. The left ventricular cavity is smaller than normal, measuring 12 mm in diameter. **B,** In the long-axis view taken during systole, papillary muscle hypertrophy is evident. These muscles are obliterating the left ventricular cavity. Systolic anterior motion of the mitral valve is obliterating the left ventricular outflow tract. Note that the left atrium is not enlarged in this young cat.

echocardiogram (see Figures 21-4 and 21-5). Spectral Doppler can be used to determine the pressure gradient across the region of subaortic stenosis produced by the SAM. The pressure gradient roughly correlates with the severity of the SAM. Consequently, the pressure gradient can be used to document the success or failure of therapy to decrease SAM. Care must be taken not to record the high-velocity mitral regurgitation jet that is positioned close to the dynamic subaortic stenosis jet. Usually, the dynamic subaortic stenosis jet is narrower than the mitral regurgitation jet, often becoming even more narrow in mid-to-late systole (see Figure 21-6). SAM is not present in all cats with HCM. Some cats develop SAM before they have any evidence of wall thickening, whereas others only have SAM as the manifestation of their disease. Within our colony of Maine coon cats with HCM, some cats with severe HCM have SAM, some cats with severe HCM have no SAM, and some cats with echocardiographic evidence of mild wall thickening have SAM. The latter cats usually have evidence of papillary muscle hypertrophy and often develop more wall thickening over time.

MILD-TO-MODERATE HCM

The diagnosis of HCM is much more difficult and controversial in cats with lesser wall thickening or only regional thickening on an echocardiogram. In human families with HCM associated with specific gene abnormalities, varying degrees of severity have been noted within the affected family members.[53] Echocardiographic findings in family members with the mutation range from no abnormalities to severe HCM. This may also be true in cats, indicating that milder forms of the disease do exist. However, distinguishing mild disease from normal or distinguishing mild-to-moderate HCM from hypertrophy secondary to other abnormalities

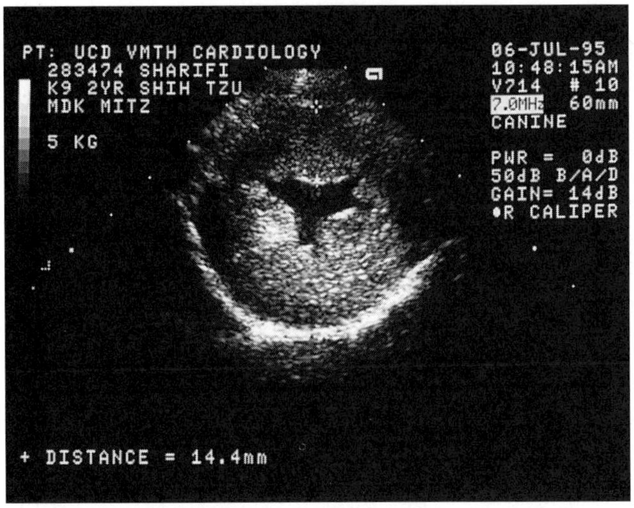

FIGURE 21-14 Cross-sectional view of the left ventricle on a two-dimensional echocardiogram from a 2-year-old Shi Tzu with hypertrophic cardiomyopathy. The dog weighed 5 kg, which means the left ventricular diastolic wall thickness should have been 5 to 6 mm. Instead it is 14 mm thick. This dog had been referred for a kidney transplant because of renal dysplasia. Cardiac ultrasound was performed after a heart murmur was detected. The dog did not have systemic hypertension.

is not easy in individual cases. In a clinical situation in which one is examining an older cat with what appears to be mild hypertrophy, one must first decide whether hypertrophy is present or not. Then one must determine if another disease is causing the hypertrophy, before making the diagnosis of feline HCM. The upper limit for normal left ventricular wall thickness is 5.0 to 5.5 mm in the cat. We consider concentric hypertrophy in the cat to be anything 6 mm or greater.

DIFFERENTIAL DIAGNOSES

Once concentric hypertrophy is diagnosed, especially in an older cat, it is best to rule out hyperthyroidism, systemic hypertension, and, possibly, acromegaly. Hyperthyroidism is usually easy to rule out. Devices to measure blood pressure in the cat, however, are not readily available, and the technique requires some practice. We prefer to measure systolic blood pressure using a pediatric inflatable cuff placed around the distal forelimb and then use a Doppler flow–sensing device placed on the ventral metacarpal region to detect flow. Most cats with systemic hypertension have an increase in systolic blood pressure, although it is theoretically possible to have just diastolic hypertension that would be missed using this technique. We have had little success with oscillometric devices in cats. We consider a systolic blood pressure greater than 150 mm Hg to be abnormally high in a nonfractious cat. If systemic arterial blood pressure cannot be measured, one should at least rule out the common causes of systemic hypertension in a cat with left ventricular concentric hypertrophy (i.e., hyperthyroidism and renal failure).

Rarely, infiltrative disease such as lymphoma produces hypertrophy that is indistinguishable from HCM on an echocardiogram. One such case is presented in Color Plate 89.[1] Pseudohypertrophy, resulting from hypovolemia must also be excluded.

Treatment

Cats that present in heart failure have clinical signs referable to pulmonary edema or pleural effusion. Consequently, therapy is generally aimed at decreasing left atrial and pulmonary venous pressures in these cats. In some cats with severe heart failure, clinical evidence of hypoperfusion (low-output heart failure) may be apparent in addition to the signs of congestive heart failure. The signs may manifest as cold extremities and total body hypothermia.

Pulmonary edema is treated with diuretics, calcium channel blockers, venodilators, and, possibly, β-adrenergic blockers and angiotensin converting enzyme (ACE) inhibitors. Thoracentesis and pleural drainage are most effective for treating cats with severe pleural effusion. However, the drugs mentioned above may be helpful in preventing recurrent effusion or clearing lesser amounts of an effusion.

SEVERE ACUTE HEART FAILURE

Cats that present with respiratory distress and are suspected of having heart failure secondary to HCM should be placed in an oxygen-enriched environment. If possible, the cat should be initially evaluated by a cursory physical examination. Care should be taken not to stress the patient during this or any other procedure. Stress or excitement tend to exacerbate the dyspnea in any cat that is already dyspneic. Escalating dyspnea in this situation often leads to death. Most cats with severe HCM that are in heart failure have a heart murmur and/or a gallop sound (gallop rhythm). A butterfly catheter should be used to perform thoracentesis on both sides of the chest to look for pleural effusion as soon as possible. Generally this should be done with the cat in a sternal position so that it does not become stressed during the procedure. If fluid is identified, it should be removed. If none is identified, a lateral or dorsoventral chest radiograph may be taken, with the veterinarian present to ensure that the cat is not stressed (i.e., make sure no one stretches the cat out or in any way interferes with its ability to breathe). If the patient struggles or appears to be stressed or fractious during or before radiographic examination, the procedure should be canceled. The patient should then be placed into an oxygen-enriched environment.

Furosemide. Furosemide (Lasix, Hoechst-Roussel, Somerville, N.J.) should be administered intravenously or intramuscularly. The route of administration depends on the stress level of the patient. Furosemide should be administered intramuscularly to cats that are very distressed and cannot tolerate restraint for an intravenous injection. Cats that can tolerate an intravenous injection may benefit from the more rapid onset of action (within 5 minutes of an intravenous injection vs. 30 minutes for an intramuscular injection). The initial furosemide dose to a cat in distress should generally be in the 2- to 4-mg/kg range. This dose may be repeated within 1 hour of an intravenous injection (duration of effect following intravenous administration is approximately 1 hour) or within 2 hours of an intramuscular injection (duration of effect following an intramuscular injection is approximately 2 hours). Dosing must be reduced sharply once the resting respiratory rate starts to decrease.

High-dose parenteral furosemide therapy commonly produces electrolyte disturbances and dehydration in both cats and dogs. Dogs generally recover readily on their own when they start to feel better and start to eat and drink. Cats are more precarious. They may be presented dehydrated and electrolyte-depleted because of anorexia. They may remain anorexic and consequently dehydrated and depleted of electrolytes once the edema or effusion is lessened. Judicious intravenous or subcutaneous fluid administration may be required to improve these cats clinically. Overzealous fluid administration will result in the return of clinical signs referable to heart failure.

Nitroglycerin. Nitroglycerin cream (Nitro-Bid, Marion Laboratories, Kansas City, Mo.; Nitrol, Adria Laboratories, Dublin, Ohio;

Nitrong, Wharton, Princeton, N.Y.; Nitrostat, Parke-Davis, Morris Plains, N.J.) may be beneficial in cats with severe edema formation secondary to feline HCM. However, no studies have examined any effects of this drug in this species. When nitroglycerin is used clinically, it is almost universally administered with furosemide, a drug known to have profound beneficial effects in congestive heart failure. Consequently it is generally impossible to tell if any observed beneficial effects are due to the furosemide or the combination of furosemide and nitroglycerin. Because of this, the numerous anecdotal reports of nitroglycerin's benefits in this situation are suspect. However, nitroglycerin is safe when administered judiciously, and some benefit may occur with its administration. Consequently, we would not dissuade anyone from administering ⅛ inch to ¼ inch of a 2% cream to the inside of an ear every 4 to 6 hours for the first 24 hours, as long as furosemide was being administered concomitantly. Nitroglycerin tolerance develops rapidly in other species and probably does so in the cat. Consequently, prolonged administration is probably of lesser benefit.

No other drugs are useful for treating acute, severe congestive heart failure secondary to HCM. Once furosemide and nitroglycerin are administered, the cat should be left to rest quietly in an oxygen-enriched environment. Care should be taken not to distress the cat by placing catheters, taking body temperature, and so on. A baseline measurement of the respiratory rate and assessment of respiratory character should be taken when the cat is resting. This should be followed at 30-minute intervals and furosemide administration continued until the respiratory rate starts to decrease (a consistent decrease of 10 breaths/min over an hour is a good general guide) or the character improves. When this occurs the furosemide dose and dosage frequency should be curtailed sharply.

Sedation or anesthesia. Some cats with severe pulmonary edema become extremely agitated because of their dyspnea or because they are stressed by a procedure. In some of these cats sedation with acepromazine (0.05 to 0.1 mg/kg IV) may be all that is required to produce anxiolysis. Oxymorphone (0.05 to 0.15 mg/kg q6h IM or IV) or butorphanol tartrate (0.1 mg/kg IV or 0.02 to 0.4 mg/kg q4h IM or subcutaneously) may also be used but are secondary choices because they can produce respiratory depression. Oxymorphone may produce excitement in some cats. The analgesic properties of butorphanol are 5 times that of morphine. However it has recently become a controlled drug and its respiratory depressant effects equal those of morphine.

In some cats, anesthesia, intubation, and ventilation are required to control the respiratory failure. Although this method is not preferred for all severely dyspneic cats, it can be life-saving in some. This procedure has the advantage of allowing the administration of 100% oxygen and the draining or suctioning of fluid from the large airways in a controlled environment.

CHRONIC HEART FAILURE

Cats that make it through their respiratory crisis or cats that present with lesser degrees of heart failure can be started on chronic drug therapy for heart failure. Many aspects of chronic therapy of HCM are controversial. All therapy is palliative and ultimately futile in most cases.

Furosemide. In cats with congestive heart failure, furosemide administration should usually be maintained. In a few cases, furosemide can be discontinued gradually once the cat has been stabilized. Sometimes furosemide may not be required because the administration of another drug has improved cardiac function (e.g., diltiazem has improved left ventricular diastolic function or decreased the amount of mitral regurgitation enough to allow decreasing the dose of or discontinuing furosemide). The maintenance dose of furosemide in cats usually ranges from 6.25 (½ of a 12.5-mg tablet) once a day to 12.5 mg q8h. The dose must be titrated carefully in each patient. Having the owner count the resting respiratory rate at home and keep a daily log of the respiratory rate is highly beneficial for making decisions regarding dosage adjustment in individual patients. We have administered higher doses (up to 37.5 mg q12h) than commonly recommended to Maine coon cats without identifying severe consequences. Cats on high-dose furosemide therapy are commonly mildly dehydrated and mildly-to-moderately azotemic. However, they often continue to act normally, eat, and drink. Lower doses have resulted in resumption of respiratory difficulty.

Diltiazem and β-adrenergic blockers. In cats with severe HCM that have or have had evidence of congestive heart failure, administration of diltiazem or a β-adrenergic blocking agent is generally indicated. Both provide symptomatic benefit in human patients. Because the idea for administering both drugs comes from their administration to human patients, comparing the human and the feline disease and the therapeutic goals in each species may be worthwhile. The pathology of HCM in humans is somewhat different from that seen in cats. The primary difference is the predominant septal hypertrophy that usually occurs in humans. Despite this difference, the pathophysiology of the disease in the two species is similar.[43] Human patients with severe disease also have marked hypertrophy, a smaller-than-normal left ventricular cavity, impaired diastolic function, and SAM of the mitral valve. These abnormalities culminate in symptoms of dyspnea, reduced exercise capability, and chest pain in humans. The dyspnea is caused by increased left ventricular diastolic pressure (interestingly, this is rarely called *congestive heart failure* in human patients with HCM). The major difference between the two species from this aspect may be the degree of the elevation in ventricular diastolic or left atrial pressure. The diastolic pressure elevations appear to be mild to moderate at rest in humans and result in mild-to-moderate left atrial enlargement. In cats, the increases in left ventricular diastolic and/or left atrial pressure are often marked, resulting in severe left atrial enlargement and pulmonary edema and pleural effusion. Consequently, drug therapy only has to reduce diastolic pressure mildly to moderately in humans to produce symptomatic benefit, whereas, in the cat, major reductions in left ventricular filling pressure must be produced. Because of this, furosemide is usually required to treat cats with heart failure secondary to HCM. In humans, diuretic administration is not used or is thought to be contraindicated because decreases in end-diastolic volume are thought to worsen SAM. Improvement in exercise capability is an important therapeutic goal in humans. Domestic cats rarely exercise, so improvement in exercise tolerance is not a therapeutic goal. Relief of chest pain is a major goal in humans. Chest pain resulting from ischemia may occur in cats, but, obviously, evidence is lacking. In summary, in the cat the major therapeutic goal is often to treat moderate-to-severe congestive heart failure, so diuretic administration is often required, along with other drugs such as diltiazem and propranolol. In humans the therapeutic goals are to treat mild heart failure and alleviate chest pain. Calcium channel blockers and propranolol are commonly used alone to achieve these goals.

Diltiazem. Diltiazem (Cardizem, Marion Merrell Dow, Inc., Kansas City, Mo.) is a calcium channel blocker documented to have beneficial effects in cats with HCM when dosed at 7.5 mg q8h.[54,55] Beneficial effects include lessened edema formation and decreased wall thickness in some cats. Exactly how these beneficial effects occur are open to debate. Only a few cats experience a clinically significant decrease in wall thickness in our experience. Diltiazem does improve the early diastolic relaxation abnormalities seen in

A 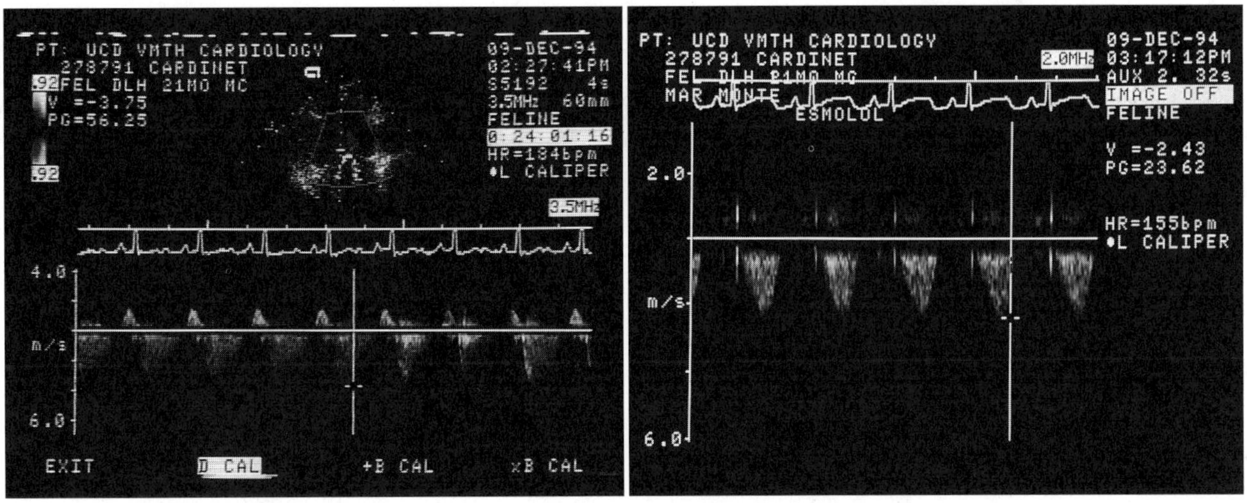 B

FIGURE 21-15 Continuous-wave Doppler echocardiograms taken from a 21-month-old domestic longhaired cat with severe hypertrophic cardiomyopathy before **(A)** and after **(B)** esmolol administration. The velocity decreased from 3.7 m/sec to 2.4 m/sec after esmolol administration. This indicates that the degree of dynamic subaortic narrowing decreased, presumably because of decreased systolic anterior motion of the mitral valve. This cat was in severe heart failure at the time of this recording and was anesthetized and on a ventilator because of severe pulmonary edema. The cat was treated with furosemide, propranolol, and diltiazem and recovered. It died suddenly 1 year later.

feline HCM.[42,55] Whether this helps decrease diastolic intraventricular pressure and so decrease edema formation is unknown. Slower myocardial relaxation can increase diastolic intraventricular pressure if the heart rate is very fast, so that the myocardium does not have time to relax. Incomplete relaxation and decreased compliance, however, are more plausible explanations for increased diastolic pressure due to diastolic dysfunction in feline HCM. In humans, diltiazem does not change left ventricular chamber stiffness and so does not alter passive diastolic function.[56] In cats it also appears not to alter late diastolic filling properties.[57] Diltiazem may decrease SAM and in so doing decrease the amount of mitral regurgitation, resulting in a decrease in left atrial pressure. However, in humans diltiazem does not reduce the left ventricular outflow tract gradient and in some patients actually increases it as blood pressure decreases.[56]

The pharmacokinetics of diltiazem have been examined in cats. Diltiazem, when administered per os at a dose of 1 mg/kg has a bioavailability of 94%, a terminal half-life of 2 hours, and a volume of distribution of 1.9 L/kg.[58] Peak serum concentration occurs 30 minutes after dosing, and the serum concentration remains in the therapeutic range (50 to 300 μg/mL) for 8 hours.

Diltiazem is also supplied as slow-release (long-acting) products. The pharmacokinetics of one long-acting product (Cardizem CD, Marion Merrell Dow, Inc., Kansas City, Mo.) have been studied.[58] The product was dosed at 10 mg/kg. The bioavailability of this product is only 38%, necessitating a much higher dose for this product than for the usual product. The half-life is much longer at 6.5 hours, and peak serum concentration does not occur until 6 hours after drug administration. Serum concentration remains within therapeutic range for 24 hours. Cardizem CD is supplied as 180-mg capsules that contain many smaller capsules. The larger capsule can be opened and the smaller capsules divided to produce an appropriate dose. We commonly divide the smaller capsules into groups of four (45 mg each) and place them in smaller gelatin capsules for administration. One capsule is then administered once per day. The other extended-release formulation that is appropriately packaged for use in cats is Dilacor XR (Rhone-Poulenc Rorer, Collegeville, Pa.). This product is supplied as 120-, 180-, and 240-mg capsules. Each large capsule can be opened to yield 2, 3, or 4 60-mg tablets. This drug produces significant decreases in heart rate and blood pressure in cats with HCM for 12 to 14 hours and appears to be effective when administered at a dose of 30 mg q12h.[59]

β-Blockers. In one third to two thirds of humans with HCM, angina, dyspnea, and exercise tolerance improve following the administration of large doses of β-adrenergic blocking agents.[60] β-Blockers may also decrease the incidence of sudden death, although this has not been proved. The β-blocker of choice in humans is propranolol. High-dose propranolol therapy is often recommended in humans, in whom doses exceeding 300 mg are used unless contraindications to its use exist. This means that human patients commonly receive more than 4 mg/kg of propranolol per day. This would be comparable to more than 1.0 to 1.5 mg/kg q8h in a cat. Maximum doses in humans appear to be in the 500- to 800-mg/day range. This would be comparable to around 3 mg/kg q8h in the cat. The mechanisms by which propranolol improves symptoms in people are not well understood. Original studies suggested improvement in diastolic function, but it is now suggested that this improvement is purely due to a slowing of the heart rate.[60] β-Blockers may prevent an exercise-induced increase in outflow tract obstruction but usually do not alter the resting obstruction in humans. The decrease in resting- or effort-induced angina is probably related to decreased myocardial oxygen consumption.

No studies of propranolol use in feline HCM have been completed. Consequently, reports of improvement or lack of improvement are anecdotal. One study has examined the effects of esmolol, a short-acting β_1-adrenergic blocking drug, in six cats with HCM and obstruction to left ventricular outflow due to systolic anterior motion.[61] In this study the degree of outflow tract obstruction decreased and the heart rate slowed. Esmolol can be administered acutely to determine the type of response that might be achieved with propranolol or atenolol (Figure 21-15). If the data on esmolol can be translated to propranolol's or atenolol's effects in cats (which seems reasonable), one would predict that propranolol or atenolol would decrease SAM in cats and in so doing decrease the amount of mitral regurgitation and degree of dynamic subaortic stenosis. We have documented this clinically in several cats. Propranolol (Inderal, Wyeth-Ayerst, Philadelphia, Pa.) is supplied as 10-, 20-, 40-, 60-, 80-, and 90-mg tablets. Only the 10- and 20-mg tablets are appropriate for use in cats. The dose in cats is generally in the 0.5- to 2.0-mg/kg q8h range, although higher doses might be beneficial, as noted earlier.

Atenolol (Tenormin, Zeneca, Inc., Wilmington, Del.) is a specific β_1- adrenergic blocking drug that should be administered twice a day, usually at a total dose of 6.25 to 12.5 mg.[59,62] We have administered this drug at a dose of 25 mg twice a day to one Maine coon cat with HCM to decrease heart rate. No untoward effects were noted. In the cat, atenolol has a half-life of 3.5 hours. Its bioavailability is high, at 90%, and the pharmacokinetic variability from cat to cat is small. When administered to cats at a dose of 3 mg/kg, atenolol attenuates the increase in heart rate produced by isoproterenol for 12 but not for 24 hours. The product is supplied as 25-, 50-, and 100-mg tablets.

We commonly use diltiazem first and then either switch to propranolol or titrate propranolol into the therapeutic regimen if the response is suboptimal or becomes suboptimal. Other veterinary cardiologists use β-blockers first and, if the response is minimal, switch to diltiazem. Occasionally we administer the two drugs concomitantly. Because most cats with HCM that are being treated are or have been in congestive heart failure and are receiving furosemide, response to diltiazem or propranolol therapy may be difficult to evaluate unless one takes the time and effort to tailor diuretic therapy and to reduce diuretic administration to the lowest possible level.

ASYMPTOMATIC CATS

Treatment of asymptomatic cats is controversial. In humans, treatment of asymptomatic patients with a definite family history of HCM with either propranolol or a calcium channel blocker is sometimes recommended in the hope of slowing the progression of the disease.[63] Similar advice might be prudent in cats. However, progression of the disease in adult humans is rare, so this recommendation may be suspect.[64] One of the authors owns a Maine coon cat with severe HCM that receives no therapy and has been followed for 6 years as an adult. No progression of the hypertrophy was noted in this cat as an adult. Consequently, this recommendation may also be suspect in cats. Diltiazem appears to produce regression of the hypertrophy in some cats.[55] Therefore it may be reasonable to administer diltiazem to an asymptomatic cat with moderate-to-severe hypertrophy for several months to see if hypertrophy regression will occur. It might make more sense to administer a drug to a young cat during the time that hypertrophy is developing. This type of study has not been performed in either cats or humans.

REFRACTORY HEART FAILURE

Treatment of heart failure resulting from HCM that is refractory to conventional drugs is also controversial. The ACE inhibitors may be beneficial or theoretically may be detrimental in this type of patient. Captopril and enalapril are efficacious drugs in congestive heart failure resulting from other diseases in the cat. ACE inhibitors are commonly classified as contraindicated in cats with HCM. The rationale for this contraindication is that ACE inhibitors cause arteriolar dilation and in so doing may increase the vigor of left ventricular contraction and increase the amount of SAM of the mitral valve. This would then increase the outflow tract gradient and potentially worsen the mitral regurgitation. This could potentially occur. However, the arteriolar dilating capabilities of the ACE inhibitors are mild. Their primary benefit appears to come from their ability to decrease plasma aldosterone concentration and in so doing decrease sodium and water retention. One small study has suggested that ACE inhibitors do not produce untoward effects in cats with HCM.[65] One of the authors has documented increases in plasma aldosterone concentration in cats with HCM and we both have observed beneficial responses to ACE inhibitors in several cats with HCM. Consequently, we do not believe that ACE inhibitor administration should be ruled out in cats with HCM that are refractory to other drugs, based on theoretical concerns. Instead, they should be used judiciously in such cases.

Captopril (Capoten, E. R. Squibb & Sons, Inc., Princeton, N.J.) is dosed at ¼ to ½ of a 12.5 mg tablet q8h PO. Enalapril (Enacard, Merck & Company, West Point, Pa.) is dosed at 0.25 to 0.5 mg/kg PO. The dosing frequency of enalapril is controversial in the cat. This is primarily because one study showed that plasma angiotensin converting enzyme activity was depressed to less than 50% of control for up to 2 to 3 days after enalapril administration in normal cats. However, generally one must suppress an enzyme system to less than 10% of control activity to produce clinical effect. Consequently, instead of administering enalapril every 2 to 3 days, we administer the drug q12h or q24h. Benazepril (Lotensin, Ciba-Geigy Pharmaceutical, Summit, N.J.) can be administered to cats at a dose of 0.5 mg/kg q24h PO.[66]

PREVENTION OF THROMBOEMBOLIC DISEASE

Prevention of thromboembolic disease in cats with HCM is controversial. Aspirin (80 mg q48h or q72h PO) is commonly prescribed to prevent the formation of intravascular thrombi in cats. Because there is little risk associated with administering this drug on this schedule to cats (other than gastric upset or erosions that rarely produce clinical signs in cats), we recommend continuing this practice. One should realize, however, that aspirin administration in no way guarantees that thromboembolic disease will not occur. In one study of the use of tissue plasminogen activator to lyse thromboemboli in cats, most of the cats rethrombosed within months of successful thrombolysis, despite the administration of aspirin.[67]

Because of the potential lack of benefit with aspirin, some veterinarians are now advocating the use of warfarin (Coumadin) to prevent the formation of intracardiac thrombi.[68] Warfarin is standard preventive therapy in humans at risk for the formation of intracardiac thrombi. To date, however, the use of warfarin to prevent the formation of intracardiac thrombi has not been adequately studied, therefore the benefit and the incidence of complications are unknown. The major risk with warfarin is hemorrhage. We have observed this complication in several cats on warfarin therapy, despite appropriate monitoring of coagulation parameters. If warfarin therapy is contemplated, we recommend that the patient be referred to a qualified specialist that can monitor prothrombin time frequently in the patient. We have also witnessed rethrombosis in cats being administered warfarin.

Besides standard antithrombotic agents, calcium channel blockers and nitrates also have antiplatelet effects.[69,70] Verapamil and diltiazem inhibit platelet aggregation induced by adenosine diphosphate (ADP), arachidonic acid, and prostaglandin H_2 in cat plasma.[71] One study, however, has suggested that diltiazem, when administered to cats at a dose of 7.5 mg q8h, does not affect platelet aggregation.[72] Nitrates inhibit platelet aggregation stimulated by ADP, collagen, adrenaline, and thrombin.[73,74] Consequently, diltiazem and nitroglycerin may do more than produce beneficial hemodynamic effects in cats with HCM.

Prognosis

The prognosis is determined by clinical presentation and echocardiographic severity of the disease. Adult cats that are asymptomatic and have mild-to-moderate disease and no-to-mild left atrial enlargement have a good short-term and possibly a good long-term prognosis. Some, however, may progress to more severe disease, and some may die suddenly. Asymptomatic cats with severe wall thickening and mild-to-moderate left atrial enlargement have a guarded prognosis for developing heart failure at some point in the future. They should have some risk for developing thromboembolism and may be at risk for sudden death. Asymptomatic cats with severe wall thickening and moderate-to-severe left atrial enlargement are at risk for developing heart failure or often already have mild-to-moderate heart failure that has gone undetected. These cats are at risk for developing thromboembolic disease and are at risk for sudden death. Cats presented in heart failure usually have a poor prognosis. In one study they had a median survival time of 3 months.[75] Most died of intractable heart failure (Color Plate 90); some developed thromboembolism, and some died suddenly. However, some cats (about 20% in this study) in this class stabilize and do well for prolonged periods for unknown reasons. Cats in the aforementioned study that had severe HCM and aortic thromboembolism had a poor prognosis, with a median survival time of 2 months.

REFERENCES

1. Brummer DG, Moise NS: Infiltrative cardiomyopathy responsive to combination chemotherapy in a cat with lymphoma, *J Am Vet Med Assoc* 195:1116, 1989.
2. Fox PR, Liu SK, Maron BJ: Echocardiographic assessment of spontaneously occurring feline hypertrophic cardiomyopathy: an animal model of human disease, *Circulation* 92:2645, 1995.
3. Liu SK, Maron BJ, Tilley LP: Canine hypertrophic cardiomyopathy, *J Am Vet Med Assoc* 174:708, 1979.
4. Thomas WP, Mathewson JW, Suter PF et al: Hypertrophic obstructive cardiomyopathy in a dog: clinical, hemodynamic, angiographic, and pathologic studies, *J Am Anim Hosp Assoc* 20:253, 1984.
5. Sisson D, Thomas WP: Dynamic subaortic stenosis in a dog with congenital heart disease, *J Am Anim Hosp Assoc* 20:657, 1984.
6. Maron BJ, Mulvihill JJ: The genetics of hypertrophic cardiomyopathy, *Ann Intern Med* 105:610, 1986.
7. Jarcho JA, McKenna W, Pare JA et al: Mapping a gene for familial hypertrophic cardiomyopathy to chromosome 14q1, *N Engl J Med* 321:1372, 1989.
8. Rosenzweig A, Watkins H, Hwang DS et al: Mutations in cardiac myosin heavy chain genes cause familial hypertrophic cardiomyopathy, *Mol Biol Med* 8:159, 1991.
9. Tanigawa G, Jarcho JA, Kass S et al: A molecular basis for familial hypertrophic cardiomyopathy: an alpha/beta cardiac myosin heavy chain hybrid gene, *Cell* 62:991, 1990.
10. Geisterfer-Lowrance AA, Kass S, Tanigawa G et al: A molecular basis for familial hypertrophic cardiomyopathy: a beta cardiac myosin heavy chain gene missense mutation, *Cell* 62:999, 1990.
11. Marian AJ, Roberts R: Recent advances in the molecular genetics of hypertrophic cardiomyopathy, *Circulation* 92:1336, 1995.
12. Watkins H, Thierfelder L, Hwang DS et al: Sporadic hypertrophic cardiomyopathy due to de novo myosin mutations, *J Clin Invest* 90:1666, 1992.
13. Thierfelder L, Watkins H, MacRae C et al: Alpha-tropomyosin and cardiac troponin T mutations cause familial hypertrophic cardiomyopathy: a disease of the sarcomere, *Cell* 77:701, 1994.
14. Watkins H, Conner D, Thierfelder L et al: Mutations in the cardiac myosin binding protein-C gene on chromosome 11 cause familial hypertrophic cardiomyopathy, *Nat Genet* 11:434, 1995.
15. Bonne G, Carrier L, Bercovici J et al: Cardiac myosin binding protein-C gene splice acceptor site mutation is associated with familial hypertrophic cardiomyopathy, *Nat Genet* 11:438, 1995.
16. Poetter K, Jiang H, Hassanzadeh S et al: Mutations in either the essential or regulatory light chains of myosin are associated with a rare myopathy in human heart and skeletal muscle, *Nat Genet* 13:63, 1996.
17. Seidman CE: A molecular biology primer for clinicians, audio tape from the 45th Annual Scientific Session of the American College of Cardiology, 1996.
18. Carrier L, Hengstenberg C, Beckmann JS et al: Mapping of a novel gene for familial hypertrophic cardiomyopathy to chromosome 11, *Nat Genet* 4:311, 1993.
19. Geisterfer-Lowrance AA, Christe M, Conner DA et al: A mouse model of familial hypertrophic cardiomyopathy, *Science* 272:731, 1996.
20. Vikstrom KL, Factor SM, Leinwand LA, Transgenic mouse model for familial hypertrophic cardiomyopathy, *Mol Biol Cell* 4:39a, 1993 (abstract).
21. Lankford EB, Epstein ND, Fananapazir L et al: Abnormal contractile properties of muscle fibers expressing beta-myosin heavy chain gene mutations in patients with hypertrophic cardiomyopathy, *J Clin Invest* 95:1409, 1995.
22. Cuda G, Fananapazir L, Zhu WS et al: Skeletal muscle expression and abnormal function of beta-myosin in hypertrophic cardiomyopathy, *J Clin Invest* 91:2861, 1993.
23. Lankford EB, Epstein ND, Fananapazir L et al: Abnormal contractile properties of muscle fibers expressing beta-myosin heavy chain gene mutations in patients with hypertrophic cardiomyopathy, *J Clin Invest* 95:1409, 1995.
24. Sweeney HL, Straceski AJ, Leinwand LA et al: Heterologous expression of a cardiomyopathic myosin that is defective in its actin interaction, *J Biol Chem* 269:1603, 1994.
25. Kittleson MD, Pion PD, Mekhamer Y: Hypertrophic cardiomyopathy in a group of highly interrelated Maine coon cats, *J Vet Intern Med* 7:117, 1993 (abstract).
26. Kittleson MD, Kittleson JA, Mekhamer Y: Development and progression of inherited hypertrophic cardiomyopathy in Maine coon cats, *J Vet Intern Med* 10:165, 1996.
27. Meurs KM, Kittleson MD, Towbin J et al: Familial systolic anterior motion of the mitral valve and/or hypertrophic cardiomyopathy is apparently inherited as an autosomal dominant trait in a family of American shorthair cats, *J Vet Intern Med* 11:138, 1997 (abstract).
28. Fananapazir L, Epstein ND: Genotype-phenotype correlations in hypertrophic cardiomyopathy: insights provided by comparisons of kindreds with distinct and identical beta-myosin heavy chain gene mutations, *Circulation* 89:22, 1994 (comments).
29. Epstein ND, Cohn GM, Cyran F et al: Differences in clinical expression of hypertrophic cardiomyopathy associated with two distinct mutations in the beta-myosin heavy chain gene: a 908Leu—Val mutation and a 403Arg—Gln mutation, *Circulation* 86:345, 1992 (comments).
30. Kittleson MD, Pion PD, DeLellis LA et al: Increased serum growth hormone concentration in feline hypertrophic cardiomyopathy, *J Vet Intern Med* 6:320, 1992.
31. Peterson ME, Taylor RS, Greco DS et al: Acromegaly in 14 cats, *J Vet Intern Med* 4:192, 1990.
32. Liu SK, Roberts WC, Maron BJ: Comparison of morphologic findings in spontaneously occurring hypertrophic cardiomyopathy in humans, cats and dogs, *Am J Cardiol* 72:944, 1993.
33. Peterson EN, Moise NS, Brown CA et al: Heterogeneity of hypertrophy in feline hypertrophic heart disease, *J Vet Intern Med* 7:183, 1993 (comments).
34. Tanaka M, Fujiwara H, Onodera T et al: Quantitative analysis of narrowings of intramyocardial small arteries in normal hearts, hypertensive hearts, and hearts with hypertrophic cardiomyopathy, *Circulation* 75:1130, 1987.
35. Maron BJ, Wolfson JK, Epstein SE et al: Intramural ("small vessel") coronary artery disease in hypertrophic cardiomyopathy, *J Am Coll Cardiol* 8:545, 1986.

36. Liu SK: The intramural coronary arterial lesions in 102 cats with hypertrophic cardiomyopathies, *US and Can Acad Path Annu Meet* 320:54A, 1995 (abstract).
37. Woolf AS, Fine LG: Genetically engineered kidneys, *Pediatr Nephrol* 7:605, 1993.
38. Maron BJ, Roberts WC: Hypertrophic cardiomyopathy and cardiac muscle cell disorganization revisited: relation between the two and significance, *Am Heart J* 102:95, 1981.
39. Maron BJ, Epstein SE: Hypertrophic cardiomyopathy: recent observations regarding the specificity of three hallmarks of the disease: asymmetric septal hypertrophy, septal disorganization and systolic anterior motion of the anterior mitral leaflet, *Am J Cardiol* 45:141, 1980.
40. Liu SK, Hsu FS, Lee RCT: *An atlas of cardiovascular pathology,* Tainan, Taiwan, 1989, Pig Research Institute of Taiwan.
41. Marian AJ, Yu QT, Mann DL et al: Expression of a mutation causing hypertrophic cardiomyopathy disrupts sarcomere assembly in adult feline cardiac myocytes, *Circ Res* 77:98, 1995.
42. Golden AL, Bright JM: Use of relaxation half-time as an index of ventricular relaxation in clinically normal cats and cats with hypertrophic cardiomyopathy, *Am J Vet Res* 51:1352, 1990.
43. Maron BJ, Bonow RO, Cannon RO et al: Hypertrophic cardiomyopathy: interrelations of clinical manifestations, pathophysiology, and therapy. II. *N Engl J Med* 316:844, 1987.
44. Saito T, Hirota Y, Kita Y et al: Evaluation of left ventricular contractility in hypertrophic cardiomyopathy from end-systolic pressure-volume relation, *Jpn Circ J* 51:511, 1987.
45. Ferrans VJ, Rodriguez ER: Evidence of myocyte hyperplasia in hypertrophic cardiomyopathy and other disorders with myocardial hypertrophy? *Z Kardiol* 76(suppl 3):20, 1987.
46. Vlahakes GJ, Lefebvre X, Guerrero JL et al: Papillary muscle displacement causes systolic anterior motion of the mitral valve: experimental validation and insights into the mechanism of subaortic obstruction, *Circulation* 91:1189, 1995.
47. Miller WS: The vascular supply of the pleura pulmonalis, *Am J Anat* 7:389, 1907.
48. McLaughlin RF, Tyler WS, Canada RO: A study of the subgross pulmonary anatomy in various mammals, *Am J Anat* 108:149, 1961.
49. Fatkin D, Kelly RP, Feneley MP: Relations between left atrial appendage blood flow velocity, spontaneous echocardiographic contrast and thromboembolic risk in vivo, *J Am Coll Cardiol* 23:961, 1994.
50. Reeder GS, Charlesworth JE, Moore SB: Cause of spontaneous echocardiographic contrast as assessed by scanning electron microscopy, *J Am Soc Echocardiogr* 7:169, 1994.
51. Maron BJ, Spirito P, Wesley Y et al: Development and progression of left ventricular hypertrophy in children with hypertrophic cardiomyopathy, *N Engl J Med* 315:610, 1986.
52. Maron BJ, Fananapazir L: Sudden cardiac death in hypertrophic cardiomyopathy, *Circulation* 85:I57, 1992.
53. Solomon SD, Wolff S, Watkins H et al: Left ventricular hypertrophy and morphology in familial hypertrophic cardiomyopathy associated with mutations of the beta-myosin heavy chain gene, *J Am Coll Cardiol* 22:498, 1993 (comments).
54. Bright JM, Golden AL, Gompf RE et al: Evaluation of the calcium channel-blocking agents diltiazem and verapamil for treatment of feline hypertrophic cardiomyopathy, *J Vet Intern Med* 5:272, 1991.
55. Bright JM, Golden AL: Evidence for or against the efficacy of calcium channel blockers for management of hypertrophic cardiomyopathy in cats, *Vet Clin North Am Small Anim Pract* 21:1023, 1991.
56. Betocchi S, Piscione F, Losi MA et al: Effects of diltiazem on left ventricular systolic and diastolic function in hypertrophic cardiomyopathy, *Am J Cardiol* 78:451, 1996.
57. Bright JM, Herrtage ME: Pulsed Doppler assessment of left ventricular diastolic function in normal and cardiomyopathic cats, *Proc Annu Vet Med Forum,* 1997, p 212.
58. Atkins C, Johnson L, Keene B et al: Diltiazem pharmacokinetics and pharmacodynamics in cats, *J Vet Intern Med* 8:144, 1994 (abstract).
59. Keene BW: Feline cardiovascular drugs: which drug/which dose? *Proc Annu Vet Med Forum,* 1997, p 155.
60. Louie EK, Edwards LC: Hypertrophic cardiomyopathy, *Prog Cardiovasc Dis* 36:275, 1994.
61. Bonagura JD, Stepien RL, Lehmkuhl LB: Acute effects of esmolol on left ventricular outflow obstruction in cats with hypertrophic cardiomyopathy, *J Vet Intern Med* 5:123, 1991 (abstract).
62. Quinones M, Dyer DC, Ware WA et al: Pharmacokinetics of atenolol in clinically normal cats, *Am J Vet Res* 57:1050, 1996.
63. Dabrowski M, Michalak E, Maurin A et al: [Results of long-term verapamil treatment of patients with hypertrophic cardiomyopathy] Wyniki przewleklego leczenia verapamilem u chorych z kardiomiopatia przerostowa, *Kardiol Pol* 32(suppl 2):6, 1989.
64. Spirito P, Maron BJ: Absence of progression of left ventricular hypertrophy in adult patients with hypertrophic cardiomyopathy, *J Am Coll Cardiol* 9:1013, 1987.
65. Rush JE, Freeman LM, Brown DJ et al: The use of enalapril in the treatment of feline hypertrophic cardiomyopathy, *J Am Anim Hosp Assoc* 34:38, 1998.
66. Tilley L, King JN, Humbert-Droz E et al: Benazepril activity in cats: Inhibition of plasma ACE and efficacy in the treatment of hypertension, *J Vet Intern Med* 10:163, 1996 (abstract).
67. Pion PD, Kittleson MD: Therapy for feline aortic thromboembolism. In Kirk RW, ed: *Kirk's current veterinary therapy, X: small animal practice,* Philadelphia, 1989, WB Saunders.
68. Harpster NK, Baty CJ: Warfarin therapy of the cat at risk of thromboembolism. In Bonagura JD, ed: *Kirk's current veterinary therapy, XII: small animal practice,* Philadelphia, 1995, WB Saunders.
69. Torfgard KE, Ahlner J: Mechanisms of action of nitrates, *Cardiovasc Drugs Ther* 8:701, 1994.
70. Zucker ML, Budd SE, Dollar LE et al: Effect of diltiazem and low-dose aspirin on platelet aggregation and ATP release induced by paired agonists, *Thromb Haemost* 70:332, 1993.
71. Lippton HL, Horwitz PM, McNamara DB et al: Influence of verapamil and diltiazem on aggregatory responses in cat and rabbit platelet rich plasma, *Prostaglandins Leukot Med* 16:121, 1984.
72. Behrend EN, Grauer GF, Greco DS et al: Comparison of the effects of diltiazem and aspirin on platelet aggregation in cats, *J Am Anim Hops Assoc* 32:11, 1996.
73. Anfossi G, Massucco P, Mularoni E et al: Effects of forskolin and organic nitrate on aggregation and intracellular cyclic nucleotide content in human platelets, *Gen Pharmacol* 25:1093, 1994.
74. Ivanova K, Schaefer M, Drummer C et al: Effects of nitric oxide-containing compounds on increases in cytosolic ionized Ca2+ and on aggregation of human platelets, *Eur J Pharmacol* 244:37, 1993.
75. Atkins CE, Gallo AM, Kurzman ID et al: Risk factors, clinical signs, and survival in cats with a clinical diagnosis of idiopathic hypertrophic cardiomyopathy: 74 cases (1985-1989), *J Am Vet Med Assoc* 201:613, 1992.

CHAPTER 22

Feline Unclassified and Restrictive Cardiomyopathy

The term *cardiomyopathy* denotes any disease of the heart muscle. Various classification schemes for cardiomyopathy have evolved over the years. The most recent recommendations in humans for the clinical classification of cardiomyopathies divide them into dilated, hypertrophic, restrictive, unclassified, and specific cardiomyopathies.[1] Dilated and hypertrophic cardiomyopathies are discussed in Chapters 20 and 21. The specific cardiomyopathies seen in cats and dogs include parvovirus myocarditis, taurine deficiency–induced myocardial failure, and carnitine deficiency–induced myocardial failure. These are discussed in Chapter 20. This leaves restrictive and unclassified cardiomyopathies. Restrictive cardiomyopathy is a specific physiologic/morphologic/pathologic diagnosis in humans. Endomyocardial fibrosis is one cause of restrictive cardiomyopathy. The term *restrictive cardiomyopathy* has often been misused in the veterinary literature to describe a poorly defined type of cardiac disease in cats.[2,3] This disease is characterized by a left ventricle that is normal to near normal in appearance on an echocardiogram with left atrial enlargement and little-to-no mitral regurgitation. Because ventricular systolic function is either normal or only mildly reduced and ventricular wall thickness is normal or only mildly increased, clinicians have often surmised that there must be abnormal diastolic ventricular function causing the moderate-to-severe abnormalities noted (i.e., atrial enlargement and heart failure). Consequently, the diagnosis of restrictive cardiomyopathy is often placed on these cats. Restrictive cardiomyopathy is "characterized by restrictive filling and reduced diastolic volume of either or both ventricles with normal or near-normal systolic function and wall thickness. Increased interstitial fibrosis may be present."[1] The clinical diagnosis of restrictive cardiomyopathy is made by identifying clinically significant diastolic dysfunction without evidence of overt concentric hypertrophy. This can be done by identifying characteristic pressure waveform abnormalities at cardiac catheterization or by identifying characteristic Doppler flow signals across the mitral valve. Recently the use of Doppler tissue imaging has emerged as a potential new modality to assess diastolic function. Cardiac catheterization is rarely performed in cats, and the characteristic Doppler patterns seen in humans often cannot be discerned in cats because of their fast heart rate. Consequently, definitive evidence of restrictive physiology often is not or cannot be identified before death. In some cases, the left ventricle in a cat with an enlarged left atrium is clearly affected with a form of disease that does produce restrictive physiology (i.e., endomyocardial fibrosis). These cats most commonly have obvious endocardial thickening or have a cavity that is smaller than normal because of excess tissue within the cavity. Making a diagnosis of restrictive cardiomyopathy in these cases is appropriate, although the latter form of the disease has, at times, been termed *obliterative cardiomyopathy*.

In the cat without clear echocardiographic evidence of endocardial scarring or cavity obliteration that does not undergo cardiac catheterization and whose heart rate does not slow enough to identify abnormal mitral valve Doppler signals, it is probably incorrect to assume that a form of restrictive cardiomyopathy is present. This is not to say that restrictive cardiomyopathy is definitively ruled out. The real diagnosis in this situation is "open," which means that the clinician does not know what is causing the cardiac problem. Veterinarians have great difficulty in saying "I do not know." Consequently, most veterinarians end up placing some term on what they observe. Intermediate, or intergrade, cardiomyopathy is a classification originally introduced by Harpster[4,5] to place a name on this disease entity and to end the misuse of the term *restrictive cardiomyopathy*. Although clinical and echocardiographic features in these cats may be similar to both dilated and hypertrophic cardiomyopathy, the terms *intermediate* and *intergrade* are probably inappropriate because they suggest that the characteristic changes seen in these cats share pathophysiologic or etiologic features of the more common cardiomyopathies. Although it is likely that some of these cats have an end-stage or variant form of hypertrophic cardiomyopathy, this situation appears to be rare. According to the WHO classification, "Unclassified cardiomyopathies include a few cases (of cardiomyopathy) that do not fit into any group."[1] Because a definitive diagnosis of a type of restrictive cardiomyopathy cannot be made in many of these cats, the term *unclassified cardiomyopathy* may be more appropriate. Placing a cat with undiagnosed cardiac disease into a specific category, regardless of its name, can be dangerous. In our clinic we have seen many cats with primary mitral regurgitation, mitral and tricuspid valve dysplasia, and hyperthyroidism placed into this category, probably because it was convenient and gave the clinician a false sense of security, allowing him or her to think a definitive diagnosis had been made.

To confuse the issue further, disease entities that could look like the clinical disease just described have been described in the pathology literature. These include endomyocarditis and endocardial fibrosis. Dr. Sam Liu first described these abnormalities more than 25 years ago.[6] Myocarditis is inflammation of the myocardium resulting from any cause. Myocarditis most commonly destroys cardiac muscle, resulting in systolic myocardial failure. Endomyocarditis is a cardiac disease in which the inflammation primarily affects the endocardium, whereas the other layers of the myocardium are affected to a lesser degree. This most commonly results in endomyocardial fibrosis that decreases the compliance of the affected ventricle. Recently a group from the University of Pennsylvania looked at this issue.[7] These cats have a nonseptic form of endomyocarditis that may lead to left ventricular endocardial fibrosis. Cats with endomyocarditis are most commonly young (less than 4 years of age) and are most commonly presented because of respiratory distress. Some have evidence of thromboembolic disease, including aortic thromboembolism. At postmortem examination the heart typically weighs more than normal. The left atrium is dilated, and the endocardium of the left ventricle is often opaque, although it is normal in some cases. Histologically, there are varying degrees of inflammation. The cellular infiltrates are primarily neutrophils and macrophages in most cats but can consist of lymphocytes and plasma cells in some. Fibroplasia is striking in most cats. An interstitial pneumonia is also common in this group and may be responsible for the dyspnea in these cats. Endomyocarditis may lead to left ventricular endomyocardial fibrosis, but this cause-and-effect relationship has not been established. Left ventricular endocardial fibrosis is more commonly observed in middle-age cats. Respiratory distress is also a common presenting clinical complaint in these cats, presumably as a result of left heart failure. At necropsy, the heart is enlarged, especially the left atrium. The left ventricular endocardium in these cats is thick and gray-white. This lesion may be generalized or localized to the left ventricular outflow tract. Histologically, marked endocardial fibrosis without inflammation is present. Mild-to-moderate fibrosis may also be present within the myocardium. Unfortunately, a good study tying the pathologic disease reported in these studies to the clinical disease described earlier has not been reported. However, there is a reasonable possibility that left ventricular endocardial fibrosis is at least one cause of the clinical entity known as *unclassified cardiomyopathy* and so truly is a form of restrictive cardiomyopathy. However, we have observed cats at postmortem examination that had echocardiographic evidence of a normal left ventricle and left atrial enlargement without any histologic evidence of endocardial fibrosis, therefore we firmly believe that not all cats with unclassified cardiomyopathy have endocardial fibrosis.

Recently, one of our residents (Dr. Brad Gavaghan) examined diastolic function in nine cats with unclassified cardiomyopathy with Doppler tissue imaging. He found that six of these cats had clear evidence of reduced diastolic left ventricular wall and mitral annular velocities. The reduction in diastolic function was comparable to that seen in a group of cats with hypertrophic cardiomyopathy and in a group of human patients with restrictive cardiomyopathy. Consequently, it appears that the pathophysiology of their disease was due to diastolic dysfunction of the left ventricle, and therefore they most likely had a form of restrictive cardiomyopathy. In the other three cats, diastolic function was somewhat abnormal, but in an atypical fashion. The echocardiograms from these nine cats appeared identical. Consequently, it appears that the abnormality responsible for the left heart dysfunction is not the same in all cats with unclassified cardiomyopathy

Feline Restrictive Cardiomyopathy (Endomyocardial Fibrosis)

Restrictive cardiomyopathy (RCM) is defined as a diverse group of myocardial conditions characterized by abnormal diastolic function and/or a restriction of diastolic filling.[2] Restrictive cardiomyopathy occurs when ventricular diastolic stretch (i.e., compliance) is impaired by endocardial, subendocardial, or myocardial fibrosis or an infiltrative disease, resulting in an increased diastolic pressure for any given diastolic volume.[3] In contrast to human medicine, specific clinical and morphologic criteria for the diagnosis have not been clearly defined in the cat. Without the use of invasive diagnostic procedures or necropsy examination, distinguishing this disorder from infiltrative diseases of the myocardium and unclassified forms of cardiomyopathy is not always possible.

PATHOPHYSIOLOGY

In their classic forms, endocardial, subendocardial, and myocardial fibrosis impede ventricular diastolic filling and so alter diastolic function. Other types of infiltrative myocardial disease may also lead to diastolic dysfunction and may be classified as "secondary" restrictive cardiomyopathies.[2] These disorders are characterized by an elevated ventricular diastolic pressure with normal-to-reduced ventricular filling volumes (decreased compliance). The elevation in diastolic ventricular pressure results in atrial enlargement and edema formation. Systolic function is usually preserved. The lesions are generally confined to the left ventricle in humans, and congestive left heart failure predominates the clinical presentation. Papillary muscle fibrosis, distortion of the mitral valve apparatus, and changes in left ventricular geometry may contribute to the development of mitral regurgitation and left heart failure. Similar pathophysiology may result from pericardial fibrosis (constrictive pericarditis) or infiltrative, neoplastic, and inflammatory diseases of the epicardium or myocardium.

PATHOLOGY

The postmortem changes are unique to this form of cardiomyopathy and may be used to differentiate it from other disorders. Patchy or diffuse endocardial, subendocardial, or myocardial deposition of fibrous tissue is a characteristic necropsy finding.[8] The endocardium may appear whitish-gray, opaque, and thickened (Color Plate 91). Endocardial fibrosis without eosinophilia is the most common form reported in the cat, whereas eosinophilic endocardial inflammation is common in humans.[2,3] Restrictive cardiomyopathy has been reported in one cat with hypereosinophilic syndrome, although it is impossible to determine whether the hypereosinophilia in this cat caused the restrictive cardiomyopathy or whether the two diseases happened to occur together in this cat.[9] Fibrous adhesions between papillary muscles and the myocardium with distortion and fusion of the chordae tendineae and mitral valve leaflets may also be noted in restrictive cardiomyopathy. In extreme cases, the left ventricular cavity may be partially obliterated. As with most cardiomyopathies, the left ventricle appears to be most severely affected, although other cardiac chambers may exhibit similar pathologic findings. Extreme left atrial and left auricular enlargement are common. A high prevalence of systemic thromboembolism is reported.[10,11]

Histologic features include extreme endocardial thickening by hyaline, fibrous, and granulation tissue.[8] Chondroid metaplasia is occasionally exhibited by the surface layer of hyaline tissue. A layer of loose fibrous tissue lies beneath this layer, with a layer of granulation tissue adjacent to the myocardium. These changes are similar but not identical to those seen in humans with restrictive cardiomyopathy.[2]

CLINICAL FEATURES

Signalment is difficult to report accurately because little agreement exists among veterinary cardiologists as to which cases fall within this classification. From a series of pathologic studies in cats, Liu reported an age range of 8 months to 19 years.[8] No breed

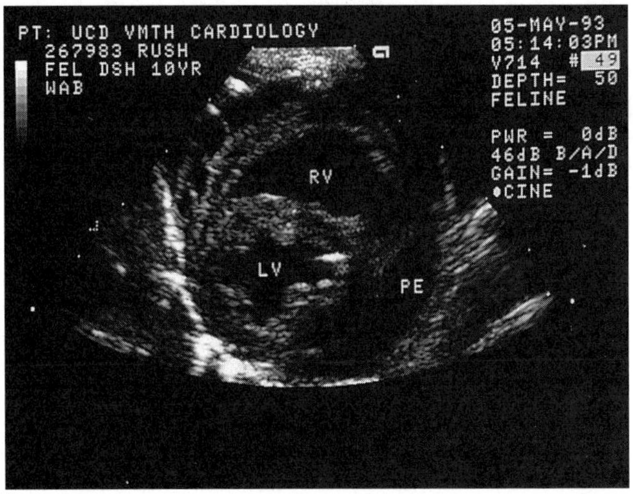

FIGURE 22-1 Right parasternal short-axis echocardiogram from a cat with restrictive cardiomyopathy. Notice the loss of left ventricular (LV) symmetry and the irregular, thickened and hyperechoic endocardium. *PE,* Pericardial effusion; *RV,* right ventricle.

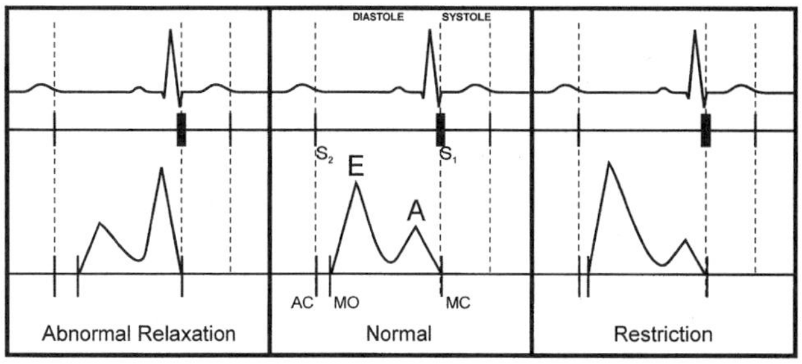

FIGURE 22-2 Schematic representation of the common transmitral Doppler flow patterns associated with abnormal relaxation or restriction. The electrocardiogram *(top),* phonocardiogram *(middle),* and transmitral Doppler tracing *(bottom)* are depicted. The first heart sound *(S_1),* second heart sound *(S_2),* aortic valve closure *(AC),* mitral valve opening *(MO),* and mitral valve closure *(MC)* are labeled. A normal transmitral flow pattern is represented by the middle figure. Characteristics of abnormal relaxation *(left figure)* compared with normal include increases in isovolumic relaxation time (time between aortic closure and mitral opening), deceleration time and flow velocity of the *A* wave *(A)* and decreases in peak *E* wave *(E)* velocity and the ratio of peak *E* wave to peak *A* wave velocity. Compared with normal, a restrictive pattern is characterized by a decrease in isovolumic relaxation time and flow velocity of the *A* wave and an increase in the ratio of peak *E* wave velocity to peak *A* wave velocity.

predisposition has been reported. Although some reports indicate a male predominance, others show an equal sex distribution.[3] In our hospital, most cats are middle-age or older. Presenting complaints and clinical signs are similar to other forms of myocardial disease, including dyspnea/tachypnea; a poor general condition; weakness; lethargy or, rarely, exercise intolerance; and anorexia. Some cats may present with acute posterior paresis or paralysis associated with systemic thromboembolism.

The physical examination is similar to other forms of cardiomyopathy seen in cats. Auscultation may detect a systolic murmur of mitral insufficiency (commonly heard at the apex), a gallop sound, or an irregular cardiac rhythm. Cats in heart failure are typically tachypneic and/or dyspneic as a result of pleural effusion or pulmonary edema. Occasionally, jugular pulses or distention is present. Hypothermia may be seen in cats with a severe reduction in cardiac output.

The electrocardiogram and thoracic radiographs are usually no different from those seen with other forms of cardiomyopathy. The electrocardiogram may be normal or may demonstrate a left axis shift. A variety of ventricular and supraventricular arrhythmias have been identified. Thoracic radiographs typically show dramatic left atrial or biatrial enlargement and enlarged and tortuous pulmonary veins. When congestive heart failure is present, pleural effusion or pulmonary edema are observed.

The echocardiographic findings in RCM are variable. Severe left atrial dilation is a common feature, and the left ventricular internal dimensions are typically mildly-to-moderately reduced, although they may be mildly enlarged. Two-dimensional echocardiography may demonstrate loss of normal left ventricular symmetry, distorted or fused papillary muscles, and mild left ventricular concentric hypertrophy. Occasionally the endocardium is notably thickened and irregular with increased echogenicity (Figure 22-1). Indices of left ventricular systolic function (e.g., shortening fraction, E-point–to–septal separation, velocity of circumferential fiber shortening) are normal or only mildly depressed. Mild mitral regurgitation may be detectable with spectral and color flow Doppler. The presence of a large jet of mitral regurgitation on color flow Doppler is more consistent with primary mitral regurgitation. Left atrial thrombi may be identified in some cases.

The role of Doppler echocardiography in the evaluation and characterization of diastolic dysfunction is a subject of much debate in both human and veterinary medicine. The accuracy of such techniques is hampered by the dynamic and complex nature of transmitral blood flow that is subject to influence by volumetric flow, ventricular preload, afterload, and heart rate.[12] Most currently employed methods involve evaluation of transmitral flow velocities and contours obtained by pulsed-wave Doppler echocardiography.[12] Two distinct patterns of mitral flow have been demonstrated in humans that suggest either abnormal relaxation or cardiac restriction (Figure 22-2). Abnormal relaxation is suggested by an increased isovolumic relaxation time (i.e., time from aortic valve closure to mitral valve opening), a slow early diastolic mitral flow acceleration (*E* wave) with or without a reduced peak velocity, and an increased peak flow velocity associated with atrial contraction (*A* wave).[13] A restrictive pattern in humans is characterized by a normal or shortened isovolumic relaxation time, an increased *E* wave peak velocity with a rapid acceleration, followed by a reduction in peak *A* wave velocity.[12,13] Interestingly, most patients with restrictive cardiomyopathy tend to have either normal mitral flow patterns or velocity contours that suggest abnormal relaxation rather than restriction. When the heart rate exceeds approximately 160 beats/min, the *E* and *A* waves merge so that they can no longer be distinguished. Because most cats have a fast heart rate at the time of examination, examination of spectral Doppler left ventricular inflow signals is severely limited. Consequently, the clinical utility of these techniques in cats with restrictive cardiomyopathy has not been evaluated.

Expected changes seen at cardiac catheterization include increased pulmonary capillary wedge pressure with a prominent *a* wave and elevated left ventricular end-diastolic pressure with a characteristic wave form that is close to zero at the onset of rapid ventricular filling followed by a rapid rise in pressure that then plateaus during middiastole ($\surd\overline{\ \ }$). Distortion of the left ventricular chamber with apical obliteration, filling defects, and an irregular endocardial surface have been demonstrated in some cats studied by angiography.[3] Other abnormalities include left atrial enlargement, prominent and tortuous pulmonary veins, mitral regurgitation, and intracardiac thrombi.

PROGNOSIS

As with other forms of cardiomyopathy, the prognosis is difficult to predict for individual cases before observing the initial response to therapy. A high incidence of serious arrhythmias, systemic thromboembolism, and refractory congestive heart failure have been reported by some authors. In our experience, cats with restrictive cardiomyopathy have a poor prognosis, with high mortality and morbidity. Although an initial response to standard therapy (see below) is possible, progressive and refractory heart failure develops in most cases.

Unclassified Feline Cardiomyopathies

In recent years, an increasing number of cats have been recognized with obviously abnormal hearts that do not fit into any recognized disease classification. It is not known whether these cases represent a single disease category, although our data suggest they do not. It is not known whether these represent congenital or acquired disease. It is not known whether these cases are afflicted by a primary myocardial disease or disease secondary to or associated with another condition. It has been proposed that cats with ill-defined cardiac disorders may represent progressive or regressive states of other known cardiomyopathic processes.[3] Although this theory cannot be refuted, no current evidence to support this conclusion exists. Due to the lack of substantiated information regarding this group of cats, we prefer to identify them as *unclassified cardiomyopathies.*

PATHOPHYSIOLOGY

The pathophysiology of unclassified cardiomyopathies in the cat is unresolved. Although some degree of systolic left ventricular dysfunction may be present and valvular insufficiency is also commonly recognized, the degree of these changes does not sufficiently explain the severe atrial enlargement and severe congestive heart failure generally identified in this group of cats. In the absence of severe myocardial failure and severe valvular disease, impairment of diastolic function is one realistic abnormality that can explain the spectrum of clinical abnormalities seen. However, again from the data presented above, this is clearly not the only explanation. If diastolic dysfunction is present, the etiology of the diastolic dysfunction is unknown. Progressive increases in left atrial and left ventricular end-diastolic pressures lead to elevated pulmonary venous and capillary pressures and pulmonary edema or pleural effusion. Many cats also display enlargement of the right atrium and ventricle. Whether or not right ventricular diastolic dysfunction is the cause of these changes is debatable. It is also possible that chronic left atrial hypertension leads to chronic pulmonary hypertension, which results in progressive enlargement of the right ventricle and elevated central venous pressure. Pulmonary edema and pleural effusion are typical manifestations of congestive heart failure in these cats. Occasionally, hepatic congestion (indicated by increased hepatic vein size on abdominal ultrasound) or, more rarely, ascites may be associated with right heart failure. Abnormal blood flow in the left atrium undoubtedly predisposes affected cats to left atrial thrombus formation and systemic thromboembolism.

PATHOLOGY

Although pathologic criteria have not been established, severe biatrial enlargement appears to be the most common feature in affected individuals.[14] The ventricle may be mildly concentrically or eccentrically hypertrophied, or may be normal. Regional thinning of the left ventricular free wall interspersed with areas of focal concentric hypertrophy have been described in some reports involving unclassified or "intermediate" cardiomyopathies.[15] In a few of these cases myocardial infarction has been reported, often at the left ventricular apex.[15] Whether or not these cases represent spontaneous coronary artery disease or myocardial infarction secondary to another underlying process is unknown. Because the etiology of the disease in these cats is unknown, it is probably most appropriate to classify them as unclassified cardiomyopathies. Systemic thromboemboli are common, and intracardiac thrombi may occasionally be seen.

CLINICAL FEATURES

Because of the absence of a discrete clinical classification scheme, no known sex, breed, or age predispositions exist. Presenting complaints, clinical findings, electrocardiographic findings, and radiographic abnormalities are similar to other forms of myocardial disease and are generally nondiscriminatory. The common radiographic findings are severe left or biatrial enlargement and a patchy pulmonary interstitial pattern resulting from pulmonary edema. Pleural effusion may be seen but appears to be less common than in other forms for feline cardiomyopathy.

The most consistent echocardiographic finding is severe dilation of the left atrium (Figure 22-3, *A*). The left ventricle is usually normal in size or only mildly eccentrically or concentrically hypertrophied. (Figure 22-3, *B*) Various patterns of mild regional myocardial hypertrophy are observed in the septum or left ventricular free wall of some cats. Enlargement of the right heart is variable, but may be marked in some cases. Echocardiography may demonstrate a mildly increased left ventricular end-systolic dimension and hence a mildly reduced left ventricular shortening, suggesting some degree of systolic dysfunction. Rarely, marked regional wall hypokinesis with or without dramatic thinning of the myocardium may be noted. (Figure 22-3, *C*) As stated above, the exact nature of these findings is uncertain but they suggest myocardial infarction. Mitral and, occasionally, tricuspid regurgitation can be detected with spectral and color flow Doppler in most affected cats but are generally mild and probably related to changes in ventricular geometry (Color Plate 92). As with cats with restrictive cardiomyopathy, abnormalities of transmitral Doppler flow signals may suggest diastolic dysfunction in some cats (Figure 22-4). In some cases, a thrombus is observed within the left atrium (Figure 22-5). In one patient in our clinic that demonstrated severe right atrial and ventricular enlargement, along with the typical left-sided abnormalities, cardiac catheterization revealed elevated diastolic pressure in all cardiac chambers and moderate-to-severe pulmonary hypertension. The etiology of the pulmonary hypertension was not defined, however, and no difference in the pulmonary arterial pressures at an FIO_2 of 21% and 100% was present. This suggests the changes were pathologic and irreversible.

Prognosis

The prognosis is generally based on clinical presentation, echocardiographic and radiographic evidence of elevated diastolic

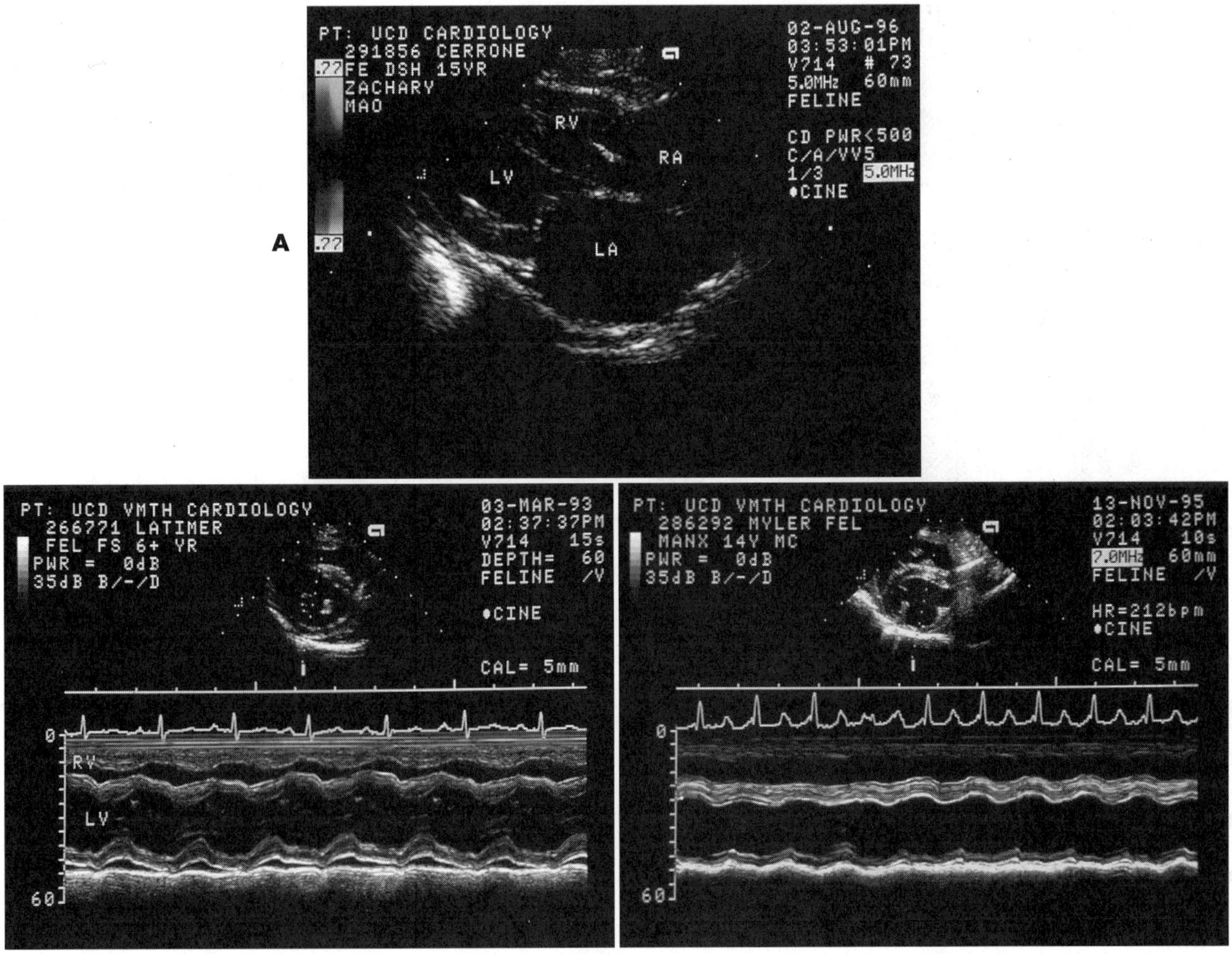

FIGURE 22-3 Echocardiograms from cats with unclassified cardiomyopathies. **A,** Right parasternal four-chamber view showing mild eccentric hypertrophy of the left ventricle *(LV)* and severe left atrial *(LA)* enlargement. **B,** LV M-mode showing mild LV eccentric hypertrophy (mildly enlarged end-diastolic dimension with normal wall thickness) and a mild reduction in LV systolic function (mildly enlarged end-systolic dimension). **C,** Left ventricular M-mode showing severe hypokinesis and thinning of the LV free wall.

pressures, and response to therapy. Asymptomatic cats with mild left atrial enlargement are believed to have a good long-term prognosis. Asymptomatic cats with marked left atrial enlargement are likely at higher risk for developing heart failure. Cats that present in heart failure generally have a poor prognosis with a short survival time (weeks to months). Cats that present in heart failure and respond favorably to therapy may do well for longer periods. Cats presenting with aortic thromboembolism usually have a poor prognosis.

Modcrator Band Cardiomyopathy

A rare and unique pathologic syndrome has been reported in cats in which bands of tissue that appear similar to moderator bands in the right ventricle have been described in the left ventricle. These bands are more commonly called *false tendons* in the left ventricle (see Chapter 1). In these cats many abnormally thickened false tendons or moderator bands bridge the left ventricular free wall, septum, or papillary muscles.[16,17] Some of the reported cats were very young,

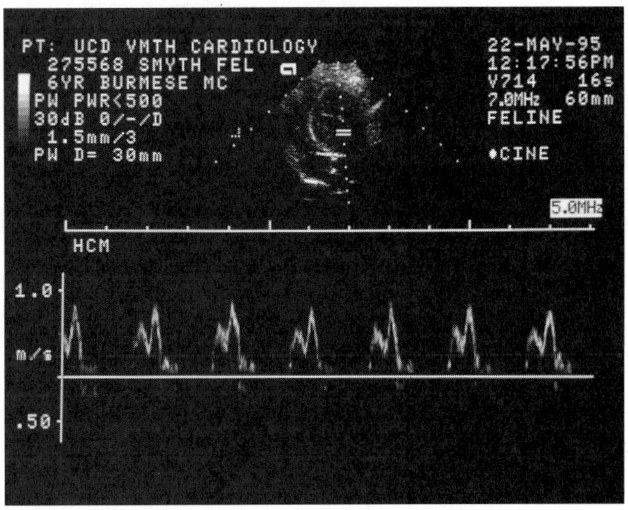

FIGURE 22-4 Transmitral Doppler tracing from a cat with unclassified cardiomyopathy. (See text for details.)

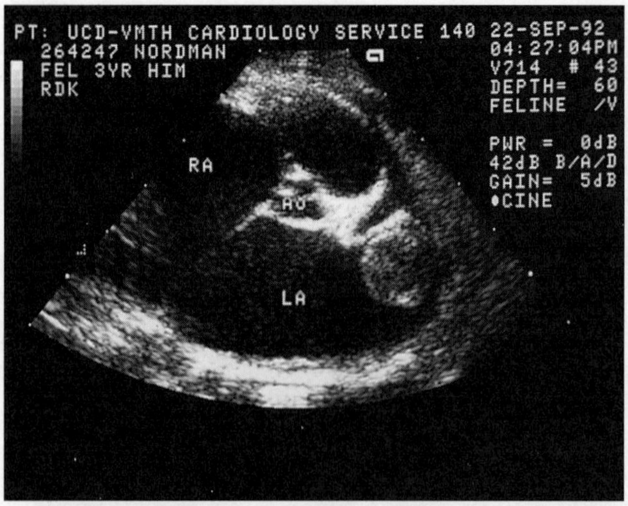

FIGURE 22-5 Right parasternal short-axis view from a cat with unclassified cardiomyopathy. Severe left atrial enlargement is noted, and there is a large thrombus within the left auricle.

suggesting a congenital malformation, while many were middle-age and older.

Clinical findings are variable yet similar to other forms of feline myocardial disease.[3] Reported findings include anorexia, depression, dyspnea, hypothermia, congestive heart failure, gallop sounds, systolic heart murmurs, systemic thromboembolism, and various arrhythmias. Reported electrocardiographic changes in 21 cats included right bundle branch block ($n = 6$), left axis shift ($n = 4$), first- and third-degree atrioventricular blocks ($n = 3$), and sinus bradycardia ($n = 4$). Cardiomegaly is typically present on the thoracic radiograph, with varying degrees of left atrial enlargement. Cardiac catheterization in two cats revealed elevated left ventricular diastolic pressure and normal systolic pressure.[16]

Pathologic changes include an irregular left ventricular endocardial contour with a rounded apex and numerous thick and irregular left ventricular false tendons (Color Plate 93). Reported heart weights are greater than normal but are less than those found in cats with hypertrophic and dilated cardiomyopathy.[17] Histologically the moderator bands are composed of central Purkinje fibers and dense or loose collagen and are covered by normal endocardium. Necropsy findings suggest that younger cats have a tendency for left ventricular concentric hypertrophy, whereas older cats have a tendency for left ventricular eccentric hypertrophy.[3]

The diagnosis of this disorder is difficult and often is made only at necropsy. Angiographic findings are insensitive because of the heterogenous nature of the structural abnormalities and the similarities with restrictive cardiomyopathy. Echocardiography has facilitated the diagnosis; however, the findings may overlap those seen in restrictive cardiomyopathy. Occasionally, a network of false tendons can be clearly imaged using two-dimensional echocardiography.

Therapy

Therapy for all these disorders is symptomatic and palliative. It is generally aimed at alleviating the signs of congestive heart failure and preventing systemic thromboembolism. Urgent care because of life-threatening pulmonary edema or pleural effusion is often necessary. If the severity of the dyspnea prevents radiographic evaluation, thoracocentesis should be attempted, and, if thoracocentesis is negative, medical therapy should be pursued. When pleural effusion is present, immediate thoracocentesis with the cat in sternal recumbency is indicated. Initial therapy for life-threatening pulmonary edema consists of supplemental oxygen and aggressive diuretic therapy (furosemide 2 to 4 mg/kg IM or IV q2-4h) with or without transdermal nitroglycerine therapy (2%, ¼ to ½ inch topically q12h). Once diuresis is observed and the respiratory rate begins to decline, the furosemide should be decreased to 1 to 2 mg/kg q6-12h. For recommendations regarding the treatment and prevention of systemic thromboembolism see Chapter 31.

Chronic therapy involves continued management and prevention of recurrent congestive heart failure. Standard therapy includes oral furosemide therapy (for dose recommendations see Chapter 10). Although no formal studies exist, the use of angiotensin converting enzyme (ACE) inhibitor therapy in these cats is indicated because of the severe nature of the congestive signs and the presence of moderate mitral insufficiency in some instances (see Chapter 10).

No specific therapy for reversing or preventing progression of these conditions currently exists; therefore therapeutic decisions beyond standard treatment for congestive heart failure are generally based on clinical experience and theoretical considerations. The clinician should be aware that if the current therapeutic plan is not sufficient, an alternative is warranted. However, it should be noted that therapy for congestive heart failure in this group of cats is not always successful.

The one consistent feature of all the atypical feline cardiomyopathies is that the primary hemodynamic abnormality is presumed to be ventricular diastolic dysfunction.[3,14] Therefore medications such as diltiazem that improve diastolic function (i.e., positive lusitropic agents) would appear to have merit in such disorders. However, in cases with restrictive and moderator band cardiomyopathy these medications probably have no theoretical or practical benefit, because the diastolic dysfunction is associated with a physical restriction within the severely diseased endomyocardium, not impaired relaxation. Although the literature contains anecdotal reports suggesting clinical improvement with positive lusitropic agents in cats with these disorders, the effects of concomitant therapies have not been adequately assessed. We have had several cats with unclassified cardiomyopathy and congestive heart failure apparently respond favorably to lusitropic support. However, because virtually 100% of these patients also receive high doses of furosemide and ACE inhibitor therapy, the added benefit of the positive lusitrope is questionable. Diltiazem (7.5 mg/cat q8h) might be considered in these cases if they exhibit signs of refractory congestive heart failure or if diuretic therapy can no longer be increased because of renal complications. Digoxin therapy (1/4 of a 0.125-mg tablet q24-48h) should be considered in cats with echocardiographic evidence of moderate-to-severe myocardial failure (shortening fraction less than 25%) or in cats with severe supraventricular arrhythmias.

REFERENCES

1. Richardson P, Meckenna W, Bristow M et al: Report of the 1995 World Health Organization/International Society and Federation of Cardiology Task Force on the Definition and Classification of Cardiomyopathies, *Circulation* 93:841, 1996.
2. Wynne J, Braunwald E: The cardiomyopathies and myocarditises: toxic, chemical, and physical damage to the heart. In Braunwald E, ed: *Heart disease: a textbook of cardiovascular medicine,* Philadelphia, 1992, WB Saunders.

3. Fox PR: Feline myocardial disease. In Fox PR, ed: *Canine and feline cardiology,* New York, 1988, Churchill Livingstone.
4. Harpster NK: Feline myocardial diseases. In Kirk RW, ed: *Kirk's current veterinary therapy, IX,* Philadelphia, 1986 WB Saunders.
5. Harpster NK: The cardiovascular system. In Holzworth J, ed: *Diseases of the cat,* Philadelphia, 1986, WB Saunders.
6. Liu SK: Acquired cardiac lesions leading to congestive heart failure in the cat, *Am J Vet Res* 31:2071, 1998.
7. Stalis I, Bossbaly MJ, VanWinkle T: Feline endomyocarditis and left ventricular endocardial fibrosis, *Vet Pathol* 32:122, 1995.
8. Liu SK: Cardiovascular pathology. In Fox PR, ed: *Canine and feline cardiology,* New York, 1988, Churchill Livingstone.
9. Saxon B, Hendrick M, Waddle JR: Restrictive cardiomyopathy in a cat with hypereosinophilic syndrome, *Can Vet J* 32:367, 1991.
10. Pion PD, Kienle RD: Feline cardiomyopathy. In Miller MS, Tilley LP, eds: *Manual of canine and feline cardiology,* ed 2, Philadelphia, 1995, WB Saunders.
11. Liu SK, Tilley LP: Animal models of primary myocardial disease, *Yale J Biol Med* 53:191, 1980.
12. DeMaria A, Wisenbaugh TW, Smith MD et al: Doppler echocardiographic evaluation of diastolic dysfunction, *Circulation* (suppl I):I, 1991.
13. Appleton CP, Hatle LK, Popp RL: Demonstration of restrictive ventricular physiology by Doppler echocardiography, *J Am Coll Cardiol* 11:757, 1988.
14. Fox PR: Restrictive cardiomyopathy, *Proc ACVIM Forum,* 1996, p 235.
15. Bonagura JD: Feline restrictive cardiomyopathy, *Proc ACVIM Forum* 1994, p 205.
16. Liu SK, Fox PR, Tilley LP: Excessive moderator bands in the left ventricle of 21 cats, *J Am Vet Med Assoc* 180:1215, 1982.
17. Liu SK: Left ventricular false tendons associated with cardiac malfunction in 101 cats, *Lab Invest* 56:44A, 1980 (abstract).

CHAPTER 23

Heartworm Infestation and Disease (Dirofilariasis)

Heartworms (*Dirofilaria immitis*) are filarial nematodes that primarily reside in the pulmonary arteries of dogs (Color Plate 94). Heartworms also reside in the right heart in unusual circumstances, such as in caval syndrome and massive infestation. They are occasionally identified as adult worms in other species, such as domestic cats, sea lions, and ferrets. Because heartworms primarily reside in pulmonary arteries and not within the heart, heartworm disease is a relative misnomer. Heartworm was so named because veterinarians for many years observed the worms in the right heart at postmortem examination. Adult heartworms are held within the pulmonary arteries by blood flow. When blood flow stops, they fall back through the pulmonic valve into the right ventricle. Consequently, this is where they are found after death. With the advent of echocardiography, it has become readily apparent that the right heart is an aberrant location for heartworms in dogs.

Heartworm disease in dogs and cats occurs worldwide. Lauro Travassos of Brazil first reported it in cats in 1921. The first reported case in a cat in the United States occurred in Virginia in 1922.

Definition

Heartworm *infestation* (dirofilariasis) is the infestation of the pulmonary arteries and, occasionally, the right heart, by the parasite *Dirofilaria immitis*. Heartworm *disease* is the pathologic and clinical findings associated with heartworm infestation. Heartworm infestation and heartworm disease are not the same. Heartworm infestation may be present without producing clinically significant disease. Evidence of heartworm disease may remain after heartworm infestation is eradicated. Heartworm infestation is usually called *heartworm infection.* Infection is the invasion of the body by microorganisms, whereas infestation is the invasion of the body by macroparasites, such as helminths. Consequently, the correct term is *heartworm infestation.*

Life Cycle

DEVELOPMENT IN THE MOSQUITO

D. immitis was the first filarial parasite to have its life cycle in a vertebrate host deciphered.[1] The life cycle of *D. immitis* must pass through a female mosquito (Figure 23-1; Table 23-1). Only female mosquitoes are bloodsuckers, and, for many, a blood meal is necessary for egg production. A mosquito ingests blood from an infested dog or other susceptible species that has circulating first stage larvae (L_1), called *microfilariae.* The microfilariae are produced by the adult ovoviviparous female worm and released into the bloodstream.[2] Mosquitoes can only harbor one to three larvae.[3] Greater numbers result in the death of the mosquito. More than 60 species of mosquitoes can transmit *D. immitis.*[4] There are more than 3000 species of mosquitoes, so obviously some cannot transmit the disease. Nonsusceptible mosquito species appear to lack anticoagulins, so the blood meal clots, trapping the larvae in the gut.[5] Larvae develop more readily in some mosquito species than in others.[6] The type of mosquito present depends on the locality. Different species have different feeding habits. Some prefer to feed during the day (e.g., *Culex* sp.), whereas others feed in the evening (e.g., *Aedes* sp.).[7] Most prefer to feed on dogs, but at least one species (*Culex pipiens*) also feeds, and may prefer to feed, on cats.[8] Once ingested, the L_1 larvae remain in the stomach and midgut for a short time, moving to the malpighian tubules within an hour in susceptible mosquito species.[5] Malpighian tubules are excretory structures in mosquitoes and are similar to kidneys. They take up waste products from the blood and pass them to the hindgut and anus. Within the malpighian tubules the larvae undergo two molts (L_1 to L_2 and L_2 to L_3) over 14 to 16 days. Under ideal conditions they are inside the cells of the malpighian tubules for the first 6 to 8 days.[9] During the first 4 days the parasite becomes immobile, shortens and thickens, and produces the so-called sausage form of larva. The first molt occurs in the malpighian tubule cells at 8 days. Following this they are found in the lumen of the tubules. During the L_2 larval stage, formation of internal organs takes place. The second molt occurs at 12 days. L_3 larvae resemble miniature adults. During the next 2 to 3 days, they increase in length, break out of the malpighian tubules, migrate through the body to the head, and accumulate in the mouthparts. The larvae penetrate the tip when the mosquito feeds and are deposited on the skin of the animal during feeding. A drop of mosquito blood protects the larvae from drying before their entry into the host. They enter the puncture site once the mosquito withdraws.

Maturation time in the mosquito depends on ambient temperature and can range from 10 days at 28° C (82° F) to 30 days at 18° C (64° F). Larvae do not mature in the mosquito when the ambient temperature averages below 14° C (57° F).[10,11] There is a linear relationship between ambient temperature and larval development such that it takes 130 days for the larvae to develop when the temperature is 1° C above 14° C, 65 days when the temperature is 2° C above 14° C, and so on.

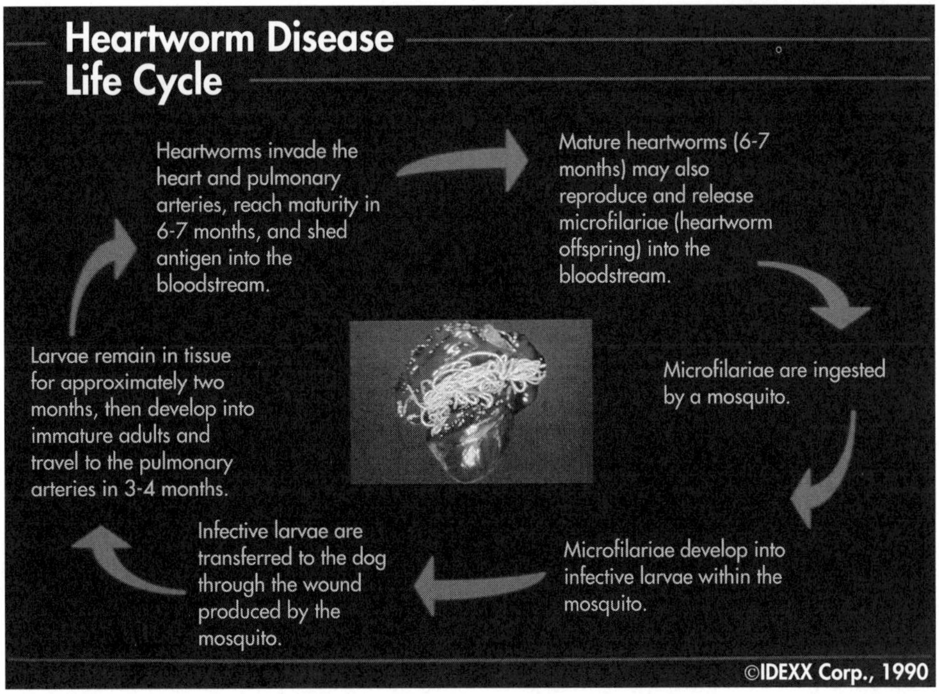

FIGURE 23-1 Life cycle of *Dirofilaria immitis*. (Courtesy Idexx Corp., Westbrook, Me.)

TABLE 23-1

Maturation times during the life cycle of *D. immitis*

Host	*Days postingestion*	*Days postinfestation*
Mosquito		
L_1 to L_3	10-14 (optimal conditions)	
Dog		
L_3 to L_4 (body tissues)		2-12
L_4 to L_5 (body tissues)		50-70
L_5 (pulmonary arteries)		70-110
L_1 (microfilariae) produced		190 minimum

DEVELOPMENT IN THE MAMMALIAN HOST

After entering the puncture site, the larvae begin their migration in the subcutaneous tissues and muscles of the host. During the migration through the tissues (67 to 80 days) the larvae molt two more times (L_3 to L_4 and L_4 to L_5).[2] The molt from the L_3 to the L_4 form is thought to start around 2 days after inoculation.[12] Almost all larvae are molted to the L_4 stage within 12 days after inoculation.[2] The molt from L_4 to L_5 occurs 50 to 70 days after inoculation.[2] L_3 larvae are about 1 mm in length; L_4 larvae start between 1 and 2 mm and attain a length of about 10 mm. L_5 larvae grow to 2.5 cm. The L_5 form penetrates a systemic vein and is carried to the pulmonary arteries by blood flow, where it lodges in terminal branches of the pulmonary artery. The distribution of the worms in the pulmonary arteries depends on distribution of pulmonary blood flow and streaming of flow in the arteries. More blood flows through the caudal lobar pulmonary arteries, and therefore more worms reside in these arteries. Blood flow tends to stream toward the larger right caudal pulmonary artery, and therefore this artery is preferentially infested with worms. In dogs the migration usually culminates in maturation and penetration of a systemic vein. In cats, fewer larvae reach maturity and more fail to penetrate a systemic vein, resulting in the more frequent presence of worms in aberrant locations.

The worms mature within the pulmonary arteries. Within 190 to 285 days after inoculation (at least 6 months in dogs and at least 7 months in cats) or within 110 to 210 days (3.5 to 7 months) after reaching the pulmonary arteries, the worms are sexually mature and capable of producing microfilariae.[13] Mature adult male worms range in size from 9.5 to 17 cm, and mature female worms range in size from 13.5 to 30.5 cm in dogs. In cats, female worms are usually less than 21 cm and male worms less than 12 cm.[10] Adult worms appear to develop more slowly in cats than in dogs.[13]

Most experimentally injected L_3 larvae develop into adults in dogs. One study has shown that 40% to 70% of injected larvae can be recovered as adults. In cats, only about 5% to 10% of L_3 larvae develop into adults.[14] Consequently, cats usually harbor only 1 to 9 worms, although up to 31 worms have been documented following experimental infestation.[15] Dogs can harbor more than 100 worms. Cats also transmit the disease poorly. Many do not have circulating microfilariae, and only about 1% of microfilariae from cats with patent infestations develop in mosquitoes.[13]

When female worms reach sexual maturity in dogs, they avidly produce microfilariae once they mate. Apparently, the males must mate with the females periodically to continue producing microfilariae.[16] The number of circulating microfilariae changes throughout the day. In the past it has been believed that peak numbers are present during the late evening and early morning hours.[17] However, more recent studies have documented midday peaks and unpredictable patterns.[18,19] Consequently, classic descriptions of periodicity cannot be applied consistently to *D. immitis*. There is no relationship between the number of microfilariae found on a concentration test and the number of adult female worms.[20] In cats, circulating microfilariae are usually absent.[13] This is due to either immune destruction of the circulating microfilariae or unisex or single-worm infestations.

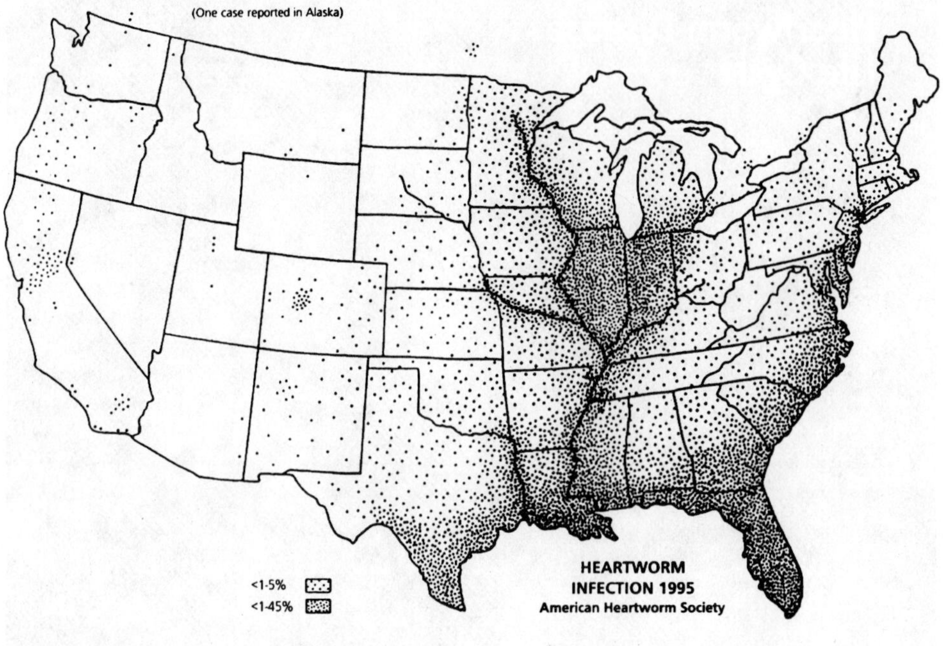

FIGURE 23-2 Map showing regions of the continental United States in which heartworm infestation has been identified. Note that all 48 states are involved.

Adult heartworms are thought to live for 5 to 7 years in dogs, although this is poorly documented and based primarily on one paper describing the life span in one dog.[21] The life span in cats apparently is much shorter, probably about 2 years.[13] Microfilariae are thought to live at least 2 years in dogs.[22] The immune system can kill microfilariae, rendering an animal amicrofilaremic. This occurs frequently in cats.[23]

Microfilariae can be passed from a mother dog to the fetus, resulting in the puppies having circulating microfilariae.[24] Based on the previous discussion, these larvae cannot develop into adult worms. The microfilariae, however, are infective to mosquitoes and therefore may contribute to the continuation of the life cycle.

Epidemiology

Heartworm disease is endemic in many regions of the United States. Figure 23-2 delineates the prevalence in these regions in 1995. Highest infestation rates are in the southeastern United States, the Atlantic coast, and along the Mississippi River and its major tributaries. The regions of infestation continue to grow. Areas of northern California, Oregon, and Canada have become infested within the past 10 to 15 years. The number of heavily infested areas appears to be decreasing with the more widespread use of heartworm preventive medications. Still, the prevalence of heartworm infestation in dogs kept outdoors and not receiving preventive drugs in the southeastern United States is greater than 50%.[23] Besides the United States, Canada, Mexico, South America, southern Europe, and countries along the Pacific rim, such as Australia and Japan, have significant prevalence of heartworm disease.[25]

The rate of transmission in an area depends on the type of mosquito population present, the density of the population that can transmit the parasite, the feeding habits of that population, the reservoir of susceptible species that carry microfilariae, and the exposure time that a susceptible host has to the mosquitoes. Some mosquitoes that have a long breeding season feed repeatedly and so transmit the disease more efficiently. Some mosquitoes, such as *Aedes vexans*, can fly long distances and so can transmit the disease to dogs that live several miles from the mosquito's breeding site.[7] Risk factors for being infested with *D. immitis* include species (wild and domestic canids are the natural host and are at least 3 times as likely to be infested as cats; wild canids such as coyotes and red foxes probably have an incidence similar to domestic dogs), sex (the male-to-female ratio is 2 to 4:1), habitat (outdoor dogs are more commonly infested than indoor dogs), and size (large dogs are more commonly infested than small dogs).[26] Because large male dogs are more commonly housed outdoors, many of these risk factors interact. Neither hair coat length nor breed appear to affect the infestation rate. Dogs of any age can become infested. Dogs less than 6 months old cannot have patent infestations, as explained by the life cycle. Because heartworm disease may take time to develop, clinical signs of disease are more common in dogs greater than 1 year of age. The incidence of infestation increases with increasing age, although this trend is eventually reversed in older dogs.[27] This may be due to the susceptible population dying over time or to protective immunity being acquired through repeated exposure. Male cats are much more commonly infested than female cats.[23]

Heartworms not only infest domestic dogs, but they also infest wild Canidae (e.g., coyotes, foxes), domestic cats, ferrets, and sea lions.[28] Wild Canidae and feral dogs serve as reservoirs of infestation in regions where heartworm disease exists. The existence of these reservoirs ensures that heartworm disease will remain in an infested region even if most of the domestic dogs are on prophylactic medication.

The incidence of heartworm disease in cats is poorly documented but appears to parallel the incidence in dogs but at a lower rate. An estimate of the prevalence is somewhere less than 30% of the incidence in dogs. Prevalence in cats in relationship to prevalence in dogs varies from region to region. Prevalence may depend on the types of mosquitoes in the region, because some mosquitoes prefer to feed on dogs, some on cats, and some feed on both.

Heartworm disease apparently continues to spread into regions where it previously did not exist. Canada is a good example of a country where new infestations have been documented over the past 15 years.[29] Heartworm clearly spreads into new regions by advancing along a front. An example is the continued advance of heartworm from the foothills of the Sierra Nevada into the eastern regions of Sacramento in northern California. It also appears that foci of infestation may develop followed by expansion within an area, as evidenced by the Canadian experience.[29]

Pathophysiology

THE RESPONSE OF THE PULMONARY ARTERIES TO HEARTWORMS

The response of pulmonary arteries to the presence of heartworms has been studied extensively. The presence of adult worms in direct contact with pulmonary arteries results in pathology in the large pulmonary arteries. The pathologic lesions start very soon after the parasite contacts the vessel intima. These lesions can be identified within 4 days using scanning electron microscopy, and lesions detectable by angiography are present within 2 to 3 weeks.[30-32] Pulmonary microvasculature and pulmonary parenchymal pathology probably occurs secondary to an adult heartworm antigen deposited in these regions.[33] Changes in the pulmonary arteries are complex. An increased pulmonary artery diameter is the most common, consistent, and readily apparent change. Endothelial and medial thickening contribute to this increase in size. Endothelial damage begins very soon (within days) after heartworm infestation and consists of swelling, sloughing, and platelet adhesion.[30] Growth factors are released by the platelets and leukocytes that invade the region. Factors such as platelet-derived growth factor stimulate multiplication of smooth muscle cells within the tunica media and migration of these cells to the intima. Their multiplication in this region produces protuberances of the pulmonary artery lining. In essence, villi are produced, which make the lining of the pulmonary arteries look like intestinal endothelium (which seems appropriate for a structure infested with worms) (see Color Plate 94). These changes start in small peripheral pulmonary artery branches, where the immature worms first lodge, and occur in more proximal segments as the worms grow.

Besides the endothelial and medial changes, pulmonary arteries also dilate, their course becomes tortuous instead of straight, and smaller arteries become obstructed because of embolization. These lead to the characteristic changes identified on radiographs of enlarged, tortuous, and blunted or pruned pulmonary arteries. These changes occur in regions where heartworms are in direct contact with the arteries. The changes may or may not lead to clinically significant pulmonary hypertension. The amount of pathologic change in the arteries depends roughly on the number of worms present in the area and on the immune or allergic response of the host to the parasite. Consequently, the worst pathologic and radiographic changes are noted in dogs with a high worm burden and in dogs with immune-mediated occult heartworm disease (i.e., dogs that mount a massive immunologic reaction to adult heartworms and microfilariae).[34] Pulmonary parenchymal disease also occurs and is primarily a local inflammatory response to the parasites. Pulmonary infiltrates consist primarily of eosinophils and neutrophils. Chronic pulmonary parenchymal inflammatory disease leads to fibrosis.

Angiograms provide more detailed information regarding the anatomy of the pulmonary artery pathology than do plain radiographs. A series of angiograms is presented in Figures 23-3 through 23-5.[32] The first series, in Figure 23-3, shows disease progression in a dog over a 21-month period after experimental infestation with L_3 larvae. The first angiogram *(A)* is relatively normal. The pulmonary artery branches become dilated, tortuous, and blunted over the next 18 months. Linear filling defects as a result of the presence of adult worms can be seen in many arteries. After 21 months of infestation the main pulmonary artery is dilated *(C)*. It should be noted that the pulmonary artery pressures at 3 months were 28/13 (systolic/diastolic) mm Hg, at 6 months were 33/19 mm Hg, and at 21 months were 28/16 mm Hg—all within normal limits or slightly elevated. In Figure 23-4, angiograms from a dog 9 and 11 months after infestation with 154 larvae are shown. At 9 months *(A)*, there are peripheral pulmonary artery changes present and the main pulmonary artery and the caudal lobar branches are mildly dilated. The dog's pulmonary artery pressures at this time were 32/22 mm Hg. Eleven months after infestation *(B)* the main pulmonary artery and the caudal lobar branches are grossly enlarged, and one can readily appreciate that the right caudal lobar artery has no flow into its branches. At this time the dog was in right heart failure and the pulmonary artery pressures were severely increased (90/55 mm Hg). In Figure 23-5, angiograms are presented from a dog 13 to 26 months after infestation. At 13 months (A), there are moderate pulmonary artery changes. Pulmonary artery pressure at this time was mildly increased (45/30 mm Hg). At 17.5 months this dog went into right heart failure, but measurements were not taken at this time. It was studied at 18.5 months, when no longer in heart failure (B). The pulmonary arteries at this time were grossly distended, but pulmonary artery pressures were only mildly increased, to 44/24 mm Hg. Blood flow to the caudal lobes is obviously slow. At 26 months, gross pulmonary artery distension was still present but caudal lung blood flow was improved (C). Pulmonary artery pressures were normal (28/20 mm Hg).

PULMONARY HYPERTENSION

The endothelial and medial thickening combined with the obstructions to blood flow in heartworm disease lead to a decrease in pulmonary vascular compliance and an increase in pulmonary vascular resistance that, if severe, will lead to increased pulmonary artery pressure (pulmonary hypertension). Of these factors, obstruction to pulmonary blood flow appears to be the most significant, as was demonstrated in Figure 23-4. This conclusion is based on the findings from the angiographic study above and from another study in which the best predictor of pulmonary artery pressure was the number of thromboemboli and the size of the pulmonary artery tree occluded with thromboemboli.[32,35] Another study in cats documented that only cats with no flow to caudal lung lobes had pulmonary hypertension.[36] Two thirds or more of the pulmonary vascular bed must be obliterated before pulmonary hypertension becomes evident at rest.[37]

Pulmonary hypertension is probably present in most dogs with radiographically apparent heartworm disease. However, the increase in pulmonary artery pressure appears to be mild in most dogs. In the angiographic/pressure study from above, in which 16 dogs were heavily infested with 145 ± 67 larvae (which means most dogs had more than 80 adults present), pulmonary artery pressures were normal to mildly increased in all but one dog (see Figure 23-4). Pressures ranged from 25/13 mm Hg to 45/30 mm Hg 6 to 42 months after infestation.[32] In a recent study, dogs with a low worm burden had an average mean pulmonary artery pressure of 14 mm Hg, which is normal, whereas dogs with a high worm burden had an average

A

B

C

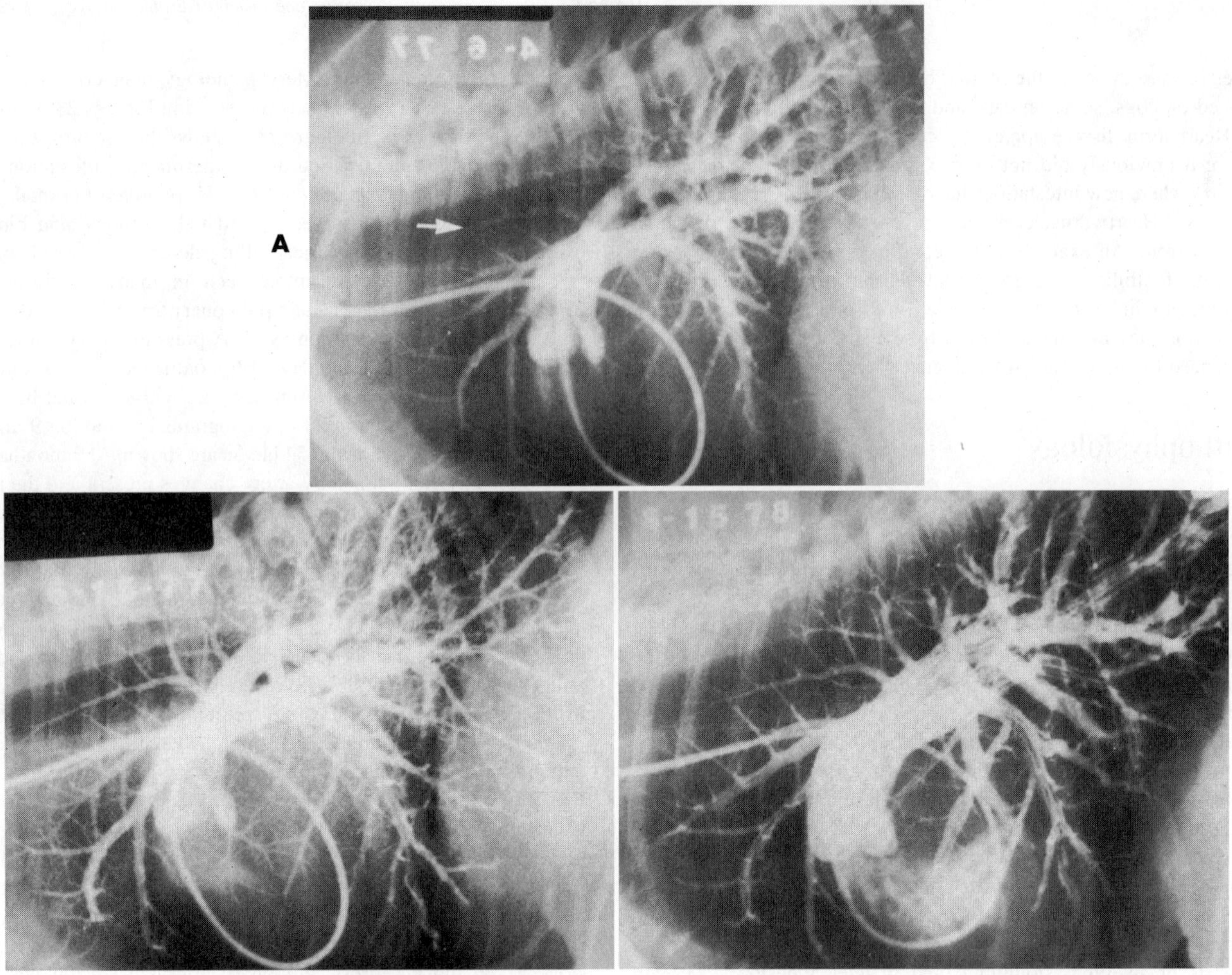

FIGURE 23-3 Pulmonary arteriograms from a dog after experimental infestation with *Dirofilaria immitis*. **A,** Arteriogram taken 3 months after infestation. The pulmonary arterial vasculature is normal. **B,** Six months after infestation, the pulmonary arteries are starting to enlarge and the distal branches are becoming tortuous. Linear filling defects caused by worms are present in some pulmonary artery branches. **C,** At the 21-month examination the main pulmonary artery and the caudal lobar branches are increased markedly in size. The distal branches are tortuous and blunted. Linear filling defects can be clearly seen in pulmonary artery branches. The dog had only mild pulmonary hypertension. (From Knight DH. In Otto GF, ed: *Proceedings of the Heartworm Symposium '80,* Batavia, Ill. 1980, American Heartworm Society.)

A

B

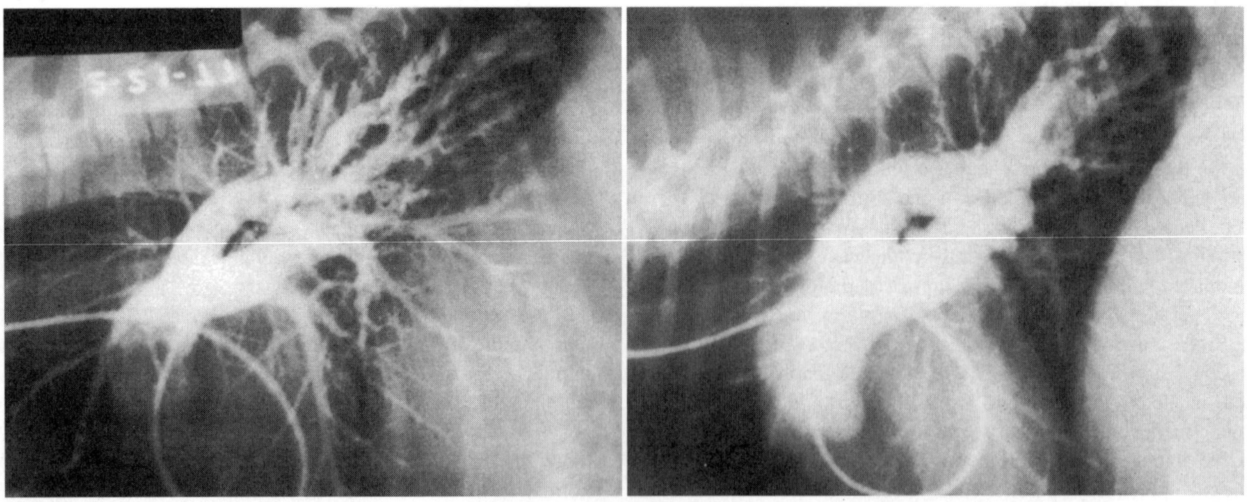

FIGURE 23-4 Pulmonary arteriograms from a dog after experimental heartworm infestation. **A,** Nine months after infestation, the main pulmonary artery and major pulmonary artery branches are mildly dilated. Some increase in vessel tortuosity and blunting of distal pulmonary artery branches are present. **B,** This arteriogram was taken when the dog was in right heart failure. The dog had severe pulmonary artery hypertension because of obstruction of flow to many areas but particularly through the right caudal pulmonary artery branch. (From Knight DH. In Otto GF, ed: *Proceedings of the Heartworm Symposium '80,* Batavia, Ill. 1980, American Heartworm Society.)

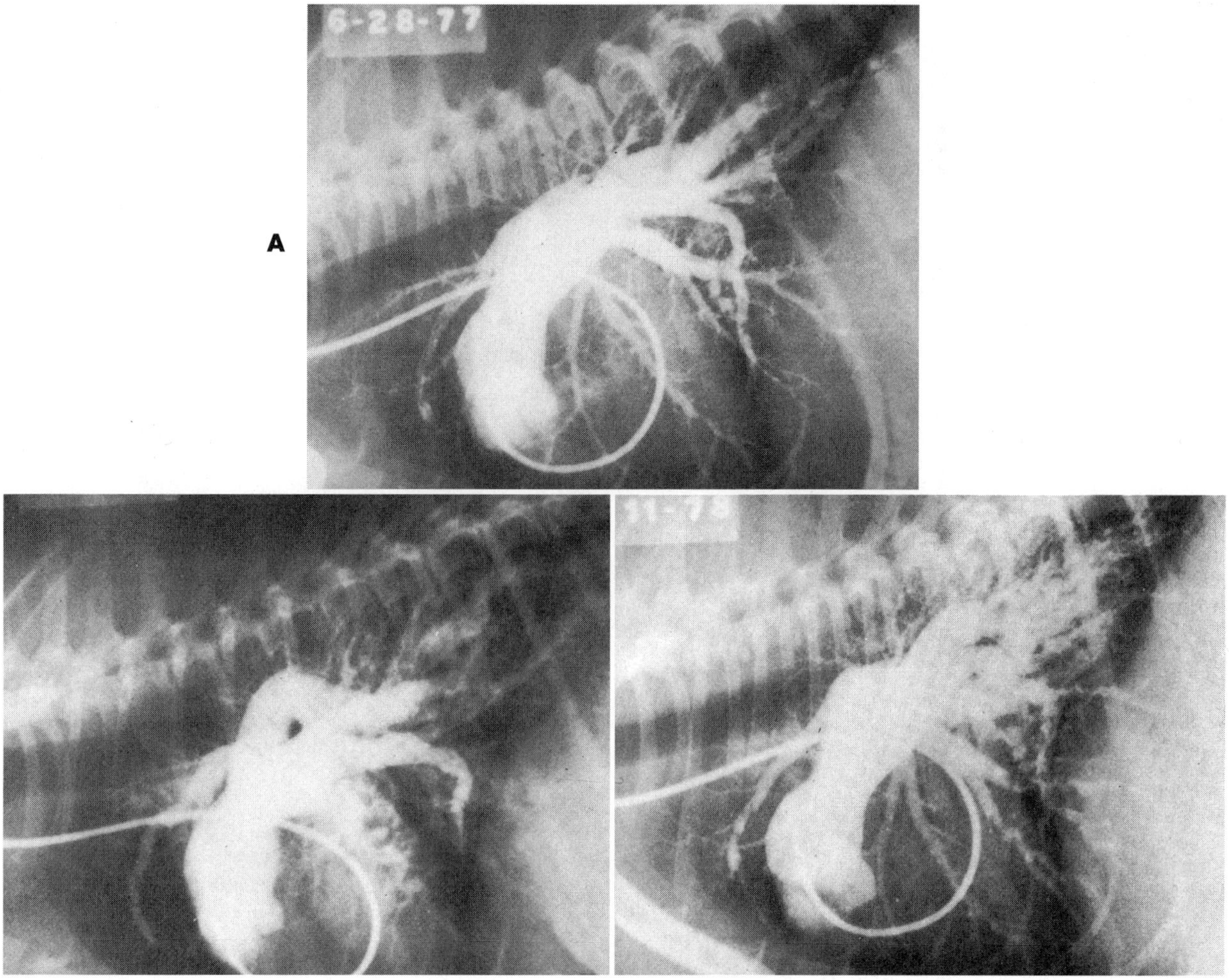

FIGURE 23-5 Set of pulmonary arteriograms from a dog after experimental infestation with *Dirofilaria immitis*. **A,** Arteriograms taken 13 months after infestation reveal moderate pulmonary artery changes with slow flow to the caudal lung lobes. **B,** The dog developed heart failure 17.5 months after infestation. The arteriogram shown here was taken 1 month later, when the dog was not in heart failure. Blood flow to the caudal lung lobes appears to be even worse than in **A. C,** Twenty-six months after infestation, caudal lung lobe flow appears to have improved. (From Knight DH. In Otto GF, ed: *Proceedings of the Heartworm Symposium '80,* Batavia, Ill. 1980, American Heartworm Society.)

mean pulmonary artery pressure of 22 mm Hg (mildly increased).[38] When these pressures are compared with the radiographic changes seen in Figures 23-3 through 23-5 it should be readily apparent that the increase in pulmonary artery size is not due to pulmonary artery hypertension in most cases and that pulmonary artery size has no correlation with pulmonary artery pressure. All of the pressures measured in different studies have been while the dogs were at rest. One can assume, however, that pulmonary vascular resistance and pulmonary vascular compliance are relatively fixed in heartworm disease. This means that it is unlikely that the pulmonary vasculature can dilate and that unused vessels can be recruited. One study documented a linear relationship between pulmonary artery pressure and flow in heartworm disease.[39] Consequently, pulmonary artery pressure probably does increase dramatically upon exercise, when pulmonary blood flow increases. Blood flow can easily increase to 3 times the baseline during exercise. This means that pulmonary artery pressure could triple. This probably contributes to the clinical sign of exercise intolerance commonly observed in dogs with heartworm disease. It may also produce syncope through stimulation of ventricular mechanoreceptors by the markedly increased intraventricular pressure.

The severity of the pulmonary artery changes and the increase in pulmonary vascular resistance and pulmonary artery pressure are thought to be correlated to the number of worms and the avidity of the immune response that an individual dog has to the worms. A recent study suggests that of these two, the severity of the immune response is the primary factor, because there was no relationship between worm number and pulmonary vascular resistance in a group of naturally infested dogs.[39] Another study has shown that dogs with severe disease have a lower antigen concentration than do dogs with mild or moderate heartworm disease.[40] The amount of exercise a dog receives may also be a factor. One study suggested that dogs that exercise develop more severe disease than do caged dogs.

RIGHT HEART ENLARGEMENT

Right heart enlargement is common in dogs with severe heartworm disease. One would assume, from general pathophysiologic principles, that the right heart would concentrically hypertrophy

A

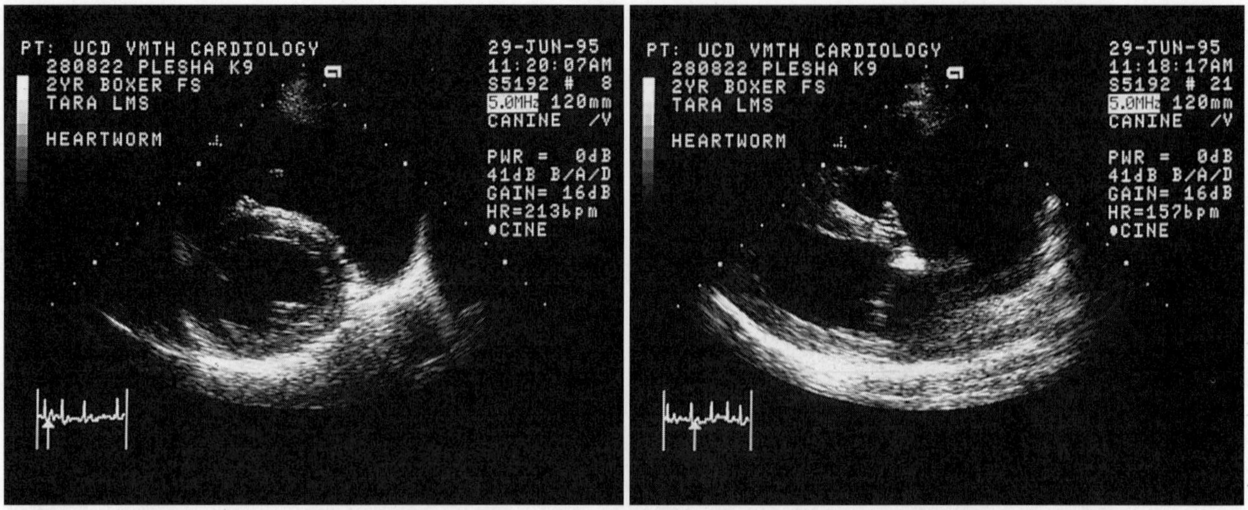

B

FIGURE 23-6 Two-dimensional echocardiograms from a 3-year-old female spayed boxer with severe heartworm disease. The dog presented 4 months previously with evidence of severe right heart failure and massive heartworm infestation. The main pulmonary artery was filled with heartworms on the echocardiogram. Despite this, the pulmonary artery pressure was normal. The worms were removed surgically. At the time the echocardiograms in this figure were obtained, the dog was presented for adulticide therapy to kill the remaining heartworms. The dog had jugular vein distension and an enlarged liver but no ascites. The right ventricle is severely enlarged. This can be best appreciated in the cross-sectional view **(A).** The right atrium is also severely enlarged in the long-axis view **(B).** This dog did not have pulmonary hypertension at the time of this examination, as evidenced by a normal tricuspid regurgitation velocity (2 m/sec).

secondary to right ventricular pressure overload caused by pulmonary hypertension. Instead, the ventricle is volume-overloaded with possibly some wall thickening in severe heartworm disease (Figure 23-6). One study found that the right ventricular free wall weighs more in dogs with severe heartworm disease.[41] However, another has found that right ventricular weight to body weight ratio is normal, even in dogs with severe right ventricular enlargement.[42] Consequently, there appears to be primarily eccentric (volume overload) hypertrophy or pure ventricular dilation with possibly some concentric (pressure overload) hypertrophy. There are at least two possible explanations for finding a volume-overloaded ventricle. First, an acquired pressure overload of the right ventricle appears to produce this pattern of hypertrophy in other diseases, and therefore this finding may be consistent with the manner in which the right ventricle responds to an acquired pressure overload. Second, because pulmonary hypertension is often not severe in cases that have right heart enlargement, the right ventricular enlargement may be due to something else. Myocardial failure may be that something else. Right ventricular myocardial failure would result in a volume-overloaded ventricle, as it does for the left ventricle. No ready explanation for why myocardial failure would develop is available. The motion of the right ventricular free wall in dogs with heartworm disease and severe right ventricular enlargement suggest, however, that myocardial failure is present.

RIGHT HEART FAILURE

Pulmonary hypertension can become severe in dogs with severe heartworm disease. Moderate-to-severe pulmonary hypertension leads to right heart enlargement and may lead to right heart failure. In one report, all dogs with ascites (n = 2) or a heart murmur had moderately-to–markedly elevated mean pulmonary artery pressure (40 to 81 mm Hg).[43] Some cases in this report, however, had moderate-to-severe pulmonary hypertension with no clinical signs. In this report, out of 41 dogs only five had moderate-to-severe pulmonary hypertension with a mean pulmonary artery pressure greater than 50 mm Hg (approximately 53 to 81 mm Hg). Consequently, it appears that moderate-to-severe pulmonary hypertension is not common in dogs with heartworm disease. In another report, mean pulmonary artery pressure ranged from 23 to 55 mm Hg in a group of dogs with no or only mild clinical signs, whereas in another report from the same laboratory, mean pulmonary artery pressure ranged from 23 to 53 mm Hg in a group of dogs with right heart failure (right atrial pressure = 13 ± 14 mm Hg).[43,44] Consequently, although one can assume that severe pulmonary hypertension can cause right heart failure, it appears that right heart failure in dogs with heartworm disease isn't necessarily caused by severe pulmonary hypertension. The cause in these dogs is unknown.

PULMONARY PARENCHYMAL DISEASE

Pulmonary parenchymal disease and resultant coughing are common in dogs with heartworm disease. Severe pulmonary arterial disease results in increased permeability of small vessels to plasma and inflammatory cells.[45] Periarterial edema and inflammation occur. They produce interstitial and alveolar infiltrates. The severity of this type of pulmonary change correlates with the severity of the pulmonary artery disease. Chronic, severe disease results in pulmonary fibrosis that is irreversible.

Thromboembolic disease also causes focal or diffuse areas of increased parenchymal density. Lesions are most commonly identified in the caudal lung lobes (Figure 23-7). Embolization may occur before or following adulticide therapy. Pulmonary abnormalities result from dead worms obstructing blood flow to lung parenchyma. The worms stimulate thrombus formation, further obstructing blood flow. In addition, the pulmonary artery disease is exacerbated with increased myointimal proliferation, villous hypertrophy, and arteritis. A ventilation/perfusion mismatch can occur, leading to hypoxemia.

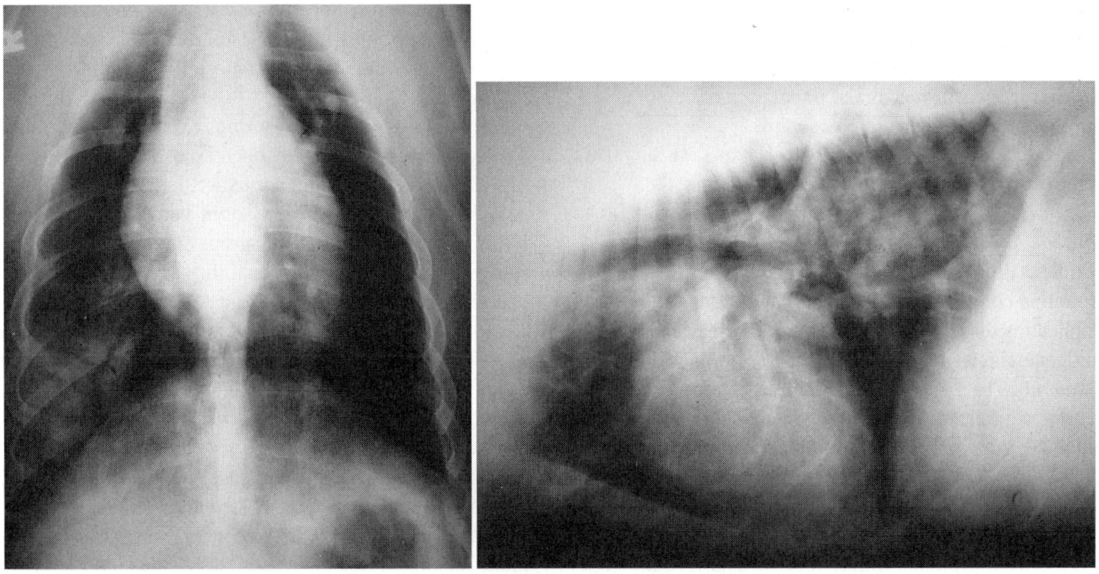

A

B

FIGURE 23-7 Thoracic radiographs from a dog with severe heartworm disease. The radiographs were taken at presentation, before any therapy. The caudal lobar pulmonary arteries on the dorsoventral view **(A)** are severely enlarged, as are the cranial lobar vessels on the lateral view. A region of lung consolidation in the right caudal lung lobe is present. This is presumably due to thromboembolic disease. This area makes it appear as if there is diffuse pulmonary fibrosis on the lateral view **(B).**

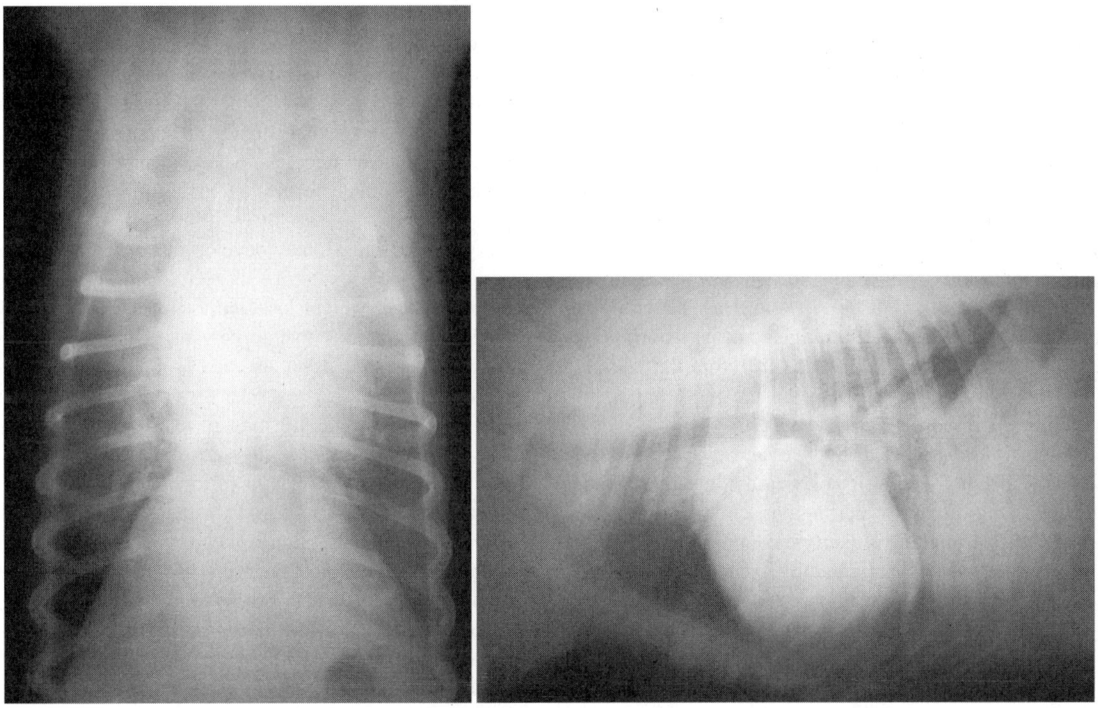

A

B

FIGURE 23-8 Thoracic radiographs from a dog with pneumonitis secondary to heartworm infestation. A heavy interstitial lung pattern is present that is not as apparent on the dorsoventral radiograph **(A)** as it is on the lateral **(B)** radiograph, where it is most prominent in the caudodorsal lung fields. This was mistaken for pulmonary edema and initially treated with furosemide. The lung pattern improved. The dog had no evidence of left heart disease and was subsequently treated with corticosteroids and thiacetarsemide.

Allergic pneumonitis is another pulmonary parenchymal disease that can occur in dogs infested with heartworms. Radiographically this presents as diffuse interstitial and alveolar infiltrates (Figure 23-8). These dogs often do not have circulating microfilariae, and it is thought that the microfilariae in this disease are trapped in the pulmonary circulation, where they produce an intense allergic reaction.[46] The radiographic pattern of this disease can be confused with pulmonary edema. Significant pulmonary artery disease and cardiomegaly are frequently absent. This disease is usually very responsive to corticosteroid administration.

Lastly, pulmonary eosinophilic granulomatosis is a rare problem associated with heartworm disease.[45] The granulomas appear as large densities on chest radiographs and may be confused with pulmonary neoplasia. The granulomas have a mixed population of mononuclear cells, neutrophils, macrophages, and eosinophils.

Cats also have extensive alveolar type 2 cell hyperplasia.[47] This may contribute to their pulmonary parenchymal disease.

RENAL DAMAGE

Organs other than the lungs and heart may be affected by heartworm infestation. Immune complex glomerular disease is one of the most common complicating diseases seen in heartworm disease.[48] Chronic low-grade antigenemia is a common cause of immune complex damage to glomeruli. The exact antigen that results in the glomerular damage in heartworm infestation is unknown and may be shed from either the adult worms or the microfilariae. Immune complex glomerulonephropathy most commonly results in proteinuria of varying severity. Less commonly it may lead to azotemia. Amyloidosis is a less common cause of glomerular damage in heartworm-infested dogs.[48] Severe proteinuria may lead to hypoalbuminemia. The plasma concentration of antithrombin III may also be reduced in patients with glomerular disease. This can lead to enhanced formation of thrombi.

Clinical Signs

DOGS

Most dogs with heartworm infestation do not have clinical signs of heartworm disease. Thoracic radiographs are normal in many dogs. In one study, out of 33 dogs with microfilariae, only 15 had radiographic changes.[42] Clinical signs commonly develop in dogs that have a large number of mature worms per body weight for months to years. Clinical signs also commonly develop in dogs that have a profound allergic response to the adult worms and microfilariae. This probably isn't much different from dogs with fleas; some dogs show clinical signs only with heavy infestation whereas others develop an allergic dermatitis with only a few fleas. Recent data suggest that worm burden (heartworm antigen concentration) does not correlate well with disease severity, and therefore the allergic response of the host to the parasite may be the most important variable in determining disease severity.[40]

Respiratory signs of coughing, tachypnea, and dyspnea are the most common clinical signs. These signs generally develop secondary to parenchymal lung disease, which is most commonly present in the caudal lung lobes. Coughing is the most common clinical sign. It is often a deep cough that is aggravated by exercise. Hypoxemia produces the respiratory signs of tachypnea and dyspnea. Mild-to-moderate hypoxemia is common in dogs with severe heartworm disease. Hypoxemia is probably due to mismatch of ventilation and perfusion, with some areas of the lung with parenchymal disease being hypoventilated. In dogs with heartworm disease, regions of hypoventilation may not be appropriately underperfused because heartworm disease interferes with the ability of pulmonary arteries to constrict in response to regional hypoxia.[49] Consequently, blood continues to flow through regions of the lung that are not ventilated, resulting in deoxygenated blood returning to the left heart and in turn being pumped through the systemic circulation. In other situations, hypoxemia may be secondary to thromboembolic disease, causing diversions to blood flow away from the embolized lung to normal lung, which causes a relative increase in flow and a ventilation/perfusion mismatch.[50]

Exercise intolerance is another common clinical sign. Hypoxemia contributes to the exercise intolerance. Reduced blood flow to working skeletal muscle also contributes to exercise intolerance. Dogs with mild-to-severe heart failure have reduced blood-pumping capacity during exercise. This, along with the hypoxemia, contributes to decreased oxygen delivery to working muscles. Increased pulmonary vascular resistance leading to pulmonary hypertension (increased right ventricular afterload) and, most likely, right ventricular myocardial failure, contribute to the reduced right ventricular pumping capability and reduced blood flow during exercise.

Syncope may occur in dogs with severe heartworm disease. It most commonly occurs secondary to exercise or excitement. The exact mechanisms responsible for syncope in this condition have not been defined. The fixed pulmonary vascular resistance in heartworm disease restricts the increase in right ventricular cardiac output required for exercise and decreases the blood return to the left heart. Although blood return is restricted to the left heart, systemic vascular resistance decreases reflexly during exercise. The combination of inadequate flow and decreased resistance could lead to hypotension during exercise in dogs with heartworm disease, resulting in syncope. More likely, the syncope is mediated by mechanoreceptors in the pulmonary vasculature and the right ventricle, which are stimulated by the high systolic pressure during exercise. The mechanoreceptors reflexly stimulate an increase in vagal tone, producing bradycardia and, possibly, systemic arteriolar dilation.[51]

Hemoptysis (coughing up blood) is the presenting clinical sign in a few dogs with severe heartworm disease. Hemoptysis probably develops secondary to small pulmonary artery rupture. Diseased pulmonary arteries may develop aneurysms, and coughing may precipitate arterial rupture in these cases. Hemoptysis may be mild but can be so severe that it leads to hypovolemic shock and death. Blood loss may be underestimated because of the dog swallowing blood. Melena may be present in dogs with subacute or chronic hemoptysis.

Right heart failure may develop in dogs with severe heartworm disease. These dogs present with ascites and hepatomegaly. They also commonly have weight loss and exercise intolerance. On physical examination, besides the ascites, one may identify jugular vein distension in some but not all cases. A split second heart sound or a systolic murmur heard best over the right apex may be ausculted in some cases. Heart failure may develop relatively acutely or may occur gradually. A more acute course of the disease may occur after a dog exercises strenuously or following adulticide therapy, when a large number of worms die and obstruct circulation to a large section of lung. Right heart failure may or may not be associated with pulmonary hypertension from the few cases in the literature from which these types of data can be extracted.[43]

Complications related to the presence of adult heartworms in aberrant locations are rare but have been reported. Heartworms have on occasion been identified in such diverse locations as the lateral ventricle of the brain, anterior chamber of the eye, peritoneal cavity, left heart, systemic arteries, intramuscular and subcutaneous cysts and abscesses, bronchi, and liver.[52,53] Clinical signs are referable to the physical presence of the worms or thrombus formation secondary to the worms. For example, a recent report described the complications associated with the presence of heartworms in the systemic arteries of five dogs.[53] Each of these dogs had worms in the aorta and, in some cases, in the femoral arteries. All of these dogs presented for hind limb abnormalities, including lameness, paresthesia, paresis, and tissue necrosis. Worms could be visualized in the aorta in some dogs. The worms were removed via femoral arteriotomies using balloon embolectomy catheters and loop stone extractors. The presence of the worms in a systemic artery could be explained by the presence of a right-to-left shunting patent ductus arteriosus in one dog. In the others the site was aberrant and may have occurred when the L_5 stage penetrated a systemic artery rather than a vein.

CATS

Many cats with heartworm disease are probably asymptomatic. Because heartworm disease is difficult to diagnose in cats, the number of asymptomatic cats in a population is unknown. On the other end of the spectrum are cats with heartworm disease that die suddenly. Any cat that dies suddenly in a region endemic for heartworm should be examined for the presence of heartworms. Death may be preceded by acute signs of severe cardiopulmonary disease, or the cat may be found dead. Cats that die suddenly may appear clinically normal up to 1 hour before death.[14] Death probably occurs most commonly secondary to acute filarial embolism and pulmonary artery occlusion. Postmortem examination has revealed as few as two worms in cats that have died suddenly.[14]

Cats with heartworm disease are most commonly identified because they are exhibiting clinical signs, because routine screening for heartworm disease is not commonly done in this species. Clinical signs of heartworm disease in cats presented to a veterinarian are often nonspecific and include lethargy, anorexia, vomiting, coughing, dyspnea, and syncope. Cats may have signs indistinguishable from asthma.[47] The reported vomiting may be true vomiting, but the owner may mistakenly identify coughing as vomiting. Coughing and vomiting are difficult to distinguish in cats, and cats may regurgitate gastrointestinal contents after coughing. In an attempt to distinguish them, any cat that presents for either one should be subjected to tracheal manipulation vigorous enough to make the patient cough in front of the owner. The response should be noted and the owner queried about the similarity of the response to what the owner has observed at home. Cats may present with acute dyspnea. Acute dyspnea resulting from acute thromboembolism is best treated with corticosteroids and oxygen. Dyspneic cats tend to die if they are stressed, therefore handling and other stressful procedures must be avoided.

Because heartworm larvae migrate throughout the body and because not every L_5 form finds a vein to penetrate, adult heartworms may, at times, be identified in aberrant locations. Clinical signs may occur secondary to the presence of these aberrantly located worms. This phenomenon appears to occur more frequently in cats than in dogs. Neurologic signs secondary to aberrant heartworm migration in the central nervous system are rare but do occur with greater frequency in cats.[14]

In the southeastern United States, almost 80% of cats with clinical signs referable to heartworm disease present to a veterinarian in the months of October through January.[54] Presumably these cats are infested in the spring, and clinical signs begin as the young adults reach the pulmonary arteries and start to mature.

Physical Examination

DOGS

The physical examination in most dogs with heartworm disease is normal. Dogs that present with a history of exhibiting clinical signs more commonly have abnormalities identified on physical examination. The most common finding is a spontaneous or easily elicited cough. Usually only dogs with severe heartworm disease have any other physical abnormalities. These abnormalities include weight loss, tachypnea, dyspnea, abnormal respiratory sounds, abnormal heart sounds, fever, and evidence of right heart failure. Significant lung pathology can be present without auscultatory abnormalities, so chest radiographs must be evaluated. Abnormal heart sounds can occur, but most dogs have normal heart sounds. A split second heart sound is commonly reported in the veterinary literature in association with heartworm disease. In our experience, however, this is an uncommon finding. A split second heart sound should be most commonly ausculted in severe pulmonary hypertension. Because severe pulmonary hypertension is uncommon, it is logical that a split second heart sound would also be uncommon. Even when a split second heart sound is present, it is subtle enough that many veterinarians cannot appreciate it. Consequently, the diagnostic accuracy of this test is extremely poor. A heart murmur due to tricuspid regurgitation may be ausculted in dogs with heartworm disease but almost never occurs in dogs with mild-to-moderate disease. It is most commonly identified in dogs with right heart failure and in dogs with caval syndrome (see below). The presence of worms in the pulmonary arteries does not result in turbulence and consequently does not produce a heart murmur. Cardiac arrhythmias may be ausculted in dogs with severe heartworm disease. Hemoptysis may also occur in severely affected dogs. Fever may be present in dogs with acute pulmonary filarial embolism.

CATS

The physical examination in cats with heartworm disease is usually normal, although nonspecific signs may be identified. A cough may be elicited. Occasionally a heart murmur, a gallop sound, or abnormal lung sounds can be identified. Right heart failure is rare.

The General Approach to Diagnosing and Treating Heartworm Infestation in Dogs

Routine screening of dogs with tests to detect circulating microfilariae or an antigen from the reproductive tract of female worms (a heartworm antigen test) is the most common means of identifying a dog with heartworm infestation. Less commonly, a dog is presented with clinical signs suggestive of heartworm disease. A dog or cat suspected of being infested with *D. immitis* should be examined carefully. Diagnostic testing should always include a thorough physical examination, blood tests to detect the worms, and a thoracic radiograph to determine the presence and the severity of heartworm disease. Once heartworm infestation is diagnosed, a complete blood count, serum chemistry panel, and urinalysis should be evaluated to detect any secondary or complicating diseases.

Drug therapy to kill the adult worms is the usual first step in treating heartworm infestation. The arsenicals, thiacetarsemide or melarsomine, are used in a manner that slowly kills the worms. As the worms die, they disintegrate in the pulmonary circulation and are carried into the terminal branches of the pulmonary arteries. Strict cage rest is advised during this stage to prevent the production of large worm emboli created by exercise during this stage. Aspirin, corticosteroids, or heparin may also help decrease complications associated with worm embolization.

Four months following adulticide therapy, a heartworm antigen test should be repeated to document clearance of the worms from the system. If the heartworm antigen test is still positive, a decision must be made whether to treat the dog again. This decision is based on the dog's response to the initial treatment, the amount of disease, and the owner's wishes. Decreasing the worm burden often results in significant clinical improvement, so adulticide treatment does not necessarily have to kill all the worms to be considered a success.

Dogs with circulating microfilariae must be treated to kill the microfilariae, because these dogs act as reservoirs for infestation of other dogs. The avermectins, ivermectin and milbemycin, are usually used for this purpose. Ivermectin can be started at a preventive dose immediately following adulticide therapy. When administered in this manner, the microfilarial numbers decrease gradually over several months. Alternatively, it can be administered at a higher dose to destroy the microfilariae more rapidly. This is most commonly done 4 to 6 weeks after adulticide therapy. The preventive dose of milbemycin is rapidly microfilaricidal and can be started any time following adulticide therapy.

Any dog in a region endemic for heartworm disease should be on a preventive medication. Choices include diethylcarbamazine (daily administration) or the avermectins (once-a-month administration). Diethylcarbamazine cannot be administered to a dog with circulating microfilariae. Administration of a heartworm prophylactic drug should start in puppies as early as possible to prevent heartworm infestation.

Diagnosis

The diagnosis of heartworm infestation in dogs is usually based on identifying the microfilariae of *D. immitis* in a blood sample or on finding adult heartworm antigen in blood, serum, or plasma. The diagnosis is occasionally made by identifying worms in the pulmonary arteries or right heart using echocardiography.

All dogs more than 6 months of age that have not been administered an avermectin for heartworm prophylaxis that undergo an initial screening for heartworm infestation should be evaluated for both circulating microfilariae and circulating heartworm antigen. Heartworm disease can be diagnosed by identifying typical radiographic changes. A positive finding on any of these tests leads to a positive diagnosis of heartworm infestation. Usually a combination of the three is used in screening asymptomatic animals and for confirming the diagnosis in symptomatic animals. Echocardiography can be helpful for diagnosing heartworm infestation in specific situations and especially in cats. One general algorithm for diagnosing and treating heartworm disease is pictured in Figure 23-9.

In cats, echocardiography is one of the more sensitive and specific means of identifying heartworm infestation.[55,56] Heartworm antibody tests are a very sensitive means of identifying heartworm infestation in this species, but cats exposed to the parasite but without adult infestation are positive on this test also. Consequently, the test is not specific for adult worm infestation. Heartworm antigen tests and tests to detect circulating microfilariae are notoriously poor at detecting heartworm infestation in cats because of the small number of worms usually present.

TESTS TO DETECT MICROFILARIAE

Techniques for detecting circulating *D. immitis* microfilariae include examining wet blood smears, examining hematocrit capillary tubes, the Knott concentration test, and the filter test. Wet blood smears and hematocrit tube examination are insensitive (more false negative tests) compared with the Knott concentration and filter tests and should not be used for definitive screening for heartworm infestation. The concentration tests concentrate the number of microfilariae in 1 mL of blood for identification. The concentration tests use either a Millipore filter (Difil Test, Filarassay-F) or centrifugation and examination of the sediment (modified Knott test) to identify microfilariae. Both techniques lyse the red blood cells and fix the microfilariae for examination. The modified Knott test is less expensive but more time-consuming than the filter tests. Identification of microfilariae in peripheral blood is about 75% sensitive at detecting patent heartworm infestations in dogs not on avermectin prophylaxis. There is no relationship between the number of microfilariae per milliliter of blood and the number of adult heartworms.[20]

Not all circulating microfilariae are those of *D. immitis*. *Dipetalonema reconditium* is a harmless subcutaneous parasite that also produces microfilariae that can be found on a blood smear. Differentiation of these microfilariae from those of *D. immitis* is crucial because identification of *D. immitis* microfilariae commonly sentences the patient to arsenical therapy. Up to 50% of cases with microfilaremia in some areas can be due to *D. reconditium*.[57] The easiest screening method for determining if microfilariae are *D. immitis* is to perform a heartworm antigen test. If the test is positive, at least some microfilariae are *D. immitis*. Because mixed infestations can occur, microfilariae of both parasites may be present in the same animal. If the antigen test is negative, the microfilariae could still be *D. immitis*, because it takes only one male and one female to produce microfilariae and two worms may be below the limit of detection for an antigen test in an animal. Although many criteria are published for anatomic differentiation of the microfilariae from these two parasites, differentiation is best accomplished by measuring the microfilarial length and width and examining the morphology of the parasite. Criteria are different whether one is using the Knott test or the filter test. With the filter test, the microfilariae of *D. immitis* are greater than 6 μm wide, 235 to 285 μm in length, and have tapered heads, whereas microfilariae of *D. reconditum* are less than 6 μm wide, 215 to 240 μm long, and have blunt heads. With the Knott test, the microfilariae of *D. immitis* are the same width (greater than 6 μm), but are greater than 290 μm in length, and the microfilariae of *D. reconditum* are less than 275 μm long and less than 6 μm wide. Veterinarians that diagnose heartworm disease frequently should become adept at differentiating these parasites. Veterinarians that only occasionally diagnose heartworm disease should rely on a trained individual, such as a parasitologist in a commercial laboratory, to make the differentiation. It should be noted that there is a very poor correlation between the number of microfilariae and the type of parasite.

Dogs and cats that harbor adult worms but do not have circulating microfilariae are said to have *occult* infestations. Animals with adult worms may not have circulating microfilariae for four possible reasons: (1) the infestation is prepatent (immature adults only are present in the pulmonary arteries), (2) there is only a single sex present, (3) the worms are sterile, or (4) there is immunologic destruction of microfilariae by the host.[58] Dogs with prepatent infestations in which the adult worms are in the pulmonary arteries but are not yet mature enough to produce microfilariae can have radiographic evidence of heartworm disease. These dogs would be expected to be asymptomatic or only symptomatic for a short time. Dogs with unisex infestations would be expected to have a low worm burden. Consequently, they may not only have a negative microfilariae examination but may also be negative on an antigen test. Female worms may be rendered sterile by drugs routinely used to treat or prevent heartworm disease. A combination of thiacetarsemide, dithiazanine, and levamisole, with levamisole the most likely culprit, has been reported to cause female worm sterility.[58]

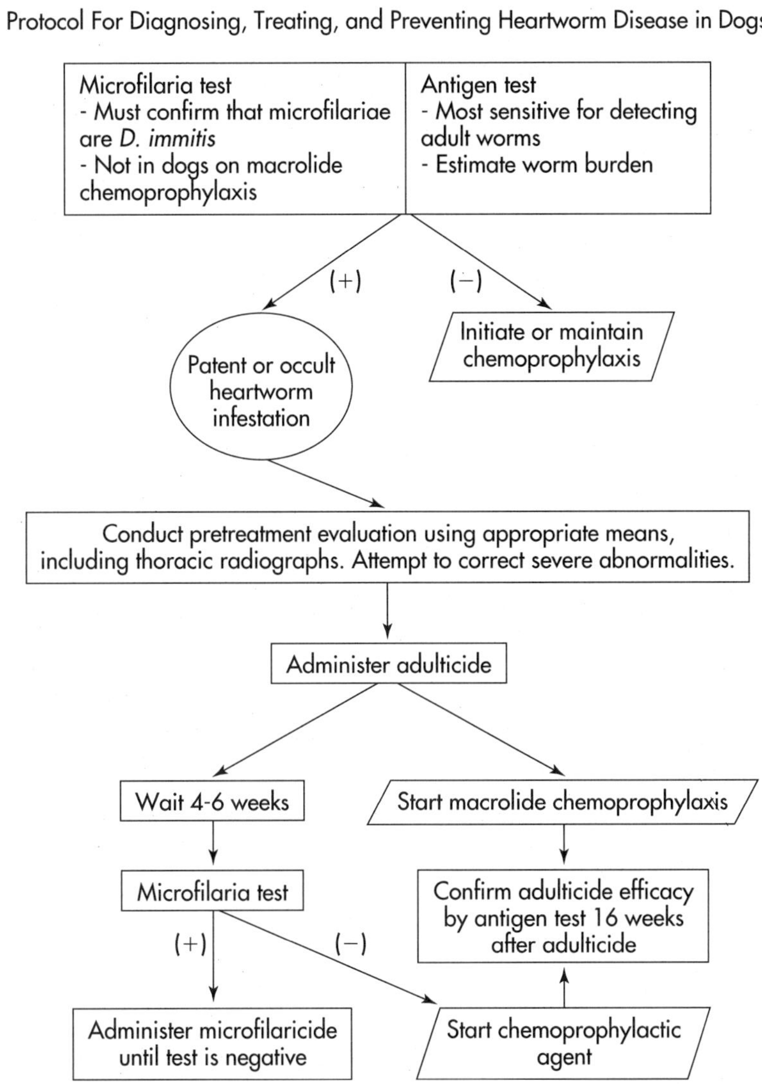

FIGURE 23-9 Diagnostic and therapeutic algorithm for a dog that has not been on a macrolide heartworm preventative.

The avermectins, ivermectin and milbemycin, reduce circulating microfilarial numbers to a very low level or to zero.[12,16] Because of the widespread use of the avermectins for heartworm prevention, the incidence of occult disease has increased within recent years. In dogs that have immunologic destruction of microfilariae, the adult females are gravid and can produce live microfilariae. The immunologic destruction occurs after the microfilariae are shed into the bloodstream. Here the microfilarial antigens are exposed to circulating immunoglobulins. Dogs that have an immunologic response to microfilariae strong enough to clear the bloodstream of microfilariae are commonly also very allergic to adult worms and commonly have severe heartworm disease present on chest radiographs. Apparently this severe disease is secondary to an intense immunologic reaction within the pulmonary arteries and pulmonary parenchyma.

Tests for detecting microfilariae are less useful in cats. Only about 20% of heartworm-infested cats have circulating microfilariae.[14] Microfilaremia usually lasts only about 1 month in experimentally infested cats and rarely persists for more than 7 months.[47] This probably is due to the cat's immune system avidly clearing any microfilariae that are produced. Worms transplanted from cats without microfilariae to heartworm-naive cats produce microfilariae. However, these cats also become amicrofilaremic within a short time. Cats also commonly have single-worm infestations. *D. reconditium* infestation has not been reported in cats.

HEARTWORM ANTIGEN TESTS

Diagnosis of heartworm infestation in dogs. Because of the problem of occult infestations, other tests to detect heartworm disease have been devised (Table 23-2). Indirect fluorescent antibody tests and enzyme-linked immunosorbent assay (ELISA)-based antibody tests have been used in the past in dogs. They detected immunoglobulins against microfilarial antigens and therefore were most likely to be positive in dogs with the immunologic form of occult heartworm disease. Antibody tests are notoriously nonspecific and insensitive in dogs.[59]

More recently, tests that detect a circulating adult heartworm antigen have been devised. These tests are very sensitive and

TABLE 23-2

Heartworm antigen test kits

Product name	*Manufacturer*	*Type**	*Format*	*Control*	*Approved for use in:*	*Type of sample***
Assure/CH	Synbiotics	ELISA	Wand	None	Dogs; cats	P, S
Uni-Tec CHW	Synbiotics	ELISA	Membrane	Positive	Dogs; cats	P, S, WB
ICT Gold HW	Synbiotics	ICT	Membrane	Positive	Dogs	P, S, WB
DiroCHEK	Synbiotics	ELISA	Microwell	Positive; negative	Dogs; cats	P, S
Snap Canine Heartworm PF	IDEXX	ELISA	Membrane	Positive; negative	Dogs; cats	P, S, WB
PetChek HTWM PF	IDEXX	ELISA	Microwell	Positive; negative	Dogs; cats	P, S
VetRED	Rhone Merieux	HA	Well	Negative	Dogs	WB

**ELISA,* Enzyme-linked immunosorbent assay; *ICT,* immunochromatographic; *HA,* hemagglutination.
***P,* Plasma; *S,* serum; *WB,* whole blood.

absolutely specific for *D. immitis* and so have supplanted the antibody tests for diagnosing heartworm disease in dogs. Currently these antigen tests are used to screen dogs for heartworm infestation, to diagnose occult heartworm infestation, and to monitor the efficacy of therapy. Some tests can be used to semiquantitate the worm burden.

Antigen tests to detect heartworm infestation are ELISA, immunochromatographic, or hemagglutination-based tests that detect an antigen shed by adult female heartworms into the circulation. They detect an antigen that is widely distributed in adult worms but is most abundant in the uteri of gravid females and eggs.[60] Because of this, antigen tests only detect female worms. A list of the products available in 1998 and some of their characteristics are outlined in Table 23-2. Test kits are constantly changing, so this table may not be current after 1998.

These tests are virtually 100% specific for *D. immitis* in commercial laboratories (i.e., there are virtually no false positives). False-positive tests do occur in veterinary practices for various reasons, but the incidence is still low. Care must be taken not to contaminate samples with other samples in the laboratory. The manufacturer's instructions must be followed to the letter. Any deviation can result in an invalid test result. The companies that manufacture heartworm antigen tests offer a confirmation service for their tests. Consequently, if there is any question about a particular test, the manufacturer should be contacted and serum, plasma, or whole blood sent to them to confirm or deny the test result.

Sensitivity of heartworm antigen tests at detecting adult heartworm infestation is good but depends on several factors. Antigen tests are virtually 100% positive in dogs with patent infestations (when live adult worms and microfilariae are present). In dogs with occult infestations resulting from immune-mediated destruction of microfilariae, the sensitivity of antigen tests is approximately 90%. Single-sex infestations most commonly occur in animals with very low worm burdens. In dogs with single-sex worm infestations, antigen tests are close to 100% sensitive at detecting dogs with female worms only and very insensitive at detecting infestations of only male worms. In one study, up to 24 male worms were transplanted into heartworm-free dogs. No antigen was detected.[61] Conversely when one or two female worms are present, ELISA-based antigen tests are now 90% to 100% sensitive, and when three or more female worms are present, antigen tests are virtually 100% sensitive.[62] Female worms must be gravid for detection. Consequently, young worms (less than 5 months of age) are generally not detected. Female worms greater than 8 months of age are almost always detected.

Because antigen tests are virtually 100% specific for heartworm infestation when performed correctly and because they are much more sensitive at detecting heartworm infestation than microfilariae detection, antigen tests should always be used for routine screening of dogs for heartworm infestation. Only about 1% of heartworm-infested dogs that are antigen-negative are microfilaremic and, as stated previously, antigen tests are virtually 100% positive in dogs with circulating microfilariae.[63] Conversely, microfilariae are present in only approximately 70% to 80% of heartworm-infested dogs. Consequently, antigen testing is far superior to microfilariae detection for diagnosing heartworm infestation. However, because 0.5% to 1% of dogs with heartworm infestation can be positive for microfilariae and negative for heartworm antigen, tests to detect microfilariae should generally be used in initial screening of dogs for heartworm disease. Because administration of ivermectin or milbemycin renders heartworms sterile, detecting microfilariae in dogs on macrolide prophylaxis is highly unlikely. Only antigen testing in these dogs is needed.

With the advent of antigen tests, not detecting a dog that has a significant heartworm infestation leading to heartworm disease is unusual. The severity of heartworm disease depends on the number of worms present and on the immune response of the animal to the worms. Dogs that have fewer than three female worms, do not have circulating microfilariae, and are not extremely allergic to the worms usually have no evidence of heartworm disease. Consequently, if this level of infestation is detected in a dog, it is questionable whether or not to treat it. Not detecting this type of dog does not affect the dog's health. If, on the other hand, a dog has a small worm burden, is microfilariae-negative, and antigen test–negative, but is very allergic to the worms, radiographic changes and clinical signs would be present and detection could still be made by examining a thoracic radiograph.

Determination of adult heartworm burden. Antigen tests not only detect infestation but also indicate the level of infestation, at least semiquantitatively (Snap, Idexx Laboratories, Westbrook, Me.). The circulating antigen concentration increases with an increasing worm burden. To take advantage of this fact, this antigen test determines if a low concentration or high concentration of the antigen is present. Dogs with a high antigen concentration and therefore a greater worm burden are at greater risk for developing disease secondary to their heartworm infestation, if they do not already have it, and for developing thromboembolic disease after adulticide therapy. The DiroCHEK heartworm antigen test (Synbiotics Corp., San Diego, Calif.) can also be used to quantitate antigen concentration, albeit in a more complex fashion. Serial dilutions of serum can be used to determine a titer. This titer is determined by making two-fold serial dilutions of serum or plasma with phosphate-buffered saline to dilutions of 1:1, 1:2, 1:4, 1:8, 1:16, 1:32, 1:64, and 1:128. Dogs that are still positive at dilutions greater than 1:32 may be at greater risk of developing postadulticide therapy thromboembolic complications.[64]

Detection of adult infestation in cats. The sensitivity of heartworm antigen tests in cats is poor. One study reported a sensitivity of only 37.5% in cats, little better than the sensitivity of a concentration test to detect microfilariae (20%).[65] Antigen tests are generally considered 100% specific for *D. immitis* in cats. In another study of 24 experimentally infested cats using an antigen test developed by the company HEska, the test was negative in all eight cats harboring 170-day-old single male infestations.[66] In 16 cats with at least one female worm (range, one to seven worms per cat), the test was positive in six cats. In another study of 13 cats harboring more (range, one to 20) female worms for a longer period (6 to 9 months), the test was 100% positive.

Assessment of adulticide efficacy using antigen tests. Antigen tests are also used to assess the efficacy of adulticide therapy in dogs. After worm death, the circulating antigen concentration gradually decreases until it is usually undetectable 3 to 5 months after adulticide therapy.[67] An antigen test usually is evaluated 4 months after adulticide therapy. If the antigen test is still positive after this time, this documents that live female worms are still present. If microfilariae are still present also, therapy should be repeated to kill off the adult worms, the source of the microfilaremia, or avermectin prophylaxis should be started to eliminate microfilariae. If microfilariae are not present, the clinician and client should discuss the advisability of re-treating with an adulticide. Adulticide therapy usually reduces the worm burden significantly.[68] In dogs that are not severely allergic to the worms, a decrease in worm number may result in significant clinical improvement. If a dog has improved clinically and did not tolerate arsenical treatment well, a decision not to re-treat is rational. Re-treatment may not be always be beneficial. Older female worms and male worms are more susceptible to arsenical therapy, whereas younger female worms are more resistant. Consequently, if a dog remains antigen-positive, it is most likely that a group of young female worms remains and they may still be resistant to arsenical therapy when a dog is retreated.

Limitations. The major limitation of current antigen tests is their inability to detect male and immature (nongravid) female worms. Tests to detect other heartworm antigens may be devised. A protein expressed by late L_4 larvae, adult male and female worms, and microfilariae has been identified and an ELISA-based test devised to detect this protein.[69] This test was positive as early as 11 weeks postinfestation and detected single male worm infestations. This test was not commercially available as of mid-1998.

HEARTWORM ANTIBODY TESTS

Dogs. Tests to detect antibodies to microfilarial or adult heartworm antibodies have been used over the past 2 decades. ELISA-based heartworm antibody tests were marketed in the first half of the 1980s. These tests were insensitive and very nonspecific.[59] The large number of false-positive tests probably resulted in many dogs with no heartworm infestation being treated with thiacetarsemide. These tests are no longer used in dogs.

Cats. Because of the poor sensitivity of antigen tests in cats, other serologic means of detecting feline dirofilariasis have been sought. An ELISA-based antibody test (Animal Diagnostics, St. Louis, Mo.) is one test available. In one study, this test was 100% sensitive at detecting dirofilariasis 6 months after inoculation.[70] However, any test that detects circulating antibodies to heartworms is often positive in cats exposed to heartworm larvae but that do not have adult heartworm infestation. In one study, this test was used to screen for heartworm infestation in 215 cats.[65] Of these, 28 (13%) were antibody-positive but only eight (4%) had live adult heartworms present. Of these eight cats, seven were antibody-positive. Consequently, this antibody test is very sensitive at detecting heartworm infestation but is not specific for the presence of adult heartworms. The false positive results may be due to the presence of an antibody to previous infestation, antibody response to circulating larvae that never develop to adults, the presence of adult worms at aberrant sites, or cross-reaction of the test to an antibody to other parasites.

Recently, another ELISA-based test to detect IgG antibodies to a proprietary heartworm antigen has been marketed (Heska Feline Heartworm Reference Lab Diagnostic, Heska Corporation, Fort Collins, Colo.). Antibodies to this antigen are produced within 50 to 60 days after a cat is infested with heartworm larvae. Preliminary evidence suggests that this test is 97% sensitive (60 of 62 cats with known heartworm infestation) and 93% sensitive in cats with a single male worm infestation.[71] As with the previously described test, a positive test does not mean that adult heartworms are present in the pulmonary arteries. When 86 cats were experimentally infested with L_3 *D. immitis* larvae, 91% developed a positive antibody response, even though 29% did not have any worms in the pulmonary arteries or heart at necropsy.[71] Cats more commonly clear their own infestations. An antibody response appears to be mounted to immature forms of the worm that fail to develop to adults. The test becomes positive 2 to 3 months after inoculation with L_3 larvae in experimental cats. The antibody titer remains elevated for approximately 9 to 12 months after the adults have been cleared. Consequently, this test is probably most useful at ruling out heartworm infestation via a negative test. A positive test appears to be helpful in a cat with clinical signs referable to heartworm disease to strengthen suspicion of heartworm disease. The test cannot, however, be used as a screening or a confirmatory test.

THORACIC RADIOGRAPHY

Dogs. Thoracic radiographs should be evaluated routinely in any dog or cat diagnosed with heartworm infestation, regardless of the clinical signs or physical examination findings. Physical examination is commonly normal in dogs with heartworm disease until the disease is severe and is no substitute for evaluating thoracic radiographs. Clinical signs are also commonly not present until heartworm disease is severe, and significant disease can be present without any clinical signs.

Both a dorsoventral or ventrodorsal and a lateral view should be obtained and evaluated. The dorsoventral view is usually most enlightening. The caudal pulmonary arteries usually have the largest worm burden. Of these, the right caudal artery is most commonly infested or most heavily infested because of a streaming effect of blood toward this branch. Consequently, the right caudal pulmonary artery is the most frequently affected pulmonary artery branch, and the left caudal artery is the next most commonly affected. Most dogs have changes in both. The caudal pulmonary arteries should be examined closely in any dog suspected of having or confirmed to have heartworm infestation. In dogs with heavier infestation, the cranial lobar arteries may also be infested and have radiographic changes, best appreciated on a lateral view. The main pulmonary artery may also be enlarged, and this enlargement may be visible on the dorsoventral or ventrodorsal radiograph.

Pulmonary artery changes observed in heartworm disease in dogs include enlargement (increased diameter), increased tortuosity, and blunting (pruning). Pulmonary artery enlargement is caused by the arteritis. The arteritis occurs in close proximity to the adult worms in dogs with mild-to-moderate heartworm disease. In dogs with severe heartworm disease, moderate-to-severe pulmonary hypertension may also be present and also contributes to the enlargement. The arteritis, if severe, also produces pulmonary artery tortuosity. Blood flow is not interrupted by live worms. Dead worms, however, produce pulmonary emboli that interrupt blood flow to lung segments, resulting in pulmonary arteries that appear to terminate suddenly when examined on a thoracic radiograph (i.e., they are blunted or pruned). All these changes are generally most severe in dogs with large worm burdens and dogs that are very allergic to heartworms.

Pulmonary parenchymal changes may also exist in dogs with heartworm disease. Radiographically, these changes can be quite varied. In dogs with mild-to-moderate parenchymal disease, increased lung densities may be observed adjacent to the affected arteries. In more severe disease, generalized densities throughout the lung fields may be observed.

Right heart enlargement is a secondary change and should only be evaluated after the pulmonary vasculature has been evaluated. In dogs with moderate-to-severe pulmonary hypertension, right heart enlargement may also be identified on thoracic radiographs. This is generally best appreciated on a dorsoventral or ventrodorsal view. Right heart enlargement is not a feature of mild heartworm disease and may not be present or apparent in dogs with moderate disease. Mild right ventricular enlargement cannot be reliably detected using thoracic radiographs.[72]

Cats. Cats with heartworm infestation often also have radiographic evidence of the infestation (heartworm disease), although the pattern is often different from that seen in dogs. Radiographic findings can include bronchointerstitial, bronchial, or alveolar lung patterns, lobar pulmonary arterial enlargement, and pulmonary hyperinflation.[55] Enlargement of the caudal lobar pulmonary arteries is a common finding during the early stages of the disease but may resolve as the disease progresses.[55] The right caudal lobar artery may be more frequently involved.[54] Pulmonary artery tortuosity and blunting are much less common in the cat than in the dog. Presence of a main pulmonary artery bulge is rare. Heart enlargement also occurs but usually appears as generalized enlargement rather than right heart enlargement, despite the presence of isolated right heart enlargement.[55] Right heart failure is rare in cats, although pleural effusion or ascites may be seen on occasion.[55] Cats that present for acute dyspnea as a result of acute thromboembolism of dead worms either before or after adulticide therapy usually have at least one large region of alveolar density, often confined to a lung lobe, usually the right caudal lung lobe.

The primary differential diagnoses for the common radiographic patterns seen in cats include *Aelurostrongylus* infestation and feline asthma. Bacterial pneumonia is rare in cats. If a transtracheal wash is performed, eosinophils may be the primary cell type identified in the first 4 to 8 months after adults arrive in the pulmonary arteries.[54] After that, macrophages are the primary cell type.

ANGIOGRAPHY

Nonselective angiography is a more invasive means of diagnosing dirofilariasis. Examples of angiograms from dogs with heartworm infestation are presented in Figures 23-3 through 23-5. Angiography is almost never used to diagnose heartworm infestation in dogs. Occasionally it is useful in cats when the diagnosis is in doubt and adulticide therapy is anticipated. Angiography is not without risk, and death is a potential outcome, albeit in a small percentage of cats. Angiography should not be performed in a dyspneic cat. The procedure is performed with the cat awake and unsedated. Administration through a jugular catheter is preferred. The cat is placed in right lateral recumbency, and 2 mL/kg of an iodinated contrast agent is injected rapidly through the catheter. The radiograph is taken at the end of the injection.

ECHOCARDIOGRAPHY

Echocardiography is usually normal in dogs with mild heartworm disease. In dogs with moderate heartworm disease, the right ventricular chamber is usually dilated and the free wall may be thickened. If a regurgitant jet across either the tricuspid or the pulmonic valves can be identified, mildly-to-moderately increased flow velocity may be identified using spectral Doppler echocardiography, indicating mild-to-moderate right ventricular systolic or pulmonary artery diastolic hypertension. Dogs with severe heartworm disease may have moderate-to-marked right ventricular chamber dilation and may have Doppler evidence of moderate-to-severe pulmonary hypertension.

Heartworms can be identified in the main pulmonary artery, proximal caudal lobar artery branches, the right heart, and the vena cavae in selected cases. Heartworms appear as two parallel linear densities with a lucent linear region between them (Figure 23-10). Usually a large number of worms must be present to visualize the worms in the main pulmonary artery or the proximal branches in dogs. In one study, 50% to 60% of dogs with heartworm infestation had worms visible in the pulmonary arteries.[73] In California, where the heartworm burden is probably less than in the eastern United States, it is less common to identify heartworms in pulmonary arteries, in our experience. Out of 66 dogs without caval syndrome, only six had a few worms visible in the right atrium and right ventricle in one report.[73] All six of these dogs were terminally ill.

In cats, heartworms can be identified in the pulmonary artery branches, the main pulmonary artery, the right ventricle, and the right atrium. They are more commonly identified in these locations in cats than they are in dogs. This makes sense because the worms are still large and the pulmonary arteries in cats are quite small. Echocardiography may be the most sensitive means of identifying

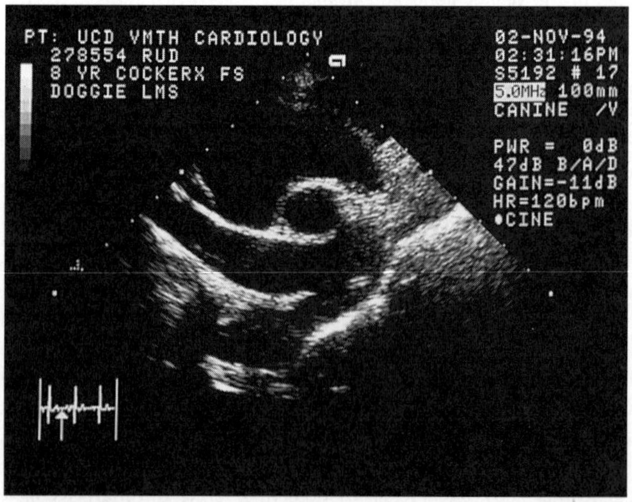

FIGURE 23-10 Two-dimensional echocardiogram from an 8-year-old female spayed American cocker spaniel cross with heartworm disease. The view is a cross-sectional view of the heart base taken from a right parasternal position. A heartworm can be visualized in the main pulmonary artery as two short parallel echodense lines separated by an echolucent line.

heartworm infestation in cats. In one study performed in Italy in a hyperendemic area for heartworm disease, heartworm infestation was identified using echocardiography in 11 of 51 cats examined.[74] Of these 11 cats, none were microfilariae-positive and only three were antigen test–positive. Radiographic evidence of the disease was present in the three antigen test–positive cats but not in the others. On echocardiography, four of the 11 cats had heartworms present in the right ventricle, one had them in the right atrium, and six had worms in the pulmonary vasculature. Of the six cats with worms in the pulmonary vasculature, four had them in the pulmonary trunk and two had them in the right caudal lobar pulmonary artery. In another study, seven of nine cats infested with adult worms were detected using echocardiography.[55] Worms were detected in all cats with three or more worms. In another study, 14 of 39 cats (36%) with confirmed heartworm disease had echocardiographic evidence of worms.[56] In 24 of these cats the echocardiogram was obtained by a cardiologist. Heartworms were found in 13 of these cats (54%). An antigen test was positive in all but two of these cats. Worms were most commonly identified in the pulmonary artery (64%). Less commonly they were identified in the right ventricle (43%) or the right atrium (36%). They were in both the right atrium and the right ventricle in four cats. One can conclude from these studies that an experienced echocardiographer can frequently identify heartworms in heartworm-infested cats.

To diagnose heartworm infestation, a right parasternal short-axis basilar view that includes the right ventricular outflow tract, pulmonic valve, main pulmonary artery, and proximal portions of the caudal lobar arteries should be obtained. This view is above the view of the aorta and left atrium. The angle to obtain this view is often obliqued from the view used to see the aorta and left atrium. This view allows visualization of about 15 to 18 mm of the right caudal lobar artery branch and 3 to 6 mm of the left branch. The portion of these branches that are large enough to accommodate an adult worm is only about 3 cm in length. Because heartworms in cats are 12 to 20 cm, it is easy to see why they can be visualized on an echocardiogram and why at least part of the worm is so frequently present in the right ventricle.

ELECTROCARDIOGRAPHY

Electrocardiography is a poor diagnostic test for dogs or cats with heartworm disease. In dogs with mild-to-moderate disease, the ECG is usually normal. In dogs with severe disease and severe right heart enlargement, the ECG usually shows evidence of right ventricular enlargement, but the enlargement is readily appreciated on chest radiographs and echocardiographic examination. Rarely does the electrocardiogram give the clinician useful additional information in this disease unless an arrhythmia is present.

CLINICAL PATHOLOGY

The hemogram is normal in most dogs with heartworm infestation.[75] However, approximately 60% of severely diseased dogs have mild anemia. The anemia is nonregenerative, except in dogs with caval syndrome (see below) that have hemolysis. The leukogram is commonly abnormal. About 20% of dogs with heartworm infestation have a neutrophilia. About 20% of these have a left shift. A mild-to-moderate lymphopenia is common and probably stress-related. Eosinophilia is also common and occurs in about 85% of dogs with circulating microfilariae and 95% of dogs that are amicrofilaremic because of immune destruction of their microfilariae. Basophils may also be seen in heartworm-infested dogs. Heartworm disease is the most common cause of a basophilia in an endemic region.

Serum chemistries are normal in most dogs with heartworms.[75] The serum alkaline phosphatase (SAP), serum alanine aminotransferase (ALT), and serum aspartate aminotransferase (AST) concentrations are normal in most infested dogs. Only about 5% to 10% have significant elevations. Neither the severity of the disease nor the likelihood of thiacetarsemide toxicity correlates with liver enzyme elevation. Azotemia is rare, occurring in less than 5% of heartworm-infested dogs. Serum globulin concentration is commonly increased. Serum albumin concentration is usually normal but may be decreased in severely affected dogs.

About 20% of the asymptomatic dogs, 30% of mildly-to-moderately affected dogs, and most severely affected dogs have proteinuria.[75] Most of the proteinuria is due to mild albuminuria. Severe proteinuria can occur, however, and lead to hypoalbuminemia and, occasionally, nephrotic syndrome.

Acid-base balance is usually normal.[75] About 15% of heartworm-infested dogs have a mild, compensated metabolic acidosis. Blood gases are usually normal. Surprisingly, only about 30% have mild hypoxemia. Dogs with severe disease may have more profound changes.

HEARTWORM DISEASE CLASSIFICATION

Dogs with heartworm disease should be classified into one of three classes for determining prognosis and treatment protocol.[76,77] Class 1 dogs are those dogs that are subclinical or have very mild clinical signs. They have no or only mild radiographic changes. They are more commonly younger dogs (an average of 3.8 years of age vs. 5.4 years for class 2 and 7.4 years for class 3 dogs in one study).[40] About 75% of them have a serum antigen concentration less than 1.7 μg/mL (note that this cutoff is different from the demarcation between "high" and "low" serum antigen concentration for the Snap antigen test).[40] Class 2 dogs have moderate disease. This is the most common class. In one study, of 322 dogs treated for heartworm infestation, 219 were in this class.[40] Dogs in class 2 most commonly have mild clinical signs, a cough, and mild-to-moderate radiographic changes. They may also experience exercise intolerance and have mild weight loss and poor hair coat condition. About 55% of them have a serum antigen concentration greater than 1.7 μg/mL. Dogs with a higher antigen concentration have a higher incidence of thromboembolic complications than those with a lower antigen concentration. Consequently, dogs with a higher antigen concentration that are in class 2 may be treated differently than those with a lower antigen concentration.[40] Class 3 dogs have severe heartworm disease. They almost always have clinical signs (e.g., persistent cough, weight loss, dyspnea), may be in right heart failure, and always have severe radiographic changes.[77] They commonly have mild anemia. Interestingly, class 3 dogs commonly have a lower antigen concentration than other classes of dogs.[40] This may be because worms have died in these dogs. Dead worms produce a more severe pulmonary reaction than live worms. This could contribute to the more severe disease in dogs in which dead worms are found. More likely, class 3 dogs are dogs that have a greater immune response to adult heartworms and so can have severe disease even with a lesser number of worms. Class 3 dogs are generally at greater risk of having complications with adulticide therapy. Conversely, they may also be the dogs that improve the most following therapy.

RECOMMENDATIONS FOR HEARTWORM TESTING

Testing dogs that have not been tested previously. Dogs less than 6 months of age do not need to be tested and can be placed on prophylactic therapy at the time of presentation. When an adult dog from a heartworm-infested region presents to a veterinarian's clinic for the first time, the veterinarian should determine the dog's heartworm prevention status and test accordingly. If a dog has not been on a preventative drug or the veterinarian cannot document to his or her satisfaction that the dog has been on an adequate program of heartworm prophylaxis and the dog is old enough to harbor adult heartworms, both an antigen test and a test to detect microfilariae should be performed. The argument put forth for performing a microfilaria detection test in this situation is because 0.5% to 1.0% of dogs can be antigen-negative but positive for microfilariae.

Testing dogs administered diethylcarbamazine prophylaxis. If a dog with circulating microfilariae is administered diethylcarbamazine, a life-threatening shock reaction can occur.[78] For this reason, any dog that is to be exposed to diethylcarbamazine must be tested for circulating microfilariae before diethylcarbamazine administration. This should be done each spring before reinstituting prophylaxis in cold climates and probably annually in warmer regions if prophylaxis is administered year-round.

Testing dogs administered macrolide prophylaxis. Almost all dogs administered ivermectin prophylaxis will be rendered amicrofilaremic within approximately 6 to 9 months if they are microfilaremic or will remain amicrofilaremic if they develop an infestation while on macrolide prophylaxis. Milbemycin renders most dogs amicrofilaremic after one prophylactic dose. Consequently, these dogs must be tested with antigen tests to detect heartworm infestation. Performing a concentration test to detect circulating microfilariae in these cases is not required, because this test is almost always negative and administering a macrolide to a dog with a low number of microfilariae produces no adverse effects.

Retesting for heartworm disease has historically been performed annually. However, if an owner administers a macrolide preventative religiously, the chances of a dog becoming reinfested are negligible. In this case, annual retesting may not be required. Of course, many owners are not religious about administering any type of medication. However, even if a macrolide preventative is administered to a dog every 2 months, the chances of reinfestation are very small. With ivermectin administration every 4 months, the number of heartworms that reach adulthood is still very small.[79] Consequently, in most cases, annual retesting may not be necessary.

TABLE 23-3

Drugs used to treat heartworm infestation in dogs

Stage	*Drug*	*Dosage*
Adult (L_5)	Thiacetarsemide	2.2 mg/kg IV twice a day for 2 days
	Melarsomine	
Microfilariae (L_1)	Ivermectin	50 µg/kg PO (single dose) 6 µg/kg/mo
	Milbemycin	500 µg/kg (single dose)
	Dithiazanine (not currently available)	6-20 mg/kg PO once a day
	Levamisole (not frequently used)	2.5 mg/kg PO once a day for 3-7 days
L_3-L_4 molt	Diethylcarbamazine	1.25 mg/kg PO once a day
L_3, L_4, immature L_5	Ivermectin	6 µg/kg PO once a mo
L_3, L_4	Milbemycin	500-999 µg/kg/mo PO

Treatment to Kill Adult Heartworms

ADULTICIDE THERAPY IN DOGS

Table 23-3 provides drug and dosage information for the various stages of heartworm infestation. Two drugs, thiacetarsemide and melarsomine, are approved for killing adult heartworms in dogs. Both products are organoarsenics. Thiacetarsemide can be used in cats. A safe dose of melarsomine for cats had not been identified at the time of this publication.

Treatment decisions and methods of treatment are always controversial. This is especially true with adulticide therapy of heartworm disease. Veterinarians that have treated dogs infested with heartworms for many years develop a sixth sense about which dogs will do well and which ones will not. They often modify their therapy based on experimentation and word-of-mouth findings from other veterinarians. This is probably to be expected, because heartworm therapy is not an exact science and no one can predict the safety or the efficacy of a drug such as thiacetarsemide in a given patient. Hopefully, the predictions will become easier and the folklore less with melarsomine.

The decision to treat with an adulticide. In general, any dog that has evidence of heartworm disease has the potential to improve if it is treated with an adulticide. In most cases, ridding the dog of its infestation ultimately results in clinical improvement. Dogs with severe heartworm disease or with severe complications to heartworm disease, however, are a challenge. They may not tolerate adulticide therapy as well as a dog with less disease and often do not tolerate the thromboembolic complications of the disease as well. In these types of patients, becoming caught between a rock and a hard place is common. That is, the dog may develop life-threatening complications if treatment is pursued and may develop life-threatening complications if it is not pursued. In most of these dogs, melarsomine is a better choice for therapy because of its lack of hepatotoxicity and the ability to give a graded dose to kill a lesser number of worms each time. However, the expense of this drug interferes with its use in some cases. In all cases, coexisting diseases should be controlled as much as possible before instituting adulticide therapy.

A dog without radiographic or clinical evidence of heartworm disease but that is repeatedly positive on a heartworm antigen test or is positive for *D. immitis* microfilariae can be handled two ways—it can be treated with an adulticide or it can be monitored. The manner in which this type of patient is managed depends on the views and wishes of the veterinarian and the client. Because no evidence of disease in such a patient is present, there is no absolute need to treat with an adulticide immediately. If the veterinarian is comfortable with not treating such a patient and if the owner prefers not to have the dog undergo treatment with an arsenical or to risk postadulticide complications, then the alternative is not to treat at the time of diagnosis and to monitor the dog for any evidence of disease. Our general recommendation in this situation is to examine the patient every 6 months and to take a radiograph each time. If any signs of disease develop on the thoracic radiographs, our recommendation is to treat at that time. If none develops, then we recommend continued monitoring every 6 months. Dogs that present with evidence of heartworm infestation but no heartworm disease generally fall into two categories—dogs that have a weak immune response to heartworms or have a small number of worms and dogs that have only recently developed a patent infestation. The dogs in the first category often go on to live normal lives without adulticide therapy, presuming that they are on a preventive drug and therefore not infested with additional worms. The dogs in the latter category may go on to develop heartworm disease and that disease has the potential of becoming severe. One can sometimes make a reasonable guess about the category into which a particular patient fits. For example, a 7-year-old dog that has been on a preventive drug for only the last 2 years and is being tested for only the second time in its life (the first being before it was placed on a preventive medication) probably had a prepatent infestation at the time of original testing and has had heartworm infestation for 2 years without developing heartworm disease. At other times no clues as to when the dog became infested are available. In these situations, one must talk to the client and outline all of the advantages and disadvantages of waiting and monitoring or treating immediately. The client then must make the choice with guidance from the veterinarian. The major potential complications associated with waiting and monitoring are rapid development of severe disease and caval syndrome. In most situations, heartworm disease does not progress rapidly. Consequently, an examination every 6 months is usually adequate. However, no guarantee that more rapid progression will not occur can be given. Although caval syndrome is rare, when it does occur it is usually a severe and potentially lethal complication to the disease. An owner that decides to wait and monitor must be willing to accept these risks just like an owner that decides to treat must accept the risks of arsenical therapy and embolic complications.

Pretreatment evaluation. Three ideal goals for pretreatment assessment of dogs infested with heartworms can be delineated. They are (1) to predict the likelihood of adulticide toxicity, (2) to identify dogs most likely to develop severe thromboembolism after adulticide therapy, and (3) to estimate reversibility of the disease.

Dogs that are to be administered melarsomine or thiacetarsemide should be evaluated to detect any serious underlying disease. Predicting thiacetarsemide toxicity in the average dog is almost impossible. In an attempt to predict the likelihood of thiacetarsemide toxicity, every dog should have a complete physical examination and blood withdrawn for evaluating the hemogram and serum chemistries. A urinalysis should also be evaluated to determine urine specific gravity and to identify proteinuria. Mild-to-moderate increases in ALT or AST are not indications for withholding arsenical therapy. Icterus, however, is a contraindication to administering thiacetarsemide. Azotemia in conjunction with an isosthenuric specific gravity (primary renal failure) is also a contraindication to the administration of thiacetarsemide. Mild-to-moderate prerenal azotemia does not appear to be a contraindication to melarsomine administration.[80] A mild anemia is commonly present in dogs with severe disease but is not a contraindication to therapy. In fact, the best treatment for this mild anemia is to kill the adult heartworms.

Dogs with large worm burdens and dogs with severe pulmonary artery or parenchymal lung changes are at greatest risk for developing complications because of thromboemboli after adulticide therapy. Consequently, an estimate of worm burden using a semiquantitative heartworm antigen test may be used in an attempt to predict postadulticide complications. Chest radiographs should be evaluated before therapy. As discussed below, dogs with severe lung disease are at greater risk for postadulticide complications. They are candidates to be treated prophylactically with drugs such as aspirin, corticosteroids, and, possibly, heparin. They should also be treated with melarsomine, using a split schedule as explained below, rather than thiacetarsemide.

Predicting the reversibility of the disease is a difficult task. Usually, the worse the disease and the longer it has been present, the less is the likelihood the radiographic pulmonary changes will reverse after adulticide therapy. Most dogs, however, improve clinically if they had clinical signs before therapy.

Thiacetarsemide. Thiacetarsemide has been used since 1947 to kill adult heartworms. It belongs to the phenylarsenoxide group of compounds. Of this group, it is the only one stable enough in an

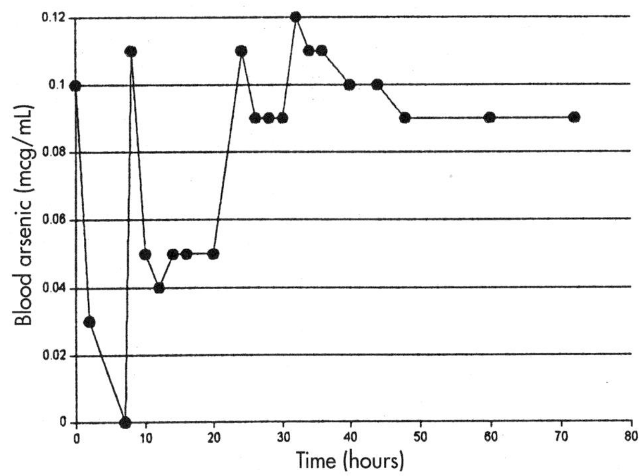

FIGURE 23-11 Blood arsenic concentration over time following the administration of four doses of thiacetarsemide 2.2 mg/kg every 8 to 16 hours starting at time 0.

aqueous solution to be stored in multidose vials. It has a steep dose-response curve and a narrow margin of safety. Its efficacy is inconsistent and it has potentially very serious side effects. Consequently, it is far from being a perfect drug.

The exact method by which thiacetarsemide kills adult heartworms is unknown. The tissue concentration of arsenic following oral or intravenous administration is similar, yet only intravenous administration results in worm death.[81] This suggests that elemental arsenic is not the ingredient that kills the worms. More likely, a metabolite of thiacetarsemide that contains arsenic is the active ingredient. Although arsenic is not the active ingredient, its concentration parallels the pharmacodynamics of thiacetarsemide.[82]

Thiacetarsemide is administered as four intravenous injections (2.2 mg/kg each) over approximately 48 hours. This dose was arrived at empirically and has been used since 1963.[83] Injections should be at least 6 and not more than 16 hours apart. All four injections must be administered to produce the desired effect. If only 1 to 3 injections are administered, usually no worms will be killed. Extreme care must be taken to ensure intravenous delivery of the drug. The drug is extremely caustic and causes severe tissue necrosis if the drug is administered extravascularly. The four-dose protocol results in slow worm death so that not all worms are killed at once. A rapid worm kill would result in severe worm embolism. Slow worm kill results in lesser degrees of worm embolism that start within 4 to 8 days after completing the four-injection series and is usually complete within 3 weeks. Doses 10% to 20% greater than the recommended dose may be associated with greater efficacy but may also produce greater toxicity.[84] Administering six doses over a 3-day period is no more efficacious and produces more postadulticide complications, presumably from a faster worm kill.[85]

Treatment efficacy is almost assuredly related to blood arsenic concentration, although in one study the differences in blood arsenic concentration between groups administered 2.2 mg/kg, 2.7 mg/kg, 2.9 mg/kg, and 3.3 mg/kg did not affect the efficacy of the worm kill.[82] However, dogs that maintain a higher concentration of arsenic in blood for a longer period have a higher worm kill.[82] Consequently, it appears that a longer exposure to a therapeutic concentration of thiacetarsemide metabolites is a major factor in determining the worm kill. One study has shown that dogs with impaired liver function and therefore slower arsenic clearance have a better worm kill than those with normal liver function.[86] As seen in the graph in Figure 23-11, blood arsenic concentration peaks immediately after each intravenous injection and then decreases rapidly. From the second dose on it remains relatively static for the 8 to 16 hours between doses. Blood arsenic concentration is maintained at approximately 0.1 μg/mL for about 30 hours after the fourth dose is administered. Consequently, it appears that the arsenic in thiacetarsemide has a very long terminal half-life. Based on this fact, it is unlikely that the exact interval between doses, be it 6 or 16 hours, makes much difference in total concentration achieved or in the total exposure of the worms to arsenic.

Thiacetarsemide is more effective at killing older worms and male worms. Immature adult worms (young L_5) are very resistant to the effects of thiacetarsemide.[87] Consequently, after thiacetarsemide treatment, many dogs are left with a population of young female worms and immature worms, if the worms were present at the time of treatment. Only about 40% of dogs are completely cleared of their infestation following thiacetarsemide therapy. Thiacetarsemide is also effective at killing heartworms at the time of their last molt from L_4 to L_5 or shortly thereafter. This means that it has some capability as a heartworm preventive.[88] However, it is not used in this fashion.

Thiacetarsemide produces toxicity in most dogs, although this toxicity is commonly not clinically apparent. Thiacetarsemide produces liver cell necrosis, resulting in leakage of hepatic enzymes in almost all cases and acute hepatic failure in some patients. Following the administration of thiacetarsemide, serum ALT and AST concentrations increase in most dogs, and in some dogs severe increases can be noted.[89] Measuring these serum concentrations is generally not indicated, because identifying marked increases in these enzymes is not indicative of the severity of the toxicity and may deter the clinician from administering further doses. This would be inappropriate. Dogs that have more severe hepatotoxicity commonly vomit repeatedly, become depressed and anorexic, and may develop hepatic failure and become jaundiced. The appearance of any of these clinical signs during thiacetarsemide treatment necessitates stopping therapy. Vomiting is not an indication to stop therapy unless it is persistent, the dog is anorexic and depressed, or icterus or azotemia develop. In this context, *icterus* is defined as clinically apparent yellowing of the mucous membranes or sclera. Identifying icteric serum or increased bilirubinuria are not indications to discontinue therapy. Hepatotoxicity is unpredictable. In one study that examined 100 dogs that were administered thiacetarsemide, less than 15% developed signs of toxicity and treatment was discontinued in only 25% of these dogs.[81] Nephrotoxicity is rare. However, thiacetarsemide can cause degeneration and necrosis of renal tubular epithelial cells.[48] In one study, administering 1.5 times the normal dose of thiacetarsemide to normal beagles produced mild increases in blood urea nitrogen (BUN), although BUN did not increase into the abnormal range.[90] Avoiding the use of thiacetarsemide in dogs with renal disease or renal failure is prudent.

If a dog develops clinically significant hepatotoxicity, intravenous fluids should be administered to correct any dehydration that occurs secondary to vomiting and to maintain hydration while the dog is not eating. Dogs can usually be discharged 24 to 48 hours after the last thiacetarsemide injection. Dogs that do not successfully complete the four-injection protocol the first time should be brought back 4 weeks later and the same four-treatment protocol repeated. These dogs will usually tolerate the protocol the second time.

Care must be taken not to inject any thiacetarsemide perivascularly, because extravasation of thiacetarsemide causes tissue necrosis, and severe tissue sloughing can result. Swelling, inflammation, and pain develop within 2 hours of injection. If it is suspected that any drug was infiltrated perivascularly or if the aforementioned clinical signs develop, the area should be infiltrated with sterile saline to dilute the compound and lidocaine given to reduce pain. Topical dimethylsulfoxide (DMSO) or DMSO combined with a corticosteroid may be applied liberally every 4 hours for 2 to 4 days. The site may also be infiltrated with dexamethasone. Hot compresses may be useful to decrease the swelling in the early stages. Pain usually subsides in 2 to 3 days, but the swelling may remain for several weeks.

Thiacetarsemide (Caparsolate, Rhone Merieux, Athens, Ga.) is marketed as a clear liquid for intravenous use. Its concentration is 10 mg/mL. The drug should be refrigerated. Presence of yellow-orange coloration or precipitates means the drug has deteriorated and should be discarded.

Melarsomine. Melarsomine dihydrochloride is a trivalent organoarsenical and a melaminyl thioarsenite supplied as a lyophilized white powder for reconstitution with sterile water. Its development for use in dogs began in 1985, and it was approved to kill adult heartworms by the Food and Drug Administration in 1995.[67] Melarsomine is very effective at killing heartworms, but the method by which it does this is not known. Because it is a new drug, it is expensive. In our hospital, melarsomine alone can cost a client that owns a large dog between $300 and $400 for a series of three injections.

The compound is administered to dogs by deep intramuscular injection into the lumbar muscles between L3 and L5. When administered in this fashion, the drug is absorbed rapidly into the systemic circulation. More than 50% is absorbed within 5 minutes.[67] Following injection, the serum concentration increases to a peak within the first 30 minutes and then rapidly decreases to maintain a low but very stable concentration for more than a day.[67] The drug is metabolized via hydrolysis in the liver and excreted in the bile. The arsenic acid derivative is excreted in the urine.

Melarsomine has several advantages over thiacetarsemide. (1) Tissue necrosis is milder with extravascular injection. (2) Hepatotoxicity and nephrotoxicity are very mild to nonexistent. (3) The percentage of worms killed is greater. (4) One dose of melarsomine results in the death of most male worms, and a two-dose regimen kills both males and females, allowing for a graded worm kill.

The dosing regimen of melarsomine depends on the severity of heartworm disease and the antigen concentration in a given patient.[40] In dogs with class 1 heartworm disease, two doses of 2.5 mg/kg melarsomine are administered into the lumbar musculature between L3 and L5 24 hours apart. The first dose should be administered on one side on the first day and the second dose on the other side the next day. The site of injection should be recorded, and administration at the same site should be avoided. This dosage regimen results in approximately 76% of dogs treated becoming heartworm antigen–negative within 4 months.[68] If a dog is not negative for the adult heartworm antigen after 4 months, administering the same dose results in almost all dogs (90% to 96%) becoming antigen-negative. In dogs with class 2 disease and a low antigen concentration, the same schedule is used and a similar result expected. Even in dogs that do not become negative on an antigen test, serum antigen concentration decreases markedly, signifying a marked decrease in the worm burden. In one study it decreased from an average concentration of 3.96 μg/mL to 0.33 μg/mL following one series of injections.[68]

In dogs with class 2 disease and a high antigen concentration and in class 3 patients, we recommended that one 2.5-mg/kg dose be administered intramuscularly initially (this is called the "Alternate Dosing Regimen" in the package insert). This regimen is not recommended for class 2 dogs by the manufacturer. We feel that this more conservative approach may be warranted, however, because of the greater worm kill with two consecutive doses of melarsomine compared with thiacetarsemide.[67] One dose of melarsomine kills approximately 90% of the male worms and only 15% to 20% of the female worms.[91] The total worm kill is 50% to 65%.[91] The one dose is followed 1 month later with the standard two-dose regimen, 24 hours apart. This results in approximately 90% of the treated dogs becoming negative on a heartworm antigen test.[68,92] About 75% of class 3 patients improve clinically after melarsomine therapy. In one study, 86% of these severely affected dogs survived adulticide therapy with melarsomine.[92] No correlation was identified between aspirin use, corticosteroid use, or cage rest and survival in these dogs.[80]

Melarsomine has a low margin of safety. The target organ of toxicologic significance appears to be the lung. Administration of 3 times the recommended dose (7.5 mg/kg) can produce pulmonary inflammation, pulmonary edema, and death. At the normal dose of 2.5 mg/kg, adverse reactions are common but usually mild. They include coughing and gagging (22%), depression and lethargy (15%), anorexia (13%), fever (7%), lung congestion (5%), emesis (5%), diarrhea (2.5%), dyspnea (2.5%), hypersalivation (2%), and panting (2%). Hypersalivation and panting are uncommon but can occur shortly after injection and can be severe. Adverse reactions can occur after the second dose even though no problems were noted after the first dose. Dogs should be observed for 24 hours after the last injection. We have seen one dog die of pulmonary edema several days following melarsomine administration. Adverse reactions, including depression and lethargy, anorexia, and vomiting occur more frequently in dogs greater than 8 years of age. Other direct systemic side effects are uncommon. One report states that no increase in hepatic enzymes was observed following melarsomine administration to 183 dogs.[93] Treatment of adverse reactions is nonspecific and supportive.

Transient swelling and pain at the injection site commonly occur. The most severe reactions apparently occur when the drug leaks back from the intramuscular site into the subcutaneous tissue. The primary reason the drug is injected into the lumbar musculature is because less leakage from muscle occurs at this site than when the drug is injected into the caudal limb musculature.[67] Digital pressure should be applied to the injection site for 1 to 2 minutes following injection to minimize leakage. Marked increases in serum creatine kinase concentration occur after the injection, indicating acute skeletal muscle necrosis. Histologically, a cellular infiltrate, necrosis, and hemorrhage occur at the injection site. This is followed by fibrosis. It has been reported that most dogs (approximately 60%) have no signs of pain or swelling following injection, about 30% have mild pain and swelling that resolve within 24 hours, and about 10% have pain and swelling for 2 to 5 days.[93] The percentage of dogs with pain and swelling is greater, in our experience. Rarely, a firm nodule may occur at the injection site and can persist indefinitely. Severe swelling is less common and abscessation is rare. The only major problem with melarsomine is that it is expensive enough to preclude therapy to all heartworm-infested dogs.

Melarsomine appears to be safe and effective in ferrets infested with heartworms.[80] Anyone anticipating using the drug in ferrets should contact the company that manufactures melarsomine before its use. Melarsomine should not be used in cats.

Melarsomine (Immiticide, Rhone Merieux, Athens, Ga.) is supplied as 50 mg of melarsomine and 33.75 mg of glycine as a lyophilized powder in vials, with 2-mL vials of sterile water for reconstitution. This provides a final concentration of 25 mg/mL and a final volumetric dose of 0.1 mL/kg. The reconstituted product is unstable but is stable up to 24 hours if refrigerated and kept in the dark.[67] As with all labeled drugs, the package insert should be read carefully before using melarsomine.

ADULTICIDE THERAPY IN CATS

The decision to treat. Treatment of heartworm infestation in cats is controversial. The administration of thiacetarsemide more frequently results in toxic complications, and thromboembolic complications, including fatal complications, are more common in cats than in dogs. Consequently, many veterinarians recommend not treating cats with thiacetarsemide and instead use symptomatic therapy to treat cats with clinical disease. Symptomatic treatment usually consists of corticosteroid administration (prednisone at 2 mg/kg/day PO, declining gradually to 0.5 mg/kg every other day within 2 weeks) to cats with mild-to-moderate symptomatology and other supportive care (oxygen, fluids, diuretics) to cats with severe disease. The rationale is that most cats tolerate worms and only become symptomatic when thromboembolism occurs. Because the worms only live for about 2 years in cats, waiting for the worms to die naturally and treating the complications of worm death as they occur might be more efficacious.[54] No controlled clinical trials on which to base decisions have been performed. Cats diagnosed with heartworm disease should be placed on a preventive drug to prevent further infestations.

Thiacetarsemide. Thiacetarsemide is the only arsenical used to kill adult worms in cats. However, complications, including fatal complications, are more common in cats than in dogs. One study has shown that thiacetarsemide administration (2.2 mg/kg q12h × four doses) to normal cats can result in fulminant pulmonary edema, usually after the second dose.[94] At necropsy, 11 of 13 cats in this study had evidence of noncardiogenic (high-protein) pulmonary edema. A high incidence of depression, anorexia, nausea, and vomiting were also observed. In another study, thiacetarsemide (2.2 mg/kg q12h × four doses) was administered in combination with ketamine (4.5 mg/kg IM) or pentothal and halothane.[95] No radiographic or clinical evidence of pulmonary edema was noted in these cats, and those conducting the study speculated that the antiserotonin activity of ketamine might protect against what appeared to be neurogenic pulmonary edema in the earlier report. Consequently, thiacetarsemide may be safe to administer to cats and may be safer if ketamine or another anesthetic agent is administered before the thiacetarsemide. However, postadulticide complications are common in cats days after thiacetarsemide administration and can be severe and can result in death.

POSTADULTICIDE PNEUMONITIS

Dogs. Following adulticide therapy, worms die and worm debris is carried by blood flow to terminal pulmonary artery branches. These worm emboli usually occlude small (usually less than 10 mm diameter) pulmonary arteries.[46] They may also stimulate regional thrombus formation, resulting in further occlusion.[96] If individual worms die and embolize small pulmonary arteries, they are degraded and phagocytized with few clinical sequelae. Radiographically, focal parenchymal densities develop around the affected arteries.[46] If many worms die simultaneously and are carried into a large pulmonary artery, clinical signs of pulmonary embolism can result. Radiographically, consolidation of the affected lung lobe can occur (Figure 23-12). Exercised dogs are at greater risk of severe postadulticide pneumonitis, presumably because larger numbers of worm fragments are carried into the lungs when blood flow increases. Massive embolization can also occur with exercise and result in sudden death. Dogs with severe heartworm disease

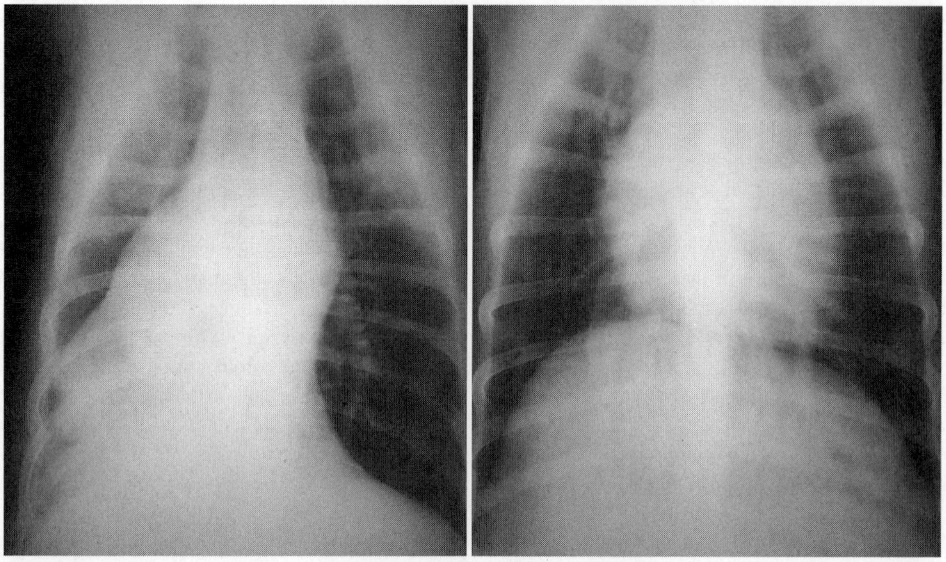

FIGURE 23-12 **A,** Thoracic radiographs taken from a dog with postadulticide pneumonitis. The dog had mild heartworm disease and had been treated with thiacetarsemide 8 days before presentation. The owner noted the dog to be depressed and anorectic. It had also developed a cough. At presentation the dog was febrile. The dorsoventral radiograph taken at presentation shows consolidation of the right caudal lung lobe, consistent with thromboembolic disease. The dog was treated with cage rest and corticosteroids. The clinical signs rapidly resolved over the next 24 to 48 hours. **B,** The thoracic radiographs taken 2 days later revealed complete resolution of the pulmonary disease.

(class 3) are more prone to postadulticide pneumonitis. Dogs with caudal pulmonary arteries 2.5 times the diameter of the ninth rib (dorsoventral radiograph) or larger are at greater risk for thromboembolic complications.[97] Dogs infested with a large number of worms are also at greater risk. Because dogs with greater numbers of worms generally have worse heartworm disease, these two factors are probably often related. Dogs with severe lung disease are at greater risk of developing clinically significant complications associated with embolization because they have less pulmonary reserve. Radiographic evaluation for severity of heartworm disease and pulmonary disease secondary to heartworm disease should be performed on all dogs before adulticide therapy. In dogs with severe lung disease, treatment with corticosteroids may be tried in an attempt to improve lung function. Often the pulmonary lesions are those of pulmonary fibrosis, however, and these cannot be reversed. A semiquantitative evaluation of the serum heartworm antigen concentration may also be useful. Dogs that are at greater risk of postadulticide complications should be considered for therapy to prevent postadulticide complications, as outlined below, and should undergo a graded worm kill with melarsomine, as outlined above.

Owners should be warned not to allow any strenuous exercise or let the dog become excited. In some dogs this means confinement to the house with leash walks outside. For others it means placing the dog in a cage at home or maybe in the hospital. If postadulticide pneumonitis does occur, most owners notice that their dog is anorexic and lethargic because of fever. Coughing is also commonly noted. Sudden death is rare but does occur. In one study, evidence of clinically significant postadulticide embolization consisted of anorexia (86% of cases); fever (71%); depression (48%); tachypnea, dyspnea, or coughing (32%); pale-to-cyanotic oral mucosa (30%); hemoptysis (19%); and disseminated intravascular coagulation (6%).[98] These clinical signs occurred between 2 and 20 days following completion of adulticide administration, but most occurred 4 to 8 days afterward (83%).[98]

Every owner should be educated about the clinical signs associated with postadulticide pneumonitis and told to have their dog examined if signs develop. Radiographs should be taken to assess the severity of the problem. Dogs with significant disease are usually treated with corticosteroids, cage rest, and antibiotics. The antibiotics play no primary role but are often administered by veterinarians. Most dogs respond just as well to corticosteroids alone. We have seen only one case of a bacterial pneumonia following adulticide therapy, and this dog had a *Pseudomonas* sp. growing in its lungs. The response to corticosteroid therapy is often dramatic (see Figure 23-12).

Cats. Cats are very prone to developing thromboembolic complications. These may occur before or after adulticide therapy. The radiographic signs are similar to those observed in dogs, but the clinical signs are often worse. Cats often develop dyspnea, which is commonly severe. Cats more frequently die of thromboembolism. They respond to corticosteroid administration but also often need oxygen administration to maintain life. Oxygen should be administered via either an oxygen cage or nasal insufflation (intranasal oxygen). Dyspneic cats can die very easily during stressful procedures. Consequently, they should be handled as little as possible and diagnostic procedures kept to a minimum.

Means of preventing postadulticide complications

Dogs. The best way to prevent postadulticide pneumonitis is to confine the dog for 3 to 4 weeks after adulticide therapy. In severe cases, such as those cases that are in right heart failure, cage rest in a veterinary hospital may be necessary for 1 week before and 3 to 4 weeks after adulticide therapy.

Aspirin has been studied extensively as an agent to reduce thromboembolic complications.[96,99-101] Unfortunately, most of these studies have been limited to dogs with very small worm burdens (8 to 10 worms). Aspirin has both antiinflammatory properties and antithrombotic properties that could be beneficial to a patient that is having worm embolization. In addition, aspirin reduces the response of the pulmonary arteries to the adult worms. One study has documented decreased myointimal proliferation in pulmonary arteries exposed to adult worms.[102] However, we do not believe that aspirin administration produces its clinically significant benefits after adulticide therapy in dogs with severe pulmonary artery disease via this mechanism. It is unlikely that severe pulmonary artery disease is readily reversible. Consequently, we reserve aspirin use for decreasing inflammation and thrombosis after the administration of either thiacetarsemide or melarsomine rather than administering it before therapy in an attempt to reduce pulmonary artery damage. We also reserve its use to dogs considered at higher risk for postadulticide complications (i.e., dogs with large pulmonary arteries or with high worm burdens). The dosage of aspirin to use is controversial. Doses as high as 25 mg/kg once a day have been used in experimental animals. More commonly, doses of 5 to 10 mg/kg once a day are used clinically.[103] In one study, a dose of 10 mg/kg once a day decreased the radiographic changes that occurred after adulticide therapy and appeared to improve the perfusion of pulmonary artery branches.[101] Aspirin therapy is not without risk. Gastrointestinal bleeding is the most common side effect in the dog. Although subclinical bleeding may occur frequently, clinically significant bleeding is uncommon, and this side effect should not dissuade veterinarians from using the drug. On the other hand, because side effects can occur, aspirin probably should not be used routinely after adulticide therapy, especially in class 1 dogs.

Corticosteroids have also been studied in dogs after adulticide therapy.[96,99,101] Corticosteroids decrease the pulmonary reaction to the dead worms after adulticide therapy better than does aspirin.[100] However, corticosteroids, when administered in large doses, either have no beneficial effect on pulmonary blood flow or worsen it.[101] One study suggests that corticosteroids may have an effect of protecting the adult worms from thiacetarsemide, because there were remaining live adult worms in the groups that were administered prednisolone and no live worms in the control dogs or the dogs that were administered aspirin.[99] Because of this fact, corticosteroids have fallen from grace for routine use after adulticide therapy. This act is almost assuredly premature, and this is a controversy that awaits further study. It is our opinion that it is probably more surprising that all of the worms were killed by thiacetarsemide in the non–corticosteroid treated groups in the aforementioned studies than is the fact that not all of the worms in the treated group were killed, knowing the propensity of thiacetarsemide not to kill all worms. The possibility of this finding resulting from chance is too great to ignore and too great to condemn the use of corticosteroids after adulticide therapy. In fact, some respected veterinarians that are active in heartworm research use low-dose, alternate-day prednisone therapy routinely following the administration of an adulticide.[104]

A combination of aspirin and prednisolone produces the most beneficial effects after adulticide therapy.[99] Pulmonary inflammation is reduced, and thrombosis is lessened. However, this combination predisposes dogs to gastrointestinal bleeding that can be severe.[105] Consequently, this combination is not recommended for routine clinical use.

Heparin has also been evaluated as an antithrombotic agent to prevent thrombus formation after adulticide therapy in dogs. In one experimental study, heparin was administered at a dose sufficient to maintain the activated partial thromboplastin time at 1.5 to 2.0 times the normal value. This dose successfully lessened the amount of pulmonary artery obstruction present on angiograms.[106] Interestingly, aspirin did not produce the same decrease in this study. In a clinical study, 75 dogs considered at high risk for postadulticide thromboembolic disease were treated with heparin (n = 45; 50 to 100 IU/kg q8-12h) or with either aspirin or indobufen (n = 34).[98] Heparin reduced the severity and the duration of the postadulticide complications compared with the aspirin and indobufen group. The survival rate was also significantly better in the dogs administered heparin. Despite these findings, heparin is not a popular agent for treating dogs at high risk of postadulticide thromboembolic complications. This probably reflects veterinarians' general inexperience with using antithrombotic agents. It should be noted that no complications directly attributed to the heparin therapy occurred in the clinical trial just described.

Cats. Aspirin administration has been studied in experimentally infested cats.[107] The standard dose of 80 to 100 mg every 3 days was not effective at altering heartworm disease. Doses tailored to maintain inhibition of platelet function in individual cats was more effective but was close to the toxic dose. Consequently, although aspirin administration is not contraindicated in cats with heartworm disease, it is not recommended for this purpose.

Corticosteroids probably have limited efficacy at preventing postadulticide complications in most cats after adulticide therapy. Still, cats can suffer severe complications once the worm or worms die. They must be watched closely for 2 weeks after therapy and treated aggressively with corticosteroids and oxygen if they become dyspneic.

FORCEPS REMOVAL OF ADULTS

A technique for removing adult heartworms from the pulmonary arteries using a flexible alligator forceps has been described and used in Japan and elsewhere.[108] The forceps (Ishihara alligator forceps, Fuji Photo Optical Ltd., Japan) are passed into the pulmonary arteries from a jugular vein access site in an anesthetized dog. The forceps are manipulated into the pulmonary arteries using fluoroscopic guidance. The technique has been described in dogs as small as 5 kg. The worm retrieval rate has been reported to be between approximately 80% and 100%. Minimal damage to cardiovascular structures has also been reported.

SURGICAL REMOVAL OF WORMS

Occasionally, surgical removal of worms in dogs without caval syndrome is indicated. We have limited surgical removal in dogs in our hospital to patients with a massive number of worms in the main pulmonary artery, as seen on echocardiography. Surgical removal of worms may be a reasonable means of treating severe heartworm disease in cats. One veterinary cardiologist has removed heartworms from four cats.[109] In each of these cats, the worms were identified on echocardiography. In two of these cats all of the worms were apparently removed and the clinical signs completely abated. In the other two, one or two worms escaped removal. The clinical signs in these cats also improved. Surgical removal is most often accomplished via a pulmonary arteriotomy using either a purse string suture or inflow occlusion.[110] A right atriotomy may be used in selected cases.

TREATMENT OF DOGS WITH RIGHT HEART FAILURE

Dogs with severe heartworm disease may also be in right heart failure. These dogs must be treated differently from dogs with less severe disease. Initially, these dogs should be stabilized with furosemide and angiotensin converting enzyme (ACE) inhibitor administration and abdominocentesis. If thiacetarsemide is used, these dogs should be cage-rested for 1 week before adulticide therapy and for 3 weeks after adulticide therapy. In addition they should be administered aspirin (5 to 10 mg/kg q24h). One study has shown that this regimen resulted in 92% survival, whereas only 69% of dogs treated in a routine manner survived.[103] Because a smaller number of worms can be killed with one dose of melarsomine, this drug is preferred for treating class 3 patients. If melarsomine is used, the dog may be cage-rested for 1 week before therapy. One injection, rather than two, should be administered initially. This should be followed 1 month later by administering the standard two-injection protocol.

Dogs in right heart failure that are successfully treated with an adulticide generally improve clinically within 2 to 3 months after therapy. It is common for them to improve to the point that they no longer require diuretic administration to control their heart failure. Mean pulmonary artery pressure decreases in dogs after heartworms are removed with flexible alligator forceps and so presumably also decreases after successful adulticide drug therapy. In one study, mean pulmonary artery pressure decreased from 48 ± 11 mm Hg to 39 ± 14 mm Hg.[43] This decrease in right ventricular afterload would be expected to improve cardiac function and therefore lessen heart failure severity.

TREATMENT OF GLOMERULONEPHROPATHY

Glomerulonephropathy is best treated by killing the adult worms and microfilariae. Dogs with clinically significant proteinuria will generally improve following successful therapy.

Microfilaricidal Therapy

Dogs that have circulating microfilariae must undergo microfilaricidal therapy (see Table 23-3). If they are not treated, they continue to serve as a reservoir for microfilariae. Although many drugs have been used to kill microfilariae, only the macrolides are currently used for this purpose. Neither ivermectin nor milbemycin is approved by the Food and Drug Administration (FDA) for this use. Dithiazanine iodide is the only microfilaricidal drug approved by the FDA. It is currently not available from the manufacturer. Levamisole has been used in the past. However, complications are more frequent than with the macrolides, and therefore it is only rarely used.

Cats rarely require drug therapy to kill microfilariae because the incidence of microfilaremia is low. Even if microfilariae are present, they are generally present in low numbers, produce few if any clinical sequelae, and are unlikely to be transmitted to another animal.[13] Macrolide administration is safe in cats and should be effective at killing microfilariae.

IVERMECTIN

When used to kill microfilariae, ivermectin is administered to dogs at a dose of 50 μg/kg, approximately 10 times the prophylactic dose.[111] This can be accomplished by administering either the prophylactic product Heartgard at a higher dose or the bovine worming product Ivomec in a diluted form. Heartgard is marketed in three tablet sizes: 68, 136, and 272 μg. One 272-μg tablet can be used to kill microfilariae in a 5-kg dog. A 25-kg dog would require five of these tablets. Treating larger dogs in this manner can be expensive. Ivomec is much less expensive (about 1% of the cost of Heartgard) if treating heartworm disease frequently. However, the concentration is too high (10 mg/mL, or 10,000 μg/mL) to use undiluted. Consequently, this product must be diluted 10 to 1 with propylene glycol before using it, such that the final concentration is 1000 μg/mL. One milliliter of the diluted product is administered per 20 kg of body weight. Although Ivomec is marketed to be administered parenterally to cattle and can be administered subcutaneously to dogs, it is usually administered orally to dogs.

Microfilarial numbers are decreased by approximately 90% within 18 hours following the administration of the aforementioned dose of ivermectin.[112] When experimental dogs are examined at this time, the microfilariae are present in capillaries throughout the body in association with red cells, white cells, and macrophages. By 3 days, the microfilariae are fragmented and being phagocytized, and by day 6 they are being incorporated in microgranulomas.[113]

Alternatively, ivermectin can be administered once a month starting soon after adulticide therapy at the prophylactic dose. Microfilariae numbers decrease gradually to or close to zero within several months. The chance of adverse reactions with this approach is minimal.

MILBEMYCIN

Milbemycin can also be used to kill microfilariae after adulticide therapy. This approach is simpler than using ivermectin, because the preventive dose of 500 μg/kg is also effective at eliminating microfilariae.[114] One study has documented that one dose eliminates more than 98% of microfilariae.[115]

Dogs should be retested for the presence of microfilariae 2 to 3 weeks after treatment. If no microfilariae are present, heartworm prophylaxis should be started. If microfilariae are still present, another microfilaricidal dose of ivermectin should be administered or milbemycin continued. If only a few microfilariae are present, the dog can be started on a monthly preventive dose of ivermectin and retested in 3 to 5 months. If microfilariae are still present after three doses of an avermectin, the presence of remaining adults should be considered. An antigen test, 4 to 5 months after adulticide therapy should be evaluated to determine if adults are still present.

COMPLICATIONS

Complications following the administration of microfilaricidal doses of macrolides to kill microfilariae can occur. Rapid death of a large number of circulating microfilariae apparently produces systemic side effects in 5% to 8% of dogs treated with 50 μg/kg of ivermectin or with prophylactic doses of milbemycin.[116] The side effects most commonly include vomiting, diarrhea, depression, and anorexia and rarely include circulatory collapse. Dogs may be observed in a veterinary hospital for 6 to 8 hours after the administration of a microfilaricidal dose of a macrolide to a dog with circulating microfilariae. Dogs that harbor a large number of microfilariae are thought be at greatest risk of this complication. If circulatory collapse (shock) occurs, corticosteroids and intravenous fluids should be administered. To decrease the chance of adverse reaction to macrolides in dogs with high microfilariae counts, levamisole administration (2.5 mg/kg for 3 to 7 days) has been advocated first to kill microfilariae, presumably at a slower rate.[117] One study has documented that administering prednisolone (1 mg/kg) simultaneously with milbemycin completely prevented any adverse effects, whereas an antihistamine and indomethacin had no beneficial effect.[118]

In one study, caval syndrome (see below) occurred in approximately 10% (8 of 85) of dogs with adult worms and microfilariae following the administration of either 1 or 5 mg/kg milbemycin.[119] All of these dogs developed a murmur secondary to tricuspid regurgitation, jugular vein pulsation, and hemoglobinuria. Echocardiograms confirmed the presence of worms at the tricuspid valve orifice. Evidence of caval syndrome spontaneously resolved in these experimental dogs 21 to 117 hours after the appearance of clinical signs.

Prophylaxis

"An ounce of prevention is worth a pound of cure." Heartworm disease can be a devastating disease, but prevention of the disease is efficacious and safe. Consequently, any client with a dog in an endemic area should be strongly encouraged to administer a heartworm chemoprophylactic agent regularly (see Table 23-3). There are still large areas of the western United States where heartworm disease is not endemic. The administration of heartworm preventives in these areas is not indicated and will never be indicated unless heartworm disease establishes itself in these regions. Continued monitoring of these sites is clearly necessary to determine if the disease is encroaching into a region. Of course, any dog that travels from a nonendemic area to an endemic area should be placed on a heartworm preventative.

Preventing the introduction of heartworm into a nonendemic region is most likely a hopeless endeavor, because feral dog and wild dog populations are most likely infested simultaneously with or before client-owned animals are infested when heartworm invades an area. The goal of heartworm prophylaxis is to prevent heartworm infestation in individual animals. Likewise, producing a heartworm-free region cannot be achieved because of inadequate owner compliance, feral dog populations, and the presence of a resident population of infested coyotes and foxes in a given region.

The length of time that heartworm prevention should be carried out during the year depends on the local climate. In all but the southernmost regions of the United States the temperature during some winter months is too low for heartworm larvae to mature to an infective stage in mosquitoes before the mosquito dies a natural death. The average daily temperature must be at least above 57° F for larval maturation to occur in time for the mosquito to pass on the larvae. This means that in many parts of the United States heartworm prevention is only required for 6 to 8 months with macrolide preventive drugs. However, many owners may elect to remain on year-round heartworm prevention because, once they are in the habit of administering a tablet monthly, maintaining that routine is easier than interrupting and reestablishing the routine each year. A map of the United States displaying the month that heartworm prevention can start and the month it can end is depicted in Figure 23-13.

Heartworm prevention can be readily accomplished with either diethylcarbamazine or the macrolides (ivermectin and milbemycin) in dogs. In puppies, either type of medication should be started at 6 to 8 weeks of age or as soon as the weather becomes warm enough to warrant heartworm prevention. One study has shown that in a heartworm-endemic area milbemycin administered to 2-month-old puppies prevents heartworm infestation.[120] If milbemycin is withheld until 4 months of age, about 15% to 20% will harbor heartworms. If milbemycin administration does not start until 6 months of age, 60% will become infested with heartworms. No testing is required before starting the medication to puppies. There has never been a report of adverse effects of administering a heartworm preventive agent to a puppy with microfilariae acquired transplacentally. Any young dog exposed to heartworm infestation for more than 6 months and presented to a veterinarian for the first time should be tested for the presence of *D. immitis* microfilariae and heartworm antigen before starting heartworm prevention. Detecting microfilariae in dogs that are to be administered diethylcarbamazine is especially crucial because diethylcarbamazine administration to a microfilaremic dog can produce a potentially fatal reaction. Any dog that has just undergone adulticide therapy should be placed on a heartworm preventive drug following successful microfilaricidal therapy.

Heartworm prophylaxis in cats can be accomplished by administering ivermectin or milbemycin. However, the dose of ivermectin is higher in cats than in dogs. Diethylcarbamazine has not been tested in cats.[47]

DIETHYLCARBAMAZINE

Diethylcarbamazine (various manufacturers) has been used to prevent heartworm disease in dogs since the early 1960s. It is a substituted piperazine compound. Several formulations are available and are equally effective. Some formulations contain other antiparasiticides, such as oxibendazole and styrylpyridium chloride, to prevent roundworm, hookworm, and whipworm infestation. Diethylcarbamazine citrate (DEC) is dosed at a minimum of 5.5 mg/kg/day. At this dose it consistently prevents heartworm larvae from maturing in the dog. It probably stops the larvae from molting from the L_3 to the L_4 stage. This occurs 1 to 12 days after the mosquito infests the dog with the L_3 form. This molt only takes a short time and occurs daily in individual larvae, so owners should be encouraged to administer the drug every day. The drug should be started at least 2 weeks before the average daily temperature is above 57° to 60° F and should continue for 2 months after the temperature has decreased below this level. Consequently, in regions where the average daily temperature is less than 60° F for only 3 months out of the year, DEC should be administered year-round. If a lapse in DEC administration occurs, ivermectin or milbemycin can be administered to kill the L_4 larvae that have developed within the past 6 to 8 weeks. Because owner compliance is always a potential problem with a drug that must be administered every day, dogs should be retested annually, even if they are on DEC continuously.

Dogs that are to be administered DEC must be tested for the presence of microfilariae before instituting or reinstituting therapy, and no dog that is microfilaremic can be administered DEC. Between 15% and 86% of dogs that are microfilaremic develop an adverse reaction to DEC administration. Microfilarial numbers do not predict the severity of the reaction. The reaction usually starts within 1 hour after administering DEC.[78] Depression, lethargy, and reduced responsiveness may occur first, followed by vomiting and diarrhea. This may be followed by bradycardia and circulatory collapse. Most dogs recover within 24 hours, but the reaction may terminate in hypovolemic shock and death. Hemoconcentration, leukocytosis, thrombocytopenia, and an elevation in liver enzymes are consistently identified. Dogs that experience this adverse effect should be treated with intravenous fluids and high-dose corticosteroid administration. Dogs that are going to survive this event generally improve within 3 to 5 hours after therapy. The lesions at postmortem examination are typical of a type I hypersensitivity reaction (anaphylactic shock).[121] Primary lesions occur in the liver and consist of centrilobular congestion and necrosis with hemorrhage in the gallbladder and periportal tissues.

DEC is safe in normal dogs, although an occasional dog will vomit or have diarrhea. Experimental evidence suggests that no reproductive abnormalities occur in dogs administered DEC, although anecdotal reports of decreased sperm motility and conception rates exist.[122] The combination of DEC and oxibendazole (Filarabits-Plus, SmithKline Beecham Animal Health, Exton, PA)

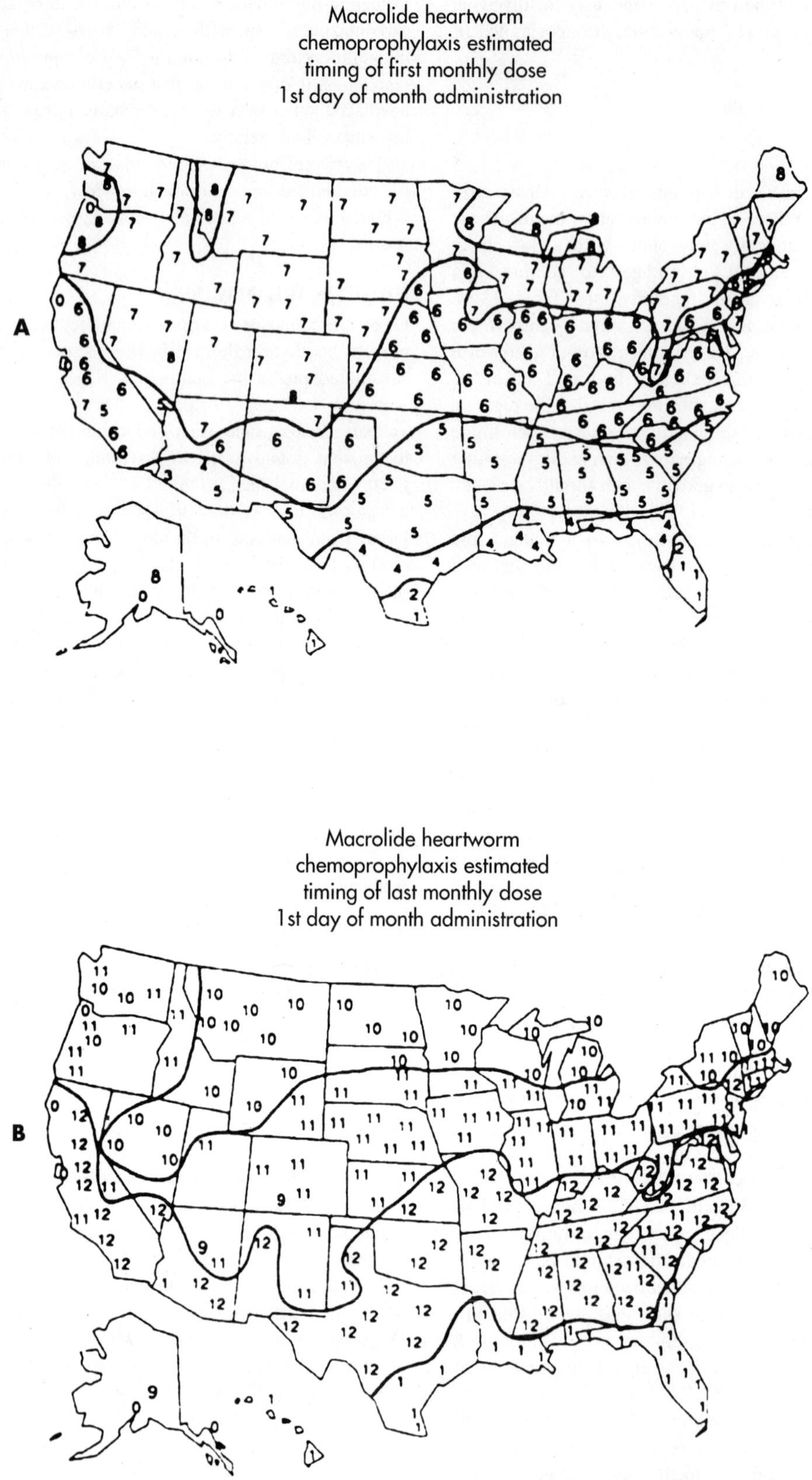

FIGURE 23-13 Maps of the United States with isotherms overlying them, delineating the month in which heartworm prevention should start **(A)** and stop **(B).** (From Knight DH, Lok JB. In Soll M, ed: *Proceedings of the Heartworm Symposium '95,* Batavia, Ill. 1995, American Heartworm Society.)

has been associated (rarely) with a periportal hepatitis, which can be fatal.[123] Concurrent phenobarbital administration may exacerbate the toxic potential of this drug combination.

IVERMECTIN

Ivermectin (Heartgard, Merck & Co., Inc., Whitehouse Station, N.J.) is an avermectin (a mixture of avermectin B_1a and B_1b). Avermectins are produced by filamentous bacteria belonging to the genus *Streptomyces*. Avermectins act by enhancing gamma-butyric acid (GABA) presynaptic release and postsynaptic binding in some invertebrates. GABA acts as an inhibitory neurotransmitter, blocking postsynaptic stimulation of the adjacent neuron (interneuron) and motor neuron transmission in nematodes and neuromuscular transmission in arthropods.[124] This causes paralysis of the parasite and eventual death. Avermectins generally do not cross the blood-brain barrier in mammals in which GABA is also a neurotransmitter.[125] Ivermectin is very effective at killing both L_3 and L_4 heartworm larvae. Because the larvae are in these stages for 67 to 80 days, ivermectin is effective when administered every 2 months. However, avermectins are most effective at preventing heartworm disease when administered every 30 to 45 days.[126] In addition, ivermectin appears to be effective at killing immature adult (L_5) worms. In one study, dogs that were administered ivermectin starting 4 months after experimental inoculation of L_3 larvae either had no adult worms 12 months later or had only two to four live worms compared with 12 to 39 live worms in the control group.[79] Ivermectin is not effective at killing mature adult heartworms.

Ivermectin is marketed as a tablet that is administered once a month for convenience and to improve owner compliance. Ivermectin is dosed at 6 to 12 μg/kg once a month in dogs. Ivermectin is also marketed in combination with pyrantel pamoate (Heartgard-30 Plus, Merck & Co., Inc., Whitehouse Station, N.J.) to control roundworm and hookworm infestations in dogs.

MILBEMYCIN

Milbemycin oxime (Interceptor, Novartis Animal Health US Inc., Greensboro, N.C.) is another avermectin. The commercial product consists of 80% milbemycin A_4 and 20% milbemycin A_3. Milbemycin is effective at killing L_3 and L_4 heartworm larvae. It is not as effective as ivermectin at killing immature adult worms.[79] It is also effective at preventing roundworm, hookworm, and whipworm infestation in dogs. The dose is 500 to 999 μg/kg once a month. Milbemycin is more effective at killing circulating microfilariae at the preventive dose than is ivermectin at the preventive dose. This means that adverse effects with this drug at the preventive dose may be more common in dogs with circulating microfilariae. Consequently, the manufacturer recommends that dogs with microfilariae be treated for the adults and the microfilariae before initiating milbemycin chemoprophylaxis. Of course, milbemycin at the preventive dose and ivermectin at 5 to 10 times the preventive dose are used as microfilaricides. Side effects with both drugs at these doses are probably comparable. Any dog harboring microfilariae that is administered these doses of an avermectin probably should be observed for 6 to 8 hours after drug administration, as outlined in the above discussion of microfilaricidal therapy, and treated appropriately if an adverse event occurs. Milbemycin oxime in combination with lufenuron (Sentinel, Novartis Animal Health US Inc., Greensboro, N.C.) prevents the same infestations as milbemycin alone and controls flea egg development.

AVERMECTINS AND MICROFILARIAE

Administration of avermectins to dogs with adult heartworms results in the disappearance of the circulating microfilariae. When administered over about 6 months, ivermectin usually renders dogs amicrofilaremic. Because microfilariae probably live longer than 6 months, the microfilariae that are present at the time the drug is first administered must be killed by the drug. However, if the female worms continue to reproduce, microfilariae should be replaced. Apparently they are not. This may be due to an effect of the avermectins on the reproductive tract of the female heartworm. Ivermectin is known to render the human parasite, *Onchocerca volvulus*, incapable of shedding microfilariae.[127] It has also been shown that ivermectin causes embryo degeneration in adult female heartworms.[128] Similarly, milbemycin, when administered at routine prophylactic doses to microfilaremic dogs with patent infestations, causes the microfilarial count to decrease to zero after 7 months of administration.[129] This may be due to a combination of microfilaricidal activity of the drug and a persistent blocking of embryogenesis in the adult females. The effects of both drugs, however, may also be due to an effect of the drugs on the ability of the male worms to produce effective sperm.[16] The sperm of male worms treated with a macrolide do not show any gross abnormalities in number or morphology. However, it has been noted that when treated female worms are transplanted into another dog along with untreated male worms microfilariae are produced. When the reciprocal of this is done, the male worms are unable to sustain microfilariae production in the female worms. Whichever is affected, the effect on the worms seems permanent in that microfilariae do not reappear for at least 10 months after discontinuing milbemycin administration.[129]

AVERMECTINS AND COLLIES

Avermectins apparently can cross the blood-brain barrier in about one-third of rough-coated collies and cause problems when administered at doses higher than that prescribed for prophylaxis. The heartworm prophylactic dose for both ivermectin (6 to 12 μg/kg) and milbemycin (500 to 999 μg/kg) is thought to be safe in collies, based on scientific studies.[130] For ivermectin, one dose of 100 μg/kg can produce toxicity in susceptible collies.[124] A dose of 50 μg/kg, however, does not produce toxicity in ivermectin-sensitive collies (4 to 8 times the prophylactic dose).[131] For milbemycin, the toxic dose in ivermectin-sensitive collies is more than 5 mg/kg (10 times the preventive dose).[132] Collies administered a toxic dose of an avermectin can develop hypersalivation, mydriasis, apparent blindness, ataxia, bradycardia, and slowed respirations and may become sedate to comatose and may die. Duration and severity of the toxicity are related to dose. An injection of 10,000 μg of ivermectin to one collie resulted in coma for 7 weeks.[133]

To illustrate the seriousness of an avermectin overdose in rough-coated collies, the following set of cases is presented. An owner of a colony of rough-coated collies in northern California obtained a collie from another breeder. This dog was infested with *Sarcoptes* and was treated, on the recommendation of his veterinarian, with 250 μg/kg of ivermectin subcutaneously (approximately 20 times the heartworm prevention dose). This dog had no adverse effects, and so the owner proceeded to treat his other 22 collies with the same dose. Ultimately, two of the dogs died. Twelve of the remaining dogs were presented to the University of California, Davis, Veterinary Medical Teaching Hospital for signs of ivermectin toxicosis. Five were mildly affected and released within 2 days. All of the remaining seven dogs were very sedate to severely obtunded. Most had evidence of mydriasis and hypersalivation. Supportive care was required for up to 3 weeks after the ivermectin administration. Supportive care included intravenous fluid administration, total parenteral nutrition, force feeding, antibiotic administration, and so on. Three dogs required ventilatory support during their hospitalization for hypoventilation. Pneumonia, sepsis, bradycardia, and decubital ulcers were common complications. The hospitalization bill for one dog was $5700. The owner sued the veterinarian that recommended treating with the ivermectin.

Other breeds can also be affected with ivermectin toxicosis at relatively low doses of ivermectin.[124] Collie crosses and Australian shepherds (which have common lineage with the collie) have been the most frequent types of dogs reported to exhibit clinical signs of toxicity at doses between 100 and 500 μg/kg. Rare instances of low-dose toxicity in other breeds have also been reported. Any dog or cat can develop avermectin toxicity if a large enough dose is administered. Inadvertent administration of the bovine and equine worming products is the most common method of producing toxicity. Doses of 2000 μg/kg ivermectin to normal dogs cause no toxic effects; 2500 μg/kg produces mydriasis; 5000 μg/kg produces tremors; 10,000 to 20,000 μg/kg produces coma; and 40,000 μg/kg produces death in some animals.[12]

HEARTWORM PROPHYLAXIS IN CATS

Although not routinely employed, ivermectin and milbemycin are also effective agents for heartworm prophylaxis in cats. Doses up to 750 μg/kg ivermectin produce no toxic effects in cats.[134] Monthly doses of 24 μg/kg ivermectin are effective at preventing heartworm disease in cats.[15,135] This protocol has been tested in more than 2500 cats and proved to be highly efficacious with no toxicity. This dose is also effective at preventing hookworm infestation.[136] Doses of 500 to 990 μg/kg milbemycin administered monthly are also effective at preventing heartworm infestation.[137] Heartworm prophylaxis in cats may become more popular because of greater recognition of the importance of this disease in cats, the popularity of cats as domestic pets, the safety of the drugs used to prevent the disease, and the convenience of once-a-month dosing. It has been estimated that the incidence of heartworm disease in highly endemic areas probably is similar to the incidence of feline leukemia virus and feline immunodeficiency virus.[54] If these diseases could be prevented by administering a pill once a month, many owners and veterinarians would opt for this choice. Ivermectin is marketed for heartworm prophylaxis in cats (Heartgard For Cats, Merck & Co., Inc., Whitehouse Station, N.J.). The recommended minimum dose is 24 μg/kg administered once a month.

Caval Syndrome

Caval syndrome is an acute manifestation of heartworm disease that occurs in association with a large number of heartworms in the right heart that entwine around and pass through the tricuspid valve apparatus. This syndrome has been reported to occur in up to 20% of heartworm cases, although the studies involved were not designed to determine this number and the incidence is almost assuredly much less than this.[138] Caval syndrome most commonly occurs in male dogs that have had no previous clinical signs of heartworm disease. It can occur in dogs infested with a moderate or large number of worms.

PATHOPHYSIOLOGY

Caval syndrome is a life-threatening presentation of heartworm disease. The outstanding features of the syndrome are severe tricuspid regurgitation with poor cardiac output and intravascular red cell lysis with resultant hemoglobinemia and hemoglobinuria. The hemoglobinuria is usually marked, resulting in dark brown to black urine.

The pathophysiology of caval syndrome may be as follows. The initiating event must be a mass of worms falling into the right ventricle (see the discussion below of etiology). Once the worms are in the right ventricle they probably can move toward the right atrium by entwining themselves in the tricuspid valve apparatus. The mass of worms in and around the tricuspid valve apparatus produces acute and severe tricuspid regurgitation (Figure 23-14). Severe pulmonary hypertension may exacerbate the amount of tricuspid regurgitation.[139] The severe regurgitation results in a decrease in forward blood flow through the pulmonary vasculature, back to the left heart. As a result, the left heart becomes volume underloaded (the left atrium and the diastolic size of the left ventricle decrease in size) and the left ventricular forward cardiac output decreases. The decrease in systemic blood flow results in clinical signs of poor perfusion (pale or ashen mucous membranes, decreased femoral pulse pressure). The acute, severe tricuspid regurgitation causes a right apical systolic murmur, right heart failure (jugular vein distension, hepatomegaly, and, potentially, ascites), and hemolysis. The right heart failure is purely secondary to the right atrial and right ventricular volume overload caused by the tricuspid regurgitation and not to occlusion of the tricuspid valve orifice because there is no pressure gradient across the tricuspid valve when this variable is measured.[140] The pathophysiology of the hemolysis is not completely understood, because hemolysis does not occur in tricuspid regurgitation resulting from other causes. However, all of the signs of caval syndrome, including hemolysis, have been reproduced by placing silicone tubes the size of heartworms across the tricuspid valve in experimental dogs.[141] Consequently, there is little doubt that the hemolysis is related to shear stresses on the red cells created by the red cells being forced to flow around the worms at a high velocity (calculated to be around 4 m/sec if the systolic pulmonary artery pressure is 65 mm Hg). In addition, there is evidence that the red cells are more fragile in dogs with caval syndrome.[142] Factors that may increase red cell fragility include altered serum free and esterified cholesterol concentrations and lecithin acyltransferase activity.

ETIOLOGY

The exact reason or reasons that a large number of heartworms invade the right heart are not completely understood. It has been noted that caval syndrome is most common in dogs with many heartworms. In one study of experimental dogs, one group of dogs with a large worm burden developed caval syndrome; whereas another group with a similar worm burden did not.[140] In this study, the group of dogs that developed caval syndrome had an average mean pulmonary artery pressure of 60 mm Hg, whereas the dogs that did not develop caval syndrome had an average mean pulmonary artery pressure of 30 mm Hg. Consequently, it appears that a large worm burden and moderate-to-severe pulmonary hypertension may be precipitating variables. It should be noted, however, that another study has documented caval syndrome in dogs with an average of only 40 worms and as few as 12 worms in one dog (range from 12 to 125 worms).[143] Also, many dogs in this study had a mean pulmonary artery pressure less than 30 mm Hg.

Statistical alterations such as these do not give any clues as to the reasons why worms end up in the right heart. There are very few ways for heartworms to get from the pulmonary arteries to the right heart. They cannot start there because there is nothing to trap them in the

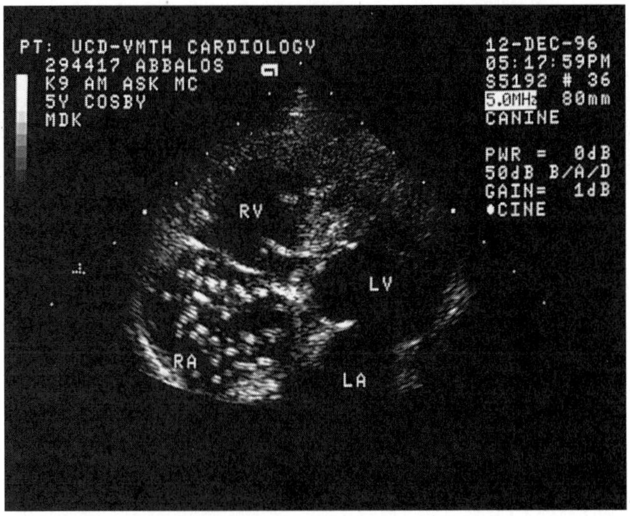

FIGURE 23-14 Two-dimensional echocardiograms from a 5-year-old male American Eskimo dog with caval syndrome. The dog was pale and icteric when presented to the referring veterinarian. It had circulating microfilaria and a positive heartworm antigen test. On presentation, hemoglobinuria and hemoglobinemia were identified. The echocardiograms reveal a mass of worms involving the tricuspid valve apparatus. This frame was taken in systole, when the worms were in the right atrium. In diastole they followed blood flow into the right ventricle. The worms look like tubular structures with two echodense lines on either side of an echolucent line. Worms were removed via a right jugular venotomy using an alligator forceps. Despite severe hypoxemia following the procedure the dog went on to do well.

right ventricle once they enter the circulation. Consequently, they have to start in the pulmonary arteries and somehow descend into the right ventricle and then ascend into the right atrium. Although heartworms can move (anyone who has watched them crawl out of a jugular vein during removal for caval syndrome can attest to this), they have nothing to grab onto in the pulmonary artery to actively move from the pulmonary artery into the right ventricle. Consequently, they must fall through the pulmonic valve. Heartworms are normally held in place against gravity in the pulmonary arteries by blood flow. Consequently, a marked decrease in blood flow would allow them to fall into the right ventricle. This happens after death and is the reason that heartworms are found in the right ventricle at postmortem examination. One study has documented that administering a large dose of a β-blocker to decrease cardiac output can result in heartworms falling back into the right heart.[144] In this study, heartworms were observed, using echocardiography, in the right ventricle and right atrium (across the tricuspid valve) in five of six dogs. A murmur of tricuspid regurgitation was audible in these dogs. In two cases the worms remained in this position throughout the experiment; in the other three dogs, the worms were expelled back into the pulmonary arteries. Another report suggests that pentobarbital administration can do the same thing.[143] These findings suggest that any hemodynamic event that results in transient or sustained pulmonary artery hypoperfusion can result in heartworms falling back into the right heart. This also suggests that hemodynamic forces may act to push heartworms back into the pulmonary artery, strengthening the argument that blood flow is the determining variable. If the worm mass is great enough, the force may not be great enough to push them back out, or, if they entwine themselves around the tricuspid valve apparatus, they may not be expelled. Once the worms are in place in the tricuspid valve orifice and tricuspid regurgitation is produced, forward blood flow is probably too low to expel the worms from the right heart. Dogs with a large worm burden more commonly have severe heartworm disease, and severe heartworm disease is more commonly associated with hemodynamic abnormalities such as moderate-to-severe pulmonary hypertension and decreased cardiac output. Dogs with severe heartworm disease may also have arrhythmias. All of these could contribute to either sustained or transient decreased pulmonary blood flow that could cause heartworms to fall into the right ventricle. The movement of heartworms from the pulmonary arteries to the right heart is commonly called *migration.* Migration infers an active moving process and so cannot be a correct term for this process. However, once the worms are in the right ventricle, they probably can migrate to the right atrium by attaching to the tricuspid apparatus and pulling themselves into the right atrium. Once they are in this structure there are no more cardiac structures for them to attach to so their migration should be complete. If large numbers were present, however, the leading worms could be forced into the vena cavae by the trailing worms.

CLINICAL SIGNS AND DIAGNOSIS

Dogs that present because of caval syndrome commonly have evidence of circulatory collapse (shock) and therefore are weak and pale and have a slow capillary refill time. Hemoglobinuria and bilirubinuria are present and are due to intravascular hemolysis. Hemoglobinemia also can usually be identified. Respiratory signs of tachypnea and dyspnea may be present. A murmur secondary to tricuspid regurgitation is ausculted over the right cardiac apex. The jugular veins are often distended, and the liver is enlarged. Ascites may be present. Laboratory abnormalities that are commonly present include microfilaremia, moderate regenerative anemia, and increases in serum AST, ALT, alkaline phosphatase, bilirubin, and urea nitrogen concentrations.[145] Urine hemoglobin concentration is increased. The laboratory abnormalities are secondary to hemolysis, acute hepatic congestion, and hypoperfusion. Thoracic radiographs are usually typical of severe heartworm disease. The electrocardiogram will have an *S* wave present in lead CV_6LU in most cases, with evidence of right heart enlargement in other leads in fewer cases. Arrhythmias may be present.

The diagnosis of caval syndrome is made based on typical clinical signs combined with echocardiographic identification of a mass of heartworms in the right atrium and right ventricle and involving the tricuspid valve apparatus (see Figure 23-14). Other echocardiographic findings include right ventricular volume overload, left ventricular volume underload with a normal-to-decreased shortening fraction, and paradoxical septal motion.[145]

The prognosis for caval syndrome is guarded to poor. Even with appropriate therapy the mortality rate is often in the 30% to 40% range. Organ failure and disseminated intravascular coagulation can develop before or after therapy and can result in death.

TREATMENT

Treatment of caval syndrome involves supportive care and removing the worms from the right atrium and possibly from the right ventricle as soon as possible. Supportive care generally should include intravenous fluid administration to improve cardiac output, prevent or help reverse disseminated intravascular coagulation, prevent hemoglobin nephropathy, and reverse lactic acidosis resulting from decreased tissue perfusion. If fluids are administered before worm removal, care must be taken not to exacerbate the right heart failure. Once the worms are removed, right heart failure abates rapidly. Consequently, fluid administration may be more aggressive at this time. Other supportive measures can include administration of corticosteroids, heparin, and, possibly, antibiotics.

Heartworm removal is accomplished by passing an instrument down the jugular vein and into the right heart, grasping or entwining the worms, and then removing them. The procedure may be accomplished with no chemical restraint if the patient is moribund, with sedation if the patient is tractable, or with anesthesia if the patient is intractable. The right lateral neck should be clipped and scrubbed in preparation for surgery. If no chemical restraint or only sedation is used, a local anesthetic should be infiltrated over the jugular vein. The skin should be incised over the jugular vein and the vein isolated using blunt dissection. A ligature should be placed around the proximal end of the vein and tied. Another piece of suture should be placed around the distal end of the vein to control bleeding. A small incision is then made in the jugular vein, through which an instrument is passed. A variety of instruments have been described for removing heartworms from dogs with caval syndrome. A long alligator forceps (20 to 40 cm and of a small diameter) is the most commonly used instrument. It has the advantages of being easy to maneuver and easy to use to grasp worms. Alligator forceps, however, are rigid instruments that can perforate vessels and cardiac chambers, and the jaws can be closed forcefully enough to macerate worms. Consequently, they must be used with extreme care. The Jackson forceps is a forceps made specifically to remove heartworms from the right atrium. It is long and cumbersome in small patients. Its jaws are long and flat. This allows for more gentle worm grasping, but at times it does not grasp worms firmly enough to result in worm removal. Endoscopic baskets used for retrieval of gastric foreign bodies, a horsehair type of brush (Tayama String brush, Kawasaki Masuda, Irakakogyo, Japan), and a flexible alligator forceps (Ishihara alligator forceps, Fuji Photo Optical LTD, Japan) have all been used with success to remove heartworms. Once the instrument is placed into the jugular vein, it must be advanced carefully. This can be done without any imaging assistance or with either fluoroscopic or echocardiographic guidance. Fluoroscopic guidance makes it easier to pass the forceps through the thoracic inlet and allows one to visualize where the catheter is in the heart. Echocardiographic guidance allows one to have some feel for the relationship between the forceps and the worms. It also allows one to identify remaining worms. If one is doing the procedure without imaging assistance, the distance between the opening made in the jugular vein and the heart should be estimated by aligning the tip of the forceps with the fourth intercostal space on the outside of the dog and noting where the jugular vein opening sits with respect to the rod portion of the forceps. Generally, going in somewhat deeper than this measurement is not a problem, because the forceps usually slides down the caudal vena cava. The thoracic inlet is the most difficult region through which to manipulate the forceps. It is not unusual for the forceps to start going down an axillary vein, into a front leg. If resistance is met in this region, the forceps should be withdrawn and the neck of the dog pulled ventrally so that the tip of the forceps is aimed more dorsally; the forceps can then be gently advanced again. Once the tip of the forceps is in the right atrium, the jaws should be opened, the forceps advanced slightly, the jaws closed, and the forceps removed. Usually 1 to 4 worms are removed. This should be repeated until 5 to 6 successive attempts are unsuccessful or until no or only a few worms are seen on the echocardiogram.

In our experience, macerating worms results in massive antigen release that results in pulmonary vasoconstriction or may precipitate disseminated intravascular coagulation. We have watched on ultrasound the right ventricle of one cat become progressively more hypodynamic and progressively distend over several minutes, presumably because of acute severe pulmonary hypertension, following the maceration of one worm during withdrawal. At times, worm maceration is unavoidable because worms may be inexorably entwined around chordae tendineae. This results in worm pieces being removed. If worm maceration has occurred, we recommend parenteral corticosteroid (antiinflammatory doses) and heparin (100 to 500 U/kg q8h) administration.

Following the removal of the adult worms, intravenous fluids should be administered. Urine color, BUN, and hematocrit should be monitored. Some dogs require oxygen therapy. The dog may be sent home once it has stabilized. When the dog's appetite, respiratory rate, BUN, and hematocrit are normal again, an adulticide should be administered to kill the remaining worms. Following the removal of the worms, the tricuspid regurgitation disappears, cardiac output increases, and right atrial pressure decreases, as expected.[143] This, however, usually takes several days.

REFERENCES

1. Kume S, Itagaki S: On the life cycle of *Dirofilaria immitis* in the dog as the final host, *Br Vet J* 111:16, 1955.
2. Kotani T, Powers KG: Developmental stages of *Dirofilaria immitis* in the dog, *Am J Vet Res* 43:2199, 1982.
3. Bemrick WJ, Sandholm HA: *Aedes vexans* and other potential mosquito vectors of *Dirofilaria immitis* in Minnesota, *J Parasitol* 52:762, 1966.
4. Otto GF: Epizootiology of canine heartworm disease. In Bradley RE, ed: *Canine heartworm disease: the current knowledge,* Gainesville, Fla, 1972, University of Florida Press.
5. Nayar JK, Sauerman DM: Physiological basis of host susceptibility of Florida mosquitoes to *Dirofilaria immitis*, *J Insect Physiol* 21:1965, 1975.
6. Tolbert RH, Johnson WE: Potential vectors of *Dirofilaria immitis* in Macon County, Alabama, *Am J Vet Res* 43:2054, 1982.
7. Hendrix CM, Bemrick WJ, Schlotthauer JC: Natural transmission of *Dirofilaria immitis* by *Aedes vexans, Am J Vet Res* 41:1253, 1980.
8. Sacco B, di Cancrini G, Genchi C et al: Study of tropism to dogs and cats of *Diptera*, potential vectors of filariasis in the province of Pavia, *XVII Congr Naz Soc Ital Parassitol,* 34:11, 1992.
9. Taylor ER: The development of *Dirofilaria immitis* in the mosquito *Aedes aegypti*, *J Helminthol* 34:27, 1960.
10. McTeir TL, McCall JW, Dzimianski MT et al: Epidemiology of heartworm infection in beagles naturally exposed to infection in three southeastern states. In Soll MD, ed: *Proceedings of the Heartworm Symposium '92,* Batavia, Ill, 1992, American Heartworm Society.
11. Fortin JF, Slocombe JOD: Temperature requirements for the development of *Dirofilaria immitis* in *Aedes triseriatus* and *Aedes vexans, Mosquito News* 41:625, 1981.
12. Campbell WC: Ivermectin and heartworm, *Sem Vet Med Surg Small Anim* 2:48, 1995.
13. Donahoe JMR: Experimental infection of cats with *Dirofilaria immitis, J Parasitol* 61:599, 1975.
14. Dillon AR: Feline heartworm disease. In Otto GF, ed: *Proceedings of the Heartworm Symposium '86,* Washington, DC, 1986, American Heartworm Society.
15. McTier TL, McCall JW, Dzimianski MT et al: Prevention of heartworm infection in cats by treatment with ivermectin at one month post-infection. In Soll MD, ed: *Proceedings of the Heartworm Symposium '92,* Batavia, Ill, 1992, American Heartworm Society.
16. Lok JB, Knight DH: Macrolide effects on reproductive function in male and female heartworms: implications for diagnosis and treatment, *Proceedings of the Heartworm Symposium '95,* Batavia, Ill, 1995, American Heartworm Society.
17. Sawyer TK, Weistein PP: Experimentally induced canine dirofilariasis, *J Am Vet Med Assoc* 143:975, 1963.
18. Church EM, Georgi JR, Robson DS: Analysis of the microfilarial periodicity of *Dirofilaria immitis, Cornell Vet* 66:333, 1976.

19. Grieve RB, Lauria S: Periodicity of *Dirofilaria immitis* microfilariae in canine and murine hosts, *Acta Trop* 40:121, 1983.
20. Otto GF, Jackson RF, Bauman PM et al: Variability in the ratio between the numbers of microfilariae and adult heartworms, *J Am Vet Med Assoc* 168:605, 1976.
21. Newton WL: Longevity of an experimental infection with *Dirofilaria immitis* in a dog, *J Parasitol* 54:187, 1968.
22. Underwood PC, Harwood PD: Survival and location of the microfilariae of *Dirofilaria immitis* in dogs, *J Parasitol* 25:23, 1939.
23. Courtney CH: Discussion 3. In Soll MD, Knight DH, eds: *Proceedings of the Heartworm Symposium '95,* Batavia, Ill, 1995, American Heartworm Society.
24. Todd KS, Howland TP: Transplacental transmission of *Dirofilaria immitis* microfilariae in the dog, *J Parasitol* 69:371, 1983.
25. Knight DH: How current knowledge has affected the diagnosis, prevention, and treatment of heartworm infection. In Soll MD, ed: *Proceedings of the Heartworm Symposium '92,* Batavia, Ill, 1992, American Heartworm Society.
26. Pappas LG, Lunzman AT: Canine heartworm in the domestic and wild canids of southeastern Nebraska, *J Parasitol* 71:828, 1985.
27. Glickman LT, Grieve RB, Breitschwerdt EB et al: Serologic pattern of canine heartworm (*Dirofilaria immitis*) infection, *Am J Vet Res* 45:1178, 1984.
28. Forrester DJ, Jackson RF, Miller JF et al: Heartworms in captive California sea lions, *J Am Vet Med Assoc* 163:568, 1973.
29. Slocombe JOD: Reflections on heartworm surveys in Canada over 15 years. In Soll MD, ed: *Proceedings of the Heartworm Symposium '92,* Batavia, Ill. 1992, American Heartworm Society.
30. Schaub RG, Rawlings CA, Keith JC: Platelet adhesion and myointimal proliferation in canine pulmonary arteries, *Am J Pathol* 104:13, 1981.
31. Keith JC, Schaub RG, Rawlings C: Early arterial injury-induced myointimal proliferation in canine pulmonary arteries, *Am J Vet Res* 44:181, 1983.
32. Knight DH: Evolution of pulmonary artery disease in canine dirofilariasis: evaluation by blood pressure measurements and angiography. In Otto GF, ed: *Proceedings of the Heartworm Symposium '80,* Edwardsville, Kan, 1980, American Heartworm Society.
33. Tarish JH, Atwell RB: Ultrastructural localization of *Dirofilaria immitis* antigen in canine lung tissue using the protein A-gold labeling technique, *Vet Parasitol* 38:23, 1991.
34. Munnell JF, Weldon JS, Lewis RE et al: Intimal lesions of the pulmonary artery in dogs with experimental dirofilariasis, *Am J Vet Res* 41:1108, 1980.
35. Sasaki Y, Kitagawa H, Hirano Y: Relationship between pulmonary arterial pressure and lesions in the pulmonary arteries and parenchyma, and cardiac valves in canine dirofilariasis, *J Vet Med Sci* 54:739, 1992.
36. Rawlings CA, Farrell RL, Mahood RM: Morphologic changes in the lungs of cats experimentally infected with *Dirofilaria immitis:* response to aspirin, *J Vet Intern Med* 4:292, 1990 (comments).
37. Yarns DA, Tashjian RJ: Cardiopulmonary changes in heartworm-infected dogs after 32-months interval, *Res Vet Sci* 2:112, 1970.
38. Rawlings CA, Raynaud JP, Lewis RE et al: Pulmonary thromboembolism and hypertension after thiacetarsemide vs. melarsomine dihydrochloride treatment of *Dirofilaria immitis* infection in dogs, *Am J Vet Res* 54:920, 1992.
39. Dillon AR, Brawner WR, Hanrahan L: Influence of number of parasites and exercise on the severity of heartworm disease in dogs, *Proceedings of the Heartworm Symposium '95,* Batavia, Ill, 1995, American Heartworm Society.
40. Dunavent B, Keister DM, Tanner PA et al: Correlation between heartworm disease classification, serum antigen concentration and associated clinical pathology parameters. In: Soll MD, Knight DH, eds: *Proceedings of the Heartworm Symposium '95,* Batavia, Ill, 1995, American Heartworm Society.
41. Wallace CR, Hamilton WR: Study of spontaneous congestive heart failure in the dog, *Circ Res* 11:301, 1962.
42. Rawlings CA, Lewis RE: Right ventricular enlargement in heartworm disease, *Am J Vet Res* 38:1801, 1977.
43. Kitagawa H, Kubota A, Yasuda K et al: Cardiopulmonary function in dogs with serious heartworm disease, *J Vet Med Sci* 54:751, 1992.
44. Ishihara K, Kitagawa H, Sasaki Y et al: Changes in cardiopulmonary values after heartworm removal from pulmonary artery using flexible alligator forceps, *Jpn J Vet Sci* 50:731, 1988.
45. Calvert CA, Rawlings CA: Pulmonary manifestations of heartworm disease, *Vet Clin North Am Small Anim Pract* 15:991, 1995.
46. Rawlings CA, Losonsky JM, Schaub RG et al: Postadulticide changes in *Dirofilaria immitis*-infected beagles, *Am J Vet Res* 44:8, 1983.
47. Atkins CE, Atwell RB, Dillon AR et al: Guidelines for the diagnosis, treatment, and prevention of heartworm (*Dirofilaria immitis*) infection in cats, *Compend Cont Educ Pract Vet* 19:422, 1997.
48. Osborne CA, Hammer RF, O'Leary TP et al: Renal manifestation of canine dirofilariasis. In Otto GF, ed: *Proceedings of the Heartworm Symposium '80,* Edwardsville, Kan, 1980, American Heartworm Society.
49. Chapleau MW, Fish RE, Levitzky MG: Regional hypoxic vasoconstriction in dogs with asymptomatic dirofilariasis, *Am J Vet Res* 46:1341, 1985.
50. West JB: *Pulmonary pathophysiology: the essentials,* Baltimore, 1978, Williams & Wilkins.
51. Kapoor WN: Syncope and hypotension. In Braunwald E, ed: *Heart disease: a textbook of cardiovascular medicine,* ed 5, Philadelphia, 1997, WB Saunders.
52. Goggin JM, Biller DS, Rost CM et al: Ultrasonographic identification of *Dirofilaria immitis* in the aorta and liver of a dog, *J Am Vet Med Assoc* 210:1635, 1997.
53. Frank JR, Nutter FB, Kyles CE et al: Systemic arterial dirofilariasis in five dogs, *J Vet Intern Med* 11:189, 1997.
54. Dillon AR: Case discussion: management of feline heartworm disease. In Soll MD, Knight DH, eds: *Proceedings of the Heartworm Symposium '95,* Batavia, Ill, 1995, American Heartworm Society.
55. Selcer BA, Newell SM, McCall JW: Radiographic and 2-D echocardiographic findings in eighteen cats experimentally exposed to *D. immitis* via mosquito bites, *Vet Radiol Ultrasound* 37:37, 1996.
56. DeFrancesco TC, Atkins CE, Meurs KM et al: Diagnostic utility of echocardiography in feline heartworm disease, *J Vet Intern Med* 11:141, 1997.
57. Patton S, Faulkner CT: Prevalence of *Dirofilaria immitis* and *Dipetalonema reconditum* in dogs: 805 cases (1980-1989), *J Am Vet Med Assoc* 200:1533, 1992.
58. Rawlings CA, Dawe DL, McCall JW et al: Four types of occult *Dirofilaria immitis* infections in dogs, *J Am Vet Med Assoc* 180:1323, 1982.
59. Sisson D, Dilling G, Wong MM et al: Sensitivity and specificity of the indirect-fluorescent antibody test and two enzyme-linked immunosorbent assays in canine dirofilariasis, *Am J Vet Res* 46:1529, 1985.
60. Weil GJ, Malane MS, Powers KG et al: Monoclonal antibodies to parasite antigens in the serum of *Dirofilaria immitis*-infected dogs, *J Immunol* 134:1185, 1985.
61. McTier TL: A guide to selecting adult heartworm antigen tests, *Vet Med* 89:528, 1994.
62. McCall J, McTier T, Supakorndej N: Evaluation of the sensitivity of heartworm antigen test kits using whole blood and/or serum from heartworm-infected dogs, *Proc Annu Meet AAVP, 1994, p 9.*
63. Courtney CH: Guidelines for the use of parasitologic and serologic screening for heartworm infection. In Soll MD, ed: *Proceedings of the Heartworm Symposium '92,* Batavia, Ill, 1992, American Heartworm Society.
64. Courtney CH, Zeng Q: Application of heartworm immunodiagnostic tests. In Otto GF, ed: *Proceedings of the Heartworm Symposium '89,* Washington, DC, 1989, American Heartworm Society.
65. McCall JW, Supakorndej N, Ryan W et al: Utility of an ELISA-based antibody test for detection of heartworm infection in cats, In Soll MD, Knight DH, eds: *Proceedings of the Heartworm Symposium '95,* Batavia, Ill, 1995, American Heartworm Society.

66. HESKA Corporation, Professional Resource Web Page, www.heska.com, 1997.
67. Keister DM, Tanner PA, Meo NJ: Immiticide: review of discovery, development, and utility. In Soll MD, Knight DH, eds: *Proceedings of the Heartworm Symposium '95,* Batavia, Ill. 1995, American Heartworm Society.
68. Miller MW, Keister MD, Tanner PA et al: Clinical efficacy of melarsomine dihydrochloride (RM340) and thiacetarsemide in dogs with moderate (class 2) heartworm disease. In Soll MD, Knight DH, eds: *Proceedings of the Heartworm Symposium '95,* Batavia, Ill, 1995, American Heartworm Society.
69. Hong XQ, Mejia JS, Nkenfou C et al: A promising recombinant antigen for the early detection of heartworm infection, In Soll MD, Knight DH, eds: *Proceedings of the Heartworm Symposium '95,* Batavia, Ill, 1995, American Heartworm Society.
70. McCall JW, Supakorndej N, Ryan W et al: Utility of ELISA-based antigen and antibody tests for detection of heartworm infection in cats, In Soll MD, Knight DH, eds: *Proceedings of the Heartworm Symposium '95,* Batavia, Ill, 1995, American Heartworm Society.
71. Donaghue AR, Mondesire RR, Porter JP: Detection of antibodies to *Dirofilaria immitis* in the cat using a highly specific recombinant antigen, *Proc North Am Vet Conf* 1997 (abstract).
72. Lombard CW, Ackerman N: Right heart enlargement in heartworm-infected dogs: a radiographic, electrocardiographic, and echocardiographic correlation, *Vet Radiol* 25:210, 1984.
73. Hagio M: Two-dimensional echocardiography for the detection of *Dirofilaria immitis* in the right heart and adjacent vessels of dogs, *J Jpn Vet Med Assoc* 39:74, 1986.
74. Venco L, Mazzacchi D, Morini S et al: The use of echocardiography as a diagnostic tool for detection of feline heartworm (*Dirofilaria immitis*) infections, personal communication, 1997.
75. Calvert CA, Rawlings CA: Diagnosis and management of canine heartworm disease. In Kirk RW, ed: *Kirk's current veterinary therapy, VII,* Philadelphia, 1983, WB Saunders.
76. Atwell RB: Aspects of natural and experimental canine dirofilariasis, PhD dissertation, Brisbane, 1983, University of Queensland.
77. DiSacco B, Vezzoni A: Clinical classification of heartworm disease for the purpose of adding objectivity to the assessment of therapeutic efficacy of adulticidal drugs in the field. In Soll MD, ed: *Proceedings of the Heartworm Symposium '92,* Batavia, Ill, 1992, American Heartworm Society.
78. Atwell RB, Boreham PFL: Studies on the adverse reactions following diethylcarbamazine to microfilaria-positive (*D. immitis*) dogs. In Otto GF, ed: *Proceedings of the Heartworm Symposium '83,* Edwardsville, Kan, 1983, American Heartworm Society.
79. McCall JW, McTeir TL, Supakorndej N et al: Clinical prophylactic activity of macrolides on young adult heartworms, In Soll MD, Knight DH, eds: *Proceedings of the Heartworm Symposium '95,* Batavia, Ill. 1995, American Heartworm Society.
80. Keister DM: Melarsomine in the dog, personal communication, 1995.
81. Hoskins JD, Hagstad HV, Hribernik TN: Complications following thiacetarsemide sodium therapy in Louisiana dogs with naturally-occurring heartworm disease, *Cornell Vet* 75:531, 1985.
82. Sundlof SF, Courtney CH, Bell JU et al: Pharmacokinetics of thiacetarsemide in relationship to therapeutic efficacy. In Otto GF, ed: *Proceedings of the Heartworm Symposium '86,* Washington, DC, 1986, American Heartworm Society.
83. Jackson RF: Two-day treatment with thiacetarsemide for canine heartworm disease, *J Am Vet Med Assoc* 142:23, 1963.
84. Courtney CH, Sundlof SF, Jackson RF: New dose schedule for the treatment of canine dirofilariasis with thiacetarsemide. In Otto GF, ed: *Proceedings of the Heartworm Symposium '86,* Washington, DC, 1986, American Heartworm Society.
85. Jackson RF, Otto GF: Thiacetarsemide reevaluation. In Otto GF, ed: *Proceedings of the Heartworm Symposium '80,* Bonner Springs, Kan, 1980, American Heartworm Society.
86. Holmes RA, McCall JW, Prasse KW et al: Thiacetarsemide sodium: pharmacokinetics and the effects of decreased liver function on efficacy against *Dirofilaria immitis* in dogs. In Otto GF, ed: *Proceedings of the Heartworm Symposium '86,* Washington, DC, 1986, American Heartworm Society.
87. McCall JW, Lewis RE, Rawlings CA: Reevaluation of thiacetarsemide as an adulticidal agent against *Dirofilaria immitis* in dogs. In Otto GF, ed: *Proceedings of the Heartworm Symposium '80,* Bonner Springs, Kan, 1981, American Heartworm Society.
88. Knight DH: Heartworm infection, *Vet Clin North Am Small Anim Pract* 17:1463, 1987.
89. Sundlof SF, Courtney CH, King RR: Laboratory methods for evaluating the effectiveness of thiacetarsemide in treating canine heartworm disease. In Otto GF, ed: *Proceedings of the Heartworm Symposium '89,* Washington, DC, 1989, American Heartworm Society.
90. Winograd H, Lorgue G, Keister DM: Thiacetarsemide toxicity in the normal dog. In Soll MD, ed: *Proceedings of the Heartworm Symposium '92,* Batavia, Ill, 1992, American Heartworm Society.
91. Keister MD, Dzimianski MT, McTier TL et al: Dose selection and confirmation of RM 340, a new filaricide for the treatment of dogs with immature and mature *Dirofilaria immitis.* In Soll MD, ed: *Proceedings of the Heartworm Symposium '92,* Batavia, Ill, 1992, American Heartworm Society.
92. Case JL, Tanner PA, Keister DM et al: A clinical field study of melarsomine dihydrochloride (RM340) in dogs with severe (class 3) heartworm disease. In Soll MD, Knight DH, eds: *Proceedings of the Heartworm Symposium '95,* Batavia, Ill, 1995, American Heartworm Society.
93. Vezzoni A, Genchi C, Raynaud JP. Adulticide efficacy of RM 340 in dogs with mild and severe natural infections. In Soll MD, ed: *Proceedings of the Heartworm Symposium '92,* Batavia, Ill, 1992, American Heartworm Society.
94. Turner JL, Lees GE, Brown SA et al: Thiacetarsemide in normal cats: pharmacokinetic, clinical, laboratory, and pathologic features. In Otto GF, ed: *Proceedings of the Heartworm Symposium '89,* Washington, DC, 1984, American Heartworm Society.
95. Dillon AR, Cox N, Brawner B et al: The effects of thiacetarsemide administration to normal cats. In Soll MD, ed: *Proceedings of the Heartworm Symposium '92,* Batavia, Ill, 1992, American Heartworm Society.
96. Keith JC, Rawlings CA, Schaub RG: Pulmonary thromboembolism during therapy of dirofilariasis with thiacetarsemide: modification with aspirin or prednisolone, *Am J Vet Res* 44:1278, 1983.
97. Calvert CA, Rawlings CA: Canine heartworm disease. In Fox PR, ed: *Canine and feline cardiology,* New York, 1988, Churchill Livingstone.
98. Vezzoni A, Genchi C: Reduction of post-adulticide thromboembolic complications with low dose heparin therapy. In Otto GF, ed: *Proceedings of the Heartworm Symposium '89,* Washington, DC, 1989, American Heartworm Society.
99. Rawlings CA, Keith JCJ, Losonsky JM et al: An aspirin-prednisolone combination to modify postadulticide lung disease in heartworm-infected dogs, *Am J Vet Res* 45:2371, 1984.
100. Rawlings CA, Keith JC, Lewis RE et al: Aspirin and prednisolone modification of radiographic changes caused by adulticide treatment in dogs with heartworm infection, *J Am Vet Med Assoc* 182:131, 1983.
101. Rawlings CA, Keith JC, Losonsky JM et al: Aspirin and prednisolone modification of postadulticide pulmonary arterial disease in heartworm-infected dogs: arteriographic study, *Am J Vet Res* 44:821, 1983.
102. Schaub RG, Keith JCJ, Rawlings CA: Effect of acetylsalicylic acid on vascular damage and myointimal proliferation in canine pulmonary arteries subjected to chronic injury by *Dirofilaria immitis, Am J Vet Res* 44:449, 1983.
103. Calvert CA, Thrall DE: Treatment of canine heartworm disease coexisting with right-side heart failure, *J Am Vet Med Assoc* 180:1201, 1982.
104. Atwell RB: Discussion 4. In Soll MD, Knight DH, eds: *Proceedings of the Heartworm Symposium '95,* Batavia, Ill, 1995, American Heartworm Society.

105. Plumb DC: *Veterinary drug handbook,* ed 2, Ames, Iowa, 1995, Iowa State University Press.
106. Luethy MW, Sisson DD, Kneller SK et al: Angiographic assessment of aspirin and heparin therapy for the prevention of pulmonary thromboembolism following adulticide therapy. In Otto GF, ed: *Proceedings of the Heartworm Symposium '89,* Batavia, Ill, 1989, American Heartworm Society.
107. Rawlings CA: Pulmonary arteriography and hemodynamics during feline heartworm disease: effect of aspirin, *J Vet Intern Med* 4:285, 1990.
108. Ishihara K, Sasaki Y, Kitagawa H: Development of a flexible alligator forceps: a new instrument for removal of heartworms in the pulmonary arteries of dogs, *Jpn J Vet Sci* 48:989, 1986.
109. Brown WA: Surgical removal of heartworms from cats with severe heartworm disease, personal communication, 1997.
110. Jackson RF: Surgical treatment of heartworm disease, *J Am Vet Med Assoc* 154:383, 1969.
111. Blair LS, Malatesta PF, Ewanciw DV: Dose-response of ivermectin against *Dirofilaria immitis* microfilariae in dogs with naturally acquired infections, *Am J Vet Res* 44:475, 1983.
112. McManus EC, Pulliam JD: Histopathologic features of canine heartworm microfilarial infection after treatment with ivermectin, *Am J Vet Res* 45:91, 1984.
113. Simpson CF, Jackson RF: Lesions in the liver and kidney of *Dirofilaria immitis*-infected dogs following treatment with ivermectin, *Z Parasitenkd* 71:97, 1985.
114. Sasaki Y, Kitagawa H: Effects of milbemycin D on microfilarial number and reproduction of *Dirofilaria immitis* in dogs, *J Vet Med Sci* 55:763, 1993.
115. Blagburn BL, Hendrix CM, Lindsay DS et al: Post-adulticide milbemycin oxime microfilaricidal activity in dogs naturally infected with *Dirofilaria immitis*. In Soll MD, ed: *Proceedings of the Heartworm Symposium '92,* Batavia, Ill, 1992, American Heartworm Society.
116. Recommended procedures for the diagnosis and prevention of heartworm (*Dirofilaria immitis*) infection in dogs, In Soll MD, Knight DH, eds: *Proceedings of the Heartworm Symposium '95,* Batavia, Ill, 1995, American Heartworm Society.
117. Wolfe A: Use of levamisole prior to macrolide administration to dogs with high microfilarial counts, personal communication, 1995.
118. Sasaki Y, Kitagawa H, Ishihara K et al: Prevention of adverse reactions following milbemycin D administration to microfilaremic dogs infected with *Dirofilaria immitis, Nippon Juigaku Zasshi* 51:711, 1989.
119. Kitagawa H, Sasaki Y, Ishihara K: Canine dirofilarial hemoglobinuria induced by milbemycin D administration, *Jpn J Vet Sci* 48:517, 1986.
120. Bater AK: Prevention of natural heartworm infection by milbemycin in puppies not receiving their initial dose until two, four and six months after birth. In Soll MD, Knight DH, eds: *Proceedings of the Heartworm Symposium '95,* Batavia, Ill, 1995, American Heartworm Society.
121. Furrow RD, Powers KG, Parbuoni EL: *Dirofilaria immitis.* II. Gross and microscopic hepatic changes associated with diethylcarbamazine citrate (DEC) therapy in dogs. In Otto GF, ed: *Proceedings of the Heartworm Symposium '80,* Edwardsville, Kan. 1980, American Heartworm Society.
122. Courtney CH, Nachreiner RF: The effect of diethylcarbamazine on fertility in the dog. In Otto GF, ed: *Proceedings of the Heartworm Symposium '77,* Bonner Springs, Kan, 1978, American Heartworm Society.
123. Ware WA: Heartworm disease. In Nelson RW, Couto CG, eds: *Essentials of small animal internal medicine,* St Louis, 1992, Mosby.
124. Lovell RL: Ivermectin and piperazine toxicoses in dogs and cats, *Vet Clin North Am Small Anim Pract* 20:453, 1990.
125. Campbell WC, Fisher MH, Stapley EO: Ivermectin: a potent new antiparasitic agent, *Science* 221:823, 1983.
126. Grieve RB, Frank GR, Stewart VA et al: Chemoprophylactic effects of milbemycin oxime against larvae of *Dirofilaria immitis* during prepatent development, *Am J Vet Res* 52:2040, 1991.
127. Shulz-Key H, Klager S, Awadzi K: Treatment of human onchocerciasis: the efficacy of ivermectin on the parasite, *Trop Med Parasitol* 36:20, 1985.
128. Anantaphruti M, Kino H, Terada M: Studies on chemotherapy of parasitic helminths. XIII. Efficacy of ivermectin against microfilariae and embryonic development in the female worm of *Dirofilaria immitis, Jpn J Parasitol* 31:517, 1982.
129. Lok JB, Knight DH, LaPaugh DA et al: Kinetics of microfilaremia suppression in *Dirofilaria immitis* infected dogs during and after a prophylactic regimen of milbemycin oxime. In Soll MD, ed: *Proceedings of the Heartworm Symposium '92,* Batavia, Ill, 1992, American Heartworm Society.
130. Paul AJ, Tranquilli WJ, Todd KS et al: Evaluating the safety of administering high doses of a chewable ivermectin tablet to collies, *Vet Med* 86:623, 1991.
131. Pulliam JD, Seward RL, Henry RT: Investigating ivermectin toxicity in collies, *Vet Med* 79:33, 1985.
132. Tranquilli WJ, Paul AJ, Todd KS: Assessment of toxicosis induced by high-dose administration of milbemycin oxime in collies, *Am J Vet Res* 52:1170, 1991.
133. Easby SM: Ivermectin in the dog, *Vet Rec* 115:45, 1984 (letter to the editor).
134. Clark JN, Pulliam JD, Alva R et al: Safety of orally administered ivermectin in cats. In Soll MD, ed: *Proceedings of the Heartworm Symposium '92,* Batavia, Ill, 1992, American Heartworm Society.
135. Paul AJ, Acre KE, Todd KS et al: Efficacy of ivermectin against *Dirofilaria immitis* in cats 30 and 45 days post-infection. In Soll MD, ed: *Proceedings of the Heartworm Symposium '92,* Batavia, Ill, 1992, American Heartworm Society.
136. Longhofer SL, Daurio CP, Plue RE et al: Ivermectin for the prevention of feline heartworm disease, *Proceedings of the Heartworm Symposium '95,* Batavia, Ill, 1995, American Heartworm Society.
137. Stewart Va, Blagburn BL, Hendrix CM et al: Milbemycin oxime as an effective preventative of heartworm (*Dirofilaria immitis*) infection in cats. In: Soll MD, ed: *Proceedings of the Heartworm Symposium '92,* Batavia, Ill, 1992, American Heartworm Society.
138. Jackson RF, Otto GF, Bauman PM et al: Distribution of heartworms in the right side of the heart and adjacent vessels of the dog, *J Am Vet Med Assoc* 149:515, 1966.
139. Atkins CE, Keene BW, McGuirk SM: Pathophysiologic mechanism of cardiac dysfunction in experimentally induced heartworm caval syndrome in dogs: an echocardiographic study, *Am J Vet Res* 49:403, 1988.
140. Atkins CE: Pathophysiology of heartworm caval syndrome. In Otto GF, ed: *Proceedings of the Heartworm Symposium '89,* Washington, DC, 1989, American Heartworm Society.
141. Kitagawa H, Sasaki Y, Ishihara K et al: Development of artificial model of caval syndrome in canine heartworm disease, *Nippon Juigaku Zasshi* 52:1029, 1990.
142. Ishihara K, Kitagawa H, Ojima M: Clinicopathological studies on canine dirofilarial hemoglobinuria, *Jpn J Vet Sci* 40:525, 1978.
143. Kitagawa H, Sasaki Y, Ishihara K et al: Cardiopulmonary function values before and after heartworm removal in dogs with caval syndrome, *Am J Vet Res* 52:126, 1991.
144. Kitagawa H, Ishihara K, Sasaki, X: Canine dirofilarial hemoglobinuria: changes in right heart hemodynamics and heartworm migration from pulmonary artery towards right atrium following $beta_1$-blocker administration, *Nippon Juigaku Zasshi* 49:1081, 1987.
145. Atkins CE: Caval syndrome in the dog, *Sem Vet Med Surg Small Anim* 2:64, 1987.

CHAPTER 24

Infective Endocarditis (and Annuloaortic Ectasia)

Literally translated, infective endocarditis is inflammation of the endocardial surface of the heart resulting from invasion by an infectious agent. In reality, almost all endocarditis that is recognized in dogs and cats involves valve tissue, and the vast majority of the infectious agents recognized are bacterial. However, in rare situations the mural endocardium can become infected, and, rarely, fungal or rickettsial organisms can cause infective endocarditis. When a bacterial organism is known to cause infective endocarditis, the appropriate name for the disease is *bacterial endocarditis.* When bacteria colonize a heart valve, they generally produce proliferative lesions (vegetations) or destroy valve tissue (Color Plate 95). Vegetations usually result in improper valve coaptation, resulting in regurgitation. The vegetations may also result in a narrowed valve orifice, creating stenosis, but this is unusual. Valve destruction results in regurgitation in all instances. Other common names for infective endocarditis are *vegetative endocarditis and acute or subacute bacterial endocarditis.* Acute bacterial endocarditis is usually associated with a virulent organism, such as Escherichia coli.[1] The diagnosis is usually made within 2 weeks of the onset of clinical signs. Subacute bacterial endocarditis is associated with organisms of low virulence, and the disease evolves over several weeks to months. Much of the disease seen in dogs and cats appears to be acute and commonly follows a malignant course.

Incidence

Although several studies have been performed to look at the incidence of infective endocarditis in dogs, most of them have severe limitations and therefore are not reported here. Suffice it to say that infective endocarditis is a rare lesion. The diagnosis of infective endocarditis was made in 45 canine patients in the University of California, Davis, Veterinary Medical Teaching Hospital between August 1, 1986, and August 1, 1996; this is approximately five cases per year. This probably means that a veterinarian in private practice will see a case of bacterial endocarditis once every several years, at most. Infective endocarditis is more common in dogs than in cats. Infective endocarditis primarily affects the mitral and aortic valves in dogs and cats. The tricuspid valve is rarely affected, and the pulmonic valve is almost never affected.[2] In the 45 canine patients from our hospital, 22 had lesions confined to the aortic valve cusps, 16 had lesions confined to the mitral valve leaflets, one had both the aortic valve and mitral valve involved, and one had tricuspid valve endocarditis. In five the valve involved could not be confirmed from the record.

Infective endocarditis is a disease of medium-size–to–large dogs and of purebred dogs. Only eight of the aforementioned 45 cases from our hospital were not purebred dogs. The most commonly affected breeds among these cases included German shepherds or German shepherd crosses, golden retrievers, and Labrador retrievers. The incidence in the retrievers probably reflects the fact that these breeds are popular and therefore we examine many of them. German shepherds appear to be overrepresented. The only two dogs under 10 kg that we saw in that same period were a Chihuahua and a toy poodle. All other dogs were greater than 15 kg. None of the cases were identified following a dentistry.

Infective endocarditis is rare in cats. During the same period that we identified 45 dogs with infective endocarditis, we diagnosed seven cats with infective endocarditis. Five of these had infective endocarditis of the aortic valve and two of the mitral valve.

Pathogenesis and Pathophysiology

BACTEREMIA

Bacteremia must occur for bacteria to colonize a heart valve. A transient bacteremia apparently is a common event. In humans, bacteremia occurs secondary to such diverse events as defecation and teeth brushing.[3] That transient bacteremia is a normal event in humans is suggested by the fact that circulating antibody titers to normal flora are identified in healthy humans.[4] Bacteria that gain entry to the bloodstream are usually rapidly removed by macrophages in the liver, bone marrow, and spleen and by neutrophils in capillaries.[5]

Physical manipulation of mucosal surfaces (urinary catheterization, dental scaling) produces bacteremia in humans.[3] Dental scaling is a primary concern of most veterinary practitioners for producing bacteremia. Consequently, the administration of prophylactic antibiotics to patients with cardiac disease that are undergoing dental procedures is commonly recommended.[6] To place this subject in perspective, one investigator documented that in humans, 40% are bacteremic after dental extractions, but 38% are bacteremic after hard chewing, and 25% are bacteremic after tooth brushing or oral irrigation.[7] Two recent studies looked at bacteremia in dogs during dental procedures. In the first, 67% of the dogs had bacteremia.[8] This study identified numerous organisms, including *Streptococcus, Staphylococcus, Pasteurella, Acinetobacter, Neisseria, Pseudo-*

monas, and both gram-positive and gram-negative anaerobic organisms. One half of these dogs were administered sodium penicillin G prophylactically, which did not reduce bacterial numbers. A subsequent study examined two groups of 30 dogs.[9] The first group was anesthetized or sedated only, and the second group was anesthetized and underwent dental scaling. Approximately 30% of the dogs in both groups were bacteremic. Five of the dogs that had the dental procedure had *Pasteurella* spp. cultured from their blood, whereas none of the other dogs did, and four of the sedated dogs had *Staphylococcus* spp. cultured.

In humans, fewer than 20% of patients with infective endocarditis have a history of a medical procedure before developing infective endocarditis. In our experience, most canine patients do not have any history of a previous medical procedure, and in many the source of the infection cannot be ascertained. In one study, however, the investigators were able to suggest or define a route of entry or a source of infection in 62% of their cases of infective endocarditis in dogs.[2]

It is our general impression that veterinarians commonly administer antibiotics prophylactically to dogs undergoing dental scaling, especially to dogs with myxomatous mitral valve disease. From the data presented above one might conclude that it makes just as much sense to administer antibiotics to all patients that are being sedated. We have not witnessed a dog with myxomatous mitral valve disease develop infective endocarditis following a dental procedure. Consequently, we question whether these patients are at a greater risk of developing endocarditis. The evidence for dentistry-induced infective endocarditis in the literature is lacking. One report states that of 61 dogs studied retrospectively, eight were greater than 7 years of age and six had evidence of myxomatous mitral valve degeneration.[2] All six dogs had endocarditis of the mitral valve. There was no mention of a past history of dental procedures in these dogs. One other report from 1979 lists lack of antibiotic prophylaxis after dentistry in two poodles diagnosed with infective endocarditis.[10] One of these dogs had a typical murmur of mitral regurgitation and a history of heart failure and survived. Its other clinical signs were a fever and an elevated white blood cell count. The other dog had no heart murmur, a fever, and an elevated white blood cell count. The diagnosis of endocarditis was based on a positive blood culture. The diagnosis could be questioned in both these dogs. We also do not believe that the antibiotics that are commonly used prophylactically with dental procedures, such as penicillin, streptomycin, and ampicillin, have a spectrum of activity broad enough to be beneficial, even if they were warranted.

BACTERIAL ISOLATES

The primary difference between the types of organisms isolated in humans and dogs with infective endocarditis is that dogs have a higher incidence of gram-negative infections. In four studies, *Staphylococcus aureus* accounted for approximately 25% of the organisms isolated, hemolytic and nonhemolytic streptococci for 20%, and *E. coli* for 25%.[2,11-13] *Corynebacterium* was isolated in 10% and *Pseudomonas* in 6%. *Erysipelothrix* sp. accounted for 3% of the cases. This unusual organism has been reported elsewhere and has recently been determined to be *Erysipelothrix tonsillarum,* not *Erysipelothrix rhusiopathiae,* the swine pathogen.[14,15] *Bartonella vinsonii,* a rickettsial organism, has been reported in dogs with culture-negative vegetative endocarditis.[16]

PREDISPOSING FACTORS

Circulating microorganisms must attach to the endocardial surface of a valve for infective endocarditis to occur. In humans, most (60% to 80%) patients with infective endocarditis have an identifiable predisposing cardiac lesion that makes it easier for the organism to attach.[3] This is not be the case in dogs and cats. Most cases of infective endocarditis in animals occur on apparently normal valves.[1,2,11,12] In one study, out of 61 dogs with infective endocarditis, only four had congenital heart defects.[2] Of these four, three had subaortic stenosis. No evidence exists to support a relationship between myxomatous degeneration of the mitral valve and infective endocarditis.[17]

In humans, platelets aggregate on valves damaged by congenital or rheumatic disease. Platelet aggregation occurs because of endothelial damage that exposes collagen fibers.[18] Microscopic platelet thrombi may stabilize to form larger lesions (so-called nonbacterial thrombotic endocarditis). Experimentally these lesions can be colonized by circulating bacteria, resulting in endocarditis.[19]

The fact that most dogs with infective endocarditis do not have underlying cardiac disease makes the canine disease distinctly different from the human disease. Why do bacteria lodge on apparently normal heart valves more readily than on other normal structures in the cardiovascular system? Multiple factors likely exist. Heart valves are subject to constant trauma as they open and close with each cardiac cycle. This trauma probably results in very minute damage to the endothelial surfaces of the valves. This may explain why valves are more prone to infective endocarditis. That trauma to valve leaflets is part of the pathogenesis of infective endocarditis is suggested by the fact that the incidence of infective endocarditis is directly related to the force placed on each valve. The mitral valve is affected in 86% of human patients and is subjected to approximately 116 mm Hg systolic pressure, the aortic valve is affected in 55% of human cases and is subjected to approximately 72 mm Hg diastolic pressure, the tricuspid valve is affected in 20% of cases and is subjected to approximately 24 mm Hg systolic pressure, and the pulmonic valve is affected in 1% of cases and is subjected to approximately 5 mm Hg diastolic pressure.[20] Normal valves may also develop nonbacterial thrombotic endocarditis. However, in humans this is more common in patients that are systemically ill, such as those with advanced malignancy, uremia, systemic lupus erythematosus, and so on.

Bacteremia is common and infective endocarditis is rare. Why then do some dogs and cats with apparently normal valves develop infective endocarditis and others do not? This is unknown. Some factors that might contribute are as follows. First, the type of organism is probably an important factor. Some virulent bacteria, such as *Staphylococcus, Streptococcus,* and *Pseudomonas,* can adhere to normal endocardial surfaces.[3] In gram-negative bacteremia, serum bactericidal activity appears to play an important role such that only serum-resistant isolates of *E. coli, Pseudomonas aeruginosa,* and *Serratia marcescens* produce bacterial endocarditis in rabbits.[21] Of course, many dogs are probably exposed to bacteremia with similar organisms, and most do not develop endocarditis. It seems likely that immune factors could play a major role in determining whether a dog or cat develops infective endocarditis. Rabbits homozygous for C_6 deficiency develop infective endocarditis more readily than normal rabbits.[19,22] Antibodies are known to protect against endocarditis by either inhibiting adhesion of the bacteria or clearing the blood of the organism more rapidly.[3] Abnormalities in antibody production or function could predispose to endocarditis. German shepherds were more commonly affected with bacterial endocarditis in the southeastern United States in the 1980s. Some type of inherited immune system abnormality might have produced this phenomenon. When one examines the breeds with infective endocarditis reported in the literature, very few mixed-breed dogs are represented. This could reflect the demographics of a referral population or it could suggest that hereditary abnormalities, such as an inherited immune system abnormality, might be involved.

Dogs with subaortic stenosis are one group of dogs with preexisting cardiac disease at risk for developing infective endocarditis.[23] In subaortic stenosis, turbulent, high-velocity blood flow develops in the subvalvular region. This jet traumatizes the aortic valve leaflets during each systolic interval. This damage is apparent from the fact that these otherwise normal valve leaflets consistently become insufficient early in life. Presumably, this injury to the valve makes it easier for bacteria to colonize on the leaflet endothelium. Dogs with subaortic stenosis should be administered prophylactic antibiotic therapy during procedures known to produce bacteremia.[11,23,24]

Administering prophylactic antibiotics to dogs with other congenital cardiac abnormalities also may be rational based on experience in humans. One author suggests that dogs that are at risk be administered penicillin G, ampicillin, or amoxicillin, based on a study that showed that the oral flora of normal dogs and dogs with dental disease consisted primarily of anaerobic bacteria.[6] However, anaerobic bacteria have been reported only once as an isolate from a dog with infective endocarditis. Another author identified aerobic organisms from dog and cat mouths.[25] Anaerobic organisms have not been isolated from any dog in the four most recent reports of dogs with IE.[1,2,11,12] Because of this and because of the high incidence of gram-negative cases of infective endocarditis in dogs, we do not feel that the aforementioned antibiotics are the best choices.

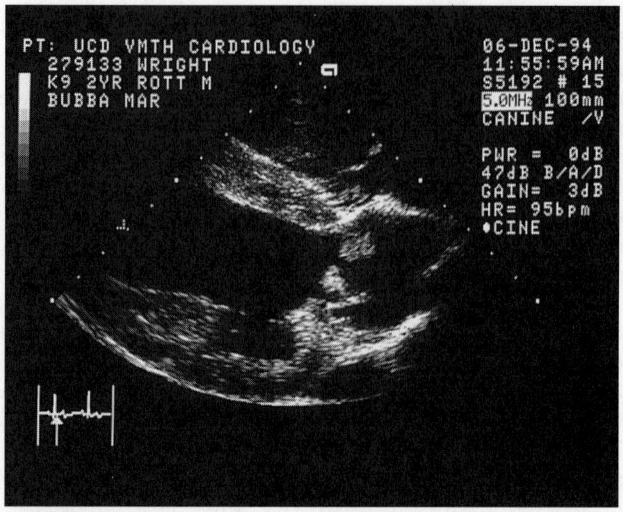

FIGURE 24-1 Two-dimensional echocardiogram using a right parasternal long-axis view of the left ventricle, aortic valve, and aorta from a 2-year-old intact male rottweiler. The echocardiogram revealed large "vegetative" lesions on the aortic valve. This dog was presented because of weight loss, reluctance to move, and vomiting. On physical examination the dog had a fever (103° F), was emaciated, and had a painful abdomen. No murmur was ausculted. He had a white blood cell count of 44,200 with a left shift. He also had hypergammaglobulinemia. Abdominal radiographs revealed discospondylitis. Abdominal ultrasonography revealed hyperechoic regions in the renal cortices, consistent with infarcts. An exudative abdominal fluid was identified. No organisms were grown from the fluid. An echocardiogram was obtained because of the possible renal infarcts. It revealed the endocarditis. Blood cultures grew *Citrobacter freundii,* a gram-negative rod sensitive only to gentamicin and amikacin. The dog was treated at home with subcutaneously administered amikacin for 4 months. Renal function was examined for evidence of amikacin toxicity periodically, with no abnormalities detected.

VEGETATIONS AND EMBOLIC DISEASE

The vegetations in infective endocarditis vary in size and shape from small, warty nodules to large cauliflower-like masses. Histologically, vegetations consist of colonies of bacteria imbedded in a fibrin-platelet matrix.[3] This matrix protects the bacteria from being phagocytized by leukocytes. The bacteria in the matrix are packed tightly (e.g., 10^9 to 10^{10} organisms per gram). Consequently, they metabolize and reproduce slowly. Slow reproduction and protection from phagocytosis make it difficult to kill bacteria in vegetations, especially with a bacteriostatic antibiotic.

Vegetative lesions commonly break free and are carried to distal sights within the arterial tree, where they lodge (embolization). In humans, 15% to 35% of patients have clinical evidence of embolization, whereas 45% to 65% have evidence of embolization at an autopsy.[3] In one report on 44 dogs with infective endocarditis that were examined at necropsy, 84% had evidence of systemic embolization.[2] The kidney had evidence of infarction in 64%, and the spleen was infarcted in 45%. Clinical signs of embolization develop more commonly in humans infected with organisms that tend to produce large vegetations that are more prone to dislodge.[3] These organisms include *S. aureus,* streptococci, and fastidious gram-negative organisms. Emboli that originate from the mitral or aortic valves lodge in numerous places in the body, including myocardium, brain, limbs, kidneys, spleen, bowel, and iliac artery.[2] Resultant clinical problems can include neurologic signs, arrhythmias, lameness (fixed or shifting), renal failure, gastrointestinal signs, abdominal pain, and posterior paresis and pain. The emboli are septic and so produce regions of infection and inflammation. This may result in exacerbation of nonspecific clinical signs at the time of embolization, especially fever.

VALVULAR REGURGITATION

Infective endocarditis usually destroys valve tissue or interferes with valve function, resulting in valvular regurgitation (Figures 24-1 through 24-3, Color Plate 96). Rarely, it results in clinically significant stenosis (Figures 24-4 and 24-5). Aortic valve endocarditis often results in severe aortic regurgitation. Both acute and chronic severe aortic regurgitation are poorly tolerated by the cardiovascular system. Dogs with severe aortic regurgitation secondary to infective endocarditis commonly present in left heart failure and usually die of this complication within a short time. In dogs with acute bacterial endocarditis, the left heart may not have time to compensate for the severe regurgitation. Consequently, bacterial endocarditis should always be a differential diagnosis when pulmonary edema is identified radiographically without left heart enlargement (Figure 24-6). Mild-to-moderate mitral regurgitation can be tolerated for prolonged periods. Even severe mitral regurgitation may be successfully managed medically for months.

IMMUNE SYSTEM ABNORMALITIES

Persistent bacteremia in infective endocarditis stimulates both the cell-mediated and humoral immune systems. This has not been well studied in dogs or cats, although hyperglobulinemia and glomerulonephritis have both been reported in dogs with infective endocarditis.[2,14] In humans, circulating immune complexes (containing IgG, IgA, IgM, and complement) are found in almost all patients with infective endocarditis that have positive blood cultures.[3] These complexes are deposited along the glomerular basement membrane and in joint capsules, where they cause glomerulonephritis and arthritis. Clinical signs associated with infective endocarditis in dogs can sometimes mimic those of immune-mediated disorders. Arthritis, either septic or nonseptic, is a common sequela to infective

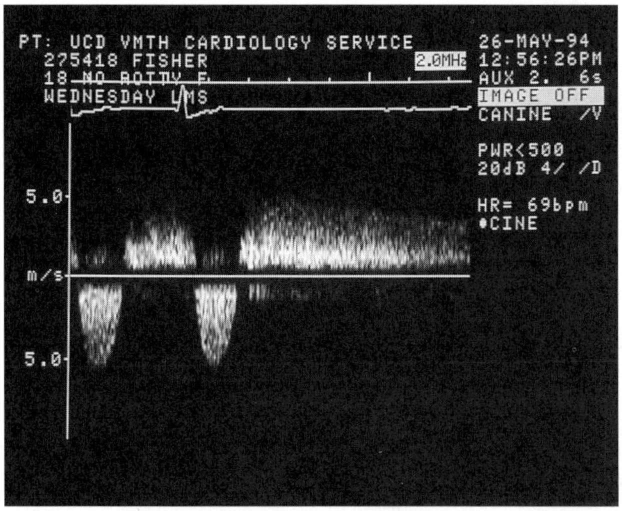

FIGURE 24-2 Continuous-wave Doppler echocardiogram from a dog with aortic regurgitation and severe subaortic stenosis. The ultrasound beam is directed across the left ventricular outflow tract and the proximal aorta from the cardiac apex. The peak systolic velocity is approximately 5 m/sec and is due to the subaortic stenosis. The tracing in diastole is a recording of the aortic regurgitation jet velocity. The velocity peaks at approximately 5 m/sec in early diastole. This means that the pressure gradient from the aorta to the left ventricle is approximately 100 mm Hg, which is normal. The velocity then gradually decreases after the second systolic interval (decrescendo), as aortic pressure decreases and left ventricular diastolic pressure increases slightly. The first diastolic interval is very short. Consequently, the jet velocity does not have time to decrease.

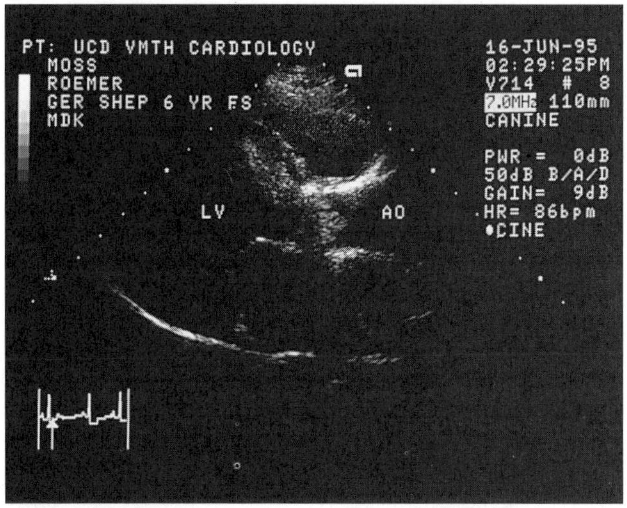

FIGURE 24-4 Two-dimensional echocardiogram using a right parasternal long-axis view of the left ventricle, aortic valve, and aorta from a 6-year-old German shepherd dog with massive vegetative lesions on the aortic valve creating valvular aortic stenosis. The frame is taken in systole and shows no evidence of valve opening. *LV,* Left ventricular chamber; *AO,* aorta.

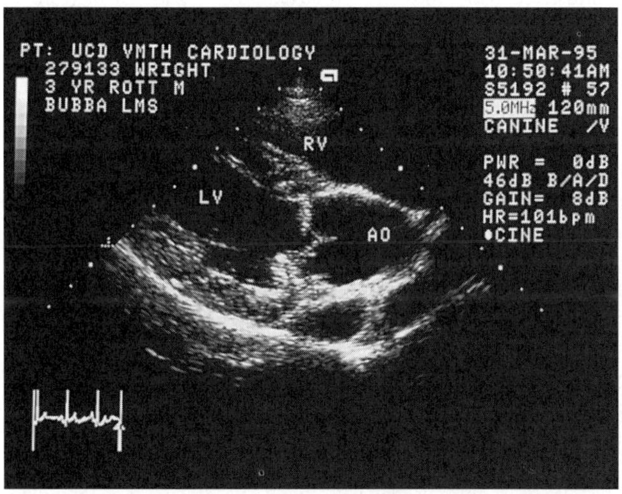

FIGURE 24-3 Two-dimensional echocardiogram from the dog shown in Figure 24-1 and Color Plate 96 after 4 months of antibiotic therapy with amikacin. The aortic valve lesions have regressed. *LV,* Left ventricular chamber; *AO,* aorta; *RV,* right ventricular chamber.

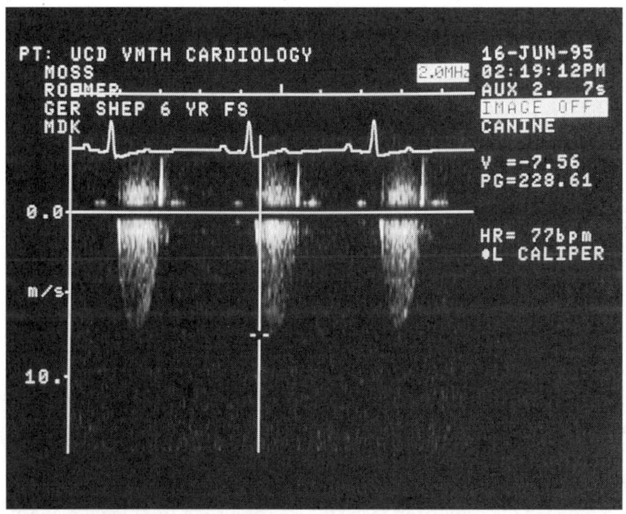

FIGURE 24-5 Continuous-wave Doppler echocardiogram taken through the stenotic region from the dog shown in Figure 24-4. The peak velocity of the blood flowing through the region of stenosis is 7.56 m/sec. This translates into a pressure gradient across the stenosis of 228 mm Hg. There was no evidence of subaortic stenosis.

endocarditis in dogs. Occasionally an antinuclear antibody test or Coombs' test is positive in a dog with infective endocarditis.[2]

RENAL FAILURE

Renal failure can be a devastating complication to infective endocarditis. It can occur secondary to immune complex glomerulonephritis or secondary to renal infarction.[14] Glomerulonephritis may result in significant protein loss and hypoalbuminemia (nephrotic syndrome).

Signalment, History, and Physical Examination

The vast majority of dogs with infective endocarditis are large dogs. Less than 10% of the dogs with infective endocarditis reported in the literature weigh less than 15 kg.[2,10-13] Most dogs are more than 4 years of age.[26] The male-to-female ratio was 2:1 in one study.[2] Most are purebred dogs. The disease is rare in cats.

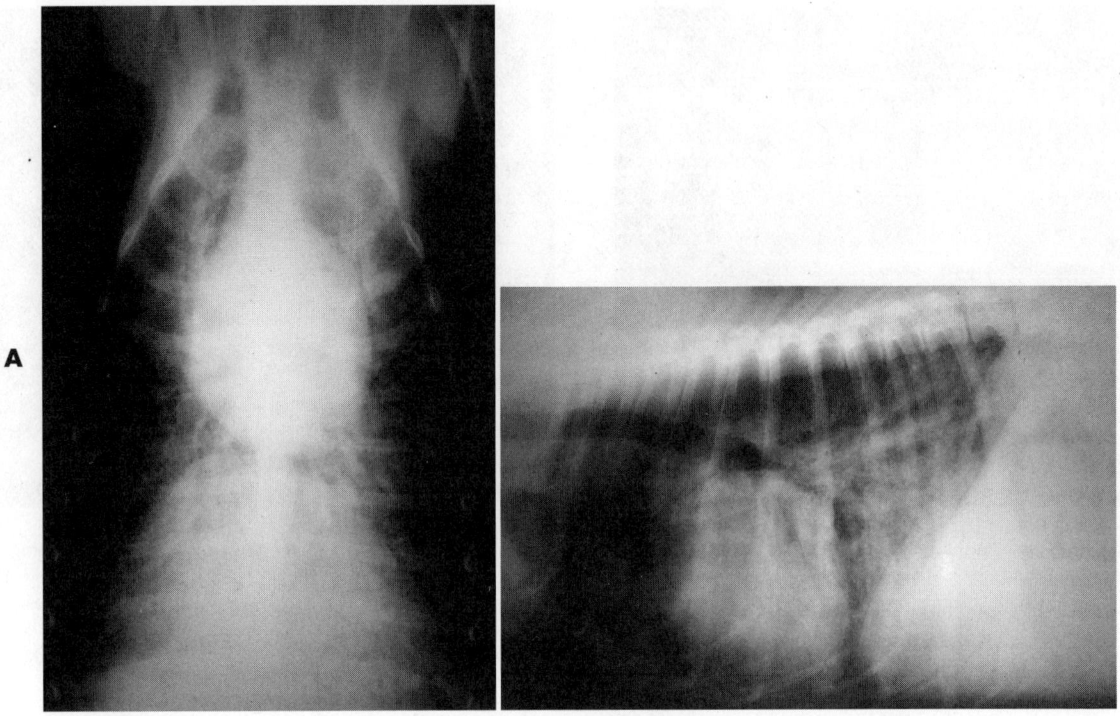

FIGURE 24-6 Dorsoventral (**A**) and lateral (**B**) thoracic radiographs from a Doberman pinscher with aortic valve endocarditis and acute, severe aortic regurgitation. The dog is in left heart failure (pulmonary edema). The cardiac silhouette is not enlarged because the left heart has not had time to enlarge.

A history of a predisposing factor (previous bacterial infection, recent dental procedure, immunosuppressive drug therapy, intravenous or urinary tract catheterization, trauma) is uncommon in canine or feline patients with infective endocarditis. Patients are most commonly presented because they appear systemically ill to the owner. They are often depressed and weak. They commonly are not eating well or not eating at all. Weight loss is frequent. They may have signs of left heart failure. The owners often note respiratory abnormalities (tachypnea, dyspnea, cough) in this situation. Concomitant discospondylitis is a common problem.

Systemic septic emboli commonly lodge in various regions of the body and can create a multitude of clinical signs. Very small emboli may take the first exit off the aorta and travel down a coronary artery, creating a small, septic myocardial infarct. This can cause sudden death or an arrhythmia. Slightly larger emboli may take the first large exit off the aorta, which is the brachiocephalic trunk. They then take the first exit off the brachiocephalic trunk (the right subclavian artery) and lodge in the right front leg. This causes a right front leg lameness. Although right front leg lameness is most common in our experience, other legs are commonly involved. Larger emboli can travel to numerous regions of the body, creating infarcts in kidney, brain, spleen, or bowel. Appropriate clinical signs are produced. Lameness is a common clinical sign in dogs with infective endocarditis.[2] It may be due to septic embolization of skeletal muscle or to arthritis. Two types of arthritis have been described in dogs with infective endocarditis.[27] One is septic arthritis, presumably secondary to bacteremia or embolization. The other is a sterile arthritis, thought to be due to immune complex deposition that occurs secondary to the bacterial antigenemia. The lameness may be stable or shift from leg to leg.

On physical examination, most canine patients will have a fever or a recent history of a fever. Patients that are already being administered antibiotics or corticosteroids or patients that are in severe heart failure may be afebrile.[17] A heart murmur is also a common finding. Discovering a new heart murmur in a patient that is febrile is the classic finding to make one suspicious of infective endocarditis. Of course, most clinicians realize that classic findings usually do not occur in most cases. In one study, only 25 out of 61 cases of dogs with infective endocarditis had a new or latent heart murmur.[2] A systolic heart murmur is the most common. In infective endocarditis the murmur can be heard with either mitral or aortic involvement. The murmur associated with mitral valve endocarditis is that of mitral regurgitation. In one report of 24 dogs with aortic valve endocarditis, 23 had a systolic heart murmur, although the intensity was not reported.[11] Presumably at least some of these systolic murmurs were due to some degree of aortic stenosis. Others may have been due to concomitant disease, such as myxomatous atrioventricular valve degeneration, or may have been flow murmurs secondary to fever-induced high cardiac output. The significance of a systolic heart murmur may be difficult to ascertain in an individual patient. If the murmur is grade 3 or louder and can be documented to be new and the patient is febrile, infective endocarditis must be a primary differential diagnosis. Being certain that a systolic heart murmur has only occurred recently, however, is often difficult. A loud heart murmur in a young dog with a fever examined previously by a veterinarian, however, should be considered a new murmur until proven otherwise. Even in an older, large-breed dog, a loud systolic heart murmur is not common. Consequently, it can be considered highly suspicious for recent valve tissue destruction if the patient has or has had a fever. A loud systolic murmur in a small-breed, geriatric dog (even one with a fever) is most commonly due to myxomatous mitral valve degeneration, not to infective endocarditis. A soft systolic murmur in a large dog can be due to infective endocarditis but can also occur with numerous other

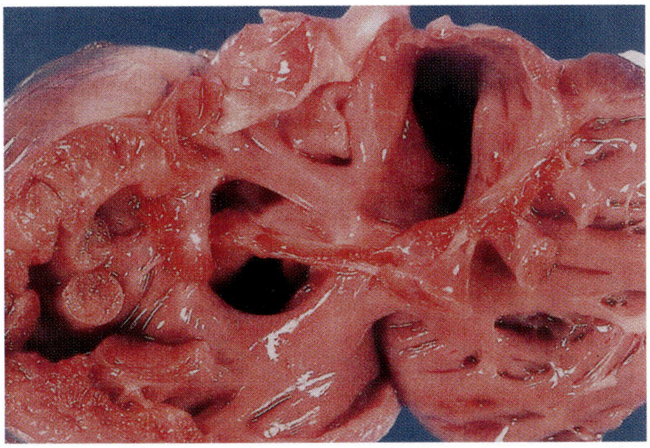

COLOR PLATE 64 Postmortem cardiac specimen from a 7-month-old male domestic shorthair cat with a complete atrioventricular (AV) canal defect. The right side of the heart has been opened, revealing a large defect that involves the upper portion of the interventricular septum and the lower portion of the atrial septum. The common AV leaflet crosses the defect and does not attach to either septum. The valve attaches directly to the papillary muscles. (From Liu SK, Hsu FS, Lee RCT: *An atlas of cardiovascular pathology,* Taiwan, 1989, Pig Research Institute)

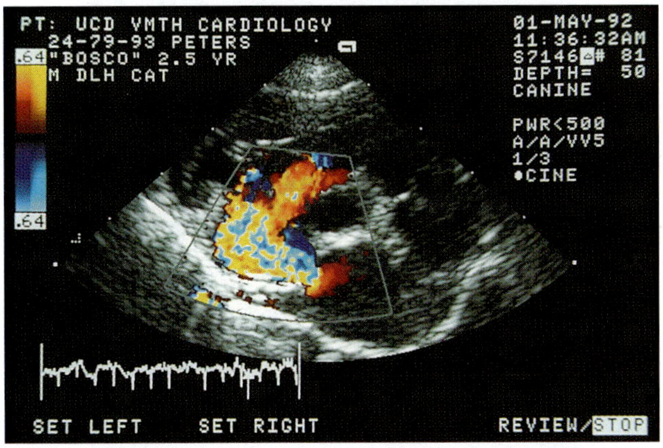

COLOR PLATE 65 Color flow Doppler echocardiogram from the cat shown in Figure 18-6, from the same view. Laminar flow (bright red) starts in LA2 and becomes turbulent as it crosses through the membrane separating LA2 from LA1.

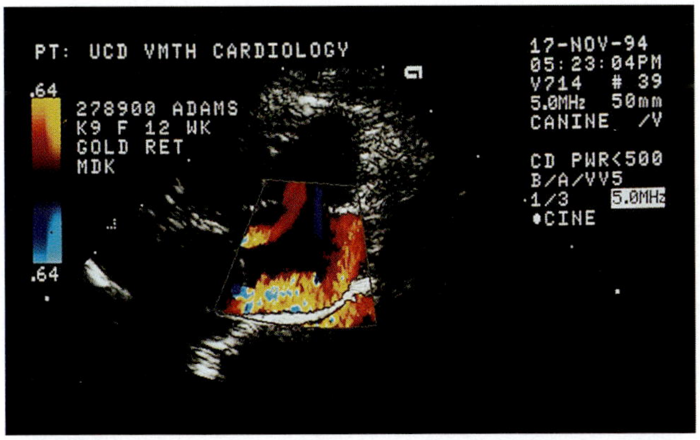

COLOR PLATE 66 Color flow Doppler echocardiogram from the dog shown in Figure 18-7. There are two perforations in the membrane that allow blood to flow from RA1 to RA2. Blood flow is turbulent. At cardiac catheterization, the pressure in RA1 was 14 mm Hg and in RA2 it was 3 mm Hg.

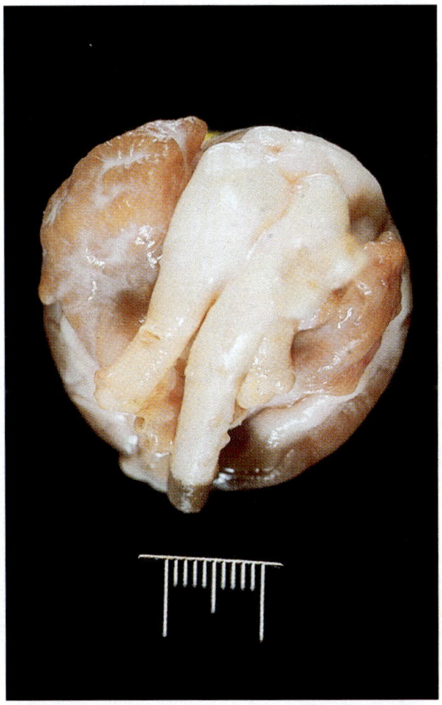

COLOR PLATE 67 Great vessels from the cat shown in Figure 18-9, viewed from above at postmortem examination. The picture is oriented with the cranial part of the heart on the top of the figure. The aorta is the large vessel on the right, and the pulmonary artery is on the left. They course parallel to each other.

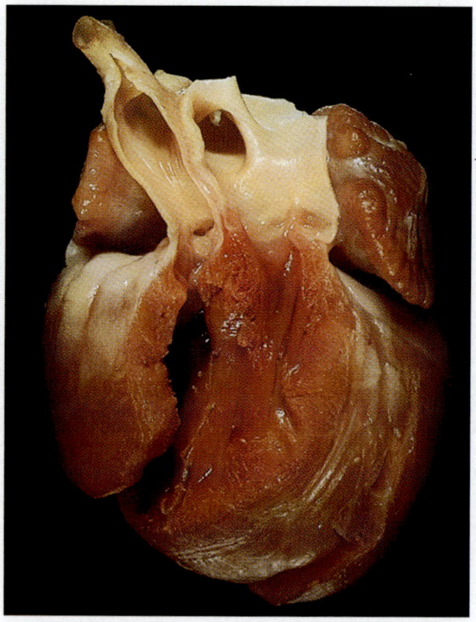

COLOR PLATE 68 The right ventricular outflow tract and right ventricle from the cat in Figure 18-9 and Color Plate 67 have been opened. The picture is taken from the front of the heart. The pulmonary artery originates normally from the right ventricular outflow tract. The aorta is malpositioned, originating from the right ventricle, to the right (anatomically) of the pulmonary artery.

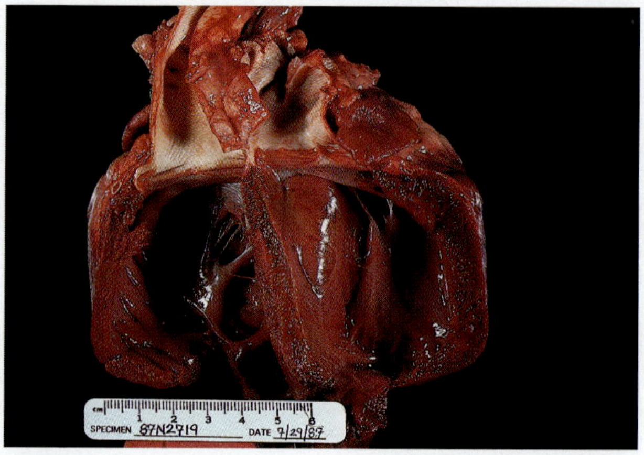

COLOR PLATE 69 Picture of a heart taken from a young llama with transposition of the great vessels. The picture is taken from the front so that the right ventricle is on the left side of the picture and the left ventricle is on the right. The pulmonary artery originates from the left ventricle and branches above the heart. The aorta originates from the right ventricle.

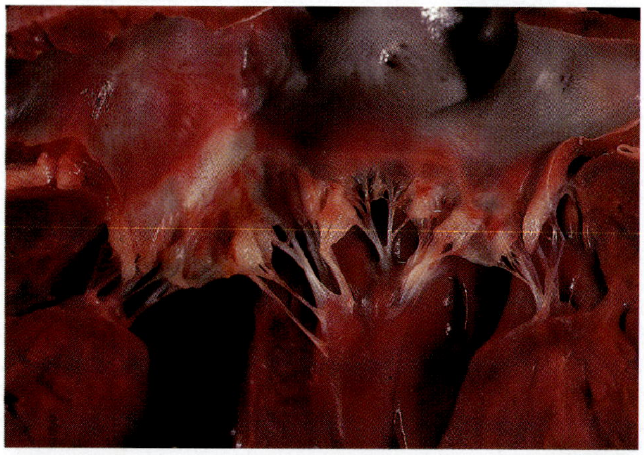

COLOR PLATE 70 Postmortem specimen of a mitral valve from a dog with moderate myxomatous mitral valve degeneration. The leaflet edges are thickened and contracted.

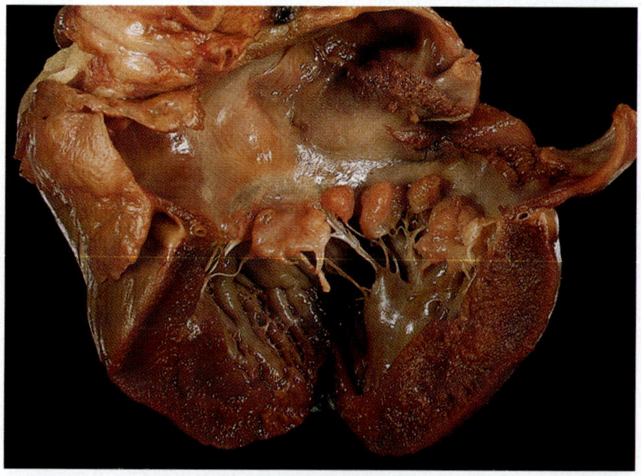

COLOR PLATE 71 Heart from a 16-year-old terrier cross with a long history of mitral regurgitation and left heart failure. The dog died acutely. There is severe myxomatous mitral valve degeneration, a fresh tear in the left atrial wall, and a partially healed left atrial tear. The primary chorda tendineae attached to the septal leaflet is ruptured, which is a lethal injury.

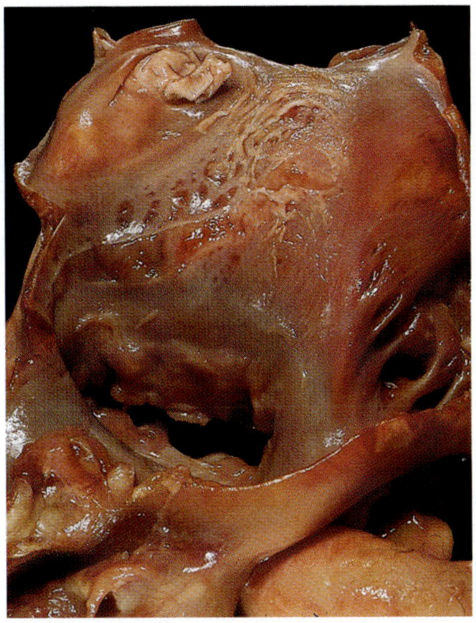

COLOR PLATE 72 Jet lesion in the left atrium from a dog with severe mitral regurgitation. The endocardial fibrous tissue that makes up the jet lesion is rippled as if pushed dorsally by the regurgitant jet. There is also a large endocardial tear.

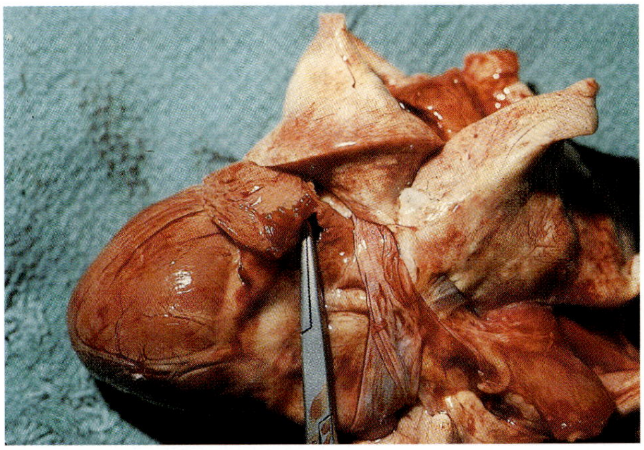

COLOR PLATE 73 Heart from a 14-year-old terrier that died suddenly. There is a large left atrial tear that resulted in acute pericardial tamponade.

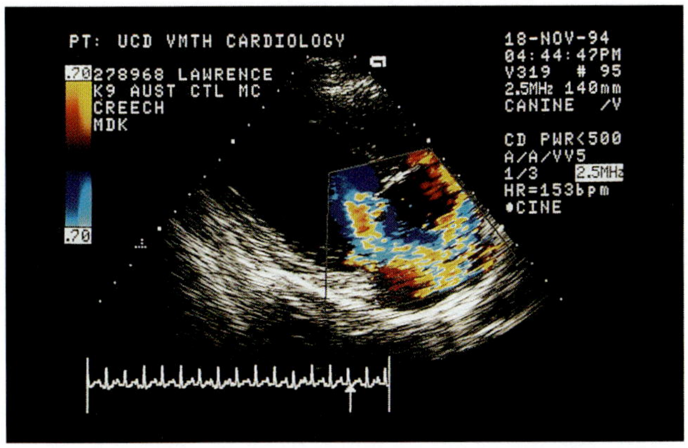

COLOR PLATE 74 Color flow Doppler echocardiogram showing severe mitral regurgitation from the dog shown in Figure 19-23. Blood flow accelerates toward the mitral valve orifice. The color jet originates at the mitral valve and strikes the dorsal wall of the left atrium during systole.

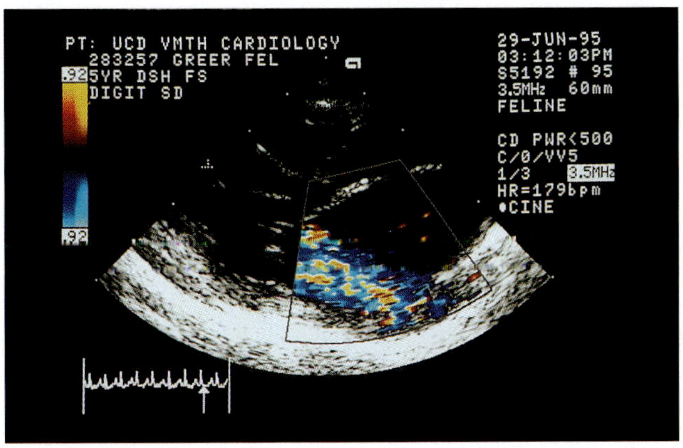

COLOR PLATE 75 Color flow Doppler echocardiogram from the cat shown in Figure 19-24 showing severe mitral regurgitation.

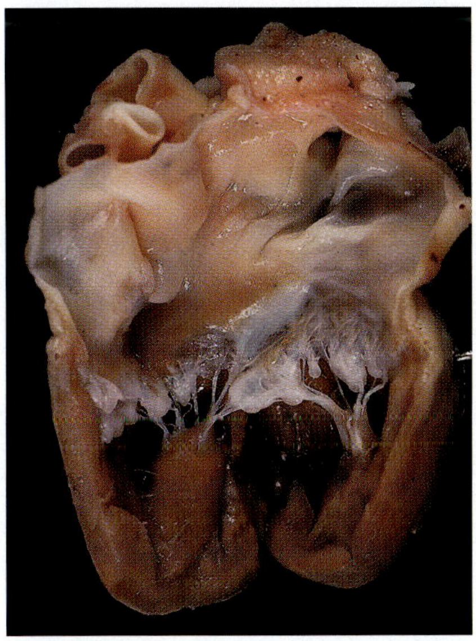

COLOR PLATE 76 Heart from the cat shown in Figure 19-24 at postmortem examination. The mitral valves are severely thickened. Histopathologic examination confirmed myxomatous degeneration.

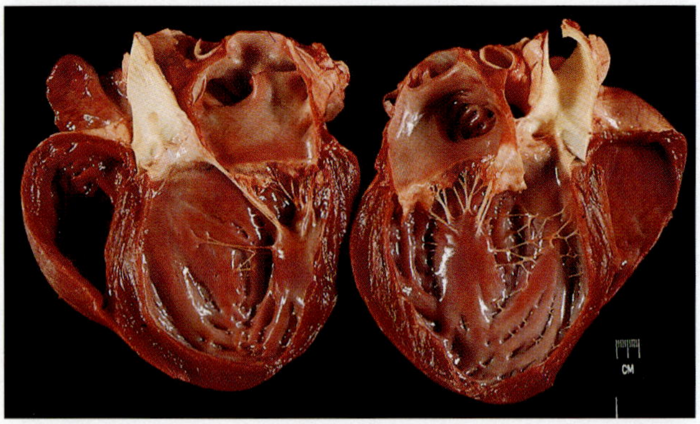

COLOR PLATE 77 Postmortem example of a heart from a great Dane with severe dilated cardiomyopathy. The left ventricular and left atrial chambers are enlarged. The left ventricular cavity has a "scooped-out" appearance.

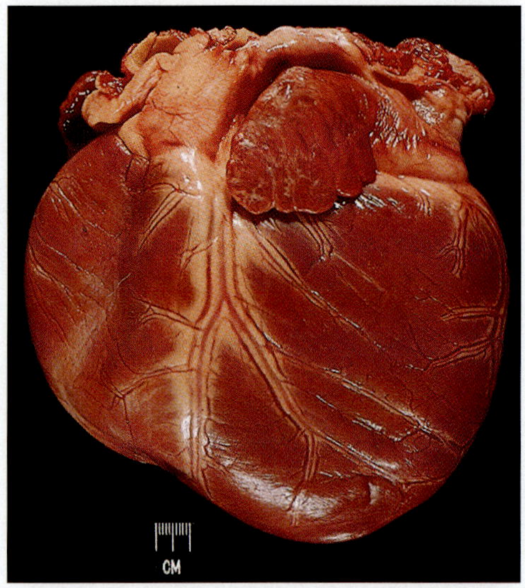

COLOR PLATE 78 Heart shown in Color Plate 77 before opening the heart. The heart does not retain its shape. Instead it has collapsed when placed on the table.

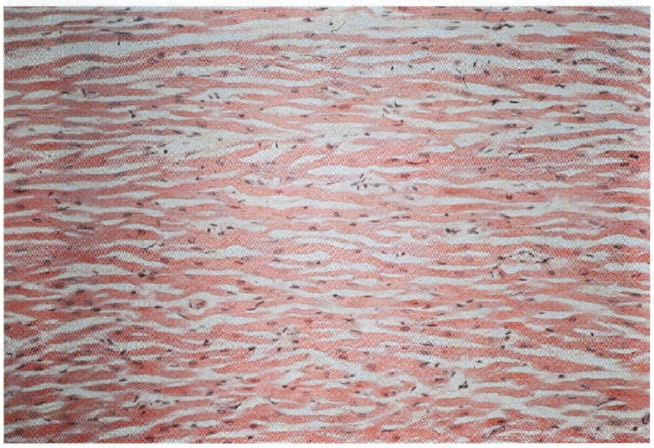

COLOR PLATE 79 Histopathologic section of myocardium from a cat with dilated cardiomyopathy. The myofibrils are longer than normal. There is no evidence of degenerative or inflammatory changes.

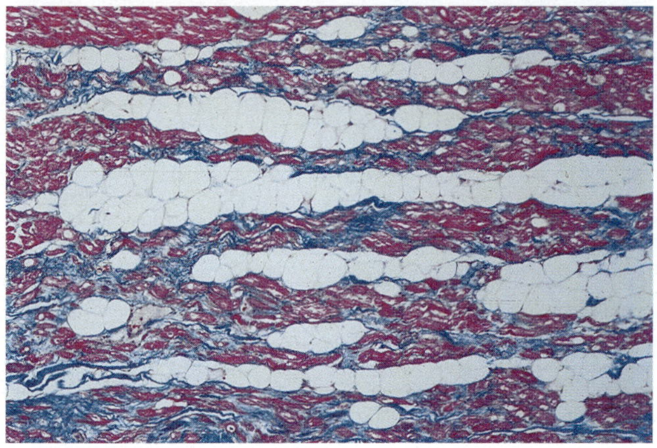

COLOR PLATE 80 Histopathologic section from a papillary muscle from a Doberman pinscher with dilated cardiomyopathy. There is marked replacement and interstitial fibrosis and fatty replacement of tissue. The tissue was stained with Masson's (trichrome) stain. Fibrous connective tissue is stained blue. (Courtesy of Dr. Lyndon Badcoe.)

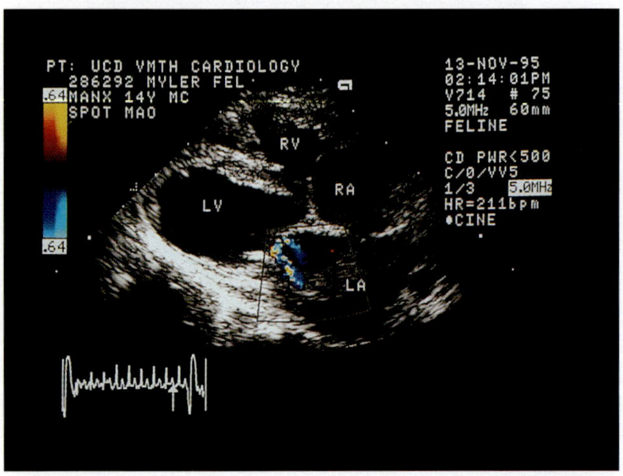

COLOR PLATE 81 Two-dimensional echocardiogram with color flow Doppler echocardiogram from a 14-year-old cat with severe myocardial failure. The frame is taken during late systole. The left ventricle and left atrium are markedly increased in size. The thickness of the interventricular septum is normal. The left ventricular free wall is thin. Mild mitral regurgitation is evident as two small turbulent color flow jets originating at the mitral valve and extending into the left atrium.

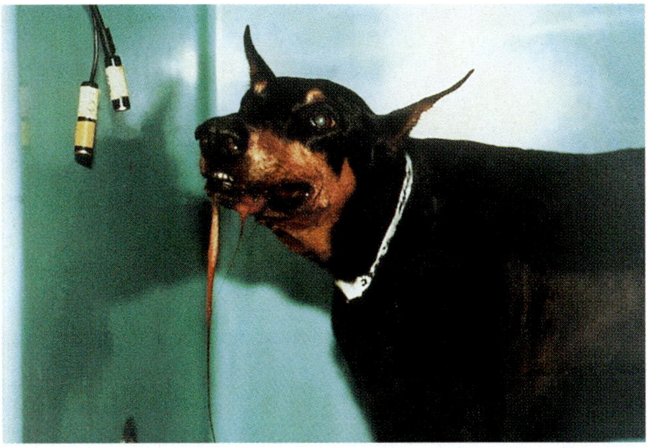

COLOR PLATE 82 Doberman pinscher that presented in fulminant heart failure. The dog was dyspneic and severely tachypneic (respiratory rate = 84 breaths/min) at presentation. Pulmonary edema fluid is dripping from his mouth. (Courtesy of Dr. Grant Guilford.)

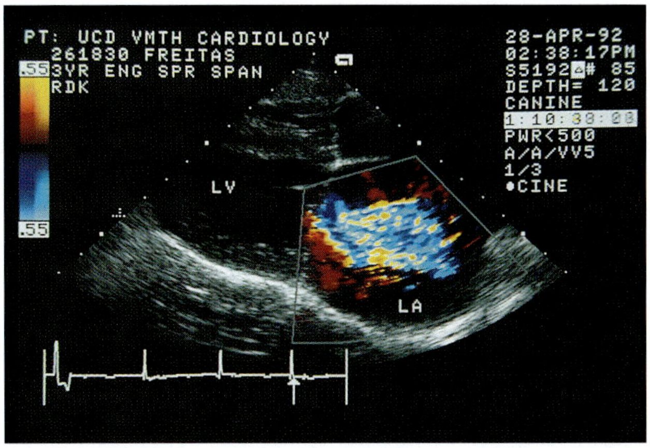

COLOR PLATE 83 Two-dimensional and color flow echocardiogram from the dog shown in Figure 20-18. There is at least moderate mitral regurgitation present. The mitral regurgitation accounts for the left ventricular volume overload hypertrophy and left atrial enlargement seen in Figures 20-18 and 20-19.

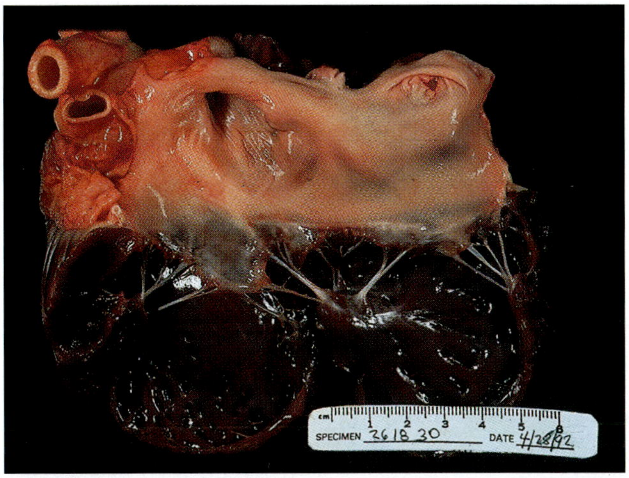

COLOR PLATE 84 Heart opened through the left atrium and ventricle from an English springer spaniel with atrial standstill, mitral regurgitation, and mild myocardial failure. Note the pinkish-white color of the left atrium, which is due to replacement of the myocardium by fibrous tissue. There is mild mitral valve degeneration.

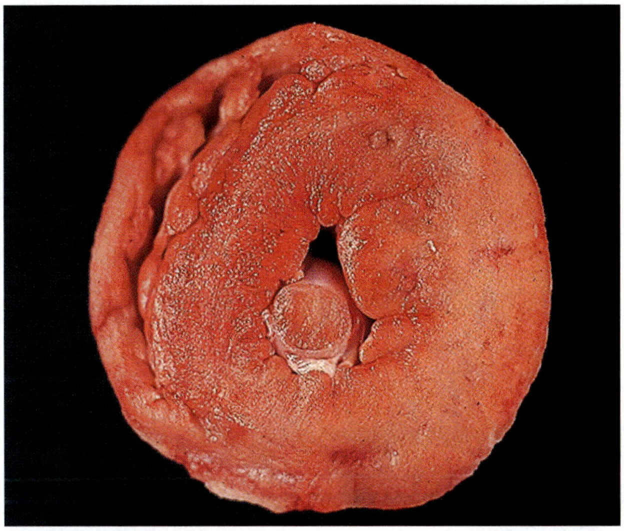

COLOR PLATE 85 Postmortem specimen of a heart from a cat with hypertrophic cardiomyopathy. The heart has been cut in cross-section at the level of the papillary muscles. The entire left ventricular wall and the papillary muscles are grossly thickened. The left ventricular chamber is small.

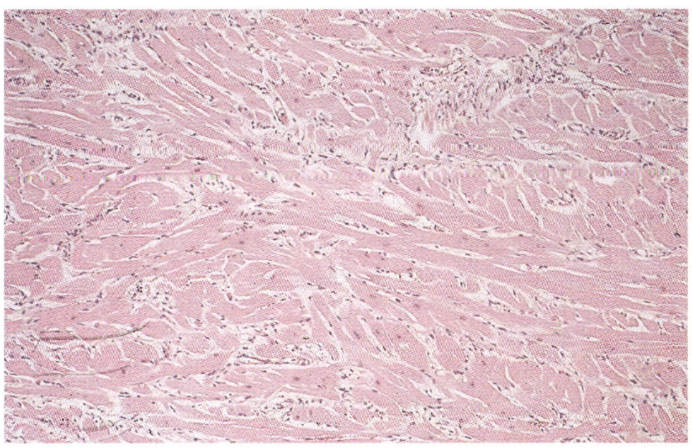

COLOR PLATE 86 Histologic section of myocardium from a Maine coon cat with hypertrophic cardiomyopathy showing myofiber disarray. This type of disarray occurs in only about 30% of cats with hypertrophic cardiomyopathy.

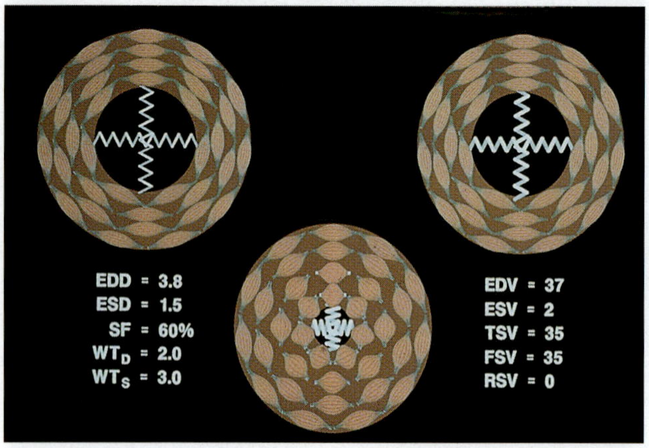

COLOR PLATE 87 Schematic diagram, similar to those seen in Chapters 2 and 9, of severe hypertrophic cardiomyopathy. The numbers correspond to those for an animal that is 25 to 30 kg (1 m^2 of body surface area) and so do not relate to normal numbers for a cat. Note that the left ventricular wall has doubled in thickness via the sarcomeres increasing in parallel. The left ventricular end-diastolic and end-systolic volumes are decreased. *EDD,* End diastolic diameter; *ESD,* end systolic diameter; *SF,* shortening fraction; WT_D, wall thickness in diastole; WT_S, wall thickness in systole; *EDV,* end diastolic volume; *ESV,* end systolic volume; *TSV,* total stroke volume; *FSV,* forward stroke volume; *RSV,* right stroke volume.

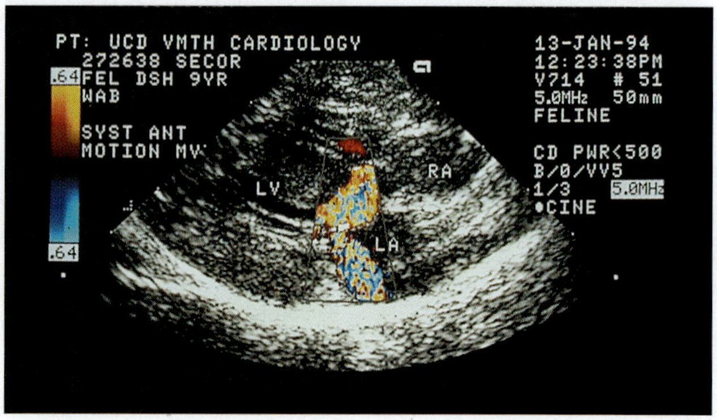

COLOR PLATE 88 Color flow Doppler two-dimensional echocardiogram from a cat with hypertrophic cardiomyopathy showing two turbulent jets, one of mitral regurgitation going into the left atrium and one of dynamic subaortic stenosis going into the aorta. *LV,* Left ventricle; *LA,* left atrium; *RA,* right atrium.

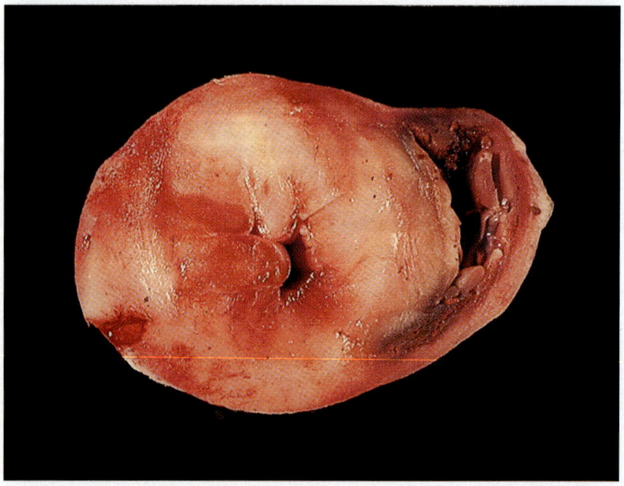

COLOR PLATE 89 Postmortem specimen of a heart infiltrated with lymphoma. The left ventricular walls are grossly thickened. The myocardium has large white patches that contain malignant lymphocytes. This 2-year-old cat was diagnosed with hypertrophic cardiomyopathy on an echocardiogram. The owner elected to euthanize the animal.

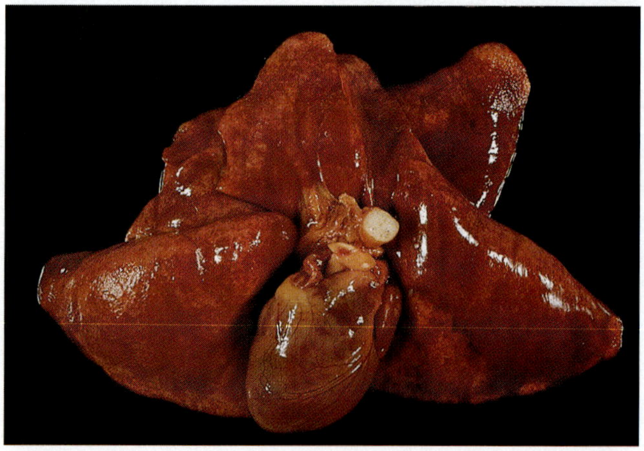

COLOR PLATE 90 Heart and lungs from a 2-year-old male Maine coon cat that died of heart failure secondary to hypertrophic cardiomyopathy. The lungs appear rounded and wet. There is pulmonary edema fluid emanating from the trachea.

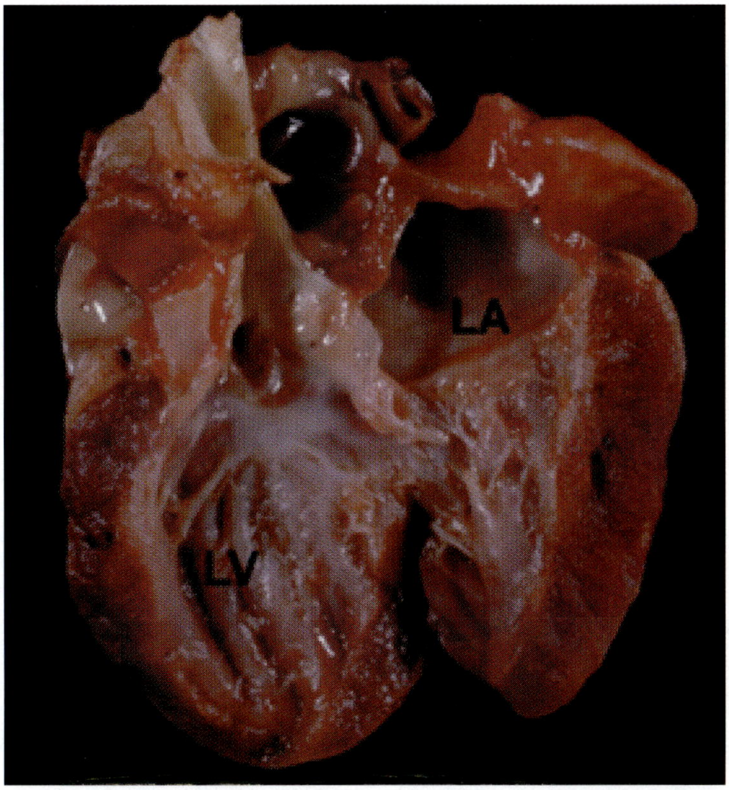

COLOR PLATE 91 The left heart from a seven-year-old cat that presented with acute rear limb pain and paralysis, along with tachypnea resulting from a terminal aortic thromboembolus and pulmonary edema, respectively. Echocardiography revealed a severely enlarged left atrium and a normal-appearing left ventricle. The cat was diagnosed with unclassified cardiomyopathy and was euthanized at the owner's request. The postmortem examination revealed the severely enlarged left atrium and endomyocardial fibrosis. The endocardium in this picture is white because of the increased fibrous tissue. *LA,* Left atrium; *LV,* left ventricle.

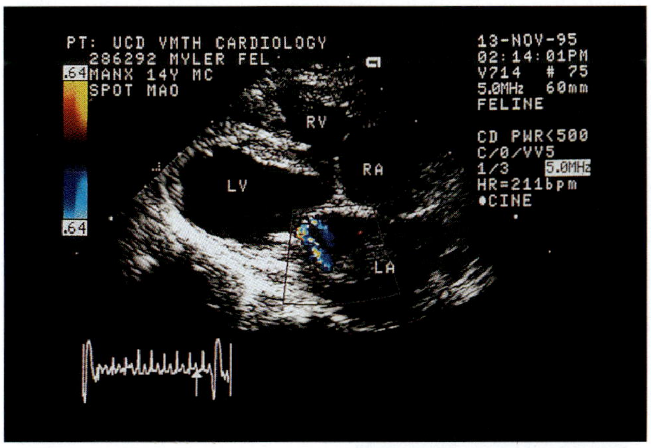

COLOR PLATE 92 Right parasternal short-axis view from a cat with unclassified cardiomyopathy. Severe left atrial enlargement is noted, and there is a large thrombus within the left auricle.

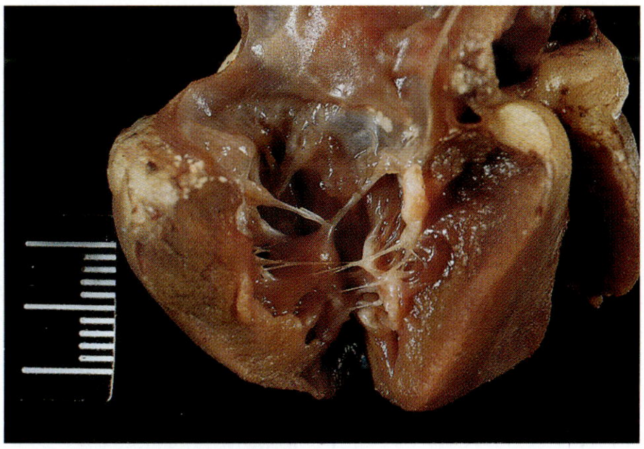

COLOR PLATE 93 Gross pathologic specimen from a cat with moderator band cardiomyopathy. The apex of the left ventricle has been opened and is viewed from the apex. Numerous thickened and irregular false tendons can be seen in the apical region of the left ventricular chamber.

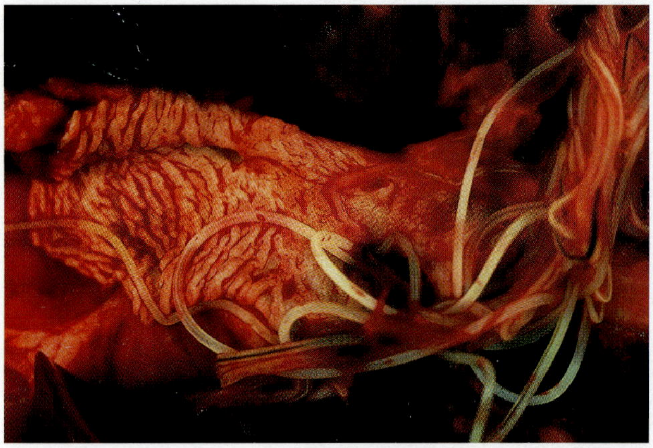

COLOR PLATE 94 Adult heartworms in the pulmonary arteries of a dog at postmortem examination. Obvious villous proliferation of the endothelium in response to the presence of adult heartworms is present.

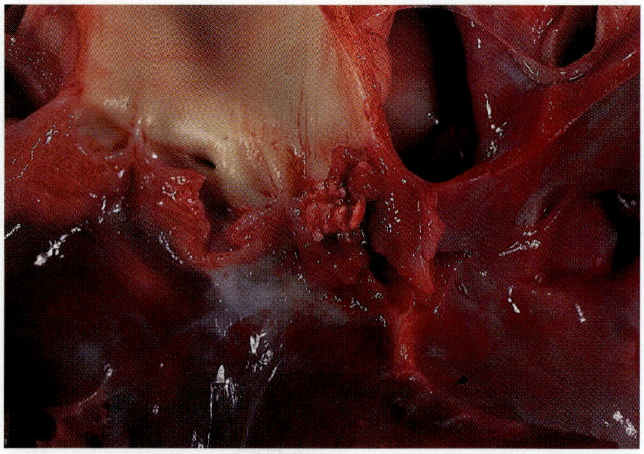

COLOR PLATE 95 Postmortem specimen of the aortic root, aortic valve, and left ventricular outflow tract from a dog with aortic valve endocarditis. The cusp on the left is thickened, the cusp in the middle has a destructive lesion, and the cusp on the right has a vegetative lesion.

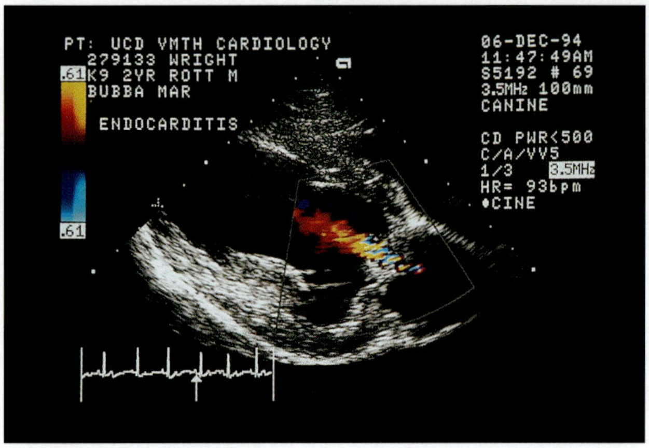

COLOR PLATE 96 Color flow Doppler echocardiogram from the dog shown in Figure 24-1. Moderate aortic regurgitation is present late in diastole.

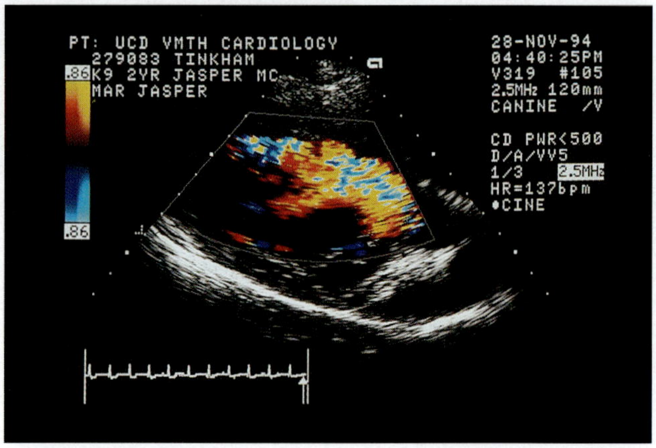

COLOR PLATE 97 Color flow Doppler echocardiogram using a right parasternal long-axis view taken from the dog shown in Figure 24-9 showing severe aortic regurgitation secondary to the aortic valve infective endocarditis.

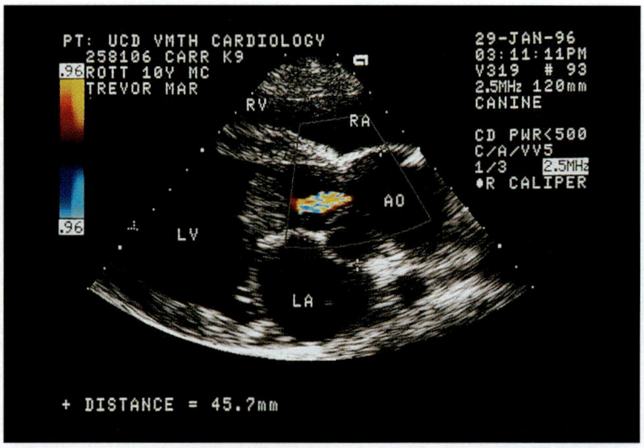

COLOR PLATE 98 Aortic regurgitation is present on the color flow Doppler echocardiogram. Although the size of the color jet is small, the left ventricular chamber is enlarged, indicating that the aortic regurgitation is moderate to severe. The dog was not in heart failure but did have a chylothorax. It also had a history of a leiomyoma of the esophagus, megaesophagus, and aspiration pneumonia. *LA* = Left atrium; *RVOT* = right ventricular outflow tract; *RA* = right atrium; *RV* = right ventricular chamber.

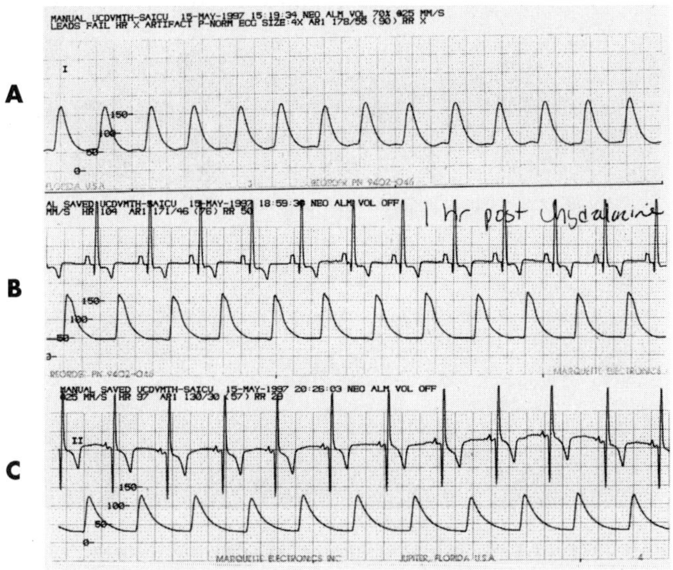

FIGURE 24-7 **A,** Recording of arterial blood pressure through an indwelling catheter from a boxer with severe aortic regurgitation secondary to infective endocarditis. The systolic pressure is approximately 175 mm Hg, and the diastolic pressure is approximately 55 mm Hg. The pulse pressure is greatly increased to 120 mm Hg. **B,** Simultaneous recordings of an ECG and arterial blood pressure following hydralazine 0.5 mg/kg PO. Pressures are essentially unchanged. **C,** The same recordings 1 hour after an additional dose of hydralazine 0.5 mg/kg PO. The pressures have decreased appropriately and the dog improved clinically.

cardiovascular lesions. It can also be due to an increased stroke volume secondary to fever.

A diastolic heart murmur due to aortic regurgitation is commonly identified in dogs with aortic valve endocarditis.[11] The murmur of aortic regurgitation is often soft and therefore difficult to identify. Consequently, one must auscult any patient suspected of having infective endocarditis very carefully in a quiet room. The murmur is heard best over the left base. It is blowing in character. It starts immediately after the second heart sound and decreases in intensity (decrescendo) through diastole. Infective endocarditis is by far the most common cause of an audible diastolic heart murmur secondary to aortic regurgitation in the dog and cat. Consequently, identification of a diastolic heart murmur heard best over the left base in a dog or cat, especially in one with a fever, should be regarded as caused by infective endocarditis until proven otherwise.

Dogs with aortic regurgitation often have an increase in pulse pressure (bounding pulse; Figure 24-7). Systolic pressure is commonly increased because of the increased stroke volume that the left ventricle must generate in systole to compensate for the leak. The diastolic pressure is decreased because of blood flowing back into the left ventricle in diastole.

Diagnosis

Before the arrival of echocardiography, the diagnosis of infective endocarditis in humans was typically based on clinical signs of infection (fever, leukocytosis, etc.) and positive blood cultures combined with a new regurgitant heart murmur. Alternatively, it was based on positive blood cultures, predisposing heart disease, and evidence of embolic disease.[28] In patients with negative blood cultures, the patient had to have a fever, a new regurgitant heart murmur, and evidence of embolic disease to be definitively diagnosed with infective endocarditis. When transthoracic echocardiography became available, it was used as an adjunctive diagnostic tool. Because transthoracic echocardiography lacked sensitivity and specificity for diagnosing infective endocarditis in humans, it was not included in listings of diagnostic criteria. Many false negative findings in humans with infective endocarditis can be attributed to the relatively poor transthoracic image produced in many adult humans. Others can be attributed to the need to use a low-frequency transducer in adult humans. The resolution of a low-frequency transducer is poorer than that of a higher-frequency transducer, resulting in a reduced ability to identify smaller vegetations. More recently, the use of transesophageal echocardiography has markedly increased the image quality in humans, and the sensitivity of identifying infective endocarditis has improved to approximately 90%.[29] Because of this documented improvement in sensitivity, more recent recommendations for diagnosing infective endocarditis have included a positive echocardiographic (transthoracic or transesophageal) finding as a major criterion for diagnosis.[29] However, even this has been disputed.[30]

In small animal veterinary medicine, higher-frequency transducers are routinely used and echocardiographic image quality is usually very good to excellent. In fact, the image quality is usually so good that, in our experience, transesophageal echocardiography usually provides no distinct advantage over transthoracic echocardiography in cats and only provides more detailed information about heart base structures in dogs. We feel that our ability to examine the aortic and mitral valves with transthoracic echocardiography in dogs and cats rivals that of transesophageal echocardiography in adult humans. Because of this and other factors mentioned later in this paragraph, echocardiography has been the major tool used to diagnose infective endocarditis in dogs and cats for the past 10 years at our institution. Most patients that we diagnose with infective endocarditis are presented with clinical signs that suggest it, and the diagnosis is made using echocardiography. Blood cultures are then used to attempt to identify the offending organism. Blood cultures are almost never used to make the definitive diagnosis of infective endocarditis because they lack sensitivity and specificity in dogs and cats. Of dogs with infective endocarditis, blood cultures are positive in 50% to 90% of the cases (lack of sensitivity). The variability in the percentage of positive cases is probably due to the variability in skill and diligence of various microbiology laboratories, as well as the criteria used for diagnosing infective endocarditis. In one previous report of dogs examined before the widespread use of echocardiography (before 1982), blood cultures were positive in 88% of cases diagnosed with infective endocarditis.[2] However, one of the primary diagnostic criteria for the diagnosis of infective endocarditis in this report was a positive blood culture. Currently, most of our cases are initially diagnosed based on clinical signs (usually fever, leukocytosis with a heart murmur, or signs consistent with systemic embolic disease) and echocardiography, and then blood cultures are obtained. In this situation, we estimate that our laboratory's success rate at identifying the offending organism is closer to 50%. This poor success rate may be related to prior antibiotic therapy (a common problem), fastidious organisms, laboratory technique, or noncontinuous shedding of organisms in dogs and cats with infective endocarditis (species difference from humans). Since the advent of the use of echocardiography as a major diagnostic tool for diagnosing infective endocarditis in humans, the number of culture negative cases has increased to as high as 41% in one series of cases.[31]

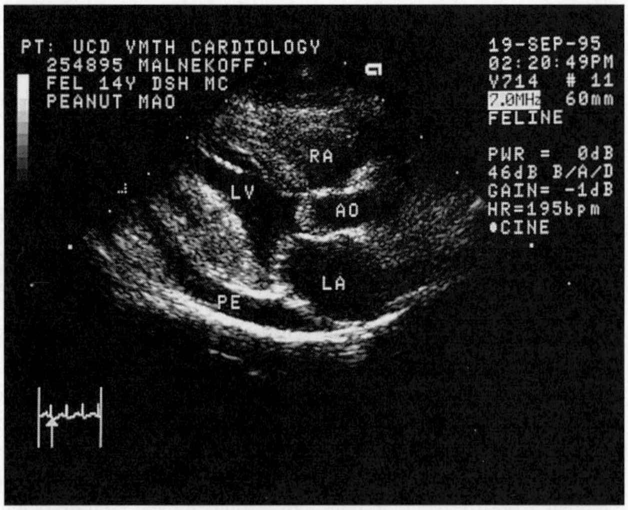

FIGURE 24-8 Two-dimensional echocardiogram from a 14-year-old cat with severe aortic valve endocarditis. Although the vegetative lesions on the aortic valve cusps are obvious and larger than 3 mm in width, one can readily appreciate structures within the vegetations and other cardiovascular structures that are 1 mm in size. *LV,* Left ventricular chamber; *LA,* left atrium; *AO,* aorta; *RA,* right atrium; *PE,* pericardial effusion.

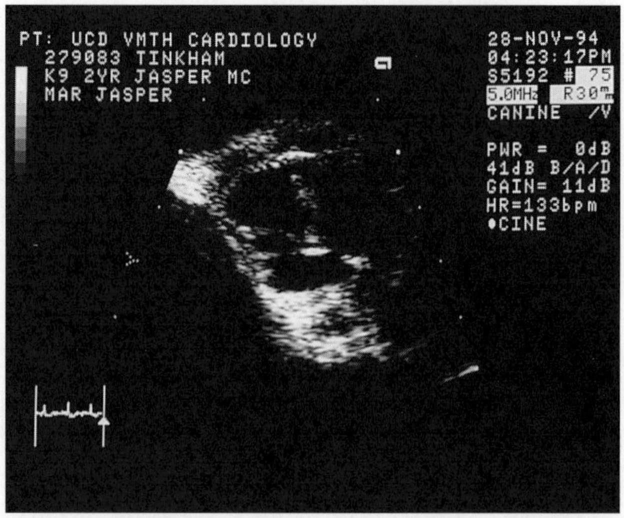

FIGURE 24-9 Two-dimensional echocardiogram using a right parasternal cross-sectional view of the aortic root and aortic valve leaflets from a 1.5-year-old Labrador retriever. There is a large defect (region of valve destruction) between the right and noncoronary cusps of the aortic valve. The dog was presented with a history of a fever, leukocytosis, and anorexia 2 weeks before admission. The referring veterinarian had administered enrofloxacin per os, and the fever had abated. Recurrence of anorexia prompted the referral. On physical examination a diastolic heart murmur, bounding femoral arterial pulses, and an arrhythmia were noted. The dog also had a right coxofemoral luxation, and the owner decided to euthanize the dog. Pathology revealed a thick, fibrillar, yellow adherent material on the aortic valve cusps and a large aortic valve perforation. Histopathologically the aortic valve lesions were consistent with infective endocarditis, although no organisms were identified. No organisms grew on culture. The lung lobes were diffusely edematous, and the trachea was filled with white-red frothy material, consistent with pulmonary edema.

Blood cultures are never used definitively to make a diagnosis of infective endocarditis because they are also positive in other diseases (lack of specificity). In one study, of 165 dogs with positive blood cultures, only 45 were diagnosed as having infective endocarditis. A similar number (42) had discospondylitis. Presumably the rest were septicemic secondary to other diseases. Critically ill animals frequently develop sepsis and have positive blood culture results.[32] Dogs with discospondylitis can have clinical signs that closely mimic infective endocarditis.

Echocardiography, however, is not 100% sensitive or specific. In humans, vegetations less than 3 mm in diameter usually go undetected.[3] Modern two-dimensional echocardiography equipment can resolve down to less than 1 mm. It is difficult to believe that in a small patient, such as a cat, a lesion 2 mm in diameter or smaller could not be visualized, because a normal left ventricular wall in a cat can be 3 mm thick (Figure 24-8). Consequently, we believe that it is incorrect to transfer statements regarding the ability to resolve or detect a lesion based on size from human texts directly to the situation in veterinary medicine. Instead, we believe that we can identify smaller lesions that are present in smaller animals with modern equipment. Besides identifying vegetations, dogs with destructive lesions of their valves but without vegetations can be diagnosed with infective endocarditis based on the presence of a regurgitant lesion and the echocardiographic appearance of the valve, especially when the aortic valve is involved (Figures 24-9, Color Plate 97). It has been stated in the human literature that the echocardiogram is positive in up to 80% of patients with infective endocarditis, but the usual sensitivity is 60%.[3] We believe that our sensitivity is greater than 90%. In fact, we think that missing the diagnosis of infective endocarditis when echocardiography is used is very unusual in our clinic. Specificity (false positive diagnoses) can sometimes be a problem. This occurs primarily in the older small breed of dog with myxomatous mitral valve disease. The degenerative lesions that involve the mitral valve in these dogs can be mistaken for vegetations. In dogs with no history of fever, lameness, and so on, the abnormal appearance to the valve is almost always due to myxomatous degenerative change. Differentiation between mitral valve degeneration and infective endocarditis in an older, small-breed dog with a fever or other evidence of infection may be impossible. However, blood cultures do not necessarily make the distinction possible either, if the patient is bacteremic or septic from another cause. In some cases, the echocardiographic appearance of a vegetative lesion is different from that of a myxomatous lesion (Figure 24-10). These cases may have a lesion or lesions that appear more isolated and echodense than myxomatous lesions. False negative findings may be a problem with tricuspid valve lesions. In one report, endocarditis lesions on the tricuspid valve were not detected in the two dogs examined.[12]

We have devised a list of diagnostic criteria used in diagnosing infective endocarditis in dogs and cats (Box 24-1). From these criteria we have devised a diagnostic scheme for diagnosing infective endocarditis in dogs and cats (Box 24-2).

Blood cultures must be obtained to try to identify the offending organism and subsequently to identify the appropriate antibiotic in patients with infective endocarditis. Although bacteremia is continuous in bacterial endocarditis in humans and therefore thought to be continuous in animals, this may not be true in dogs and cats. It certainly does not translate into a 100% success rate at identifying the offending organism in veterinary patients with endocarditis. The bacterial numbers are usually small (less than 100 bacteria/mL of blood) and can be very small (less than 10 bacteria/mL of blood) in humans and are probably the same or less in veterinary patients.[3] The bacteria are collected, in this situation, in blood that contains

A 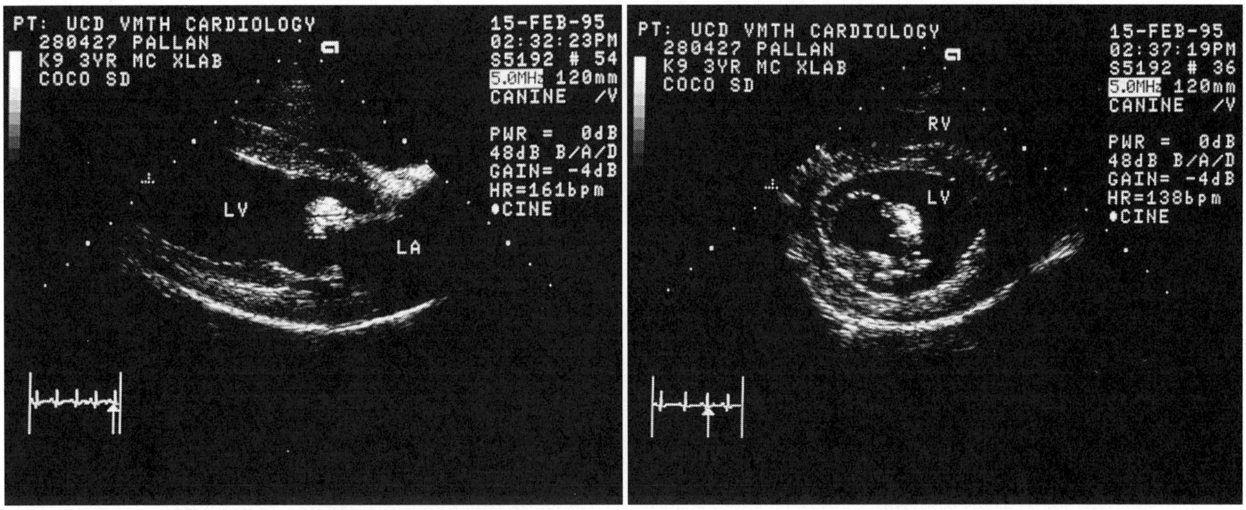 B

FIGURE 24-10 Two-dimensional echocardiograms from a 3-year-old Labrador retriever with mitral valve endocarditis. The dog was a castrated male. **A,** In the right parasternal long-axis view, the septal leaflet of the mitral valve is markedly thickened and could be mistaken for a myxomatous lesion. However, the dog is young and a large breed, which makes this diagnosis unlikely. In addition, the lesion is more echodense than most myxomatous lesions. **B,** In the short-axis view, a discrete, echodense lesion can be identified on the septal leaflet. These findings are compatible with endocarditis. This dog had been presented to the referring veterinarian for lameness and a fever. A polyarthritis had been diagnosed. The arthritis did not respond to tetracycline, so corticosteroids were administered. This resulted in transient improvement followed by return of the fever. A loud left apical systolic heart murmur was identified, and the dog was referred. The endocarditis, a pneumonia, and spinal lesions were diagnosed. Bacterial cultures of the blood and joints were negative. The dog was initially treated with ampicillin and amikacin. This was followed by amoxicillin and clavulanic acid. Two months later the dog had improved clinically, and the valvular lesions were improved. Antibiotics were continued. Two months following that examination, however, the dog presented in left heart failure. The dog was treated with furosemide and lisinopril and lost to follow-up. *LV,* Left ventricular chamber; *LA,* left atrium; *RV,* right ventricular chamber.

BOX 24-1

Diagnostic criteria for the diagnosis of infective endocarditis in dogs and cats

I. Major Criteria
   A. Positive echocardiographic findings
      - Vegetative lesions
      - Destructive lesions
      - Thickened aortic valve leaflets
   B. Positive blood cultures in the absence of diskospondylitis or obvious sepsis
      - At least three positive cultures when common skin contaminants are cultured
      - Preferably at least two positive blood cultures with other organisms
   C. The recent onset of a diastolic heart murmur or evidence of more than trivial aortic regurgitation on a Doppler echocardiographic examination in the absence of subaortic stenosis or annuloaortic ectasia

II. Minor Criteria
   A. Fever
   B. Large (greater than 15 kg) dog
   C. New or worsening systolic heart murmur

III. Supporting Evidence
   A. Embolic disease
      - Lameness
      - Renal failure; hematuria
   B. Immunologic disease
      - Lameness
      - Glomerulonephritis
      - Positive immunologic test (ANA, Coombs')
   C. Subaortic stenosis in a dog greater than 5 years of age

BOX 24-2

Criteria for the diagnosis of infective endocarditis in dogs and cats

I. Definite or Very Probable Infective Endocarditis
   A. Pathologic criteria
      - Microorganisms demonstrated by culture or histology in a vegetation
      - Pathologic lesions confirmed by histology to show active endocarditis
   B. Clinical criteria (see Box 24-1)
      - Two major criteria, or
      - Positive echocardiographic finding plus one minor criterion, or
      - Three minor criteria

II. Possible Infective Endocarditis
   A. One major criterion
   B. Two minor criteria
   C. Supporting evidence with at least two minor criteria

III. Not Infective Endocarditis
   A. Identification of alternative diagnosis to explain signs compatible with infective endocarditis
   B. Resolution of clinical signs with short-term antibiotic therapy
   C. No pathologic evidence of infective endocarditis

elements that normally inhibit bacterial growth (e.g., complement) or destroy bacteria (e.g., granulocytes).[33] Consequently, expecting to be able to identify all patients that are bacteremic is unreasonable. If one combines the data from the four largest and most recent reports of infective endocarditis in dogs in which a positive blood culture was not a prerequisite for the diagnosis, out of 78 dogs, 57 (73%) had a positive blood culture and 21 (27%) had a negative blood culture.[2,11-13] Because a positive blood culture strengthens the diagnosis and not all of these dogs had echocardiograms, we believe that these data are probably optimistic if used to predict the number of veterinary patients with infective endocarditis that will have a positive blood culture. Even so, this leaves at least 25% of patients that must be treated without the benefit of a positive culture and a determination of microbial antibiotic sensitivity.

To maximize the chance of identifying the bacteremia through the use of blood cultures in a patient with infective endocarditis, the veterinarian must pay attention to technique. More than one blood culture should always be taken because this increases the chance of success.[2] Preferably the patient should not be on antibiotic therapy at the time of culture, but positive blood cultures can still be obtained, and therefore antibiotic therapy is not an absolute contraindication.[2] It is often stated in the veterinary literature that presence or absence of fever at the time of culture makes no difference. However, in one study 88% of the febrile canine patients had a positive blood culture, whereas only 50% of afebrile patients had a positive blood culture.[2] Obtaining blood cultures from an afebrile patient at the time of echocardiographic diagnosis and then waiting seems prudent. One can then take further cultures if the patient develops a fever, if immediate antibiotic treatment is not required. Commercial vacuum bottles for collecting the blood samples, supplied by a laboratory, should be used. These bottles usually contain a tryptic digestion of protein. An additive such as the anticoagulant sodium polyanetholsulfonate increases the chances of isolating bacteria by anticoagulating the sample and interfering with complement and granulocyte activity.[33] The venipuncture site must be prepared for aseptic collection by clipping the region over the vein and alternately wiping it with povidone iodine and alcohol. The area cannot be touched with an ungloved finger during venipuncture or the chances of culturing a skin contaminant increases greatly. As much blood as possible should be collected, because the more blood that there is in the bottle, the more organisms that are present. This can be a problem in a cat or small dog. At least nine volumes of medium per one volume of blood should be used to dilute the complement and the granulocytes.[33] The blood should be placed in two bottles after collection. One should be left unvented for anaerobic culture, and the other must be vented to produce an aerobic environment. In patients with subacute endocarditis that are not in immediate danger, three separate venous blood cultures should be taken on the first day, at least 1 hour apart. If no growth is obtained by the second day, two more should be taken. If there still is no growth, and the diagnosis is still likely, two more cultures should be taken.[3] If the patient has already been administered antibiotics, three more cultures can be taken over the following week. For patients with acute bacterial endocarditis that have evidence of sepsis or appear to have rapid destruction of valve tissue, three blood cultures should be taken over a 3-hour span and empirical antibiotic therapy should be started. Cultures should be incubated for at least 3 weeks, and Gram's stains should be made at intervals, even if no growth is apparent.[3]

CLINICAL PATHOLOGY

Leukocytosis with a left shift is present in approximately 80% of dogs with infective endocarditis.[2] An increase in the absolute number of monocytes is seen in approximately 90% of cases and is usually greater than 1500 cells/mL.[2] Anemia is also common (60%) and is usually normocytic and normochromic. Severe azotemia occurs in about 10% of cases. If glomerulonephritis is present, proteinuria is present and the patient may be or may become hypoalbuminemic. Hypergammaglobulinemia can occur secondary to the chronic immune stimulation.

Treatment

ANTIMICROBIAL THERAPY

Ideally, antibiotic therapy is chosen based on culture of the offending organism from blood and on identifying an antibiotic to which the organism is sensitive. Every patient suspected of having infective endocarditis should have its blood cultured before antibiotic therapy is instituted. The time that it takes to collect the samples for blood culture does not alter the course of the disease. Antibiotics selected to treat a patient with infective endocarditis must be bactericidal. The bacteria are growing slowly within the vegetations, and the vegetations prevent leukocytes from phagocytizing cells. Consequently, a bacteriostatic agent will not successfully sterilize the vegetation. Optimally, the serum concentrations of the antibiotics should be in the high end of therapeutic range for weeks. In humans, antibiotics are administered intravenously every 4 to 8 hours for 4 to 6 weeks.[3] Presumably this type of aggressive approach would also be preferred in dogs and cats. This approach, however, is often not economically feasible. Teaching an owner to administer antibiotics via intramuscular or subcutaneous injection may be an alternative approach. Usually, we try to hospitalize a patient for 1 to 2 weeks to administer antibiotics parenterally. If the disease appears to be controlled after that period, the patient is usually discharged and the antibiotics are administered parenterally or orally at home.

Basing antibiotic therapy on blood culture results often is not feasible, either because the blood culture is negative or because the blood culture does not identify the organism early enough in a patient with acute bacterial endocarditis. A combination of ampicillin (a broad-spectrum antibiotic) and nafcillin or oxacillin (for β-lactamase-producing bacteria) and gentamicin or amikacin (for gram-negative bacteria) may be administered to these patients. Special care must be taken with gentamicin or amikacin because both are nephrotoxic. Usually, therapy with these agents should be limited to 1 to 2 weeks, if possible. Patients with preexisting renal disease or renal failure must be approached with extreme caution. Furosemide potentiates the renal toxicity of the aminoglycosides.

Fluoroquinolones (e.g., enrofloxacin) may be an alternative antibiotic class to the aminoglycosides for treating confirmed or suspected gram-negative infective endocarditis. They are bactericidal, concentrate well in heart valves and myocardium, and are effective against *E. coli* and *Pseudomonas aeruginosa* in experimental models of infective endocarditis.[34,35] At least seven fluoroquinolones have been studied in experimental models of infective endocarditis.[36] They have been found effective against staphylococcal, enterococcal, and gram-negative infective endocarditis. Three quinolones have been studied in experimental models of gram-negative bacillary infective endocarditis. In all cases, the quinolones were equivalent to or superior to comparison drugs, including gentamicin and amikacin. In humans with prosthetic valve endocarditis, the fluoroquinolones may resolve bacteremia and therefore reduce fever and clinical signs, but they do not sterilize the vegetation.[37] The only comparable situation in veterinary medicine would be endocarditis associated with a pacemaker lead.

The treatment for *Bartonella* species is aminoglycoside antibiotics. Ciprofloxacin may also be effective, because it is reported to be more effective than aminoglycosides for *Bartonella henselae* (cat-scratch fever).[38]

HEART FAILURE THERAPY

Congestive heart failure is one of the most common complications of infective endocarditis and is the most common cause of death.[17] Aortic valve endocarditis often produces severe heart failure that is difficult to manage. Standard heart failure therapy with furosemide, an angiotensin converting enzyme inhibitor, and digoxin is warranted. In addition, a more potent arteriolar dilator, such as hydralazine, can be very beneficial in a patient that has acute, severe pulmonary edema or that is refractory to the other drugs (see Figure 24-7). Hydralazine reduces peripheral vascular resistance and so reduces the amount of regurgitation in both aortic and mitral regurgitation. This results in decreased diastolic intracardiac pressures and a rapid reduction in pulmonary edema formation. Care must be taken not to produce profound hypotension when administering hydralazine along with an angiotensin converting enzyme inhibitor. Blood pressure monitoring and careful drug titration are crucial to prevent this complication.

CONTRAINDICATIONS TO CORTICOSTEROID THERAPY

Corticosteroids are administered with some frequency to dogs with infective endocarditis, presumably either to control the fever or to treat signs mistaken for an immune-mediated disease.[2] Corticosteroid administration exacerbates the clinical signs and worsens the prognosis in patients with infective endocarditis. The patient may feel better for 24 to 48 hours but then usually deteriorates. Patients that have occult infective endocarditis usually develop clinical signs rapidly following corticosteroid administration. For these reasons, corticosteroid administration is contraindicated in a patient with infective endocarditis.

Prognosis

The prognosis for dogs and cats with active infective endocarditis is poor. In one study, of 45 dogs proven to have infective endocarditis by either fulfillment of clinical diagnostic criteria or necropsy, only 20% survived.[2] In a second study of 45 dogs, the survival rate was identical (20%).[1] Dogs with large aortic valve lesions commonly develop severe left heart failure and die as a result. In one study, all dogs with aortic valve endocarditis died.[11] Dogs with severe mitral valve endocarditis may follow a similar course but generally have a better prognosis, depending on the severity of regurgitation. No definitive treatment for valve destruction (i.e., prosthetic valve replacement) exists in veterinary medicine. Consequently, once severe regurgitation is produced, heart failure and death are ultimately the expected result. Other patients die of embolic complications, especially renal infarction and failure. Other patients die of sepsis or infective complications.

Annuloaortic Ectasia

Annuloaortic ectasia is idiopathic dilation of the proximal aorta and aortic annulus. It is a rare cause of aortic regurgitation in dogs. In humans, severe degenerative change, usually cystic medial necrosis, in the wall of the aorta is the pathologic feature of this disease.[39] About one fourth to one half of human patients have other evidence of Marfan's syndrome or have relatives with Marfan's syndrome. Consequently, connective tissue disorders are suspected to cause this abnormality in humans. The cause in dogs is unknown.

When the media weakens, the aorta dilates. This places traction on the annulus, pulling it apart. This results in the aortic valve cusps being drawn apart, causing aortic regurgitation.

Aortic regurgitation severity ranges from mild to severe in canine patients with annuloaortic ectasia. Severe aortic regurgitation can result in left heart failure. It can also cause a bounding pulse. A diastolic, decrescendo heart murmur may be identified at the left heart base. A dog with annuloaortic ectasia is presented in Figure 24-11 and Color Plate 98.

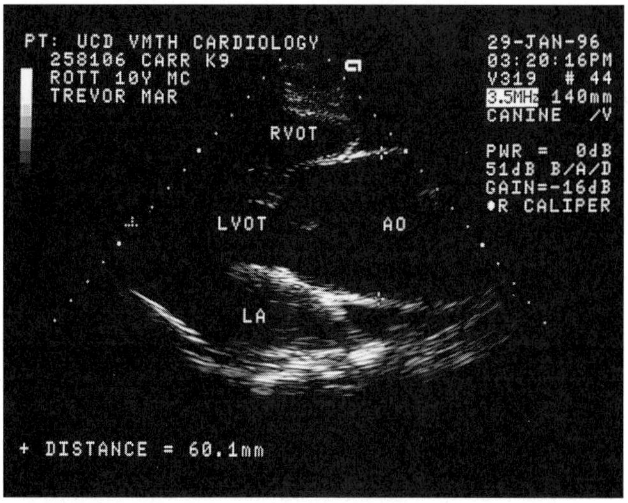

FIGURE 24-11 Echocardiograms from a 10-year-old rottweiler dog with annuloaortic ectasia. The two-dimensional echocardiogram shows the markedly dilated proximal aorta *(AO)*. The aortic annulus, just above the left ventricular outflow tract *(LVOT)* is much smaller than the proximal aorta.

REFERENCES

1. Calvert CA, Greene CE, Hardie EM: Cardiovascular infections in dogs: epizootiology, clinical manifestations, and prognosis, *J Am Vet Med Assoc* 187:612, 1985.
2. Calvert CA: Valvular bacterial endocarditis in the dog, *J Am Vet Med Assoc* 180:1080, 1982.
3. Korzeniowski OM, Kaye D: Infective endocarditis. In Braunwald E, ed: *Heart disease: a textbook of cardiovascular medicine,* ed 4, Philadelphia, 1992, WB Saunders.
4. Loesche WJ: Indigenous human microflora and bacteremia. In Kaplan EL, Taranta AV, eds: *American Heart Association Symposium: infective endocarditis,* Dallas, 1977, American Heart Association.
5. Petersdorf RG: Disorders caused by biologic agents. In Wintrobe MM, Thorn GW, Adams R, eds: *Principles of internal medicine,* New York, 1974, McGraw-Hill.
6. Wilcke JR: Use of antimicrobial drugs to prevent infections in veterinary patients, *Probl Vet Med* 2:298, 1990.
7. Guntheroth WG: How important are dental procedures as a cause of infective endocarditis? *Am J Cardiol* 54:797, 1984.
8. Black AP, Crichlow AM, Saunders JR: Bacteremia during ultrasonic teeth cleaning and extraction in the dog, *J Am Anim Hosp Assoc* 16:611, 1980.
9. Harari J, Besser TE, Gustafson SB et al: Bacterial isolates from blood cultures of dogs undergoing dentistry, *Vet Surg* 22:27, 1993 (comments).
10. Drazner FH: Bacterial endocarditis in the dog, *Compend Cont Educ* 1:918, 1979.
11. Sisson D, Thomas WP: Endocarditis of the aortic valve in the dog, *J Am Vet Med Assoc* 184:570, 1984.

12. Elwood CM, Cobb MA, Stepien RL: Clinical and echocardiographic findings in 10 dogs with vegetative bacterial endocarditis, *J Small Anim Pract* 34:420, 1993.
13. Lombard CW, Buergelt CD: Vegetative bacterial endocarditis in dogs; echocardiographic diagnosis and clinical signs, *J Small Anim Pract* 24:325, 1983.
14. Eriksen K, Fossum K, Gamlem H et al: Endocarditis in two dogs caused by Erysipelothrix rhusiopathiae, *J Small Anim Pract* 28:117, 1987.
15. Takahashi T, Tamura Y, Yoshimura H et al: *Erysipelothrix tonsillarum* isolated from dogs with endocarditis in Belgium, *Res Vet Sci* 54:264, 1993.
16. Breitschwerdt EB, Kordick DL, Malarkey DE et al: Endocarditis in a dog due to infection with a novel *Bartonella* subspecies, *J Clin Microbiol* 33:154, 1995.
17. Sisson DD: Bacterial endocarditis. In Bonagura JD, Lemkuhl LB, eds: *The 18th Annual Waltham Symposium for the Treatment of Small Animal Diseases,* Columbus, Ohio, 1994, Waltham.
18. Durack DT: Infective and noninfective endocarditis. In Hurst JW, ed: *The heart,* ed 7, New York, 1990, McGraw Hill.
19. Baddour LM, Christensen GD, Lowrance JH et al: Pathogenesis of experimental endocarditis, *Rev Infect Dis* 11:452, 1989.
20. Lepeschkin E: On the relation between the site of valvular involvement in endocarditis and the blood pressure resting on the valve, *Am J Med Sci* 224:318, 1952.
21. Yersin B, Glauser MP, Guze PA et al: Experimental *Escherichia coli* endocarditis in rats: roles of serum bactericidal activity and duration of catheter placement, *Infect Immun* 56:1273, 1988.
22. Durack DT: Experimental bacterial endocarditis. IV. Structure and evolution of very early lesions, *J Pathol* 115:81, 1975.
23. Kienle RD, Thomas WP, Pion PD: The natural clinical history of canine congenital subaortic stenosis, *J Vet Intern Med* 8:423, 1994.
24. Muna WF, Ferrans VJ, Pierce JE et al: Discrete subaortic stenosis in Newfoundland dogs: association of infective endocarditis, *Am J Cardiol* 41:746, 1978.
25. Rayan GM, Downard D, Cahill S et al: A comparison of human and animal mouth flora, *J Okla State Med Assoc* 84:510, 1991.
26. Thomas WP: Update: Infective endocarditis. In Kirk RW, Bonagura JD, eds: *Kirk's current veterinary therapy, XI: small animal practice,* Philadelphia, 1992, WB Saunders.
27. Bennett D, Taylor DJ: Bacterial endocarditis and inflammatory joint disease in the dog, *J Small Anim Pract* 29:347, 1987.
28. von Reyn CF, Levy BS, Arbeit RD et al: Infective endocarditis: an analysis based on strict case definitions, *Ann Intern Med* 94:505, 1981.
29. Durack DT, Lukes AS, Bright DK: New criteria for diagnosis of infective endocarditis: utilization of specific echocardiographic findings: Duke Endocarditis Service, *Am J Med* 96:200, 1994 (comments).
30. von Reyn CF, Arbeit RD: Case definitions for infective endocarditis, *Am J Med* 96:220, 1994 (editorial; comments).
31. Bayer AS, Ward JI, Ginzton LE et al: Evaluation of new clinical criteria for the diagnosis of infective endocarditis, *Am J Med* 96:211, 1994 (see comments).
32. Dow SW, Curtis CR, Jones RL et al: Bacterial culture of blood from critically ill dogs and cats: 100 cases (1985-1987), *J Am Vet Med Assoc* 195:113, 1989.
33. Hirsh DC, Jang SS, Biberstein EL: Blood culture of the canine patient, *J Am Vet Med Assoc* 184:175, 1984.
34. Krcmery VJ, Goljer J: [Quinolones in the treatment of bacterial endocarditis] Chinolony v liecbe bakterialnej endokarditidy, *Cas Lek Cesk* 129:1043, 1990.
35. Mertes PM, Voiriot P, Dopff C et al: Penetration of ciprofloxacin into heart valves, myocardium, mediastinal fat, and sternal bone marrow in humans, *Antimicrob Agents Chemother* 34:398, 1990.
36. Scheld WM: Evaluation of quinolones in experimental animal models of infections, *Eur J Clin Microbiol Infect Dis* 10:275, 1991.
37. Daikos GL, Kathpalia SB, Lolans VT et al: Long-term oral ciprofloxacin: experience in the treatment of incurable infective endocarditis, *Am J Med* 84:786, 1988.
38. Raoult D, Fournier PE, Drancourt M et al: Diagnosis of 22 new cases of *Bartonella* endocarditis, *Ann Intern Med* 125:646, 1996.
39. Eagle KA, De Sanctis RW: Diseases of the aorta. In Braunwald E, ed: *Heart disease: a textbook of cardiovascular medicine,* ed 4, Philadelphia, 1992, WB Saunders.

CHAPTER 25

Pericardial Disease and Cardiac Neoplasia

Pericardial diseases are commonly overlooked or mistaken for other cardiac and noncardiac disorders.[1,2] This is due to the fact that they comprise a relatively small portion of clinically important cardiovascular diseases in dogs and cats and because the physical findings may be relatively indistinct.[1-6] Pericardial disorders are one of the most important underlying causes responsible for the development of right heart failure in dogs and must be reliably distinguished from other causes, such as valvular or myocardial disease.[3,5] Clinically important pericardial disease is extremely uncommon in cats and is usually associated with other illness.[2,3,6] Clinical signs of pericardial disease may be subtle, yet the consequences can be dramatic and life-threatening. Because the pathophysiology and treatment of these conditions are distinct, it is important for the veterinary clinician to have a firm understanding of the more common pericardial disorders.

The Normal Pericardium

MICROSCOPIC ANATOMY

The gross anatomy of the pericardium is described in Chapter 1. Microscopically, the fibrous layer of the pericardium is composed primarily of compactly arranged, wavy collagen fibers in a complex, multilayered orientation and less abundant elastin fibers oriented at right angles to the collagen fibers. The serosal layer is composed of a single cell layer of mesothelial cells overlying a lamina propria containing connective tissue and elastic fibers. Ultrastructurally, the serosal layer possesses exuberant microvilli and long, single cilia to increase the surface area, enhance fluid transport, and facilitate movement of the serosal surfaces over each other during the movement of the heart.[7,8]

The pericardium receives its blood supply from the pericardial branches of the aorta and internal thoracic and musculophrenic arteries.[7] The pericardium is innervated by the vagus nerve, the left recurrent laryngeal nerve, and the esophageal plexus and has rich sympathetic innervation from the stellate and first dorsal root ganglions.[9] The phrenic nerves are embedded in the dorsal aspect of the parietal pericardium and may also supply sensory fibers to the pericardium.[7,8]

MECHANICAL (VISCOELASTIC) PROPERTIES

Because of its composition, the pericardium is much like a plastic bag that is very distendible when first filled but becomes relatively indistendible when full.[10] Thus a curve relating pericardial pressure to pericardial volume has an initial flat portion during which volume increases with little or no change in pressure, followed by a transition to a rapid pressure increase with little or no increase in volume (Figure 25-1). However, there is an adaptive pericardial response to chronic increases in volume (e.g., chronic effusions, cardiac hypertrophy). Under these conditions, the pressure-volume relationship shifts markedly to the right and its slope decreases, indicating an increase in pericardial reserve volume and an increase in compliance (see Figure 25-1). This increase in intrapericardial volume allows the pericardial pressure to remain lower at any given volume. Although a portion of this response is due to pericardial stretch, the majority of the adaptation occurs as a result of pericardial hypertrophy (i.e., growth of the pericardium), with a resultant increase in compliance.[8,10]

Normal intrapericardial pressure is generally thought to parallel intrapleural pressure and so remain subatmospheric throughout most of the cardiac cycle.[9-11] Small fluctuations in intrapericardial pressure are influenced by the events of the cardiac cycle, with intrapericardial pressure reaching its nadir during ventricular ejection. The *fluid* pressure in the pericardial cavity is actually lower than the pericardial *surface* pressure, as measured by an intrapericardial balloon. This may more accurately reflect pericardial restraint on the heart.[7,10]

FUNCTION

Although the pericardium is thought to serve several important functions, it is not essential for normal cardiovascular function and no adverse effects occur with congenital absence or surgical removal.[9,11] The true physiologic role of the pericardium remains controversial. The primary roles of the pericardium are to fix the heart anatomically, to maintain optimal functional shape of the heart, and to prevent excessive movement of the heart with changes in body position.[7,8,11] The pericardium also reduces friction between the moving heart and surrounding organs and provides a physical barrier to infection and malignancy from contiguous structures.[9] The thin layer of pericardial fluid reduces friction and is thought to equalize gravitational forces over the surface of the heart so that transmural cardiac pressures do not dramatically change or differ regionally.[8,11] Other physiologic functions that investigators have attributed to the pericardium include prevention of overdilation of the heart (pericardial restraint), regulation of the interrelation between the stroke volumes of the two ventricles (ventricular coupling), and positive influences on right ventricular function, especially in the face of elevated diastolic pressure.[7,9,11-13]

Pathophysiology

PATHOPHYSIOLOGY OF CARDIAC TAMPONADE

Cardiac tamponade may be considered to be an impairment of ventricular filling as a consequence of increased intrapericardial pressure caused by the accumulation of fluid within the pericardial

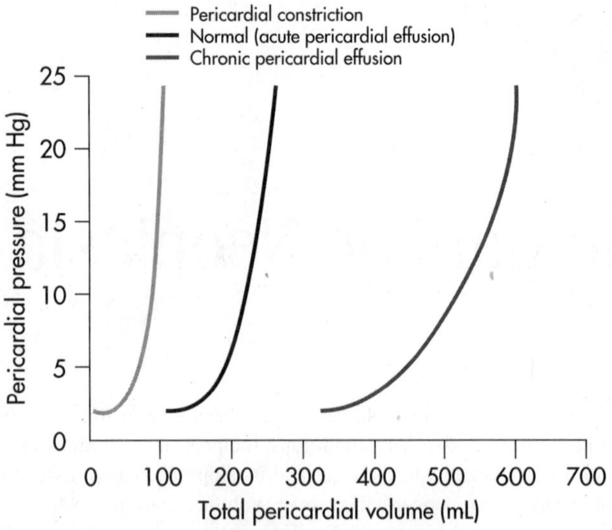

FIGURE 25-1 Representative pressure-volume relationships of the parietal pericardium in a normal dog and dogs with constrictive pericarditis, acute pericardial effusion (normal curve), and chronic pericardial effusion. (See text for details.) (Modified from Freeman G, LeWinter MM: Pericardial adaptations during chronic dilation in dog, *Circ Res* 54:294, 1984.)

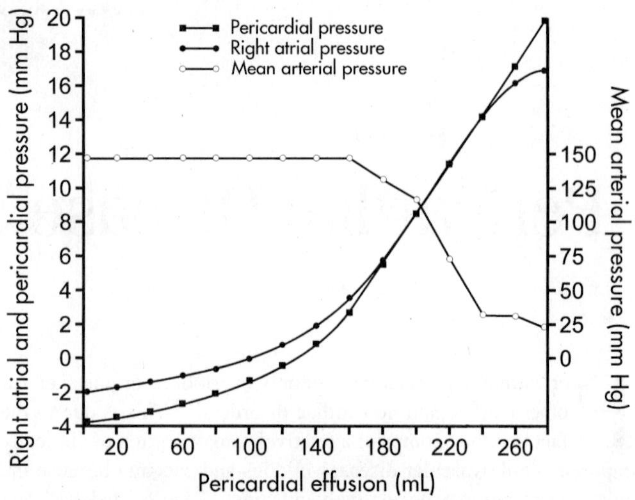

FIGURE 25-2 Graphic representation of acute cardiac tamponade. Rapid and progressive accumulation of pericardial fluid causes right atrial and intrapericardial pressures to equalize and rise steeply, leading to an abrupt decline in mean arterial pressure. (Modified from Fowler NO: Physiology of cardiac tamponade and pulsus paradoxus. II. Physiologic, circulatory, and pharmacologic responses in cardiac tamponade, *Mod Concept Cardiovasc Dis* 47:115, 1978.)

cavity.[7,14] It occurs clinically in two forms—acute and chronic. Cardiac tamponade is characterized by elevation of intracardiac diastolic pressures (congestive heart failure), and progressive limitation of ventricular filling leading to a reduction of stroke volume and cardiac output (forward, or low-output, heart failure).[7,8] Congestive right heart failure (increased right ventricular diastolic pressure) predominates in chronic cardiac tamponade, whereas low cardiac output and shock predominate in acute tamponade. Cardiac tamponade is actually a continuum that ranges from subclinical disease to fulminant heart failure. Patients with chronic pericardial tamponade often show a gradual onset of the above impairment. The development of increased pericardial pressure secondary to pericardial effusion depends on several factors, including the volume of the effusate, the rate of fluid accumulation (i.e., acute vs. chronic), and the physical nature of the pericardium. The pericardium in the dog normally contains 2.5 to 15 mL of fluid and can accommodate the rapid accumulation of only an additional 50 to 150 mL (in a 20-kg dog) of fluid without a significant increase in intrapericardial pressure and subsequent decline in systemic arterial pressure (Figure 25-2). However, if the additional fluid accumulates slowly, the pericardium hypertrophies and stretches such that it may be able to accommodate several hundred milliliters of fluid without a clinically significant increase in pressure (see Figure 25-1).

When the intrapericardial pressure equilibrates with right atrial and right ventricular diastolic pressures, the transmural distending pressure is zero and cardiac tamponade begins. Further accumulation of fluid causes intrapericardial pressure, right atrial pressure, and right ventricular diastolic pressure to rise in concert to the level of left atrial and left ventricular diastolic pressures. Subsequently, all pressures rise together.[15] Because systemic capillaries leak badly at pressures between 10 and 15 mm Hg and pulmonary capillaries do not leak badly until the pressure is approximately 30 mm Hg, patients with chronic cardiac tamponade always present with right heart failure (most commonly ascites) rather than left heart failure.

Acute cardiac tamponade, usually caused by trauma and bleeding into the pericardial space, is uncommon in dogs and cats. Several hemodynamic consequences result from acute cardiac tamponade, some compensatory and some deleterious. Equalization of intracardiac and intrapericardial pressures results in a diminished transmural distending pressure and diastolic volumes of both ventricles. This in turn leads to a reduction in cardiac stroke volume.[15] These alterations are initially counteracted by reflex increases in adrenergic tone (increased heart rate and contractility) that initially help maintain forward cardiac output.[16] In response to the increased sympathetic activity, systemic vascular resistance also increases. Although this initially helps to maintain systemic blood pressure, it does so at the expense of cardiac output. In patients that present with acute cardiac tamponade, cardiac output is often reduced. However, unless there is preexisting left ventricular disease, ventricular systolic function is unimpaired in cardiac tamponade, and the reduced cardiac output in cardiac tamponade reflects a reduction in diastolic volume, not systolic pump failure [8,16] As the severity of the compression increases, these compensations are no longer able to counteract the decline in ventricular filling and stroke volume. Consequently, first cardiac output and then systemic blood pressure decrease precipitously in concert with the increased systemic venous and pulmonary venous pressure (Figure 25-3).[7,16]

Cardiac tamponade alters the dynamics of systemic venous return and cardiac filling. Normally, one surge of venous flow occurs during ventricular systole coincident with the *x* decent of the venous pressure pulse, and a second surge occurs during right atrial emptying with the opening of the tricuspid valve, coincident with the *y* descent. Cardiac tamponade results in compression of the heart throughout the cardiac cycle. This prevents rapid emptying of the right atrium when the tricuspid valve opens. During ventricular ejection, total intracardiac volume decreases, resulting in a transient fall in intrapericardial and right atrial pressures. This is accompanied by a surge of systemic venous return. However, in early diastole the total volume within the pericardial space remains elevated despite opening of the tricuspid valve. During this phase of the cardiac cycle, intrapericardial pressure remains elevated and is equal to or exceeds right atrial pressure, so that transmural distending pressure is zero or

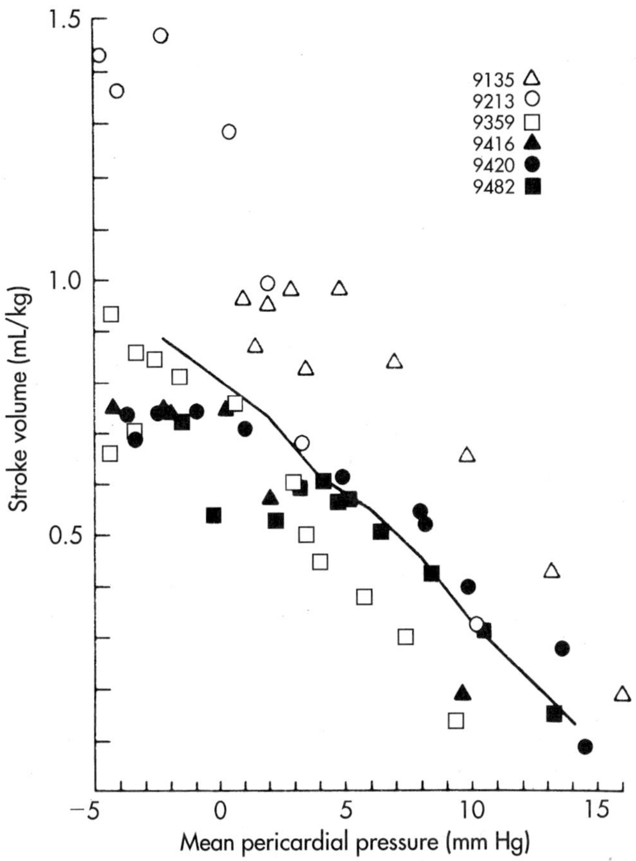

FIGURE 25-3 The effects of cardiac tamponade on ventricular performance (stroke volume). In this graph, stroke volume versus intrapericardial pressure is plotted. Increasing pericardial pressure causes a nearly linear decrease in stroke volume. Symbols represent individual dogs. (From Reed JR, Thomas WP: Hemodynamics of progressive pneumopericardium in the dog, *Am J Vet Res* 45:308, 1984.)

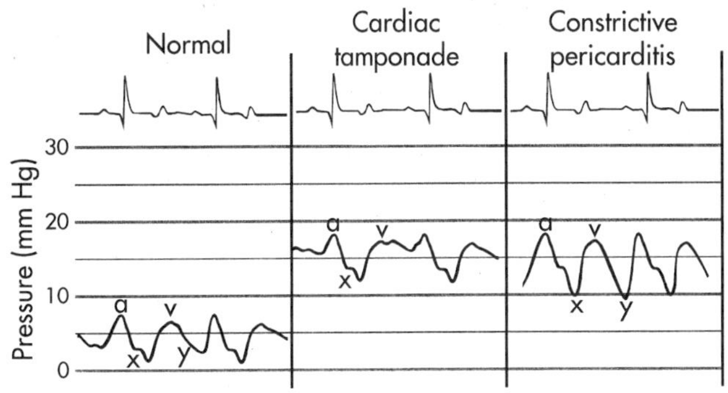

FIGURE 25-4 Representative right atrial pressure tracings from a normal dog, a dog with cardiac tamponade, and a dog with constrictive pericarditis. In the tracing depicting cardiac tamponade there is elevation of right atrial pressure with an attenuation of the diastolic *y* descent. In the tracing depicting constrictive pericarditis there is both a prominent *x* descent and *y* descent. (See text for details.)

even negative. As a result, the normal surge of systemic venous return during early ventricular diastole is attenuated, right atrial emptying is impeded, and the right atrium is compressed or even collapsed during diastole.[7,17] These events are reflected in right atrial or systemic venous pressure tracings as an increase in mean pressure, a prominent systolic *x* descent, and an attenuated or absent diastolic *y* descent (Figure 25-4).[17] The ultimate effect of altered systemic venous return clinically manifests as congestive right heart failure.

Cyclic alterations in systemic arterial pressure are also characteristic of cardiac tamponade. Normally there is a slight decline (less than 10 mm Hg) in systemic arterial pressure during inspiration. In patients with cardiac tamponade, there is an abnormally profound inspiratory decline in aortic blood flow velocity and a decrease in left ventricular stroke volume, producing a more dramatic decline (greater than 10 mm Hg) in systolic arterial blood pressure.[14,16,17] Blood pressure then increases again on expiration. This phenomenon, pulsus paradoxus, may be identified by a waxing and waning arterial pulse pressure in response to inspiration and expiration in patients with pericardial effusion. For a detailed description on the pathophysiology of pulsus paradoxus see Box 25-1.

PATHOPHYSIOLOGY OF PERICARDIAL CONSTRICTION

Pericardial constriction occurs when the parietal or visceral (epicardium) pericardium are histologically altered by a disease process that produces fibrosis or fusion of the two layers, resulting in decreased pericardial compliance or an actual decrease in intrapericardial volume, causing constriction.[7] In some cases the pericardial space is obliterated by complete fusion of the parietal and visceral layers (true constrictive pericarditis); in others a small fluid space remains (constrictive-effusive pericarditis). With constrictive pericarditis, the pericardium constricts the chambers, resulting in increases in atrial and diastolic ventricular pressures. With constrictive-effusive pericarditis the normal pressure-volume relationship is altered so that minimal increases in pericardial volume cause dramatic increases in pericardial pressure (see Figure 25-2). Usually the changes are symmetric and global so that both ventricles are equally affected, however, in a minority of cases constriction develops asymmetrically so that one ventricle is more dramatically affected than the other.[21] The pathophysiology is similar to cardiac tamponade in that the main consequences are a limitation of diastolic ventricular volume, elevation and equilibration of diastolic pressures throughout the heart, and, ultimately, the development of congestive right heart failure.[16,17] The diseased pericardium directly interferes with diastolic filling of all chambers and determines the total diastolic volume of the heart.[7] In a minority of cases, the disease process may also affect the ventricular myocardium, causing an impairment of myocardial contractility that may further decrease performance.[17]

The nature of the histologic changes in the pericardium influences the timing of ventricular filling and the resulting hemodynamic changes.[17] Pericardial constriction does not limit ventricular filling in early diastole but produces an abrupt cessation in middiastole.[7] The result is a characteristic diastolic dip-and-plateau pressure waveform (the square root sign) in both the right and left ventricles.[7] The early diastolic dip corresponds to the period of excessively rapid diastolic filling that occurs when the intracardiac volume is less than that defined by the stiff pericardium, whereas the plateau phase corresponds to the period in mid-to-late diastole when little additional ventricular volume expansion occurs. Because of equilibration of atrial and ventricular pressures, the jugular venous waveform and right and left atrial waveforms show both a prominent and deep early diastolic (*y*) descent that corresponds to early, rapid ventricular filling (see Figure 25-4).[7,17] The *x* descent usually is present, giving these waveforms a characteristic W-shaped configuration.

Certain major differences are apparent when cardiac tamponade is compared with pericardial constriction. The most consistent difference is the waveform configuration of atrial and venous pressure tracings. The prominent *y* descent is a consistent feature in

BOX 25-1

The "paradoxical" pulse

Under normal conditions, systemic arterial pressure and blood flow fluctuate with the respiratory cycle, falling slightly with inspiration and rising with expiration.[18] These fluctuations may be exaggerated by conditions that alter pleural pressure (e.g., asthma, pulmonary embolism) or by conditions that increase the interactive coupling between the ventricles (e.g., cardiac tamponade). When the inspiratory decrease in systolic arterial pressure is greater than 10 mm Hg, it is referred to as *pulsus paradoxus* or the *paradoxical pulse* (see accompanying figure of a dog with pericardial effusion; mean femoral artery and pulse pressure decrease with normal inspiration).[18] This name is a misnomer because pulsus paradoxus is not paradoxical but is an exaggeration of the normal pulse character. The physical identification of pulsus paradoxus by arterial palpation depends on the absolute reduction in the pulse and its total amplitude. Small fluctuations, especially with a narrow pulse pressure, can be difficult to detect, and, in many patients with pericardial effusion and cardiac tamponade, pulsus paradoxus cannot be confidently identified upon physical examination. Although pulsus paradoxus was originally described in human patients with constrictive pericarditis, it is now thought to be an uncommon finding in that disorder compared with pericardial effusion and cardiac tamponade.[18]

In cardiac tamponade, the changes in pleural pressure during the respiratory cycle and the transmission of those changes to the pericardial space are thought to alter left ventricular and right ventricular dynamics in such a way as to produce an exaggeration of the normal respiratory fluctuations in arterial pressure.[16-18] The exact pathophysiology of this phenomenon, even after decades of scientific research, is still a matter of substantial debate. In lieu of the controversy and the large number of well-designed studies with conflicting conclusions, there is probably no single mechanism responsible for pulsus paradoxus. Instead, it is likely the result of several contributing hemodynamic alterations induced by respiration in the presence of pericardial disease.

Several prevailing theories have been proposed to explain the paradoxical pulse.[7,8] It is generally accepted that, during inspiration, systemic venous return, right ventricular (RV) filling, and pulmonary blood flow increase and left ventricular (LV) filling and systemic blood flow decrease. It has been shown that when RV systemic venous return is experimentally held constant, pulsus paradoxus fails to occur.[11] Based on these principles and numerous studies, three major factors that are responsible for impaired LV filling have

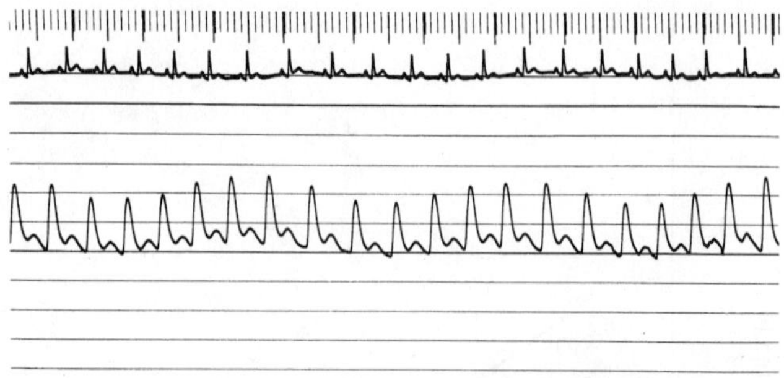

been proposed as the "primary" cause of pulsus paradoxus. The most widely accepted theory is that the inspiratory increase in RV filling physically shifts the interventricular septum leftward and reduces the LV chamber dimension in diastole.[7,18,19] This is thought to occur secondary to a fixed total ventricular volume imposed by the pericardial fluid. Consequently, increased RV filling must occur at the expense of LV filling. This reduction in LV preload subsequently leads to a reduced LV stroke volume and a decreased systolic arterial pressure. Others have shown experimentally that the inspiratory increase and expiratory decrease in RV filling are delayed in time by passage through the pulmonary vasculature, resulting in changes in LV filling and output that are 180 degrees out of phase with respiration.[16-18] In other words, the augmented filling of the RV is not transferred to the LV for several beats and tends to occur during the subsequent expiration. Consequently, blood must be stored in the pulmonary vasculature during inspiration and expelled into the left heart during expiration. This leads to the third proposed theory with widespread support that the inspiratory fall in pulmonary venous pressure is greater than the fall in LV diastolic pressure because of decreased transmission of pleural pressure changes to the pericardium and heart.[7,18,19] As a result, blood flows into and is stored in the pulmonary venous system. This reduces LV venous return and subsequently limits LV stroke volume. Also, the LV may be operating on the steep portion of the ascending limb of the Starling curve, so that any inspiratory reduction in LV filling results in marked depression of LV stroke volume.[20]

---

constrictive pericarditis, but not in cardiac tamponade, in which the *y* descent is attenuated or absent. In pericardial constriction, pulsus paradoxus is an uncommon clinical finding.[22] This relates to the fact that the most plausible theories of pulsus paradoxus rely on the changes in intrapleural pressure to be transmitted to the interior of the heart (see Box 25-1). With pericardial effusion this transmission occurs normally because the pericardium is still flexible.[16] However, with constrictive pericardial disorders, the increase in venous return with inspiration may not occur to a normal degree because the pericardium takes the form of a rigid shell and intrathoracic pressure variations are not transferred to the heart.[22] In some patients with constrictive pericarditis, there may be a decrease in systemic venous return during inspiration, with a resultant increase in systemic venous and right atrial pressures.[7] This finding, known as *Kussmaul's sign*, is not pathognomonic for constrictive pericardial disease. However, it is not an expected finding in patients with cardiac tamponade.[7,22]

INTRAPERICARDIAL MASS LESIONS

The physiologic effects of a mass lesion within the pericardial space are influenced by its etiology, size, and location, and the presence of effusion or pericardial fibrosis. Most intrapericardial tumors produce pericardial effusion, usually in large quantities. Consequently, most clinical disease associated with intrapericardial mass lesions is produced by concurrent pericardial effusion and chronic cardiac tamponade.[2] Small masses without pericardial effusion are generally clinically silent. Very large masses may produce clinical consequence by invasion or compression of cardiac structures or great vessels. Signs of venous congestion may manifest if a mass impairs venous return. Compression of the cranial vena cava tends to cause edema of the head and forelimbs, whereas compression of the caudal vena cava usually results in venous congestion of the abdominal organs and ascites. Obstruction of the outflow tracts or great vessels of one or both ventricles may lead to ventricular hypertrophy and result in signs related to reduced cardiac output or syncope.

Classification of Pericardial Disorders

Pericardial disorders may result from multiple etiologies. Pericardial disorders reported in dogs and cats are presented in Box 25-2. Pericardial effusion resulting from pericarditis, along with cardiac and pericardial neoplasia account for the vast majority of clinically important pericardial disorders in dogs. Although multiple potential causes exist, most effusions in dogs are hemorrhagic regardless of etiology.[3,5] Clinically significant pericardial disease is rare in cats.[6,23]

Only a few of the conditions listed in Box 25-2 are commonly

BOX 25-2

Pericardial diseases of dogs and cats

Congenital disorders

Pericardial defects†

Peritoneopericardial diaphragmatic hernia†

Pericardial cyst (?)

Acquired disorders

Pericardial effusion

- Hydropericardium (transudate)†
  - Congestive heart failure
  - Hypoalbuminemia
  - Peritoneopericardial diaphragmatic hernia
- Pericarditis (exudate)
  - Infectious (bacterial, fungal)
  - Sterile (idiopathic, metabolic, viral)
- Hemopericardium (hemorrhage)
  - Neoplastic
  - Traumatic
  - Cardiac rupture (especially left atrial)
  - Idiopathic

Pericardial mass lesions (± effusion)

- Pericardial cyst
- Neoplastic
- Granulomatous (actinomycosis, coccidioidomycosis)
- Pericardial abscess

Constrictive pericardial disease

- Idiopathic
- Infectious
- Pericardial foreign body
- Neoplastic

†Conditions that rarely compromise cardiac function.
Modified from Thomas WP: Pericardial disorders. In Ettinger SJ, ed: *Textbook of small animal internal medicine,* ed 3, Philadelphia, 1989, WB Saunders.

encountered in clinical practice. General statements may be made in regard to signalment, although exceptions do occur: (1) young animals most commonly have congenital or infectious disorders; (2) middle-age, large-breed dogs most frequently have idiopathic hemorrhagic pericardial effusion; (3) older dogs more commonly have neoplastic effusions. It should also be kept in mind that most but not all patients with pericardial disease or space-occupying lesions develop obvious pericardial effusion.

CONGENITAL DISORDERS

Pericardial cysts. Pericardial cysts are developmental abnormalities that are rarely encountered in dogs and have not been reported in cats.[24-26] In humans, four types of pericardial cysts are identified: pericardial cysts arising from anomalous pericardial development (coelomic), pericardial cysts from lymphatic elements (lymphangiomatous; springwater), bronchial cysts, and teratomas.[7] Pericardial cysts reported in dogs do not meet gross pathologic and histologic criteria of any of the above categories. Instead, they appear to resemble acquired cystic hematomas.[24] However, pericardial cysts occur primarily in young dogs, suggesting a developmental or congenital anomaly. Congenital cysts are thought to be the result of incarcerated omentum or abnormal development of mesenchymal tissue during fetal development.[26] They may be located in the right or left costophrenic angle and usually have a pedicular attachment to the apex of the parietal pericardium, with the rest of the cyst lying free within the pericardial cavity. Pericardial cysts in humans are usually unilocular and filled with clear fluid, whereas in dogs they may be either unilocular or multilocular and usually contain a bloody, brown-tinged opaque fluid.[24,25] Histologically, pericardial cysts in dogs are characterized by broad bands of organized connective tissue lined by reactive mesothelial cells.[24]

The clinical presentation and signs in dogs with pericardial cysts are similar to those of other pericardial diseases. Presenting complaints include fatigue, abdominal distention, and dyspnea. Depending on the size of the cysts, the heart sounds may be muffled on auscultation. If cardiac tamponade is present, jugular venous distension, hepatomegaly, and ascites may be detectable. In one report of six dogs, electrocardiograms demonstrated small-amplitude *R* waves (less than 1 mV) without electrical alternans, in all leads.[24] Cardiomegaly is typical on thoracic radiographs, and the heart may assume a spherical shape or the contour of the cardiac silhouette may be interrupted by an abnormal protrusion. Pneumopericardiography or echocardiography are necessary for definitive diagnosis, although other imaging techniques, such as computed tomography or magnetic resonance imaging, may also be employed.[8,24] Surgical removal of the cyst and its pedicle, followed by subtotal pericardiectomy, results in resolution of clinical signs.[24,27]

Peritoneopericardial diaphragmatic hernia. Peritoneopericardial diaphragmatic hernia (PPDH) is the most frequent congenital pericardial anomaly reported in dogs and cats.[28-30] This anomaly consists of a persistent communication between the pericardial and peritoneal cavities, allowing abdominal contents to enter the pericardial cavity while the pleural space remains intact (Color Plate 99). Although usually considered a result of abnormal fusion of the septum transversum with the pleuroperitoneal folds during embryonal development, it is thought that postnatal injuries may also cause formation of acquired PPDH.[27] The size of the defect may vary from a clinically silent, small communication involving herniation of the omentum to very large defects with herniation of other abdominal organs.[31] The liver and gallbladder are herniated most frequently, followed by the small intestines, spleen, and stomach.[28] Hernias in the cranioventral abdominal wall and caudal sternebrae abnormalities commonly occur in association with congenital PPDH.[26,29] In one report, male dogs were affected more often than females and 18% of the cases were Weimaraners.[28]

Although in the majority of cases the hernia is present from birth, clinical signs may occur at any age or not at all.[30] In reported cases, the age at the onset of clinical signs ranges from 4 weeks to 15 years, with most diagnoses being made within the first year of life.[28] In many instances, the PPDH is identified as an incidental radiographic finding while evaluating other problems or is first identified at necropsy. Although clinical signs are commonly absent, when they are present they are primarily related to the gastrointestinal system and the respiratory tract. Clinical signs include vomiting, diarrhea, weight loss, exertional fatigue, dyspnea/tachypnea, and cough. Rarely, pericardial effusion accompanies the hernia, and signs of cardiac tamponade may predominate. Physical findings may be normal with smaller defects. With larger defects findings may include diminished or displaced heart sounds, umbilical or abdominal hernias, caudal sternal deformities, inability to palpate abdominal organs, and, rarely, signs of cardiac tamponade and congestive right heart failure.

Electrocardiograms may demonstrate reduced amplitudes as a result of the addition of abdominal contents into the pericardial sac, and the mean electrical axis may be shifted because of cardiac displacement. The diagnosis of PPDH is usually made by radio-

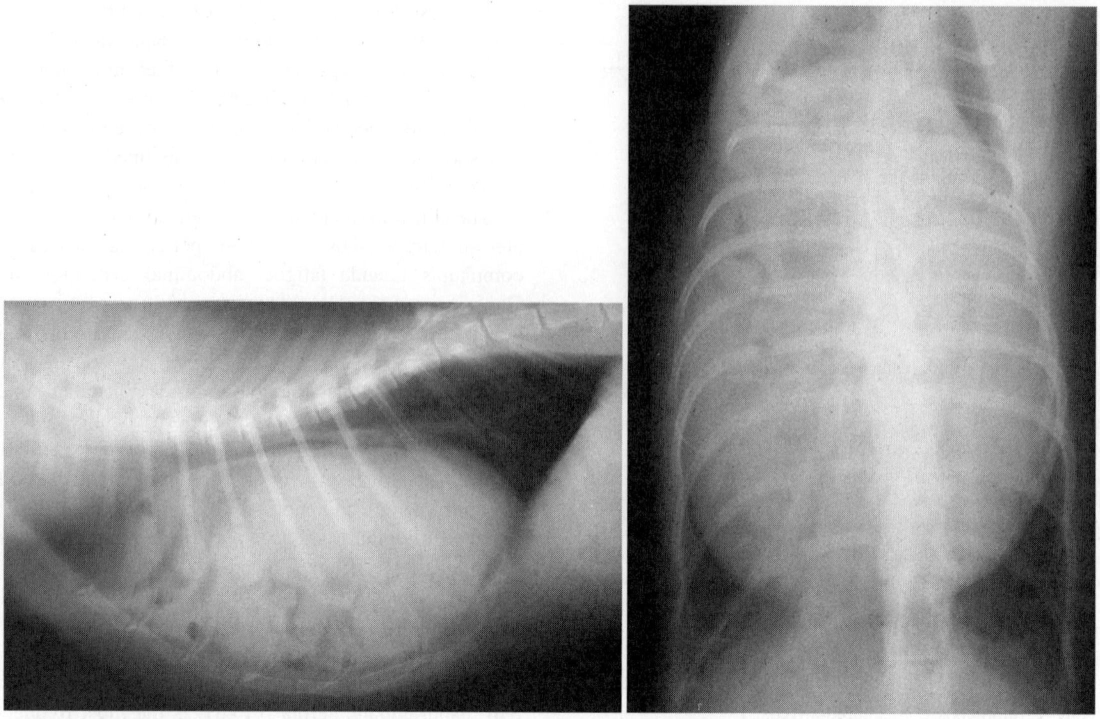

FIGURE 25-5 Thoracic radiographs from a cat with a pericardioperitoneal diaphragmatic hernia. **A,** In the lateral projection, severe cardiomegaly and tracheal elevation is apparent. The cardiac silhouette consists of heterogeneous densities and gas patterns, suggesting the presence of abdominal contents in the pericardial space. **B,** Dorsoventral projection showing the same findings as in **A.**

graphic examination.[29,30] Survey thoracic radiographs characteristically show cardiac enlargement, dorsal displacement of the trachea, and silhouetting of the caudal heart border and the diaphragm.[28] In some cases, regions of the cardiac silhouette may have a heterogeneous density of soft tissue, gas, or fat because of the varied contents of the pericardial cavity (Figure 25-5). The silhouette of the heart may be seen in some cases, especially when it is surrounded by fat. Although thoracic radiographs may be diagnostic, in many cases the findings are merely suggestive. Abdominal radiographs may show a smaller-than-normal liver. In extreme cases the peritoneal cavity may appear to be devoid of organs. In some cases gastrointestinal gas patterns may be seen extending from the peritoneal cavity into the pericardial cavity. Two-dimensional echocardiography may allow direct visualization of an extracardiac, intrapericardial mass that displaces the heart with or without a small amount of pericardial effusion (Figure 25-6).[30,32,33] Occasionally the discontinuity in the diaphragm can be seen, and herniated tissue may appear to be continuous with abdominal contents. If echocardiography is not available, fluoroscopy, nonselective angiocardiography, upper gastrointestinal barium studies, or pneumopericardiography may also be helpful to establish the diagnosis.[2,30] A definitive diagnosis can also be established by placing an iodinated radiopaque contrast agent (not barium) or a radionuclide-tagged substance in the peritoneal cavity, elevating the dog's caudal body, and determining if the substance flows forward into the pericardial space.

Surgical correction via laparotomy or thoracotomy is the recommended treatment (Color Plate 100).[26,31] In asymptomatic adult patients in which the PPDH was an incidental finding and in asymptomatic patients with small hernias, treatment may not necessarily be indicated. The postoperative prognosis for most patients is excellent.

Pericardial defects. Pericardial defects have been infrequently reported in dogs and cats and are rare in clinical practice.[29,34-37] Most are identified incidentally upon postmortem examination for other disorders. Although pericardial defects are thought to be congenital in origin, trauma could not be ruled out as the underlying cause in most reported cases. Pericardial defects commonly involve the left side of the pericardium as round or oval communications between the pericardial cavity and the pleural space, and a portion of the heart may be herniated or incarcerated through the defect.[2,29] Although such defects are usually clinically silent, variable clinical signs or abnormal findings on diagnostic studies may occur. The most common abnormality that we have noted is an abnormal bulge on the cardiac silhouette, where a portion of the heart bulges through the defect (Figure 25-7). This can be mistaken for a tumor. The severity of clinical consequences is generally related to the area and degree of cardiac strangulation. Congenital complete absence of the pericardium is rare and generally asymptomatic.[2]

Pericardial Effusion Resulting from Acquired Disease

The syndrome of pericardial effusion is by far the most common pericardial disorder encountered in dogs and cats and is the most likely pericardial disorder to lead to cardiac tamponade and congestive heart failure.*

Because the common causes of pericardial effusion produce similar if not identical clinical signs, it is appropriate to discuss these

* References 1, 2, 5, 6, 27, 31.

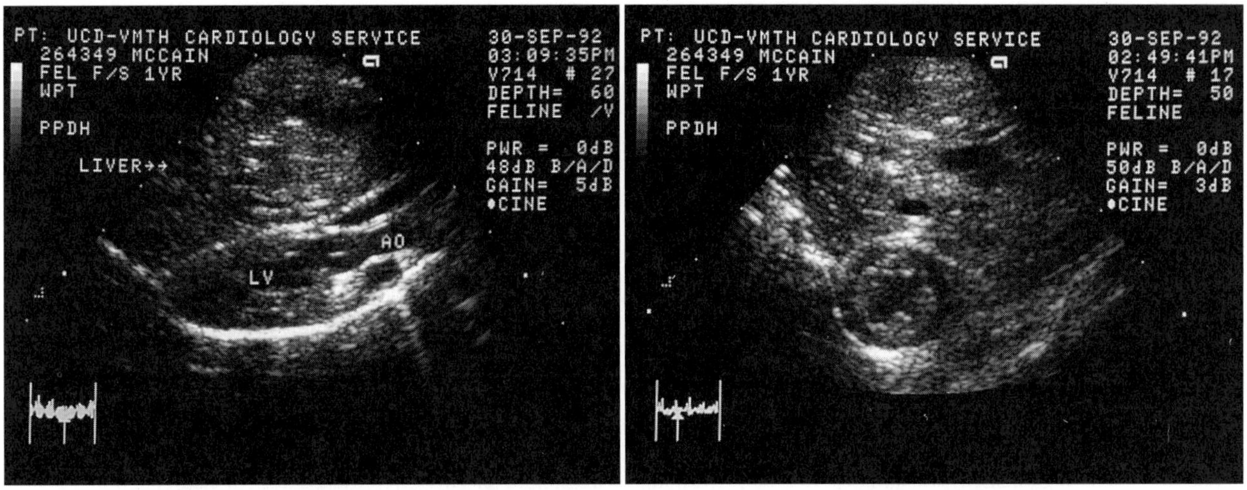

FIGURE 25-6 Two-dimensional echocardiograms from the cat shown in Color Plate 99. **A,** Right parasternal long-axis view showing the liver within the pericardial sac between the heart and the right chest wall. **B,** Right parasternal short-axis view from the same cat. *LV,* Left ventricle, *AO,* aorta. (From Kienle RD, Thomas WP: Echocardiography. In Nyland TG, Mattoon JS, eds: *Veterinary Diagnostic Ultrasound,* Philadelphia, 1995, WB Saunders.)

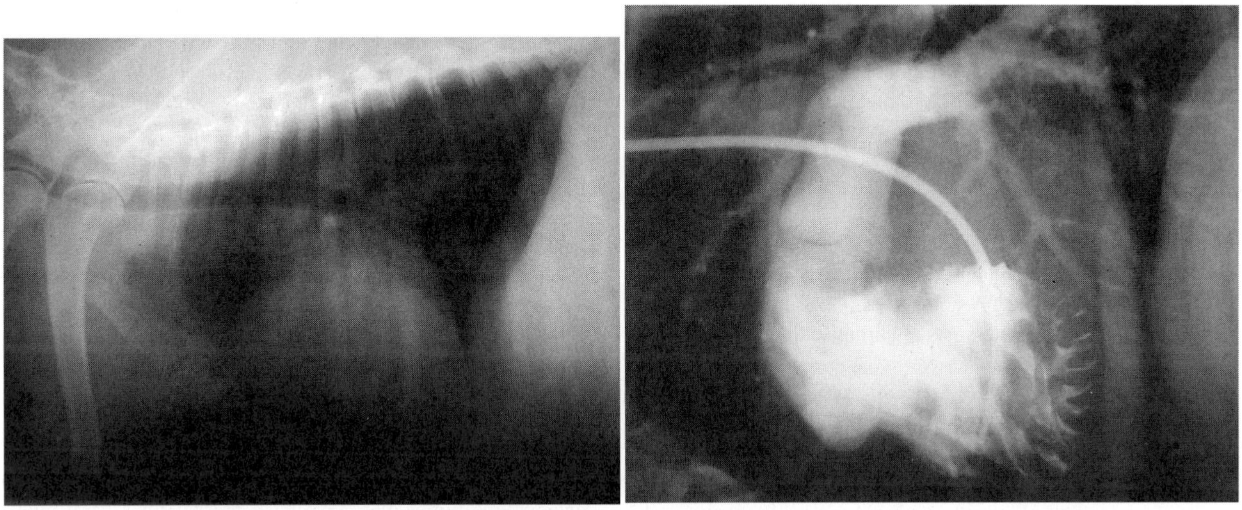

FIGURE 25-7 Pericardial defect in a dog. **A,** Lateral thoracic radiograph. There is an unusual contour to the cranial border of the cardiac silhouette in the area of the right ventricular outflow tract. **B,** Lateral right ventricular angiogram demonstrating bulging of the right ventricular outflow tract through a pericardial defect.

disorders as a syndrome with a variety of specific etiologies. The effusion may be the primary manifestation of the disorder or may simply be an incidental manifestation of the overall disease process.

ETIOLOGY

Virtually any disease process that affects the pericardium can lead to the development of pericardial effusion and, subsequently, cardiac tamponade (see Box 25-2). However, the frequent causes are few. Pericardial effusions may be classified by the etiology or by the physical characteristics of the fluid. As with any other body cavity, the four types of potential fluid composition include transudate, modified transudate, exudate (inflammatory, noninflammatory), and hemorrhage (sanguinous or serosanguinous). Occasionally, chylous pericardial effusions are encountered.[2] The type of effusion is classified based on appearance and laboratory characteristics (Table 25-1). The majority of effusions in dogs are sanguinous (hemorrhagic) or serosanguinous, noninflammatory or mildly inflammatory, and nonseptic. More than 90% of dogs with pericardial effusion have either idiopathic (hemorrhagic) pericardial effusion or cardiac or pericardial neoplasia. The most common form of nonneoplastic pericardial effusion in dogs is idiopathic (hemorrhagic) pericardial effusion.[2,26,27] It is most likely due to pericardial inflammation (i.e., pericarditis). Neoplastic pericardial effusion represents the largest group of pericardial disorders (with and without effusion).[2,26,27] Other reported but less common causes include left atrial rupture secondary to chronic mitral valvular disease, trauma, pericardial masses other than neoplasia, and uremia.[2] In cats the most common causes of pericardial effusion are feline infectious peritonitis, septic pericarditis, and neoplasia.[6,23]

Idiopathic (hemorrhagic) pericardial effusion. Idiopathic (hemorrhagic) pericardial effusion (IHPE) is one of the more common causes of pericardial effusion in dogs, second in frequency

TABLE 25-1
Characteristics of effusions

Parameter	*Transudate*	*Modified transudate*	*Exudate*	*Hemorrhage*
Specific gravity	<1.018	1.018-1.025	>1.025	>1.025
Protein (g/dL)	<2.5	2.5-6.0	>2.5	>2.5
Appearance	Clear and watery	Clear to serosanguinous	Turbid; Serosanguinous; serofibrinous	Serosanguinous; sanguinous
Cellularity (cells/mm^3)	<1000	>2500	>5,000	>5000
Cytology	Macrophages, mesothelial cells, and occasional neutrophils	Macrophages, mesothelial cells, and occasional neutrophils and erythrocytes	Variable	Primarily erythrocytes

only to neoplastic disorders.[38-41] Many terms have been applied to this condition including: *benign idiopathic pericardial effusion, hemopericardium, benign pericardial effusion,* and *idiopathic pericardial hemorrhage.* The term *benign* may be misleading, because the condition is potentially life-threatening. The cause is unknown, but an inflammatory condition secondary to viral or immune-mediated causes is the most plausible suspect. The exact prevalence of IHPE is unknown. It has been reported to account for 20% to 75% of the cases of pericardial effusion in dogs.[40, 41] Dogs with IHPE are most commonly large or giant breeds, predominantly male, and most frequently middle-age (range 9 months to 14 years).[38-41] The breeds reported to be frequently affected include the great Pyrenees, great Dane, Saint Bernard, and golden retriever.[38] Although the disease process is probably inflammatory in nature, the effusion is generally hemorrhagic, without specific inflammatory cells present. Histologically it appears that the blood vessels and lymphatics of the pericardium are the primary targets of a mononuclear inflammatory process with fibrosis. These damaged blood vessels appear to be the source of the effusion.[38] The effusion generally accumulates slowly, and dogs typically present with signs of chronic cardiac tamponade and right heart failure. The effusion may be self-limiting, with spontaneous resolution following pericardiocentesis, or may recur for several years.[2] Constrictive pericarditis is an uncommon late sequela to this disease.

Cardiac neoplasia. Tumors of the heart are sporadic occurrences in small animals, with an incidence of 0.17% in dogs in one report.[42] Although cardiac neoplasms may occur on the extracardiac surface and not cause pericardial effusion or may occur as isolated intracardiac masses, the vast majority of cardiac neoplasms are present on the surface of the heart or great vessels and most cause pericardial effusion. Severe pericardial effusion with cardiac tamponade and right heart failure are the most common abnormalities in dogs with cardiac neoplasia. The majority of animals with cardiac neoplasms are middle-age to geriatric, although younger animals are occasionally affected. The most common tumors reported in dogs are hemangiosarcoma of the right atrium and chemodectoma or ectopic thyroid carcinoma at the heart base. The most commonly reported cardiac tumor in cats is lymphosarcoma. Hemangiosarcomas and heart base tumors are rare in cats. Although intrapericardial tumors may be suspected based on radiographic abnormalities, special procedures (usually echocardiography) are required for definitive diagnosis and characterization of their exact origin.[43,44]

Hemangiosarcoma. Most tumors originating form the right atrium or surrounding tissues in dogs are hemangiosarcomas (Color Plate 101).[42] There appears to be a higher incidence of hemangiosarcomas in German shepherds and golden retrievers.[43,45,46]

Signs of congestive right heart failure are the most common reason for an owner to present a dog for examination. Hemangiosarcomas commonly hemorrhage. Slow hemorrhage produces chronic pericardial tamponade, but acute bleeding may produce signs of acute cardiac tamponade.[42] There is often significant metastasis at the time of diagnosis, and dogs may be systemically ill. Generalized weakness is a common complaint.[47] Some dogs have episodes of collapse, and acute incidents are often associated with pallor and other signs, suggesting acute hemorrhage into the pericardial space.[47] Common metastatic sites include the lungs, liver, spleen, and kidney.[43] Common laboratory findings include neutrophilia, a mild nonregenerative anemia, and large numbers of circulating nucleated and immature red blood cells.[47-49]

Heart base tumors. Heart base masses are usually neoplasms classified as *chemoreceptor cell tumors* (aortic body tumor, chemodectoma, nonchromaffin paragangliomas) or *ectopic thyroid carcinomas.*[42,48,50] The thyroid carcinomas are usually not functional and so do not produce thyroid hormone. Heart base tumors appear to originate around the perimeter of the proximal ascending aorta, between the aorta and pulmonary artery (Color Plate 102). When tumors are large, it is impossible to determine their exact origin. Although metastasis to other organs is reported, it is a rare and late occurrence.[42] Most commonly the mass becomes very large and produces clinical problems by causing pericardial effusion. By the time congestive right heart failure secondary to pericardial effusion develops, the tumor may have been present for several months to years. Occasionally, heart base tumors may become invasive and infiltrate or penetrate other areas of the heart.

Brachycephalic breeds have a greater tendency to develop heart base tumors, and males are more commonly affected in those breeds.[51] Clinical signs are usually only apparent when significant pericardial effusion is present.

Mesothelioma. Pericardial mesothelioma is a lethal and fortunately rare cardiac neoplasm.[52] The tumor arises from serous membranes such as the pleura, pericardium, peritoneum, and tunica vaginalis of the testes. Mesothelioma is generally a diffuse neoplastic process. When it involves the pericardium it produces a hemorrhagic pericardial effusion without masses large enough to be identified by two-dimensional echocardiography.[53]

Clinical signs are generally related to pericardial or pleural effusion and include weakness, dyspnea, and tachypnea. Ascites is commonly present secondary to chronic pericardial tamponade. Clinical features and results of diagnostic studies depend on the location and extent of the tumor. Pericardial effusion and pleural effusion without ascites in an older dog should raise an index of suspicion for pericardial or pleural mesothelioma. Although cytologic examination of fluid samples may demonstrate large numbers of clustered

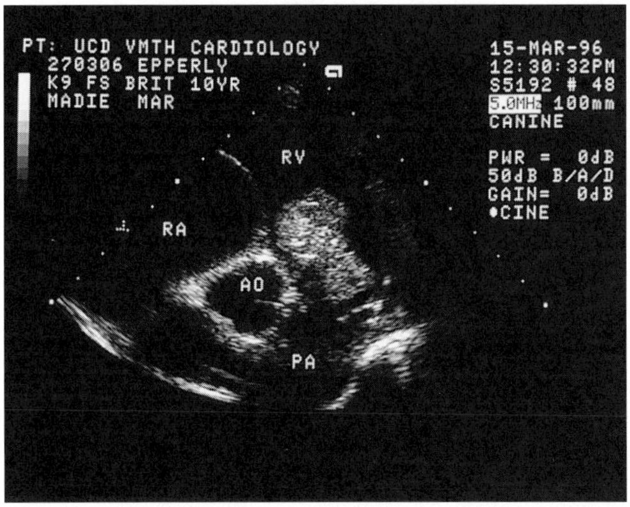

FIGURE 25-8 Tumor causing right ventricular outflow obstruction in a dog. Right parasternal short-axis echocardiographic image from the level of the aortic valve. A soft tissue mass can be seen within the right ventricular outflow tract just below the pulmonic valve. *RA,* Right atrium; *AO,* aorta; *PA,* pulmonary artery; *RV,* right ventricle.

mesothelial cells, differentiation from reactive mesothelial cells is impossible. Neoplastic effusions may be differentiated from non-neoplastic effusions using analysis of pH, and mesothelioma may be further suspected based on hyaluronic acid concentration.[54-56] The definitive diagnosis requires exploratory thoracotomy and biopsy.[42] Often mesothelioma must be differentiated from metastatic carcinomas using special immunohistochemical staining.[53]

Other. Other types of primary tumors involving the heart are rare in dogs. Other primary cardiac tumors reported include myxoma, fibrosarcoma, intracardiac ectopic thyroid tumor, squamous cell carcinoma, cardiac carcinomatosis, chondrosarcoma, and rhabdomyosarcoma.[42,57-60] In most reports the tumors involve right heart structures. Reported metastatic tumors include lymphoma and various sarcomas and carcinomas.[42,61] Clinical signs and features depend on the location and severity of the lesion. Atypical tumors are more likely to produce obstruction to blood flow or myocardial dysfunction than the more common tumors described above (Figure 25-8, Color Plate 103).

Pericardial infection. Exudative effusions are infrequently diagnosed in dogs primarily because infective pericarditis is uncommon.[5] In contrast, septic pericarditis is one of the common causes of significant pericardial effusion in cats, although the incidence is rare because pericardial effusion is uncommon in this species.[2,6,23] Pericardial exudates are usually purulent, serofibrinous, or serosanguinous, and cytology usually identifies the inflammatory process and occasionally an offending organism. Infective pericarditis in dogs and cats has been associated with bacterial and fungal infections, including tuberculosis, coccidioidomycosis, actinomycosis, nocardiosis, and various bacterial organisms.[2,62-64] Coccidioidomycosis, actinomycosis, and nocardiosis secondary to foxtail migration are the most common causes in our clinic. Clinically significant, sterile, inflammatory pericardial effusion has also been reported in cats with feline infectious peritonitis, and small incidental sterile effusions have been reported in dogs with leptospirosis or distemper.[2,5,65,66] Rarely, chronic uremia leads to small amounts of a sterile serofibrinous or serosanguinous effusion.[67]

Left atrial rupture. Left atrial perforation is an infrequent complication of chronic degenerative mitral valve disease.[2,68,69] Increased left atrial pressure and left atrial enlargement, with or without jet lesions, may lead to endocardial tears in dogs with advanced valvular disease.[70] These are usually only partial-thickness tears, although left atrial rupture occurs. Acute cardiac tamponade, usually resulting in cardiogenic shock or sudden death, results from severe hemorrhage into the pericardial space. Small-breed dogs predisposed to acquired mitral valve disease are primarily affected. Left atrial rupture in association with acquired mitral valve disease is apparently more frequent in male poodles, dachshunds, and cocker spaniels.[68] (See Color Plate 71.)

HISTORY AND PHYSICAL EXAMINATION

Animals are often presented for vague clinical signs of lethargy, weakness, anorexia, abdominal enlargement, and, possibly, collapse. In chronic cases, weight loss and cachexia may be observed. In animals with severe congestive right heart failure there may be dyspnea and tachypnea secondary to either severe pleural or peritoneal effusion. Signs of the underlying disease may be present and may dominate the clinical history, especially when neoplasia or systemic infection is involved.

A small effusion is generally not detectable by routine physical examination. When a large effusion is encountered, a constellation of clinical findings (Beck's triad) is often present.[14] The combination of jugular venous distention and/or pulsation (increased systemic venous pressure), weak and variable femoral pulse quality (decreased pulse pressure and pulsus paradoxus), and muffled heart sounds on thoracic auscultation are highly suggestive of a pericardial effusion.[2] However, there are many stages of disease between small and large effusions that may have a variable combination of clinical findings, and the consistency of these physical findings even in patients with large effusions is variable.

Muffled heart sounds may be accompanied by a decreased palpable precordial impulse, and the lung sounds may also be diminished if pleural effusion is present. Muffled heart and lung sounds may also be detected in patients with pleural effusions from other causes, intrathoracic masses, low cardiac output, or obesity and are not pathognomonic for pericardial effusion in isolation. Other abnormal auscultatory findings are usually absent, although dogs with left atrial rupture may have a systolic murmur of mitral regurgitation that is reduced in intensity compared with previous examinations.[68] Cardiac arrhythmias may be detected in some cases, with sinus tachycardia secondary to decreased cardiac output being the most common.

Jugular venous distention, pulsation, and a positive hepatojugular reflex are usually present but often overlooked. However, failure to identify abnormalities of the jugular veins does not preclude the diagnosis of pericardial effusion. In patients in which jugular veins are difficult to evaluate or if physical abnormalities of the jugular veins are not detected, measurement of central venous pressure will document the presence or absence of systemic venous hypertension. Measures of central venous pressure are usually abnormal in patients with pericardial effusion (greater than 5 mm Hg) and exceed 10 to 12 mm Hg in most with signs of right heart failure resulting from any cause. Abdominal distension from hepatomegaly and ascites are common in patients with cardiac tamponade and congestive right heart failure, but are usually absent with acute effusions in which signs of cardiogenic shock predominate.

As a result of a reduced left ventricular stroke volume, the arterial pulse is often weak and abrupt. In patients with acute effusions or in the face of severe chronic cardiac tamponade, peripheral arterial pulses may be difficult to detect because of the severe reduction in stroke volume and systemic hypotension. Pulsus paradoxus may occur but is less frequently detected, probably because many dogs do not breathe evenly and deeply (see Box 25-1).

ELECTROCARDIOGRAPHY

Although electrocardiographic findings are neither sensitive nor specific for pericardial effusion, several are supportive of the diagnosis. Diminished QRS voltages (less than 1 mV in all limb leads in dogs) are a common finding (50% to 60%), especially compared with previous tracings or tracings obtained after pericardiocentesis (Figure 25-9).[71,72] Other causes of diminished QRS voltages include obesity, pleural effusion, hypothyroidism, and large thoracic masses.[71,72] Occasionally, diminished QRS voltages may be identified in otherwise normal dogs. The normal low amplitude of QRS complexes recorded in cats makes recognition of this finding difficult unless compared with previous tracings.[71]

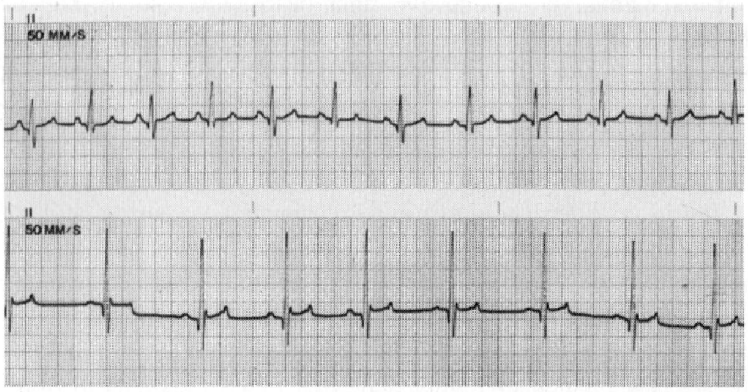

FIGURE 25-9 Electrocardiogram taken from a dog with pericardial effusion (lead II, 50 mm/sec, 1 cm = 1 mV). **A,** QRS amplitudes are reduced (less than 1 mV), and there is a mild beat-to-beat variation in the wave amplitude of both the *R* and *S* waves (electrical alternans). **B,** Electrocardiogram from the same dog taken after pericardiocentesis. The electrocardiogram is now normal.

Electrical alternans, defined as a beat-to-beat variation in QRS or *T* wave height or configuration, may also be recorded from as many as 50% of dogs with pericardial effusion (see Figure 25-9).[2,21] Most commonly this is seen as the *R* wave height in lead II varying with every other beat. Electrical alternans is produced by swinging of the heart within the fluid-filled pericardial space and is usually only present with large effusions. It has been shown in an experimental model that electrical alternans is rate-dependent and is most likely to occur at relatively normal heart rates in dogs (90 to 144 beats/min).[74] Although not highly sensitive, electrical alternans is quite specific for pericardial effusion. Arrhythmias other than sinus tachycardia are uncommon. Although others have suggested that ventricular or supraventricular arrhythmias may occur in up to 40% of cases, these studies were based on patients with inflammatory pericarditis.[21,75] Nonspecific ST segment deviations have been reported in dogs with pericardial effusion, but are usually mild and inconsistent.[2,21,71]

RADIOGRAPHY

Thoracic radiographs are usually abnormal in dogs and cats with pericardial effusion. However, as with other examinations, small effusions may cause no recognizable change. Many of the consistent findings on survey thoracic radiographs are nonspecific. The earliest noticeable changes are generalized cardiac enlargement and loss of the normal chamber contours.[29] As the effusion becomes more pronounced, generalized cardiac enlargement becomes dramatic, and the cardiac silhouette assumes a spherical shape (Figure 25-10). Dogs with left atrial perforation may still display left atrial enlargement.[68] The degree of cardiomegaly depends on the amount of the effusion, as well as the rate of accumulation. Consequently, the shape of the heart is more important than the overall size of the heart in recognizing the presence of pericardial effusion. Because other

A

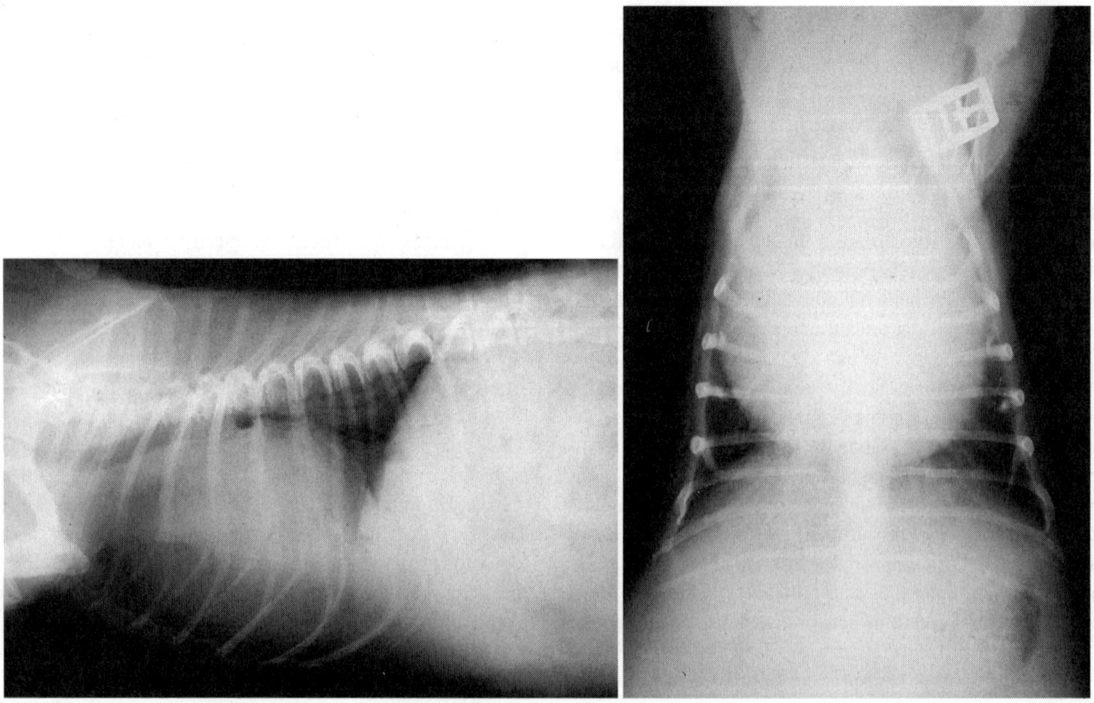

B

FIGURE 25-10 Thoracic radiographs from dogs with pericardial effusion. **A,** Lateral projection. **B,** Dorsoventral projection. (See text for details.)

conditions may produce similar findings when cardiomegaly is severe (e.g., dilated cardiomyopathy, tricuspid dysplasia), the radiographic diagnosis of pericardial effusion must be interpreted along with clinical data from other examinations, especially the physical examination and echocardiography. In patients with cardiac tamponade and congestive right heart failure, an enlarged caudal vena cava is evident on thoracic radiographs and hepatomegaly and ascites are usually evident on abdominal radiographs. Pleural fluid may be present in some dogs and may obscure evaluation of the cardiac silhouette. Pleural effusion in the absence of other signs of congestive right heart failure (e.g., jugular distension, ascites, etc.) may signify the presence of thoracic mesothelioma, some other diffuse neoplastic process, or other systemic illness. Occasionally a mass lesion produces an abnormal bulge in the cardiac outline if pericardial effusion is not present or deviates the trachea dorsally or laterally.[47] Pulmonary infiltrates suggestive of pulmonary metastasis may also be present.

Other radiographic procedures that may supplement survey radiography include fluoroscopy, angiocardiography, and pneumopericardiography. These procedures have largely been supplanted by echocardiography and are generally only of historical interest. Fluoroscopy typically shows an enlarged cardiac silhouette and relatively motionless cardiac borders.[2] Nonselective and selective angiocardiography may display normal-size cardiac chambers displaced within the large heart shadow and may be used to outline cardiac masses that have invaded the cardiac chambers, especially right atrial hemangiosarcomas and heart base tumors.[76-78]

PNEUMOPERICARDIOGRAPHY

When echocardiography is not available, pneumopericardiography is a relatively simple and helpful diagnostic aid that may provide similar information.[79] However, it is rarely performed. If done, it should be performed immediately following pericardiocentesis, using the same catheter, primarily to rule out the presence of intrapericardial mass lesions (Figure 25-11). The technique involves replacing approximately three quarters of the fluid removed (using the same needle and catheter that was used for pericardiocentesis) with room air or, preferably, CO_2.[80] Thoracic radiographs are then obtained in right lateral, left lateral, ventrodorsal, and dorsoventral positions.[79,80] The lateral views are generally the most helpful, and positional horizontal beam projections may be used to better visualize specific regions of interest.[79] Particular attention is paid to the right atrium and auricle and the heart base because of the prevalence of tumors in these locations (see below). Hemangiosarcomas are usually associated with the right atrium or auricle and are best visualized on the left lateral view, whereas heart base tumors are outlined near the ascending aorta.[2] As with any other technique, care must be taken not to overinterpret normal findings.

ECHOCARDIOGRAPHY

Echocardiography is the most sensitive diagnostic technique for detecting pericardial effusion and is crucial for identifying small or asymmetric effusions. The two-dimensional examination displays the effusion as a hypoechoic space surrounding the heart between the pericardial sac and the ventricular walls (Figure 25-12).[81-83] A small echocardiographic free space denotes a small effusion. As the amount of pericardial fluid increases, the echocardiographic free space becomes larger. Other findings include diminished right ventricular and left ventricular internal dimensions and a swinging motion of the heart within the effusion.[32] The effusion, diminished chamber dimensions, and swinging of the heart may also be observed with M-mode imaging (see Figure 25-12), but mass lesions cannot be

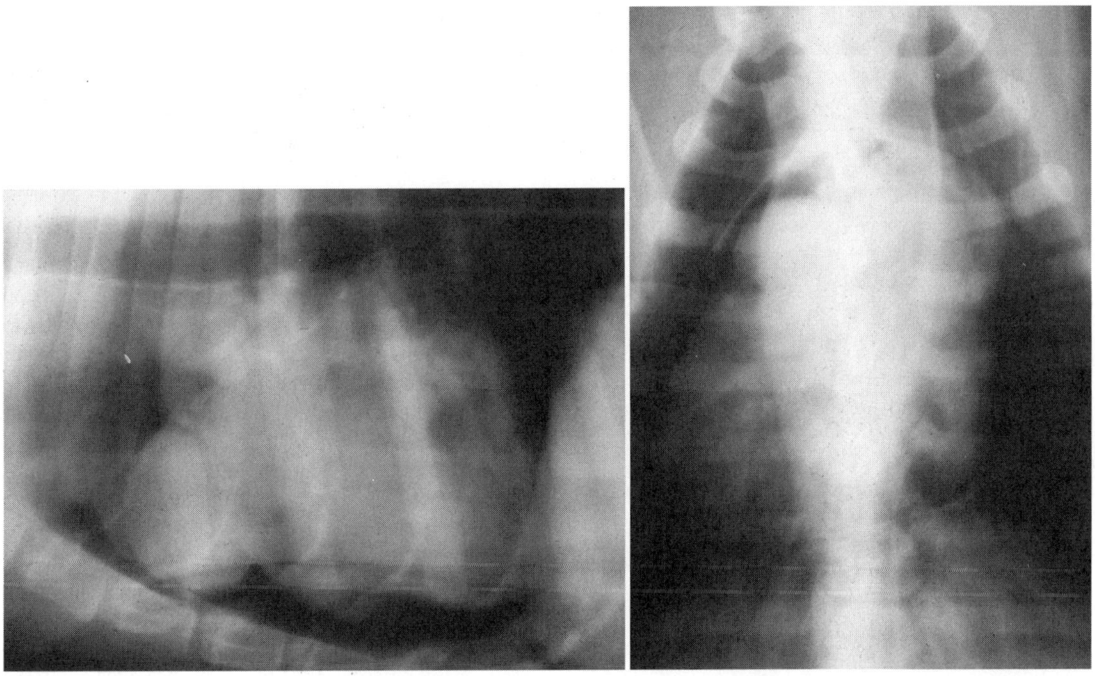

A

B

FIGURE 25-11 Pneumopericardiography in a dog with right atrial hemangiosarcoma. **A,** Lateral projection. The cardiac silhouette is outlined by a gas density, and a large soft tissue mass can be seen extending craniodorsally from the region of the right atrium. **B,** Dorsoventral projection. In this view the mass is seen overlying the right cranial portion of the cardiac silhouette, confirming its association with the right atrium. The thin parietal pericardium can also be seen surrounding the heart in this view. (Courtesy Paul D. Pion.)

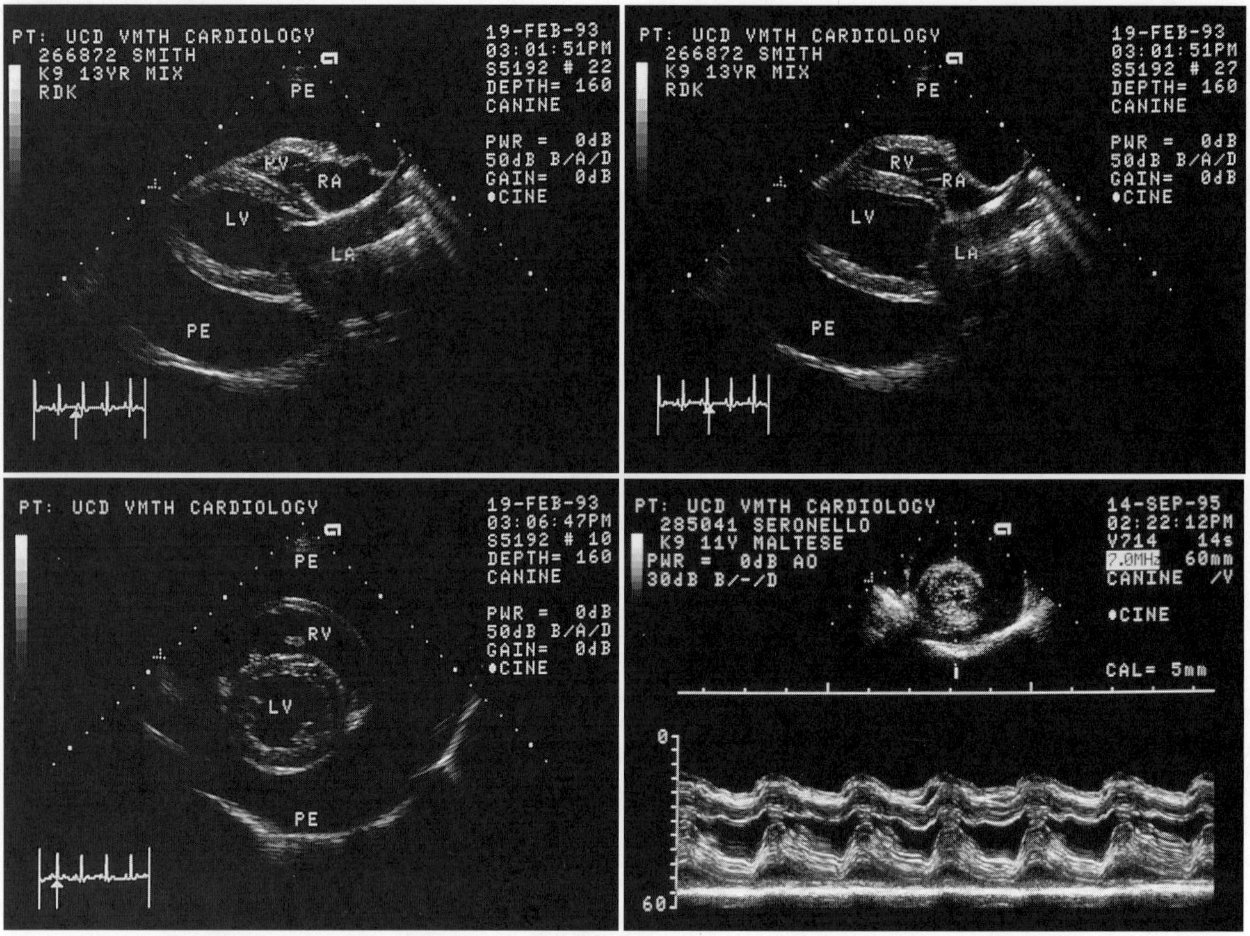

FIGURE 25-12 Echocardiograms from dogs with pericardial effusion *(PE).* **A,** Right parasternal long-axis view recorded in late diastole, showing the large, hypoechoic effusion around the heart. The right atrial wall position is normal. **B,** Same view as in **A,** recorded in systole, showing systolic collapse of the right atrium *(RA).* **C,** Right parasternal short-axis view, showing the large effusion and a small left ventricular chamber. **D,** M-mode echocardiogram at the ventricular level, showing the hypoechoic space, small left ventricular chamber dimension, swinging motion of the heart, and paradoxical septal motion characteristic of pericardial effusion. *RV,* Right ventricle; *LA,* left atrium; *LV,* left ventricle.

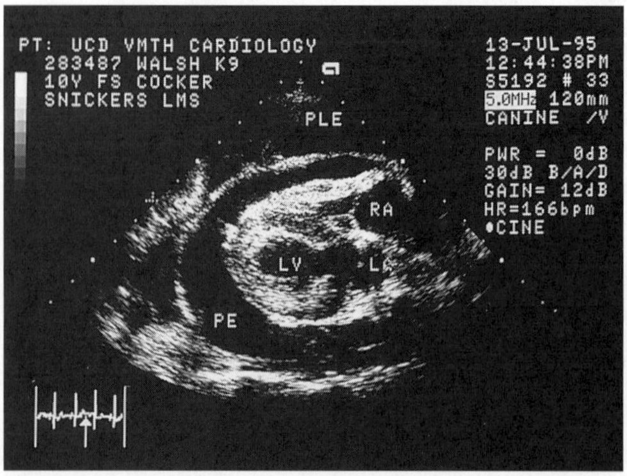

FIGURE 25-13 Two-dimensional echocardiogram from a dog with pericardial and pleural effusion (PLE). The pericardium is outlined by the fluid on both sides, allowing visualization of its true thickness. The pericardium is normal to mildly thickened in this patient, suggesting the cause of the effusion is not from a lesion in the pericardium itself. Abbreviations as in Figure 25-12.

easily identified with this modality. Because of the large mismatch in tissue types at the pericardium-lung interface, ultrasound avidly reflects from the pericardium and the pericardium always looks bright and thick on echocardiography. Consequently, echocardiography cannot be used to assess the thickness of the pericardium in most circumstances. If pleural effusion is present, the pericardium may be outlined and may be evaluated for thickness and symmetry (Figure 25-13). It may be difficult to distinguish pleural from pericardial effusion using M-mode echocardiography, but a skilled examiner can almost always make the distinction using two-dimensional echocardiography. Pleural effusion is more diffuse and often has mediastinal pleura and the edges of lung lobes within it. It is usually present between the heart and the diaphragm, and tags of fibrin can often be seen floating in the fluid. Fibrin tags are rare in pericardial effusion. Pericardial effusion is contained within a circular region around the heart and provides contrast that outlines cardiac structures such as the auricles. In most cases, pericardial effusion is more abundant at the cardiac apex and scant or absent behind the left atrium.[84]

Cardiac tamponade can be recognized using two-dimensional echocardiography as early diastolic or systolic collapse of the right atrium or right ventricular walls.[85,86] Diastolic collapse of the caudal

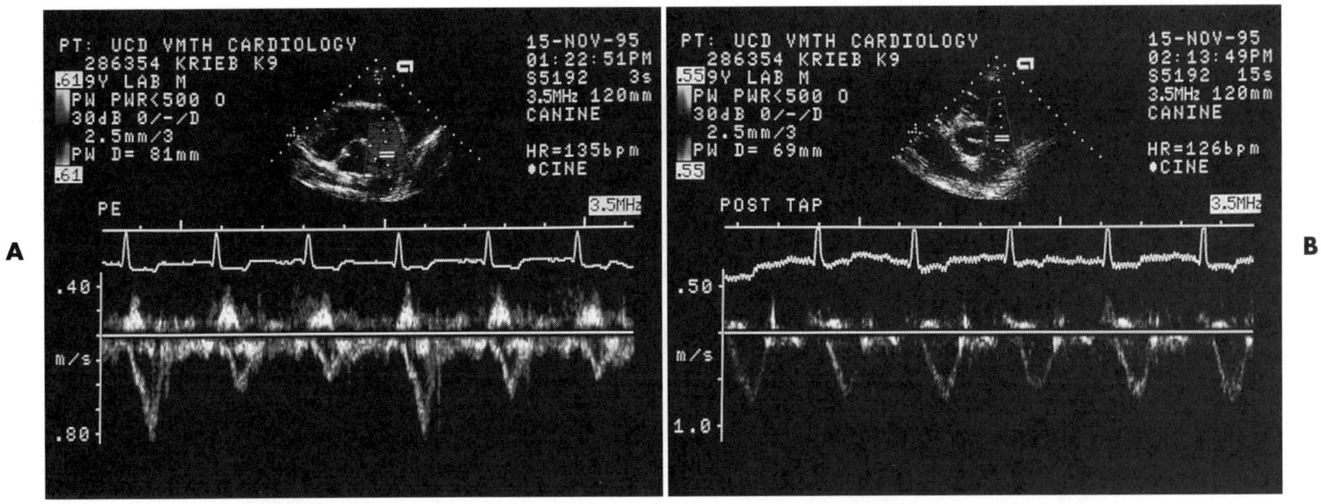

FIGURE 25-14 Pulsed-wave Doppler echocardiograms taken from a dog with pericardial effusion and cardiac tamponade. **A,** This tracing was taken from the main pulmonary artery in a dog with pericardial effusion. Notice the cyclic variability in peak flow velocity resulting from the respiratory variation in right ventricular filling (pulsus paradoxus). **B,** This tracing was taken from the same location immediately after pericardiocentesis. The peak velocities are normal, demonstrating only the mild variation that occurs with normal respiration.

vena cava has been found to be a sensitive indicator of cardiac tamponade in humans, but has not been reported in dogs and cats.[87] Diastolic or systolic collapse of the right atrium is usually seen best in the right parasternal, long-axis views (see Figure 25-12). In severe cardiac tamponade, the reduction in left ventricular chamber filling increases left ventricular wall thickness but not total mass (pseudo-hypertrophy).[88] The degree of left ventricular wall thickening correlates with the reduction in chamber size and the degree of hemodynamic compromise, but should not be misinterpreted as concentric hypertrophy.[88] M-mode examination may demonstrate some of these findings, but diastolic collapse is more difficult to recognize, especially if the heart is swinging.

Doppler echocardiographic parameters to determine the degree of cardiac tamponade have been evaluated in humans and canine experimental models, but have not been reported in dogs and cats with spontaneous disease.[86] Doppler studies may be useful in patients with equivocal or absent two-dimensional abnormalities and eventually may be helpful in quantifying the degree of hemodynamic compromise. The most notable findings on Doppler examination are marked respiratory variations in blood flow velocities, especially in the aorta and pulmonary artery (Figure 25-14). Typically, tricuspid valve and pulmonary artery flow velocities increase during inspiration and decrease during expiration, and mitral valve and aortic flow velocities decrease during inspiration and increase during expiration.[86]

In patients with IHPE, echocardiography demonstrates the consistent features of pericardial effusion and cardiac tamponade described above. No mass lesions or anatomic abnormalities can be demonstrated.[10] Therefore IHPE is a diagnosis of exclusion, in which a hemorrhagic or serosanguinous pericardial effusion is found, but no mass lesion or other etiology is identified by echocardiography or any other examination technique. Pericardial mesothelioma is a diffuse neoplastic process that usually produces hemorrhagic pericardial effusion without masses large enough to be identified by two-dimensional imaging, often resulting in a misdiagnosis of IHPE.[53] Intrapericardial thrombi have been reported in one dog with IHPE and if present can be mistaken for neoplastic masses during echocardiographic evaluation.[38] This, however, is rare.

Two-dimensional echocardiography is the most accurate technique available for detection and localization of cardiac and pericardial masses and may be useful in predicting surgical accessibility of these lesions.[50] Pericardial effusion provides contrast around the heart that improves visualization of normal and abnormal structures. Because mass lesions, especially small ones, may be much harder to identify in the absence of a surrounding effusion, a complete echocardiographic examination should be performed before pericardiocentesis, if possible. Masses may be large and easily imaged or small and difficult to distinguish from normal structures, such as pericardial or periaortic fat. Systematic examination using multiple planes is required to identify the origin and extent of most masses. The three types of lesions usually identified in dogs are right atrial masses, heart base masses, and other masses within the pericardial sac. However, failure to identify a mass does not exclude the possibility of a neoplastic disease, particularly a diffuse process such as mesothelioma.[53]

Right atrial masses may arise from the right auricle, the right atrial lateral wall, or the junction between the right atrium and right ventricle (Figure 25-15). Large hemangiosarcomas are usually readily evident upon echocardiographic examination, whereas small or cystic tumors may be more difficult to identify.[32,89] Right atrial or auricular masses are often imaged best from the right parasternal long-axis and short-axis views, or the left apical four-chamber view. The left cranial long-axis and short-axis views of the tricuspid valve and right atrium are especially valuable for detecting masses confined to the right auricle. Most right atrial masses project into the pericardial space and are accompanied by pericardial effusion, but they sometimes also project into the right atrial chamber, where large masses may obstruct tricuspid flow. Small, hypoechoic cavities are commonly seen within hemangiosarcomas, giving the lesions a mottled appearance (see Figure 25-15).[32,89]

Heart base tumors may be readily apparent on echocardiographic examination or may be difficult to image because of their typically dorsal location (Figure 25-16). Their full extent should be determined using multiple long-axis and short-axis views from both sides of the thorax. Pericardial effusion is present in most, but not all, cases. Heart base tumors commonly originate from the left cranial aspect of the aorta and lie between the aorta and main pulmonary artery. However,

A

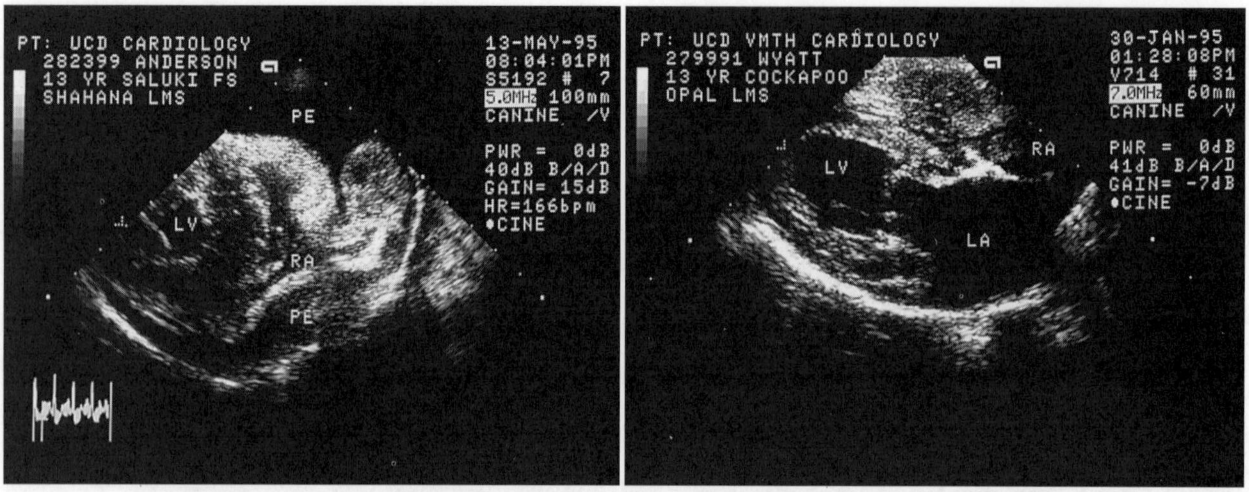

B

FIGURE 25-15 Echocardiograms from dogs with hemangiosarcoma and pericardial effusion. **A,** Off-plane left cranial view showing a soft tissue mass associated with the right auricle. Notice the "punched-out" region within the center of the mass, suggesting a cavitation filled with blood. **B,** Right parasternal four-chamber view showing a large soft tissue mass associated with the right atrioventricular junction and a smaller mass within the right atrium. Abbreviations as in Figure 25-12.

A

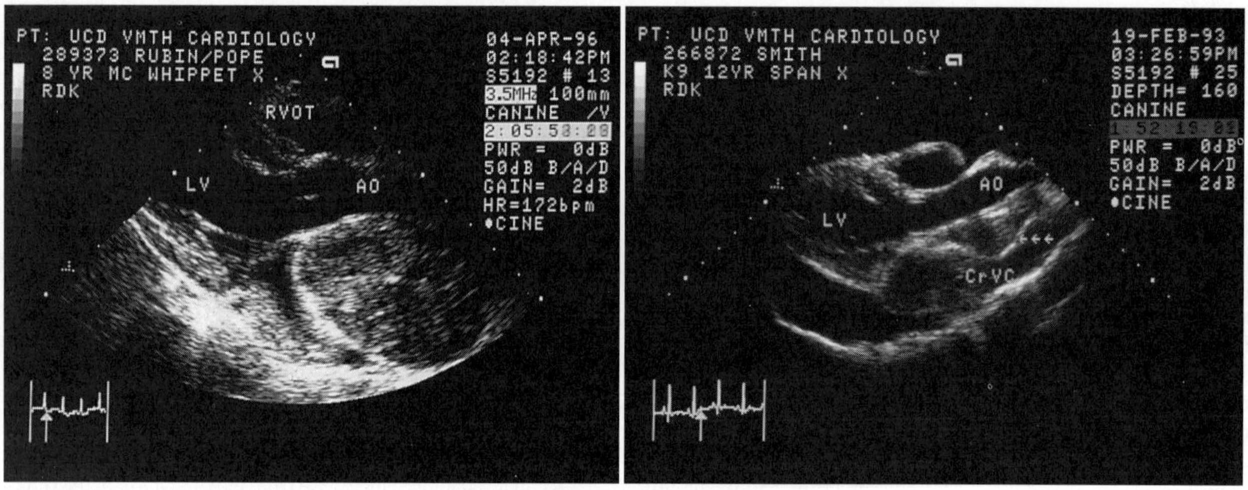

B

FIGURE 25-16 Echocardiograms from dogs with heart base tumors. **A,** Right parasternal long-axis view showing a large soft tissue mass caudal to the ascending aorta and dorsal to the left atrium. Note the absence of pericardial effusion in this dog. **B,** Right parasternal long-axis view showing a "relatively" small soft tissue structure associated with the caudal aspect of the ascending aorta. Notice the large amount of pericardial fluid. Abbreviations as in Figure 25-12.

any mass located and originating around the aortic root is suggestive of a heart base tumor. Occasionally, heart base tumors infiltrate the right atrium, making a definitive distinction from hemangiosarcoma impossible. Compared with hemangiosarcomas, heart base tumors tend to appear as more homogeneous soft tissue structures without hypoechoic regions, although this is not universally true.

Other mass lesions within the pericardial space, including abscesses, cysts, granulomas and neoplasms, may be imaged using two-dimensional echocardiography. In one report, pericardial abscesses in two dogs appeared as ovoid masses with thin outer walls and large hypoechoic centers, located over and compressing the right ventricle and atrium.[50] In another review, pericardial cysts appeared as single large hypoechoic regions or multicystic masses.[24]

PERICARDIOCENTESIS

Pericardiocentesis is an important diagnostic and therapeutic technique that should be pursued in all patients with pericardial effusion. Pericardiocentesis provides a fluid sample for analysis, reduces pericardial pressure, improves cardiac filling, and relieves clinical signs, at least temporarily. The technique of pericardiocentesis is described in Box 25-3. Unfortunately, in contrast to human medicine, the diagnostic potential of pericardiocentesis is limited in dogs and cats.[90] In many cases, other than providing definitive proof of the presence of pericardial fluid, pericardiocentesis offers no diagnostic advantage. However, because the technique may provide valuable information in some cases, such as infectious causes, laboratory evaluation of pericardial fluid should be routinely performed. The

BOX 25-3

Pericardiocentesis

Pericardiocentesis is indicated as a means of obtaining a fluid sample in all patients with pericardial effusion. Pericardiocentesis is also indicated for the initial clinical stabilization of dogs and cats with cardiac tamponade. When properly performed, pericardiocentesis is relatively easy, safe, and therapeutically effective. If the animal is critically unstable, fluid support just before and during pericardiocentesis may be warranted (see discussion of pericardiocentesis). Preparation of the patient involves shaving and surgically preparing the right hemithorax (sternum to midthorax; third to eighth ribs). Local anesthesia, including the intercostal muscles and parietal pleura, is usually adequate, but mild general sedation may be used in anxious patients. Electrocardiographic and echocardiographic monitoring are helpful but not mandatory.

Technique

Pericardiocentesis should always be performed with the patient in left lateral recumbency, and the area of the right precordium should be used to avoid laceration of extramural coronary vessels on the left side (Color Plate 104). The right lung lobes also have a larger cardiac notch, so trauma to lung tissue is minimized. The site of needle insertion can be determined in several ways. Generally, somewhere between the fourth and sixth intercostal spaces is used for pericardiocentesis, although the catheter may be inserted at the fifth intercostal space, a few inches dorsal to the costochondral junction. Also, with the patient relaxed on the table, the right forelimb can be flexed at the elbow and rotated at the shoulder in a caudal direction. The point a few inches dorsal to where the elbow crosses the costochondral junction is a good "rule-of-thumb" location for insertion of the catheter. If echocardiography is available, the site can be determined by scanning the patient from above while it is in left lateral recumbency. The site with the largest amount of effusion between the thoracic wall and the heart is chosen. Echocardiographic guidance is usually unnecessary once the site of insertion has been chosen. Several different catheter types may be used. We prefer a 14- to 16-gauge, 5- to 6-inch, over-the-needle, radiopaque catheter with one to three extra side-holes cut near the tip. Extra side-holes are cut using a no. 11 scalpel blade, taking care not to leave burrs on the edges of the cut holes. The catheter needle is connected to a three-way stopcock, extension tubing, and a large (30 to 60 mL) syringe. After surgical preparation and infiltration with local anesthetic, the catheter is inserted through a small skin incision and is slowly advanced. Once the catheter enters the thorax, mild suction is applied to the syringe and the catheter is slowly advanced toward the heart. As the catheter is advanced and contacts the pericardium, a scratching sensation may be detected, and minimal further advancement will result in penetration of the pericardium. In other instances, the actual penetration of the pericardium is not detected. When pleural effusion is present, it will often enter the catheter immediately upon entering the thoracic cavity. Pleural effusion is most commonly clear to serosanguinous or pale yellow and generally acellular. If pleural effusion is encountered, the needle should be further advanced until pericardial fluid is obtained. Pericardial effusion is generally hemorrhagic with a "port wine" appearance. When fluid is obtained, the catheter is advanced over the needle into the pericardial space, the needle is removed, and the stopcock is connected directly to the catheter. As much pericardial fluid as possible should be removed. Gently altering patient or catheter position may aid in removing remaining fluid as the pericardial space collapses.

Complications

Pericardiocentesis, when performed as described, is a safe procedure and serious complications are rare. The degree of risk is inversely related to the amount of effusion present. In patients with small effusions and without clinical signs the risks of pericardiocentesis may outweigh the benefits. Complications include cardiac puncture, hemorrhage, arrhythmias, coronary artery or tumor laceration, and dissemination of neoplasia or infection throughout the thorax.

Cardiac puncture usually occurs when the catheter is advanced too quickly or too aggressively and is inserted into the right ventricular chamber. This usually is not a serious complication if the catheter is immediately removed and repositioned. If right ventricular puncture is not recognized, a large amount of peripheral blood may be removed from the patient, leading to cardiogenic and hypovolemic shock. Pericardial effusion usually can be differentiated from peripheral blood in that it rarely clots unless it is the result of very recent hemorrhage. Also, the packed cell volume of pericardial fluid is usually significantly lower than peripheral blood, and the supernatant of pericardial effusion after centrifugation is usually xanthochromic.[5] Once fluid is obtained, a sample should be immediately placed in a glass tube. The tube should be rotated every 30 seconds and examined for clot formation. Blood will usually clot within 5 minutes, but occasionally this time will be prolonged. Commercial glass tubes that contain thrombin can also be used. Blood clots form almost immediately upon exposure to thrombin. Ventricular arrhythmias usually are evident when the catheter is placed into the right ventricle, and the catheter usually will "bounce" as the heart contracts. Further manipulation of the catheter within the right ventricle may lead to laceration of the wall and fatal hemorrhage into the pericardial space.

Advancing the needle too far may result in contact with the epicardium. This usually is evident by a scratching or tapping sensation and commonly results in ventricular arrhythmias. In most cases, these arrhythmias are not serious, and repositioning of the catheter leads to resolution. Rarely, antiarrhythmic medications (i.e., lidocaine) are necessary to resolve residual arrhythmias. The patient should be monitored for hemorrhage or arrhythmias for a few hours after pericardiocentesis.

---

routine evaluation of pericardial fluid should include complete white and red blood cell counts, protein content, and careful cytologic examination.[2] Bacterial culture and sensitivity are indicated if cytologic examination demonstrates bacterial organisms.

Pericardial fluid analysis generally allows accurate identification of transudative, septic, and chylous pericardial effusions.[90] However, the differentiation of serosanguinous and sanguinous effusions (i.e., neoplastic vs. nonneoplastic) is precluded by the overlap in the ranges of cell counts and biochemical properties. Also, because many intrapericardial neoplastic disorders do not readily exfoliate and high numbers of reactive mesothelial cells occur in all pericardial fluid samples, accurate cytologic identification of neoplastic effusions is difficult to impossible.[21] Consequently, caution should be exercised when evaluating the cellular component of pericardial fluid for neoplastic cells. In one report, 74% of neoplastic effusions were not detected based on cytology, and 13% of nonneoplastic effusions were falsely reported as consistent with neoplasia.[90]

In human patients, and more recently in dogs, pericardial fluid pH has been evaluated as a means of differentiating neoplastic from inflammatory disorders.[54,91] Although it has never gained widespread use in humans, the technique appears to have some valuable clinical utility in dogs, although further study is warranted. Using an acid-base analyzer in 11 dogs, Edwards[54] found that with spontaneous pericardial effusion dogs with inflammatory (vs. neoplastic) pericardial effusion, most dogs had pericardial fluid that was notably more acidic than peripheral blood. Using a reagent strip for urinalysis to determine pericardial pH values in 40 dogs with spontaneous pericardial effusion, he found that dogs with inflammatory disorders generally had pH values in the acidic range (6.5 to 7.0), and dogs with neoplastic effusions tended to have pericardial pH values in the alkaline range (7.0 to 7.5).[54] Combining both data sets, Edwards reported that a pericardial pH of 7.0 or greater had a 93% accuracy for correctly identifying neoplastic disorders and a pericardial pH of less than 7.0 had a 78% accuracy for correctly identifying non-neoplastic disorders.[54]

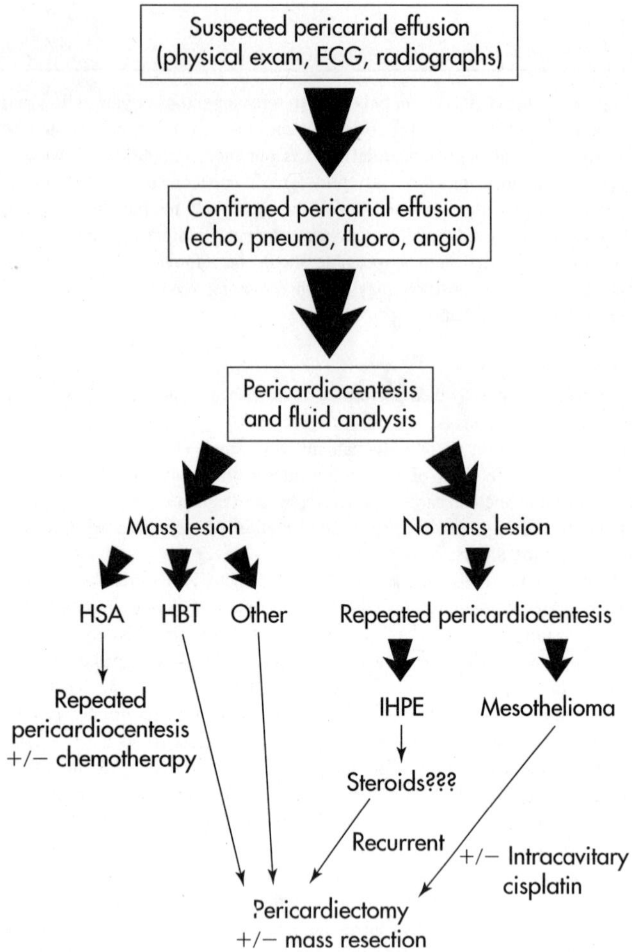

FIGURE 25-17 Flow chart for the diagnosis and treatment of sanguinous pericardial effusion in the dog. (See text for details.)

DIFFERENTIAL DIAGNOSIS

The differential diagnosis of pericardial effusion includes other causes of congestive right heart failure (or biventricular failure), such as dilated cardiomyopathy, tricuspid insufficiency (congenital or acquired), cor pulmonale, and pulmonary hypertension. Other disorders that lead to abdominal distension, pleural effusion, diminished heart sounds, and similar radiographic and electrocardiographic changes must also be considered.

Of considerable clinical importance is the fact that most pericardial effusions in dogs are sanguinous or serosanguinous, have variable and overlapping laboratory characteristics, and are generally not etiologically distinguishable. Consequently, neither the age and breed of the dog nor the physical appearance of the fluid should be used to diagnose a neoplastic pericardial disorder without a more definitive diagnosis being established, usually by echocardiography.

THERAPEUTIC STRATEGIES

The most important therapy for the clinical effects of pericardial effusion with cardiac tamponade is pericardiocentesis (see Box 25-3).[2,21] Subsequent therapy depends on the underlying disorder and in some cases involves surgical intervention. Most patients show dramatic clinical improvement following pericardial drainage, with reduction in jugular pulsation and distension, increased arterial pulse quality and resolution of pulsus paradoxus, and a reduction in the heart rate. Subsequently, the patient's general attitude improves, often immediately, and the ascites and pleural effusion resolve over the next several days. Pericardial drainage also results in an increase in the QRS complex amplitude and resolution of electrical alternans on the ECG (see Figure 25-9). Aggressive medical therapy for signs of congestive right heart failure may be tempting but should be avoided before pericardiocentesis. Because elevated venous pressure is critical for maintaining filling pressure in the compressed ventricles, diuretic and vasodilator therapy may dramatically diminish stroke volume and cardiac output by lowering venous pressure, leading to weakness or collapse.[2,16] If a patient shows signs of weakness and collapse and pericardiocentesis is not pursued, then a more rational medical therapy would be aggressive fluid expansion and *immediate* referral for pericardiocentesis. Although fluid administration will lead to increased ascites and pleural effusion in the long run, in the short run, volume expansion will maintain high venous pressures and will augment ventricular filling and cardiac output. This approach should not be taken without caution and should not be pursued when pericardiocentesis will be delayed.

Infective pericarditis should be treated with appropriate antimicrobial drugs, combined with continuous or intermittent pericardial drainage. There is a high potential for pericardial fibrosis and constriction secondary to infectious pericarditis, and pericardiectomy is almost always indicated once the patient is stabilized.[2,7] Pericardiectomy also allows retrieval of foreign objects. Acute hemopericardium or left atrial rupture should be initially relieved with pericardiocentesis. However, surgical exploration may be necessary.[68-70,92] Surgical repair of left atrial rupture secondary to severe mitral regurgitation can be attempted but is usually unsuccessful.[68-70]

Treatment of sanguinous or serosanguinous effusions, following pericardiocentesis, should be based on probable etiology as defined by pertinent diagnostic studies.[2,26] Figure 25-17 outlines the diagnostic and therapeutic approaches to sanguinous effusions in the dog. If a presumptive diagnosis of IHPE is made, the therapeutic approach is generally conservative and consists of frequent follow-up examination and pericardiocentesis, if necessary. Occasionally, pericardiocentesis is curative in dogs with IHPE. About half of the dogs with IHPE have recurrence of the effusion following pericardiocentesis within several days to several years. Oral, intrapericardial, and parenteral corticosteroids have been advocated in humans, but their use has not been validated in dogs.[7] Dogs with recurrent effusion from IHPE (usually after three or more isolated episodes) should probably undergo subtotal pericardiectomy to prevent recurrent signs of cardiac tamponade and to decrease the risk of pericardial fibrosis and constriction.[2,5,26,39,40]

Several treatment options exist in animals with an identified intrapericardial mass. The most aggressive approach involves exploratory thoracotomy with subtotal pericardiectomy and attempted mass resection. This approach is rational in patients with nonneoplastic masses and is often curative.[2,26] Surgical therapy is considered palliative in most patients with heart base tumors, often allowing several months to a year or two of symptom-free life.[26,93] Because many heart base tumors grow slowly, metastasize late, and do not bleed, pericardiectomy is a reasonable alternative to euthanasia or repeated pericardiocentesis. On the other hand, prognosis and outcome are generally not affected by surgery in patients with right atrial hemangiosarcomas because metastasis is usually already present at the time of diagnosis.[26,45,94,95] In fact, subtotal pericardiectomy may be contraindicated in patients with right atrial hemangiosarcoma because it may lead to direct spread of the tumor and may allow fatal hemorrhage to occur if the tumor ruptures. However, leaving the pericardium intact would limit the amount of hemorrhage.[2] Recently, chemotherapy has been shown to improve survival in dogs with hemangiosarcoma (splenic and right atrial) compared with clinical controls, although average survival is still less than 1 year and the improved survival time was only a couple of months.[93-98]

Treatment for pericardial mesothelioma is generally palliative. Repeated pericardiocentesis is generally the preferred means of therapy. However, surgery is often performed because the clinician cannot differentiate mesothelioma from IHPE and a surgical biopsy is the only way to make a definitive diagnosis. Although subtotal pericardiectomy relieves signs of recurrent cardiac tamponade, dissemination of the tumor to the pleural space (if not already present) and a grave prognosis prevent performing of the procedure. Intracavitary cisplatin has shown promise for producing extended periods of remission in dogs with pleural and peritoneal mesothelioma, but has not been evaluated in dogs with isolated pericardial mesothelioma.[99]

Recent reports on humans suggest that percutaneous pericardial balloon dilation may be an alternative to pericardiectomy for certain pericardial disorders.[100,101] The procedure is performed by placing a guide wire and balloon catheter across the parietal pericardium following pericardiocentesis. When the balloon is inflated the pericardium ruptures, forming a pericardial "window" that allows continuous drainage of pericardial fluid into the pleural space. Pericardial balloon dilation has not been evaluated in dogs and cats.

Constrictive and Constrictive-Effusive Pericarditis

Restriction of cardiac filling may occur as a result of reduced pericardial compliance involving the parietal pericardium, the visceral pericardium (epicardium), or both. In some cases, a small amount of pericardial fluid, although not enough to cause signs of tamponade if the pericardium were normal, may accompany constrictive pericarditis (constrictive-effusive pericarditis). In our experience the latter form is more frequently recognized in dogs. Constrictive pericarditis usually occurs as a result of thickening and fibrosis of the parietal pericardium secondary to an inflammatory process (Color Plate 105). With time the epicardium also becomes thickened and fibrotic and may fuse with the parietal pericardium, causing obliteration of the pericardial space. Reported causes in dogs include recurrent IHPE, intrapericardial foreign bodies, chronic septic pericarditis, intrapericardial neoplasia, and traumatic pericardial hemorrhage.[2,75,102-104] Constrictive pericarditis has been reported in a cat with dilated cardiomyopathy.[105] The cause of constrictive pericarditis cannot be determined in most cases at the time of diagnosis. In humans, most constrictive pericardial disease is the result of an infectious process or neoplasia.[7]

HISTORY AND PHYSICAL EXAMINATION

Presenting complaints and physical findings are quite similar to pericardial effusion. Ascites is the most common. Less common clinical signs include dyspnea, tachypnea, fatigue, weakness, syncope, and weight loss. Most reported cases have involved middle-age, large-breed dogs.[75] The clinical signs have often been present for weeks to months. Occasionally there is a history of previous IHPE. The most consistent clinical findings are ascites and jugular venous distension, although jugular distension is not a consistent feature.[26,75] The femoral pulse is often weak, but pulsus paradoxus is rarely observed.[7,26,75] Diminished heart sounds may be identified but less commonly than with pericardial effusion. Other auscultatory findings may include a gallop sound, a systolic murmur, or a systolic click.

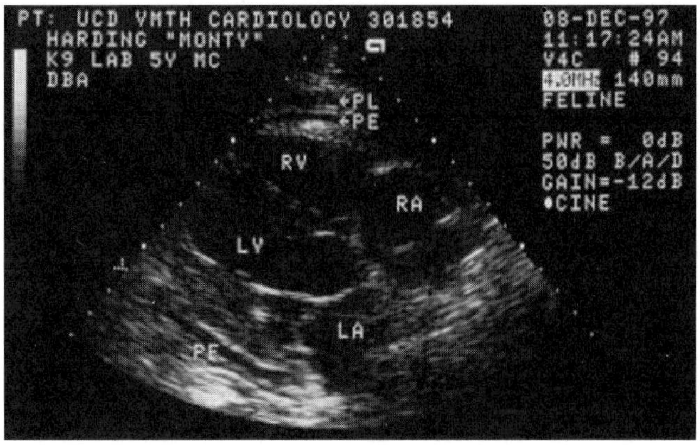

FIGURE 25-18 Long-axis two-dimensional echocardiogram from a 5-year-old dog with constrictive-effusive pericarditis presented in right heart failure (i.e., ascites) with evidence of chronic cardiac tamponade but only a small amount of pericardial effusion *(PE)*. Right ventricular diastolic pressure was characteristic of constrictive pericarditis. The massively thickened pericardium was successfully removed at surgery. *PL,* Pleural effusion; *RA,* right atrium; *RV,* right ventricle; *LA,* left atrium; *LV,* left ventricle.

These usually are not due to the constrictive pericarditis but are related to concurrent disease.[26,75] The prominent pericardial knock commonly heard in humans is uncommonly detected in dogs.[7,21,75]

ELECTROCARDIOGRAPHY, RADIOGRAPHY, AND ECHOCARDIOGRAPHY

The electrocardiographic findings in constrictive pericarditis are nonspecific, yet may aid in the diagnosis. Pericardial fibrosis tends to diminish QRS voltage, similar to pericardial effusion, although to a lesser degree and with less consistency.[75] Electrical alternans has not been reported in dogs with constrictive pericarditis. A right ventricular hypertrophy pattern has been reported in one dog with coccidioidomycosis and is a common electrocardiographic feature in human patients.[2,21] Tachycardia is the most commonly reported arrhythmia in dogs although other supraventricular arrhythmias are common in humans.[2,7]

Thoracic radiographs may or may not aid the diagnosis of constrictive pericarditis. Mild cardiomegaly may be identified with or without rounding of the cardiac silhouette. However, these findings are neither as dramatic nor as frequently identified as with pericardial effusion.[2,21,26] The caudal vena cava is commonly dilated, especially in dogs with moderate-to-severe ascites. Pleural effusion may be present.[75] As with pericardial effusion, fluoroscopic evaluation may demonstrate diminished or absent motion of the cardiac borders.

The echocardiographic diagnosis of constrictive pericarditis without an effusion is very difficult, and cardiac catheterization is usually required for an accurate diagnosis. In most cases, the diagnosis is based on the presence of clinical signs of cardiac tamponade, with only a very small amount of pericardial effusion identified echocardiographically. If pleural effusion is present and the pericardium is outlined, it may appear thickened (Figure 25-18). Subtle abnormalities on the M-mode tracing have been reported in humans with constrictive pericarditis, including flattened diastolic left ventricular posterior wall motion and abnormal systolic septal motion, but these findings have not been evaluated in dogs or cats.[106,107] Doppler echocardiography may be helpful for identifying constrictive physiology and may be able to distinguish pericardial and myocardial disease. Pulsed-wave Doppler evaluation of systemic venous, hepatic, or pulmonary venous flow often shows characteristic changes in blood flow velocity in humans.[108]

CARDIAC CATHETERIZATION

Although noninvasive studies may be supportive, the definitive diagnosis of constrictive pericarditis often requires cardiac catheterization. Central venous pressure is invariably elevated, and mean atrial and diastolic ventricular pressures are usually high. Simultaneous recordings of atrial and ventricular pressures often show equilibration and superimposition of diastolic pressures. In some dogs, a prominent early diastolic dip and middiastolic plateau may infrequently be identified on ventricular pressure tracings. The lack of consistency of this finding compared with findings in humans may reflect the fact that many dogs with constrictive pericarditis have a small amount of pericardial fluid (constrictive-effusive pericarditis). Some dogs show surprisingly normal catheterization studies, and the above findings are only evident after rapid fluid loading with a crystalloid solution.

THERAPY AND PROGNOSIS

The temporary benefits and potential adverse effects of medical therapy (diuretics and venodilators) provide little value for the treatment of constrictive pericarditis. Successful treatment invariably requires surgical removal of the fibrotic pericardium. When the epicardium is minimally involved, subtotal pericardiectomy is relatively easy and highly successful for controlling the clinical signs of congestive right heart failure.[75] However, when the epicardium is also fibrotic and thickened, epicardial stripping, a more difficult procedure, is required. There is a high degree of morbidity and mortality associated with epicardial stripping, and the results are generally less favorable than those controlled by pericardiectomy alone.[21,75]

REFERENCES

1. Miller MW, Fossum TW: Pericardial disease. In Kirk RW, Bonagura JD, eds: *Kirk's current veterinary therapy, XI: small animal practice,* Philadelphia, 1992, WB Saunders.
2. Thomas WP: Pericardial disorders. In Ettinger SJ, ed: *Textbook of small animal internal medicine,* ed 3, Philadelphia, 1989, WB Saunders.
3. Buchanan JW: Causes and prevalence of cardiovascular diseases. In Kirk RW, Bonagura JD, eds: *Kirk's current veterinary therapy, XI: small animal practice,* Philadelphia, 1992, WB Saunders.
4. Detweiler DK, Patterson DF: The prevalence and types of cardiovascular disease in dogs, *Ann NY Acad Sci* 127:481, 1965.
5. Berg RJ, Wingfield WE: Pericardial effusion in the dog: a review of 42 cases, *J Am Anim Hosp Assoc* 20:721, 1984.
6. Rush JE, Keene BW, Fox PR: Pericardial disease in the cat: a retrospective evaluation of 66 cases, *J Am Anim Hosp Assoc* 26:39, 1990.
7. Lorell BH, Braunwald E: Pericardial disease. In Braunwald E, ed: *Heart disease: a textbook of cardiovascular medicine,* ed 4, Philadelphia, 1992, WB Saunders.
8. Shabetai R: Diseases of the pericardium. In Hurst JW, Schlant RC, Rackley CE et al, eds: *The heart, arteries and veins,* ed 7, New York, 1990, McGraw Hill.
9. Holt JP: The normal pericardium, *Am J Cardiol* 25:455, 1970.
10. Watkins MW, LeWinter MM: Physiologic role of the pericardium, *Ann Rev Med* 44:171, 1993.
11. Shabetai R, Mangiardi L, Bhargava V et al: The pericardium and cardiac function, *Prog Cardiovasc Dis* 22:(2)107, 1979.
12. Harasawa H, Li KS, Nakamoto T, Coghlan L: Ventricular coupling via the pericardium: normal versus tamponade, *Cardiovasc Res* 27:1470, 1993.
13. Burger W, Straube M, Behne M et al: Role of pericardial constraint for right ventricular function in humans, *Chest* 107:46, 1995.
14. Fowler NO: Physiology of cardiac tamponade and pulsus paradoxus. II. Physiologic, circulatory, and pharmacologic responses in cardiac tamponade, *Mod Concepts of Cardiovasc Dis* 47:115, 1978.
15. Reed JR, Thomas WP: Hemodynamics of progressive pneumopericardium in the dog, *Am J Vet Res* 45:(2)308, 1984.
16. Shabetai R: The pathophysiology of cardiac tamponade and constriction, *Cardiol Clin* 7:67, 1976-89.
17. Shabetai R, Fowler NO, Guntheroth WG: The hemodynamics of cardiac tamponade and constrictive pericarditis, *Am J Cardiol* 26:480, 1970.
18. Savitt MA, Tyson GS, Elbeery JR et al: Physiology of cardiac tamponade and paradoxical pulse in conscious dogs, *Am J Physiol* 265:H1996, 1993.
19. Lorell BH, Grossman W: Profiles in constrictive pericarditis, restrictive cardiomyopathy, and cardiac tamponade. In Grossman W, Baim DS, eds: *Cardiac catheterization, angiography and intervention,* ed 4, Philadelphia, 1991, Lea & Febiger.
20. Friedman HS, Sakuri H, Lajam F: Pulsus paradoxus: a manifestation of marked reduction of left ventricular end-diastolic volume in cardiac tamponade, *J Thorac Cardiovasc Surg* 79:74, 1980.
21. Miller MW, Sisson DD: Pericardial disorders. In Ettinger SJ, Feldman EC, eds: *Textbook of veterinary internal medicine: diseases of the dog and cat,* ed 4, Philadelphia, 1995, WB Saunders.
22. Hancock FW. On the elastic and rigid forms of constrictive pericarditis, *Am Heart J* 100:(6)917, 1980.
23. Owens JM: Pericardial effusion in the cat, *Vet Clin North Am Small Anim Pract*; 7:373, 1977.
24. Sisson DD, Thomas WP, Reed JR: Intrapericardial cysts in the dog, *J Vet Intern Med* 7:364, 1993.
25. Marion J, Schwatrz A, Ettinger SJ: Pericardial effusion in a young dog, *J Am Vet Med Assoc* 157:1055 1979.
26. Reed JR: Pericardial diseases of the dog and cat. In Bonagura JD, ed: *Contemporary issues in small animal practice: cardiology,* New York, 1987, Churchill Livingstone.
27. Bouvy BM, Bjorling DE: Pericardial effusion in dogs and cats. I. Normal pericardium and causes and pathophysiology of pericardial effusion, *Compend Contin Educ Pract Vet* 13:(3)417, 1991.
28. Evans SM, Biery DN: Congenital peritoneopericardial diaphragmatic hernia in the dog and cat: a literature review and 17 additional case histories, *Vet Radiol* 21:108, 1980.
29. Suter PF: *Thoracic radiography: a text atlas of thoracic diseases of the dog and cat,* Wetswil, Switzerland, 1984, Peter F Suter.
30. Hay WH, Woodfield JA, Moon MA: Clinical, echocardiographic, and radiographic findings of peritoneopericardial diaphragmatic hernia in two dogs and a cat, *J Am Vet Med Assoc* 195:(9)1245, 1989.
31. Howell LD, ed: Pericardial disease in the dog and cat, 1985; 79-86.
32. Kienle RD, Thomas WP: Echocardiography. In Nyland TG, Mattoon JS, eds: *Veterinary diagnostic ultrasound,* Philadelphia, 1995, WB Saunders.
33. Schulman AJ, Lusk R, Lippincott CL: Congenital peritoneopericardial diaphragmatic hernia in a dog, *J Am Anim Hosp Assoc* 21:655, 1985.
34. van der Gaag I, van der luer RJT: Eight cases of pericardial defects in the dog, *Vet Pathol* 14:14, 1977.
35. Detweiler DK: Wesen und Haufigkeit von Herzkrankheiten bei Hunden, *Zentralbl Veterinarmed* 9:317, 1962.
36. van den Ingh TS: Perikarddefekt mit Einklemmung des Herzens bei einem Hund, *Schweiz Arch Tierheilkd* 119:473, 1977.
37. Milli UH, Unsuren H: Incarceration of the heart resulted from pericardial rupture in the dog, *Vet Fakult Dergisi Ankara Univ* 29:214, 1982.
38. DeMadron E, Prymak C, Hendricks J: Idiopathic hemorrhagic pericardial effusion with organized thrombi in a dog, *J Am Vet Med Assoc* 191:(3)324, 1987.
39. Matthiesen DT, Lammerding J: Partial pericardiectomy for idiopathic hemorrhagic pericardial effusion in the dog, *J Am Anim Hosp Assoc* 21:41-46, 1985.

40. Berg RJ, Wingfield WE, Hoopes PJ: Idiopathic hemorrhagic pericardial effusion in eight dogs, *J Am Vet Med Assoc* 185:(9)988, 1984.
41. Gibbs C, Gaskell CJ, Darke PG: Idiopathic pericardial hemorrhage in dogs: a review of fourteen cases, *J Small Anim Pract* 2:483, 1982.
42. Ware WA: Cardiac neoplasia. In Kirk RW, Bonagura JD, eds: *Kirk's current veterinary therapy, XII: small animal practice,* Philadelphia, 1995, WB Saunders.
43. Holt D, Van Winkle T, Schelling C et al: Correlation between thoracic radiographs and postmortem findings in dogs with hemangiosarcoma: 77 cases (1984-1989), *J Am Vet Med Assoc* 200:1535, 1992.
44. DeMadron E: Malignant pericardial effusion in dogs: seven cases, *Prat Med Chir Anim Cie* 23:(1)59, 1990.
45. Aronsohn M: Cardiac hemangiosarcoma in the dog: a review of 38 cases, *J Am Vet Med Assoc* 187:922, 1985.
46. Srebernik N, Appleby EC: Breed prevalence and sites of haemangioma and haemangiosarcoma in dogs, *Vet Rec* 129:408, 1991.
47. Kleine LJ, Zook BC, Munson TO: Primary cardiac hemangiosarcomas in dogs, *J Am Vet Med Assoc* 157:326, 1970.
48. Cobb MA, Brownlie SE: Intrapericardial neoplasia in 14 dogs, *J Small Anim Pract* 33:309, 1992.
49. Hosgood G: Canine hemangiosarcoma, *Compend Contin Educ Pract Vet* 13:(7)1065, 1991.
50. Thomas WP, Sisson DD, Bauer TG et al: Detection of cardiac masses by two-dimensional echocardiography, *Vet Radiol* 25:(2)65, 1984.
51. McFadden ER, Braunwald E: Cor pulmonale. In Braunwald E, ed: *Heart disease: a textbook of cardiovascular medicine,* ed 4, Philadelphia, 1992, WB Saunders.
52. Thrall DE, Goldschmidt MH: Mesothelioma in the dog: six case reports, *Vet Radiol* 19:107, 1978.
53. McDonough SP, MacLachlan NJ, Tobias AH: Canine pericardial mesothelioma, *Vet Pathol* 29:256, 1992.
54. Edwards NJ: The diagnostic value of pericardial fluid pH determination, *J Am Anim Hosp Assoc* 32:63, 1996.
55. Petterson T, Froseth B, Riska H: Concentration of hyaluronic acid in pleural fluid as a diagnostic aid for malignant mesothelioma, *Chest* 1988; 94:(5)1037-1039.
56. Takeda K, Ohba H, Hyodo H et al: Pericardial mesothelioma: hyaluronic acid in pericardial fluid, *Am Heart J* 110:(2)486, 1985.
57. Southerland EM, Miller RT, Jones CL: Primary right atrial chondrosarcoma in a dog, *J Am Vet Med Assoc* 203:1697, 1993.
58. Krotje LJ, Ware WA, Niyo Y: Intracardiac rhabdomyosarcoma in a dog, *J Am Vet Med Assoc* 197:368, 1990.
59. Ogilvie GK, Sundberg JP, O'Banion MK et al: Papillary squamous cell carcinoma in three young dogs, *J Am Vet Med Assoc* 192:933, 1988.
60. Vicini DS, Didier PJ, Ogilvie GK: Cardiac fibrosarcoma in a dog, *J Am Vet Med Assoc* 189:1486, 1986.
61. Ogilvie GK, Brunkow CS, Daniel GB et al: Malignant lymphoma with cardiac and bone involvement in a dog, *J Am Vet Med Assoc* 194:793, 1989.
62. Fisher EW, Thompson H: Congestive cardiac failure as a result of tuberculous pericarditis, *J Small Anim Pract* 12:629, 1971.
63. Chastain CB: Pericardial effusion from granulomatous pleuritis and pericarditis in a dog, *J Am Vet Med Assoc* 164:1201, 1974.
64. Lorenzana R: Infectious pericardial effusion in a dog, *J Am Anim Hosp Assoc* 21:725, 1985.
65. DeMadron E: Pericarditis with tamponade secondary to feline infectious peritonitis in a cat, *J Am Anim Hosp Assoc* 22:65, 1986.
66. Vacirca G, Mantelli F, Ferro E et al: Pericardial effusion with feline infectious peritonitis, *Comp Anim Pract* 19:(8)25, 1989.
67. Madewell BR, Norrdin RW: Renal failure associated with pericardial effusion in a dog, *J Am Vet Med Assoc* 167:1091, 1975.
68. Buchanan JW, Kelly AM: Endocardial splitting of the left atrium in the dog with hemorrhage and hemopericardium, *Vet Radiol* 5:28, 1964.
69. Sadanaga KK, MacDonald MJ, Buchanan JW: Echocardiography and surgery in a dog with left atrial rupture and hemopericardium, *J Vet Intern Med* 4:216, 1990.
70. Buchanan JW: Spontaneous left atrial rupture in dogs, *Adv Exp Med Biol* 22:315, 1972.
71. Edwards NJ: *Bolton's handbook of canine and feline electrocardiography,* ed 2, Philadelphia, 1987, WB Saunders.
72. Bonagura JD: Electrical alternans associated with pericardial effusion in the dog, *J Am Vet Med Assoc* 178:574, 1981.
73. Kienle RD, Pion PD, Bruyette D: The effects of thyroid hormone and thyroid dysfunction on the cardiovascular system, *Vet Clin North Am Small Anim Pract* 24:495, 1994.
74. Sacks E, Widman LE: Nonlinear heart model predicts range of heart rates for 2:1 swinging in pericardial effusion, *Heart Circ Physiol* 33:h1716, 1993.
75. Thomas WP, Reed JR, Bauer TG et al: Constrictive pericardial disease in the dog, *J Am Vet Med Assoc* 184:(5)546, 1984.
76. Cantwell HD: Angiographic diagnosis of heart base tumor in the dog, *J Am Anim Hosp Assoc* 18:83, 1982.
77. Buchanan JW: Selective angiography and angiocardiography in dogs with acquired cardiovascular disease, *Vet Radiol* 6:5, 1965.
78. Bohn FK, Rhodes WH: Angiograms and angiocardiograms in dogs and cats: some unusual filling defects, *Vet Radiol* 11:21, 1970.
79. Reed JR, Thomas WP, Suter PF: Pneumopericardiography in the normal dog, *Vet Radiol* 24:(3)112, 1983.
80. Ticer JW, Pneumopericardiography. In Ticer JW, ed: *Radiographic technique in small animal practice,* Philadelphia, 1975 WB Saunders.
81. Moise NS: Echocardiography. In Fox PR, ed: *Canine and feline cardiology,* New York, 1988, Churchill Livingstone.
82. Bonagura JD, Pipers FS: Echocardiographic features of pericardial effusion in dogs, *J Am Vet Med Assoc* 179:49, 1981.
83. Anonymous: The heart and arteries. In Evans HE, ed: *Miller's anatomy of the dog,* ed 3, Philadelphia, 1993, WB Saunders.
84. Bonagura JD, Herring DS: Echocardiography: acquired heart disease, *Vet Clin North Am Small Anim Pract* 15:1209, 1985.
85. Berry CR, Lombard CW, Hager DA: Echocardiographic evaluation of cardiac tamponade in dogs before and after pericardiocentesis: four cases (1984-1986), *J Am Vet Med Assoc* 192:1597, 1988.
86. Chandraratna PA: Echocardiography and Doppler ultrasound in the evaluation of pericardial disease, *Circulation* 84(suppl I):I-303, 1991.
87. Fowler NO, Gabel M: The hemodynamic effects of cardiac tamponade: mainly the result of atrial, not ventricular, compression, *Circulation* 71:(1)154, 1985.
88. DiSegni E, Feinberg MS, Sheinowitz M et al: Left ventricular pseudohypertrophy in cardiac tamponade: an echocardiographic study in a canine model, *J Am Coll Cardiol* 21:1286, 1993.
89. Fruchter AM, Miller CW, O'Grady MR: Echocardiographic results and clinical considerations in dogs with right atrial/auricular masses, *Can Vet J* 33:171, 1992.
90. Sisson DD, Thomas WP, Ruehl WW et al: Diagnostic value of pericardial fluid analysis in the dog, *J Am Vet Med Assoc* 184:(1)51, 1984.
91. Kindig JR, Goodman MR: Clinical utility of pericardial fluid pH determination, *Am J Med* 75:1077, 1983.
92. Straw BE, Ogburn P, Wilson JW: Traumatic pericarditis in a dog, *J Am Vet Med Assoc* 174:501, 1979.
93. Brownlie SE, Clayton Jones DG: Successful removal of a heart base tumor in a dog with pericardial hemorrhagic effusion, *J Small Anim Pract* 26:191, 1985.
94. Brown NO, Patnaik AK, MacEwen EG: Canine hemangiosarcoma: retrospective analysis of 104 cases, *J Am Vet Med Assoc* 186:56, 1985.
95. Brown NO: Hemangiosarcomas, *Vet Clin North Am Small Anim Pract* 15:569, 1985.
96. Sorenmo KU, Jeglum KA, Helfand SC: Chemotherapy of canine hemangiosarcoma with doxorubicin and cyclophosphamide, *J Vet Intern Med* 7:370, 1993.
97. Hammer AS, Couto CG, Filppi J et al: Efficacy and toxicity of VAC chemotherapy (vincristine, doxorubicin, and cyclophosphamide) in dogs with hemangiosarcoma, *J Vet Intern Med* 5:160, 1991.

98. de Madron E, Helfand SC, Stebbins KE: Use of chemotherapy for treatment of cardiac hemangiosarcoma in a dog, *J Am Vet Med Assoc* 190:887, 1987.
99. Moore AS, Kirk C, Cardona A: Intracavitary cisplatin chemotherapy experience with six dogs, *J Vet Intern Med* 5:227, 1991.
100. Ziskind AA, Pearce AC, Lemmon CC et al: Percutaneous balloon pericardiotomy for the treatment of cardiac tamponade and large pericardial effusions: description of technique and report of the first 50 cases, *J Am Coll Cardiol* 21:1, 1993.
101. Palacios IF, Tuzcu EM, Ziskind AA et al: Percutaneous balloon pericardial window for patients with malignant pericardial effusion and tamponade, *Cathet Cardiovasc Diagn* 22:244, 1991 (comments).
102. Schwartz A, Wilson GP, Hamlin RL et al: Constrictive pericarditis in two dogs, *J Am Vet Med Assoc* 159:763, 1971.
103. Ader P, Hansen J: Constrictive pericarditis in a dog, *Canine Pract* 7:16, 1980.
104. Neer TM: Chronic constrictive pericarditis in an American Staffordshire, *J Am Anim Hosp Assoc* 18:595, 1982.
105. Bunch SE, Bolton GR, Hornbuckle WE: Pericardial effusion with restrictive pericarditis associated with congestive cardiomyopathy in a cat, *J Am Anim Hosp Assoc* 17:739, 1981.
106. Feigenbaum H: *Echocardiography,* ed 4, Philadelphia, 1986, Lea & Febiger.
107. Engel PJ, Fowler NO, Tei CW et al: M-mode echocardiography in constrictive pericarditis, *J Am Coll Cardiol* 6:471, 1985.
108. Hatle LK, Appleton CP, Popp RL: Differentiation of constrictive pericarditis and restrictive cardiomyopathy by Doppler echocardiography, *Circulation* 79:357, 1989.

CHAPTER 26

Pulmonary Arterial and Systemic Arterial Hypertension

Pulmonary Hypertension

NORMAL PULMONARY CIRCULATION

The lung serves several important physiologic functions. During passage of blood through the lungs, hemoglobin is normally saturated by oxygen and the blood is cleansed of particulate matter and bacteria. In addition, the lungs serve an important role in acid-base balance by excreting carbon dioxide, and the vascular endothelium participates in synthesizing and degrading various hormones and vasoactive substances.[1-3] Normal pulmonary function depends on several factors, including the rate of pulmonary blood flow, the physical properties of the alveolar membrane, capillary and interstitial hydrostatic pressure gradients, and the physical properties of the blood.[4] Any of these factors may be adversely affected in patients with pulmonary artery hypertension (PAH).

Pulmonary blood flow describes the amount of blood per unit time that passes from the pulmonary arteries, through the pulmonary capillaries, and to the pulmonary veins. Normally, pulmonary blood flow is roughly equal to cardiac output and systemic blood flow. The lungs also receive an oxygenated blood supply from the bronchial circulation. This is part of the systemic circulation and does not traverse the alveolar capillary network.[3] Bronchial arteries ramify into a capillary network drained by bronchial veins that primarily empty into the pulmonary veins. Therefore the bronchial circulation constitutes a physiologic right-to-left shunt, and, consequently, the left ventricular output is slightly greater than right ventricular output. In the normal individual, bronchial circulation accounts for only about 1% to 2% of total cardiac output, and the resulting desaturation of arterial blood is trivial.[3,4] In some disease states, however, bronchial blood flow may increase and clinically significant arterial desaturation may occur.[5]

The pulmonary circulation is a low-pressure, low-resistance, high-capacitance vascular bed.[3] Normal pulmonary arterial pressure must be considered in relation to the setting in which it is being measured. Most veterinary patients require at least heavy sedation for right heart catheterization. This may alter the accuracy of pressure measurements. Also, pulmonary artery pressure is highly influenced by altitude. The lower partial pressure of atmospheric oxygen at higher altitudes promotes pulmonary vasoconstriction. This elevates pulmonary artery pressure (see below). Thus different normal reference ranges must be established at different altitudes. Normal awake dogs at sea level have a peak systolic pulmonary artery pressure between 15 and 25 mm Hg, end-diastolic pressure between 5 and 10 mm Hg, and mean values ranging from 10 to 15 mm Hg.[6]

The pressure within the pulmonary artery is directly related to the pulmonary venous pressure, right ventricular cardiac output, and pulmonary vascular impedance. Pulmonary vascular resistance (PVR) is the dominant factor in impedance and is mathematically quantified, using Ohm's law, as the ratio of mean driving pressure (mean pulmonary artery pressure − mean left atrial pressure; ΔP in mm Hg) to mean flow (cardiac output; Q in L/min).[5] Vascular resistance is expressed as mm Hg/L/min or may be converted to metric units (dynes sec cm^{-5}) by multiplying by 80.[5] In normal human adults, PVR is 67 ± 23 dynes sec cm^{-5} In dogs and cats, PVR decreases as body size increases because pulmonary artery pressure remains constant as pulmonary blood flow increases. PVR can be indexed to body size by multiplying by the body surface area.

Vascular resistance reflects several factors that include the cross-sectional area of small muscular arteries and arterioles. The main determinants of PVR are the activity of vascular smooth muscle in these small arteries and arterioles, the intravascular pressure, and the extravascular pressure.[3] Other determinants of vascular resistance include blood viscosity, total lung mass, and the presence or absence of proximal vascular obstruction.[3,5]

The normal pulmonary vascular bed is highly distensible.[7] Thus the cross-sectional area of the bed varies directly with transmural pressure and flow. Even with large increases in pulmonary blood flow (e.g., during exercise) only minimal increases in pulmonary artery pressure occur as a result of a passive decrease in PVR (Figure 26-1).[3,5,8] The reduction in PVR is partly due to an increase in the effective radius of distensible vessels secondary to the increased flow and partly due to recruitment of vessels not used at rest.[5,7,8] It is apparent from the Poiseuille relationship (see Chapter 2) that PVR can be significantly altered by even small changes in the radius of the vessels.

ETIOLOGY AND PATHOGENESIS

The pulmonary vascular system is vulnerable to several pathologic conditions that can precipitate PAH (Table 26-1). The anatomic site of these abnormalities ranges from the main pulmonary artery to the left ventricle during diastole. In the clinical setting, moderate-to-severe PAH usually results from an increase in pulmonary blood flow or an increase in PVR. Often, multiple abnormalities lead to the development of PAH.

Increased pulmonary blood flow. So called hyperkinetic pulmonary hypertension results from large increases in pulmonary blood flow.[5,9,10] In patients with large left-to-right shunts, PAH may occur simply because of increased pulmonary blood flow. Congenital

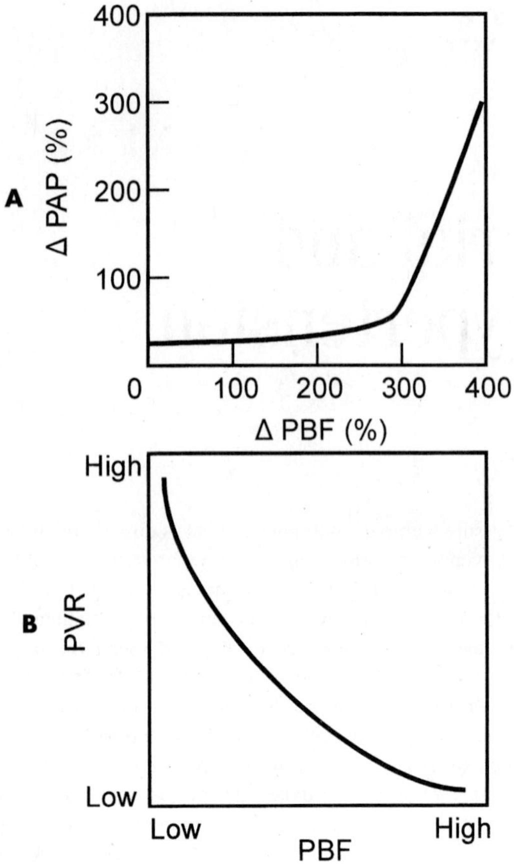

FIGURE 26-1 Pulmonary pressure-flow and resistance-flow relation. **A,** At any given lung volume a hyperbolic relationship exists between pressure and flow in which large changes in pulmonary blood flow are associated with only small elevations in pulmonary artery pressure. **B,** The net result is that as flow increases, pulmonary vascular resistance decreases. *PAP,* Pulmonary artery pressure; *PBF,* pulmonary blood flow; *PVR,* pulmonary vascular resistance.

TABLE 26-1

Mechanisms and causes of pulmonary hypertension

Mechanism	*Clinical cause*
Increased pulmonary blood flow	Congenital left-to-right shunts, increased cardiac output
Increased blood viscosity	Polycythemia
Increased pulmonary vascular resistance	
Increased resistance to pulmonary venous drainage	Prolonged left atrial hypertension Prolonged elevated left ventricular end-diastolic pressure Pulmonary venous obstruction Congenital anomalies of pulmonary veins and/or left atrium
Loss of pulmonary vessels	Pulmonary embolism: heartworm disease, hyperadrenocorticism, immune-mediated hemolytic anemia, sepsis, neoplasia, nephrotic syndrome Severe parenchymal disease (cor pulmonale)
Luminal narrowing	
Anatomic	Eisenmenger's syndrome Heartworm disease (mild-to-moderate arteriopathy) Primary pulmonary hypertension
Pulmonary vasoconstriction	High altitude disease Severe parenchymal disease (cor pulmonale) Hypoventilation: neuromuscular disease, obesity, chest wall deformities

anomalies, including atrial septal defect, ventricular septal defect, and patent ductus arteriosus, are the most common causes of increased pulmonary blood flow in veterinary patients. Animals with an elevated cardiac output from almost any underlying cause (e.g., anemia, fever, exercise) may theoretically develop PAH. However, the hypertension is generally mild, and clinical recognition of this abnormality is uncommon. In many cases, the increased flow may be accompanied by a passive reduction in PVR and little increase in pulmonary artery pressure occurs.[7,8] However, many disease states reduce the compliance of the pulmonary vasculature so that even modest increases in cardiac output can elevate the pulmonary artery pressure. If pulmonary blood flow exceeds the capacity of the pulmonary vascular bed to accommodate the extra flow, PAH occurs. As long as PVR is normal or low, indicating normal pulmonary vasculature, the shunt or other underlying cause may be corrected and normal pulmonary vascular physiology restored.[9] Prolonged exposure to increased flow and pressure may result in pulmonary artery pathology that leads to a permanent increase in PVR. This can ultimately result in a right-to-left shunt, as seen in Chapters 12 and 13.

Increased blood viscosity. Increased blood viscosity is an often overlooked cause of PAH, primarily because it is infrequently encountered in clinical practice. Diseases that cause hypoxemia (e.g., tetralogy of Fallot) result in an increase in erythropoietin secretion and an expansion of the red blood cell mass. If the resultant increase in hematocrit exceeds 55%, a rise in blood viscosity occurs. This increases PVR and exacerbates the PAH.[8] The resultant decrease in pulmonary blood flow and increase in right-to-left shunting may actually offset any improvement in local tissue oxygen delivery brought about by the polycythemia. Other diseases that increase blood viscosity have similar effects. Correction of the polycythemia can improve pulmonary blood flow, decrease the amount of right-to-left shunt, and reduce hypoxemia.

Increased resistance to pulmonary venous drainage. Many diverse conditions cause so-called postcapillary (pulmonary veins, left atrium, mitral valve, left ventricle) obstruction to pulmonary blood flow and increased resistance to pulmonary venous drainage.[5,8,10] Most are diseases of the left heart that result in left heart failure. These conditions lead to chronic elevations in pulmonary artery diastolic pressure and to pulmonary capillary hypertension. Pulmonary capillary hypertension has a physiologic or symptom-limited ceiling (approximately 25 mm Hg) determined by Starling's forces. Reaching or exceeding that ceiling produces pulmonary congestion or overt pulmonary edema. An elevation of pulmonary venous and capillary pressures produces an obligatory increase in diastolic pulmonary artery pressure (Figure 26-2). In fact, the pulmonary artery diastolic pressure is virtually identical to the increased downstream mean capillary pressure. The magnitude of this pressure increase is only mild to moderate in most dogs, because

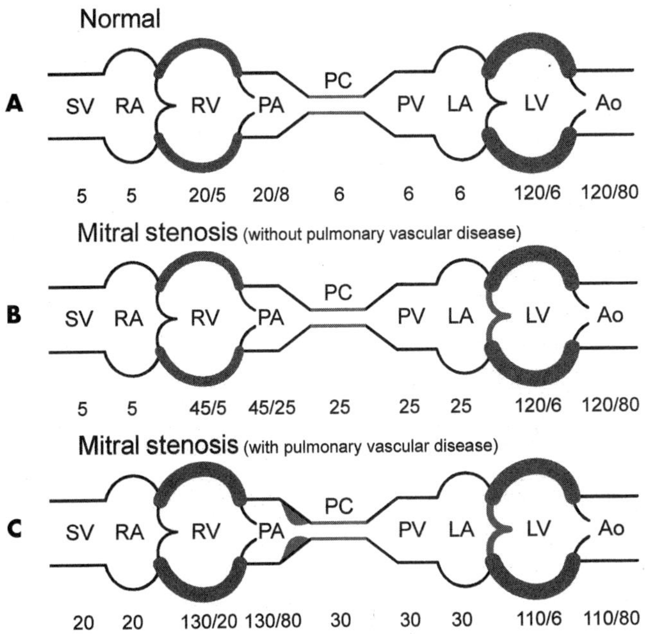

FIGURE 26-2 Schematic diagram of cardiopulmonary circulation in patients with mitral stenosis (postcapillary obstruction). **A,** Normal cardiopulmonary circulation. **B,** Severe mitral stenosis without pulmonary arterial changes. **C,** Severe mitral stenosis with pulmonary arterial changes (vasoconstriction and/or structural changes). Pressures (mm Hg) are listed below the diagrams. Note that with pulmonary vascular disease severe pulmonary hypertension and right heart failure develop. *SV,* Systemic veins; *RA,* right atrium; *RV,* right ventricle; *PA,* pulmonary artery; *PC,* pulmonary capillary; *PV,* pulmonary vein; *LA,* left atrium; *LV* left ventricle; *Ao,* aorta.

the maximal increase in pulmonary capillary pressure is approximately 40 mm Hg. This finding suggests that there is no significant precapillary obstruction to flow in these patients.[9] In human patients, a more dramatic increase in pulmonary artery pressure is often identified. In these patients, a chronic elevation of pulmonary capillary pressure leads to an increase in precapillary resistance characterized by a disproportionate increase in pulmonary artery pressure (including diastolic pressure) compared with pulmonary capillary wedge pressure (see Figure 26-2).[5,9] This so called secondary hypertension, which was first described in human patients with mitral valve stenosis, may accompany any disorder associated with chronic left-sided heart failure or other postcapillary anatomic obstructions. This, however, is unusual in dogs. The mechanism by which postcapillary obstruction elicits this precapillary response is not clearly defined but is believed to reflect arteriolar vasoconstriction because of its partial reversibility in patients with corrected mitral stenosis. This paradoxic response is thought to be a protective mechanism against pulmonary congestion and edema.[5] Clinical evidence suggests that the obstruction tends to be progressive and may lead to irreversible pulmonary vascular damage when prolonged. This vasoconstriction may be, at least in part, stimulated by increased endothelin concentrations in patients with heart disease.[11]

Decreased cross-sectional area of the pulmonary vascular bed. Many abnormalities that produce PAH do so by decreasing the cross-sectional area of the precapillary resistance vessels in the pulmonary vascular bed. This may occur because of anatomic abnormalities (e.g., stenosis of pulmonary artery branches), may be the result of physical destruction or obstruction of pulmonary vessels (e.g., pulmonary thromboembolism), may be secondary to vasoconstriction (e.g., secondary to endothelin stimulation), or may be the result of structural disease in the pulmonary vessel wall (e.g., intimal or medial hypertrophy).

Loss of pulmonary vessels. This category of disorders produces an increase in precapillary resistance to pulmonary blood flow not elicited by an associated postcapillary obstruction. In these disorders the pulmonary arteries or arterioles are physically destroyed or obstructed. The most common group of disorders in this category seen in veterinary medicine are those that produce pulmonary embolism (see Chapter 31).

Pulmonary embolism is a common sequel[9] to heartworm disease, especially after adulticide therapy.[12] Otherwise it is an uncommon complication of numerous systemic diseases in dogs, including cardiac disease, neoplasia, pancreatitis, disseminated intravascular coagulopathy, autoimmune hemolytic anemia, sepsis, glomerular disease, and hyperadrenocorticism.[13,14] No matter the cause or the composition of the embolus (thrombus, air, fat, etc.), pulmonary embolism causes obliteration of pulmonary blood flow by direct obstruction of the vessel and by the release of vasoactive mediators such as thromboxane A_2, histamine, and serotonin.[9,10] Although histamine is primarily thought to promote vasodilation, the attenuation of PVR in dogs with pulmonary embolism given antihistamines suggests it influences the increase in PVR seen with pulmonary embolism.[15] The exact role of histamine in the pathophysiology of pulmonary hypertension remains unclear.[5] Hypoxemia-induced pulmonary vasoconstriction (see below) and endothelial damage may lead to a reduction in local vasodilatory mediators in patients with pulmonary embolism.[16,17] Embolism of a small or distal artery may produce no change in pulmonary artery pressure and have no clinical sequelae. However, if multiple emboli occlude numerous small pulmonary arteries or a large embolus lodges in a major arterial branch or in the main pulmonary artery, the increase in PVR and resultant PAH can be severe.

Luminal narrowing. In the group of disorders that cause luminal narrowing, a precapillary increase in PVR is caused by a generalized decrease in the cross-sectional area of the pulmonary arterioles without physical loss or obstruction. This may occur because of functional vasoconstriction or may be the result of a pathologic condition that irreversibly damages the vessel.

It is well known that acute hypoxia elicits profound pulmonary vasoconstriction, and there is general agreement that this response, at least in part, is a compensatory mechanism for adjusting capillary perfusion to alveolar ventilation. However, great species variability in the magnitude of this response exists. It is quite intense in cattle, intermediate in humans and pigs, and comparatively mild in dogs and sheep.[5] There is also variability within a given species, and younger animals tend to have a more profound response. The mechanism remains unclear. However, evidence suggests a hypoxic-induced local release of histamine, and other mediators, such as endothelial-derived relaxing factor (nitric oxide) and endothelin, may play an important role.[5] Because the pulmonary vascular bed can recruit numerous other vessels, localized hypoxic vasoconstriction does not cause PAH. On the other hand, disorders that lead to generalized hypoxia cause generalized hypoxic pulmonary artery vasoconstriction and the development of PAH.

In some patients with congenital cardiac shunts, a true increase in PVR contributes to the PAH.[5,18-20] *Eisenmenger's syndrome* is a term applied to patients with cardiac shunts and severe PAH in whom reversal of a left-to-right shunt has occurred.[21] This may be in part a functional vasoconstriction or may be due to permanent pathologic

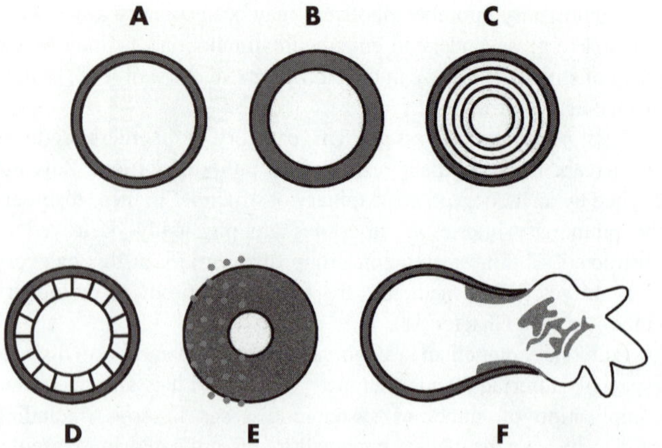

FIGURE 26-3 Schematic diagram of progressive pathologic lesions associated with pulmonary vascular obstructive disease. **A,** Normal. **B,** Medial hypertrophy. **C,** Cellular intimal proliferation. **D,** Concentric laminar intimal fibrosis. **E,** Fibrinoid necrosis with or without arteritis. **F,** Plexiform lesions.

BOX 26-1

The right ventricle in pulmonary hypertension

The right ventricular (RV) response to PAH varies depending on several variables, including congenital versus acquired obstruction, and, in the latter case, whether the obstruction occurs early or late in life; the acuteness and rapidity of progression; the severity of vascular obstruction; and the activity status of the patient.[9,24]

The ability of the RV to increase its wall thickness in response to a pressure overload is greater in the fetus and in early life.[9] This is probably because the myocardium can thicken through both hypertrophy (increased cell size) and hyperplasia (increased cell number). As a result, patients that develop PAH in utero demonstrate striking degrees of concentric hypertrophy.[9] In many cases, the hypertrophy can compensate for even marked elevations of RV systolic pressure, and RV myocardial failure is held at bay until late in life.

Conversely, acute increases in pulmonary artery pressure in adult animals, such as seen with acute pulmonary embolism or high altitude disease, are poorly tolerated by the RV because of its inability to develop and sustain the high wall tension and stress imposed by the increased afterload.[9] In this situation, the RV acutely dilates, which further increases wall tension, and acute RV failure characterized by a decrease in cardiac output and elevated end-diastolic pressure may occur.

Between the two extremes of chronic hypertrophy and acute dilation is a spectrum of pathophysiologic circumstances that relate both to the rate of development and progression and the magnitude of vascular obstruction. In general, the earlier in life and the more gradual the progression, the more likely it is that the compensatory hypertrophy can accommodate the increased workload.[9,23] However, when PAH is progressive and severe, eventual RV failure is inescapable.

The hemodynamic alterations in patients with PAH also vary greatly. Most patients with mild PAH, without severe hypoxemia, have normal mean right atrial (RA) and RV end-diastolic pressures and normal cardiac output at rest.[23] With progressive increases in RV afterload, elevations in RA and RV end-diastolic pressure follow. Cardiac output is usually still normal at rest but only increases slightly with exercise.[5] As pulmonary artery pressure and resistance reach systemic levels, failure of the RV is imminent, with an increase in circulating blood volume and chronically elevated RV filling pressures and a decrease in cardiac output.[23]

---

changes associated with the state of high pulmonary blood flow. Relatively late in the course of the disease, irreversible pathologic changes lead to decreased cross-sectional area of the pulmonary vascular bed. Irreversible PAH gradually develops, ultimately leading to shunt reversal when PVR exceeds systemic vascular resistance. In some patients, PAH is present from birth because of a partial or delayed involution of the fetal pulmonary arteries, resulting in persistently high PVR. It is unclear whether veterinary patients with right-to-left shunts and PAH (e.g., right-to-left patent ductus arteriosus) have persistently high PVR from birth or whether the lesion is initially left-to-right, with gradual development of PAH and shunt reversal.[18,20] Studies reporting pathologic lesions in dogs with right-to-left shunts and PAH have shown permanent arterial changes consistent with those in human reports of Eisenmenger's syndrome.[18-20]

In patients with heartworm disease without significant pulmonary embolism, mild-to-moderate PAH may still occur.[12] The physical presence of the adult worms in the pulmonary arteries leads to villous hypertrophy of the intima of the pulmonary arteries. In some patients these inflammatory responses reduce the cross-sectional area of the pulmonary vascular bed and lead to PAH. Extension of the inflammation into the parenchyma may further aggravate the process by producing reduced lung compliance and hypoxemia, leading to hypoxic-induced pulmonary vasoconstriction.[12]

The extent of reversibility of pulmonary vascular obstructive disease varies and depends on the degree of structural changes in pulmonary arterioles.[5,22] Although many disorders may lead to structural damage of the pulmonary vasculature, the related histopathologic lesions are nonspecific and limited to a small range of lesions (Figure 26-3 and Color Plate 106). In general, reversible conditions are those limited to medial hypertrophy of the pulmonary arterioles and vasoconstriction, whereas irreversibility is associated with necrotizing arteritis and plexiform lesions.[22] In human medicine, the classification of Heath and Edwards of six grades of structural changes is employed, primarily in congenital heart disease, to assess the potential reversibility of pulmonary vascular disease.[9]

The term *cor pulmonale* describes the pathologic effects of lung dysfunction on the heart, namely the right ventricle. The link between the lungs and right-sided heart disease is moderate-to-severe PAH. This form of secondary heart disease occurs as a late manifestation of many diseases of the lung and is characterized by a combination of hypertrophy and dilatation of the right ventricle. Although right heart failure can occur, it is not essential to the diagnosis. This classification encompasses many disease states with diverse etiologies, pathogenesis, and clinical characteristics. Although it has long been thought that a physical destruction of vessels is essential in the pathogenesis of cor pulmonale, recent evidence suggests that anatomic loss of vessels does not play a major role in the development of PAH.[23] Other mechanisms, although not completely understood, that lead to an increased PVR include arteriolar constriction resulting from hypoxemia, acidosis, and other mediators, increased blood viscosity resulting from secondary polycythemia, and increased pulmonary blood flow.[23,24] Persistent PAH may lead to intimal and medial hypertrophy and inflammatory changes of the pulmonary arterioles that further aggravate the process. The exact relative influences of these factors has not been clearly defined and probably vary from patient to patient.

Right ventricular response to pulmonary hypertension. The basic mechanisms that provoke right ventricular alterations in patients with PAH are similar to those that provoke left ventricular alterations in systemic hypertension. However, unlike systemic hypertension, the clinical significance of PAH usually involves both the cardiovascular and respiratory systems. Chronically elevated PA pressure leads to an increased impedance to right ventricular emptying, with a resultant right ventricular pressure overload that, if

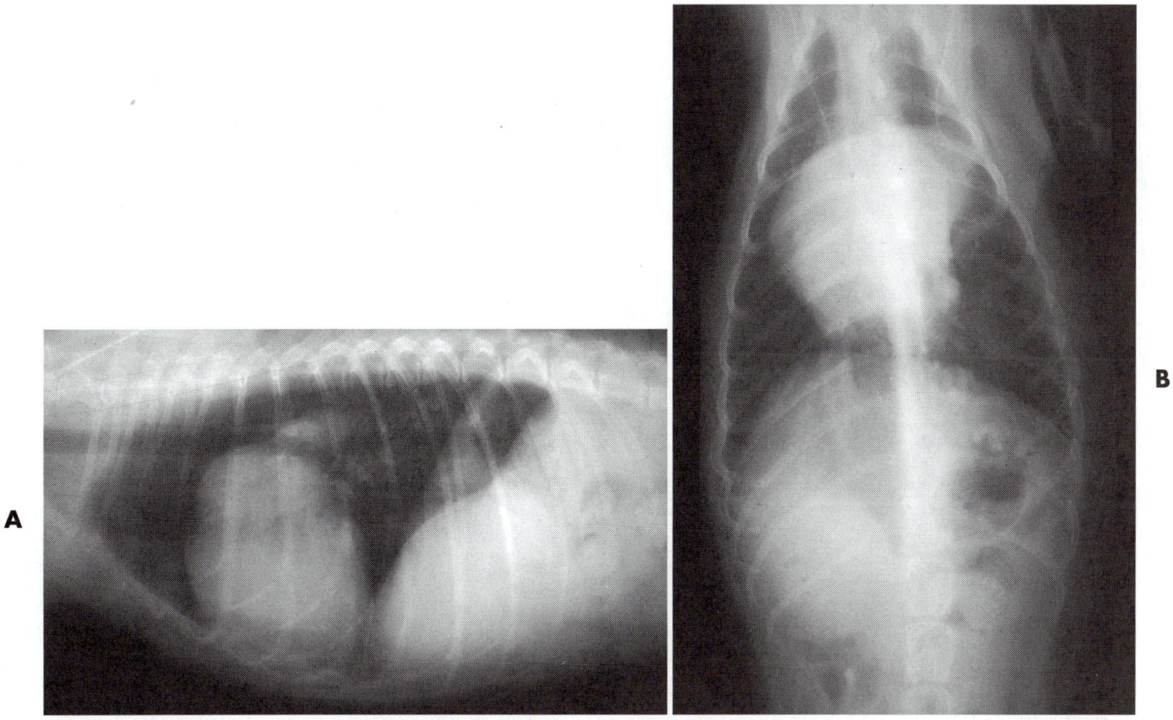

FIGURE 26-4 Thoracic radiographs from a dog with cor pulmonale and pulmonary hypertension of unknown etiology. **A,** Lateral thoracic radiograph. Moderate generalized cardiomegaly is present, and the main pulmonary artery is notably enlarged, as evidenced by the loss of the cranial cardiac waist. Right ventricular enlargement is less apparent in this projection. **B,** Dorsoventral thoracic radiograph. The main pulmonary artery and its main branches are enlarged. Right atrial enlargement and right ventricular enlargement are also evident.

severe, can ultimately lead to right heart failure.[8] Some patients with PAH may have an increased cardiac output secondary to hypoxemia. This may lead to a significant volume overload of both ventricles.[8] Diseases of the pulmonary vascular bed that may result in PAH may either lead to or result from true pulmonary disease that may further be responsible for the development of pulmonary atherosclerosis, decreased lung compliance, and intrapulmonary venous admixture.[5,9] Therefore many patients with PAH also have clinical signs relating to the respiratory system.

The actual physiologic abnormalities that result in right heart failure remain nebulous, but likely relate to either tricuspid valve incompetence resulting from right ventricular remodeling or failure of the right ventricular myocardium.[9,24] In general, the thin-walled right ventricle is better able to compensate for an increased volume load than an increase in afterload. Consequently, the primary cause of right ventricular myocardial failure is chronic elevation of afterload.[24] The exact response of the right ventricle and the hemodynamic findings in PAH depend, to some extent, on the cause, duration, acuteness, and severity of the pressure overload. For a more detailed description of the right ventricular changes in PAH see Box 26-1. As pulmonary hypertension reaches critical levels, reduced filling of the left ventricle may result because of a decrease in right ventricular cardiac output. This may lead to a reduction in systemic cardiac output with resultant clinical signs.

PRIMARY PULMONARY HYPERTENSION

When a meticulous diagnostic search fails to define an underlying cause for PAH, a presumptive diagnosis of primary or idiopathic pulmonary hypertension is appropriate.[5,25] Primary pulmonary hypertension is considered a rare and enigmatic disorder in dogs and humans. The frequency of this diagnosis in veterinary medicine, although not reported, has increased with the widespread availability of Doppler echocardiography in clinical practice. The etiology is of course unknown, and in dogs the pathology and pathophysiology have not been studied. In human medicine, however, most researchers agree that an acquired condition produces PAH through precapillary vascular obstruction (i.e., the pulmonary capillary pressure is normal), which is a complex, multifactorial syndrome.[9] It has been proposed that a vascular endothelial dysfunction that provokes pulmonary vasoconstriction, platelet activation, and thrombin formation may be involved in humans with primary PAH.[26] The presence of thrombosis in human patients with primary pulmonary hypertension has been demonstrated. It seems to have a relationship with a vascular endothelium-dependent coagulation abnormality.[26] It has further been suggested that most human patients with primary pulmonary hypertension have chronic unresolved microemboli.[25] There is no specific vascular lesion. In fact, the arteriopathy of primary pulmonary hypertension in humans is virtually identical to that seen in Eisenmenger's syndrome and other forms of pulmonary vascular obstructive disease with or without thrombotic lesions.[9,25]

CLINICAL FEATURES

Clinical manifestations of PAH usually develop late in the disorder because mild-to-moderate PAH is usually clinically silent.[9] Most patients with PAH present with clinical features reflecting the underlying heart or lung disease. These features may be more dramatic during exercise. The most prominent clinical manifestations, however, often relate to the effects of the PAH on the right heart. Patients with severe PAH often demonstrate clinical signs related to right heart failure (fatigue, ascites, etc.). Dyspnea and

A B C D

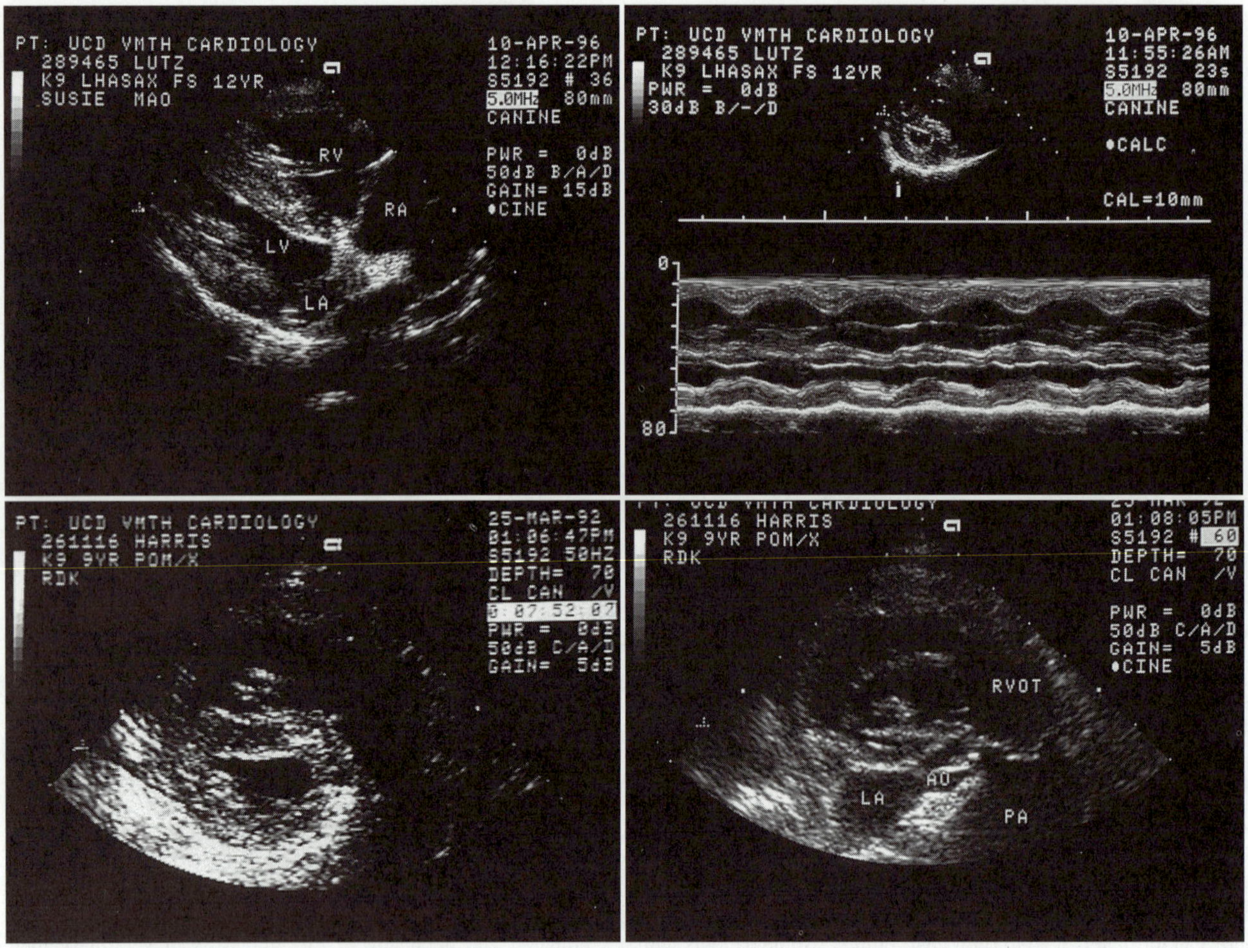

FIGURE 26-5 Echocardiograms from dogs with pulmonary artery hypertension. **A**, Right parasternal four-chamber view from a dog with primary pulmonary hypertension. Note the combined eccentric and concentric hypertrophy of the right ventricle and right atrial enlargement. **B**, M-mode echocardiogram at the level of the left ventricular papillary muscles from the dog shown in **A**, showing the right ventricular eccentric and concentric hypertrophy. **C**. Right-parasternal short-axis view at the level of the left and right ventricle from a dog with cor pulmonale. Note the flattening of the interventricular septum in response to the elevated right ventricular systolic pressure. **D**, Right parasternal short-axis view at the level of the aorta from the dog shown in **C**. Note the severe enlargement of the root of the pulmonary artery.

exercise intolerance are common manifestations when PAH is severe. Other nonspecific respiratory signs, such as tachypnea, cough, and, occasionally, hemoptysis, are also common but are usually due to an underlying respiratory abnormality rather than specifically to the PAH. On rare occasions, syncope is the main presenting complaint.[5]

Physical signs of right heart failure may be present and include abdominal distention, jugular distention and pulsation, increased right-sided precordial impulse, and cachexia. Pulmonary auscultation is variable and related to the underlying disorder. Cardiac auscultation often reveals a loud and/or split second heart sound, a right-sided systolic murmur of functional tricuspid regurgitation, and, occasionally, a gallop sound related to right ventricular hypertrophy.[8-10]

DIAGNOSIS

Routine diagnostic testing usually supports the diagnosis. However, to establish the presence of PAH, pulmonary artery pressure must be directly measured or estimated by Doppler echocardiography. The electrocardiogram is not a sensitive test, but patients with severe PAH may have tall, peaked *P* waves in lead II, a right ventricular enlargement pattern, and a right axis deviation. Thoracic radiographs usually demonstrate enlargement of the main pulmonary artery and its major branches and right ventricular enlargement (Figure 26-4). Radiographic evidence of right atrial enlargement is variable.[9,10] Other findings on thoracic radiographs may suggest a possible underlying cause.

When PAH is present from birth, M-mode and two-dimensional echocardiography usually demonstrate moderate-to-severe right ventricular concentric hypertrophy with or without right atrial enlargement. When PAH is acquired, the right ventricular response usually includes both eccentric (dilation) and concentric (increased wall thickness) right ventricular hypertrophy, rather than the pure concentric hypertrophy of congenital PAH (Figure 26-5). Paradoxical septal motion (M-mode) and systolic septal flattening (two-dimensional, short-axis) are commonly observed, and the main pulmonary artery and its branches usually appear mildly-to-moderately dilated (see Figure 26-5).[27] The degree of dilation of the main pulmonary artery and its branches is usually greater with acquired PAH. Examination of the right ventricular outflow tract and pulmonary

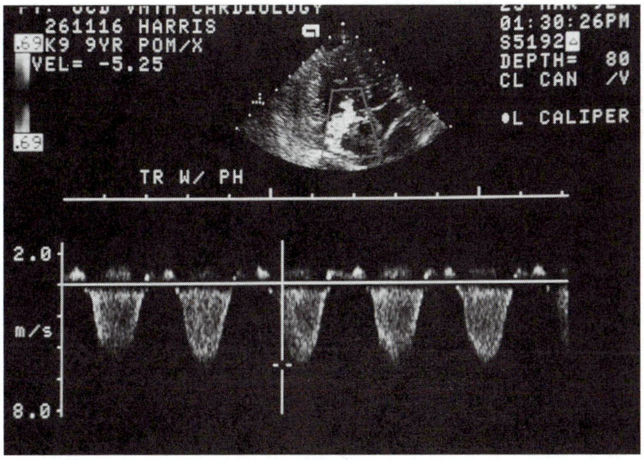

FIGURE 26-6 Continuous-wave Doppler tracing of tricuspid insufficiency from a dog with cor pulmonale. The peak systolic velocity of the tricuspid insufficiency is 5.25 m/sec. Using the Bernoulli equation (see Chapter 6), the systolic pressure gradient is 110 mm Hg. This patient was not in heart failure, so using 5 mm Hg as an estimate of right atrial pressure, the estimated right ventricular and pulmonary arterial systolic pressure is 115 mm Hg, indicating severe pulmonary hypertension.

valve region shows no evidence of pulmonic stenosis. This should be confirmed by Doppler echocardiography. In cases of severe PAH, the left ventricular internal dimensions may be reduced secondary to reduced filling and the left ventricular wall and interventricular septum may be falsely thickened (pseudohypertrophy).

Spectral Doppler echocardiography provides a means for estimating right ventricular systolic pressure or pulmonary arterial systolic and diastolic pressures noninvasively.[28,29] To estimate right ventricular and pulmonary artery systolic pressures, a tricuspid regurgitation jet is sought and its peak velocity measured by continuous-wave Doppler.[28] Because only a small valvular leak is required, clinically significant tricuspid regurgitation need not be present, and a normal, physiologic leak may be sufficient. The peak velocity and the modified Bernoulli equation are used to calculate the systolic pressure gradient across the tricuspid valve (See Chapter 6). This value is added to the estimate of right atrial pressure (5 mm Hg in a patient without right heart failure and 10 to 15 mm Hg in a patient with right heart failure) to predict the right ventricular systolic pressure (Figure 26-6). Without pulmonic stenosis, this value is also the pulmonary artery systolic pressure. Similarly, the peak velocity of a pulmonic valve regurgitant jet and an estimate of right ventricular diastolic pressure can be used to predict pulmonary artery diastolic pressure.[29] In either case, the peak regurgitant velocity is usually well above the 1.5- to 2.5-m/sec peak velocity expected if pulmonary artery, right venticular, and right atrial pressures are normal.

Cardiac catheterization is still considered the definitive diagnostic procedure to document the presence of PAH. However, this usually requires sedation or anesthesia. Patients with PAH are probably at a higher risk for anesthesia- and catheterization-related complications. Consequently, in most situations, information from Doppler echocardiographic evaluation is considered diagnostic.[9] However, additional objective information may be gained from right heart catheterization that may be important for classifying the underlying condition, determining a prognosis, or designing therapy.[8] Cardiac catheterization allows measurement of cardiac output and measurement of variables used to calculate PVR and allows testing of pharmacologic agents (see below). These data may help identify patients with reversible lesions. Pulmonary arteriograms are useful in excluding the presence of pulmonary embolism, although the risks of this procedure may outweigh its benefits (see Chapter 31).[8]

Other tests may be necessary to further define or stage the underlying disease process. Arterial blood gas analysis is helpful to establish the presence of severe pulmonary disease or pulmonary embolism. Nuclear perfusion and ventilation scans are also helpful in the diagnosis of pulmonary embolism.

TREATMENT AND PROGNOSIS

The treatment of PAH often is unsuccessful. It is most successful when the underlying disorder can be identified and controlled before the pulmonary vasculature is permanently damaged.[5] In patients in which the underlying cause cannot be removed or is not known, therapy is usually directed at decreasing PVR and controlling right ventricular pressure overload.

When decreased cross-sectional area of the pulmonary vascular bed is responsible for the PAH, pulmonary vasodilators may be attempted. However, they are only effective when active vasoconstriction of small muscular vessels contributes significantly to the PAH. Some of the vasodilators used in the acute and chronic management of PAH include oxygen, hydralazine, phentolamine, isoproterenol, calcium channel blockers, β-blockers, and ACE inhibitors.[10] The effectiveness of these agents is variable, and the ultimate choice is usually reached by clinical experience and clinical experimentation. It is common practice in human medicine to assess the acute response to a variety of agents during catheterization and to use the results to design chronic therapy.[5,9,30,31] Unfortunately, in many patients with PAH, vasodilators cause more profound systemic vasodilation than they do pulmonary vasodilation. If pulmonary vascular resistance is fixed, cardiac output cannot increase appropriately with systemic vasodilation and systemic hypotension may result.[8]

In humans, heart and lung transplantation is often the definitive therapy for patients with severe, uncontrolled PAH.[8] Recent evidence suggests that pulmonary microemboli may be a common underlying cause in all forms of PAH in humans.[25] Consequently, anticoagulation is becoming a universally accepted therapy, even in patients without proven pulmonary embolism.[5] Hypoxemia-induced pulmonary vasoconstriction may be palliated with supplemental oxygen administration.

Even when PAH can be neither cured nor improved, the ability of the cardiovascular system to tolerate the right ventricular pressure overload may be improved by controlling the right heart failure using standard therapy (diuretics, ACE inhibitors). The use of diuretics is also helpful when a component of passive PAH resulting from left atrial hypertension is present. The reduction in central volume with diuretics may cause a reduction in cardiac output; therefore diuretic use should be cautious and limited to patients with elevations in central venous pressure severe enough to produce ascites.[8]

Systemic Arterial Hypertension

Systemic hypertension is an increase in systemic arterial blood pressure. This increase can be defined as a pressure that is higher than normal or a pressure that results in clinical or pathologic sequelae. In human medicine, in which systemic hypertension is common, strict criteria for systemic hypertension have been established by following thousands of subjects over decades of life to define populations that are at risk of developing diseases secondary to systemic hypertension. Comparable data do not exist in veterinary medicine. Consequently, there is no strict definition of borderline or mild systemic hypertension in dogs and cats.

Systemic hypertension is most significant in dogs and cats with renal failure, in which it can accelerate the progression of the renal disease, and in dogs and cats with hypertension severe enough to cause secondary consequences, most commonly retinal hemorrhage, retinal detachment, and blindness. Unfortunately, because systemic blood pressure is not easy to measure and the equipment is not readily available or is expensive, many veterinarians do not have the expertise or the equipment to accurately assess systemic blood pressure. In addition, the treatment of systemic hypertension in dogs and cats has been suboptimal for many years. Consequently, even severe systemic hypertension is not treated in many veterinary patients. This problem is not limited to veterinary medicine. In one study in human medicine, only 12% of hypertensive health care workers with insurance had their hypertension adequately controlled.[32] Fortunately, blood pressure measuring devices and trained personnel are becoming more available in veterinary medicine, and drug therapy is improving.

Systemic hypertension is generally divided into essential (primary) and secondary hypertension. Although essential hypertension is common in humans, it is rare in dogs and cats, and most of the hypertension in dogs and cats is secondary to other systemic diseases. The more common causes of systemic hypertension include renal disease, hyperadrenocorticism, hyperthyroidism, and diabetes mellitus. Because systemic hypertension is secondary to primary diseases in dogs and cats, the most effective means of treating hypertension in some situations (e.g., hyperthyroidism) is to treat the underlying disease. If the underlying disease cannot be controlled or reversed, drug therapy may be warranted.

The diagnosis and treatment of systemic hypertension depends on the veterinarian's ability to accurately and reliably measure systemic blood pressure and on a knowledge of normal values for systemic blood pressure. Blood pressure in dogs remains fairly constant over the day but increases in the presence of a veterinarian and in response to stress and pain. Consequently, systemic blood pressure changes markedly from dog to dog in a clinical or laboratory setting. These factors make it difficult to identify normal values for systemic blood pressure. As a result, identifying mild systemic hypertension is generally beyond our ability. Fortunately, mild systemic hypertension is not as clinically significant in dogs and cats as it is in humans.

BLOOD PRESSURE MEASUREMENT

Pulsatile blood pressure changes continuously throughout the cardiac cycle. Measurements are taken at the peak of systole (systolic blood pressure), when the pressure is highest, and at the end of diastole (diastolic blood pressure), when the pressure is lowest. Mean blood pressure is the average of the pressures throughout the cardiac cycle. Systemic arterial pressures are usually depicted as "systolic over diastolic" pressures. A patient with a systolic pressure of 120 mm Hg and a diastolic pressure of 80 mm Hg has a systemic arterial blood pressure of 120/80 mm Hg.

Direct blood pressure measurement. Direct blood pressure measurement was first performed in a horse by Stephen Hales, an English pastor, in 1733. He exposed an artery in the horse's leg and tied it off. He then introduced a brass pipe into the artery and connected the pipe to a 9-foot glass tube. The blood reached a height of 8 feet, 3 inches and pulsed with each heart beat.[33] This height corresponds to a blood pressure of approximately 185 mm Hg. A primitive method of indirectly determining blood pressure was reported in 1555 by Joseph Struthius.[34] He described measuring blood pressure by placing objects on an artery and measuring the weight it took to suppress pulsations.

The science of blood pressure measurement has progressed in veterinary medicine in the past 260 years, yet it is an inexact science. The use of an inflatable cuff and detection of Karotkoff sounds is a well-established and accurate method of determining systemic blood pressure in humans. However, the most accurate means of determining systemic arterial blood pressure in dogs is still direct arterial puncture, albeit with a needle rather than a brass pipe. Although direct arterial puncture in an awake dog is an accurate means of determining blood pressure in that artery at that time, it may not reflect the blood pressure in the aorta or the patient's "true" blood pressure during the rest of the day when it is not in pain. Arterial pressure, especially systolic pressure, increases progressively advancing further distally in the arterial tree; therefore blood pressure measured in an artery in a limb will be higher than the pressure in the aorta.[35] Fear and pain induce catecholamine release, which increases cardiac output and raises arterial blood pressure.

Direct blood pressure measurement is accomplished by connecting a needle directly to a pressure transducer and advancing the needle into a systemic artery. The calibrated waveform is then displayed on an oscilloscope and printed on paper. The needle must be large enough so that the pressure waveform is not overdamped. We prefer a 20-gauge, 1-inch needle. The artery is then compressed manually for at least 5 minutes after the needle is withdrawn. In animals with bleeding tendencies, either the procedure should not be done or the artery should be compressed for a longer time.

Errors can occur in blood pressure measurement when direct methods are used.[36] Certain fluid dynamic properties exist within any fluid-filled pulsatile system that can alter the amplitude and shape of the pressure pulse. These include resonance, damping, and impedance mismatch.[35] The first two exert their effects primarily within the recording system as artifactual changes when fluid-filled systems are used. The latter is primarily an intraarterial property. The effect of resonance is to magnify the amplitude of certain components of the pressure pulse, especially higher-frequency components such as the initial systolic upstroke and the dicrotic notch. Resonance primarily artifactually increases systolic pressure, whereas diastolic pressure is unaffected. The tubing that connects the intraarterial cannula or needle to the transducer has the greatest influence on resonance of a recording system. The degree of resonance is determined by the tubing's internal diameter, length, and stiffness. Resonance is minimized by using a large-bore, short, stiff tube. Connecting the needle directly to the transducer obviates this problem. The presence of small air bubbles in a system greatly increases the chance of increased resonance.[36] The degree of signal amplification of a given system can be modified by a second hydraulic property damping. *Damping* describes the tendency of oscillating systems to stop oscillating because of frictional forces. An overdamped system dampens the pressure waveform, obliterating the high-frequency components and decreasing systolic pressure. Using a 25-gauge needle to record blood pressure would be an example of using a system that overdamps the signal. An underdamped system allows resonance to occur unchecked. Another factor that can produce artifactual waveforms is the use of end-hole catheters. When end-hole catheters are advanced retrograde, they face the impact of oncoming blood. This results in a falsely high pressure because of kinetic energy. The opposite occurs when an end-hole catheter is placed with its opening facing away from blood flow. Fortunately, the error produced is small, usually less than 5 mm Hg.[37]

Indirect blood pressure measurement. Indirect blood pressure measurement has been of interest to investigators in basic research for several decades.[38] Clinicians became interested a short time later in the mid-1970s, when it was documented that dogs with advanced renal disease had systemic hypertension.[39,40] Indirect blood pressure measurement has become a popular means of estimating systemic arterial blood pressure within the past 15 years. Unfortunately, the accuracy of these devices, especially in cats, is still less than optimal. Popular devices include the Dinamap Model 8300 (Critikon, Tampa, Fla.), the Ultrasonic Doppler Flow Detector Models 811 and 812 (Parks Electronics, Aloha, Ore.), the Number 1022A Ultrasonic Doppler Machine (Kontron Medical Instruments, Watford, United Kingdom), and the Finapres 2300 (Ohmeda Corp., Louisville, Colo.). All devices employ an inflatable cuff that is placed around a distal limb to occlude flow. The proximal portions of the limbs cannot be used because of their shape. Cuff width is important in determining systemic blood pressure.[38] If it is too wide, a falsely low pressure will be recorded, and, if it is too narrow, a falsely high pressure will be recorded. In the dog, the cuff width should be approximately 40% of limb circumference.[41] Although a cuff width of 40% has also been used in cats, some investigators have suggested that a cuff width of 30% of the circumference of the limb is more appropriate in this species.[42]

The machine made by Parks uses a piezoelectric crystal to send and receive an ultrasound signal to detect blood flow in an artery distal to an inflatable cuff. The hair is clipped just above the palmar metacarpal or plantar metatarsal pad, ultrasound gel is applied, and the Doppler probe is used to identify arterial blood flow in the superficial palmar or plantar arterial arch supplied by the common digital branches of the radial or caudal tibial arteries. When the correct location is identified, the probe is held or taped snugly in place (Color Plate 107). An encircling cuff with an attached gauge to read the pressure in the cuff is inflated proximal to the recording site until there is no blood flow (no Doppler signal). It is then deflated while the crystal is used to detect the onset of flow. The appearance of the Doppler signal corresponds to systolic blood pressure. In our opinion this is generally the most accurate of the noninvasive devices, especially in cats, in which the other devices are always questionable.[43] The major problem with this device is that it only measures systolic blood pressure reliably, although experienced operators may be able to determine diastolic blood pressure in many patients.[44] Diastolic pressure coincides with an abrupt muffling of the Doppler signal. Systolic and diastolic blood pressures are both increased or isolated systolic blood pressure is increased in most canine and feline patients with systemic hypertension, so an inability to recognize diastolic blood pressure is usually not a critical factor.[45] In one study of cats, out of 314 total readings, the Parks device was within 10 mm Hg of the true systolic blood pressure 152 times and within 20 mm Hg 266 times.

The Kontron machine uses an ultrasound beam and the Doppler shift to detect movement of the arterial wall. In this device, the crystal is placed over an artery, such as the medial metatarsal artery, and under an inflatable cuff attached to a gauge. Systolic pressure is then recorded as the first audible sound as blood flow begins when the cuff is gradually deflated. Diastolic blood pressure is recorded when the flow sound becomes muffled.[46] Because the change in sound associated with diastolic pressure is subjective, diastolic pressure measurements with this machine are more inaccurate than the systolic measurements, especially in awake animals. In one study in cats, the correlation coefficient (*r* value) was 0.94 between measuring systolic blood pressure with this noninvasive device and invasive measurements and was 0.82 for the diastolic measurements.[46] In anesthetized dogs, one group of investigators found correlation coefficients of 0.98 and 0.99 between direct measurements of systolic and diastolic pressure and indirect measures using a similar device to the Kontron machine.[47]

The oscillometric technique is another popular means to measure blood pressure. This technique is based on the physical principle that the vessel underneath a cuff oscillates when it is partially occluded. The largest oscillations in a partially occluded vessel occur when the cuff pressure equals mean arterial blood pressure (the same principle is used when palpating pulse pressure in a femoral artery). You can feel the oscillations as a "pounding" beneath the cuff when someone takes your blood pressure. It can also be seen as an oscillation in the mercury column if a sphygmomanometer with a mercury column is used. With an oscillometric machine, an inflatable cuff is placed over a systemic artery. The machine inflates the cuff to a suprasystemic pressure to completely occlude the vessel so that no vessel movement occurs. The cuff pressure is gradually released. When cuff pressure decreases below systolic pressure, blood starts to flow through the vessel again at a force that expands the vessel wall. A computer detects the oscillations that transmit from the cuff through the air hose to a sensor in the machine. Oscillations start when cuff pressure equals systolic blood pressure, become maximal when cuff pressure is the same as mean arterial pressure, and stop after cuff pressure equals diastolic blood pressure. A computer in the machine determines mean arterial blood pressure and then calculates the slope of the increase and decrease in oscillation height on either side of the maximum oscillation to calculate systolic and diastolic blood pressure. Consequently, mean blood pressure should be the most accurate of the three pressures. In one study in anesthetized dogs, the correlation coefficient between recorded pressures using an oscillometric machine (Dinamap) and pressures recorded directly were 0.93 for mean blood pressure and 0.91 for systolic and diastolic blood pressures.[48] However, lines of identity in this study did not pass through unity. The Dinamap is less accurate in cats than in dogs. Often, no reading is obtained. In one study, readings could be obtained only about 65% of the time.[49] When readings were obtained, only about 60% were within 20 mm Hg of the direct measurement. In our experience, use of the Dinamap is an art. It takes experience to learn how tight to wrap the cuff and how to alter variables when the machine does not provide a measurement or the measurement is clearly inaccurate. We generally do not attempt to use this device in cats or small dogs. The cuff is usually placed around the distal radius and ulna, the distal metatarsal bones, or the base of the tail.

The Finapres machine uses photoplethysmography to determine blood pressure. The device measures relative arterial blood volume by attenuation of infrared radiation. Arterial blood volume is maintained at a constant volume by a microcomputer-based servosystem. The cuff of this device can be placed around the caudal limb just distal to the hock or base of the tail. This device has only been evaluated in cats.[49] In this study, this methodology appeared to have no benefit over the Doppler technique.

In summary, noninvasive blood pressure measurement is fraught with difficulties. An experienced examiner can usually obtain a reading on a large dog, but data suggests that many times this measurement is inaccurate. Obtaining a measurement on a small dog or cat is difficult and more prone to error. Measuring systolic blood pressure with a Parks unit usually gives sufficient information and is our favorite means of measuring systemic arterial blood pressure. All noninvasive techniques are probably better for measuring trends in blood pressure rather than for one-time determinations. Invasive blood pressure measurement is technically difficult, requires expensive equipment, and is prone to error because the pressure is recorded in a patient that is frightened or in pain.

NORMAL VALUES

Defining an upper limit of "normal" for systolic and diastolic systemic arterial blood pressures in dogs and cats is difficult. These values have been determined in detail in human populations. In general, a diastolic arterial blood pressure in a resting human greater than 90 mm Hg is considered evidence of diastolic systemic arterial hypertension. Even a mild increase in diastolic pressure is associated with increased risk of cardiovascular morbidity and mortality in humans.[50] Most humans, however, develop cardiovascular disease associated with mild hypertension over decades, a period longer than most dogs and cats live. Consequently, it is probably less important to identify mild systemic hypertension in dogs and cats and probably less important to identify precise values for the upper limits of blood pressure in dogs and cats.

There are numerous studies in the literature that have examined blood pressure in normal dogs. Because there is no accurate noninvasive means of determining systemic arterial blood pressure in resting dogs, many studies that have determined normal blood pressures have done so using invasive means, although noninvasive studies have also been done. The variety of situations in which blood pressure has been measured and the variety of methodologies that have been used make it very difficult to define a normal range for systemic arterial blood pressure in dogs.[40] Rather, upper limits of normal seem to have evolved based on clinical experience and common sense. An upper limit of normal for diastolic blood pressure in dogs is often considered to be 100 mm Hg.[39,51] Mild-to-moderate increases in diastolic blood pressure can be considered to be in the 100- to 120-mm Hg range. A diastolic blood pressure greater than 130 mm Hg in humans is considered severely high, always necessitating immediate therapy.[50] It's unlikely that this cutoff is too much different in dogs and cats. Systolic blood pressure is even more labile than diastolic pressure and is influenced to a greater degree by fright and stress. Consequently, it should be interpreted differently in a patient that appears frightened or agitated than in an outwardly calm animal and may be different in the dog and cat. For example, we consider a systolic blood pressure greater than 150 mm Hg in a resting cat to be abnormal if the measurement was taken noninvasively. We consider 180 mm Hg to still be within the normal range in a dog that is frightened and having its blood pressure measured by advancing a needle into the femoral artery. Certainly any systolic pressure greater than 180 mm Hg is elevated. However, even this limit is only valid if the blood pressure measurement is accurate and the patient is reasonably calm. There are numerous examples of normal dogs in various studies in the literature that have systolic blood pressures greater than 200 mm Hg and diastolic blood pressures greater than 120 mm Hg.[40] Any blood pressure measurement should be interpreted with caution and reevaluated before any conclusion is made.

PATHOPHYSIOLOGY

Systemic arterial blood pressure is tightly controlled by numerous variables. Pressure receptors (baroreceptors) within the arterial system, volume receptors within the cardiovascular system (mechanoreceptors), and flow receptors within the kidney (e.g., the macula densa) exert a marked influence on the cardiovascular system to maintain systemic blood pressure within a fixed range. These receptors influence the adrenergic and cholinergic systems, the renin-angiotensin-aldosterone system, antidiuretic hormone release, and endothelin release. In so doing, they influence vascular, renal, and endocrine function to maintain blood pressure within a narrow range.

Blood pressure is the lateral force per unit area of vascular wall. *Force* is defined as the energy that alters motion, either producing or inhibiting motion. Pressure is expressed in units of dynes/cm^2 in the metric system. Clinically, it is expressed in millimeters of mercury, where 1 mm Hg = 1.36 cm H_2O = 1332 dynes/cm^2. Cardiovascular pressures are recorded using atmospheric pressure as the zero reference level. Intravascular pressures are further referenced to the level of the heart by placing the transducer at the level of the heart or by adding or subtracting the hydrostatic pressure of the column of blood above or below the heart. Blood pressure is usually measured with the patient in lateral recumbency, so that the heart and the systemic artery in which pressure is measured are at the same level.

In simple terms, pressure is determined by flow and resistance. In a tube in which there is constant flow, pressure can be increased by either increasing the flow rate or increasing the resistance to flow, much like voltage can be increased by increasing current or increasing resistance in a direct-current circuit. For example, when using a garden hose that is partially occluded by one's fingers, pressure in the hose can be increased by opening the faucet more to increase flow or by occluding the hose further with one's fingers to increase resistance. The cardiovascular system does not have a constant flow. Rather, it is a pulsatile system that is comparable to an alternating-current system in an electrical circuit. Consequently, the hemodynamics are somewhat different (see Chapter 2). Systemic arterial blood pressure is determined primarily by the blood volume within the arterial vascular space in diastole, the amount and rate of flow into the arterial space with each beat, arteriolar vascular resistance, and aortic compliance. Diastolic arterial blood volume is a theoretical variable because it cannot be currently measured. However, it must be a determinant. If there was no blood in the arterial system before the left ventricle ejected a quantity of blood, certainly blood pressure would be lower than if a normal blood volume existed before ejection. The mechanisms that control this volume are poorly understood, but they are probably similar to the mechanisms that control total blood volume.

Alterations in blood volume, blood flow, peripheral vascular resistance, and aortic compliance can result in systemic hypertension. Total blood volume can alter systemic arterial blood volume and directly alter systemic arterial blood pressure. Blood volume can alter systemic venous and pulmonary venous blood volume and so alter preload, stroke volume, and cardiac output and consequently cause a secondary alteration in systemic arterial blood pressure. Blood volume is controlled primarily by fluid intake and fluid excretion. Fluid intake is controlled by multiple mechanisms, including hormonal systems that include antidiuretic hormone and angiotensin II. Fluid excretion is primarily controlled by the kidneys. Renin secretion by the juxtaglomerular apparatus is a primary response to decreased renal blood flow. Resultant aldosterone secretion is a major contributor to renal sodium and water retention. Antidiuretic hormone (vasopressin) is a major factor in water retention. Blood flow (stroke volume and cardiac output) also has multiple determinants, as discussed in Chapter 2. Peripheral vascular resistance is determined primarily by cross-sectional area of the systemic arteriolar vascular bed. The radius of each individual systemic arteriole contributes to this cross-sectional area. Arteriolar radius is controlled by multiple factors, including local regulation, sympathetic and parasympathetic innervation, and circulating hormones such as angiotensin II, vasopressin, and endothelin. Alterations in the control of any of these variables could theoretically result in systemic hypertension. Aortic compliance is determined primarily by age, disease, autonomic innervation, and hormones such as angiotensin II.

Numerous diseases alter the aforementioned variables and so

produce systemic hypertension. Acute oliguric or anuric renal failure is an example of a disease that results in an increase in circulating blood volume and systemic hypertension. Hyperthyroidism increases stroke volume and cardiac output, resulting in systemic hypertension. Aortic compliance decreases with aging. When the left ventricle ejects a normal quantity of blood into a stiffer aorta, systolic blood pressure increases but diastolic blood pressure stays within the normal range. Pheochromocytoma is an example of a disease that can produce vasoconstriction to cause systemic hypertension. Systemic hypertension commonly is caused by multiple mechanisms. Pheochromocytoma is also a good example of this because secretion of catecholamines by this type of tumor not only causes vasoconstriction but also results in increased contractility and, probably, increased blood volume, which results in an increase in stroke volume and cardiac output.

ETIOLOGY

By far the most common cause of systemic hypertension in dogs is renal disease. Renal disease and hyperthyroidism are the two most common causes of systemic hypertension in cats. The incidence of systemic hypertension in cats with renal failure ranges from 61% to 73%.[45,46,52] Systemic hypertension ranges from mild to severe, with most cats in the mild-to-moderate range (systolic pressure from 151 to 180 mm Hg; diastolic pressure from 101 to 120 mm Hg). Of the 39 cats with hyperthyroidism reported from one study, 87% ($n = 34$) had systemic hypertension. None of the cats with renal failure or hyperthyroidism in these reports had isolated diastolic hypertension. All had isolated systolic hypertension or both systolic and diastolic hypertension. In a study of dogs with renal disease, 61% had systemic hypertension.[41] Of those that had glomerular disease, 80% had systemic hypertension. In this same study, 59% of dogs with hyperadrenocorticism had systemic hypertension. Recent findings suggest that about 70% of dogs with diabetes mellitus have elevated systemic pressures.[53] At our hospital, however, only about 50% have systemic hypertension.[54] Hypertension in these dogs has been significantly correlated to the duration of the diabetes mellitus and glycemic control. Pheochromocytoma is a rare cause of systemic hypertension in dogs. Resting systemic arterial blood pressure may be elevated or it may be normal in these cases. Digital manipulation of the adrenal gland tumor during surgery may markedly increase systemic blood pressure.[52]

Renal failure. The mechanisms by which renal failure causes systemic hypertension in dogs and cats have not been adequately studied. In the only study of the renin-angiotensin-aldosterone system in cats with renal failure, plasma renin activity was low, normal, or high, and plasma aldosterone concentration was usually increased.[55] In humans, an inability to excrete appropriate amounts of sodium and water with resultant hypervolemia appears to be the primary mechanism early in the course of renal disease, although increased systemic vascular resistance may predominate in chronic renal failure.[50] Reduced renal blood flow or localized renal ischemia leading to increased renin secretion also probably plays a role in some patients. Inadequate production of vasodilator substances, such as prostaglandins and components of the kallikrein-kinin system, by diseased kidneys has also been postulated.[46,56] An inability to excrete sodium and water should be countered easily by administering a diuretic and systemic hypertension in humans is often responsive to diuretic administration or dialysis.[50] Excess renin secretion with resultant aldosterone-mediated sodium and water retention should be responsive to the administration of an angiotensin converting enzyme inhibitor. Some human patients with chronic renal failure and hypertension are responsive to these agents. However, dogs and cats with renal failure rarely have a clinically significant response to diuretic administration and administration of an angiotensin converting enzyme inhibitor often produces no response or only a very mild response (less than 10 mm Hg decrease in systemic blood pressure). Dogs and cats with systemic hypertension secondary to renal failure, generally are more responsive to and often require agents that dilate systemic arterioles. Amlodipine is currently the favorite drug for treating cats with systemic hypertension resulting from renal failure. Prazosin, hydralazine, and, possibly, amlodipine are the most effective agents used in dogs to treat systemic hypertension due to renal failure. Consequently, it appears in dogs and cats with chronic renal failure that the primary mechanism for systemic hypertension is systemic vasoconstriction, not systemic volume overload.

Hyperthyroidism. It is easy to see why hyperthyroidism causes systolic systemic hypertension. Hyperthyroidism increases myocardial contractility, stroke volume, and velocity of ejection. The increased volume delivered into the arterial system in a shorter-than-normal period should increase systolic systemic arterial blood pressure unless the aorta is able to relax and become more compliant to accommodate this increased delivery of blood. Hyperthyroidism is a disease of older cats and it is presumed that the aorta is stiffer in older cats. Diastolic systemic hypertension is also frequently present in cats with hyperthyroidism.[46] The mechanism for this is less well understood. The fact that diastolic blood pressure decreases following successful treatment of hyperthyroidism strongly suggests that hyperthyroidism is the primary reason for the diastolic hypertension in these cats. Increased renin secretion may be the answer. Stimulation of β-adrenergic receptors on the juxtaglomerular apparatus stimulates renin release. Thyroid hormone increases β-adrenergic receptor sensitivity and therefore may increase renin secretion in hyperthyroid patients.[57] This has been demonstrated in human patients.[58]

Miscellaneous causes. Pheochromocytoma increases systemic blood pressure by elaborating norepinephrine and epinephrine. These neurohormones increase contractility and peripheral vascular resistance. Secretion may be normal or markedly elevated at rest and may increase remarkably with stimulation, especially digital manipulation.[59] Consequently, systemic arterial blood pressure may be normal to increased in a particular patient.

Diabetic nephropathy is a well-recognized disease in humans. Systemic arterial hypertension is an early feature of diabetic nephropathy in humans.[60] In one study, aggressive treatment with hydralazine, a β-blocker, and furosemide decreased the rate of decline in renal function in human patients with insulin-dependent diabetes mellitus.[61] The mechanism of systemic hypertension in canine diabetes mellitus has not been studied.

Hyperadrenocorticism causes systemic hypertension through a variety of mechanisms in humans. Increased mineralocorticoid secretion may occur along with the cortisol excess. Cortisol may stimulate renin substrate synthesis and increase the expression of angiotensin II receptors.[62,63] The mechanism has not been studied in dogs.

CONSEQUENCES

The consequences of prolonged mild-to-moderate systemic hypertension in humans are well known. If left untreated, about 50% of patients will die of coronary artery disease or congestive heart failure, 33% will die of a stroke, and 10% to 15% will die of renal failure.[50] The consequences of mild-to-moderate systemic hypertension in dogs and cats are less well understood. Progressive nephron damage and loss can occur.[64] The profound effects on the cardiovascular system that are observed in human patients are rarely seen in dogs and cats. Retinal lesions occur in cats with moderate systemic hypertension. Lesions consist of focal hemorrhage, diffuse or focal retinal edema, focal retinal detachments, and arterial tortuosity.[52] In one study, 80% of the cats with systemic hypertension secondary to renal failure had this type of hypertensive retinopathy.[52] None of the cats had complete retinal detachment and none were blind. Only one of three cats with hyperthyroidism had retinal lesions in this study.

The consequences of severe systemic hypertension can be more dramatic. In cats, ocular abnormalities are the most common sequela of severe systemic hypertension.[65,66] Retinal hemorrhage, retinal detachment, retinal atrophy, hyphema, perivasculitis, retinal artery tortuosity, and vitreal hemorrhage all occur in cats with severe systemic hypertension. Cats with these abnormalities are usually blind and present with bilateral mydriasis.[66] With successful treatment of the hypertension, the ocular lesions may regress, but many remain blind. Time is a factor in recovery. If systemic hypertension is allowed to remain for more than 48 hours after the onset of blindness, vision usually does not return despite the resolution of the ocular lesions.[67] Neurologic signs can also occur secondary to systemic hypertension in cats.[66] In one report, two cats with neurologic signs subjected to postmortem examination had multifocal cerebral arteriosclerosis with focal hemorrhage (stroke). Left ventricular hypertrophy also occurs in cats with systemic hypertension.[65,66] We are unaware of any cat developing left ventricular disease secondary to systemic hypertension severe enough to cause heart failure. Left ventricular hypertrophy in cats with systemic hypertension has been documented in one study.[45] The degree of left ventricular hypertrophy in this study, however, did not correlate with systemic blood pressure so one cannot say that the two were causally related. In another study, of 12 cats with systemic hypertension, 10 had left ventricular hypertrophy.[66] In another study, left ventricular mass increased by approximately 34% in experimental cats with systemic hypertension.[68] This translates into an increase of 1 mm in wall thickness in a cat. Because the range of normal for left ventricular wall thickness for cats is from 3.0 to 5.5 mm, in many cats the wall thickness will still be within the normal range. In others it will only be mildly increased in thickness. Although systemic hypertension should be ruled out whenever left ventricular hypertrophy is identified, in our experience, it is unusual to identify systemic hypertension in a cat with severe left ventricular hypertrophy.

The consequences of systemic hypertension in dogs are less well documented. Retinal hemorrhage, retinal detachment, and hyphema have also been reported in dogs with severe systemic hypertension.[69] However, in our experience the incidence of ocular abnormalities in dogs is less than that observed in cats. That left ventricular mass increases in dogs with moderate-to-severe systemic hypertension is well documented.[70] However, it is generally mild.[69] Systemic hypertension is only occasionally clinically significant or relevant to the cardiovascular system. The most common scenario is a dog with mitral regurgitation and renal failure with systemic hypertension in which the increased afterload contributes to the severity of the mitral regurgitation. Neurologic signs and epistaxis have also been observed in dogs with systemic hypertension.

Because systemic hypertension is most commonly observed in dogs and cats with renal disease and failure, the fact that systemic hypertension can contribute to progressive renal damage is particularly important. This may be the primary reason for treating systemic hypertension in dogs and cats with renal failure. It is well established that chronic renal insufficiency progresses to end-stage renal failure without the primary disease causing any further reduction in renal mass (i.e., the process becomes self-perpetuating).[64] Systemic hypertension is a well-recognized risk factor in humans for this occurrence. In normal animals, renal blood flow is regulated by the afferent arterioles such that renal blood flow remains stable at systemic blood pressures ranging from 70 to 150 mm Hg. In renal failure, instead of glomerular afferent arteriolar tone increasing to maintain a normal renal blood flow when blood pressure increases, it actually decreases. That is, the kidney loses its ability to autoregulate renal blood flow. Inability to autoregulate renal blood flow occurs in experimental dogs at blood pressures greater than 100 mm Hg when three fourths of the functioning renal mass is gone and is markedly altered when seven eighths of renal mass has been destroyed.[71] Glomerular efferent arteriolar tone also decreases in this situation but not to the same degree. This results in glomerular blood flow increasing when afferent arteriolar tone decreases, and in glomerular capillary pressure increasing as blood flow increases more than efferent arteriolar tone (resistance) decreases. The increased glomerular capillary pressure in the surviving nephrons results in increased glomerular filtration in these nephrons. The increase in single nephron glomerular filtration rate compensates for the loss of the other nephrons in renal disease and results in an increase in global renal glomerular filtration rate back toward normal. In this regard, the changes just described are beneficial to the patient. However, it appears to be detrimental to the kidney and so, in the long-term, detrimental to the patient in that it decreases survival time. The primary detrimental effect appears to be to the glomeruli. Intraglomerular hyperperfusion and hypertension lead to glomerular hypertrophy and, ultimately, to glomerular sclerosis.[72] This leads to proteinuria and nephron loss. Nephron injury occurs as a result of enhanced endothelial cell release of vasoactive substances, such as thromboxanes, lipid deposition, and intracapillary thrombosis. Mesangial cell proliferation occurs secondary to accumulations of injurious macromolecules. Epithelial injury also occurs. This augments basement membrane permeability, which leads to proteinuria. The cumulative effect of these changes is glomerular sclerosis and progressive nephron destruction.

That systemic and intraglomerular hypertension is a primary factor in progressive renal injury has been demonstrated by administering antihypertensive therapy and noting that the progressive glomerular changes are ameliorated. In one study that used experimentally uninephrectomized, diabetic dogs, lisinopril, an angiotensin converting enzyme inhibitor, was administered at an average dose of 0.7 mg/kg/day PO for 1 year.[72] Renal hemodynamics in these dogs were compared with those of a control group of dogs and a group of uninephrectomized, diabetic dogs that were not administered lisinopril. Mean arterial blood pressure in the dogs that were not administered lisinopril was mildly increased (116 mm Hg on average vs. 106 mm Hg for the control group). Lisinopril decreased mean arterial blood pressure back to normal. This did not result in a decrease in renal blood flow because lisinopril most likely dilated the afferent arteriole further. It did not decrease single nephron glomerular filtration rate either. It did, however, decrease glomerular capillary pressure. This means lisinopril dilated the efferent arteriole more than it did the afferent arteriole. The net result was a lesser increase in glomerular volume (less glomerular hypertrophy) and therefore less glomerular damage. An experimental calcium channel blocker also reduced glomerular injury in this study. It did not, however, decrease glomerular capillary pressure nor did it decrease single nephron glomerular filtration rate. Its exact mechanism of benefit is undetermined. In a study performed in hypertensive rats, amlodipine, a calcium channel blocker, did not prevent glomerular damage.[73]

SIGNALMENT AND HISTORY

Most dogs and cats with systemic hypertension are middle-age–to–geriatric animals. There is no breed predilection recognized clinically. Males may be at greater risk than females.[51] Obese animals may have higher systemic arterial pressures than animals that are not obese, but the increase is not clinically significant. Most animals present because of clinical signs referable to their underlying disease (e.g., renal failure) or because of acute blindness. A history of neurologic abnormalities suggestive of a cerebrovascular event is rare.

PHYSICAL EXAMINATION

Physical examination findings directly referable to systemic hypertension are often nonexistent. The femoral artery pulse character is usually normal. Pulse strength is determined by pulse pressure, which is the difference between systolic and diastolic pressure. Consequently, an animal with a systemic arterial blood pressure of 240/180 mm Hg will have the same pulse strength as an animal with a pressure of 130/70 mm Hg.

Examination of the retina may reveal lesions typical of systemic hypertension. In one study, 80% of cats with systemic hypertension had retinal lesions, including retinal hemorrhage, diffuse or focal retinal edema, focal retinal detachments, and arterial tortuosity.[52] Retinal examination may be a reasonable method for screening for end-organ damage in cats with systemic hypertension. Animals that are presented for blindness secondary to systemic hypertension have retinal detachments and retinal hemorrhages.

Animals may have physical examination findings referable to other diseases that are causing the systemic hypertension. For example, dogs with hyperadrenocorticism may have typical alopecia, an enlarged abdomen, weight gain, or signs referable to diabetes mellitus.

LABORATORY FINDINGS

Evidence of renal failure, hyperthyroidism, or hyperadrenocorticism is commonly identified. A definitive diagnosis of systemic hypertension, however, can only be made by measuring systemic arterial blood pressure. Because of the inaccuracy of most of the noninvasive devices, this may be difficult. We generally are comfortable with the diagnosis of systemic hypertension if an animal has evidence of a typical underlying disease or evidence of end-organ disease (e.g., retinal detachment and hemorrhage) and a systolic blood pressure greater than 150 to 180 mm Hg (depending on the animal's attitude) recorded with a Park's Doppler device in a dog or cat or a consistent recording of pressures greater than 170/100 mm Hg with a Dinamap device in a medium-size to large dog. Direct femoral artery puncture may be used for confirmation of systemic hypertension in dogs. This procedure is usually not feasible in a cat. Treatment of systemic hypertension has been recommended when the systolic blood pressure exceeds 170 mm Hg or diastolic blood pressure exceeds 100 mm Hg in cats.[74]

TREATMENT

The decision to treat systemic hypertension with antihypertensive drugs may be difficult. We use the following general guidelines. If systemic blood pressure is increased in a patient that does not have any of the common underlying diseases and has no evidence of end-organ damage, we do not treat unless we can document that the measurement is repeatable over time and the hypertension is severe. In patients with typical underlying diseases, we prefer that we have at least two and preferably three measurements that suggest the patient has hypertension to diagnose systemic hypertension. The decision to treat with antihypertensive drugs depends on the underlying disease. In cats with hyperthyroidism, we prefer to treat the underlying disease because systemic arterial blood pressure will usually normalize when the hyperthyroidism is controlled.[46] In dogs and cats with renal disease, treatment is generally warranted, and an angiotensin converting enzyme inhibitor should slow the progression of the renal disease. Treatment may also be warranted in dogs with hyperadrenocorticism or diabetes mellitus, although blood pressure may normalize when the underlying disease is controlled. Dogs or cats that have evidence of end-organ damage require therapy.

The treatment of systemic hypertension in dogs and cats is poorly documented. This probably stems from the fact that, at least in dogs, there is no single drug or drug class that is uniformly effective. Although lists of drugs that are effective in humans with systemic hypertension are commonly placed in the veterinary literature as suggestions for therapy, many of these drugs are either not effective or are only occasionally effective. The mainstays for treating systemic hypertension in humans are the diuretics and low-sodium diets. These are rarely effective in dogs or cats with systemic hypertension.

In cats with renal disease, there has been one report of amlodipine being effective at decreasing systemic arterial blood pressure.[75,76] This finding has recently been corroborated by a placebo-controlled trial.[77] Clinically, amlodipine does appear to be very effective in cats and has gained widespread popularity for this use. Its rapid acceptance as a therapeutic agent in this disease attests to its efficacy. Amlodipine (Norvasc, Pfizer Laboratories, New York) is supplied as 2.5-, 5-, and 10-mg tablets. The dose in cats is 0.625 to 1.25 mg q24h PO.[77] In one study of 12 cats with renal failure and systemic hypertension, amlodipine decreased systolic systemic arterial blood pressure from an average of 198 mm Hg to 155 mm Hg.[76] Amlodipine is a second-generation calcium channel blocker. It is similar in structure and action to nifedipine. The primary effect of this class of calcium channel blocker is to relax vascular smooth muscle in systemic arterioles, which reduces systemic vascular resistance. In humans, the half-life of amlodipine is 35 to 48 hours, and it is administered once a day.[73] The pharmacokinetics of amlodipine in the cat are unknown. Its administration to cats with renal failure does not cause any change in serum creatinine concentration, serum potassium concentration, or body weight.[75] Because of its long half-life, amlodipine usually takes 1 to 2 days to reach maximum effect. The effect in cats does not diminish over time, lasting at least 120 days and most likely much longer.[76] During therapy, body weight does not decrease and serum creatinine concentration does not change.

There currently are no published studies that document the efficacy or that have determined relative efficacies of drugs for the treatment of systemic hypertension in dogs with renal failure. The following recommendations are those of Dr. Larry Cowgill from University of California, Davis, one of the few recognized authorities on systemic hypertension in canine renal failure patients (Table 26-2).[53] The first thing to remember when treating systemic hypertension is that no drug is effective all of the time and in all patients. Consequently, following drug administration, a response or lack of response must be documented. If there is no response or if the response is very small, either the dose must be increased, another drug must be tried, or another drug must be added into the therapeutic regimen. Currently, first-line drugs are prazosin, diltiazem, and angiotensin converting enzyme inhibitors. Amlodipine will probably be added to this list in the near future. Prazosin (Minipress, Pfizer Laboratories, New York) is an α_1-adrenergic blocking drug. It is supplied as 1-, 2-, and 5-mg capsules. The dose must be titrated

TABLE 26-2

Drugs used in the management of systemic hypertension

Drug	Line	*Success %* *(estimate)*	*Expected decline*
ACE inhibitor	1st	50%	<10 mm Hg
Diltiazem	1st	50%	<10 mm Hg
Prazosin	1st	50%	10-20 mm Hg
β-Blocker	2nd	?	?
Furosemide	2nd	?	?
Hydralazine	3rd	>90%	10-50 mm Hg
Amiodipine	1st (Cats); 3rd (dogs)	>90% (cats)	40 mm Hg (average decrease in SBP)

SBP, Systolic blood pressure.

starting at 0.5 mg per dog q8-12h PO and increasing to a maximum dose of 2 mg per dog q8-12h PO. Diltiazem (Cardizem, Marion Laboratories, Inc., Kansas City, Mo.) is a calcium channel blocker that has negative inotropic, negative chronotropic, and arteriolar dilating properties. Its arteriolar dilating properties, however, are much less than that of amlodipine. It is supplied as 30-, 60-, 90-, and 120-mg tablets. The dose of diltiazem that is effective in dogs with systemic hypertension is not known. Doses in cardiovascular medicine generally range between 0.5 and 1.5 mg/kg q8h, although doses as high as 3 mg/kg q8h have been required. The most commonly used angiotensin converting enzyme inhibitor is enalapril. Enalapril (Enacard, Merck Agvet, Rahway, N.J.) is supplied as 1-, 2.5-, 5-, 10-, and 20-mg tablets. The dose of enalapril is 0.5 mg/kg q12-24h PO. Each of these drugs or drug classes produces a clinically significant decrease in systemic arterial blood pressure in about 50% of cases. Prazosin generally decreases systemic pressure by 10 to 20 mm Hg, whereas diltiazem and angiotensin converting enzyme inhibitors more commonly only decrease pressure by 5 to 10 mm Hg. β-Blockers are most commonly used as second-line drugs, usually in combination with a first-line drug if the first-line drug is not effective. Diuretics are sometimes used in the same manner. β-Blockers and diuretics are rarely effective as sole agents. Hydralazine is very efficacious but is usually used as a third choice. However, it is being used more commonly at University of California, Davis, as clinicians gain more experience with the drug. Hydralazine commonly produces a reflex tachycardia, a reflex increase in contractility, and an increase in plasma renin activity and plasma aldosterone concentration. The reflex tachycardia and increase in contractility can increase cardiac output to the point that systemic arterial blood pressure returns to pretreatment values. Consequently, the administration of a β-blocker is generally required in conjunction with hydralazine. Administration of a diuretic may be needed to counter the reflex effects on the renin-angiotensin-aldosterone system. Hydralazine (Apresoline, Ciba, Summit, N.J.) is available as 10-, 25-, 50-, and 100-mg tablets. The dose must be titrated starting at 1 mg/kg q12h and increasing gradually to as high as 3 mg/kg q12h. Titration should start at 0.5 mg/kg q12h in animals that are already being administered an angiotensin converting enzyme inhibitor.

There currently is little clinical experience with amlodipine in dogs. However, our initial experience with the drug is positive. The pharmacokinetics of amlodipine have been studied in dogs.[78] Bioavailability is about 90%, compared with bioavailability in humans of about 65%. Time-to-peak plasma concentration is 6 hours in the dog and 8 hours in humans. Following IV or oral administration, about 45% of the drug is excreted in the feces and 45% in the urine as metabolites in dogs. Only 2% of the drug is excreted unchanged.[79] Initial metabolism involves oxidation of the dihydropyridine ring to the pyridine analogue. Further metabolism involves side-chain oxidation and hydrolysis of one or both side-chain ester groups. Plasma half-life is similar to humans at about 30 hours following IV administration. Volume of distribution is also similar to humans at 25 L/kg. Approximately 95% of amlodipine is protein bound in all species studied. Because the pharmacokinetics of amlodipine are similar in dogs and humans, the oral dose in dogs may be similar to that used in humans, which is approximately 0.05 to 0.2 mg/kg/day. Because of the long half-life, amlodipine may take 1 to 2 days to reach maximum effect. We have received a report of one veterinary internist who used amlodipine in four dogs with systemic hypertension.[80] The drug was effective at normalizing systemic blood pressure in each case. The dose used ranged from 0.1 to 0.2 mg/kg/day PO, with the effective dose range usually being between 0.15 and 0.2 mg/kg/day PO. We have also successfully used this dose in our hospital in a limited number of patients.

Even though angiotensin converting enzyme inhibitors do not decrease systemic arterial blood pressure in many dogs and only produce a mild decrease in most of the remaining dogs, their administration may still be indicated in dogs with chronic renal failure. The ability of these drugs to reduce intraglomerular pressure and decrease glomerular damage in experimental animals strongly suggests that they may be beneficial in clinical patients. A long-term blinded and placebo-controlled clinical trial should be performed to determine if this effect translates into slower deterioration of renal function and in longer survival time in patients with renal failure.

REFERENCES

1. Comroe JH: The main functions of the pulmonary circulation, *Circulation* 33:146, 1966.
2. Mathew R, Altura BM: Physiology and pathophysiology of pulmonary circulation, *Microcirc Endo Lymph* 6:211, 1990.
3. Milnor WR: Pulmonary circulation. In Milnor WR, ed: *Cardiovascular physiology,* New York, 1990, Oxford University Press.
4. Guyton AC: The pulmonary circulation. In Guyton AC, ed: *Textbook of medical physiology,* ed 7, Philadelphia, 1986, WB Saunders.
5. Grossman W, Braunwald E: Pulmonary hypertension. In Braunwald E, ed: *Heart disease: a textbook of cardiovascular medicine,* ed 4, Philadelphia, 1992, WB Saunders.
6. Gross DR: Normal cardiovascular parameters from intact, awake animals. In Gross DR, ed: *Animal models in cardiovascular research,* ed 2, Boston, 1994, Kluwer.
7. Maseri A, Caldini P, Harward P: Determinants of pulmonary vascular volume: recruitment versus distensibility, *Circ Res* 21:218, 1972.
8. Paraskos JA: Pulmonary heart disease including pulmonary embolism. In Chatterjee K, Karliner J, Rapaport E et al, eds: *Cardiology: an illustrated text/reference,* Philadelphia, 1991, JB Lippincott.
9. Kuida MD: Primary and secondary pulmonary hypertension: pathophysiology, recognition, and treatment. In Hurst JW, Schlant RC, Rackley CE et al, eds: *The heart, arteries and veins,* ed 7, New York, 1990, McGraw Hill.
10. Perry LA, Dillon AR, Bowers TL: Pulmonary hypertension, *Compend Contin Educ Pract Vet* 13:226, 1996.
11. Sakai S, Miyauchi T, Sakurai T et al: Pulmonary hypertension caused by congestive heart failure is ameliorated by long-term application of an endothelin receptor antagonist: increased expression of endothelin-1 messenger ribonucleic acid and endothelin-1-like immunoreactivity in the lung in congestive heart failure in rats, *J Am Coll Cardiol* 28:1580, 1996.
12. Calvert CA, Rawlings CA: Pulmonary manifestations of heartworm disease, *Vet Clin North Am Small Anim Pract* 15:991, 1995.

13. Larue MJ, Murtaugh RJ: Pulmonary thromboembolism in dogs: 47 cases (1986-1987), *J Am Vet Med Assoc* 197:1368, 1990.
14. Keyes ML, Rush JE, Knowles KE: Pulmonary thromboembolism in dogs, *Vet Emerg Crit Care* 3:23, 1991.
15. Tucker A, Weir EK, Reeves JT: Pulmonary microembolism: attenuated pulmonary vasoconstriction with prostaglandin inhibitors and antihistamines, *Prostaglandins* 11:31, 1976.
16. Vanhoutte PM: The endothelium modulator of vascular smooth muscle tone, *N Engl J Med* 319:512, 1988.
17. Dennis JS: The pathophysiologic sequela of pulmonary thromboembolism, *Compend Contin Educ Pract Vet* 13:1811, 1991.
18. Nishida K, Wakao Y, Watanabe T et al: A case of the Eisenmenger syndrome in a dog, *J Jap Vet Med Assoc* 41:263, 1988.
19. Pyle RL, Park RD, Alexander AF et al: Patent ductus arteriosus with pulmonary hypertension in the dog, *J Am Vet Med Assoc* 178:565, 1981.
20. Oswald GP, Orton EC: Patent ductus arteriosus and pulmonary hypertension in related Pembroke Welsh Corgis, *J Am Vet Med Assoc* 202:761, 1996.
21. Feldman EC, Nimmo-Wilkie JS, Pharr JW: Eisenmenger's syndrome in the dog: case reports, *J Am Anim Hosp Assoc*17:477, 1981.
22. Kirk GR, Smith DM, Hutcheson DP et al: Postnatal growth of the dog heart, *J Anat* 119:461, 1975.
23. McFadden ER, Braunwald E: Cor pulmonale. In Braunwald E, ed: *Heart disease: a textbook of cardiovascular medicine,* ed 4, Philadelphia, 1992, WB Saunders.
24. Newman JH, Ross JC: Chronic cor pulmonale. In Hurst JW, Schlant RC, Rackley CE et al, eds: *The heart, arteries and veins,* ed 7, New York, 1990, McGraw Hill.
25. Fuster V, Steele PM, Edwards WD et al: Primary pulmonary hypertension: natural history and the importance of thrombosis, *Circulation* 70:580, 1984.
26. Collados Larumbe MT, Borbolla Escoboza JR: Hemostatic system factors and endothelial function in primary pulmonary hypertension, *Rev Invest Clin* 46:421, 1994.
27. Kienle RD, Thomas WP: Echocardiography. In Nyland TG, Mattoon JS, eds: *Veterinary diagnostic ultrasound,* Philadelphia, 1995, WB Saunders.
28. Currie PJ, Seward JB, Chan KL et al: Continuous wave Doppler determination of right ventricular pressure, *J Am Coll Cardiol* 6:750, 1985.
29. Zhimming GE: Pulmonary artery diastolic pressure: a simultaneous Doppler echocardiography and catheterization study, *Clin Cardiol* 15:818, 1992.
30. McGoon MD, Vliestra RE: Vasodilator therapy for primary pulmonary hypertension, *Mayo Clinic Proc* 59:672, 1984.
31. House EW, Ederstrom HE: Anatomical changes with age in the heart and ductus arteriosus in the dog after birth, *Anat Rec* 160:289, 1968.
32. Stockwell DH, Madhavan S, Cohen H et al: The determinants of hypertension awareness, treatment, and control in an insured population, *Am J Public Health* 84:1768, 1994 (comments).
33. Davis GPJ, Park E: In Pinchot RB, ed: *The heart: the living pump,* New York, 1984, Torstar Books, Inc.
34. Schott A: An early account of blood pressure measurement by Joseph Struthius (1510-1568), *Med Hist* 21:305, 1977.
35. Kittleson MD, Olivier NB: Measurement of systemic arterial blood pressure, *Vet Clin North Am Small Anim Pract* 13:321, 1983.
36. Rothe CF, Kim KC: Measuring systolic arterial blood pressure: possible errors from extension tubes or disposable transducer domes, *Crit Care Med* 8:683, 1980.
37. Young SS, Bentivoglia LG, Maranhao V et al: *From cardiac catheterization data to hemodynamic parameters,* ed 2, Philadelphia, 1978, FA Davis.
38. Valtonen MH, Eriksson LM: The effect of cuff width on accuracy of indirect measurement of blood pressure in dogs, *Res Vet Sci* 11:358, 1970.
39. Weiser MG, Spangler WL, Gribble DH: Blood pressure measurement in the dog, *J Am Vet Med Assoc* 171:364, 1977.
40. Spangler WL, Gribble DH, Weiser MG: Canine hypertension: a review, *J Am Vet Med Assoc* 170:995, 1977.
41. Kallet A, Cowgill LD: Hypertensive states in the dog, *Proc ACVIM,* 1982, p 79 (abstract).
42. Grandy JL, Dunlop CL, Hodgson DS: Evaluation of the Doppler ultrasonic method of measuring systolic arterial pressure in cats, *Am J Vet Res* 53:1166, 1992.
43. McLeish I: Doppler ultrasonic arterial pressure measurement in the cat, *Vet Rec* 100:290, 1977.
44. Crowe DT, Spreng DE: Doppler assessment of blood flow and pressure in surgical and critical care patients. In Bonagura JD, ed: *Kirk's current veterinary therapy, XII: small animal practice,* Philadelphia, 1995, WB Saunders.
45. Lesser M, Fox PR, Bond BR: Assessment of hypertension in 40 cats with left ventricular hypertrophy by Doppler-shift sphygmomanometry, *J Small Anim Pract* 33:55, 1992.
46. Kobayashi DL, Peterson ME, Graves TK et al: Hypertension in cats with chronic renal failure or hyperthyroidism, *J Vet Intern Med* 4:58, 1990.
47. Wessale JL, Smith LA, Reid M et al: Indirect auscultatory systolic and diastolic pressures in the anesthetized dog, *Am J Vet Res* 46:2129, 1985.
48. Hamlin RL, Kittleson MD, Rice D et al: Noninvasive measurement of systemic arterial pressure in dogs by automatic sphygmomanometry, *Am J Vet Res* 43:1271, 1982.
49. Binns SH, Sisson DD, Buoscio DA et al: Doppler ultrasonographic, oscillometric sphygmomanometric, and photoplethysmographic techniques for noninvasive blood pressure measurement in anesthetized cats, *J Vet Intern Med* 9:405, 1995.
50. Kaplan NM: Systemic hypertension: mechanisms and diagnosis. In Braunwald E, ed: *Heart disease: a textbook of cardiovascular medicine,* ed 4, Philadelphia, 1992, WB Saunders.
51. Littman MP, Drobatz KJ: Hypertensive and hypotensive disorders. In Ettinger SJ, Feldman EC, eds: *Textbook of veterinary internal medicine,* ed 4, Philadelphia, 1995, WB Saunders.
52. Stiles J, Polzin DJ, Bistner SI: The prevalence of retinopathy in cats with systemic hypertension and chronic renal failure or hyperthyroidism, *J Am Anim Hosp Assoc* 30:564, 1994.
53. Cowgill LD: Incidence and treatment of systemic hypertension, personal communication, Feb 1996.
54. Struble AL, Feldman EC, Nelson RW: Hypertension and proteinuria in canine diabetes mellitus, *Proceedings of the Nineteenth Annual House Officer Seminar Day at UCDavis,* Davis, Calif, 1997, University of California, Davis (abstract).
55. Henik RA, Jensen J, Brownfield M: Plasma renin activity, angiotensin I, and aldosterone concentrations in normal and hypertensive cats, 1996, P228.
56. Stoff JS: Prostaglandins and hypertension, *Am J Med* 80:56, 1986.
57. Ganong WF: Thyroid hormones and renin secretion, *Life Sci* 30:561, 1982.
58. Resnick LM, Laragh JH: Plasma renin activity in syndromes of thyroid hormone excess and deficiency, *Life Sci* 30:585, 1982.
59. Dehn BJ, von, Nelson RW, Feldman EC et al: Pheochromocytoma and hyperadrenocorticism in dogs: six cases (1982-1992), *J Am Vet Med Assoc* 207:322, 1995.
60. Parving HH, Andersen AR, Smidt UM et al: Diabetic nephropathy and arterial hypertension, *Diabetologia* 24:10, 1983.
61. Parving HH, Andersen AR, Smidt UM et al: Early aggressive antihypertensive treatment reduces rate of decline in kidney function in diabetic nephropathy, Lancet 1:1175, 1983.
62. Sato A, Suzuki H, Nakazato Y et al: Increased expression of vascular angiotensin II type 1A receptor gene in glucocorticoid-induced hypertension, *J Hypertens* 12:511, 1994.
63. Sato A, Suzuki H, Murakami M et al: Glucocorticoid increases angiotensin II type 1 receptor and its gene expression, *Hypertension* 23:25, 1994.
64. Anderson S, Brenner BM: Progressive renal disease: a disorder of adaptation, *Q J Med* 70:185, 1989.
65. Morgan RV: Systemic hypertension in four cats: ocular and medical findings, *J Am Anim Hosp Assoc* 22:615, 1986.
66. Littman MP: Spontaneous systemic hypertension in 24 cats, *J Vet Intern Med* 8:79, 1990.
67. Reed JR: Hypertension in small animal medicine, *Calif Vet* Jan/Feb:7-10, 1997.

68. Kanatsuka H, Lamping KG, Eastham CL et al: Coronary microvascular resistance in hypertensive cats, *Circ Res* 68:726, 1991.
69. Littman MP, Robertson JL, Bovee KC: Spontaneous systemic hypertension in dogs: five cases (1981-1983), *J Am Vet Med Assoc* 193:486, 1988.
70. Salcedo EE, Gockowski K, Tarazi RC: Left ventricular mass and wall thickness in hypertension: comparison of M mode and two dimensional echocardiography in two experimental models, *Am J Cardiol* 44:936, 1979.
71. Brown SA, Finco DR, Navar LG: Impaired renal autoregulatory ability in dogs with reduced renal mass, *J Am Soc Nephrol* 5:1768, 1995.
72. Brown SA, Walton CL, Crawford P et al: Long-term effects of antihypertensive regimens on renal hemodynamics and proteinuria, *Kidney Int* 43:1210, 1993.
73. Dworkin LD, Tolbert E, Recht PA et al: Effects of amlodipine on glomerular filtration, growth, and injury in experimental hypertension, *Hypertension* 27:245, 1996.
74. Henik RA: Diagnosis and treatment of feline systemic hypertension, *Compend Cont Educ Pract Vet* 19:163, 1997.
75. Henik RA, Snyder PS, Volk LM: Amlodipine besylate therapy in cats with systemic arterial hypertension secondary to chronic renal disease, *J Vet Intern Med* 8:145, 1994 (abstract).
76. Henik RA, Snyder PS, Volk LM: Treatment of systemic hypertension in cats with amlodipine besylate, *J Am Anim Hosp Assoc* 33:226, 1997.
77. Snyder PS: Blinded clinical trial of amlodipine in cats with hypertension, *J Vet Intern Med* 11:139, 1997 (abstract).
78. Stopher DA, Beresford AP, Macrae PV et al: The metabolism and pharmacokinetics of amlodipine in humans and animals, *J Cardiovasc Pharmacol* 12(suppl 7):S55, 1988.
79. Beresford AP, Macrae PV, Stopher DA: Metabolism of amlodipine in the rat and the dog: a species difference, *Xenobiotica* 18:169, 1988.
80. Burgener D: Use of amlodipine in four dogs with systemic hypertension, personal communication, March 1997.

CHAPTER 27

Diagnosis and Treatment of Arrhythmias (Dysrhythmias)

An arrhythmia is a disturbance in the rate, regularity, or site of cardiac electrical impulse formation. Consequently, any heart rhythm that does not originate from the sinus node at a normal rate and at regular interval is classified as an arrhythmia. An arrhythmia can produce a heart rate that is too fast or too slow and can be regular or irregular. Conduction abnormalities may or may not produce an arrhythmia. First-degree atrioventricular (AV) block and bundle branch blocks do not alter the normal sinus rhythm. Second-degree AV block produces an arrhythmia by producing an irregular heart rate. Third-degree AV block is also a type of arrhythmia because it produces a heart rate that is too slow (bradycardia). Note that in third-degree AV block, the heart rate (the ventricular rate) is usually regular.

Arrhythmia literally means "no rhythm." Because of this, some prefer the term *dysrhythmia.* However, *arrhythmia* is the commonly used term and is used in this book to describe any abnormal heart rhythm.

Mechanisms of Arrhythmogenesis

The mechanisms of arrhythmia formation primarily include disorders of cardiac electrical impulse conduction and electrical impulse formation. Conduction abnormalities commonly result in conduction delays and blocks but can also contribute to the formation of ectopic tachyarrhythmias (premature depolarizations) by producing a substrate for reentry. Abnormalities of impulse formation produce both bradyarrhythmias and tachyarrhythmias.

DISORDERS OF ELECTRICAL IMPULSE CONDUCTION

Almost all cardiac tissues depolarize during systole and help conduct the depolarization wave from site to site. Disease of cardiac tissue can result in regions of conduction delay or conduction block. Conduction delays or blocks can result in bradyarrhythmias or tachyarrhythmias.

Conduction abnormalities leading to bradyarrhythmias. Conduction abnormalities that lead to bradyarrhythmias are due to conduction delays or conduction blocks within the specialized conduction system. The conduction system starts in the tissues surrounding the sinus node and terminates in the Purkinje network in the ventricles. Slowed conduction from the sinus node to the internodal tracts (first-degree sinoatrial block) does not cause any perceptible abnormality on an ECG because it occurs before the *P* wave is inscribed. An intermittent conduction block in this region (second-degree sinoatrial block) results in the heart rhythm stopping, usually only for one beat, because of the lack of a P-QRS-T complex on the ECG. Complete blockage of conduction from the sinus node to the internodal tracts and atria theoretically results in atrial standstill and forces the AV node to take over the pacing function of the heart at a slower rate. In reality, other regions of automaticity (e.g., tissue around the coronary sinus) in the atria probably take over the function of the sinus node in this situation.

Slowed conduction through the AV conduction system results in a prolongation in the P-R interval (first-degree AV block). This conduction delay can occur in the proximal AV bundle, the AV node, the bundle of His, or the bundle branches (if both the left and right bundle branches are affected). It theoretically also may occur in the internodal tracts. An intermittent complete block of conduction results in the intermittent loss of a QRS-T complex (second-degree AV block). Third-degree AV block occurs when conduction is completely blocked through the AV node, bundle of His, or both bundle branches. Complete block of conduction through the internodal tracts is also reported to produce complete AV block (third-degree AV block) in dogs.[1]

Conduction abnormalities leading to tachyarrhythmias. Normally, the cardiac electrical impulse spreads throughout the heart in an orderly fashion. Cardiac cells depolarize and in turn depolarize cells next to them. The cells that the original cells depolarize cannot normally "turn around" and in turn depolarize the original cells because the original cells are still in a depolarized state (they are refractory to stimulation). Because of this, the wave of depolarization normally proceeds in one direction and terminates.

Conduction through abnormal or diseased cardiac tissue may behave very differently than through normal cardiac tissue and may result in a condition termed *reentry.* For example, myocardial damage often results in damage to the sarcolemma (cell membrane). When the sarcolemma is damaged, the resting membrane potential commonly becomes less negative. Because of complex features of myocardial cells, these cells are electrically stable at only three resting membrane potentials: –70 to –90 mV, –40 to –60 mV, and 0 mV. When the cells are normal, the resting membrane potential is in the –70- to –90-mV range, depolarization occurs normally, and conduction velocity is normal. If cells are partially damaged, a less negative resting membrane potential of –40 to –60 mV is common for the cells in this region. At this voltage, rapid depolarization is impossible. Instead, slow depolarization, probably via slow calcium and slow sodium channels, occurs. This results in slowed conduction through a region. If conduction through this region is slowed enough or if the region of damaged myocardium is long enough, reentry may occur (Color Plate 108). In this situation, the depolarization wave coming down from the sinus node depolarizes the abnormal tissue and the adjoining normal tissue. The depolarization wave travels through the normal tissue rapidly, but travels through the abnormal tissue very slowly or fails to conduct at all through this tissue. In the first scenario, depolarization through the diseased tissue travels so slowly that by the time the depolarization wave reaches the end of the diseased tissue, the normal tissue on the other end has had time to depolarize and then fully repolarize. Consequently, the slow depolarization wave traveling through the diseased tissue finds the normal tissue ready to be stimulated again (it reenters it). If this new depolarization wave occurs before a new wave of depolarization can descend from the sinus node to the diseased site, a new depolarization wave occurs, and it occurs before the sinus beat. The early depolarization is called a *premature depolarization* or *premature beat.* This may occur only once or the premature depolarization may reexcite the proximal end of the diseased myocardium, traveling around again to reexcite the myocardium and producing repetitive premature depolarizations. This is called *functional reentry.* In the second scenario (in which depolarization fails to conduct through the diseased tissue), the depolarization that travels through the normal tissue enters the diseased tissue from the other side and conducts retrograde slowly back to reenter normal tissue. Here it reexcites the normal tissue, producing a premature depolarization. This is called *anatomic reentry.*

In another form of anatomic reentry, two pathways are present. The best example of this is the proposed mechanism for supraventricular tachycardia using the AV node for the reentrant pathway. As seen in Figure 27-1, reentry is initiated by an atrial premature depolarization that encounters two pathways in the AV node (called α and β). These two pathways have different conduction characteristics and different refractory periods, with the β pathway having the longer refractory period and slower conduction. Because the premature depolarization tries to depolarize the AV junction early, it finds the β pathway still refractory. Consequently, conduction is blocked from proceeding down the β pathway, whereas it proceeds normally down the α pathway. These two pathways converge at some point in the AV junction. By this time the β pathway has had time to repolarize fully, so the electrical impulse can conduct back up the nondepolarized β pathway. This pathway normally conducts very slowly; therefore, by the time the electrical impulse reaches atrial myocardium again, the atrial myocardium has had time to fully repolarize (it is not refractory). Consequently, it is depolarized again by the reentrant depolarization. This new depolarization finds the α pathway ready to conduct again, and the process may start over to become repetitive.

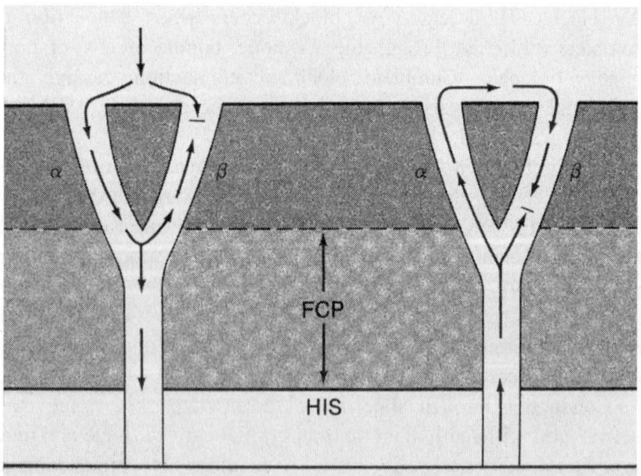

FIGURE 27-1 Schematic representation of reentry in the AV node. A premature depolarization from the atria produces a wave of depolarization that attempts to enter both α and β pathways. Because the β pathway has a longer refractory period, it is not ready to be depolarized. Conduction proceeds normally in the α pathway. When it reaches the final common pathway (FCP), it finds that the β pathway has not been depolarized. Consequently, depolarization proceeds antegrade to the ventricles through the FCP and retrograde through the β pathway to the atria. This produces a supraventricular premature depolarization. If this premature depolarization comes back to the AV node and finds the same circumstance, reentry occurs again. Consequently, the premature depolarizations become repetitive, producing a supraventricular tachycardia. (From Braunwald E: *Heart disease: a textbook of cardiovascular medicine,* ed 4, Philadelphia, 1992, WB Saunders.)

Reentry probably causes many types of tachyarrhythmias, including supraventricular and ventricular premature depolarizations and tachycardias, atrial and ventricular flutter, and atrial and ventricular fibrillation. Fibrillation is most commonly due to numerous small reentrant circuits.

DISORDERS OF IMPULSE FORMATION

Disorders of impulse formation encompasses enhanced or depressed impulse formation by abnormal pacemaker cells and abnormal impulse formation by cells that are normally not automatic.

Depressed normal automaticity. A depression in normal automaticity results in a decrease in the discharge rate of an automatic site. This can be due to disease of the automatic tissue or depression of automatic tissue as a result of diverse influences, such as the parasympathetic nervous system, electrolyte disturbances (e.g., hyperkalemia), endocrine abnormalities (e.g., hypothyroidism), and hypothermia. To be manifested as a bradyarrhythmia, the sinus node must be affected, either by itself or in combination with subsidiary pacemaker sites. For example, if the automatic cells within the AV node are suppressed by stimulation of the left vagus such that their inherent rate decreases from 50 to 30 beats/min, but the sinus node continues to depolarize at a rate of 100 beats/min, the fact that the AV nodal cells are depressed will never be identified because the faster sinus nodal rate continues to control the heart rate. If, however, the right vagus is stimulated, decreasing the sinus node rate to 45 beats/min, the AV node may take over the heart rate and maintain it at 50 beats/min. If both vagal nerves are stimulated such that the sinus rate decreases to 35 beats/min and the AV nodal rate decreases to 40 beats/min, the heart will only beat at 40 beats/min. Normal automaticity can also be depressed by disease. Sick sinus syndrome is a disease in which the sinus node tissue is diseased and destroyed. When most of the sinus node tissue is destroyed, it loses its ability to automatically produce depolarizations.

Enhanced normal automaticity. Enhanced normal automaticity results in tachyarrhythmias. Sinus tachycardia is an example of enhanced normal automaticity in which the normal sinus node is stimulated to depolarize at a rate faster than normal. Similarly, AV nodal cells can be stimulated to discharge at a rate faster than the sinus node, producing nodal premature depolarizations. Other subsidiary pacemakers (pacemakers that normally have a rate slower than that of the sinus node) that can be stimulated to usurp control of the heart's rhythm include cells in several parts of the atria, the coronary sinus, the AV valves, the AV junction, and the His-Purkinje system. Obviously, it is easier for premature depolarizations to manifest themselves if the sinus rate is slow.

Abnormal automaticity. Abnormal automaticity is another mechanism for producing premature depolarizations and tachycardias (tachyarrhythmias). It is a process by which cells that are not normally automatic (e.g., myocardial cells) are made into automatic cells or cells that are normally automatic but have a very slow rate (Purkinje fibers) are made into cells with a faster rate. This abnormality produces premature depolarizations through damage to the cell membrane that results in a lesser resting membrane potential.[2,3] Similar to the explanation for slow conduction in reentry, damaged myocardial cells can have a resting membrane potential of approximately –40 to –60 mV instead of the normal –70 to –90 mV. This membrane potential can be stable (such as happens when it contributes to reentry) or it may spontaneously depolarize, probably through slow inward movement of sodium and calcium ions. The action potentials from such tissue resembles that of normal automatic cells (Figure 27-2). Spontaneous depolarization to a threshold potential results in depolarization and initiation of a depolarization wave from the abnormal (ectopic) site. If the rate of depolarization of an ectopic site is faster than the sinus rate, the abnormally automatic site manifests, producing premature depolarizations or tachycardia. Recently it has been shown that cell swelling can induce a chloride current in canine atrial cells.[4] This current results in a decrease in resting membrane potential and in abnormal automaticity.

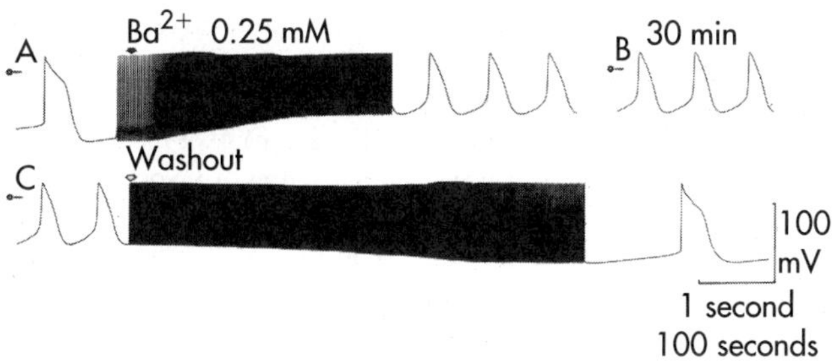

FIGURE 27-2 Action potentials recorded from an isolated Purkinje fiber in a saline bath. The initial action potential **(A)** is normal and recorded at a fast paper speed. The paper speed is slowed, and barium chloride (Ba^{2+}) is added to the saline bath. Subsequently the resting membrane potential increases from –90 mV to about –55 mV, and the resting membrane potential depolarizes at a fast rate. This abnormal automaticity is sustained **(B)** until the barium chloride is washed out of the tissue by replacing the saline bath with fresh material after **C.** (From Fox PR: *Canine and feline cardiology,* New York, 1988, Churchill Livingstone.)

Catecholamines enhance the amplitude of this current. Theoretically this type of abnormality could occur whenever myocardial cells are damaged and swell, such as occurs in numerous myocardial diseases or diseases that affect the myocardium.

It has been demonstrated that abnormal automaticity is an important mechanism for producing tachyarrhythmias, especially ventricular tachyarrhythmias. A good example is one study in which ventricular tachycardia was induced by delivering a low-energy (30 J) shock to the endocardium of the left ventricle of experimental dogs.[3] All dogs had ventricular tachycardia 1 day after shock delivery. In some dogs, the injured region was mapped electrophysiologically, studied in an isolated, perfused heart preparation, and examined histologically on day 1. Identical studies were performed on the other dogs on day 4, after the ventricular tachycardia was no longer present. In the dogs studied on day 1, a region of subendocardial injured tissue was present. The site of origin for the ventricular tachycardia was determined to be subendocardial Purkinje fibers that were in a border zone surrounding a central necrotic (dead) region. These cells had a mean resting membrane potential of –58 mV that depolarized spontaneously at a rate faster than normal (Figure 27-3). Their upstroke velocity was very slow, characteristic of cells that depolarize via slow calcium channels. All these findings are characteristic of abnormal automaticity. Histology of this region revealed swollen and necrotic cells. Presumably the arrhythmia originated from the damaged (swollen) cells. Normal cells next to this region had a mean resting membrane potential of –78 mV and normal upstroke velocity. In the dogs studied on day 4, it was difficult to identify action potentials from the same region, but those identified were normal. Histology confirmed that the cells in the region now had been replaced by fibrous tissue.

Abnormal automaticity is thought to produce the ventricular arrhythmias that occur within 24 hours of coronary artery ligation in experimental dogs.[5] Because coronary artery disease is only rarely seen in dogs, it may appear that this model has no bearing on clinical disease. However, other myocardial diseases seen in veterinary medicine are caused by myocardial hypoxia and ischemia. A good example is the myocardial lesion observed in dogs that have suffered from gastric dilatation-volvulus.[6] This lesion appears to be due to ischemia created secondary to the profound central hypovolemia caused by the distended stomach occluding the caudal vena cava. In addition, other myocardial lesions that produce accelerated idioventricular rhythms (slow ventricular tachycardias) are thought to result from abnormal automaticity.[7] Consequently, it appears that this mechanism is a very common and important cause of the clinical

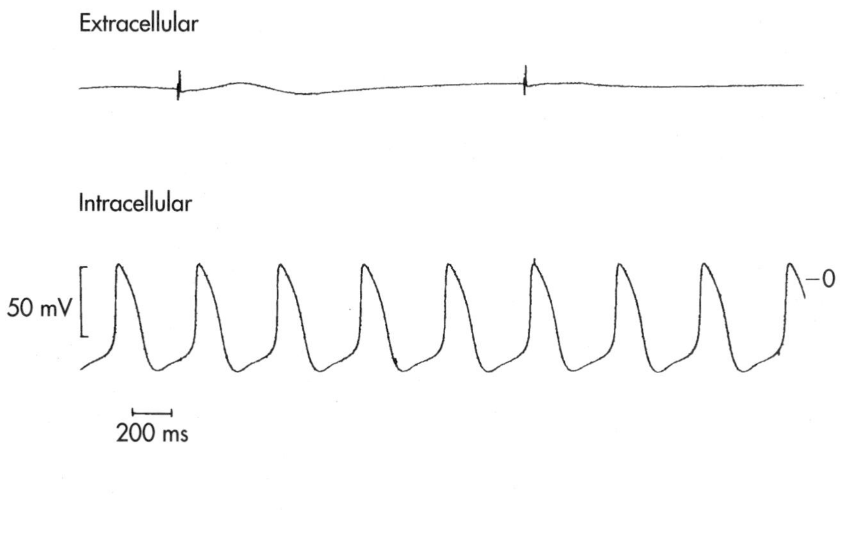

FIGURE 27-3 Intracellular recording of electrograms from a dog ventricular myocardial cell 1 day following the application of DC shocks. The resting membrane potential is decreased to –62 mV. Spontaneous depolarization occurs during phase 4 (i.e., the cell is now automatic). This is giving rise to an accelerated idioventricular rhythm with a rate of 150 beats/min (cycle length = 400 ms). This is an example of abnormal automaticity. (From Hauer RNW, deBakker JMT, de Wilde AAM, et al: Ventricular tachycardia after in vivo DC shock ablation in dogs, *Circulation* 84:276, 1991.)

ventricular tachyarrhythmias seen in dogs with acute disease syndromes that are commonly seen in an intensive care type of setting.

Triggered activity. Triggered activity is similar to abnormal automaticity in that tissue that is not normally automatic (e.g., myocardium) attains the ability to depolarize on its own. However, instead of producing an action potential similar to a normally automatic cell, triggered activity must be triggered by a preceding normal action potential. Automaticity is the property of cardiac cells to depolarize spontaneously. Consequently, triggered activity is not a form of abnormal automaticity. Two types of triggered activity have been identified: early afterdepolarizations and delayed afterdepolarizations. Afterdepolarizations are oscillations of membrane potential that attend or follow the action potential. They depend on the preceding action potential for their production.

Early afterdepolarizations (EADs) interrupt repolarization during phases 2 and 3 of the action potential. During these phases, instead of depolarization and repolarization proceeding smoothly, the action potential oscillates to a threshold and depolarizes the cell again (Figure 27-4). The mechanism underlying EADs is poorly understood.[8] However, EADs have been observed in vitro in response to drugs that decrease the availability of potassium currents for repolarization (quinidine, procainamide, bretylium, sotalol), that increase the availability of transarcolemmal calcium currents (Bay K 8644, catecholamines), and that delay sodium current activation (aconitine).[8] They occur more readily in environments low in potassium. They occur most readily at low stimulation rates (low heart rates). They are more readily produced in conducting tissue, such as Purkinje fibers, than in myocardial tissues. EADs have never been reported in superficial epicardial or endocardial syncytial tissue. They have, however, been observed in single myocardial cells. This suggests that EADs can only be produced in a discrete or isolated population of cells. Recently, the existence of a unique subpopulation of cells has been described in the deep subepicardial region of the canine ventricular free wall and the deep subendocardial regions of the interventricular septum, papillary muscles, and trabeculae.[8,9] These cells are called M cells and have electrophysiologic properties midway between myocardium and conduction tissue. Their primary distinguishing characteristic is their ability to prolong their action potential greatly when the heart rate decreases. These cells may be responsible for the U wave on the ECG and for EADs. An example of an arrhythmia thought to be due to EADs is torsade de pointes, a type of fast ventricular tachycardia in which the QRS complexes rhythmically increase and decrease in size. This arrhythmia is commonly associated with many of the factors known to produce EADs and is commonly associated with a long Q-T interval in humans. The one canine patient with torsade de pointes described in the veterinary literature had a long Q-T interval.[10] Quinidine toxicity can produce EADs and torsades de pointes in humans and in dogs with experimentally induced complete AV block.

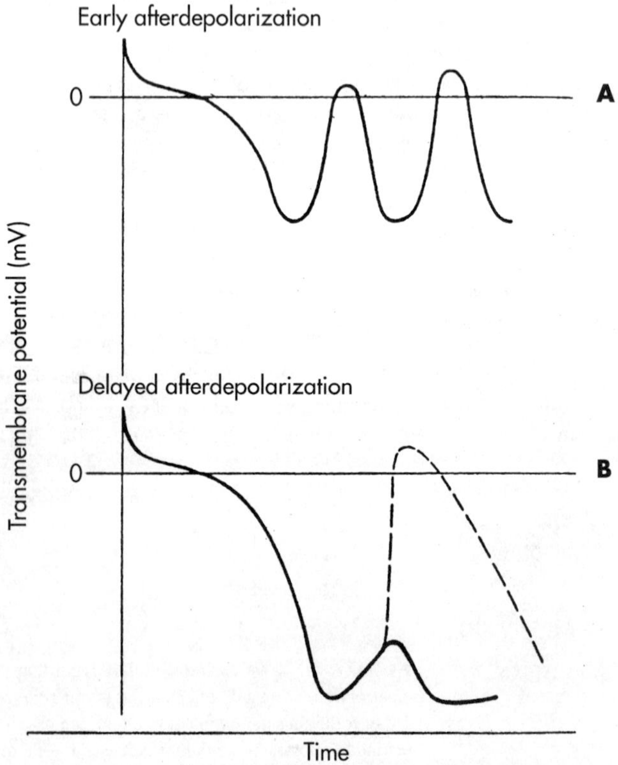

FIGURE 27-4 Drawings of abnormal action potentials. The top potential **(A)** exhibits early afterdepolarizations in which the membrane potential spontaneously depolarizes in late phase 2 and phase 3 of the action potential. The bottom potential **(B)** is an example of delayed afterdepolarization. The resting membrane potential, instead of remaining steady, oscillates to the threshold potential and depolarizes spontaneously. (From Tilley LP: *Essentials of canine and feline electrocardiography,* ed 3, Philadelphia, 1992, Lea & Febiger.)

EADs are apparently the mechanism by which the arrhythmias in German shepherds with inherited ventricular tachycardia are produced.[11] In these dogs, it appears that sympathetic innervation of regions of myocardium is deficient, especially to the cranial portion of the interventricular septum and portions of the left ventricular free wall. Sympathetic innervation is necessary for channel development. These dogs have markedly reduced cellular density of the membrane channels responsible for phase 1 repolarization of myocytes. These channels are denoted I_{to} and carry a transient outward current. Lack of these channels could prolong the action potential duration in these dogs or could initiate action potential oscillations characteristic of EADs. The EADs in this situation arise from Purkinje fibers.

Delayed afterdepolarizations (DADs) occur when the fully repolarized resting membrane potential oscillates to a threshold potential and depolarizes (see Figure 27-4). These are thought to be due to transient inward currents caused by oscillatory release of calcium from the sarcoplasmic reticulum in diastole.[12] Calcium overload appears to be the primary inciting cause of DADs. The classic method of producing DADs is to produce an intracellular calcium overload with a digitalis glycoside. It appears that DADs are also produced primarily in M cells.[13]

Evaluation of the Heart Rhythm

Determining cardiac rhythm is the most important reason for evaluating an ECG. Determining the type of abnormal cardiac rhythm from an ECG is much like solving a puzzle. Some veterinarians enjoy solving these puzzles, whereas others do not, just like some people like to work crossword puzzles and others have never completed one. If one enjoys solving ECG puzzles, our recommendation is that he or she record ECGs whenever indicated and practice making rhythm diagnoses as often as possible. If one finds this type of activity frustrating, we recommend that she or he have someone else make these determinations. Making consistently accurate diagnoses takes practice, patience, and perseverance.

To solve an ECG puzzle, one has to know the basics of impulse formation and conduction. Then one must know which questions to ask and how to answer these questions. Four basic questions should be asked and answered when evaluating cardiac rhythm. First, what are the atrial and ventricular rates? If the rate is too fast, a tachycardia is present. If it is too slow, a bradycardia is present. A finite number of reasons for tachycardias and bradycardias exist. Second, are the atrial and ventricular rhythms regular or irregular? Now there are two criteria, and the number of reasons for a fast regular rhythm or a fast irregular rhythm are less than for just a fast heart rate. If the rhythm is irregular, is it irregular because beats are occurring too fast (premature beats) or too slow (escape beats)? Third, are the *P* waves and QRS complexes normally configured and are they of normal width or too wide? *P* waves that are negative when they should be positive may indicate that they originate from an abnormal site (a site other than the sinus node). If ventricular depolarization produces a QRS complex that is of normal width, it must be using the intraventricular conduction system. Consequently, it must enter the ventricles through or from the AV node and transmit through the bundle of His, bundle branches, and Purkinje network. Consequently, it must originate in the sinus node, atrial muscle, or AV junction (the supraventricular sites) and travel to other regions of the AV node. Conversely, QRS complexes that are too wide can be generated by left ventricular hypertrophy, a bundle branch block, or an ectopic pacemaker originating in a bundle branch or ventricular myocardium. A bundle branch block and a ventricular premature depolarization set up a depolarization wave that must travel slowly from muscle cell to muscle cell and so produce a QRS complex that is wider than normal. If a QRS complex is too wide because of left ventricular hypertrophy or a bundle branch block, a *P* wave should be visible in front of each QRS complex with a constant P-R interval. If it is originating from a ventricle, there should be no *P* wave in front of the QRS complex or it should not have the same relationship as any sinus beats that are present. Fourth, are there *P* waves present, and what is the relationship between the *P* waves and the QRS complexes? Are there more *P* waves than QRS complexes? Are there more QRS complexes than *P* waves? Is there a constant P-R interval or are the *P* waves and QRS complexes dissociated? Characteristics of the common arrhythmias are listed in Table 27-1.

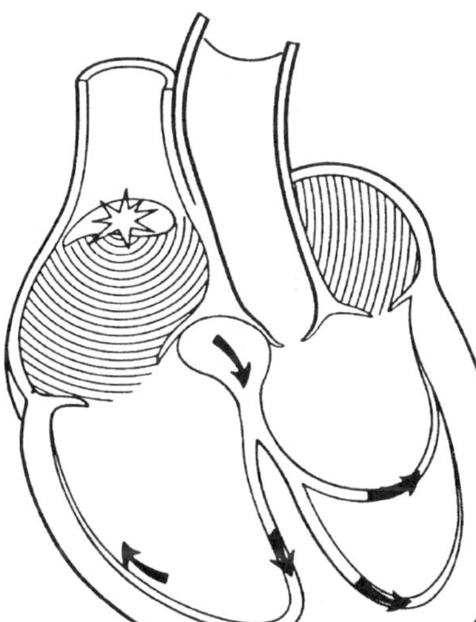

FIGURE 27-5 Drawing depicting sinus rhythm. The sinus node depolarizes followed by the atrial depolarization wave, atrioventricular nodal conduction, and bundle branch conduction. Ventricular depolarization would follow. (From Phillips RE, Feeney MK: *Cardiac rhythms: a systematic approach to interpretation,* ed 3, Philadelphia, 1990, WB Saunders.)

Specific Arrhythmias

SINUS RHYTHMS

Normal sinus rhythm. Normally the sinus node depolarizes at a rate faster than other automatic tissues in the heart, and there are no sites of ectopic depolarization. Therefore the sinus node acts as the pacemaker of the normal heart and controls heart rate and rhythm. When the sinus node controls the rate and rhythm there is a normal order of depolarization and repolarization of all cardiac tissues (Figure 27-5). The range for the normal sinus node rate (and so the heart rate) for the dog is extremely wide. Large dogs that are sleeping often have a sinus rate that is 35 to 40 beats/min or even slower, whereas a small excited dog can have a normal sinus rate of 180 beats/min. Excited cats can have sinus rates up to 240 beats/min, whereas resting heart rate may be as slow as 100 beats/min. Consequently, interpretation of the sinus node rate depends on evaluating not just the heart rate but also the type of patient and the environment. Whereas a heart rate of 170 beats/min in an examination room is acceptable for a miniature poodle, it is too fast (tachycardia) for a great Dane. The sinus rate is primarily regulated by the autonomic nervous system. Sympathetic nervous system stimulation increases the sinus node rate and parasympathetic nervous system stimulation decreases the sinus node rate.

The ECG criteria for sinus rhythm are a normal heart rate, a regular rhythm, an upright *P* wave in leads I, II, III, and aV_F, a *P* wave for every QRS complex, a QRS complex for every *P* wave, and a constant P-R interval (Figure 27-6).

Sinus arrhythmia. In sinus arrhythmia, the rhythm originates from the sinus node but is not regular. Sinus arrhythmia is normal in dogs but not in cats. In the classic case, the heart rate varies with respiration in a regular pattern, increasing on inspiration and decreasing on expiration. However, this classic pattern is not observed in dogs that do not breathe regularly while the ECG is recorded. In these cases, sinus arrhythmia is diagnosed whenever

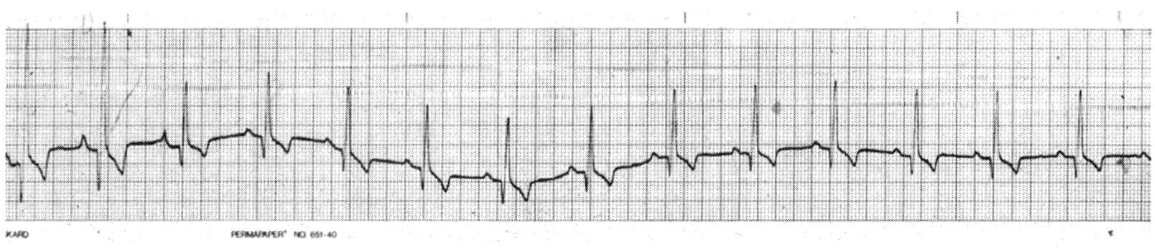

FIGURE 27-6 Lead II ECG tracing recorded from a 13-year-old miniature French poodle with mild mitral regurgitation. The rhythm is normal sinus rhythm. The heart rate is 140 beats/min. The first two complexes are taken at a normal calibration of 1 cm = 1 mV. The remaining complexes are recorded at "half sensitivity" (5 mm = 1 mV). The *R* wave height is greater than normal, which probably indicates left ventricular hypertrophy. (Paper speed = 50 mm/sec.)

TABLE 27-1
Arrhythmia characteristics

Rhythm	*P wave rate (bpm)*	*P wave rhythm*	*P wave configuration*	*QRS complex rate*	*QRS complex rhythm*	*QRS configuration*	*P-QRS relationship*
Sinus	Normal	Regular	Normal	Same as *P*	Regular	Normal	1:1
Sinus bradycardia	<Normal	Regular	Normal	Same as *P*	Regular	Normal	1:1
Sinus tachycardia	>Normal	Regular	Normal	Same as *P*	Regular	Normal	1:1
Sinus arrhythmia	Normal	Irregular	Normal or wandering	Same as *P*	Irregular	Normal	1:1
Supraventricular tachycardia	>Normal	Regular	Positive, negative, absent, or buried	Same as *P*	Regular	Normal	1:1
Atrial flutter	>350	Regular	Positive (sawtooth)	Less than *P* wave rate	Regular or irregular	Normal	More Ps than QRSs
Atrial fibrillation	>500	Irregular	None to baseline undulation (f waves)	Less than *P* wave rate (100-280)	Irregular	Normal	No *P* waves; more undulations than QRSs
Accelerated idioventricular rhythm	Normal	Regular	Normal (often buried in QRS)	70-150	Fairly regular; may be irregular	Wide	Dissociated; more QRSs than Ps
Ventricular tachycardia	Normal	Regular	Normal (often buried in QRS)	150-350	Regular or irregular	Wide	Dissociated; more QRSs than Ps
Ventricular flutter	Normal	Regular	Not discernible	>350	Regular	Sine wave	Dissociated; more QRSs than Ps
Ventricular fibrillation	Normal	Regular	Not discernible	>400	Grossly irregular	No QRS complexes	Dissociated; no QRSs
Second-degree AV block	Normal	Regular	Normal	<*P* wave rate	Irregular	Normal or wide	More Ps than QRSs
Third-degree AV block	Normal	Regular	Normal	20-60	Regular	Normal or wide	Dissociated; more Ps than QRSs; irregular P-R interval

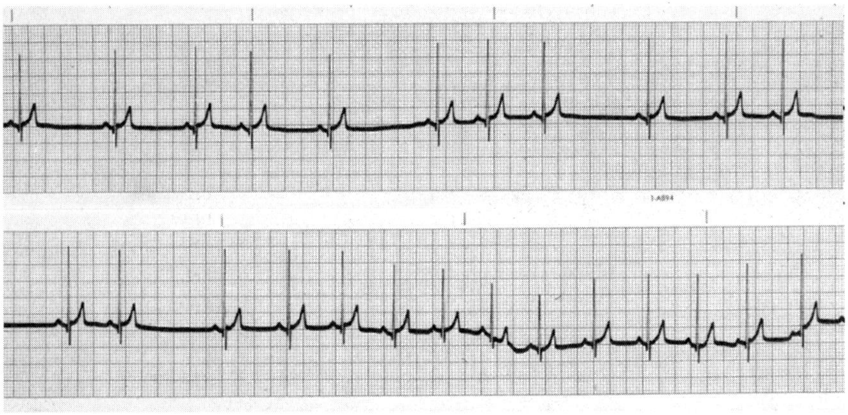

FIGURE 27-7 Lead II ECG tracing recorded from a normal 8-year-old Labrador retriever. The rhythm in the top tracing is sinus arrhythmia. The dog was not breathing slowly and steadily. Consequently, the rhythm is not regularly irregular. There is, however, a normal heart rate (it varies from approximately 50 to 100 beats/min), a *P* wave for every QRS complex and a QRS complex for every *P* wave, and the complexes are configured normally. At the end of the bottom tracing the dog became excited by its owner entering the room, producing sinus rhythm with a heart rate of approximately 100 beats/min. (Paper speed = 50 mm/sec; 1 cm = 1 mV.)

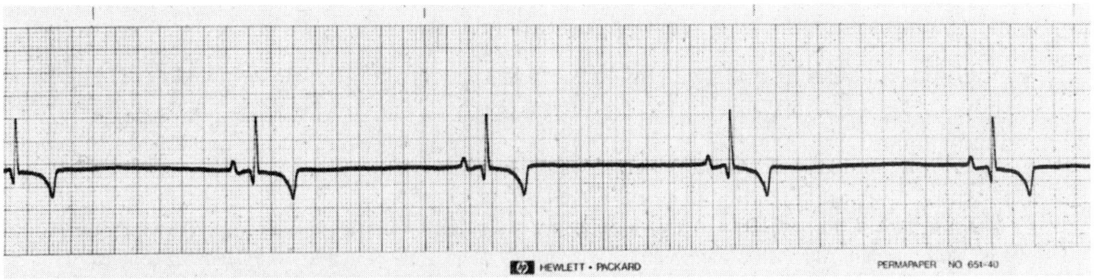

FIGURE 27-8 Lead II ECG tracing recorded from a golden retriever while it was excited. The heart rate is 55 beats/min and originates in the sinus node. Sinus bradycardia was diagnosed. The heart rate only increased to 75 beats/min after atropine administration. An inherent sinus node dysfunction (sick sinus syndrome) was diagnosed. (Paper speed = 50 mm/sec; 1 cm = 1 mV.)

there are alterations in the distance between P-QRS-T complexes (the rhythm is irregular), but all of the other criteria for sinus rhythm are present. Sinus arrhythmia is exaggerated in some dogs. This most commonly occurs in dogs that are sleeping or in dogs with chronic respiratory disease. An exaggerated sinus arrhythmia is presented in Figure 27-7.

Sinus bradycardia. Sinus bradycardia is a regular rhythm that originates from the sinus node but at a rate that is too slow for a given situation. A sinus rate less than 60 beats/min in an awake dog in an examination room is generally considered too slow (Figure 27-8). As mentioned previously, however, the sinus rate can be as slow as 20 beats/min in a normal dog that is sleeping. A heart rate less than 100 to 120 beats/min in a cat is generally too slow, although it may produce no clinical signs. Sinus bradycardia is an uncommon rhythm disturbance in clinical veterinary practice. It is most commonly identified during an anesthetic overdose. Other causes include increased vagal tone, sick sinus syndrome, hypothermia, severe hypothyroidism, and administration of vagomimetic or sympatholytic drugs, such as xylazine, digoxin, and β-blockers. Sick sinus syndrome is discussed below.

Treatment. Treatment of sinus bradycardia is unnecessary unless clinical signs are evident and depends on the underlying cause. If drug administration is precipitating the problem, it should be discontinued. If the problem is peracute, such as in a patient under anesthesia, atropine should be administered in an attempt to increase the heart rate. If this is unsuccessful, a β-adrenergic agonist, such as isoproterenol, can be administered. Conscious patients that have no apparent underlying cause should be administered atropine (0.04 mg/kg SC) and an ECG repeated 30 minutes later. In a dog with a normal sinus node, the heart rate should increase to 140 to 200 beats/min. If a normal response is identified, the diagnosis of increased vagal tone is made. If the dog is symptomatic, chronic anticholinergic therapy can be initiated. If there is no response or if the response is only partial (heart rate increases to 70 to 130 beats/min), sick sinus syndrome is most likely present.

Sinus tachycardia. Sinus tachycardia is diagnosed when all the criteria for sinus rhythm are present but the heart rate is too fast (Figure 27-9). There clearly is overlap between sinus rhythm and sinus tachycardia. For example, although veterinarians consider a heart rate of 220 beats/min in a cat undergoing an examination to be normal, most likely it is actually sinus tachycardia induced by stress and fear. Generally if a veterinarian was in a dentist's chair and his or her heart rate was 120 beats/min, it would be considered sinus tachycardia rather than normal sinus rhythm. For sinus tachycardia to be present, there generally should be an underlying reason for it to be present. Sympathetic nervous stimulation from extreme excitement in an examination room or pain are two of the most common reasons for sinus tachycardia. Fever, hyperthyroidism, hypovolemia, cardiac tamponade, and heart failure are examples of abnormalities that increase sympathetic stimulation in an attempt to increase cardiac output to meet the bodies increased (fever, hyperthyroidism) or normal (hypovolemia, cardiac tamponade, and heart failure) demands for oxygen. Drugs such as catecholamines and atropine increase the sinus node rate.

The major differential diagnosis for sinus tachycardia is supraventricular tachycardia (SVT), a tachycardia in which an ectopic pacemaker is firing faster than the sinus node, taking over the heart rhythm. An SVT may look identical to a sinus tachycardia on an ECG. Several clues may suggest the presence of an SVT rather than a sinus tachycardia. First, if the heart rate is too fast for a given patient and a given situation, SVT is a possible diagnosis. Second, if the patient has underlying heart disease, SVT is much more likely than

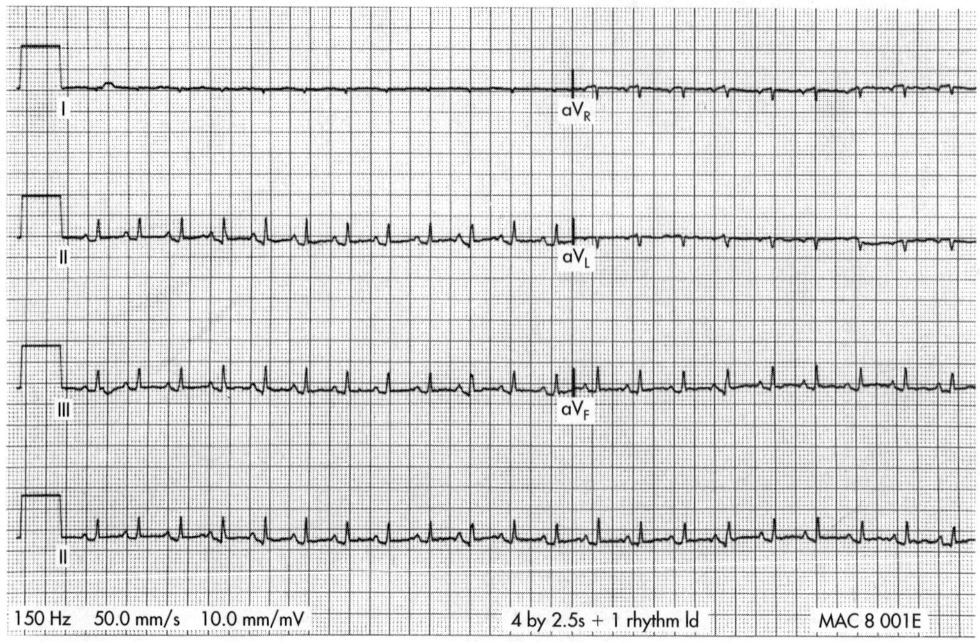

FIGURE 27-9 Recordings of six limb leads from a 6-year-old cat with unexplained tachycardia. The heart rate is 280 beats/min. Although a supraventricular (ectopic) tachycardia cannot be completely discounted, the heart rate tended to speed and slow gradually for the owner at home, making the most likely diagnosis a sinus tachycardia.

if no cardiac disease is present. A patient with cardiac disease, however, can also have sinus tachycardia, especially if it is in heart failure. The best means of differentiating sinus tachycardia from SVT is to perform a precordial thump (see discussion of supraventricular tachycardia).

There generally is no indication to treat sinus tachycardia definitively. Instead, the underlying cause should be corrected. In some cases it is contraindicated to slow the heart rate before the underlying abnormality is corrected. For example, slowing the heart rate in a dog with hypovolemia before replacing fluid volume would be detrimental.

Sinoatrial block and sinus arrest

Sinoatrial block. Sinoatrial block occurs when the tissue surrounding the sinus node fails to conduct the depolarization to the atria and ventricles. Some, but not all, depolarizations are conducted in a second-degree sinoatrial block. This is the most commonly diagnosed type of sinoatrial block. Second-degree sinoatrial block is diagnosed on an ECG when a pause occurs after a sinus beat and the interval between beats is an exact multiple (e.g., 2 or 3 times) of the normal P-P interval. In Figure 27-10, the normal interval between *P* waves (P-P interval) is 0.6 seconds (sinus rate = 100 beats/min). The longer P-P intervals are exactly 1.2 seconds (sinus rate = 50 beats/min). This indicates that the sinus node most likely depolarized at its normal rate, but the depolarization was intermittently blocked from conducting to the atria and internodal tracts (Figures 27-10 and 27-11). Consequently, no *P* wave and no QRS-T complex were produced.

Sinus arrest. Sinus arrest is a cessation of sinus node activity for a short period (Figure 27-12). Although sinus arrest is commonly described as a pause in the sinus rhythm that lasts for more than two normal R-R intervals, this can also be seen with severe sinus arrhythmia (see Figure 27-7). Consequently, there is a "gray zone" between severe sinus arrhythmia and sinus arrest in the dog.

Sinus arrest in dogs most commonly is due to either sinus node dysfunction or increased vagal tone. Sinus node dysfunction usually is due to end-stage sinus node disease and is commonly called *sick sinus syndrome.* Histologic analysis of the sinus node in canine patients with sinus node dysfunction is rarely performed. In the one dog that we have observed (a miniature schnauzer), the sinus node was completely replaced by fibrous tissue. Sinus node dysfunction in dogs can produce other arrhythmias, including sinus bradycardia and the so-called tachycardia-bradycardia syndrome. A supraventricular tachycardia can sometimes be seen with sick sinus syndrome, presumably because of reentry in or around the diseased sinus node. However, sinus arrest is the most common manifestation of end-stage sinus node disease in dogs.[14] Increased vagal tone can also produce periods of sinus arrest and can, on occasion, produce pauses long enough to cause syncope. Vagal tone can be increased secondary to chronic respiratory disease or secondary to systemic disease (e.g., gastrointestinal disease). In humans, vagal tone is increased in hypersensitive carotid sinus syndrome. In this syndrome, external pressure on the carotid sinus causes prolonged periods of sinus arrest or AV block, resulting in syncope. We have suspected this syndrome in some dogs, but the syndrome has not been proved in dogs. In most dogs with increased vagal tone, sinus arrest, and syncope, the cause is unknown.

Escape beats. Sinus arrest can last for a short period (less than 1 second in a dog) and be terminated by the sinus node depolarizing again. Sinus arrest can also last for a period long enough that a subsidiary pacemaker, such as the AV node, takes over the heart rhythm. When the AV junction or the Purkinje fibers take over the heart rhythm because the sinus node is markedly slowed or stopped or if the sinus depolarizations cannot reach the ventricles (third-degree AV block), QRS complexes occur after a pause or occur at a rate between 20 and 60 beats/min. Depolarizations that occur after a pause are called *escape beats* and the slow rhythms are called *escape rhythms.* An example of sinus arrest terminated by an escape beat is shown in Figure 27-12. Escape beats normally originate either from the AV junctional region or from Purkinje fibers. Because the rate for these two sites differ, one can determine the origin of an escape beat

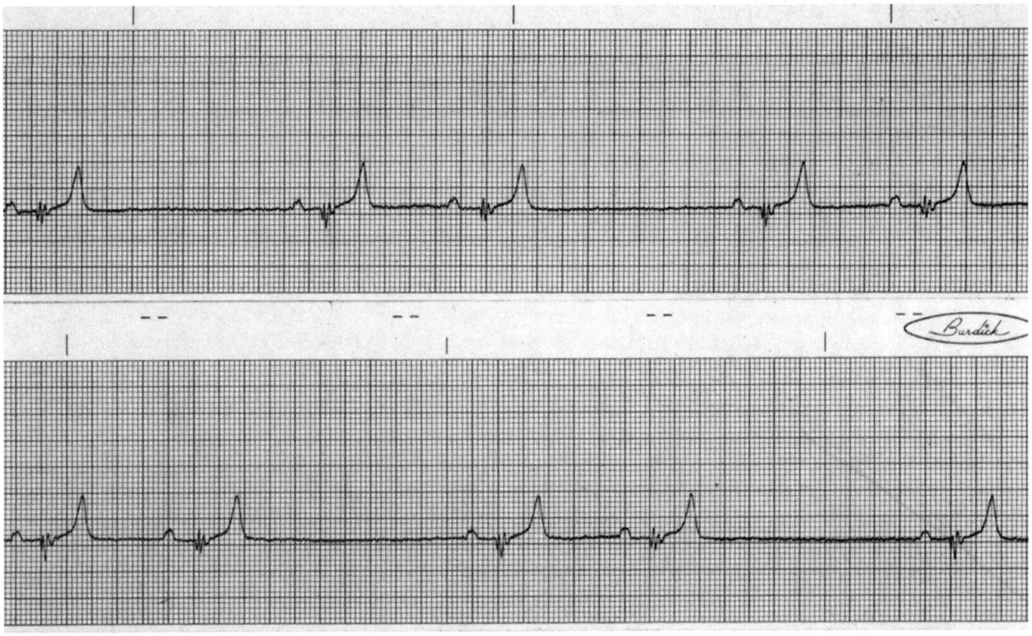

FIGURE 27-10 Continuous lead II ECG tracing recorded from a 7-year-old English springer spaniel with an irregular heart rhythm. The rhythm is a sinus rhythm with periods of second-degree sinoatrial block. In the top tracing, the second and fifth sinus depolarizations have been blocked from depolarizing the atria and internodal tracts. Consequently no electrical activity is recorded. However, the next *P* wave occurs at exactly twice the interval (1.2 seconds) of the normal P-P interval (0.6 seconds). (Paper speed = 50 mm/sec; 1 cm = 1 mV.)

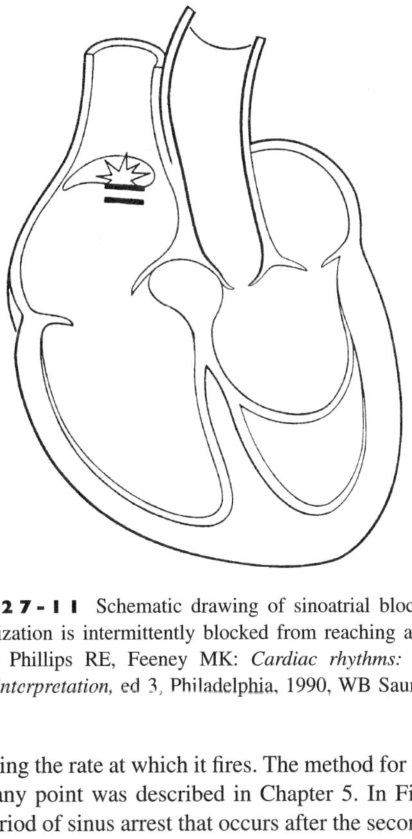

FIGURE 27-11 Schematic drawing of sinoatrial block. The sinus node depolarization is intermittently blocked from reaching atrial myocardium. (From Phillips RE, Feeney MK: *Cardiac rhythms: a systematic approach to interpretation,* ed 3, Philadelphia, 1990, WB Saunders.)

by determining the rate at which it fires. The method for determining the rate at any point was described in Chapter 5. In Figure 27-12, there is a period of sinus arrest that occurs after the second P-QRS-T complex. This pause lasts for 1.26 seconds. If it lasted for exactly 1 second (if the heart depolarized once every second) the heart rate would be 60 beats/min. The rate that the escape focus fires in this patient is 48 beats/min (60 sec/min ÷ 1.26 sec/beat). Because we know that the AV node depolarizes (fires) at a rate of 40 to 60 beats/min in the dog, we know that the escape focus in this patient is within the AV node. The configuration of this complex is compatible with a nodal escape beat. The QRS complex is narrow, so it must originate from a supraventricular focus, and the *P* wave is negative, which is compatible with the depolarization originating from a nodal focus and depolarizing the atria in a retrograde fashion. In Figure 27-13, *A,* the QRS complexes of the escape beats are wider than normal, have a different orientation from normal (they are negative), and are followed by a very abnormal-appearing T wave. All of these suggest that they originate from the Purkinje fibers in the ventricles. The rate of the escape focus, however, is 57 beats/min. This tells us that it is most likely not ventricular in origin. Consequently, something else must be occurring. In this dog, most likely the right bundle branch is not conducting after this prolonged pause. This is a so-called phase 4 conduction disturbance. Here, the right bundle branch could depolarize spontaneously during diastole (phase 4) to such a degree that the cells were hypopolarized.[15] When the cardiac electrical impulse reached these cells, they were unable to conduct normally because they were hypopolarized. In summary, this dog had periods of sinus arrest that were terminated by escape beats that originated from the AV node, but the escape beats were conducted in a right bundle branch block pattern. This dog had severe respiratory disease with chronic moderate dyspnea but no syncope. Thirty minutes following atropine administration (0.04 mg/kg SC), the dog was in sinus rhythm with a heart rate of 170 beats/min. This confirmed that the arrhythmia was vagally induced (Figure 27-13, *B*).

Dogs with diffuse conduction system disease or with increased vagal tone to both the sinus node and the AV node may have more prolonged periods of sinus arrest because the subsidiary pacemakers are either suppressed or dysfunctional. If a period of sinus arrest lasts for more than approximately 6 seconds, weakness and syncope will occur.[14] An ECG from a dog with sinus node disease (sick sinus syndrome) is presented in Figure 27-14. This dog had periods of sinus arrest that lasted up to 2.15 seconds. The periods of sinus arrest were not terminated by escape beats but instead by sinus beats as the diseased sinus node finally recovered function. In essence the dog

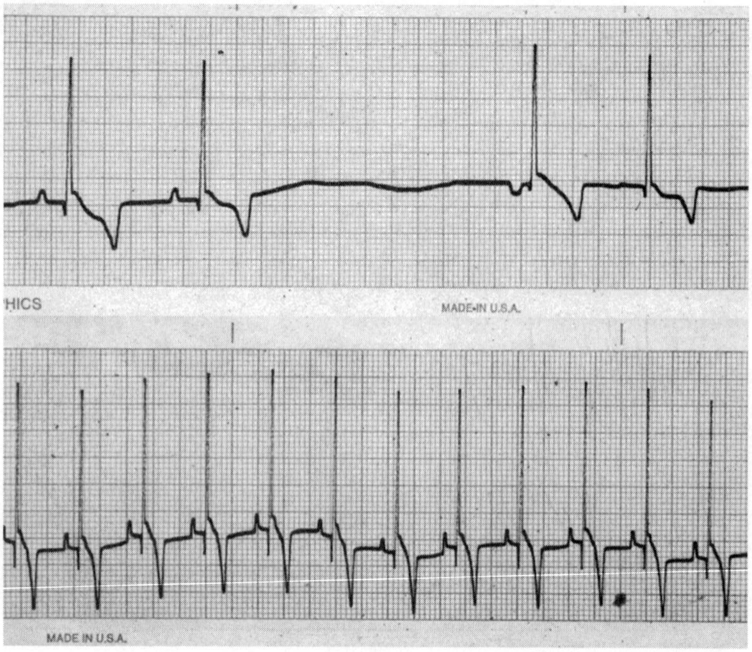

FIGURE 27-12 Lead II ECG tracings recorded from a 10-year-old Lhasa apso with an irregular heart rate. The first two beats in the first tracing are sinus beats. These are followed by a period of sinus arrest. The sinus arrest is terminated by an escape beat. The escape beat occurs after a 1.26-second pause. This means the escape focus is depolarizing at a rate of 48 beats/min (60 sec/min ÷ 1.26 sec/beat). This rate is compatible with a nodal escape beat. The *P* wave is negative, and the QRS complex is normal. These are also compatible with a nodal origin. The second tracing was recorded 10 minutes after atropine 0.04 mg/kg SC was administered. The rhythm is a sinus rhythm, and the heart rate is 130 beats/min. The periods of sinus arrest have been abolished. Twenty minutes later the heart rate was 175 beats/min, indicating that the arrhythmia was vagally mediated. (First tracing paper speed = 50 mm/sec. Second tracing speed = 25 mm/sec; 1 cm = 1 mV.)

A

B

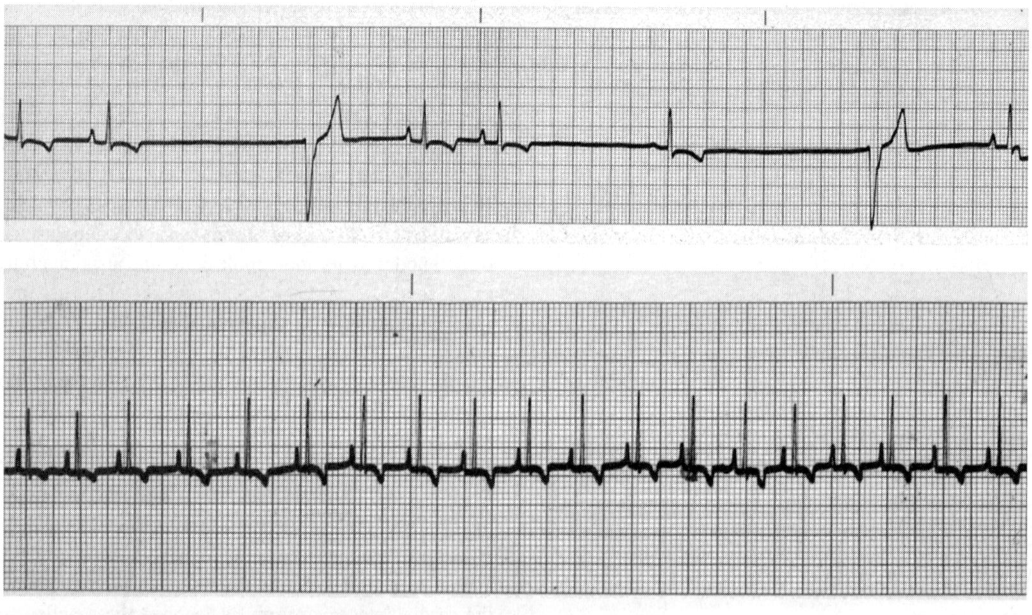

FIGURE 27-13 **A,** Lead II ECG tracing recorded from a 12-year-old Maltese with chronic upper and lower airway disease. The basic rhythm is a pronounced sinus arrhythmia with periods of sinus arrest. The periods of sinus arrest are terminated by escape beats that are depolarizing at a rate of approximately 50 beats/min, suggesting a nodal origin for the escape focus. The QRS complexes, however, are wide, oriented in the opposite direction of normal, and followed by a large T wave. These characteristics suggest that the escape focus is in the Purkinje fibers (ventricular in origin). However, based on the rate, it is more likely that the nodal escape beat is finding the right bundle branch refractory to stimulation. This results in a right bundle branch block that occurs only with the escape beats (so-called phase 4 block). (Paper speed = 50 mm/sec; 1 cm = 1 mV.) **B,** Lead II ECG tracing recorded from the dog shown in **A,** 30 minutes after atropine 0.04 mg/kg SC was administered. The rhythm is now sinus rhythm with a heart rate of 150 beats/min. This documented that the arrhythmia was vagally mediated. (Paper speed = 25 mm/sec; 1 cm = 1 mV.)

had episodes of severe sinus bradycardia with a sinus rate of only 28 beats/min (60 sec/min ÷ 2.15 sec/beat). The arrhythmia partially responded to atropine in that the number of periods of sinus arrest decreased. Because the heart rate did not respond normally into the 140- to 200-beats/min range, a bradycardia caused purely by increased vagal tone was discounted.

The last dog is compared with another that presented for syncope and whose resting ECG is presented in Figure 27-15, *A*. In this dog, sinus rhythm was abruptly terminated for 6.5 seconds. This dog's ECG following atropine administration is presented in Figure 27-15, *B*. The dog no longer had any periods of sinus arrest, and the heart rate had increased to 150 beats/min, suggesting that the cause of the periods of sinus arrest were due to increased vagal tone.

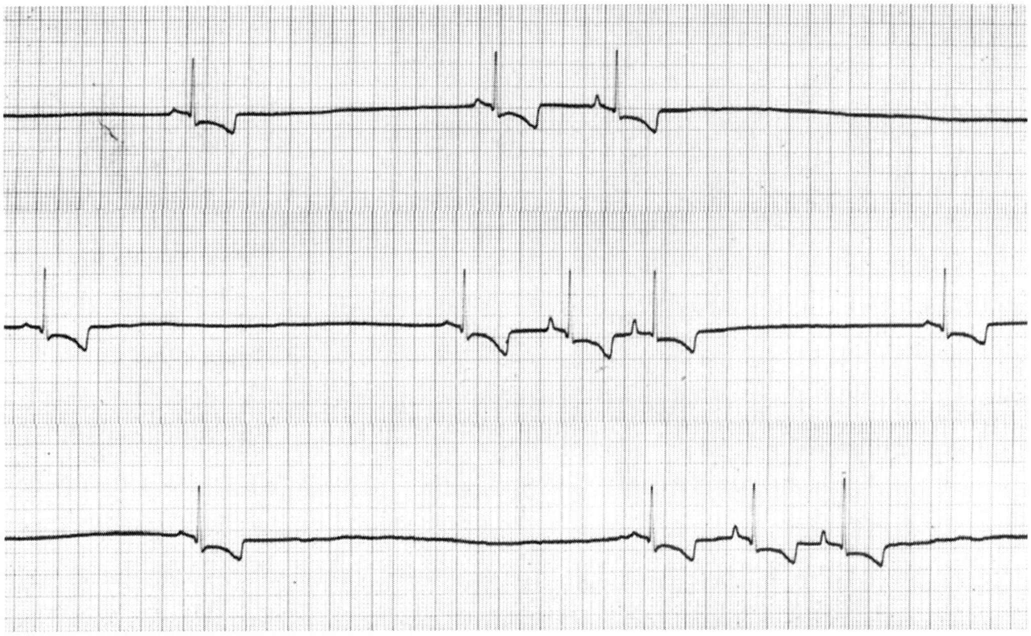

FIGURE 27-14 Lead II ECG tracing recorded from a 10-year-old miniature schnauzer presented for syncope. The rhythm can be considered either a severe sinus bradycardia (heart rate = 30 beats/min at times) or periods of sinus arrest (approximately 2 seconds) without any evidence of an escape rhythm. Atropine administration produced little change. The diagnosis was sick sinus syndrome. Implantation of an artificial pacemaker was successful at relieving the dog's clinical signs. (Paper speed = 50 mm/sec; 1 cm = 1 mV.)

A

B

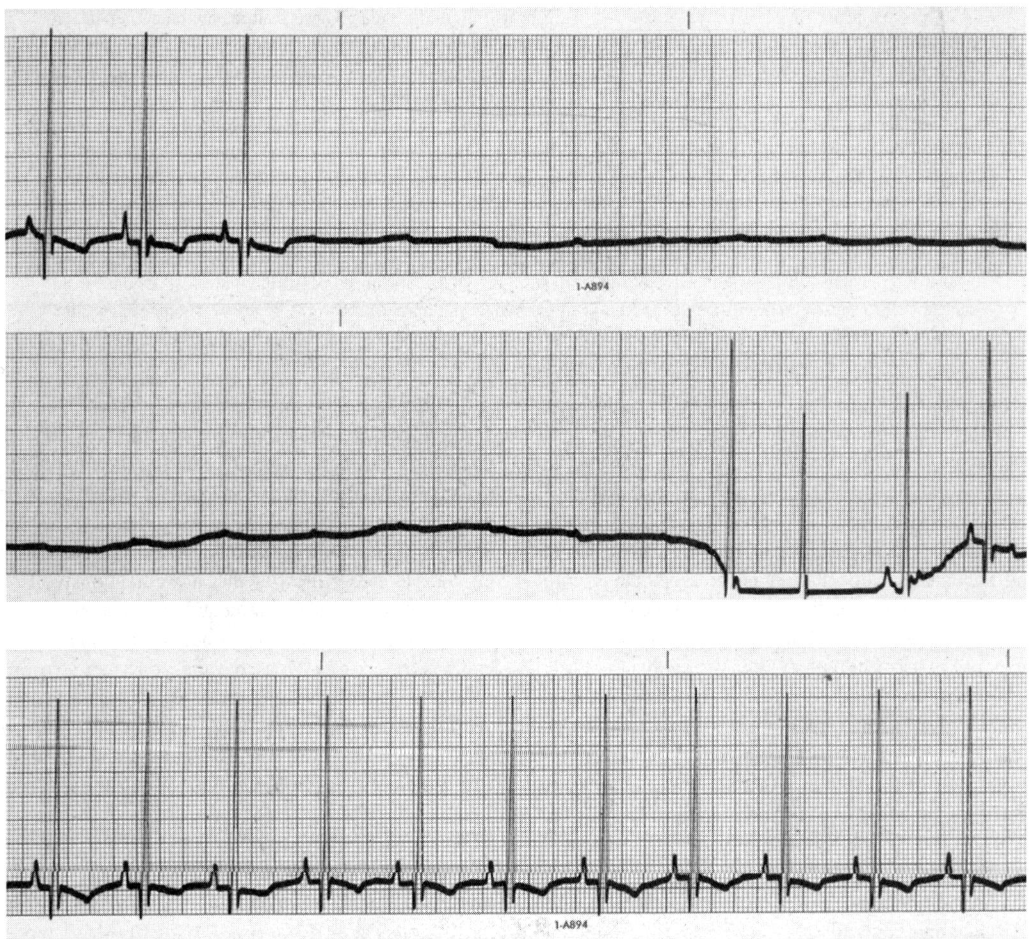

FIGURE 27-15 **A,** Lead II ECG tracing recorded from a 12-year-old American cocker spaniel. The dog was "fainting" 3 times a week. A prolonged period (6.5 seconds) of sinus arrest occurs after the third sinus beat. **B,** Atropine 0.04 mg/kg SC was administered, and another ECG tracing was recorded 30 minutes later. The rhythm was a sinus rhythm, and the heart rate was 150 beats/min.

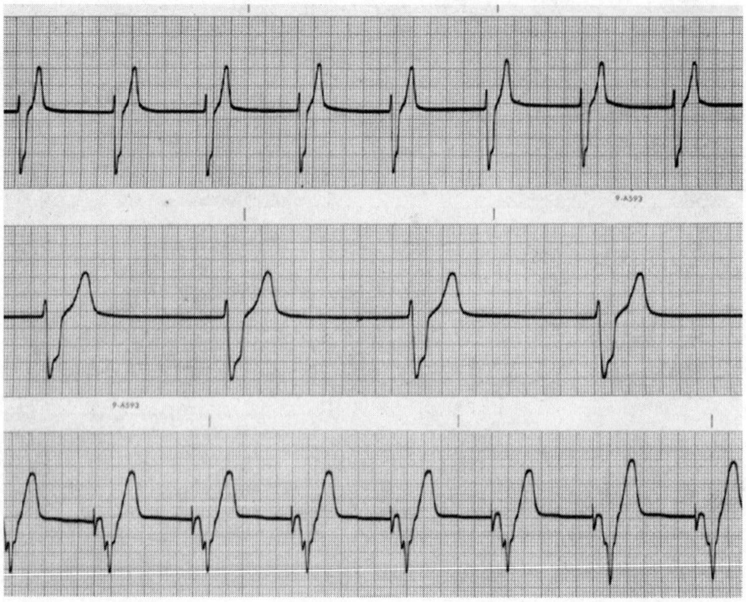

FIGURE 27-16 Lead II ECG tracings from a 2-year-old English springer spaniel that the owner presented because the dog had been lethargic for 1 month and had ascites for the previous 2 weeks. The heart rate was 50 to 60 beats/min on auscultation. There was no jugular vein distension. A soft gallop sound was ausculted, and a grade 2/6 systolic murmur was heard best over the left apex. An echocardiogram revealed moderate mitral regurgitation with a moderately enlarged left ventricle and moderately enlarged left atrium. The end-systolic diameter was increased, indicating myocardial failure. The shortening fraction was 24%. There are no P waves visible in the top and middle tracings. The top tracing is recorded at 25 mm/sec, and the middle trace is recorded at 50 mm/sec paper speed. The ventricular rate is 55 beats/min and regular. These features are characteristic of atrial standstill. (See Color Plate 83.) The QRS complexes are wide and bizarre in appearance. The configuration of the QRS complexes indicates that the escape focus in this dog is either in Purkinje fibers (ventricular escape beats) or in the AV junctional tissue and not conducted in the right bundle branch (nodal escape rhythm with a right bundle branch block). Because the rate is consistent with a nodal escape rhythm, the escape focus is most likely in the atrioventricular junctional tissue. The bottom tracing was recorded at 50 mm/sec after pacemaker implantation. The pacemaker lead was a bipolar lead and was placed in the right ventricular apex. The generator was set at a rate of 100 beats/min. A sharp deflection precedes each QRS complex. This is a so-called pacemaker spike, which occurs when the generator produces its electrical signal. The pacemaker spikes are exactly 0.6 seconds apart, indicating that the set rate (100 beats/min) is being produced. The QRS complexes are wide and bizarre in appearance because the wave of depolarization originates within myocardium and must conduct from muscle cell to muscle cell. Although the lead is implanted in the apex of the right ventricle, the negative QRS complex orientation appears as if the depolarization wave is conducting from left to right. (1 cm = 1 mV.)

Treatment. Dogs with sick sinus syndrome generally require the implantation of an artificial pacemaker to control syncope (see Chapter 30). Occasionally, a dog that is partially responsive to atropine administration can be treated chronically with an anticholinergic or a sympathomimetic agent. However, the disease usually progresses to the point that the arrhythmia becomes unresponsive to drug therapy, and pacemaker implantation is required. Dogs with vagally induced sinus arrest only require therapy if clinical signs of episodic weakness or syncope occur. Anticholinergic or sympathomimetic therapy should be tried initially. Choices of anticholinergic agents that can be administered on a chronic oral basis include atropine, isopropamide, Darbazine (prochlorperazine plus isopropamide), and propantheline. Atropine tablets are no longer manufactured, although some pharmacies still have them in stock. Otherwise, the parenteral form of atropine can be administered per os or subcutaneously at 0.04 mg/kg q6-8h. Parenteral atropine is extremely bitter and must be diluted with a sweet substance, such as corn syrup. Isopropamide and propantheline are weak anticholinergic agents compared with atropine and generally are not as effective. Anticholinergic agents can produce side effects, including mydriasis and constipation. However, in our experience these side effects are usually not present or are tolerable by the patient and the owner. Alternatively, a sympathomimetic agent can be administered. Terbutaline and albuterol syrup are the two choices. Sympathomimetics act indirectly by counteracting the effects of increased vagal tone. Sympathomimetics can produce side effects, including hyperactivity and tachycardia. Dose adjustment may reduce the side effects while still maintaining efficacy (see Chapter 29). Dogs that have intolerable side effects or that are unresponsive to medical therapy can have a pacemaker implanted. The pacemaker will alleviate any clinical signs that occur secondary to sinus arrest. However, in humans, bouts of increased vagal tone can also produce acute and profound systemic vasodilation that can cause syncope. The syncope in this case is not responsive to pacemaker implantation. For this reason we believe that it is prudent to attempt treatment of these dogs with medical therapy before implanting a pacemaker.

ATRIAL STANDSTILL

Definition, causes, and ECG findings. Atrial standstill is the rhythm diagnosis when no *P* waves are visible on the ECG and atrial fibrillation is not evident (Figure 27-16). Atrial standstill occurs when the atrial myocardium is unable to depolarize. This occurs for two broad general reasons: either the atrial muscle is destroyed by disease or the serum potassium concentration is increased to a level that

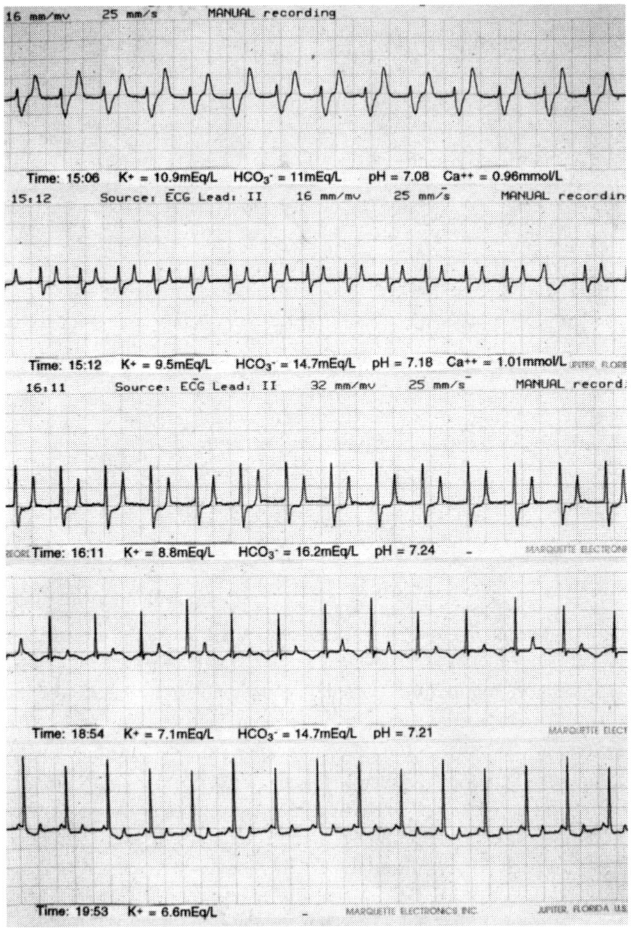

FIGURE 27-17 Sequential ECG tracings from a cat with anuric renal failure, severe hyperkalemia, and metabolic acidosis before (top tracing), during (middle three tracings), and after (bottom tracing) hemodialysis. The top tracing (serum potassium concentration = 10.9 mEq/L) shows a slow heart rate or approximately 100 beats/min, a wide QRS complex, and no *P* waves. As the potassium concentration decreases, the QRS complex duration decreases, the heart rate increases, and the *T* waves become large and "tented." The QRS complexes and *T* waves normalize at a potassium concentration of 7.1 mEq/L, and *P* waves reappear when the potassium concentration reaches 6.6 mEq/L.

results in the resting membrane potential of atrial cells being so low that they no longer depolarize. In the former, a particular type of cardiomyopathy or myocarditis destroys atrial myocardium and replaces it with fibrous tissue. This disease is discussed in Chapter 20. In this disease, the internodal tracts and the sinus node apparently are also destroyed. Consequently, the AV junctional tissue takes over the pacing function of the heart. These dogs present with heart rates usually in the 40- to 60-beats/min range. A pacemaker can be implanted to control signs of episodic weakness or syncope. Pacemaker implantation may also improve signs of heart failure by increasing cardiac output through the increase in heart rate (Figure 27-16). Long-term prognosis for these dogs is usually poor because of progressive AV valve regurgitation and ventricular myocardial dysfunction.

In dogs or cats with moderate-to-severe hyperkalemia, the atrial myocardium loses its ability to depolarize (Figure 27-17). The sinus node and ventricular myocardium retain the ability to depolarize until even higher potassium concentrations are achieved. Moderate-to-severe hyperkalemia results in a sinoventricular rhythm in which the

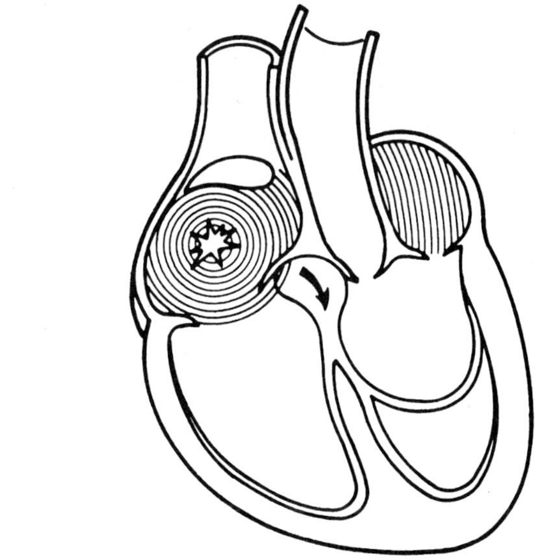

FIGURE 27-18 Schematic drawing of an atrial premature depolarization. An ectopic site in atrial myocardium has depolarized before the sinus node, resulting in depolarization of the atria and subsequently the ventricles earlier than expected (premature). (From Phillips RE, Feeney MK: *Cardiac rhythms: a systematic approach to interpretation,* ed 3, Philadelphia, 1990, WB Saunders.)

sinus node controls the electrical activity of the heart. Sinus node depolarization is carried through the internodal tracts to the AV node and the ventricles. Because the atrial myocardium does not depolarize, no *P* waves are generated on the ECG, and atrial contraction does not occur. Hyperkalemia also causes slowed depolarization of the sinus node and ventricular myocardium, resulting in a sinus bradycardia and prolonged QRS complexes.

SUPRAVENTRICULAR TACHYARRHYTHMIAS

The supraventricular tachyarrhythmias are supraventricular premature depolarizations, supraventricular tachycardia, atrial flutter, and atrial fibrillation. The primary abnormality in all these arrhythmias is the presence of premature (early) depolarizations that originate from an abnormal (ectopic) site somewhere above the ventricles. Supraventricular sites for ectopic depolarization include atrial myocardium and junctional (proximal AV bundle, AV node, bundle of His) tissue. Often, reentrant arrhythmias encompass both. Ectopic premature depolarizations can be single (premature depolarizations) or repetitive (supraventricular tachycardia, atrial flutter, atrial fibrillation). The primary difference between tachycardia, flutter, and fibrillation is the rate at which the ectopic focus depolarizes ("fires"). The rate for supraventricular tachycardia in the dog ranges between approximately 150 beats/min and 350 beats/min. Rates greater than approximately 350 beats/min in the dog can usually be considered atrial flutter, although the rate can go much higher. The atrial rate in atrial fibrillation is generally greater than 500 beats/min, although the rate of this chaotic activity is difficult to count. The other distinguishing characteristic between flutter and fibrillation is the mechanism. Atrial flutter probably originates from one site of reentry. Atrial fibrillation has many reentrant sites responsible for its chaotic atrial rhythm.

Supraventricular premature depolarizations

Definition and causes. Premature depolarizations are also called *premature beats* and *premature complexes,* and these terms are used interchangeably. Premature depolarizations occur when an ectopic site depolarizes at a rate faster than the sinus node (Figure 27-18).

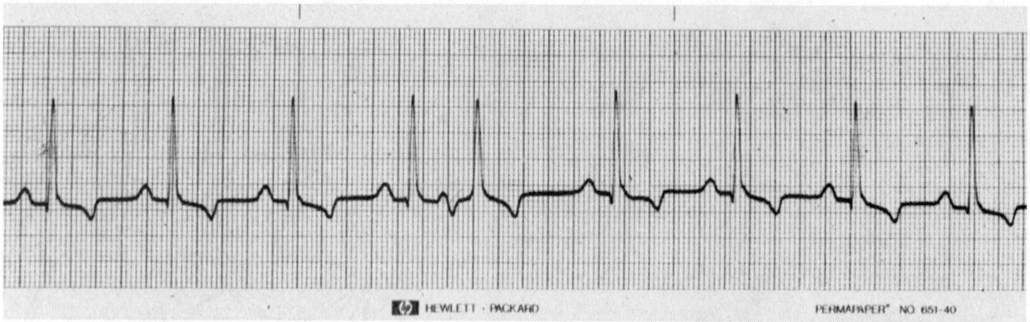

FIGURE 27-19 Lead II ECG tracing recorded from a 14-year-old German shepherd with severe pulmonary thromboembolism. There is no evidence of right atrial or right ventricular enlargement. The basic rhythm is sinus. The fifth QRS complex is premature, and the configuration of this complex is normal. Consequently, this is a supraventricular premature beat. There is an upright (positive) *P* wave in the preceding ST segment and the first part of the preceding *T* wave. The configuration of this *P* wave appears to be different from the normal *P* waves. Although this is generally considered to indicate that the focus is in an atrium, nodal premature beats can also produce a positive *P* wave (see text for details). (Paper speed = 50 mm/sec; 1 cm = 1 mV.)

Supraventricular premature depolarizations (SPDs) are also known as *atrial or nodal (junctional) premature beats, complexes,* or *depolarizations.* They can be due to reentry, abnormal automaticity, or triggered activity. However, reentry is thought to be the most common mechanism. SPDs are rare in normal dogs and cats. They occur most commonly in dogs with chronic mitral regurgitation. In this situation, they probably originate in diseased atrial muscle (most commonly left atrial myocardium). SPDs are usually identified by hearing a premature beat on auscultation or by identifying them on a diagnostic ECG.

ECG findings. On an ECG, SPDs are characterized by a normal-appearing QRS complex that occurs too early (premature) (Figure 27-19). The QRS complex is usually normal because the cardiac electrical impulse is able to take advantage of the normal specialized conduction system and depolarize the ventricles in a normal fashion. The QRS complex may or may not have a *P* wave preceding it, and the *P* wave may be normally oriented (upright in leads I, II, III, and aV_F) or be opposite in polarity to normal (negative in leads I, II, III, and aV_F). There are no absolute criteria to distinguish an atrial ectopic site from a nodal (junctional) ectopic site. Consequently, it is preferred to call premature depolarizations of this type supraventricular rather than atrial or nodal. There are three reasons why a *P* wave may not occur with an SPD. First, if the SPD originates from atrial myocardium, the premature depolarization may occur so early that it is buried either in the previous QRS complex or T wave. Second, if it originates from the AV junctional region, retrograde depolarization to the atria may not occur. Third, if it originates from the AV junction, the electrical impulse may reach the atria and the ventricles simultaneously. Because the QRS complex is larger, the P wave will be buried in the QRS complex and so not be seen in this situation. Consequently, the lack of a *P* wave does not distinguish between an atrial and a nodal (or junctional) premature depolarization. Occasionally a normally oriented *P* wave may be present in front of the premature QRS complex. Usually this *P* wave is configured differently than the normal *P* wave. This finding is generally thought to be diagnostic of an atrial premature depolarization. However, it has been shown that when the right ventricle is paced in the dog heart, depolarization can pass retrograde through the AV junction, up the interatrial septum (presumably in the cranial internodal tract) to the region of Bachmann's bundle, and then spread across the atria normally, producing positive *P* waves.[16] Presumably, depolarizations originating from the AV junction can do this also. At other times, a negative *P* wave (in leads I, II, III, and aV_F) may occur before the premature QRS complex. In this situation, the atrial wave of depolarization must conduct either from caudal to cranial or from left to right. The two potential ectopic sites from which such a wave can originate are the AV junction and the left atrium.[16] Consequently, identifying a negative *P* wave does not distinguish between an atrial premature depolarization and a nodal premature depolarization. At times, a *P* wave may follow the QRS complex in an SPD. We have observed both negative and positive *P* waves in this situation. Most likely, *P* waves that follow the QRS complex in association with SPDs originate in the AV junction and conduct retrograde to the atria. In this situation, conduction time through the AV junction is longer in the pathway that reaches the atria than in the pathway to the ventricles.

Compensatory and noncompensatory pauses on the ECG. The time following an SPD before a sinus depolarization occurs is variable and depends on several factors. The premature depolarization may occur at a time that the sinus node has fully repolarized and so is not refractory. Here, the depolarization wave initiated by the premature depolarization can conduct into the sinus node and depolarize it. The sinus node will then go through an entire new cycle and depolarize at its normal time following the premature complex. On the ECG, the interval between the last sinus beat (normal P-QRS-T complex) and the premature complex will be less than normal (premature), and the interval between the premature complex and the next sinus beat will be normal. This is most common and is termed a *noncompensatory pause.* Less commonly, the sinus node or the pathways to it are refractory so that the premature depolarization does not depolarize it. In this situation the sinus node depolarizes at its original rate. If the atrial muscle is still refractory when the sinus node depolarizes, no P-QRS-T complex will be generated. The sinus node depolarization following the nonconducted depolarization will generate normal cardiac activation. The distance between the premature complex and the next sinus complex will then be greater than a normal cycle length. This is termed *a fully compensatory pause.* If the sinus depolarization following the premature depolarization can conduct through the atria and ventricles, the premature complex will be interpolated between two normal sinus beats.

Supraventricular premature depolarizations and bundle branch blocks. At times, an SPD can produce a wide and bizarre QRS

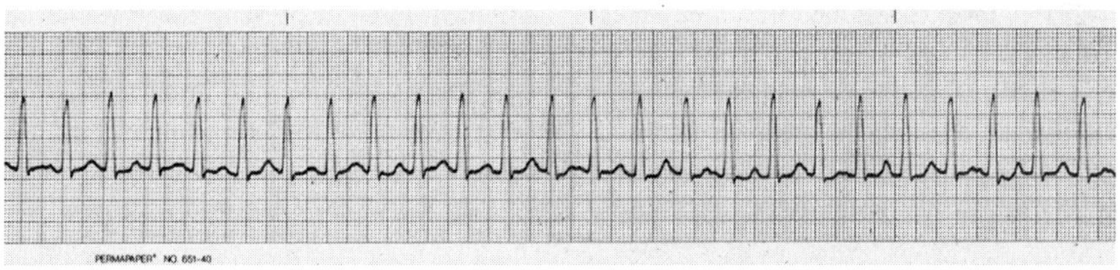

FIGURE 27-20 Lead II ECG tracing recorded from a 14-year-old Labrador retriever during recovery from anesthesia. The dog had no other indication of cardiac disease. The heart rate is 270 beats/min, indicating the presence of a tachycardia. The rhythm is extremely regular, and the QRS complexes are not wide (narrow) and appear normal. These are all characteristics of a supraventricular tachycardia. (Paper speed = 50 mm/sec; 1 cm = 1 mV.)

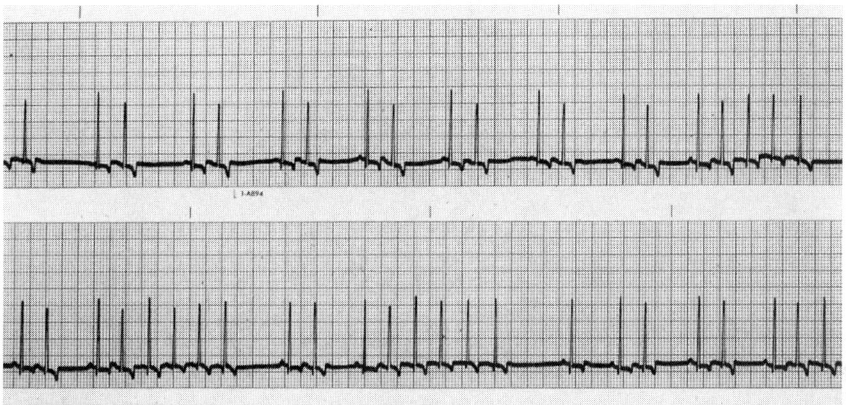

FIGURE 27-21 Lead II ECG tracing recorded from a 6-year-old German shorthaired pointer that the owner presented for an ovariohysterectomy. An arrhythmia was ausculted. The dog tested positive for heartworms. Thoracic radiographs and cardiac ultrasound were normal. The initial part of the first tracing shows a sinus rhythm with every other depolarization being premature (bigeminy). The premature beats have a normal configuration (albeit slightly shorter than normal) and appear to have P waves in front of them. Consequently, the diagnosis is supraventricular bigeminy. At the end of the first tracing, four supraventricular premature beats occur in a row. In the second tracing this recurs, but with five premature beats in a row occurring twice. These are short runs of supraventricular tachycardia. This 40-kg dog was treated with diltiazem per os. The dog initially was administered 30 mg q8h, with no response. The dose was titrated upward over the next 2 days, first to 60 mg q8h, then to 90 mg q8h, and, finally, to 120 mg (3 mg/kg) q8h. The arrhythmia was abolished at the last dose. (Paper speed = 25 mm/sec; 1 cm = 1 mV.)

complex. This occurs when the premature depolarization reaches the bundle branches before one of them has time to repolarize or when one of them is partially depolarized, resulting in a functional bundle branch block. If this occurs each time and no *P* wave is present, distinguishing an SPD from a ventricular premature depolarization can be difficult to impossible. Generally the right bundle branch has a longer refractory period than the left bundle branch. Consequently, a right bundle branch block pattern is more common in this scenario. Fortunately, this situation appears to be uncommon.

Treatment. In humans, SPDs cause palpitations. SPDs do not cause clinical signs in dogs or cats. Consequently, no treatment is required for SPDs unless they precipitate runs of supraventricular tachycardia. SPDs may be a harbinger of atrial fibrillation, although this has not been proved. Also, no proof exists that treating or abolishing SPDs delays the onset of atrial fibrillation. SPDs can usually be suppressed with digoxin, β-blockers, or calcium channel blockers (see Chapter 29).

Supraventricular tachycardia

Definition and causes. Supraventricular tachycardia (SVT) is repetitive SPDs. As with SPDs, SVT can originate from atrial myocardium or AV junctional tissue. They most commonly occur in humans because of reentry, although automatic SVT can occur. Reentrant SVT produces a constant heart rate (the interval between QRS complexes is regular). SVT originating from an automatic focus in atrial myocardium can be irregular. Few electrophysiologic studies have been performed in dogs, but response to therapy (most SVTs respond to calcium channel blocker administration) suggests that reentry is also the most common mechanism underlying SVT in the dog. In most humans, the reentrant pathway is within the AV node or uses the AV junctional tissue as part of the reentrant circuit. Again, this has not been studied in dogs. However, most cases of SVT seen in dogs present with a regular rhythm, and most are responsive to drugs that specifically alter conduction and refractoriness in the AV junctional tissue. Consequently, most cases of SVT in dogs are likely also the result of AV junctional reentry. One case report in the veterinary literature has described an electrophysiologic study in a dog with tricuspid valve dysplasia and an incessant atrial tachycardia that was due to reentry in the right atrium.[17]

ECG findings. Most SVT in veterinary medicine occurs in dogs. The rate of the ectopic focus varies widely in dogs. We have seen rates as low as 150 beats/min and as high as 350 beats/min. On an ECG, most SVTs are regular (the R-R interval is constant) and many occur for prolonged periods (Figure 27-20). Some dogs, however, can have very short runs of SVT (Figure 27-21). Rarely, the rhythm will be irregular (Figure 27-22). In most cases, the QRS complexes are typical of supraventricular complexes, narrow and upright in lead II. In some cases there is a coexisting bundle branch block that makes it difficult to impossible to differentiate an SVT from a ventricular tachycardia by examining the ECG (Figure 27-23). As with SPDs, there may or may not be *P* waves accompanying the QRS complexes and, if present, the *P* waves can be positive or negative in lead II (Figure 27-24).

Clinical features. SVTs commonly occur secondary to organic heart disease or serious systemic disease. Dogs with slow SVT exhibit no clinical signs. Dogs with sustained fast SVT (heart rate greater than 300 beats/min) generally present for weakness or

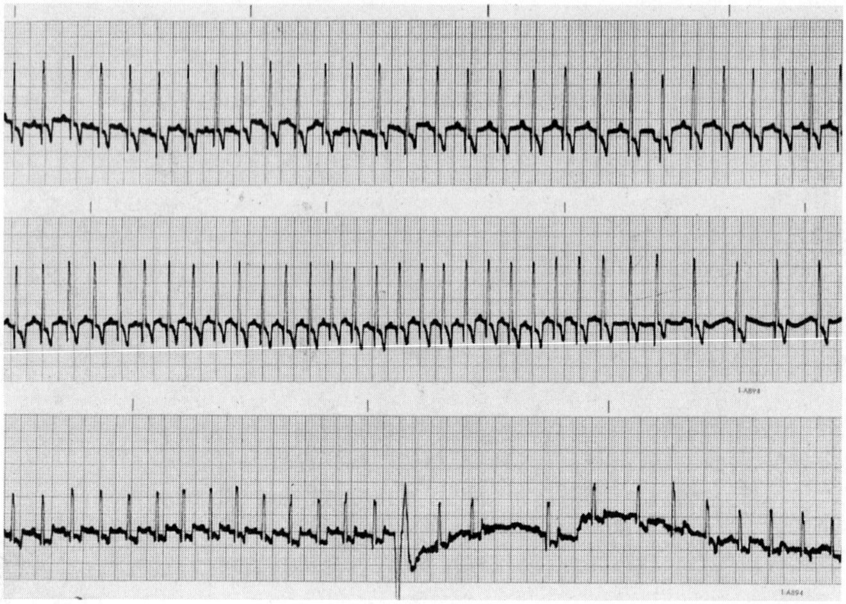

FIGURE 27-22 Lead II ECG tracing recorded from a 6-year-old great Dane with dilated cardiomyopathy (end-systolic diameter = 63 mm; shortening fraction = 14%). The dog was not in heart failure at presentation. The dog's heart rate was 180 beats/min. The ECG tracing revealed a supraventricular rhythm (normal QRS complex configuration and width). There was a *P* for every QRS complex and a QRS complex for every *P* wave. The rate was too fast (heart rate = 170 to 210 beats/min) for this size dog, even in an examination room. The rate gradually increased and decreased over time. The differential diagnoses were sinus tachycardia and supraventricular tachycardia. At the end of the second tracing, the heart rate decreased and then suddenly decreased further into what appeared to be a sinus rhythm with a heart rate of 110 beats/min. This occurred with no change in the dog's attitude and was not in response to any stimulus. This suggested that the preceding rhythm was a supraventricular tachycardia. To prove or disprove this, a precordial thump was delivered while recording the dog's ECG. This occurred in the middle of the third tracing and produced a ventricular premature beat. Immediately after this, the heart rate slowed dramatically for 5 to 6 beats and then returned to the original rate. This proved that the rhythm was not sinus in origin. Consequently, it had to be originating from an ectopic site and via an abnormal mechanism; that is, it was a supraventricular tachycardia. (Paper speed = 25 mm/sec; 1 cm = 1 mV.)

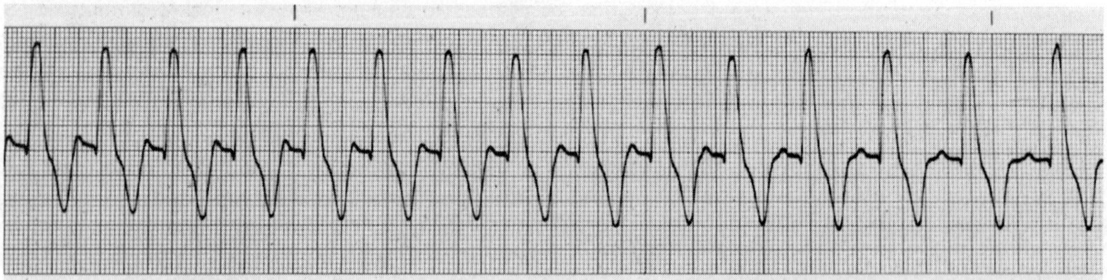

FIGURE 27-23 Lead II ECG tracing recorded from a 13-year-old German shepherd with a splenic hemangiosarcoma. No evidence of cardiac neoplasia was present. The dog's heart rate at admission was 200 beats/min. Consequently, an ECG was recorded, which revealed a wide-QRS-complex tachycardia. Differential diagnoses were ventricular tachycardia, supraventricular tachycardia with a left bundle branch block, and sinus tachycardia with a left bundle branch block. Careful examination of the ECG revealed *P* waves at the end of each *T* wave that had a consistent relationship with the QRS complexes. This ruled out ventricular tachycardia. A precordial blow produced a slower sinus rhythm for two beats (not presented). This confirmed that the rhythm was a supraventricular tachycardia. (Paper speed = 50 mm/sec; 1 cm = 1 mV.)

collapse. On physical examination they have evidence of poor peripheral perfusion with pale mucous membranes, a prolonged capillary refill time, and weak pulses. This occurs because of inadequate diastolic filling. When viewed on an echocardiogram during bursts of SVT, the left ventricle has a normal end-systolic diameter and a very small end-diastolic diameter, resulting in a decreased shortening fraction because of inadequate filling.

Treatment. SVT is a medical emergency in dogs that present for weakness and collapse. Numerous physical maneuvers and drugs can be used to terminate an SVT (see Chapter 29). Some maneuvers and drugs, however, are much more effective than others. In our experience, vagal maneuvers (ocular pressure, carotid sinus massage) are often unsuccessful. Delivering a precordial thump, on the other hand, is very successful (greater than 90% of the time) at terminating an SVT in dogs (Figure 27-25). However, this maneuver may only break the rhythm for a beat or two. At other times the rhythm will stay converted. To perform a precordial thump, the dog should be placed on its right side and the left apex beat located. This region should then be thumped with a fist while recording the ECG. The strength of the blow required to terminate an SVT depends on the size

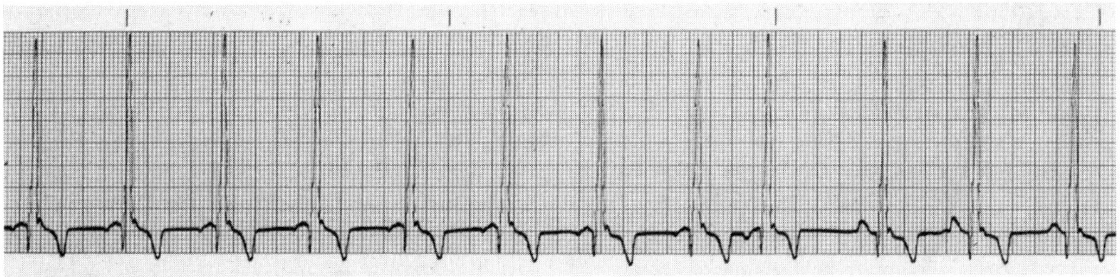

FIGURE 27-24 Lead II ECG tracing recorded from a 10-year-old Afghan hound with severe primary mitral regurgitation. At presentation the dog's heart failure was well controlled and the heart rate was 150 beats/min. The ECG was recorded to determine the source of the tachycardia. It revealed a supraventricular rhythm (normal QRS complex orientation and width), with negative P waves preceding each QRS complex. This confirmed that the site of origin for these complexes had to be ectopic, either in the atrioventricular junctional tissue or in the left atrium. This dog had a tremendously enlarged left atrium. Consequently, it was presumed that the ectopic site was in the left atrial myocardium. The diagnosis was supraventricular tachycardia. At the end of the tracing, it appears that another site in the left atrium depolarizes even more prematurely (focus depolarizing rate = 200 beats/min) than the other site. This premature depolarization appears to stop the original site from depolarizing long enough that another focus predominates. This focus depolarizes at a rate almost identical to the original focus, but the *P* waves formed from the depolarizations from this site are positive. It could not be determined whether these originated from the sinus node or another ectopic supraventricular site. It was felt that this dog was prone to developing atrial fibrillation based on his atrial size and his multiple ectopic sites. He was discharged on digoxin and returned 2 months later in atrial fibrillation. The QRS complexes appear abnormal because of a stylus malfunction. (Paper speed = 50 mm/sec; 1 cm = 1 mV.)

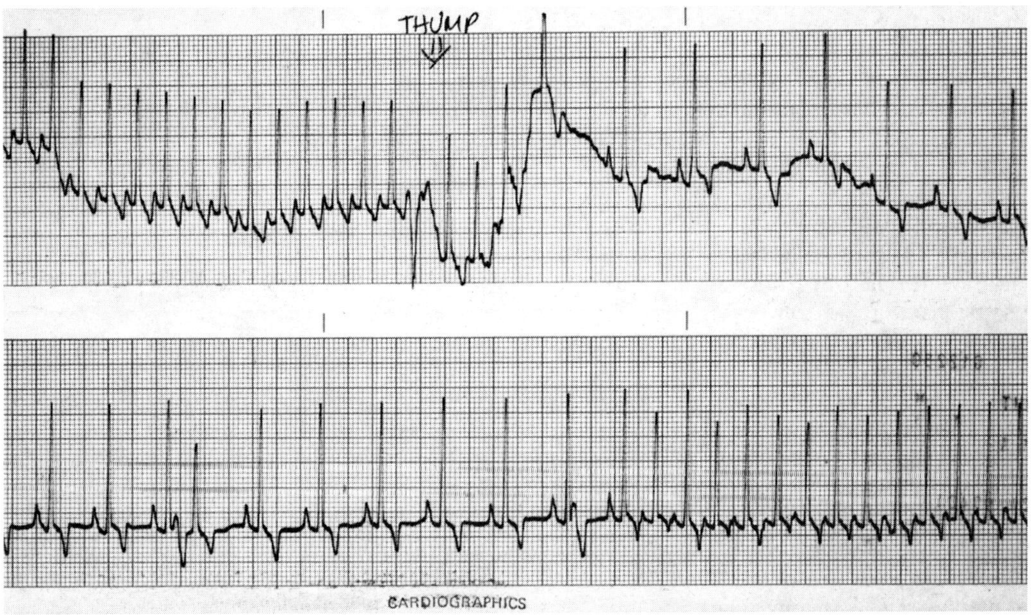

FIGURE 27-25 Lead II ECG tracing recorded from a dog with supraventricular tachycardia (SVT). The initial heart rate is 250 beats/min. In the center of the first tracing a precordial thump was delivered to the left apex. This produced a ventricular premature beat followed by sinus rhythm until the second half of the second tracing, when the SVT abruptly returned. (Paper speed = 25 mm/sec; 1 cm = 1 mV.)

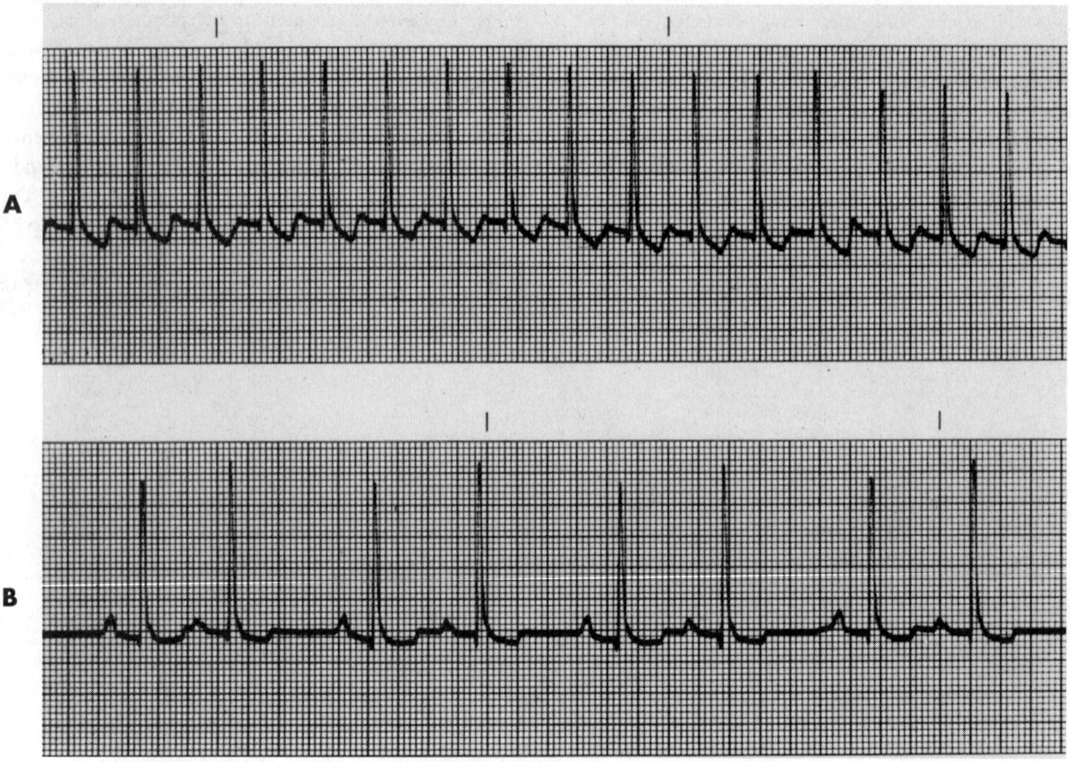

FIGURE 27-26 Lead II ECG tracing recorded from a dog that presented for weakness and collapse. **A,** The heart rate is 285 beats/min and very regular (0.21 seconds between each QRS complex). The QRS complex duration is normal. *P* waves are not visualized and are probably "buried" in preceding QRS complexes or *T* waves. The diagnosis is supraventricular tachycardia. **B,** Two minutes after the administration of a second dose of verapamil 0.05 mg/kg IV (a total dose of 0.1 mg/kg) the rhythm is a sinus rhythm with supraventricular bigeminy. The supraventricular premature depolarizations stopped 1 minute later, leaving sinus rhythm with a heart rate of 140 beats/min. (Paper speed = 50 mm/sec; 1 cm = 1 mV.)

of the patient. A forceful blow is required in large dogs. The strength of the initial blow should be similar to striking one's left palm with one's right fist hard enough to produce a sound that is comparable in intensity to a normal speaking voice. If the initial thump is unsuccessful, a firmer thump should be applied. Smaller dogs and cats require softer blows. A precordial thump delivers about a 5-J "shock" to the myocardium. At times it produces a premature ventricular depolarization. The depolarization that occurs effectively breaks up the reentrant circuit in SVT, breaking the arrhythmia. A precordial thump may also be used as a diagnostic test to differentiate sinus tachycardia from SVT when the heart rate is in the 150- to 250-beats/min range (see Figure 27-22). A precordial thump will usually stop the SVT for at least one or two beats; whereas a sinus tachycardia will not be affected (or it may get worse if the thump is forceful enough to cause pain).

Calcium channel blockers are also very effective at terminating an SVT. In a study that we reported, 12 out of 14 dogs with SVT responded to the acute administration of verapamil.[18] Verapamil is administered as 0.05-mg/kg boluses administered over 3 to 5 minutes up to 3 times (0.15 mg/kg total dose) over a total of 15 to 30 minutes while monitoring the ECG (Figure 27-26). Acute administration of verapamil can produce cardiovascular collapse if it is administered too rapidly, if an overdosage is administered, or if the patient has underlying moderate-to-severe myocardial failure. The cardiovascular depressant effects of verapamil can be countered by administering calcium intravenously or infusing a catecholamine. Diltiazem can be administered at a dose of 0.05 to 0.25 mg/kg IV over 5 to 15 minutes and appears to be as effective as verapamil in dogs.

Other drugs can also be administered to "break" an SVT. Intravenous administration of a β-adrenergic blocking drug, such as propranolol (0.02 mg/kg slow IV boluses up to a total dose of 0.1 mg/kg) or esmolol (0.25 to 0.5 mg/kg slow IV bolus administration) may be effective. The effect of esmolol is short-lived. The drug may be administered as a constant-rate infusion (50 to 200 (μg/kg/min) following the initial bolus. Moderate-to-severe myocardial failure is a relative contraindication to the administration of a β-blocker at these doses. Many pharmacologic interventions used in the past have been supplanted by calcium channel blockers and β-blockers. Older interventional therapy includes the administration of phenylephrine, methoxamine, edrophonium, and neostigmine.

Chronic therapy of SVT includes the administration of digoxin, a β-adrenergic blocker, and/or a calcium channel blocker. All three of these drugs or drug classes prolong conduction time and prolong the refractory period in the AV junctional tissue. For chronic control of SVT, digoxin can be administered at a maintenance dose or the maintenance dose can be doubled for the first day to produce a therapeutic serum concentration more rapidly. Propranolol or atenolol can be administered at doses ranging between 0.5 mg/kg and 2.0 mg/kg, as long as the patient does not have moderate-to-severe underlying myocardial failure. Diltiazem is the calcium channel blocker of choice for chronic control of SVT. A dosage required for this drug to control SVT has not been reported in the dog. Diltiazem is more frequently used to control the ventricular rate in patients with atrial fibrillation at a dosage of 0.5 to 1.5 mg/kg q8h. In our clinic, we generally start in this dosage range but almost

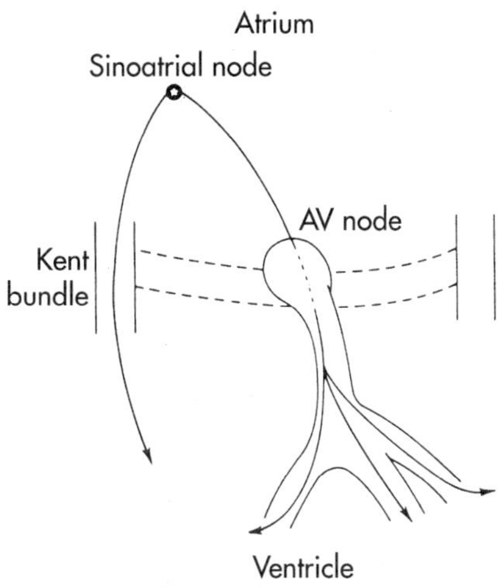

FIGURE 27-27 Drawing of an accessory pathway (Kent bundle) that bypasses the atrioventricular (AV) node. This pathway conducts the atrial depolarization more rapidly than does the AV node, resulting in a portion of the ventricular myocardium being "preexcited." This pathway can conduct anterograde and retrograde. It commonly sets up a reentrant circuit to produce premature depolarizations. (From Tilley LP: *Essentials of canine and feline electrocardiography,* ed 3, Philadelphia, 1992, Lea & Febiger.)

always find it necessary to increase the dose into the 2.0- to 3.0-mg/kg q8h dosage range to affect control (see Figure 22-21). Lastly, class I antiarrhythmic agents such as quinidine and procainamide can be tried in situations in which the aforementioned drugs are ineffective or when the SVT is thought to be due to an automatic, rather than a reentrant, rhythm. SVT caused by an automatic atrial focus may produce an irregular rhythm (as opposed to the regular rhythm observed in most cases of SVT) and may be refractory to conventional drug therapy.

Preexcitation syndrome (accessory pathways)

Definition and causes. Normally the atria and ventricles are electrically isolated from each other by the fibrous base of the heart. The only structures that normally traverse this fibrous tissue are the AV node and bundle of His. Rarely, a congenital abnormality exists in which a strip of aberrant myocardium bridges the fibrous base, allowing the cardiac electrical impulse to pass over this accessory atrioventricular pathway from an atrium to a ventricle or the bundle of His. Most commonly the bypass tract passes from atrial to ventricular myocardium and is called a *Kent bundle* (Figure 27-27). Preexcitation syndrome has been reported in dogs and cats.[19] Interestingly, six of the nine cats in one report had hypertrophic cardiomyopathy.

ECG findings. In ventricular preexcitation, if the bypass tract conducts anterograde, it conducts more rapidly than does AV junctional tissue. Consequently, the electrical impulse that traverses this bypass tract reaches a ventricle before the cardiac electrical impulse that traverses the AV junction reaches the ventricles. This is termed *ventricular preexcitation.* Ventricular preexcitation may result in a shorter-than-normal P-R interval and an abnormally shaped QRS complex. The QRS complex may have a slurred upstroke, termed a *delta wave.* The delta wave is produced by the portion of the ventricle that is activated early. The remainder of the QRS complex is a hybrid complex, because the ventricles are depolarized by the depolarization wave that originates normally from the conduction system and by the depolarization wave that originates from the bypass tract. The short P-R interval and the delta wave produce no clinical sequelae. The bypass tract can conduct both anterograde (from an atrium to a ventricle) and retrograde (from a ventricle to an atrium) or can conduct only retrograde or only anterograde. Patients with only retrograde conduction have a normal-appearing ECG during sinus rhythm.

Supraventricular tachycardia caused by preexcitation. The most serious problem associated with ventricular preexcitation is reentrant tachycardia. Both atrial and ventricular premature beats can initiate a tachycardia. An atrial premature beat can be premature enough that the cardiac impulse finds the accessory pathway refractory to conduction so that conduction only proceeds through the normal conduction system. During ventricular depolarization, the bypass tract has not been depolarized and is able to conduct the electrical impulse back to the atria and then back through the AV node to the ventricles again. This reentrant cycle then continues or terminates. In another scenario, a ventricular premature beat can find the AV junctional region refractory to conduction but conduct retrograde through the bypass tract to the atria. The electrical impulse can then conduct to the ventricles through the AV junctional tissue and then reenter the accessory pathway.

An example of ventricular preexcitation is presented in Figure 27-28. This animal had bouts of tachycardia. On the ECG there are two different P-QRS-T configurations. In one, the P-R interval is very short (0.04 seconds) and the initial portion of the QRS complex is slurred (the delta wave). In the other, the P-R interval is normal (0.09 seconds) and the QRS complex does not have a delta wave. Immediately following each of these latter QRS complexes, however, is a negative *P* wave that lies within the ST segment. In this animal, atrial activation at times resulted in conduction of the electrical impulse from the atria to the ventricles through both the AV junction and the bypass tract. This produced the short P-R interval and the delta wave. At other times, the bypass tract did not conduct anterograde, so the electrical impulse could only reach the ventricles through the AV junction. This resulted in a normal P-R interval and disappearance of the delta wave. In this situation, however, the bypass tract could conduct retrograde. Consequently, following ventricular activation, the electrical impulse conducted back through the bypass tract and stimulated the atria again, producing the negative *P* wave. Sometimes, the cycle ended here because the AV junction was refractory to being depolarized again so early in the cardiac cycle. However, at other times the AV junction could conduct, setting up a reentrant pathway and creating a tachycardia (third tracing).

In the previous example, the pattern is easy to recognize; in other cases it may not be as easily recognizable. A Labrador retriever has been reported in the literature that had prolonged periods of sustained SVT at a rate of 240 to 340 beats/min that developed heart failure during the tachycardic episodes.[20] This dog did not have a short P-R interval nor did it have a delta wave on its ECG. Sophisticated intracardiac electrophysiologic testing was required to diagnose the dog's problems. It was discerned that the dog had a bypass tract that only conducted in a retrograde direction. Thus the circuit was in place for setting up a reentrant tachycardia, but the bypass tract was concealed.

Treatment. There are multiple methods of terminating the tachycardia that occurs secondary to preexcitation (see Chapter 29). Theoretically, administering a drug that prolongs the conduction time or refractory period of the AV junction can alter the reentrant circuit and so terminate the arrhythmia. Also, administering a drug that alters the conduction and refractory properties of the myocardium in the bypass tract can do the same thing. There are very few reports of treating preexcitation-induced tachycardia in dogs or cats.[19] In one, a precordial thump was effective at terminating the arrhythmia for a short time.[20] Intravenous diltiazem administration repeatedly termi-

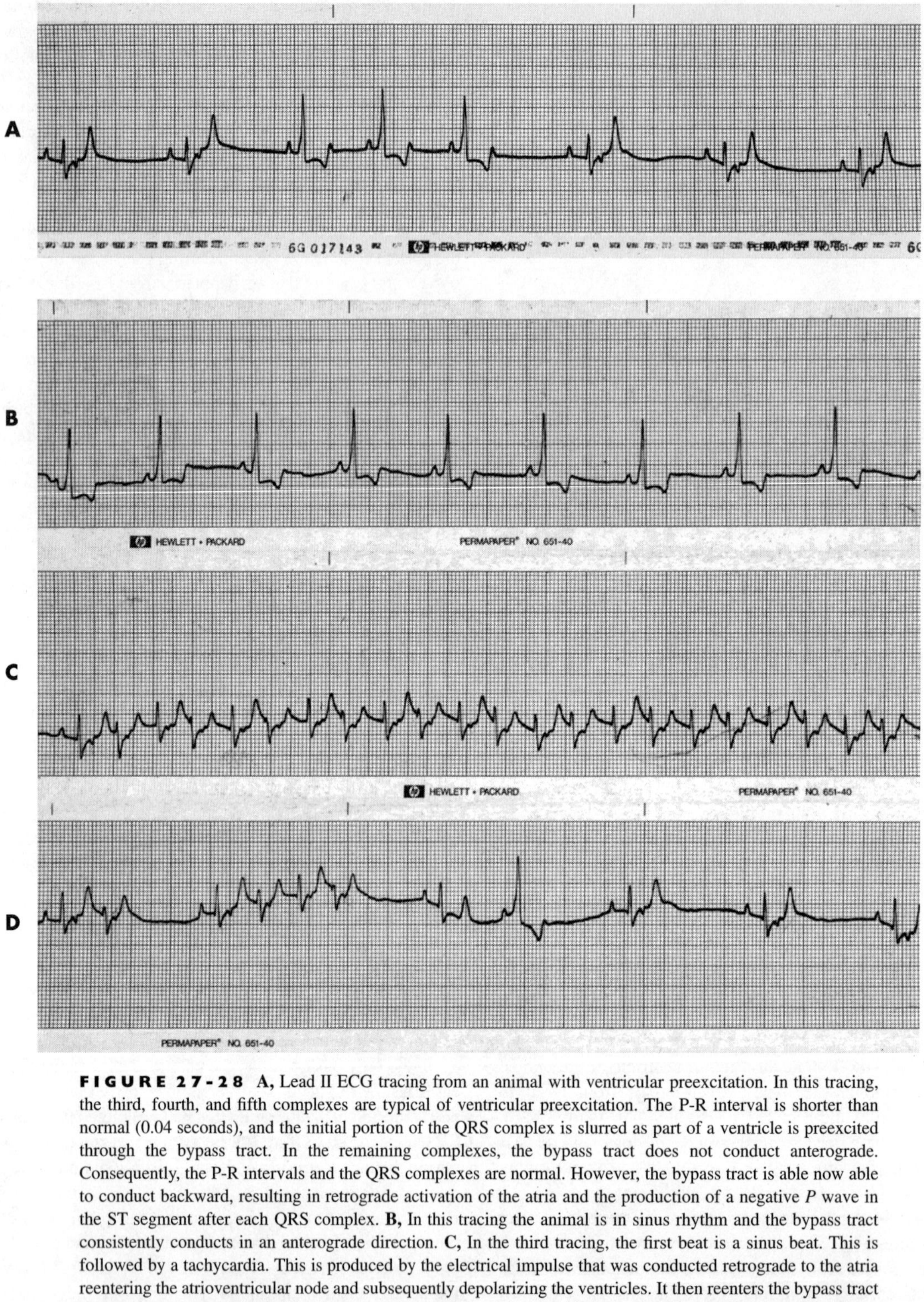

FIGURE 27-28 **A,** Lead II ECG tracing from an animal with ventricular preexcitation. In this tracing, the third, fourth, and fifth complexes are typical of ventricular preexcitation. The P-R interval is shorter than normal (0.04 seconds), and the initial portion of the QRS complex is slurred as part of a ventricle is preexcited through the bypass tract. In the remaining complexes, the bypass tract does not conduct anterograde. Consequently, the P-R intervals and the QRS complexes are normal. However, the bypass tract is able now able to conduct backward, resulting in retrograde activation of the atria and the production of a negative *P* wave in the ST segment after each QRS complex. **B,** In this tracing the animal is in sinus rhythm and the bypass tract consistently conducts in an anterograde direction. **C,** In the third tracing, the first beat is a sinus beat. This is followed by a tachycardia. This is produced by the electrical impulse that was conducted retrograde to the atria reentering the atrioventricular node and subsequently depolarizing the ventricles. It then reenters the bypass tract to start the process again. **D,** The bottom tracing shows an echo beat (the second QRS complex) in which reentry occurred once and then stopped. This is followed by a short run of reentrant supraventricular tachycardia. The seventh complex is an example of the depolarization wave not reentering the bypass tract, such that no negative *P* wave follows the QRS complex. The remaining complexes are as above. (Paper speed = 50 mm/sec; 1 cm = 1 mV.)

nated the arrhythmia in this dog, and intravenous and oral procainamide administration abolished the arrhythmia short-term and long-term, respectively. In human medicine, class Ia, Ic, and III antiarrhythmic drugs are most effective at controlling tachycardia.[21] Digoxin may also be effective in controlling the tachycardia associated with preexcitation but it is not the drug of choice. However, digoxin has been reported to be effective in four dogs or cats with preexcitation.[19] Quinidine has also been effective in one case and propranolol in two cases.[19] We have treated one case successfully with procainamide.

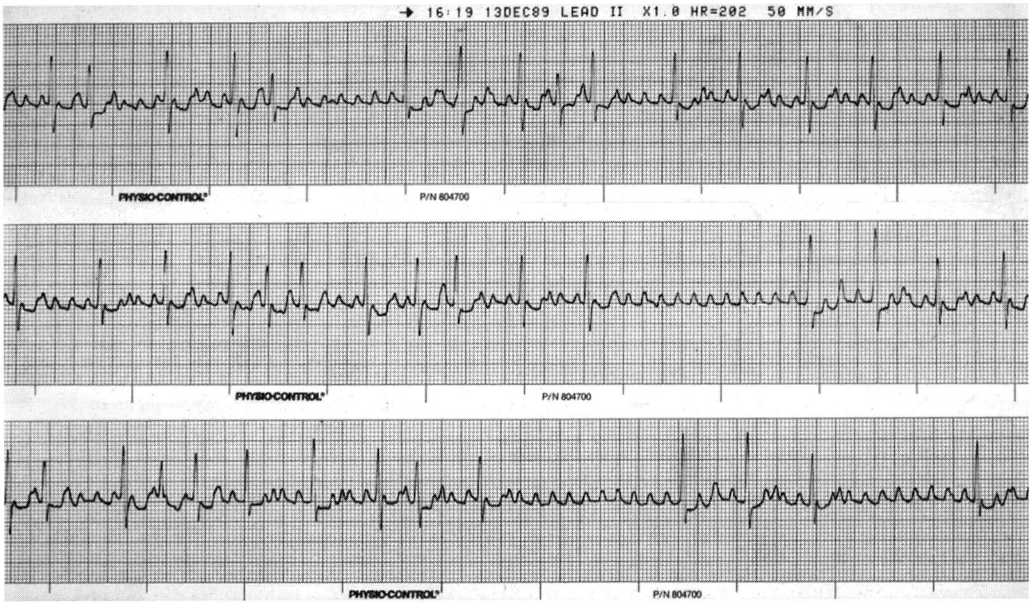

FIGURE 27-29 Lead II ECG tracing recorded from a 14-year-old miniature schnauzer that presented as an emergency patient with fulminant pulmonary edema. The dog had a loud left apical systolic heart murmur. A ruptured chorda tendineae was suspected but not proved. The heart rate was very irregular. The ECG revealed an irregular supraventricular rhythm with a very fast atrial rate. In this tracing, the distance between *P* waves is approximately 4 mm. The paper speed is 50 mm/sec, so the interval between *P* waves is 0.08 seconds. This translates into an atrial rate of 750 beats/min. The atrioventricular (AV) junctional tissue acts as a filter and only allows some of these depolarizations through to the ventricles. Because of the tremendous atrial rate, the AV junctional tissue conducts the atrial depolarizations to the ventricles irregularly (see text for details). Consequently, the ventricular rhythm is very irregular. Although the atrial rate is the same as that seen with atrial fibrillation, the fact that distinct *P* waves can be seen makes the diagnosis atrial flutter. (Paper speed = 50 mm/sec; 1 cm = 1 mV.)

Atrial flutter

Definition and ECG findings. Atrial flutter is a rare arrhythmia in the dog. We have not documented this rhythm abnormality in a cat. It has been stated that atrial flutter has never been adequately defined in human medicine.[22] The same can be said for veterinary medicine. Essentially, atrial flutter is a very fast SVT. When an SVT attains a certain rate, the refractory period of the AV node is longer than the cycle length (P-P interval) of the SVT. This results in some atrial depolarizations being blocked from traversing the AV node (functional second-degree AV block). Generally at this time the arrhythmia is termed *atrial flutter* rather than *SVT.* In humans this occurs at rates between 240 and 320 beats/min, but rates of 430 beats/min can be achieved.[22] In dogs, the rate at which functional AV block occurs is probably between 350 and 400 beats/min, although most atrial flutters have atrial rates that exceed this number. In atrial flutter, *P* waves can usually be discerned either as discrete P waves or as a "saw-toothed" baseline (Figure 27-29). The conduction pattern to the ventricles in atrial flutter is variable. In some cases every other atrial depolarization produces a ventricular depolarization (2:1 conduction ratio), producing a regular ventricular rhythm, whereas at other times the conduction pattern appears random, resulting in a very irregular ventricular rhythm that can mimic atrial fibrillation.

Treatment. Atrial flutter is probably due to reentry in most cases.[23] Treatment with digoxin, β-blockers, and calcium channel blockers should be tried, either to terminate the rhythm or, more likely, to slow the ventricular rate, if it is elevated. Procainamide at doses of 16 mg/kg and 32 mg/kg IV has successfully terminated atrial flutter in experimental dogs.[24] (See the discussion of treatment in Chapter 29.)

Atrial fibrillation

Definition and mechanisms. Atrial fibrillation is caused by numerous small reentrant pathways creating a very rapid and very disorganized depolarization pattern in the atria. It results in cessation of atrial contraction. The depolarization rate of the atria in atrial fibrillation usually exceeds 500 depolarizations/min, although the multitude of waveform configurations and the fast rate often make it difficult to ascertain the exact rate (Figure 27-30). These depolarizations continuously bombard the AV junctional tissue. The AV junction acts as a filter and does not allow all of the depolarizations to conduct to the ventricles (if all did reach the ventricle, this would cause ventricular fibrillation). The AV junction always allows conduction through it in an irregular fashion; that is, at one point five atrial depolarizations may occur before one gets through to the ventricles, the next time conduction may occur after three atrial depolarizations, and the next time after four atrial depolarizations (Figure 27-31). Many atrial depolarizations activate only a part of the atria because portions of the atria are refractory as a result of the rapid rate and thus are unable to reach the AV junction. Other atrial impulses penetrate into the AV junctional tissue but are not robust enough to penetrate the entire length. These blocked impulses affect the conduction properties of the AV junctional tissue, altering conduction of subsequent electrical impulses. This results in electrical impulses being conducted through the AV junction irregularly and produces an irregular ventricular rhythm. The total number of impulses that reach the ventricles primarily depends on the refractory period of the AV node and to a lesser extent its conduction characteristics.[25] These variables are markedly influenced by autonomic tone. If vagal tone is high and sympathetic tone is low, a lesser number of atrial depolarizations reach the ventricles. If vagal tone is

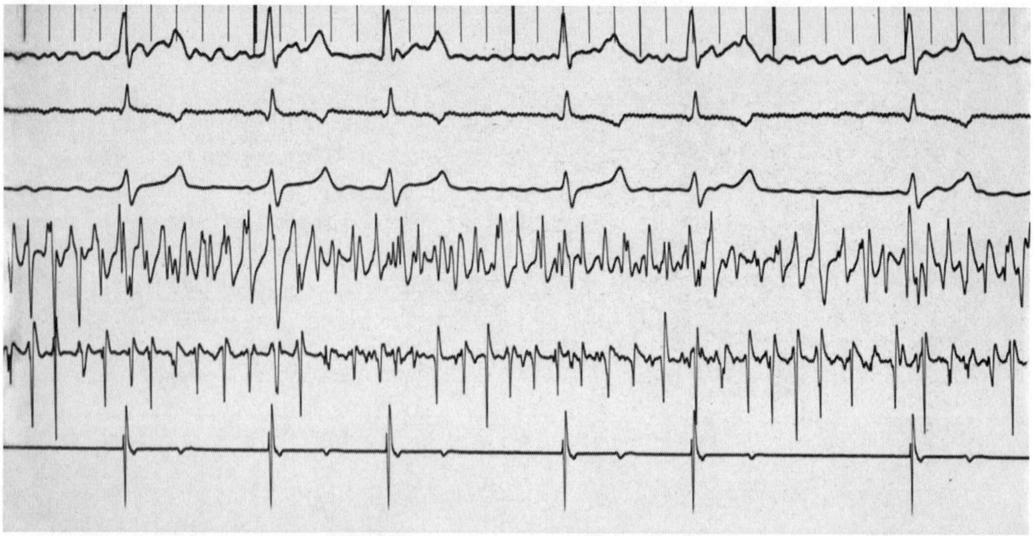

FIGURE 27-30 Surface electrocardiographic tracings and recordings of intracavitary electrograms from a 5-year-old German shepherd treated for incessant supraventricular tachycardia for 2 years. An electrophysiologic study was performed, and it was determined that the dog had a region of reentry in atrial myocardium. During the electrophysiologic study, atrial fibrillation was produced via catheter stimulation of atrial myocardium. The top three tracings in the figure are standard limb leads (leads I, II, and III), which show a fast, irregular supraventricular rhythm with fibrillation waves on the baseline. The fourth tracing is recorded from an electrode catheter placed against the right atrial myocardium. The fifth tracing is from an electrode catheter placed in the great cardiac vein. The sixth tracing is from an electrode catheter placed in the right ventricle. The fourth tracing demonstrates the electrical activity produced by atrial fibrillation. It appears much like ventricular fibrillation. The depolarizations are very fast, very erratic, and probably result from multiple small regions of reentry. The atrial depolarization rate is impossible to determine exactly, although it appears to be between 750 and 800 depolarizations/min. (Paper speed = 50 mm/sec.)

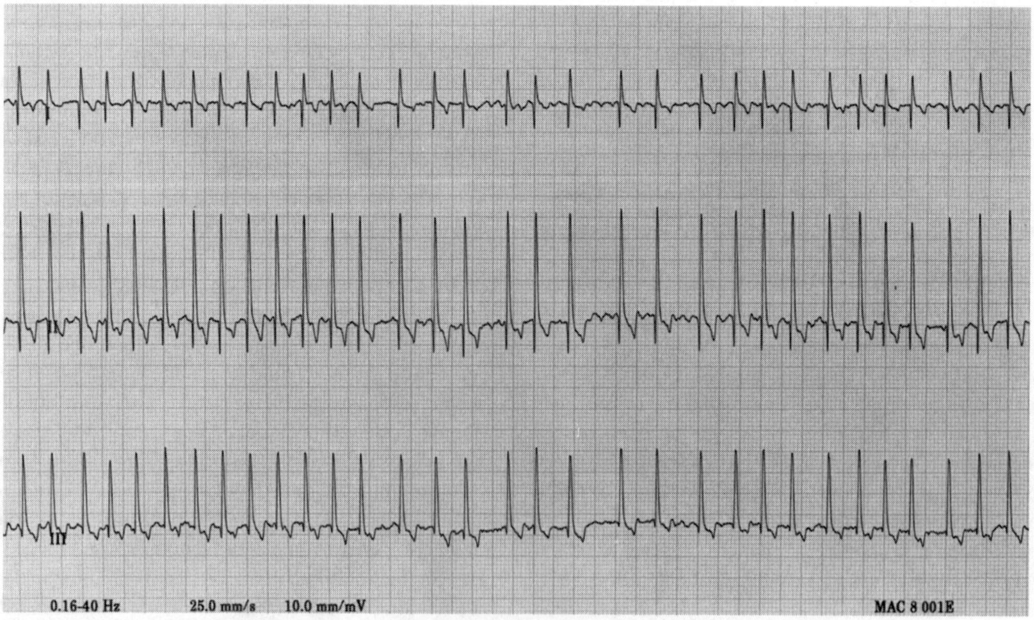

FIGURE 27-31 Lead II ECG tracing recorded from a 14-year-old Australian shepherd with severe mitral regurgitation. The heart rate is very fast (average heart rate = 250 beats/min) and very irregular (the heart rate varies from 200 to 275 beats/min). The QRS complex duration and configuration are normal. In summary, the rhythm is fast, irregular, and supraventricular in origin. This makes atrial fibrillation the primary consideration. The baseline has fibrillation waves and is devoid of *P* waves, confirming the diagnosis of atrial fibrillation. (Paper speed = 50 mm/sec; 1 cm = 1 mV.)

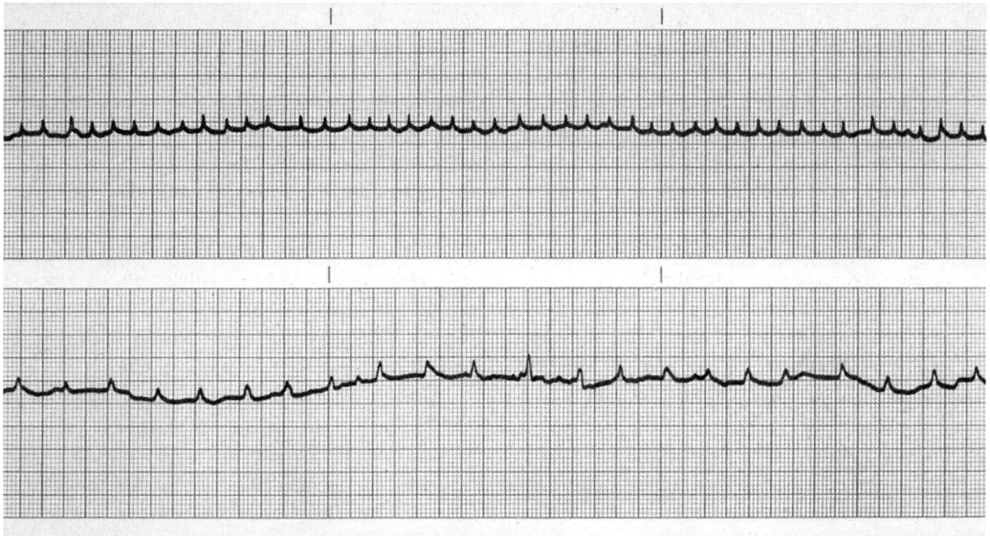

FIGURE 27-32 Lead II ECG tracings recorded from a 4-year-old female Maine coon cat with end-stage hypertrophic cardiomyopathy. The cat was in heart failure, had a markedly enlarged left atrium, and had evidence of myocardial failure on her echocardiogram. The average heart rate is 300 beats/min. The rhythm is irregular. The QRS complexes are small, but QRS complex duration is within normal limits (0.04 seconds). There are no discernible *P* waves. The diagnosis is atrial fibrillation. (*Top,* Paper speed = 25 mm/sec; 1 cm = 1 mV. *Bottom,* Paper speed = 50 mm/sec; 1 cm = 1 mV.)

low and sympathetic tone is high, as in patients in heart failure, a greater number reach the ventricles.

Causes. Atrial fibrillation is one of the most common arrhythmias seen in small animal veterinary practice. It occurs most commonly secondary to serious underlying heart disease. The most common underlying diseases are dilated cardiomyopathy and severe mitral regurgitation. The reason it occurs most frequently in these situations is because atrial fibrillation requires a certain atrial surface area or mass to propagate. In experimental studies in which atrial fibrillation is present, decreasing the atrial surface area results in cessation of atrial fibrillation.[26]

Cats may also develop atrial fibrillation. Atrial fibrillation occurs less frequently in cats and always in association with severe enlargement of at least one atrium. Consequently, the development of atrial fibrillation is also a very poor prognostic sign in cats. The electrocardiographic diagnosis can be difficult because of the very fast rate and small complexes (Figure 27-32). The same rules apply in cats as in dogs. If the rate is very fast, the rhythm originates from a supraventricular focus, and if the rhythm is irregular, atrial fibrillation is the most likely diagnosis.

Forms of atrial fibrillation and ECG diagnosis. The two forms of atrial fibrillation are primary ("lone") and secondary. Primary atrial fibrillation is a rare disease that occurs in large dogs with no or mild underlying cardiac disease. Secondary atrial fibrillation occurs in dogs and cats secondary to severe underlying cardiac disease. Dogs and cats with secondary atrial fibrillation are often in heart failure. In heart failure the resting sympathetic tone to the body and so to the AV junctional tissue is high and the parasympathetic tone is low. Consequently, the ventricular rate is high, usually between 180 and 240 beats/min in dogs and greater than 220 beats/min in cats (see Figures 27-31 and 27-32). Electrocardiographically, secondary atrial fibrillation is characterized as a fast, irregular supraventricular rhythm; that is, the ventricular rate is fast, the interval between QRS complexes is irregular, and the QRS complexes usually appear normal, not wide and bizarre. In addition, no *P* waves are present. The baseline may be flat or may have small irregular undulations (*f* waves). Baseline characteristics vary tremendously from patient to patient, and it is not unusual for some baseline undulations to look like P waves. Consequently, when reading an ECG from a patient suspected to have atrial fibrillation, it is recommended that the other characteristics of the ECG pattern be evaluated first. If the rhythm is fast, supraventricular, and irregular, usually the patient has atrial fibrillation. Once these criteria are identified, the examiner should look at the baseline to make sure that no clearly demonstrable *P* waves are present.

In primary atrial fibrillation, the patient is not in heart failure, so resting sympathetic tone is low and vagal tone is high. Consequently, the ventricular rate in these dogs is usually in the 100- to 140-beats/min range. These large dogs apparently develop atrial fibrillation spontaneously. Most of them have no evidence of underlying heart disease, although some may go on to develop dilated cardiomyopathy.

Hemodynamic consequences of atrial fibrillation. The development of atrial fibrillation in a patient with severe underlying cardiac disease is usually a serious sequela. It results in loss of atrial systolic contraction and therefore decreased late diastolic ventricular filling. In dogs, this results in a decrease in stroke volume and cardiac output, with a resultant increase in left ventricular diastolic pressure.[27] It is common for a patient to deteriorate clinically at the time atrial fibrillation commences because of these alterations in hemodynamics. In addition, the increase in heart rate results in deterioration in myocardial function. In experimental dogs that undergo rapid ventricular pacing at rates between 200 and 260 beats/min, myocardial failure is produced that is severe enough to cause heart failure within 3 to 6 weeks.[28] Because of this, one of the primary therapeutic goals in patients with atrial fibrillation and a fast ventricular response is to reduce the ventricular rate. The other argument made for decreasing the heart rate in dogs with atrial fibrillation is that the shorter diastolic filling interval at faster heart rates results in decreased ventricular filling and therefore a reduction in cardiac output. Of course, the converse may also be true. Cardiac output is calculated by multiplying stroke volume times heart rate. Therefore decreasing the heart rate in a dog with atrial fibrillation could also decrease cardiac output. Evidence exists that either can occur. In one pilot study, the respiratory rate decreased in dogs treated with drugs to slow the heart rate.[29] In our clinic, we have observed decreases in venous oxygen tension following pharmacologic reduction in the heart rate. This presumably is due to a decrease in cardiac output. Regardless, the clinical experience of most veterinarians suggests that slowing the heart rate in atrial fibrillation does not result in clinical deterioration. We know that a heart rate greater than 200 beats/min causes myocardial failure. Consequently, slowing the ventricular rate in atrial fibrillation is always a primary therapeutic goal in a patient that has atrial fibrillation with a fast ventricular response.

Clinical features. On auscultation, patients with atrial fibrillation have a very erratic heart rhythm, best described as sounding like "tennis shoes in a dryer." Auscultation is not pathognomonic for atrial fibrillation. Other erratic arrhythmias, most commonly ventricular tachyarrhythmias, can be mistaken for atrial fibrillation. The heart sounds heard with atrial fibrillation are admixtures of first, second, and third heart sounds. A fourth heart sound cannot occur in atrial fibrillation because no atrial contraction is present. The first heart sound intensity in atrial fibrillation is variable. A primary determinant of first heart sound intensity is the position of the mitral and tricuspid valves at the onset of systole. If they are wide open, they have time to accelerate to a greater velocity than if they are partially closed, resulting in a louder sound. If they are partially closed, a softer sound is produced. In atrial fibrillation in which the diastolic intervals are very irregular, maximum mitral valve opening varies from beat to beat, as does the first heart sound intensity. The second heart sound is present on some beats but not on others in patients with atrial fibrillation. Beats that have a short diastolic interval between them result in inadequate ventricular filling. This results in the ventricle not pumping out any blood with that beat. If there is no stroke volume, the aortic and pulmonic valves do not open. If they do not open, they cannot close. Consequently, no sound is produced with the beat following a short diastolic interval. A second heart sound is produced on beats with longer diastolic intervals. Along with the first and second heart sounds, third heart sounds may also be present. These occur in early diastole during rapid ventricular filling into an overdistended or stiff ventricle.

Along with the auscultatory abnormalities, patients with atrial fibrillation also have pulse abnormalities. These are usually described as *pulse deficits,* but patients with atrial fibrillation also have pulses that alternate in intensity. This occurs because of the fast irregular heart rhythm. The strength of the femoral pulse again depends on the diastolic interval preceding the pulse. Beats with a very short diastolic interval preceding them may not produce any pulse (a pulse deficit) because filling is so poor that the ventricle has nothing to eject. Other beats have a long diastolic interval preceding them, resulting in good ventricular filling and a good pulse. Other beats are between and produce pulses of lesser intensity (Figure 27-33).

Treatment. Patients with fast (secondary) atrial fibrillation are treated medically to slow the ventricular rate (see Chapter 29). Converting the atrial fibrillation to sinus rhythm would be ideal. However, attempts at this are futile in patients that have severe underlying cardiac disease and severe left atrial enlargement. In these

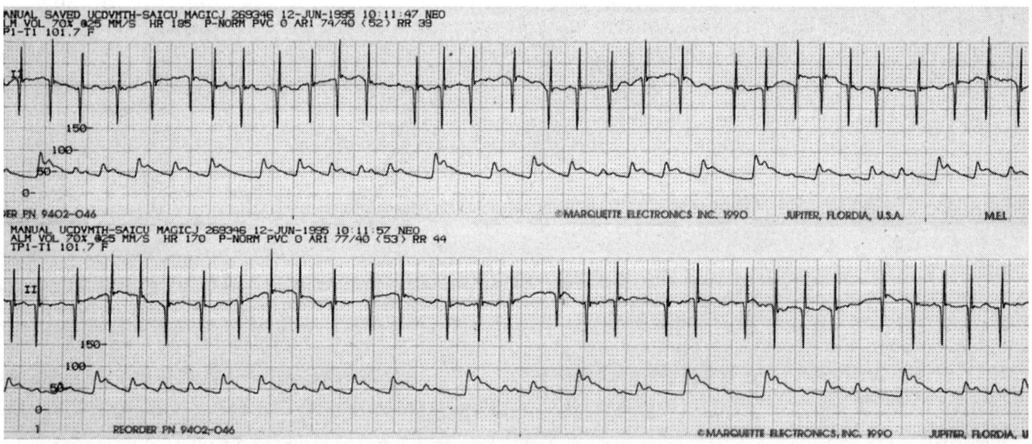

FIGURE 27-33 A monitoring lead ECG tracing and a pressure tracing from a peripheral artery from a 10-year-old golden retriever with severe mitral stenosis. The average heart rate is approximately 190 beats/min. The systemic arterial blood pulse pressure is highly variable. There is approximately a 0.1-second delay between the QRS complex and the upstroke of the pressure tracing. To examine the effect of atrial fibrillation on pulse pressure (the pressure felt when palpating a systemic artery), start at the seventeenth QRS complex from the end of the second tracing. This QRS complex occurs after a delay of almost 0.5 seconds (heart rate = 120 beats/min at that point). This long delay allows the ventricle to fill completely, which produces a maximum stroke volume and a maximum pulse pressure of approximately 60 mm Hg, which is normal. This is followed by a much faster beat that occurs only 0.28 seconds later (heart rate = 214 beats/min at that point). With this short delay and the dog's restriction to filling, the ventricles fill so inadequately that only a very small amount of blood is ejected into the aorta, producing a very small deflection on the pressure tracing. This would not be felt if one were palpating a femoral artery. This is termed a pulse deficit. The next QRS complex occurs even sooner, 0.24 seconds later (heart rate = 250 beats/min). However, now the left ventricle has had two diastolic intervals to fill and is able to generate a larger stroke volume than on the beat before this one. Consequently, a pulse pressure of 30 mm Hg (70 mm Hg systolic blood pressure and 40 mm Hg diastolic blood pressure) is generated. This results in a weak femoral pulse. These alterations continue randomly and would be felt as variable pulses with pulse deficits.

patients, conversion is usually unsuccessful. Even if it is successful, these patients usually only remain converted for hours to several days. Drugs that prolong AV junctional refractory period and slow conduction decrease the number of atrial depolarizations that conduct to the ventricles in patients with atrial fibrillation and slow the ventricular rate. Digoxin, β-adrenergic blockers, and diltiazem are frequently used for this purpose. Digoxin increases vagal tone to the AV junctional tissue. In so doing, it increases the refractory period of tissues in the AV junction and prolongs the conduction characteristics of this tissue. The net result is fewer atrial depolarizations reaching the ventricles. β-Adrenergic blockers perform a similar task by decreasing sympathetic stimulation of the AV junction. Because the AV junctional tissue depolarizes via slow calcium channels, calcium channel blockers also prolong conduction and prolong the refractory period of this region. In most patients with severe underlying cardiac disease, digoxin is administered first. It is not the most efficacious drug at decreasing heart rate in atrial fibrillation, but it can be effective and has no negative inotropic properties. It is not mandatory to administer digoxin for its positive inotropic properties before administering a β-adrenergic blocker or a calcium channel blocker. Digoxin is a very weak positive inotrope, and β-blockers and calcium channel blockers, when used at low doses, do not have any appreciable negative inotropic effects. However, digoxin is still usually used initially in an attempt to slow the ventricular rate. Digoxin's effect on the ventricular rate in patients with atrial fibrillation is highly variable. In some patients it produces no effect. In others the heart rate will promptly decrease from 200 to 240 beats/min to 140 to 160 beats/min. Most patients, however, have a midrange response, with ventricular rate decreasing by 10 to 30 beats/min. In those patients in which no response or a midrange response is produced, a β-adrenergic blocker or a calcium channel blocker should be added. β-Blockers and calcium channel blockers should not be administered together. Most of our experience is with propranolol and diltiazem. Both drugs work well, and we have no preference of one over the other. We start with one and if an adequate response is not identified, we switch to the other. Propranolol is initially administered at a dose of 0.1 mg/kg to 0.2 mg/kg q8h. The dose is then titrated upward until an adequate response is identified. We do not exceed a dose of 0.5 mg/kg q8h. For diltiazem, an initial dose of 0.5 mg/kg q8h is initially administered, and the dose is titrated up to a maximum of 1.5 mg/kg q8h or until an adequate response is identified. The definition of an adequate heart rate response varies from clinician to clinician but in dogs is generally between 140 beats/min and 160 beats/min (Figure 27-34).

In a dog that has atrial fibrillation and no or minimal underlying heart disease and a normal-to-mildly–enlarged left atrium (primary atrial fibrillation) the clinician must decide whether to attempt to convert the atrial fibrillation to sinus rhythm. This decision ideally should be made using risk vs. benefit analysis. Unfortunately we do not know the risks of leaving a dog in atrial fibrillation, and we are only superficially aware of the risks of conversion. In most of our cases, we try to convert to sinus rhythm at least once. Other veterinary cardiologists routinely leave these cases untreated. In some of the dogs we have examined, conversion has been unsuccessful, and in a few we have not attempted conversion. Some of these dogs have remained normal, whereas others have developed evidence of dilated cardiomyopathy over time. It is doubtful that the atrial fibrillation produced the dilated cardiomyopathy, and we doubt that we have hastened the progression of these dogs' disease by allowing them to remain in atrial fibrillation. We use either quinidine or electrical cardioversion to convert these dogs into sinus rhythm. We have administered quinidine at doses as high as 20 mg/kg PO q2h to as low as 12.5 mg/kg q6h. One dog administered 20 mg/kg q2h converted after two doses, with no toxicity. Another dog needed 10 doses at a dose of 12.5 mg/kg q6h, as did a dog administered 10 mg/kg q4h. The signs of quinidine toxicity that we have seen include weakness, ataxia, and seizures. Seizures are readily controlled with the administration of diazepam intravenously. We have not observed prolongation of the Q-T interval or the QRS duration before the onset of more serious signs of toxicity, as is reported in humans.[22] Electrical (DC) cardioversion is the application of a transthoracic electrical shock delivered at a specific time in the

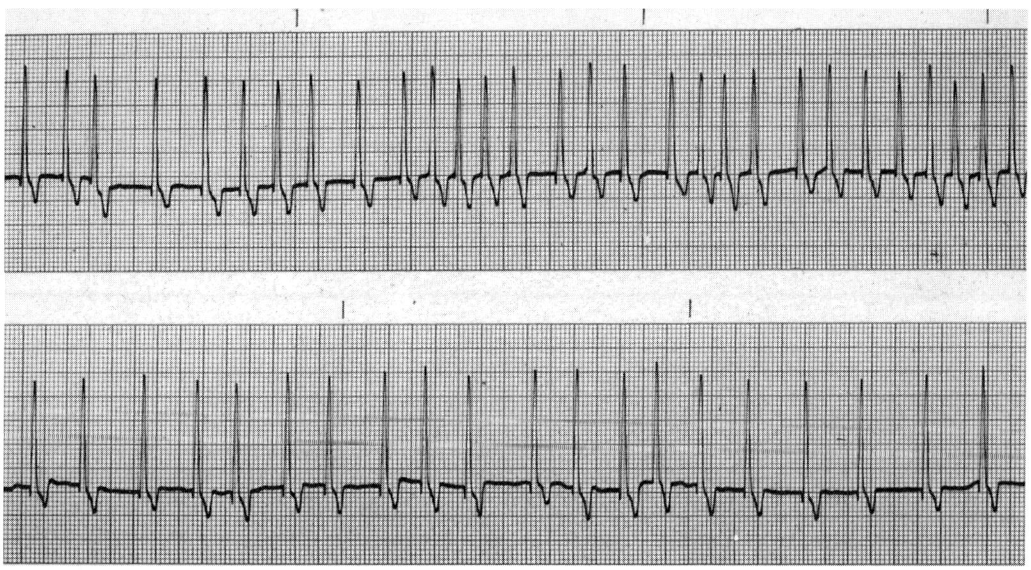

FIGURE 27-34 Lead II ECG tracing recorded from a 7-year-old Saint Bernard with dilated cardiomyopathy. The rhythm is atrial fibrillation. In the top tracing, before therapy, the average heart rate is 210 beats/min. At the time of the second recording, the dog was being administered digoxin and diltiazem. The average heart rate has been reduced to 140 beats/min. (Paper speed = 25 mm/sec; 1 cm = 1 mV.)

cardiac cycle, usually timed to occur along with the QRS complex on an ECG. The specific timing is required to avoid delivering an electrical shock on the downslope of the T wave, producing ventricular fibrillation. Electrical cardioversion requires special equipment and so must be done by or done with an experienced individual. Anesthesia is usually required. We have converted one conscious dog with a very small (10 J) electrical shock, but most require much higher power (100 to 250 J). Our procedure involves anesthetizing the dog and placing it on its back or sternum. An area is shaved on both lateral thoracic walls at the fifth to sixth intercostal spaces, midway between the thoracic spine and the sternum. We have tried delivering the shock lower on the thoracic cage with less success. We place the defibrillator paddles over this region and start with a 50-J shock while recording the ECG. If this is unsuccessful, we then increase the current by 50-J increments until conversion occurs (Figure 27-35). Dogs that are successfully converted with either quinidine or DC cardioversion may stay in sinus rhythm or may develop atrial fibrillation again within hours to months. In dogs that develop atrial fibrillation again, chronic therapy with quinidine (8 to 16 mg/kg q8h) or quinidine and digoxin may be required. These drugs are started for 2 to 3 days before reconversion and maintained after reconversion.

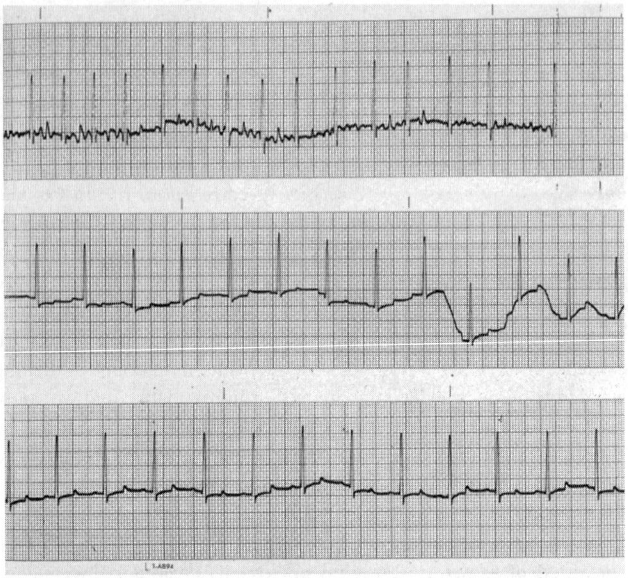

FIGURE 27-35 Lead II ECG tracings recorded from a 7-year-old bull mastiff. An arrhythmia had been ausculted by the referring veterinarian. An ECG confirmed atrial fibrillation with a heart rate of 110 beats/min. No abnormalities were noted on an echocardiogram. Primary atrial fibrillation was diagnosed. The dog was anesthetized for DC cardioversion. Cardioversion was attempted initially with 50 J and then 100, 150, and 200 J. The first 90% of the top tracing is before cardioversion. The average heart rate is 130 beats/min. At the end of the tracing, a 200-J DC electrical shock was delivered across the chest. The shock was synchronized with the ECG to deliver the charge at the same time as the QRS complex, which can be seen on the ECG. The second and third tracings were recorded immediately after cardioversion. The rhythm is a sinus rhythm. (Paper speed = 25 mm/sec; 1 cm = 1 mV.)

We have had two dogs develop ventricular fibrillation during electrical cardioversion (Figure 27-36). Both were successfully resuscitated. Quinidine was being administered to both dogs at the time of attempted conversion. Of the other approximately five dogs that we have successfully cardioverted, none have been on quinidine and none have developed ventricular fibrillation. Whether this association is causally related or a chance occurrence is unknown. Box 27-1 presents a case example of a dog with primary atrial fibrillation.

Other drugs are used in human medicine to convert atrial fibrillation to sinus rhythm. Procainamide was used successfully to convert George Bush in 1991. Class IC drugs such as flecainide, encainide, and propafenone are effective agents in humans.[30] So are the class III antiarrhythmic drugs, amiodarone and sotalol. Experience with these drugs in veterinary medicine is extremely limited at this time.

VENTRICULAR TACHYARRHYTHMIAS

When ventricular myocardium is diseased or damaged, a region of myocardium may develop the ability to depolarize, setting up a new pacemaker at an abnormal site (an ectopic pacemaker). The methods by which this occurs were outlined above. If the ectopic pacemaker site depolarizes at a rate faster than the sinus node, it can express itself and dominate the cardiac rhythm. Ventricular

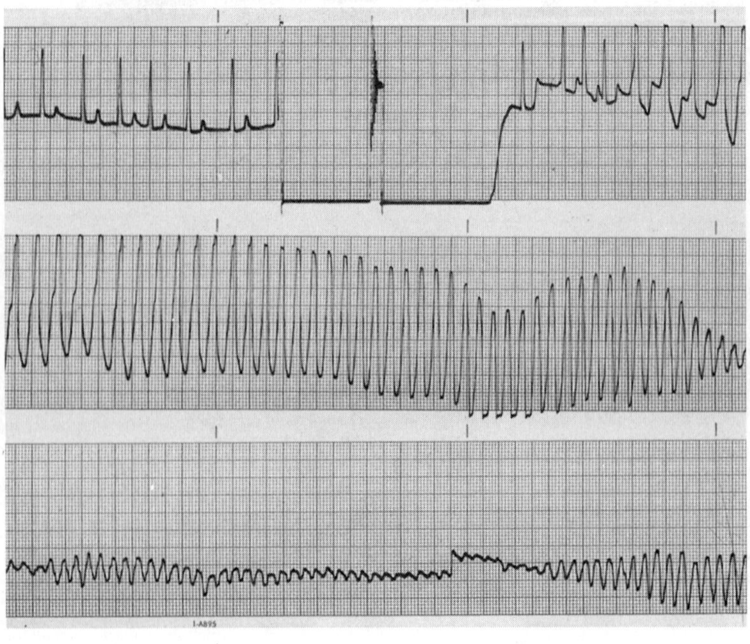

FIGURE 27-36 Lead II ECG tracings recorded from a 9-year-old Anatolian shepherd with primary atrial fibrillation during attempted cardioversion. The tracings are continuous. Digoxin and quinidine were administered before cardioversion. Medical conversion of the atrial fibrillation with oral quinidine administration had been attempted 1 week before this attempt and was unsuccessful. The initial rhythm is atrial fibrillation. A 300-J shock was delivered on the eighth QRS complex. There is an artifact on the ECG tracing immediately after delivery of the shock that lasts for approximately 2.5 seconds. Following the cardioversion attempt, the rhythm is still irregular and then degenerates into a fast ventricular tachycardia at a rate of approximately 270 beats/min on the first part of the middle tracing. This degenerates further into ventricular flutter in the middle of the middle tracing. The rate is now approximately 320 beats/min. The rhythm quickly degenerates further at the end of the middle tracing to produce the rhythm on the bottom tracing. This rhythm is characterized by small complexes that alternately decrease and increase in size. This is characteristic of torsades de pointes. The rhythm is indistinguishable from ventricular fibrillation in the middle of the tracing. Ventricular fibrillation occurred soon after. The dog was successfully defibrillated, resuscitated, and sent home.

BOX 27-1

Case example of a dog with atrial fibrillation

A 5-year-old male Irish wolfhound was presented as a referral from a veterinarian who had heard a heart murmur and suspected dilated cardiomyopathy. On physical examination the dog had a grade 2/6 left apical systolic heart murmur and an irregular heart rhythm. The ECG revealed atrial fibrillation with a ventricular rate of 100 beats/min. The left ventricle on the echocardiogram was essentially normal, with an end-diastolic diameter of 52 mm and an end-systolic diameter of 39 mm (shortening fraction = 27%). There was mild left atrial enlargement. Mild mitral regurgitation was suspected. Color flow Doppler was not available at the time this dog was examined. The dog weighed approximately 80 kg. He was administered 1000 mg quinidine (12.5 mg/kg) q6h starting at 8:00 PM. There was no change the following day, and quinidine was continued. On the morning of the third day, the dog was ataxic and had caudal limb tremors but was in sinus rhythm with a heart rate of 130 beats/min. He had first-degree AV block but no increase in QRS complex duration and a normal Q-T interval. A total of six doses of quinidine had been administered. The serum quinidine concentration was 3.2 μg/mL (assumed therapeutic range = 2 to 6 μg/mL). The serum concentration was measured at least one half-life after the last dose. Consequently, it was assumed that the peak serum concentration was at least twice that measured. The dog was sent home on 0.5 mg digoxin q12h, but this was discontinued by the owner after several days. On reexamination 2 weeks later, the dog was normal but the heart rate was 220 beats/min. A supraventricular tachycardia was diagnosed, which was controlled by administering 0.5 mg digoxin q12h again. Three weeks later the dog was in normal sinus rhythm with a normal P-R interval. The owner had again discontinued administering the digoxin. Five months later the dog presented for reexamination and was again in atrial fibrillation, with a ventricular rate of 120 beats/min. The echocardiogram was unchanged. Quinidine, 1000 mg q6h, was again administered, but this time 10 doses were required before the atrial fibrillation was converted to sinus rhythm. At the time of conversion the P-R interval on the ECG was 0.16 seconds (normal = 0.06 to 0.13 seconds), and so the dog had first-degree AV block again. By that afternoon the P-R interval was 0.14 seconds. The dog was again sent home on 0.5 mg digoxin q12h. One week later the serum digoxin concentration taken 6 hours after the last dose was 0.7 ng/mL (normal range = 0.5 to 2.0 ng/mL). Two months later the dog again presented in atrial fibrillation and again was converted with 10 doses of quinidine, using the same schedule as before. The digoxin dose was halved while the dog was being administered quinidine, because quinidine usually doubles the serum concentration of digoxin. Serum quinidine concentration 8 hours after the last dose of quinidine was 4 μg/mL. The digoxin dose was increased to 0.5 mg q12h when the dog was sent home, and 1 week later the serum digoxin concentration was 1.6 ng/mL. It was suspected that the owner may not have been administering the digoxin as directed previously. One month later the dog was in sinus rhythm, and the echocardiogram was unchanged. Two months later the dog presented for signs of systemic disease and was diagnosed with diabetes mellitus. He was again in atrial fibrillation. It was elected not to treat his atrial fibrillation again. His heart rate was 120 beats/min. His diabetes mellitus was controlled with insulin injections, and the dog did well for the next 5 months. At that time he was presented for a right foreleg lameness and was diagnosed with a bone tumor of the right humerus. He was euthanized. At postmortem examination, the heart was mildly enlarged, with mild myxomatous degeneration of both the mitral and aortic valves. In retrospect, it could be questioned whether this dog needed to be converted. His heart rate was always slow, and his cardiac disease was mild and did not progress.

tachyarrhythmias are the most common type of rhythm disturbance seen in dogs and cats.

Ventricular premature depolarizations

Definition and ECG diagnosis. Ventricular premature depolarizations (VPDs) are also known as *ventricular premature contractions, premature ventricular contractions,* and *ventricular premature beats.* These terms are used interchangeably in the literature.

A VPD is characterized by the early appearance (premature) of a wider-than-normal QRS complex and an accompanying *T* wave that is large and opposite in polarity to the QRS complex. Together they produce a QRS-T complex that is bizarre in appearance. There is no associated *P* wave (Figure 27-37). These are premature depolarizations. Consequently, they appear too early on the ECG (the distance between the last sinus QRS complex and the QRS complex generated by the VPD is shorter than the normal QRS-to-QRS interval generated by the sinus node), producing an irregularity in the heart rhythm (Figure 27-38). Ventricular tachyarrhythmias originate distal to the bifurcation of the bundle of His, in the distal regions of the specialized conduction system, and in ventricular myocardium. Because depolarization starts within a bundle branch or lower in ventricular myocardium, the depolarization cannot use any or all of the specialized conduction system in the ventricles. Instead, depolarization must occur from myocardial cell to myocardial cell. This takes longer than normal to depolarize the ventricles, resulting in a QRS complex that is wider than normal. Repolarization is also always abnormal, resulting in a large, bizarre *T* wave following the wide QRS complex. This abnormal *T* wave is commonly mistaken for a part of the QRS complex because it commonly begins immediately after the QRS complex (there is no or little ST segment). Artifacts can sometimes be generated, most commonly by movement or leads touching each other, that simulate VPDs. These can usually be

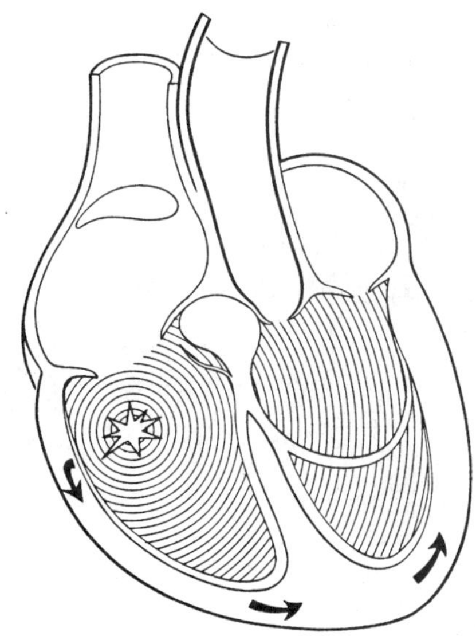

FIGURE 27-37 Schematic drawing of a ventricular premature depolarization. An ectopic site in ventricular myocardium has depolarized before the sinus node has depolarized. Consequently, it appears on the ECG before the next expected sinus beat (i.e., it is premature). The depolarization wave cannot take advantage of the intraventricular conduction system. Instead, the wave of depolarization must travel slowly from muscle cell to muscle cell. In the drawing, the depolarization originates from the right ventricle. Consequently, it spreads in the normal direction—from right to left. Consequently, the QRS complex on the ECG would be upright, albeit wider than normal. (From Phillips RE, Feeney MK: *Cardiac rhythms: a systematic approach to interpretation,* ed 3, Philadelphia, 1990, WB Saunders.)

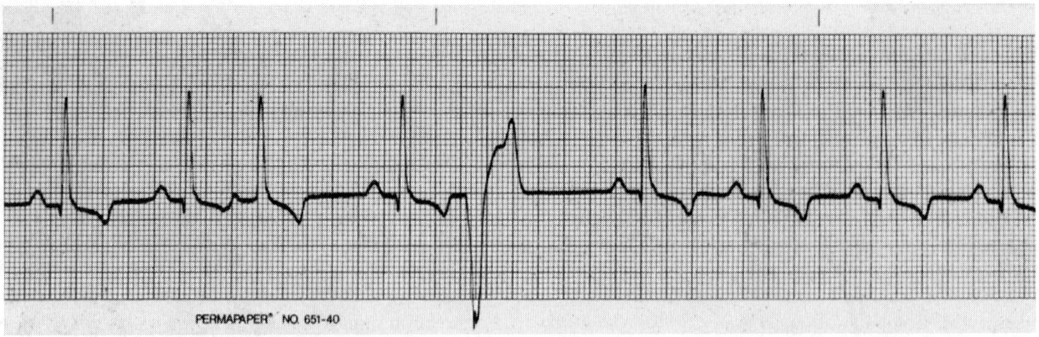

FIGURE 27-38 Lead II ECG tracing recorded from the dog shown in Figure 27-19. The third complex is a supraventricular premature depolarization. The fifth complex is also premature. However, the QRS complex is negative and its duration is prolonged. The *T* wave is opposite in polarity and very large. These are characteristics of either a premature ventricular depolarization or a supraventricular premature depolarization combined with a bundle branch block. There is no definitive way of absolutely distinguishing between these two possibilities on an ECG. However, it is almost assuredly a ventricular premature depolarization. No *P* wave occurs before or immediately after this premature depolarization. This makes a supraventricular focus less likely. A compensatory pause occurs after this premature depolarization (see text for details). The interval between *P* waves of sinus beats is 0.46 to 0.50 seconds. The interval between the *P* wave preceding the premature depolarization and the *P* wave following it is 0.95 seconds. This is twice the normal P-P interval. This occurred because the depolarization was unable to conduct back to the sinus node and reset it. Instead, the sinus node depolarized at its normal time (the *P* wave from this depolarization is presumably buried in the *T* wave of the premature depolarization) and then depolarized again at the normal time to produce the next normal QRS complex. This most likely occurred because this premature depolarization originated in a ventricle and passed part of the way into the atrioventricular (AV) junctional tissue but was unable to pass retrograde through the AV node to the atria. The atrial depolarization then found the AV junctional region refractory to conduction and so did not conduct to the ventricles to produce a QRS complex. This is opposed to the supraventricular depolarization, in which the interval between the *P* wave preceding and the *P* wave following the premature depolarization is almost the same as the normal P-P interval. This has occurred because the supraventricular depolarization has conducted back to the sinus node, depolarized it, and so reset it. Therefore the sinus node was depolarized and able to repolarize and then undergo a normal phase 4 diastolic depolarization and reach threshold at the same time after it depolarized normally on its own (0.53 seconds in this case). The fact that the second premature depolarization has a compensatory pause makes it more likely that it is ventricular in origin but still does not prove it. However, everything together makes it very likely that this is a ventricular premature depolarization. If so, the QRS complex is oriented opposite to normal, meaning the ventricular depolarization wave must be conducting left to right rather than the normal right to left. This means the premature depolarization most likely originated in the left ventricle. (Paper speed = 50 mm/sec; 1 cm = 1 mV.)

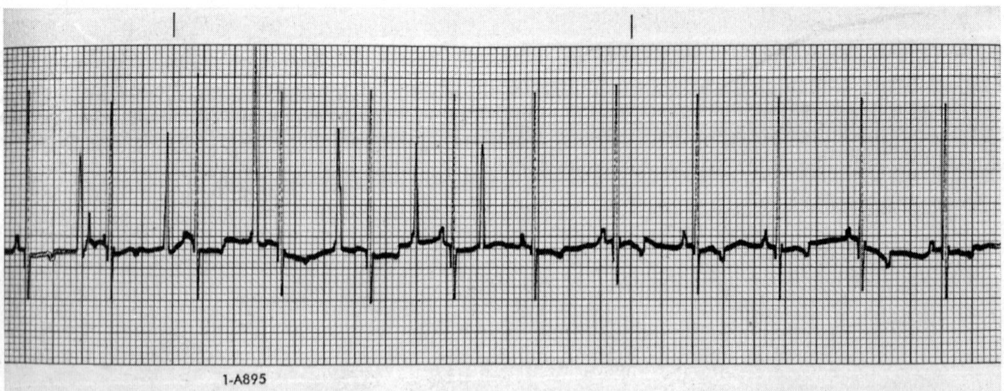

FIGURE 27-39 Lead II ECG tracing recorded from a dog. At the end of the tracing the rhythm is a sinus rhythm. At the beginning of the tracing, the *P* waves and the QRS complexes and the intervals between them are the same as at the end of the tracing. However, deflections occur in between the normal complexes. They look like premature QRS complexes. However, these deflections do not alter the underlying rhythm and have no *T* waves following them. They are artifacts generated by electrodes touching each other intermittently.

differentiated from VPDs because they do not have a *T* wave following them (Figure 27-39). A supraventricular premature depolarization can mimic a VPD if an accompanying *P* wave is not obvious and intraventricular conduction is abnormal (e.g., a bundle branch block is present; see Figure 27-23).

A VPD can originate from any part of the ventricular myocardium. If it originates from the right ventricle and spreads from right to left, the wave of depolarization advances toward the positive poles of leads I, II, III, and aV_F, the QRS complexes in these leads are upright, and the mean electrical axis is normal (Figure 27-40). These

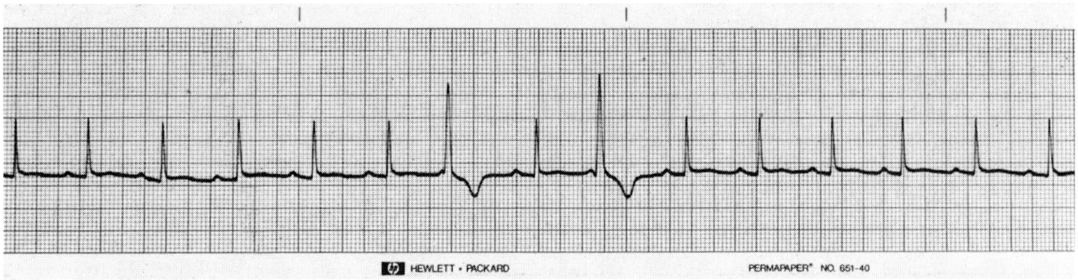

FIGURE 27-40 Lead II ECG tracing recorded from a 14-year-old cat with hypertrophic cardiomyopathy. The seventh and ninth QRS complexes are premature and wide and followed by larger-than-normal *T* waves. A *P* wave is barely visible before the first premature QRS complex and is more readily visible before the second premature complex. The P-R interval is too short for there to be any relationship between the *P* waves and the QRS complexes. This means that the atria and ventricles are dissociated during these beats, with the ventricular rate being faster than the atrial rate. A compensatory pause occurs following each premature depolarization. These features are diagnostic of premature ventricular depolarizations. The premature depolarization is oriented normally, which means it most likely originated from the right ventricle. This cat was treated with propranolol 5 mg q8h, and the premature depolarizations subsided. (Paper speed = 50 mm/sec; 1 cm = 1 mV.)

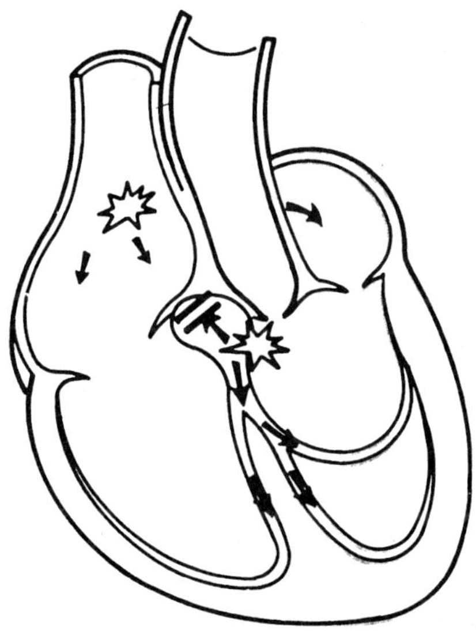

FIGURE 27-41 Schematic drawing of a ventricular premature depolarization originating high on the interventricular septum that does not conduct retrograde through atrioventricular (AV) node to depolarize the atrial myocardium and the sinus node. Consequently, the sinus node continues to depolarize. However, it finds the AV node refractory and so does not depolarize the ventricles. This creates a compensatory pause in the rhythm. (From Phillips RE, Feeney MK: *Cardiac rhythms: a systematic approach to interpretation,* ed 3, Philadelphia, 1990, WB Saunders.)

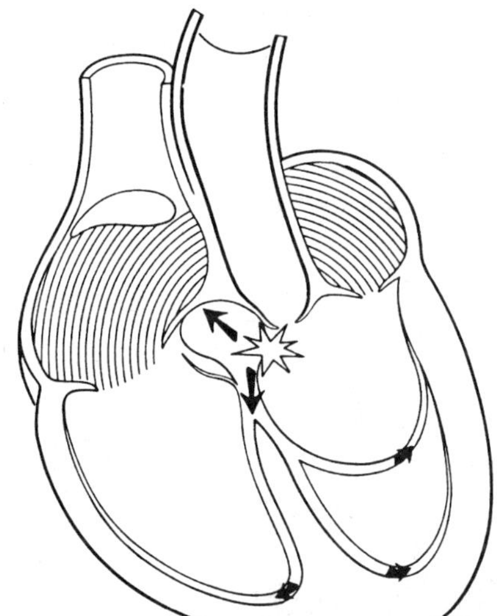

FIGURE 27-42 Same drawing shown in Figure 27-41, except in this instance the depolarization does conduct retrograde through the atrioventricular (AV) node. Consequently, the atrial myocardium and sinus node are depolarized by the ventricular premature depolarization. This resets the sinus node to depolarize at its inherent rate after being depolarized by the ventricular premature depolarization. This produces a noncompensatory pause. The same may occur with a supraventricular premature depolarization. (From Phillips RE, Feeney MK: *Cardiac rhythms: a systematic approach to interpretation,* ed 3, Philadelphia, 1990, WB Saunders.)

QRS complexes look identical to those generated by a left bundle branch block. If the VPD originates from the left ventricle, the wave of depolarization spreads from left to right, toward the negative poles of these leads. This results in QRS complexes that are negative, so that a right axis deviation exists for the abnormal beats (see Figure 27-38). These complexes look like those generated by a right bundle branch block.

The timing between the sinus depolarizations and the VPD vary on an ECG. Most commonly the VPD depolarizes the ventricular myocardium but does not conduct retrograde through the AV junction to depolarize the atria and sinus node (Figure 27-41). At the same time, the sinus node depolarization cannot depolarize the ventricles because the electrical impulse is blocked in the AV junction. This occurs because it has been depolarized by the VPD and therefore is refractory or because the ventricular myocardium is refractory. The sinus node continues to depolarize at its inherent rate, and therefore the next sinus beat appears at its normal time. When measured, the time between the two sinus beats (with the VPD in the middle) is twice the normal sinus-beat-to-sinus-beat interval, and the time from the VPD to the following sinus beat is more than the normal sinus-beat–to–sinus-beat interval (see Figure 27-38). This results in a pause after the VPD, which is called a *compensatory pause.* At times, however, the depolarization can conduct retrograde to the sinus node so that a noncompensatory pause can be produced, as described in the discussion of supraventricular depolarizations (see Figures 27-38 and 27-42). At other times the VPD depolarizes the myocardium and it repolarizes in time for the next sinus impulse to depolarize the heart again. In this situation the VPD does not interrupt

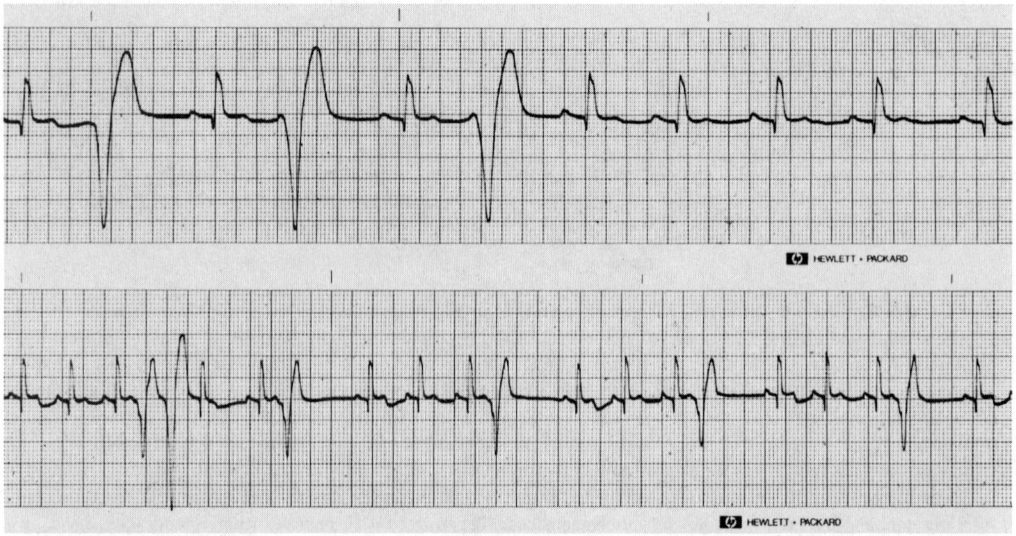

FIGURE 27-43 Lead II ECG tracings recorded from a 7-year-old Doberman pinscher with bacterial endocarditis of the aortic valve. The top tracing is recorded at 50 mm/sec. The initial rhythm is ventricular bigeminy, with every sinus beat followed by a ventricular premature depolarization. The interval between a sinus beat and a premature beat is approximately 0.35 seconds. This means that the ventricular focus is depolarizing at a rate of approximately 170 beats/min. The second tracing is recorded at 25 mm/sec. The pair of ventricular premature depolarizations is approximately 0.24 seconds apart, which means that this focus is now depolarizing at a rate of 250 beats/min. Although the second QRS complex is not yet melded with the previous *T* wave, it is close. For these reasons this dog was treated with antiarrhythmic therapy. (1 cm = 1 mV.)

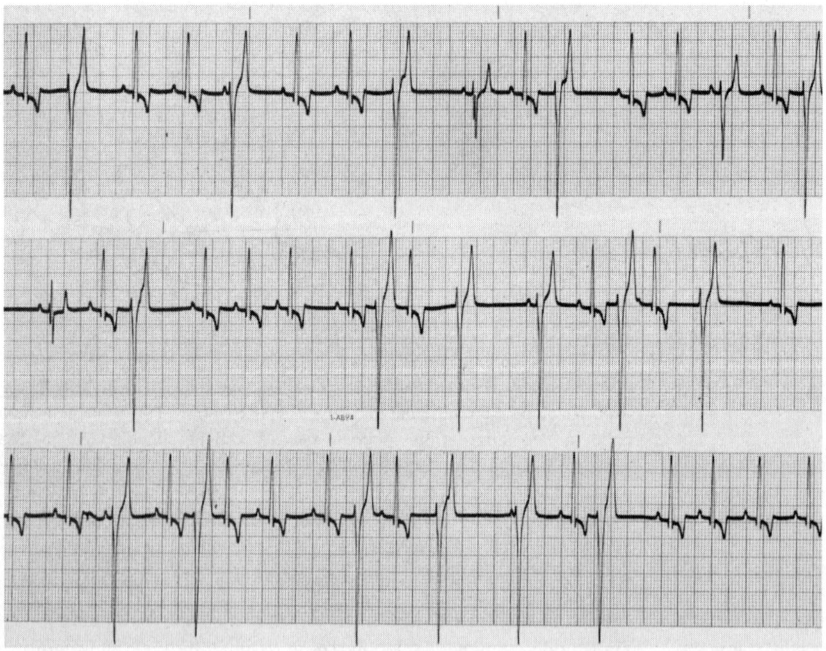

FIGURE 27-44 Lead II ECG tracing recorded from a 7-year-old rottweiler with severe subaortic stenosis. Ventricular premature depolarizations are present throughout the three tracings. Many of these premature depolarizations are 0.96 seconds apart. The intervals between others (e.g., the first two) are twice the shortest interval; whereas others are 3 times the shortest interval. The ninth and fourteenth ventricular depolarizations in the top tracing are fusion beats. These occur when the sinus depolarization and the ectopic depolarization depolarize the ventricle simultaneously, resulting in a hybrid QRS complex. The diagnosis is ventricular parasystole (see text for details). (Paper speed = 25 mm/sec; 1 cm = 1 mV.)

the normal heart rhythm. This is called an *interpolated* depolarization or beat.

VPDs can appear in patterns. The most common is called *ventricular bigeminy.* In ventricular bigeminy, each sinus beat is followed by a VPD for some period (Figure 27-43). Ventricular trigeminy (every third depolarization is a VPD) is less common. VPDs can also occur as pairs. An unusual pattern is for VPDs to occur totally independent of the sinus rhythm, so that they look similar to the sinus rhythm of a dog that has a fixed-rate pacemaker with no sensing capabilities implanted (Figure 27-44).This is called *parasystole.* It occurs when a ventricular ectopic focus is present that is protected by the tissue around it from being depolarized by the normal sinus beat (an entrance block). The tissue surrounding the ectopic focus may not let all of the ectopic depolarizations out to depolarize the ventricles either (exit block), but obviously some are able to penetrate and depolarize the myocardium. This results in VPDs that occur with no relationship to the sinus beats (no fixed coupling interval with the sinus beats). However, a fixed relationship between the VPDs is present. Consequently, at times a fixed interval between them is present. At other times the interval may be 2 or more times the shortest interval. Another common characteristic is the presence of "fusion" beats. These occur when the VPD and the sinus depolarization reach the ventricular myocardium simultaneously, resulting in an altered wave of ventricular depolarization and a "hybrid" QRS configuration. Fusion beats also occur with other forms of ventricular tachyarrhythmias and so are not diagnostic of parasystole.

Ventricular premature depolarizations may or may not have a constant coupling interval with the previous sinus beat. A constant coupling interval is commonly thought to signify that reentry is causing the ectopic rhythm. However, triggered activity and abnormal automaticity can also produce a constant coupling interval. Consequently, the coupling interval is meaningless with regard to mode of propagation. The faster the ectopic focus fires, the shorter the coupling interval will become. If the focus depolarizes at a very fast rate, the VPD will appear during the downslope of the *T* wave. This is called the *R-on-T phenomenon.* The downslope of the *T* wave is called the *vulnerable period* because depolarization during this stage can induce ventricular fibrillation.

Causes. Ventricular premature depolarizations can occur in many settings. They are rare in normal dogs and cats. They are common in hospitalized patients, occurring, for example, after trauma, after surgery, in association with gastric-dilatation volvulus, and secondary to systemic disease. VPDs are common in the presence of anesthetic agents. One of the most common situations is to observe ventricular bigeminy following the administration of a thiobarbiturate.[31] VPDs also occur in dogs and cats with primary myocardial disease. Doberman pinschers and Boxers with dilated cardiomyopathy commonly have VPDs present on an ECG.

The reason for VPDs in many patients is clear. Dogs and cats with primary myocardial disease have myocardial damage that can produce reentry, abnormal automaticity, or triggered activity. Determining the exact mechanism responsible is impossible from a surface ECG. Understanding how myocardial toxins, such as anesthetic agents, can produce VPDs is easy. These arrhythmias are exacerbated by administration of catecholamines and vagolytic agents.[32,33] Dogs with gastric dilatation-volvulus have regions of microscopic ischemia in their myocardium, probably associated with hypovolemia.[6] The reason for VPDs in other patients is unclear. Dogs with systemic disease, abdominal disease, or prostatitis develop VPDs with no evidence of cardiac disease other than the arrhythmia. Acid-base and electrolyte disturbances may exacerbate the arrhythmias in these patients but are not severe enough in the vast majority of patients to produce VPDs.

Clinical features. Patients with isolated VPDs have no clinical signs. Syncope or episodic weakness may be present if periods of fast ventricular tachycardia are admixed with the VPDs. Auscultation reveals an arrhythmia. The premature beat interrupts the rhythm because it comes in too early. The intensity of the sounds associated with the VPD can be normal or softer than normal depending on how premature the beat is and so on the time allowed for ventricular filling. Beats that occur very early allow less time for filling, resulting in a less forceful contraction and a softer first heart sound. If the beat comes in very early, the contraction may be so weak that no blood is ejected, resulting in the lack of a second heart sound. The beat following the VPD is often more forceful than normal. This is called *postextrasystolic potentiation* and is due to a longer filling period and a longer time for the sarcoplasmic reticulum to sequester calcium. The increased force of contraction results in a louder-than-normal first heart sound. Humans describe feeling this enhanced beat. This feeling is called a palpitation.

Treatment. Treatment of VPDs depends on the setting in which they are identified. Isolated VPDs in hospitalized patients with disease of other organ systems generally do not need to be treated. The ventricular arrhythmia will disappear once the underlying problem is corrected. Ventricular bigeminy associated with thiobarbiturate administration is usually self-limiting. It can often be eliminated by ventilating the patient. In dogs with myocardial disease, the presence of VPDs is often a clue that more serious ventricular arrhythmias exist. More prolonged ECG recordings (e.g., a Holter monitor recording) may be indicated to determine the extent and severity of the other ventricular tachyarrhythmias. (See the discussion of treatment of VPDs in Chapter 29.)

In humans, VPDs are commonly treated to alleviate symptoms of lightheadedness, palpitations, chest pain, dyspnea, fatigue, and lethargy. Dogs and cats rarely demonstrate any of these abnormalities. Consequently, treating VPDs in dogs to alleviate clinical signs is generally not warranted. The major reason to treat VPDs is to prevent sudden death.

In 1971, Lown and Wolf[34] proposed a system to grade ventricular arrhythmias in the hospital phase of acute myocardial infarction (Table 27-2). This grading system remains popular in human medicine today, not only for grading ventricular arrhythmias in patients with coronary artery disease but also other disease. This system is commonly carried over into the veterinary literature for grading ventricular arrhythmias in dogs and cats. This system, however, has never been studied in veterinary medicine with respect to its ability to predict sudden death in any patient population. It is often used inappropriately to grade veterinary patients with benign ventricular arrhythmias so that a decision to treat can be made. For example, in human medicine it is known that the frequency of VPDs is an independent risk factor in a patient with ischemic heart disease secondary to coronary artery atherosclerosis.[35] The greater the number of VPDs per hour, the greater is the risk for sudden death (Lown grade 1 vs. Lown grade 2). These criteria have been placed repeatedly in the veterinary literature to suggest that this is a reason to start administering antiarrhythmic drugs to dogs and cats. However, even in human medicine, the importance of VPD numbers in forms of cardiac disease other than coronary artery disease is largely unknown, and the number of VPDs in patients without cardiac disease has no apparent relationship with the propensity for sudden death.[36,37] In our experience, the number of VPDs in dogs and cats without myocardial disease is not predictive of sudden death. Sudden death is extremely rare in this population, even when the number of VPDs are greater than sinus beats. In addition to this, the number of VPDs recorded on a 24-hour ECG recording (Holter monitor) varies so much from day to day in humans that to document suppression of

TABLE 27-2

The Lown grading system for ventricular arrhythmias

Grade	*Criteria*
0	No VPDs
1	<30 VPDs/hr
2	>30 VPDs/hr
3	VPDs with more than one configuration (multiform)
4A	Two consecutive VPDs (pair or couplet)
4B	Three or more consecutive VPDs (ventricular tachycardia)
5	R on T (fast rate)

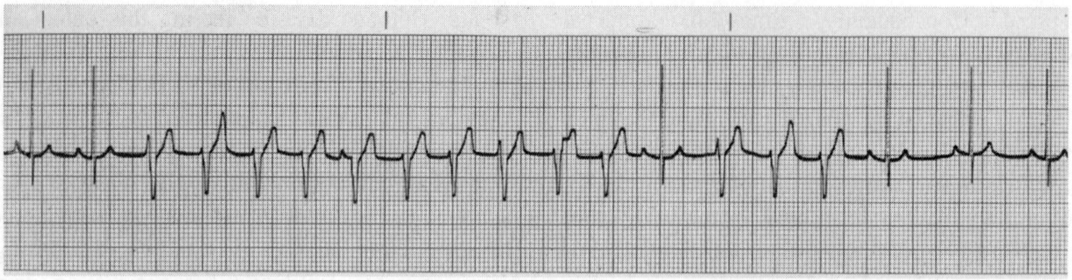

FIGURE 27-45 Lead II ECG tracing recorded from a dog with idiopathic vestibular disease and an arrhythmia. The initial rhythm is a sinus rhythm with a heart rate of 110 beats/min (R-R interval = 0.54 seconds). This is interrupted by a ventricular premature beat that depolarizes at a rate of 130 beats/min (R-R interval = 0.46 seconds) and then becomes repetitive, achieving a rate of approximately 140 beats/min. In the middle of the tracing, the ectopic focus either slows to a rate less than 120 beats/min (the interval from the last tachycardic beat to the sinus beat) or stops. This allows the sinus node to gain control of the rhythm again. Immediately, however, another premature depolarization takes over and repeats 3 times, after which it slows or stops again, allowing sinus rhythm to take over. This is accelerated idioventricular rhythm, a slow and benign form of ventricular tachycardia. No therapy was administered to this dog, because the rhythm did not alter hemodynamics to a clinically significant degree and because the risk of sudden death from this arrhythmia is minimal. The last supposition is based on the fact that the rate of ectopic depolarization is slow and on the fact that the dog has no underlying primary cardiac disease. Note that *P* waves are still being generated (one is clearly seen between the fourth and fifth premature complexes) while the ventricular tachycardia is present. This occurs because the ventricular depolarizations are not being conducted back through the atrioventricular (AV) junction to the atria (AV dissociation). (Paper speed = 25 mm/sec; 1 cm = 1 mV.)

VPDs by antiarrhythmic drugs, at least an 80% reduction must be identified before it can be called significant.[38] The frequency of VPDs on a 30- to 60-second ECG recording from minute to minute, hour to hour, and day to day is even worse. The primary risk factor for sudden death in human medicine and apparently in veterinary medicine is the presence of myocardial disease. Even in dilated cardiomyopathy in humans, there is contradictory information regarding the significance of the Lown classification and its ability to predict sudden death.[39] In Doberman pinschers, the number of VPDs per day increases as the disease progresses and so is a measure of disease progression and severity. Complex ventricular arrhythmias (Lown class 3 or higher) may predict sudden death in this breed.[40] In boxers with category 2 cardiomyopathy, VPDs are often numerous but are often admixed with fast runs of ventricular tachycardia. It is most likely these fast runs that degenerate into ventricular flutter and fibrillation that produce syncope and sudden death in this population. Although the number of VPDs may predict the occurrence of ventricular tachycardia, this is unknown. There are no data in other breeds with dilated cardiomyopathy or in dogs with other myocardial disease. Treatment of VPDs in patients with myocardial disease is the same as for ventricular tachycardia, outlined below.

Ventricular tachycardia

Definition and ECG features. Ventricular tachycardia is the presence of three or more VPDs in a row. As for other tachyarrhythmias, reentry, abnormal automaticity, and triggered activity can all cause ventricular tachycardia. Enhanced normal automaticity is probably a rare cause of ventricular tachycardia in dogs and cats. Autonomic modulation of abnormal impulse formation and conduction is probably important in many settings.

Ventricular tachycardias differ in morphology, rate, regularity, and duration. Of these, the rate is probably the most important when deciding whether to treat the ventricular tachycardia. Rates vary from approximately 70 beats/min to greater than 500 beats/min in dogs.[41] Semantics become a problem when one thinks about this definition, because a heart rate of 70 beats/min in a dog or cat is not a tachycardia. However, because the ventricular focus in this situation is firing at a rate faster than a normal ventricular escape focus should fire and to become evident it must depolarize at a rate faster than the sinus node, it is still defined as a tachycardia. In general, the slower the ventricular rate, the more benign is the ventricular tachycardia, and the faster, the more malignant. In humans, a ventricular tachycardia that depolarizes at a rate between 70 and 110 beats/min is not considered a tachycardia because it is not depolarizing at a rate faster than a sinus rate can potentially depolarize in a normal person. Consequently, a ventricular tachycardia that depolarizes at this rate is often called an *accelerated idioventricular rhythm*. This definition is arbitrary in that both a ventricular tachycardia and an accelerated idioventricular rhythm are generated by abnormalities in ventricular myocardium that set up mechanisms for generating ectopic rhythms, as explained above. The only difference between the two is the rate at which the ectopic focus depolarizes. However, accelerated idioventricular rhythm (a slow ventricular tachycardia) and a fast ventricular tachycardia often have a different prognosis, so the demarcation between the two is important. The exact demarcation between an accelerated idioventricular rhythm and ventricular tachycardia is not known in dogs and cats. We do know, experimentally, that abnormalities that generate accelerated idioventricular rhythms in humans generate accelerated idioventricular rhythms in dogs that have rates that vary from at least 66 to 132 beats/min and probably go even higher.[7,42] In one study of experimental dogs in which formalin was injected into myocardium, an accelerated idioventricular rhythm was reliably produced with an average rate of 127 beats/min.[7] However, 1 standard deviation above this mean was a rate of 179 beats/min. Because one usually considers defining a population based on 95% confidence intervals and a 95% confidence interval is approximately the mean ± 2 standard deviations, including only 1 standard deviation above a mean is very conservative. Whereas the upper limit for a normal sinus rate is 100 beats/min in a human, the upper limit of normal in a dog is usually considered to be around 180 beats/min. Because of the findings in the last study and because ventricular tachycardia is defined in humans based on the upper limit for the normal sinus rate, we consider a ventricular tachycardia that depolarizes at a rate less than 180 beats/min an accelerated idioventricular rhythm in dogs (Figures 27-45 and 27-46). We consider rates faster than 180 beats/min to be a true ventricular tachycardia (Figure 27-47). This division is somewhat

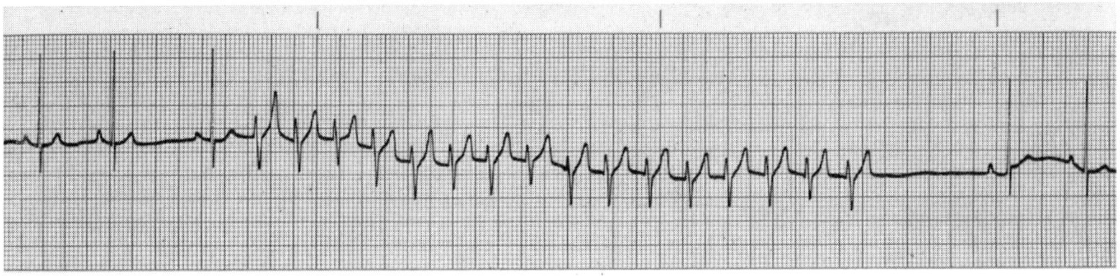

FIGURE 27-46 Lead II ECG tracing recorded a few minutes later from the dog shown in Figure 27-45. The rhythm disturbance is similar to the previous one, but the rate is faster (approximately 170 beats/min). Instead of an accelerated idioventricular rhythm, this might be called a *ventricular tachycardia.* However, this arrhythmia occurred in a dog without primary underlying cardiac disease, and the rate is slow enough that there is a clear "shelf" between the *T* waves and the QRS complexes, that is, there is no R-on-T phenomenon. These facts still make this a benign arrhythmia that does not warrant antiarrhythmic therapy unless hemodynamics are compromised. This dog had no evidence of clinically significant hypoperfusion, and no antiarrhythmic drugs were administered. It was sent home with no cardiovascular sequelae. Note that no P waves are visible in association with this rhythm. In addition, a pause occurs after the ventricular tachycardia stops. It appears that the ventricular depolarizations in this dog and at this time are being conducted back to the atria and sinus node, resulting in suppression of the sinus node. The period of sinus arrest after the tachycardia ceases is probably a functional arrest (there is no sinus node pathology). Instead, the sinus node has undergone so-called overdrive suppression. However, it does appear to take longer than normal to recover. (Paper speed = 25 mm/sec; 1 cm = 1 mV.)

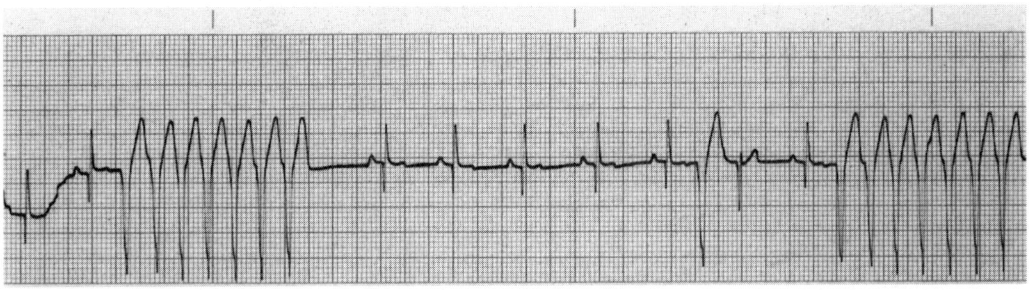

FIGURE 27-47 Lead II ECG tracing recorded from a 6-year-old Doberman pinscher with dilated cardiomyopathy. The first two beats are sinus beats that depolarize at a rate of 110 beats/min. The second sinus beat is followed by a ventricular premature beat that depolarizes at a rate of 230 beats/min. The ventricular focus immediately becomes repetitive and increases its rate to approximately 270 beats/min. This is nonsustained ventricular tachycardia. This arrhythmia is definitely associated with an increased risk of sudden death. This supposition is based on the fact that the dog has an underlying cardiac disease that is commonly associated with sudden death and on the fact that the focus is firing at a rapid rate. The rate is so rapid that the QRS complexes are very close to the preceding *T* waves (R-on-T phenomenon). This dog was treated with procainamide 25 mg/kg q8h. This appeared to decrease the severity of the arrhythmia, but the dog died suddenly 3 weeks later. (Paper speed = 25 mm/sec; 1 cm = 1 mV.)

arbitrary and probably false in identifying underlying mechanisms and assessing the potential malignancy of an arrhythmia. The important things to remember are that the slower the focus depolarizes, the more benign is the arrhythmia and the faster it fires, the more likely it is to produce ventricular fibrillation. No one would argue that a dog with an accelerated idioventricular rhythm depolarizing at a rate of 100 beats/min has a benign arrhythmia. Also, no one would argue that a dog with a ventricular focus that depolarizes at a rate of 400 beats/min is at risk for sudden death. Between, however, there is much room for controversy.

Accelerated idioventricular rhythm is a common arrhythmia in hospitalized patients without underlying primary cardiac disease. It is observed most commonly in dogs following gastric dilatation-volvulus surgery, in dogs with abdominal disease (e.g., splenic disease, pancreatitis, prostatitis), in dogs that have been hit by a moving vehicle, and in dogs with neurologic disease (see Figures 27-45 and 27-47).[43,44] At times, the sinus rate and the rate of the accelerated idioventricular rhythm are similar and compete for the heart rhythm, with the accelerated idioventricular rhythm manifesting only when the sinus rhythm slows below the inherent rate of the ventricular focus (Figure 27-48).

The morphology of the QRS complexes in ventricular tachycardia depends on the site of origination and the conduction pathway from this site. Ventricular tachycardias can be uniform (all of the QRS complexes are one shape) or multiform. Uniform complexes invariably suggest that there is one focus from which all of the complexes originate. Multiform complexes are often called *multifocal,* with the supposition that different forms mean different sites of origin. However, multiple morphologies may be formed by depolarizations originating from the same or closely adjacent sites and taking different conduction pathways (Figure 27-49).

Ventricular tachycardias can last for very short or very long periods. Ventricular tachycardias that last for less than 30 seconds are arbitrarily termed *nonsustained ventricular tachycardias* in humans. Those lasting longer than 30 seconds are termed *sustained ventricular tachycardias.* The same convention is usually used in small

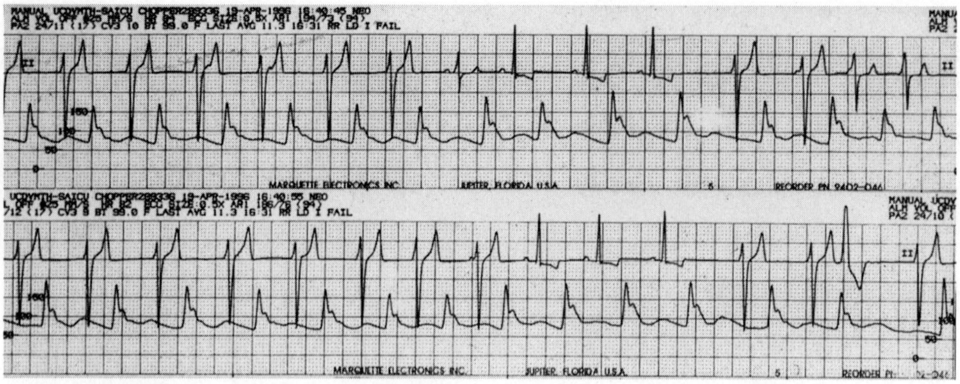

FIGURE 27-48 Simultaneous recordings of an ECG and an arterial pressure tracing from a dog with an accelerated idioventricular rhythm. The sinus node and the ectopic ventricular focus compete for control of the heart rate. Whenever the sinus rate slows, the ventricular focus assumes control. The sinus rate varies from about 78 to 95 beats/min; whereas the ventricular focus rate is more constant, at a rate of approximately 80 beats/min. Fusion beats occur (eighth complex in the top tracing and fourth complex in the bottom tracing). Blood pressure and pulse pressure are normal during both sinus rhythm and during the ventricular tachyarrhythmia. Pulse pressure tends to be mildly better during sinus rhythm. (Paper speed = 25 mm/sec; 1 cm = 1 mV.)

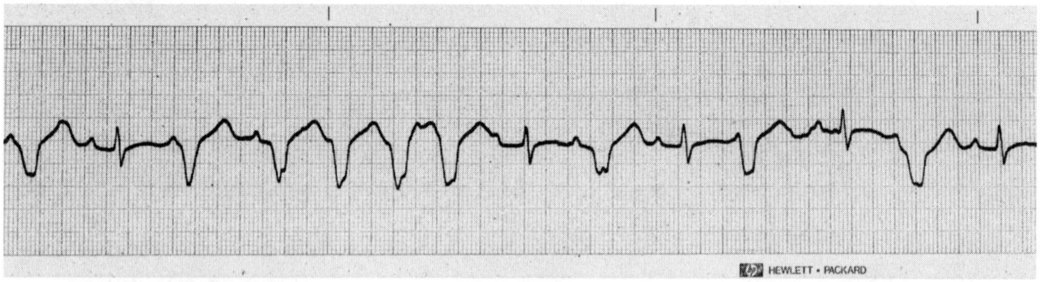

FIGURE 27-49 Lead II ECG tracing recorded from a cat with dilated cardiomyopathy. The first depolarization is a ventricular premature depolarization followed by a sinus beat, a short run of nonsustained ventricular tachycardia, and then ventricular bigeminy. The fastest that the ventricular focus depolarizes is approximately 270 beats/min between the last two complexes of the run of ventricular tachycardia. Note that the last QRS complex in this run of tachycardia clearly occurs before the *T* wave from the previous QRS complex returns to baseline (R-on-T phenomenon). The complexes also vary in morphology (multiform complexes). Some of the change in morphology may be due to the presence of fusion beats. This should be considered a malignant arrhythmia. The cat also has a first-degree atrioventricular block (PR interval = 0.12 seconds). (Paper speed = 50 mm/sec; 1 cm = 1 mV.)

animal veterinary medicine. Ventricular tachycardia can also be paroxysmal (sudden) or nonparoxysmal.

Although many ventricular tachycardias are regular (R-R interval is always the same), they can also be irregular. There does not appear to be any prognostic significance to either form.

Ventricular tachycardia can result in one form of atrioventricular (AV) dissociation. In this form, the ventricular focus is depolarizing at a rate greater than the sinus node (as opposed to third-degree AV blocks, in which the sinus rate is greater than the ventricular rate). In this scenario, the ventricular depolarizations are not being conducted retrograde through the AV node to the atria. The ventricular depolarizations partially penetrate the AV node and so make it refractory to conducting the sinus node depolarizations and resultant atrial depolarizations through the AV node to the ventricles. Consequently, one observes the ventricular tachycardia on the ECG with *P* waves that most commonly appear irregularly in the ST segment or between the *T* wave and the following QRS complex. Retrograde conduction to the atria can also occur, resulting in sinus node suppression and an absence of *P* waves.

Clinical features. Accelerated idioventricular rhythm and ventricular tachycardia are most commonly identified in two populations of dogs—those with and those without underlying primary cardiac disease. In those without primary disease, accelerated idioventricular rhythm predominates. In dogs with cardiomyopathy, dogs with subaortic stenosis, and cats with hypertrophic cardiomyopathy, either form may predominate. Accelerated idioventricular rhythm in dogs without primary cardiac disease is benign, Any ventricular tachyarrhythmia in a patient with underlying primary cardiac disease has the potential to become malignant and produce sudden death.

Clinical signs associated with ventricular tachycardia depend on the ventricular rate, the duration of the tachycardia, and the presence and extent of the underlying cardiac disease. Most ventricular tachycardia that occurs in dogs without underlying cardiac disease is not exceedingly rapid and usually does not result in clinical signs unless the cardiovascular system is compromised by conditions such as anesthesia or severe systemic disease. Very fast ventricular tachycardia (usually at a rate greater than 300 beats/min) results in a severe decrease in cardiac output. This can lead to hypotension and syncope if the tachycardia lasts longer than 6 to 8 seconds. This is a common occurrence in boxers and Doberman pinschers with cardiomyopathy. It is usually a warning that sudden death will occur if the tachycardia is left untreated.

Auscultation of a patient with ventricular tachycardia may reveal bursts of nonsustained tachycardia. If the arrhythmia is sustained, only a faster-than-normal heart rate will be evident.

The decision to treat. The decision to treat a patient with ventricular tachycardia depends on several factors. The only reasons to treat ventricular tachycardia are to improve hemodynamics and to prevent sudden death. In veterinary medicine, the vast majority of patients with ventricular arrhythmias that require therapy are dogs. Dogs with ventricular tachycardia can be divided into the following three broad general categories: (1) dogs with severe underlying cardiac disease, (2) hospitalized dogs with no underlying cardiac disease but with moderate disease or trauma to other body systems, and (3) dogs under anesthesia or with severe systemic disease. In general, dogs with ventricular tachycardia and severe underlying cardiac disease are at risk for sudden death and warrant therapy. Dogs with no underlying cardiac disease that have abnormalities in other body systems usually have benign arrhythmias that do not predispose them to sudden death and do not alter hemodynamics to a clinically significant degree. Consequently, they usually do not require treatment. Dogs and cats that are being administered an anesthetic agent or that have severe systemic disease may experience hemodynamic compromise with ventricular tachycardia and may be more predisposed to developing life-threatening arrhythmias. Consequently, antiarrhythmic therapy is commonly warranted. Lidocaine is the drug of choice.

The primary reason to treat a cardiac patient with ventricular tachycardia is to prevent sudden death. A few select groups of patients that develop ventricular arrhythmias that lead to sudden death exist in veterinary medicine. These groups include Doberman pinschers and boxers with dilated cardiomyopathy, dogs with severe subaortic stenosis, German shepherds with inherited ventricular arrhythmias, and cats with hypertrophic cardiomyopathy.[41] Consequently, severe cardiac disease is the greatest risk factor for dying suddenly from a ventricular arrhythmia. This is regardless of ventricular focus firing rate, numbers of premature beats, or whether the QRS complexes are uniform or multiform. Approximately 20% of Doberman pinschers with dilated cardiomyopathy die suddenly as a result of their disease. Usually, sudden death is due to ventricular tachycardia deteriorating into ventricular fibrillation. In this population, the Lown grade of arrhythmia may be important. In general, it appears that Doberman pinschers with Lown grade 4 or greater arrhythmia may be at greater risk for sudden death. This is discussed in more depth in Chapter 20.

In the vast majority of patients with primary cardiac disease, ventricular tachycardia does not alter hemodynamics enough to cause clinical signs. We see Doberman pinschers with dilated cardiomyopathy that frequently have very serious ventricular arrhythmias that appear clinically normal or are in heart failure but have no evidence of episodic weakness or syncope. Severe ventricular tachycardia (heart rate greater than 300 beats/min) that lasts for 10 seconds or more can result in episodic weakness or syncope, acute forms of severe hemodynamic compromise; we do observe this situation in dogs with dilated cardiomyopathy. We prefer to term this condition *aborted sudden death.* The true reason to treat this type of patient is to prevent sudden death, although preventing the syncopal events is often important to the owner.

The primary reasons to treat a hospitalized patient that has ventricular tachycardia but not severe underlying cardiac disease are also to improve hemodynamics and to prevent sudden death. Slow ventricular tachycardias (accelerated idioventricular rhythm) in canine patients are commonly treated with antiarrhythmic drugs to suppress the ventricular tachyarrhythmia, no matter the cause or rate.[44] Our impression is that most of these arrhythmias are treated because they appear worrisome to the veterinarian or the veterinary technician. We do know that in our intensive care unit, technicians and new residents worry more about these arrhythmias than do experienced veterinary clinicians. Clinicians commonly worry that the arrhythmias will cause sudden death or progressive and irreversible cardiac injury.[44] Consequently, it is commonly recommended that these arrhythmias be treated aggressively.[44] In our experience, nothing could be further from the truth. We routinely withhold antiarrhythmic therapy from this population. From this experience we have concluded that the vast majority of these arrhythmias are benign in that they do not result in sudden death, they do not cause any further cardiac injury, and they subside spontaneously within 48 to 72 hours after they start. It should be noted that even in human medicine, VPDs and accelerated idioventricular rhythms secondary to systemic disorders are usually not treated with antiarrhythmic drugs.[45,46] Therapy is considered in humans with accelerated idioventricular rhythm if: (1) the AV dissociation results in hemodynamic compromise, (2) the accelerated idioventricular rhythm occurs in association with a faster ventricular tachycardia, (3) the accelerated idioventricular rhythm starts with a VPD that has a short coupling interval such that it discharges in the vulnerable period of the preceding T wave (R-on-T phenomenon), (4) the ventricular rate is too rapid and produces symptoms, and (5) ventricular fibrillation develops as a result of the accelerated idioventricular rhythm. In humans, ventricular fibrillation secondary to accelerated idioventricular rhythms is rare.[46] We believe this to be true in dogs as well. In humans, if the sinus rate is slow, atropine administration or atrial pacing is sometimes used to increase the supraventricular rate to a rate greater than the rate of the accelerated idioventricular rhythms. This effectively suppresses the accelerated idioventricular rhythms. We have done the same things using atropine in dogs on occasion.

There is no apparent hemodynamic compromise in the vast majority of the dogs with accelerated idioventricular rhythm in our experience. To warrant therapeutic intervention because of hemodynamic compromise the patient must first have evidence that the cardiovascular system is compromised. Second, there must be a high index of suspicion that the ventricular arrhythmia is contributing to the hemodynamic compromise. The variables that determine whether the arrhythmia compromises cardiac function enough to cause clinical signs of hemodynamic impairment are: (1) whether the arrhythmia is nonsustained or sustained, (2) the rate of the ventricular tachycardia, and (3) the status of the rest of the cardiovascular system. Dogs commonly have sustained slow ventricular tachycardia with a rate of 70 to 180 beats/min, show no clinical evidence of the arrhythmia, and do not need therapeutic intervention. In a patient with ventricular tachycardia that has evidence of hemodynamic compromise, if the ventricular tachycardia is nonsustained and occurs at a rate less than 180 beats/min, it is unlikely that it is the cause of hemodynamic instability unless the cardiovascular system is severely compromised by another factor, such as anesthesia. If it is sustained at a rate greater than 200 beats/min, antiarrhythmic therapy is warranted to determine if abolishing the arrhythmia improves cardiovascular function.

Treatment. Lidocaine is the drug of choice to treat ventricular arrhythmias in hospitalized patients that have severe systemic disease or are anesthetized, if warranted. It is the most effective ventricular antiarrhythmic. It must be administered intravenously. It can be administered over a wide dose range. Other class I agents, such as procainamide and quinidine, may also be used. The addition of a β-blocker may be beneficial in patients refractory to the administration of a class I agent alone. Correction of underlying electrolyte and acid-base abnormalities may reduce the rate or frequency of a ventricular arrhythmia and may provide a more appropriate environment for antiarrhythmic drug effect. For example, many of the antiarrhythmic drugs are more effective when the serum potassium concentration is within the normal or the upper end of normal range than when it is low. (See the discussion of treatment in Chapter 29.)

Ventricular arrhythmias associated with dilated cardiomyopathy have been primarily treated in the past with class I antiarrhythmic agents such as procainamide, quinidine, and tocainide. These drugs have commonly failed to prevent sudden death in these dogs, in our experience. In human medicine, class 1 antiarrhythmic agents are rapidly being abandoned because of evidence that they are ineffective at preventing sudden death and often increase the incidence of sudden death.[47] Instead, class III agents (amiodarone, sotalol) and β-blockers are being used more frequently to accomplish sudden death prevention. Veterinary cardiologists and veterinarians have very little experience with the use of class III antiarrhythmic drugs, and high-dose β-adrenergic blockade is generally contraindicated in patients with severe myocardial failure. There is some evidence that mexiletine, an orally active lidocaine derivative, may be useful for controlling ventricular arrhythmias and, possibly, at preventing sudden death in Doberman pinschers; this is the easiest and safest drug choice at this time.[40] Consequently, mexiletine may be used as first-line antiarrhythmic therapy in Doberman pinschers with dilated cardiomyopathy and ventricular arrhythmias. If this is unsuccessful, amiodarone might be the next choice. However, we do not have enough experience to recommend its routine use. If one chooses to use amiodarone, one must keep in mind that this drug has an extremely long half-life and that it has many potential side effects, some of which can be serious. We have some experience with sotalol. We and others have primarily used it in boxers with severe ventricular arrhythmias, with or without severe myocardial failure.[48] In most of these dogs, sotalol has reduced the number of ventricular arrhythmias or eliminated them. In dogs that were syncopal, the syncope has not recurred. Sotalol generally does not suppress left ventricular function in humans with myocardial failure, although cardiac output can be decreased because of a decrease in heart rate that can, on occasion, be profound.[49-51]

The primary mode of therapy in human patients with dilated cardiomyopathy that are at risk for ventricular fibrillation is implantation of an automatic defibrillator. Devices are now becoming available that can be implanted via a transvenous approach, much like a pacemaker (see Chapter 30). Although cost of these devices currently precludes their use in most veterinary patients, devices will become available as they exceed shelf-life and from human cadavers, making it likely that a few will be implanted in veterinary patients in the future. These devices have been successfully implanted experimentally in German shepherds with inherited ventricular arrhythmias.[41] Automatic implantable defibrillators are similar to pacemakers in that they have a lead implanted in the right ventricle attached to a device that senses cardiac depolarization. When the device senses ventricular fibrillation, it passes a burst of current down the lead to defibrillate the heart.

Approximately 70% of dogs with severe subaortic stenosis die suddenly within the first 3 years of life.[52] Consequently, a method of preventing sudden death in these dogs could have a tremendous impact on the natural history of this disease. β-blockers are commonly administered to these dogs in the hope that they will prevent sudden death. Unfortunately, no studies have been performed to determine if they provide any benefit. Until such a study is performed, however, we recommend that dogs with severe subaortic stenosis be treated prophylactically with propranolol 1 to 2 mg/kg q8h or atenolol 1 to 2 mg/kg q12h.

Ventricular flutter/fibrillation

Causes and ECG findings. These arrhythmias represent severe electrical derangement of the ventricles. *Ventricular flutter* is defined as a ventricular tachycardia that is so fast that the QRS complexes and the *T* waves cannot be distinguished, giving the rhythm a sine wave appearance (see Figure 27-36). Ventricular flutter often degenerates rapidly into ventricular fibrillation. Ventricular fibrillation is recognized as irregular baseline undulations of varying contour and amplitude (Figure 27-50). There are no discernible P-QRS-T complexes. Ventricular fibrillation is a terminal rhythm that results in no ventricular contractions and so is a form of cardiac arrest. It is due to multiple microreentrant circuits within the ventricular myocardium. Ventricular fibrillation occurs in a variety of clinical settings. It most commonly occurs as the terminal event in a patient with severe systemic or cardiac disease. It also occurs unexpectedly during various procedures, such as during the induction phase of anesthesia, during cardiac surgery, and during an endomyocardial biopsy.

Treatment. The only effective treatment of prolonged ventricular flutter or ventricular fibrillation is electrical defibrillation. Bursts of ventricular flutter may be controlled with standard antiarrhythmic agents. Sotalol appears to be effective for this use in boxers. When ventricular fibrillation is the terminal event in a patient with severe systemic or cardiac disease, treatment is usually unsuccessful. Even if defibrillation is successful in this setting, fibrillation commonly recurs within seconds to a few hours. Consequently, defibrillation and resuscitation in this situation often are not indicated. In patients that are otherwise healthy and in which fibrillation has occurred unexpectedly (e.g., the patient undergoing anesthesia), defibrillation should be carried out immediately. The shorter the time between fibrillation and defibrillation, the more successful the outcome. Cardiac resuscitation procedures should not be carried out before defibrillation unless it takes time to locate and charge the defibrillator. If an ECG is not being used to monitor the patient at the time of cardiac arrest, defibrillation should be performed before determining the underlying heart rhythm. Defibrillation will not harm a patient that is in asystole and may cause the asystolic heart to start discharging again. Unfortunately, many veterinary clinics do not own a defibrillator, and many veterinarians have no experience using a defibrillator. Other means of converting ventricular fibrillation, such as chemical defibrillation and cardiopulmonary resuscitation are usually futile.

Defibrillation (nonsynchronized DC electrical shock) is carried out in the unconscious patient by placing the paddles on either side of the chest, approximately one fourth to one third the way up the chest from the sternum, over the fifth to sixth intercostal spaces. Placing the patient on its back is generally easiest. Adequate coupling gel should be placed on the paddles and on the patient, avoiding placement of gel on the operator's hands. Solutions of alcohol must be avoided because they are flammable. The initial energy dose should be approximately 5 J/kg. This means that in a patient that is 10 kg or less (small dogs and cats), the initial energy should be 50 J. A 100-J shock should be administered to medium-size dogs. In large dogs, we start at 200 J. If the initial defibrillation attempt is unsuccessful, a series of shocks at the same dose within a short period can be tried or the dose can be increased (usually twice the previous dose). Intubation, ventilation, and cardiac massage are needed if the first attempts at defibrillation are unsuccessful. Metabolic acidosis

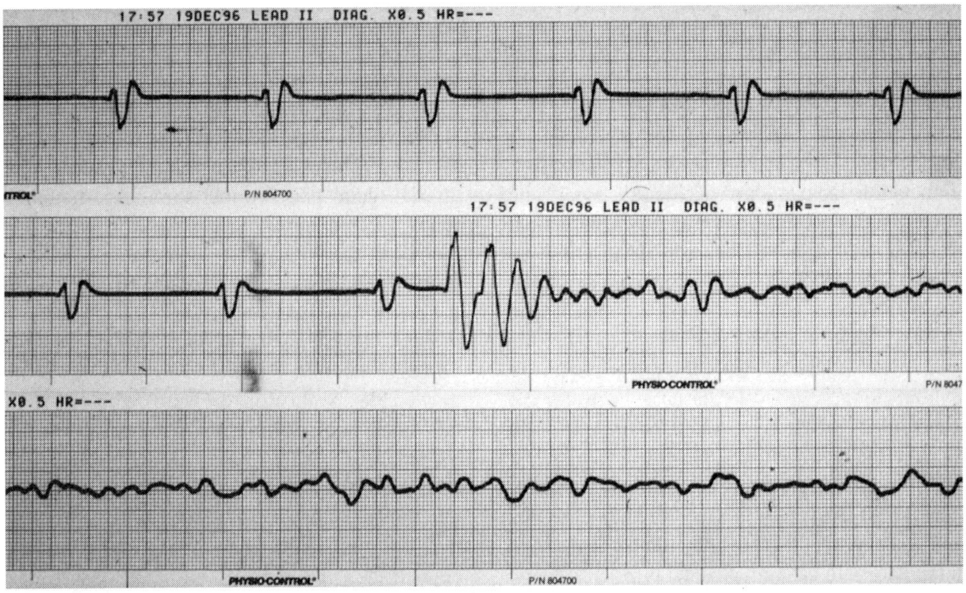

FIGURE 27-50 ECG tracing from an 8-year-old Labrador retriever with dilated cardiomyopathy. The dog arrested during a precordial thump. The initial rhythm is an idioventricular rhythm. The heart rate is 38 beats/min. There was no mechanical activity associated with the depolarizations (electromechanical dissociation). In the middle of the middle trace, several premature ventricular depolarizations occur, followed immediately by ventricular fibrillation. Resuscitation was unsuccessful. (Paper speed = 25 mm/sec; 1 cm = 0.5 mV.)

quickly follows cardiac arrest. Sodium bicarbonate may be administered if the cardiac arrest lasts longer than 2 to 3 minutes, as long as ventilation is adequate. If defibrillation is unsuccessful, epinephrine or lidocaine may be administered before subsequent attempts. Lidocaine can be administered after successful defibrillation to prevent recurrent ventricular fibrillation, especially if ventricular arrhythmias are present after defibrillation.

Torsades de pointes

Definition and ECG diagnosis. Torsades de pointes (turning about a point) is a rare arrhythmia in the dog. It has never been reported in the cat. Torsades de pointes was first reported in humans by Desertenne[53] in 1966. It is a form of polymorphic ventricular tachycardia or flutter in which the amplitude of the complexes increases and decreases in size so that they appear to twist around the baseline (see Figure 27-36). The rhythm can revert spontaneously to sinus rhythm or degenerate into ventricular fibrillation. Human patients with torsades de pointes are at risk for sudden death. The one case reported in the veterinary literature had an episode of ventricular fibrillation treated successfully with open-chest resuscitation and internal defibrillation.[10]

Mechanism. Torsades de pointes is thought to be due to early afterdepolarizations.[8] Therefore it is commonly associated with a long QT interval in humans. The one report in the veterinary literature of a canine patient with torsades de pointes also had a long QT interval.[10] The example in Figure 27-36 did not have a prolonged QT interval. Humans most commonly have a long QT interval because of inherited ion channel disease, electrolyte disturbances (hypokalemia, hypocalcemia, hypomagnesemia), or drug therapy.[54] Common drugs known to induce a long QT interval and torsades de pointes in humans are the class Ia antiarrhythmic drugs, such as quinidine and procainamide. Experimental canine models of long QT interval leading to torsades de pointes have been studied. Most of these models use either toxic doses of quinidine, quinidine plus myocardial infarction, or exotic drugs.[55-58] One potentially clinically relevant study examined the effect of quinidine, administered at a dose to produce a serum concentration within the therapeutic range, and 1% halothane in dogs anesthetized with pentobarbital.[59] In these dogs, quinidine did prolong the QT interval, and three of 20 dogs developed torsades de pointes when quinidine and halothane were administered together. We have never measured a prolonged QT interval in a dog that was being administered quinidine, even when the dogs were showing clinical signs of toxicity (e.g., ataxia, seizures). Consequently, we believe that the prolonged QT interval in this study must have been due to a combination of the anesthesia and the quinidine or other unknown factors. However, dogs administered halothane while they are being administered quinidine should probably be monitored closely with an ECG during the anesthetic period.

Treatment. In human patients with torsades de pointes resulting from a prolonged QT interval, treatment consists of administering agents that shorten the QT interval. Class Ia antiarrhythmic drugs (e.g., quinidine and procainamide), and class III drugs (e.g., amiodarone, bretylium) are avoided because they prolong the QT interval. Class Ib antiarrhythmic drugs (e.g., lidocaine), magnesium, and isoproterenol are more commonly effective.[58] Magnesium (1 to 2 mg/kg/min for 20 to 30 minutes) is successful at suppressing cesium-induced torsades de pointes in experimental dogs.[58] The one dog in the literature with torsades de pointes was treated with 150 mg/kg magnesium administered over 5 hours. When the QT interval is normal, standard antiarrhythmic therapy is employed.

IDIOVENTRICULAR RHYTHM

An idioventricular rhythm is the presence of only ventricular escape beats on an ECG tracing. It is usually a terminal rhythm that occurs when the sinus node and the AV junction are no longer functional. The last pacing cells to die in this situation are the Purkinje fiber cells. They depolarize at a rate approximately between 20 and 40 beats/min, although they can sometimes depolarize at a slightly faster rate if stimulated by catecholamine administration (see Figure 27-50). An idioventricular rhythm may be accompanied by electromechanical dissociation (no evidence of myocardial contraction during electrical stimulation).

ISORHYTHMIC ATRIOVENTRICULAR DISSOCIATION

Definition and ECG diagnosis. Atrioventricular dissociation is the atria and ventricles being controlled by separate pacemakers. Examples of AV dissociation include third-degree AV block and nodal or ventricular tachycardia without retrograde AV conduction. The term isorhythmic atrioventricular dissociation (IAVD) is used when the rates of the sinus node pacemaker and a nodal or ventricular pacemaker approximate each other and the sinus rate speeds and slows such that the P wave appears to be "marching" through the QRS complex (Figure 27-51).[60] Older terms for this phenomenon are accrochage and synchronization.[61] In IAVD, the pacemaker for the atria is usually the sinus node and the pacemaker for the ventricles can be within the AV junction or a ventricle. However, in cats and dogs, it is usually within the AV junction. This rhythm abnormality is uncommon but occurs most frequently in cats. We have observed it in apparently normal cats, in cats with cardiovascular disease, in anesthetized cats, and in cats with calcium channel blocker toxicity. Isorhythmic atrioventricular dissociation has also been reported in dogs with digitalis intoxication.[62] The rhythm appears essentially to be a nodal (junctional) tachycardia in which the sinus rate is responding in some manner to the nodal tachycardia in a rhythmic fashion.[60] From experimental studies, it appears that the sinus node rate in this abnormality fluctuates in response to hemodynamic changes initiated by the AV dissociation and then maintained by the rhythmic changes.[63] It appears that to initiate this type of abnormality, the ectopic nodal pacemaker rate and the sinus rate must be similar, with the nodal pacemaker being slightly faster. When the nodal pacemaker is slightly faster than the sinus node, ventricular depolarization and sinus depolarization, instead of being synchronized with atrial contraction occurring before ventricular contraction, become fused together (the *P* wave and the QRS complex occur at the same time on the ECG). When this occurs, atrial contribution to ventricular filling is lost because the atria contract at the same time that the ventricles contract. When the atrial contribution is lost to filling, stroke volume on subsequent beats decreases. When the atria contract against closed AV valves, atrial pressure increases. It appears that the decrease in stroke volume results in a decrease in systemic arterial blood pressure that stimulates the baroreceptor stimulation reflex.[64] This increases sympathetic tone to the sinus node and increases the sinus rate. Simultaneously, the increase in atrial pressure stretches atrial muscle and sinus node tissue, which also increases the sinus node rate. Consequently, the sinus node rate increases, bringing atrial contraction out before ventricular contraction again and the P wave before the QRS complex. Stroke volume now increases and atrial pressure decreases, resulting in a slowing of the sinus rate, starting the cycle over. The electrocardiographic diagnosis of IAVD is based on identifying *P* waves in front of the QRS complexes at some time and then observing the *P* waves move into the QRS complexes and disappear and then reappear in front of the QRS complexes. Sometimes the *P* waves may move all the way beyond the QRS complexes instead of just into them.

Treatment. The hemodynamic consequences of IAVD are related purely to the rate of the ectopic pacemaker. If the rate is within the normal range, the arrhythmia is hemodynamically insignificant and therefore no therapy is required. We have observed several cats with this rhythm for months to years. If the rate is very fast, antiarrhythmic therapy may be warranted. We have very little experience treating this arrhythmia because usually the rate is within normal limits. In human patients, both β-blockers and atropine have been effective at disrupting the arrhythmia, probably by disrupting the pathways influenced by baroreceptor and atrial receptor stimulation in this abnormality.[65,66] The administration of magnesium is also effective in humans.[67] If an underlying abnormality such as heart failure is present, treating the abnormality may result in regression of the arrhythmia.

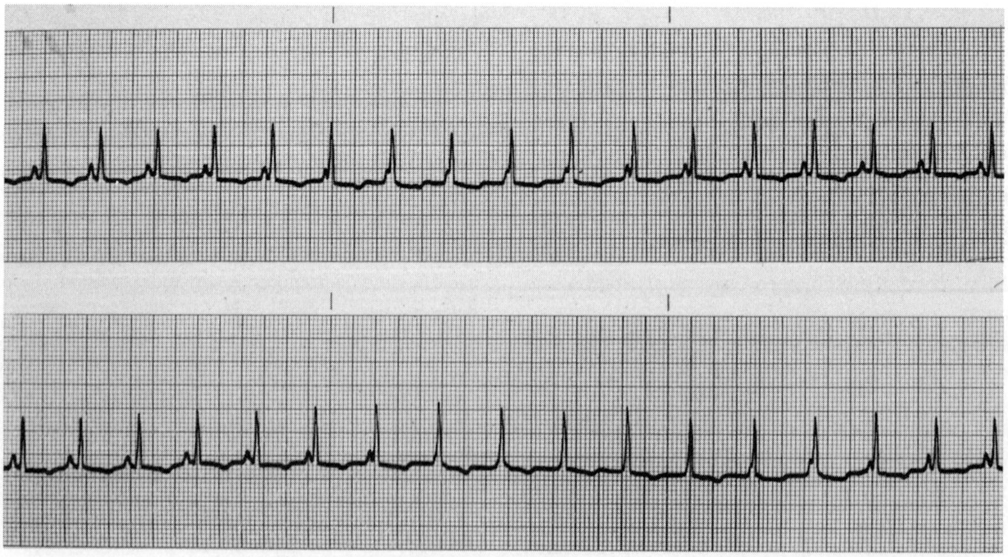

FIGURE 27-51 Lead II ECG tracing recorded from a 1-year-old cat with cauda equina syndrome, mild hypertrophic cardiomyopathy, and systolic anterior motion of the mitral valve. The cat has a supraventricular rhythm with the *P* waves "marching" in and out of the QRS complexes. This is isorhythmic atrioventricular (AV) dissociation in which there is a nodal tachycardia, and the sinus node is depolarizing at a very similar rate to the AV nodal (junctional) tissue. The sinus rate varies slightly in response to changing hemodynamics. (See text for details.) (Paper speed = 25 mm/sec; 1 cm = 1 mV.)

ATRIOVENTRICULAR BLOCKS

Atrioventricular (AV) block refers to conduction disturbances that alter conduction of the cardiac electrical impulse from the sinus node to the ventricles. Altered intraatrial conduction, altered AV junctional conduction, altered bundle of His conduction, and altered conduction in both bundle branches simultaneously can result in altered AV conduction (Figure 27-52). AV blocks are classified as first-, second-, and third-degree AV blocks. First-degree AV block is prolonged conduction, second-degree AV block is intermittent conduction, and third-degree AV block is lack of conduction. AV conduction is assessed by examining the relationship between the *P* waves and the QRS complexes. First-degree AV block is characterized by a prolonged P-R interval. Second-degree AV block is characterized by atrial depolarizations (*P* waves) intermittently failing to reach the ventricles. In third-degree AV block, AV conduction does not occur (complete block), and the atria and the ventricles are controlled by separate pacemakers (a form of AV dissociation).

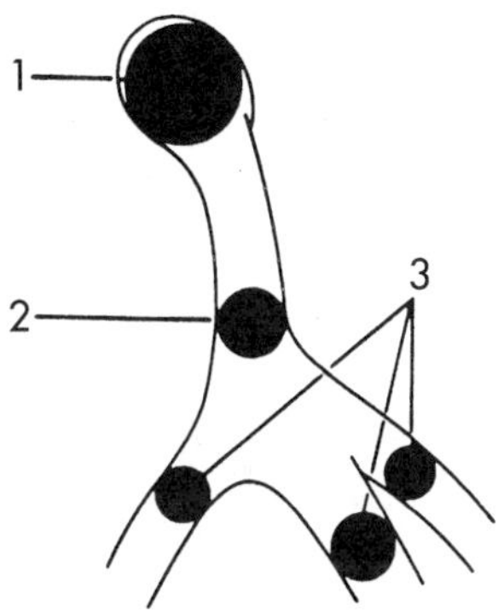

FIGURE 27-52 Schematic drawing of the AV node (1), bundle of His (2), and bundle branches (3). Disease in each of these three areas can result in various grades of atrioventricular block. (From Tilley LP: *Essentials of canine and feline electrocardiography,* ed 3, Philadelphia, 1992, Lea & Febiger.)

First-degree atrioventricular block

Definition and ECG diagnosis. First-degree AV block is a prolongation in the P-R interval. It does not result in an arrhythmia but is included in this chapter for continuity. First-degree AV block is diagnosed when the P-R interval is greater than 0.13 seconds in a dog and greater than 0.09 seconds in a cat. It can occur as an isolated abnormality or be present in conjunction with second-degree AV block (Figure 27-53). First-degree AV block occurs when the conduction time from the sinus node to the ventricles is prolonged beyond normal. An impulse originating in the sinus node must traverse the internodal tracts, the AV node, the bundle of His, and the bundle branches. Conduction delays in any of these regions are common causes of first-degree AV block in humans.[68] The exact site of conduction delay cannot be discerned from a surface ECG, and studies have not been performed to determine the exact regions of block in canine and feline patients. Electrophysiologic testing in which intracardiac electrograms are recorded is required to determine the exact location. In humans, prolongation of conduction wave propagation through the atria causing a wide *P* wave can cause a first-degree AV block. This is very unusual in dogs and cats.

Causes. First-degree AV block can occur because of degenerative or inflammatory disease of the conduction system. It can also occur secondary to drug administration (e.g., digitalis glycosides, β-blockers, calcium channel blockers), hyperkalemia, and increased vagal tone. Although quinidine and procainamide are listed as drugs that can prolong the P-R interval in humans, we have only ever noted such an increase in dogs with quinidine toxicity.

Prognosis. The prognosis for first-degree AV block is good to guarded. First-degree AV blocks that occur secondary to drug administration and electrolyte abnormalities disappear when these abnormalities are corrected. First-degree AV blocks secondary to increased vagal tone result in no clinical sequelae. Degenerative disease of the conduction system mild enough to produce only

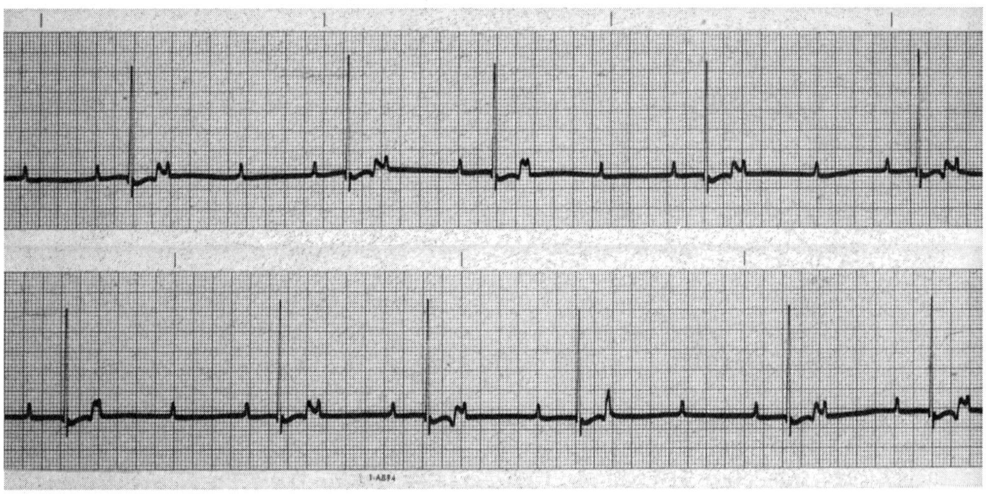

FIGURE 27-53 Lead II ECG tracing recorded from a 12-year-old Rhodesian ridgeback presented because of three episodes of syncope over the previous 10 months. The P-R interval is markedly prolonged to 0.36 seconds (first-degree atrioventricular [AV] block). The rhythm is a second-degree AV block that varies between 3:1 and 2:1 second-degree AV block. The atrial rate is reasonably constant at approximately 80 beats/min. When there is a 2:1 block, the ventricular rate is approximately 40 beats/min. When the block is 3:1 it is approximately 27 beats/min. This is an example of first-degree AV block and high-grade second-degree AV block. Atropine administration increased the atrial rate but did not change the ventricular rate. A pacemaker was implanted. (Paper speed = 25 mm/sec; 1 cm = 1 mV.)

first-degree AV block often does not progress. However, it may, on occasion, progress to higher degrees of AV block. No treatment is necessary for first-degree AV block.

Second-degree atrioventricular block

Definition and ECG diagnosis. Second-degree AV block occurs when some sinus depolarizations conduct through the AV junction to reach the ventricles while others do not. On auscultation it is heard as "dropped beats." Second-degree AV block produces an abnormal heart rhythm and is one cause of cardiac arrhythmia. Second-degree AV block can range in severity from only an occasional P wave not followed by a QRS complex on the ECG to most P waves being blocked. Second-degree AV block is divided into type I, type II, and high-grade blocks. In a type I (Mobitz type I), or Wenckebach, second-degree AV block, the P-R interval progressively prolongs before the block (Figure 27-54). The P-R interval before the block may be normal or too long (first-degree AV block). Type II (Mobitz type II) second-degree AV block is characterized by sudden failure of conduction without alteration in the P-R interval (Figure 27-55). The P-R interval may be normal or prolonged. Second-degree AV blocks are commonly labeled with the number of *P* waves followed by the number of QRS complexes generated. For example, if every other sinus depolarization is blocked from reaching the ventricles, this is called a *2:1 second-degree AV block.* Similarly, if every fourth *P* wave is not followed by a QRS complex, it is called a *4:3 AV block* (four *P* waves and three QRS complexes). Any block that is 2:1 or greater cannot be classified as type I or type II because there is no chance to determine whether progressive prolongation is occurring or not. Consequently, it is called a *high-grade block* (see Figure 27-53).

Mechanisms. Second-degree AV block can be a normal finding (functional second-degree AV block). The normal AV node prevents rapid impulses from being transmitted to the ventricles. This type of functional block is extremely important in patients with atrial fibrillation or atrial flutter. If the AV junction was not present, atrial fibrillation and flutter would conduct 1:1 to the ventricles, resulting in ventricular fibrillation and immediate death. This functional block is commonly ascribed to a physiologic property of the AV node called *decremental conduction.* Decremental conduction is the attenuation of action potential amplitude as it progresses through the AV node and therefore a reduction in its efficacy to stimulate adjoining cells. More recently, however, it has been shown to be due to changes in

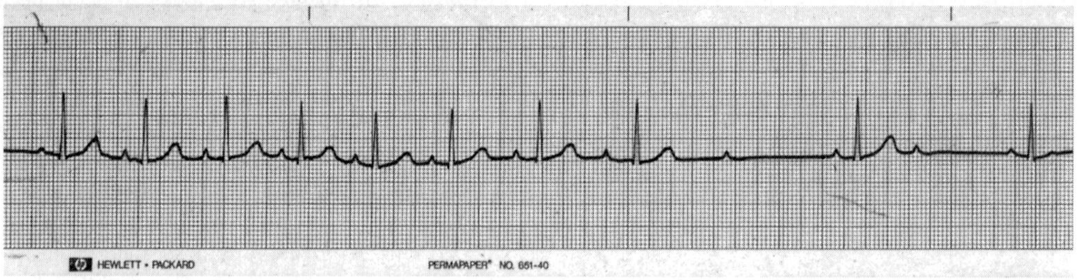

FIGURE 27-54 Lead II ECG tracing recorded from a dog with chronic respiratory disease and an arrhythmia. The ninth *P* wave is not followed by a QRS complex. Before this "dropped beat" the P-R interval prolongs and then shortens immediately after the block. This is an example of a Mobitz type I (Type I or Wenckebach) second-degree atrioventricular (AV) block. This type of AV block is usually vagally induced and can be abolished with atropine administration. (Paper speed = 50 mm/sec; 1 cm = 1 mV.)

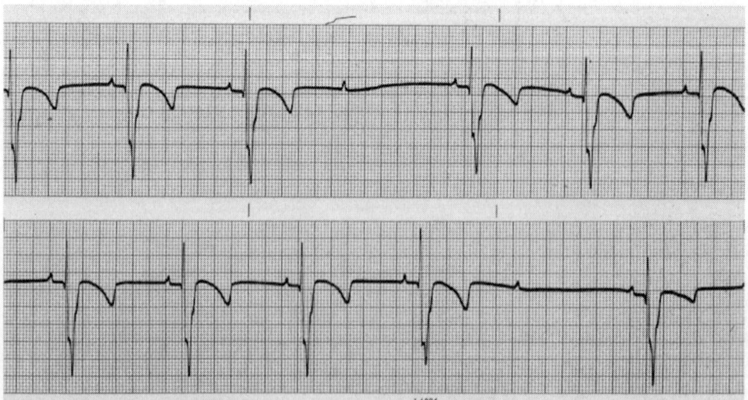

FIGURE 27-55 Lead II ECG tracing recorded from a 14-year-old mixed-breed dog with an arrhythmia. The rhythm is a sinus rhythm with intermittent periods of second-degree atrioventricular (AV) block. The P-R interval does not change before or after the block, so this is a Mobitz type II (Type II) second-degree AV block. The QRS complex configuration is abnormal (deep and wide S waves), and the complexes are too wide. The mean electrical axis and the terminal axis were shifted to the right. Consequently, the diagnosis was a type II second-degree AV block with a right bundle branch block. In humans, this type of pattern is consistent with disease of both bundle branches and is likely to progress to a high-grade second-degree AV block or third-degree AV block. This dog progressed to a third-degree AV block, developed syncope, and had an artificial pacemaker implanted. (Paper speed = 50 mm/sec; 1 cm = 1 mV.)

excitability of normal nodal cells during the cardiac cycle.[69] Briefly, AV nodal cells have a slow recovery of excitability. This slow recovery is exacerbated as heart rate increases. This results in a progressive decrease in upstroke velocity of phase 0 of depolarization on the action potentials of AV nodal cells. This translates into a progressive decrease in conduction velocity, which progresses to a point at which the cells are less excitable and produce a very small action potential that does not conduct, resulting in the conduction block.[70] AV nodal cells also have another unique property—the refractory period of AV nodal cells lasts well into diastole.[69] This prolonged refractory period results in the AV node not allowing atrial depolarizations to reach the ventricles when the atrial rate is very fast. This is called a functional second-degree AV block. It occurs most frequently in patients with atrial fibrillation.

As with first-degree AV block, conduction abnormalities in any region of the conduction system can create second-degree AV block. Few studies have been performed to delineate the exact sites of block in dogs or cats with second-degree AV block. In humans, type I second-degree AV block is rarely or uncommonly caused by abnormalities in intraatrial, His bundle, or bundle branch conduction.[68] Most type I second-degree AV blocks are caused by drug toxicity, physiologic changes, or disease within the AV node itself. One study in dogs, however, has documented type I second-degree AV block in dogs with His bundle pathology created by ischemia.[70] Type II blocks in humans, on the other hand, are almost never due to intraatrial or AV nodal abnormalities. Instead, the vast majority are due to disease of the His bundle or bundle branches. Concomitant bundle branch block patterns to the QRS complexes are more common with type II and high-grade second-degree AV blocks because the site of second-degree block is often in the bundle branches.

Causes. Second-degree AV block can be observed in normal dogs, especially in puppies 8 to 11 weeks of age.[71] This normal finding only occurs when dogs are at rest and is a Mobitz type I block. The presence of second-degree AV block in a dog in an examination room is almost always abnormal. Second-degree AV block can occur secondary to increased vagal tone. The AV node is richly innervated with vagal fibers. Consequently, increased vagal tone usually produces a type I rather than a type II second-degree AV block. Chronic respiratory disease is a common cause of second-degree AV block secondary to increased vagal tone in dogs. Digitalis intoxication is an example of a drug that can produce second-degree AV block, primarily through its ability to increase vagal tone. Other drugs that can cause second-degree AV block via vagal stimulation include xylazine and intravenous atropine. The increase in vagal tone with intravenous atropine occurs before the decrease in vagal tone and is transient. Second-degree AV block can also be due to conduction system disease. The classic example is hereditary stenosis of the bundle of His in pugs. Although this condition is rarely observed, it has been well described in the literature in a small group of related dogs.[72] These dogs were studied because they experienced episodes of syncope and died suddenly. At necropsy, no lesions were found in any part of the conduction system except the bundle of His, which was markedly narrowed and abnormally fibrotic at its midpoint. The authors of this study attempted to attribute all of their findings to this anatomic abnormality. However, the second-degree AV block in these dogs was a type I block. In addition, the syncope and sudden death were due to periods of sinus node inactivity or permanent sinus node inactivity, and the periods of sinus arrest and AV block were abolished with atropine administration. Consequently, it appears that there must have been additional abnormalities in these dogs and that the clinical picture is due to more complex phenomena than just the His bundle abnormality. Recently, we identified a very young pug with third-degree AV block that could be due to the same type of abnormality or to unrelated disease. In humans, type II second-degree AV block is more likely to progress to third-degree AV block. This is unknown in dogs or cats. The fact that ischemia to the His bundle can create a type I second-degree AV block in dogs suggests that a type I second-degree AV block may not always be a benign lesion.[70]

Treatment. Patients with type I or type II second-degree AV blocks generally do not exhibit any clinical signs. Consequently, usually no treatment is necessary for these patients except to remove an inciting cause if one exists. Dogs with high-grade second-degree AV block may not exhibit any clinical signs or may have signs identical to dogs with third-degree AV block (primarily syncope and weakness). Treatment for these patients is outlined below.

An ECG from a 12-year-old Rhodesian ridgeback with frequent bouts of syncope and exercise intolerance is presented in Figure 27-53. A 3:1 (high-grade) second-degree AV block is present, along with first-degree AV block (P-R interval = 0.36 seconds). The owner reported that the heart rate in this dog varied from 35 to 50 beats/min at home. Medical therapy with metaproterenol (sympathomimetic), propantheline (anticholinergic), and aminophylline had been tried without success. An artificial pacemaker was implanted. There were no more syncopal events, and the owners reported that the dog was more "lively."

Third-degree atrioventricular block

Definition and ECG diagnosis. Third-degree AV block (complete heart block) occurs when there is no conduction between the sinus node and the ventricles (Figures 27-56 and 27-57). This can be produced experimentally in dogs by injecting 95% alcohol into the AV junction.[73] In third-degree AV block, the sinus node depolarizes at its own inherent rate, depolarizing the atria and producing *P* waves, whereas the ventricles are depolarized by a subsidiary pacemaker (either the AV node or Purkinje fibers) that depolarizes at a slower rate, depolarizing the ventricles and producing QRS complexes. On the ECG, there is no relationship between the *P* waves and QRS complexes (AV dissociation), resulting in varying P-R intervals from beat to beat. Because the sinus node depolarizes at a rate faster

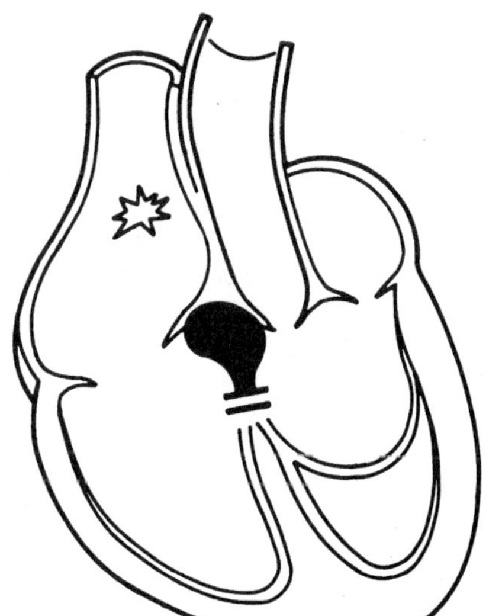

FIGURE 27-56 Schematic drawing of third-degree atrioventricular block. (From Edwards NJ: *Bolton's handbook of canine and feline electrocardiography,* ed 2, Philadelphia, 1990, WB Saunders.)

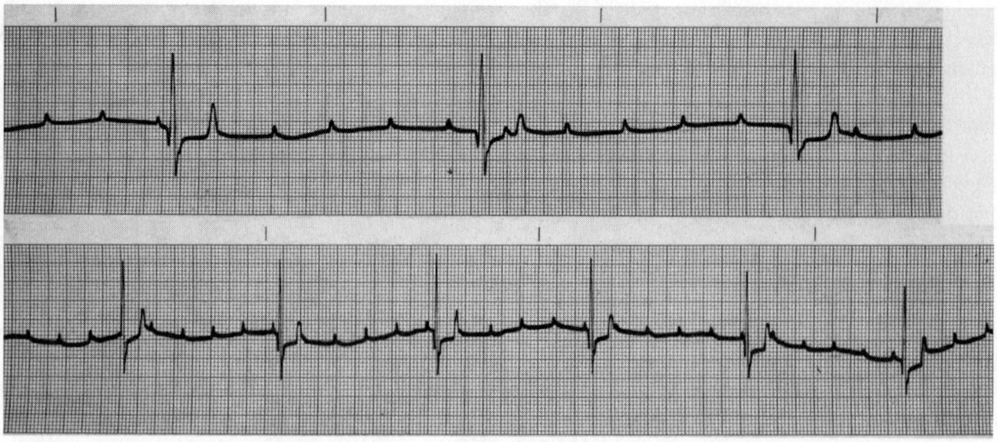

FIGURE 27-57 Lead II ECG tracings recorded from a dog presented for syncope. The P waves and the QRS complexes are dissociated (atrioventricular (AV) dissociation), as evidenced by the varying P-R intervals. The sinus rate (approximately 180 beats/min) is faster than the ventricular rate (35 beats/min). These characteristics are diagnostic of third-degree AV block. The ventricular rate suggests that the escape rhythm originates in the Purkinje fibers. The QRS duration, however, is normal, which means that the escape focus must be in the AV junction. (Top, Paper speed = 50 mm/sec; 1 cm = 1 mV. Bottom, Paper speed = 25 mm/sec; 1 cm = 1 mV.

than the subsidiary pacemaker, the atrial rate is faster (the P-P interval is shorter) than the ventricular rate (the R-R interval is longer) (Figure 27-57). The atrial rate and the ventricular rate are often constant such that the P-P intervals and the R-R intervals are constant.

Mechanisms. No studies have been performed to delineate the site of the conduction block in dogs with third-degree AV block. In humans, the blockage site is commonly in the AV node, the bundle of His, or the bundle branches (a so-called trifascicular block). It has been stated that third-degree AV block occurs if all three atrial internodal tracts are sectioned in experimental dogs.[68] This is surprising because this is not known to occur in humans and suggests that atrial myocardium is electrically isolated from the conduction system in dogs.

Causes. The cause of third-degree AV block in almost all cases is unknown. Most canine and feline patients with third-degree AV block are middle-age–to–geriatric patients. This may suggest a degenerative disease of the conduction system. Rarely, a dog less than 1 year of age will present with third-degree AV block that may be congenital, as in the pug described above. Third-degree AV block has been reported in one dog with myocarditis that was seropositive for Lyme disease.[74] AV block also has been described in humans with Lyme carditis. The AV block in this disease is usually transient. Occasionally, third-degree AV block in dogs will spontaneously resolve or resolve after corticosteroid administration, suggesting an inflammatory lesion in the conduction system.[75] It is interesting to speculate that this situation could be secondary to Lyme carditis, but there is no evidence to support this possibility at this time. AV nodal disease has been described in dogs that have died suddenly. Lesions described include mineralization of the crest of the interventricular septum, with degeneration and fibrosis of the AV conduction fibers and cartilage and bone formation in the central fibrous body.[76] Doberman pinschers appear to be overly represented in the group of dogs described with these findings.[77]

Clinical signs. Dogs with third-degree AV block generally either have no clinical signs or are presented because they are having episodes of syncope. Most cats have no clinical signs of their disorder. In general, clinical presentation depends on the underlying heart rate. Dogs generally fall into two categories—those with a ventricular rate between 40 and 60 beats/min and those with a heart rate between 20 and 40 beats/min. His bundle escape rhythms typically have a rate of 35 to 65 beats/min, so the AV node is likely the site of the block in dogs with this type of heart rate (see Figure 27-57). The subsidiary pacemaker cells in the bundle of His produce a relatively stable rhythm, and a heart rate of 40 to 60 beats/min is adequate for dogs that do not exercise strenuously. Consequently, third-degree AV block in these dogs is commonly diagnosed as an incidental finding when a bradycardia is ausculted and a subsequent ECG performed. There may or may not be a concomitant bundle branch block. Pacemaker cells in the bundle branches and distal Purkinje fibers depolarize at a slower rate (20 to 40 beats/min) than the bundle of His. On the ECG, the ventricular rate is slow and the QRS complexes are wide, indicating a bundle branch block (when the subsidiary pacemaker is a bundle branch) or a ventricular origin to the QRS complexes (when the subsidiary pacemaker is a Purkinje fiber) (Figure 27-58). The site of the conduction system blockage in these dogs is most likely in the bundle of His or the bundle branches. Diffuse disease of the bundle branches and Purkinje network is the most common cause of clinically important third-degree AV block in adult humans.[78] Dogs with this type of rhythm may show no clinical signs, but most are presented because they are fainting or weak. There are at least three explanations for why these dogs have syncopal events. We have witnessed each of these. First, the pacemaker cells in the bundle branches and Purkinje fibers are less stable and often diseased; therefore they spontaneously cease to fire, resulting in periods of asystole. Second, dogs with conduction system disease may also have episodes of tachyarrhythmia from an ectopic site. When pacemaker cells are depolarized repetitively by a faster focus of depolarization, it takes them time to recover their normal inherent rate once the faster focus ceases to fire (overdrive suppression). It appears that diseased pacing cells can take prolonged periods to recover, as seen in Figure 27-59. Prolonged periods of ventricular asystole can result. Third, when a dog with a fixed rate and slow ventricular rate becomes excited and starts to exercise, systemic arterioles dilate and, if cardiac output cannot increase, systemic arterial blood pressure decreases. If it decreases to a level less than required for cerebral perfusion, syncope occurs.

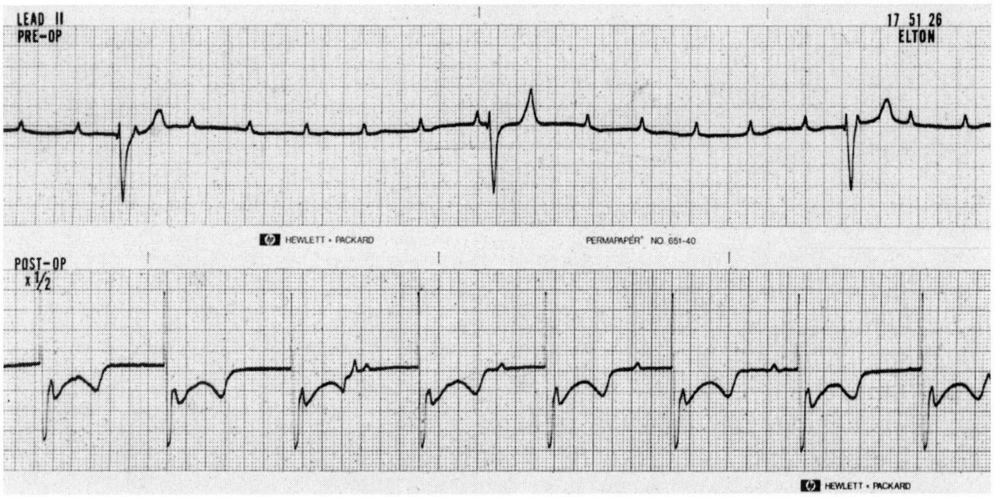

FIGURE 27-58 *Top,* Lead II ECG tracing recorded from an 8-year-old toy poodle presented for syncope. The rhythm is third-degree atrioventricular block. The ventricular rate is 30 beats/min, and the QRS complexes are wide and bizarre. This is typical of a ventricular (Purkinje fiber) escape rhythm. *Bottom,* Another lead II ECG tracing after pacemaker implantation. The pacemaker rate is set at 90 beats/min. The lead was placed transvenously and in the right ventricular apex. The initial sharp deflection is the generator depolarizing ("a pacemaker spike"). This is followed by a very bizarre-appearing QRS complex followed by a bizarre *T* wave. (Paper speed = 50 mm/sec; 1 cm = 1 mV.)

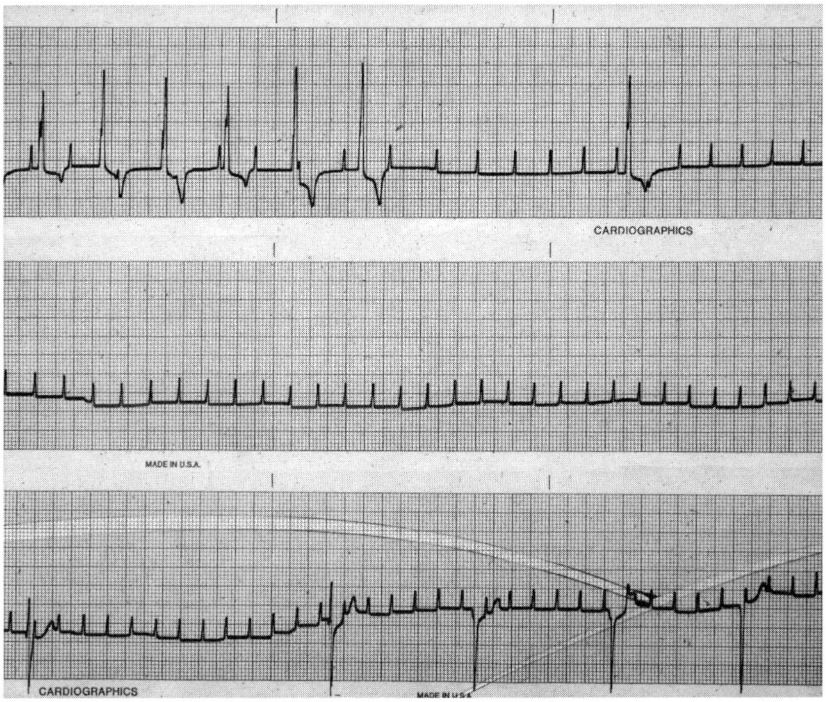

FIGURE 27-59 Continuous lead II ECG tracings recorded from a 12-year-old Pekingese that was having episodes of syncope every 3 to 7 minutes on presentation. The basic rhythm is third-degree atrioventricular block. The initial rhythm appears to be a supraventricular ectopic rhythm that depolarizes at a rate of 85 beats/min. This ectopic focus abruptly terminates and is followed by a prolonged period in which the escape focus is suppressed (overdrive suppression). This results in a long period (14.4 seconds) in which very little ventricular activity occurs. Consequently, there is a long period of cerebral hypoperfusion. The dog had a syncopal episode that started about the middle of the second tracing. It started to regain consciousness at the end of the last tracing. (Paper speed = 25 mm/sec; 1 cm = 1 mV.)

Apparently, the subsidiary pacemakers in cats depolarize at a faster rate than those of dogs and humans. Cats with third-degree AV block generally present with a ventricular rate of 80 to 130 beats/min on their ECG (Figure 27-60). Because cat's ventricular rates are generally quite fast and because cats are usually sedentary, those with third-degree AV block usually do not exhibit any clinical signs.

Clinical findings. On physical examination, most dogs with third-degree AV block appear normal between syncopal events. However, in some dogs the heart rate is slow enough to produce signs of weakness. In dogs that appear weak, we usually measure whole blood lactate concentration. In many of these dogs it is increased, signifying inadequate oxygen delivery to systemic tissues because of a low cardiac output.

On auscultation, the heart rate is slow and the first heart sound may be loud. By listening carefully in a quiet room, one can often identify soft fourth heart sounds in the background. These sounds are generated each time the atria contract. Cannon a waves may be generated in the jugular veins when atrial contraction occurs during a time that the mitral valve is closed. On echocardiography, the left

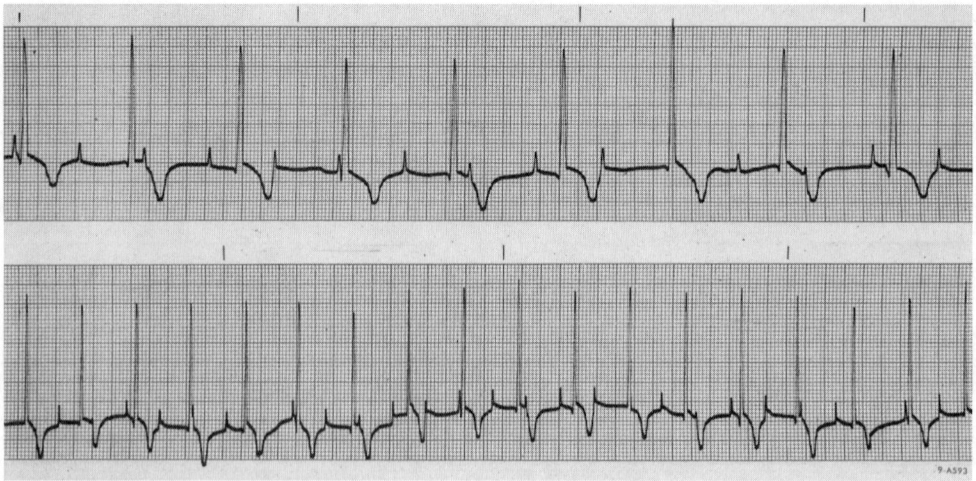

FIGURE 27-60 Lead II ECG tracings recorded from a 12-year-old cat. The referring veterinarian had ausculted a heart rate of 100 beats/min and obtained an ECG. She had correctly diagnosed third-degree atrioventricular (AV) block. The atrial rate is 170 beats/min, and the ventricular rate is 100 beats/min. The QRS complex width is normal. Consequently, the escape rhythm is a nodal escape rhythm. Apparently, the nodal pacemaker in cats depolarizes at a rate of 80 to 130 beats/min, as opposed to 35 to 65 beats/min in dogs. This cat was asymptomatic, as most cats with third-degree AV block are, and so no treatment was attempted. (*Top,* Paper speed = 50 mm/sec; 1 cm = 1 mV. *Bottom,* Paper speed = 25 mm/sec; 1 cm = 1 mV.)

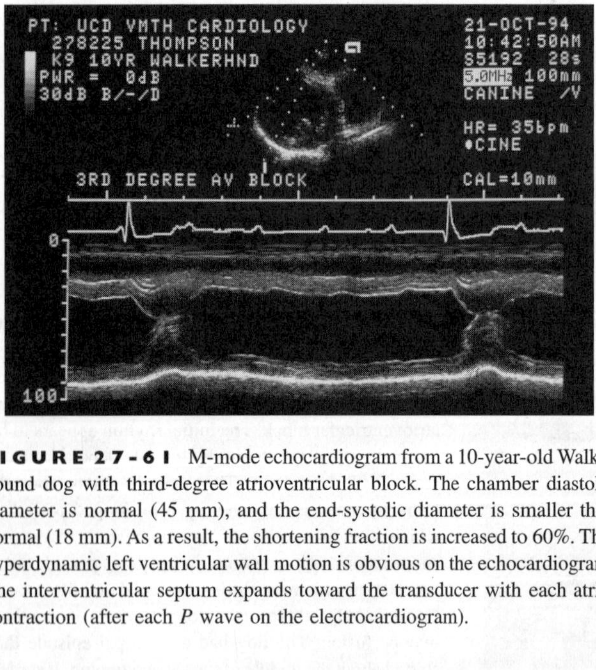

FIGURE 27-61 M-mode echocardiogram from a 10-year-old Walker hound dog with third-degree atrioventricular block. The chamber diastolic diameter is normal (45 mm), and the end-systolic diameter is smaller than normal (18 mm). As a result, the shortening fraction is increased to 60%. This hyperdynamic left ventricular wall motion is obvious on the echocardiogram. The interventricular septum expands toward the transducer with each atrial contraction (after each *P* wave on the electrocardiogram).

ventricular chamber is commonly mildly-to-moderately increased in size in diastole (Figure 27-61). During systole, the ventricle is hyperdynamic, contracting down to a smaller-than-normal end-systolic diameter. Consequently, an increased stroke volume is produced. During diastole, the left ventricular chamber can be seen to increase slightly in size after each atrial contraction (i.e., after each *P* wave on the electrocardiogram).

Treatment. The treatment of third-degree AV block is implantation of an external pacing generator and lead ("artificial pacemaker") (see Figure 27-58). (See the discussion of treatment in Chapter 30.) We generally administer atropine at the time of presentation, but it is rare to observe any improvement in AV conduction. Usually the only thing that happens is that the atrial rate increases while the ventricular rate remains constant. Some dogs with very slow heart rates (usually less than 30 beats/min) are very weak, and some are unable to stand at presentation. In these dogs, we measure a blood lactate concentration. If it is increased, we place a temporary pacemaker, implant a permanent pacemaker on an emergency basis, or administer isoproterenol as a constant-rate intravenous infusion to increase the heart rate until a permanent pacemaker can be implanted. Isoproterenol infusion is generally safe but tachyarrhythmias and hypotension secondary to systemic arteriolar dilation can be produced.

REFERENCES

1. Irisawa H, Noma A, Matsuda H: Electrogenesis of the pacemaker potentials as revealed by atrioventricular nodal experiments. In Sperelakis N, ed: *Physiology and pathophysiology of the heart,* ed 3, Boston, 1995, Kluwer.
2. Hoffman BF, Rosen MR: Cellular mechanisms for cardiac arrhythmias, *Circ Res* 49:1, 1981.
3. Hauer RN, de Bakker JM, de Wilde AA et al: Ventricular tachycardia after in vivo DC shock ablation in dogs: electrophysiologic and histologic correlation, *Circulation* 84:267, 1991.
4. Sorota S: Swelling-induced chloride-sensitive current in canine atrial cells revealed by whole-cell patch-clamp method, *Circ Res* 70:679, 1992.
5. Vos MA, Gorgels AP, Leunissen JD et al: Further observations to confirm the arrhythmia mechanism-specific effects of flunarizine, *J Cardiovasc Pharmacol* 19:682, 1992.
6. Muir WW, Weisbrode SE: Myocardial ischemia in dogs with gastric dilatation-volvulus, *J Am Vet Med Assoc* 181:363, 1982.
7. Ilvento JP, Provet J, Danilo PJ et al: Fast and slow idioventricular rhythms in the canine heart: a study of their mechanism using anti-arrhythmic drugs and electrophysiologic testing, *Am J Cardiol* 49:1909, 1982.
8. Antzelevitch C, Sicouri S: Clinical relevance of cardiac arrhythmias generated by afterdepolarizations: role of M cells in the generation of U waves, triggered activity and torsade de pointes, *J Am Coll Cardiol* 23:259, 1994.
9. Sicouri S, Fish J, Antzelevitch C: Distribution of M cells in the canine ventricle, *J Cardiovasc Electrophysiol* 5:824, 1994.

10. Baty CJ, Sweet DC, Keene BW: Torsades de pointes-like polymorphic ventrifcular tachycardia in a dog, *J Vet Intern Med* 8:439, 1994.
11. Moise NS, Gilmour RF, Riccio ML et al: Diagnosis of inherited ventricular tachycardia in German shepherd dogs, *J Am Vet Med Assoc* 210:403, 1997.
12. Rosen MR, Gelband H, Merker C et al: Mechanisms of digitalis toxicity: effects of ouabain on phase four of canine Purkinje fiber transmembrane potentials, *Circulation* 47:681, 1973.
13. Sicouri S, Antzelevitch C: Drug-induced afterdepolarizations and triggered activity occur in a discrete subpopulation of ventricular muscle cells (M cells) in the canine heart: quinidine and digitalis, *J Cardiovasc Electrophysiol* 4:48, 1993.
14. Hamlin RL, Smetzer DL, Breznock EM: Sinoatrial syncope in miniature schnauzers, *J Am Vet Med Assoc* 161:1022, 1972.
15. Elizari MV, Lazzari JO, Rosenbaum MB: Phase-3 and phase-4 intermittent left bundle branch block occurring spontaneously in a dog, *Eur J Cardiol* 1:95, 1973.
16. Waldo AL, Vitikainen KJ, Hoffman BF: The sequence of retrograde atrial activation in the canine heart: correlation with positive and negative retrograde P waves, *Circ Res* 37:156, 1975.
17. de Madron E, Kadish A, Spear JF et al: Incessant atrial tachycardias in a dog with tricuspid dysplasia: clinical management and electrophysiology, *J Vet Intern Med* 1:163, 1987.
18. Kittleson M, Keene B, Pion P et al: Verapamil administration for acute termination of supraventricular tachycardia in dogs, *J Am Vet Med Assoc* 193:1525, 1988.
19. Hill BL, Tilley LP: Ventricular preexcitation in seven dogs and nine cats, *J Am Vet Med Assoc* 187:1026, 1985.
20. Atkins CE, Kanter R, Wright K et al: Orthodromic reciprocating tachycardia and heart failure in a dog with a concealed posteroseptal accessory pathway, *J Vet Intern Med* 9:43, 1995.
21. Chatterjee K: Digitalis, catecholamines, and other positive inotropic agents. In Chatterjee K, Cheitlin MD, Karliner J et al, eds: *Cardiology: an illustrated text reference,* Philadelphia, 1991, JB Lippincott.
22. Marriot HJL, Myerburg RJ: Recognition of cardiac arrhythmias and conduction disturbances. In Hurst JW, Schlant RC, Rackley CE et al, eds: *The heart,* ed 7, New York, 1990, McGraw-Hill.
23. Allessie MA, Lammers WJ, Bonke IM et al: Intra-atrial reentry as a mechanism for atrial flutter induced by acetylcholine and rapid pacing in the dog, *Circulation* 70:123, 1984.
24. Wu KM, Hoffman BF: Effect of procainamide and N-acetylprocainamide on atrial flutter: studies in vivo and in vitro, *Circulation* 76:1397, 1987.
25. Toivonen L, Kadish A, Kou W et al: Determinants of the ventricular rate during atrial fibrillation, *J Am Coll Cardiol* 16:1194, 1990.
26. Landymore R, Kinley CE: Staple closure of the left atrial appendage, *Can J Surg* 27:144, 1984.
27. Sisson D, Brown W, Riepe R: Hemodynamic effects of atrial fibrillation in dogs with experimentally induced mitral regurgitation, *J Vet Intern Med* 9:200, 1995 (abstract).
28. Wilson JR, Douglas P, Hickey WF et al: Experimental congestive heart failure produced by rapid ventricular pacing in the dog: cardiac effects, *Circulation* 75:857, 1987.
29. Hamlin RL: What is the best heart rate for a dog in atrial fibrillation? *Proc Annu Vet Med Forum,* 1995, p 325.
30. Brand FN, Abbott RD, Kannel WB et al: Characteristics and prognosis of lone atrial fibrillation: 30-year follow-up in the Framingham Study, *JAMA* 254:3449, 1985.
31. Muir WW: Electrocardiographic interpretation of thiobarbiturate-induced dysrhythmias in dogs, *J Am Vet Med Assoc* 170:1419, 1977
32. Muir WW: Effects of atropine on cardiac rate and rhythm in dogs, *J Am Vet Md Assoc* 172:917, 1978.
33. Bednarski RM, Muir WW: Arrhythmogenicity of dopamine, dobutamine, and epinephrine in thiamylal-halothane anesthetized dogs, *Am J Vet Res* 44:2341, 1983.
34. Lown B, Wolf M: Approaches to sudden death from coronary heart disease, *Circulation* 44:130, 1971.
35. Multicenter Postinfarction Research Group: Risk stratification and survival after myocardial infarction, *N Engl J Med* 309:331, 1983.
36. Anderson JL: Clinical implications of new studies in the treatment of benign, potentially malignant and malignant ventricular arrhythmias, *Am J Cardiol* 65:36B, 1990.
37. Anderson KP, Freedman RA, Mason JW: Use of antiarrhythmic drugs: general principles. In Chatterjee K, Cheitlin MD, Karliner J et al, eds: *Cardiology: an illustrated reference,* Philadelphia, 1991, JB Lippincott.
38. Thomas LJJ, Miller JP. Long-term ambulatory ECG recording in the determination of antidysrhythmic drug efficacy. In Lucchesi BR, Dingell JV, Schwarz RPJ, eds: *Clinical pharmacology of antiarrhythmic therapy,* New York, 1984, Raven.
39. von Olshausen K, Schafer A, Mehmel HC et al: Ventricular arrhythmias in idiopathic dilated cardiomyopathy, *Br Heart J* 51:195, 1984.
40. Calvert CA: Diagnosis and management of ventricular arrhythmias in Doberman pinschers with cardiomyopathy. In Bonagura JD, ed: *Kirk's current veterinary therapy, XII: small animal practice,* Philadelphia, 1995, WB Saunders.
41. Moise NS, Meyers-Wallen V, Flahive WJ et al: Inherited ventricular arrhythmias and sudden death in German shepherd dogs, *J Am Coll Cardiol* 24:233, 1994 (comments).
42. Vassalle M, Knob RE, Cummins M et al: An analysis of fast idioventricular rhythm in the dog, *Circ Res* 41:218, 1977.
43. Muir WW, Lipowitz AJ: Cardiac dysrhythmias associated with gastric dilatation-volvulus in the dog, *J Am Vet Med Assoc* 172:683, 1978.
44. Macintire DK, Snider TG: Cardiac arrhythmias associated with multiple trauma in dogs, *J Am Vet Med Assoc* 184:541, 1984.
45. Myerburg RJ, Kessler KM: Clinical assessment and management of arrhythmias and conduction disturbances. In Hurst JW, Schlant RC, Rackley CE et al, eds: *The heart,* ed 7, New York, 1990, McGraw-Hill.
46. Zipes DP: Specific arrhythmias: diagnosis and treatment. In Braunwald E, ed: *Heart disease: a textbook of cardiovascular medicine,* ed 5, Philadelphia, 1997, WB Saunders.
47. Smith TW, Kelly RA, Stevenson LW et al: Management of heart failure. In Braunwald E, ed: *Heart disease: a textbook of cardiovascular medicine,* ed 5, Philadelphia, 1997, WB Saunders.
48. Brown WA, DeLellis LA: Sotalol administration in boxer dogs with dilated cardiomyopathy and syncope, personal communication, 1996.
49. Alboni P, Razzolini R, Scarfo S et al: Hemodynamic effects of oral sotalol during both sinus rhythm and atrial fibrillation, *J Am Coll Cardiol* 22:1373, 1993.
50. Winters SL, Kukin M, Pe E et al: Effect of oral sotalol on systemic hemodynamics and programmed electrical stimulation in patients with ventricular arrhythmias and structural heart disease, *Am J Cardiol* 72:38A, 1993.
51. Hohnloser SH, Zabel M, Krause T et al: Short- and long-term antiarrhythmic and hemodynamic effects of d, l-sotalol in patients with symptomatic ventricular arrhythmias, *Am Heart J* 123:1220, 1992.
52. Kienle RD, Thomas WP, Pion PD: The natural clinical history of canine congenital subaortic stenosis, *J Vet Intern Med* 8:423, 1994.
53. Desertenne F: La tachycardia ventriculaire a deux foyers opposes variables, *Arch Mal Coeur Vaiss* 59:263, 1966.
54. Vukmir RB: Torsades de pointes: a review, *Am J Emerg Med* 9:250, 1991.
55. Bardy GH, Ungerleider RM, Smith WM et al: A mechanism of torsades de pointes in a canine model, *Circulation* 67:52, 1983.
56. Habbab MA, el-Sherif N: TU alternans, long QTU, and torsade de pointes: clinical and experimental observations, *Pacing Clin Electrophysiol* 15:916, 1992.
57. el-Sherif N: Early afterdepolarizations and arrhythmogenesis: experimental and clinical aspects, *Arch Mal Coeur Vaiss* 84:227, 1991.
58. Bailie DS, Inoue H, Kaseda S et al: Magnesium suppression of early afterdepolarizations and ventricular tachyarrhythmias induced by cesium in dogs, *Circulation* 77:1395, 1988.
59. Gallagher JD: Effects of halothane and quinidine on intracardiac conduction and QTc interval in pentobarbital-anesthetized dogs, *Anesth Analg* 75:688, 1992.
60. Patel A, Pumill R, Goldman D et al: Isorhythmic atrioventricular dissociation revisited, *Am Heart J* 124:823, 1992 (editorial).

61. Ettinger S, Buergelt CD: Atrioventricular dissociation (incomplete) with accrochage in a dog with ruptured chordae tendineae, *Am J Vet Res* 29:1499, 1968.
62. Edwards NJ: *Bolton's handbook of canine and feline electrocardiography,* ed 2, Philadelphia, 1987, WB Saunders.
63. Levy MN, Zieske H: Mechanism of synchronization in isorhythmic dissociation. I. Experiments on dogs, *Circ Res* 27:429, 1970.
64. Paulay KL, Damato AN: Atrioventricular interaction in man during pacing-induced isorhythmic dissociation, *Am Heart J* 83:5, 1972.
65. Knuttgen D, Doehn M: [Pindolol in intraoperatively developing isorhythmic AV dissociation] Pindolol bei intraoperativ auftretender isorhythmischer AV-Dissoziation, *Anaesthesist* 36:431, 1987.
66. Knuttgen D, Hossmann V, Doehn M: [Atropine in intraoperative isorhythmic AV dissociation] Atropin bei intraoperativ auftretender isorhythmischer AV-Dissoziation, *Anasth Intensivther Notfallmed* 22: 124, 1987.
67. Knuttgen D, Weidemann D, Doehn M: Restoring sinus rhythm after intraoperatively occurring isorhythmic AV dissociation by the use of K-Mg aspartate or Mg aspartate, *Magnes Trace Elem* 9:303, 1990.
68. Josephson ME: *Clinical cardiac electrophysiology: techniques and Interpretation,* ed 2, Malvern, Pa, 1993, Lea & Febiger.
69. Hoshino K, Anumonwo J, Delmar M et al: Wenckebach periodicity in single atrioventricular nodal cells from the rabbit heart, *Circulation* 82:2201, 1990 (erratum 83[2]:714, 1991).
70. Lazzara R, el-Sherif N, Scherlag BJ: Disorders of cellular electrophysiology produced by ischemia of the canine His bundle, *Circ Res* 36:444, 1975.
71. Branch CE, Robertson BT, Williams JC: Frequency of second-degree atrioventricular heart blocks in dogs, *Am J Vet Res* 36:925, 1975.
72. James TN, Robertson BT, Waldo AL et al: De subitaneis mortibus. XV. Hereditary stenosis of the His bundle in pug dogs, *Circulation* 52:1152, 1975.
73. Wessale JL, Geddes LA, Fearnot NE et al: Cardiac output versus pacing rate at rest and with exercise in dogs with AV block, *Pacing Clin Electrophysiol* 11:575, 1988.
74. Levy SA, Duray PH: Complete heart block in a dog seropositive for Borrelia burgdorferi: similarity to human Lyme carditis, *J Vet Intern Med* 2:138, 1988.
75. Reed JR: Resolution of third degree AV block following corticosteroid administration in dogs, personal communication, 1995.
76. Liu ŞK, Hsu FS, Lee RCT: *An atlas of cardiovascular pathology,* Tainan, Taiwan, 1989, Pig Research Institute of Taiwan.
77. James TN, Drake EH: Sudden death in Doberman pinschers, *Ann Intern Med* 68:821, 1968.
78. Rosen KM, Dhingra RC, Loeb HS et al: Chronic heart block in adults: clinical and electrophysiological observations, *Arch Intern Med* 131:663, 1973.

CHAPTER 28

Syncope

Syncope is a sudden and transient loss or depression of consciousness and postural tone resulting from a transient and diffuse cerebral malfunction.[1] When consciousness is lost, the patient's muscle tone becomes flaccid, usually resulting in the patient becoming laterally recumbent. If consciousness is only altered, the patient may appear ataxic, may become sternally recumbent, or may become laterally recumbent but remain aware of its surroundings. *Episodic weakness* may be a more appropriate term to describe this type of event, depending on the clinical manifestation. Not all patients that lose consciousness remain flaccid. Localized or generalized tonic spasms may occur, and the patient may become incontinent. When spasms and incontinence occur, a syncopal event may be difficult or impossible to differentiate from a seizure, based on history alone. Seizures may occasionally also mimic syncope (so-called akinetic seizure). Syncopal events usually last only a matter of seconds, whereas seizures may persist for a few minutes. Also, following the event, the patient commonly recovers rapidly and appears normal to the observer within seconds, rather than displaying the postictal symptoms typical of seizures.

Pathophysiology

Syncope usually occurs because of a sudden, severe, and transient decrease in oxygen delivery to the brain. Oxygen delivery is determined by blood flow, systemic arterial oxygen tension, and hemoglobin concentration. Alterations in these three variables can theoretically result in syncope. The vast majority of syncopal events result from a transient reduction in brain blood flow, specifically a reduction in blood flow to the brainstem reticular activating system. Transient decreases in brain oxygen delivery resulting from severe and transient hypoxemia can occur but are rare. They may, however, occur in dogs with laryngeal paralysis or other forms of very severe upper airway disease and obstruction. Arterial oxygen tension probably must decrease abruptly to a level of less than 20 to 30 mm Hg to result in loss of consciousness.[2] This level of hypoxemia produces obvious cyanosis. Hypercyanotic spells are described in children with congenital right-to-left shunting lesions.[1] These are most often associated with crying. There is no counterpart to crying in animals, and these spells are extremely rare to nonexistent in dogs and cats with cyanotic congenital heart disease. Sudden, severe and transient anemia does not occur. Loss or alteration of consciousness can also occur when there is lack of delivery of an essential nutrient, such as glucose, to the brain. This more commonly results in the patient seizing, becoming weak, collapsing, or becoming ataxic rather than a transient loss of consciousness. In one study, only three of 27 dogs (11%) with hypoglycemia presented for signs of syncope.[3]

As stated previously, the vast majority of syncopal events are due to a transient reduction in brain blood flow. A sudden and severe decrease in blood flow occurs primarily for two general reasons in dogs and cats. First, the heart may stop pumping blood or decrease blood flow markedly for a short time, resulting in cessation or marked reduction of brain blood flow. Severe systemic hypotension results. Second, systemic arterioles may dilate for a short time, resulting in severe hypotension. In studies performed in humans, acute cessation of blood flow to the brain produced by rapid inflation of a cuff around the neck to 600 mm Hg resulted in loss of consciousness within 5 to 15 seconds.[4] Tonic spasms and incontinence generally occur in humans with more prolonged brain hypoxia. Mean systemic blood pressure at the time of syncope is generally less than 25 mm Hg.

Etiologies

Syncopal episodes can be categorized into those that occur as a result of cardiac causes, those resultng from noncardiac causes, and those that cannot be determined. In studies reported in humans, indeterminate causes commonly constitute about 40% of the cases seen.[5]

SYNCOPE ASSOCIATED WITH CARDIAC DISEASE

Most of the cases of syncope that occur in dogs are due to cardiac causes, and most of these are due to rhythm disturbances. The rhythm disturbances occur because of inherent cardiac disease or are secondary to autonomic disturbances, most commonly excessive vagal tone. Increased vagal tone resulting in syncope is classified as a noncardiac cause because an extracardiac abnormality initiates the event, and the increase in vagal tone can either initiate sinus arrest or systemic vasodilation.

Rhythm disturbances that result in syncope are either severe bradyarrhythmias or severe tachyarrhythmias. Bradyarrhythmias that result in cessation of cardiac electrical activity for more than 6 to 8 seconds result in altered or lost consciousness. Nonsustained severe tachyarrhythmias, usually nonsustained ventricular tachyarrhythmias that depolarize at rates greater than 300 beats/min, result in inadequate time for ventricular filling and a sudden and marked decrease in cardiac output.

The three most common cardiac causes of syncope are third-degree atrioventricular block, sick sinus syndrome, and fast ventricular tachyarrhythmias in dogs with cardiomyopathy (see Chapter 20). Third-degree atrioventricular block results in a ventricular bradycardia because an escape pacemaker must take over to depolarize the ventricles. The ventricular rate in dogs is 40 to 65 beats/min if a nodal escape focus is still active and 20 to 40 beats/min if Purkinje fibers must maintain a cardiac rhythm. Syncope associated with third-degree atrioventricular block is rare in cats, probably because the nodal escape rate is faster and more stable than in dogs. Dogs with heart rates between 40 and 65 beats/min may be presented for syncope or may have no clinical signs and be identified on a routine physical examination. Dogs that have heart rates between 20 and 30 beats/min may be presented because of signs of low cardiac output and may be weak and depressed. The blood lactate concentration in these dogs may be elevated. These dogs also commonly are presented because of syncope. The exact mechanism of syncope is often not identified in dogs with third-degree atrioventricular block. Instead, a pacemaker is implanted that alleviates the bradycardia and the syncope without any further diagnostic evaluation. There are probably two possible explanations for the syncope noted in dogs with third-degree atrioventricular block. One is that the subsidiary pacemaker in these dogs is unstable and stops for a period, during which syncope occurs. The other is that a nonsustained tachyarrhythmia originates from an ectopic site that results in overdrive suppression of the subsidiary pacemaker. When the ectopic pacemaker stops depolarizing, the overdrive suppression of the diseased subsidiary pacemakers results in a period of ventricular asystole before the subsidiary pacemakers function again. Whatever the mechanism, these dogs commonly faint, and the syncopal events are often what prompts the owner to take the dog in for an examination. Most of these dogs have a stable but slow rhythm at the time of examination, with no evidence of syncope or periods of ventricular asystole during the examination or subsequent hospitalization. Sudden death is rare in this population.

Sick sinus syndrome in dogs commonly results in periods of sinus arrest that terminate in syncope (Figure 28-1). In general, the sinus arrest must last for more than 5 or 6 seconds to result in syncope. Anticholinergic or β-adrenergic agents sometimes shorten or abolish the periods of sinus arrest and therefore alleviate the signs of syncope. However, these measures are usually short-lived, and signs commonly recur as the disease progresses. Although the administration of an anticholinergic agent, such as atropine, may alter the periods of sinus arrest and increase the sinus node rate, the sinus node rate never increases into the range one expects after atropine administration with this disease. Pacemaker implantation is the only effective long-term solution to alleviate this problem. Sudden death is rare with sick sinus syndrome.

Dogs with myocardial disease may also be presented because they have had syncopal episodes. They are most commonly boxers and Doberman pinschers. Boxers may or may not have evidence of primary myocardial failure (dilated cardiomyopathy), whereas Doberman pinschers almost always have myocardial failure that is often severe. The syncopal events in these dogs are due to periods of very fast nonsustained ventricular tachyarrhythmias. Ventricular tachycardia with rates greater than 300 beats/min is the most common, although occasionally short periods of ventricular flutter and even ventricular fibrillation occur. When this type of malignant arrhythmia occurs in a dog with myocardial disease, the arrhythmia may spontaneously convert back to sinus rhythm or it may persist and degrade into sustained ventricular fibrillation. The former results in syncope, and the latter results in sudden death. Syncope in this situation may be better termed *aborted sudden death.* These dogs are at great risk for dying suddenly during a subsequent episode.

Occasionally, dogs with outflow obstruction, particularly subaortic stenosis, are presented because they faint with exertion. In humans, up to 40% of patients with severe aortic stenosis have syncopal events.[6] The percentage appears to be much lower in dogs. Syncope with pulmonic stenosis in dogs is rare. The mechanism for syncope associated with outflow obstruction is controversial. The classic explanation is as follows. Exercise results in reflex vasodi-

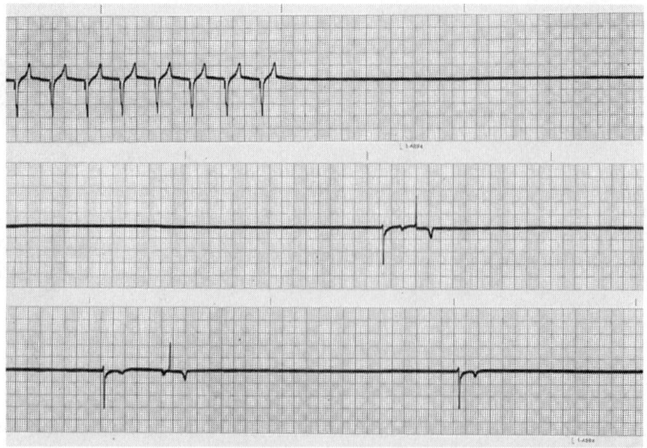

FIGURE 28-1 Lead II ECG tracing from an 11-year-old West Highland white terrier. The owner presented the dog because it was having episodes of syncope 5 times a day. The baseline ECG was similar to that seen in Figure 27-14, and there was no response to atropine. A temporary pacemaker was placed, and the dog was anesthetized for pacemaker implantation. Before implanting the permanent pacemaker, the temporary pacemaker rate was set at approximately 100 beats/min for 1 minute and then abruptly turned off. This was followed by a long period of sinus arrest. Atropine was then administered (0.04 mg/kg IV), and the procedure repeated 15 minutes later. As seen in the tracing in this figure, long periods of sinus arrest are still present, verifying that the dog has sick sinus syndrome. (Paper speed = 25 mm/sec; 1 cm = 1 mV.)

lation of systemic arterioles. Because of the fixed obstruction to flow, cardiac output cannot increase appropriately. This results in systemic hypotension and syncope. Many dogs that we see with severe subaortic stenosis perform activities that result in moderate exertion with no clinical signs. In other words, they do not have evidence of exercise intolerance, although they are not usually asked to perform heavy exercise. Consequently, it is difficult to believe that they are unable to increase cardiac output enough to maintain blood pressure. The current theory, which seems more plausible, is as follows. During exercise, contractility increases, cardiac output increases, and so flow through the fixed stenosis increases. This results in a greater pressure gradient between the left ventricle and the aorta and, more importantly, an increase in systolic left ventricular pressure. The abrupt and severe increase in intraventricular pressure overstimulates left ventricular mechanoreceptors, resulting in a reflex activation of cardiac afferent vagal fibers. The increase in parasympathetic tone to the heart and systemic blood vessels results in bradycardia and vasodilation, which culminate in syncope. Alternatively, because some dogs with severe subaortic stenosis have evidence of ventricular arrhythmias and often die suddenly, syncope may occur because of a fast, nonsustained ventricular tachyarrhythmia.

Pulmonary hypertension can result in syncope.[7] One example is a dog we observed with severe pulmonary hypertension that was presented because of exercise-induced syncopal events. This dog had pulmonary arterial pressures equivalent to systemic arterial pressures. The dog also had severe lung disease with moderate-to-severe hypoxemia (arterial oxygen tension = 51 mm Hg). Severe heartworm disease, presumably with pulmonary hypertension, can also cause syncope, especially during exercise.

Humans with hypertrophic cardiomyopathy are prone to experiencing syncopal events. This is extremely rare in cats but may occur in dogs.[8] Enhanced outflow tract obstruction resulting from systolic anterior motion of the mitral valve and subsequent increased intraventricular pressure with activation of ventricular mechanoreceptors is the most likely explanation for syncope in this population.

Rarely, syncope can occur because of acute and transient obstruction to blood flow. This is most commonly due to an intracardiac thrombus or tumor transiently obstructing blood flow through a valve orifice. This occurs more frequently in cats when a left atrial thrombus occludes the mitral valve orifice. However, this more commonly results in sudden death. When syncope is the presenting sign, the thrombus or tumor is mobile and shifts back into the cardiac chamber, allowing blood flow to recommence. One dog with a right ventricular outflow tract obstruction caused by a tumor has been reported with exertional syncope.[9] Whether the syncope was due to the tumor producing greater obstruction to blood flow, resulting in cessation of blood flow during exercise or to increased right ventricular pressure and mechanoreceptor stimulation is unknown.

Canine patients with tetralogy of Fallot may experience syncopal or collapsing episodes. Of the 19 cases of tetralogy of Fallot that we diagnosed in one 10-year period, three had syncope or episodic collapse as part of their history. The mechanism for syncope is unknown. The syncope is most commonly associated with exercise or excitement, in our experience. We have observed it in patients that are severely polycythemic and in patients that are not severely polycythemic. Stimulation of ventricular mechanoreceptors is a plausible explanation for the syncope observed in this group. The severe hypoxemia may also be involved.

Although syncope may be observed in patients with heart failure, heart failure itself is not a cause of syncope and syncope is not a sign of heart failure. Patients with heart failure commonly have a reduced cardiac output. The reduction in cardiac output can cause exercise intolerance and, if severe, can cause weakness and even collapse. The event, however, is not transient. Loss of consciousness in this situation, if it occurs, is a terminal event, and the patient does not regain consciousness unless emergency intervention occurs. Although heart failure is commonly listed as a cause of syncope in veterinary texts, it is not listed in any of the modern human cardiology texts.[1,4,6]

SYNCOPE RESULTING FROM NONCARDIAC CAUSES

There are numerous noncardiac causes of syncope in humans that do not occur or are exceedingly rare in dogs and cats. They include vasovagal or vasodepressor syncope (the common faint), orthostatic hypotension, micturition syncope, defecation syncope, sneeze syncope, swallow syncope, atherosclerotic cerebrovascular disease, glossopharyngeal neuralgia-induced syncope, anxiety-induced hyperventilation, migraine, and psychiatric illness. One of us has observed orthostatic hypotension in one dog being treated with hydralazine. This German shorthaired pointer was friendly and would elevate its head by placing its front legs in the lap of one of the authors. He would stay there to be petted but then would appear to become dizzy. He would then lower himself to stand on all four legs and recover within seconds. Syncope did not occur. We have an anecdotal report of an instance of an excitement induced syncopal event in one dog.[10] In this instance the owner reported that when the dog became very excited it "passed out." The dog was placed on an ultrasound table, and an ECG and echocardiogram were recorded and the femoral pulse palpated when the owner entered the room and excited the dog. The ECG and echocardiogram did not change, but the femoral pulse became undetectable. It was presumed that the dog experienced vasodepressor syncope in which increased vagal tone to the peripheral vasculature produced vasodilation and profound hypotension. Drugs are commonly mentioned as causes of syncope in the human literature and include hallucinogens, barbiturates, and narcotics.[1] Cocaine, especially crack cocaine, can lead to syncope through the induction of ventricular arrhythmias that can also lead to sudden death. Antiarrhythmic drugs can potentially exacerbate ventricular arrhythmias and produce syncope or sudden death. We have never observed syncope secondary to drug administration. We have, however, observed weakness to the point of collapse occur in dogs overdosed with arteriolar dilators. These dogs retain consciousness and are weak for several hours. Consequently, they are not experiencing syncope. It should be mentioned that overdoses of some antiarrhythmic drugs, such as lidocaine and quinidine, produce grand mal seizures.

We have observed vagally-mediated syncope in dogs, and it has been reported in humans.[11] These dogs often have bradycardia, exaggerated sinus arrhythmia, and periods of sinus arrest on a resting electrocardiogram (Figure 28-2). Their resting ECGs are usually indistinguishable from those of a patient with sick sinus syndrome. In dogs with a vagally-induced bradyarrhythmia, administration of atropine 0.04 mg/kg SC results in a profound increase in the heart rate within 15 to 30 minutes. The heart rate always increases in these dogs to a rate greater than 160 beats/min and usually to a rate greater than 180 beats/min. Most of these are small-breed dogs. Most have no apparent reason for their obvious increase in vagal tone. Some have chronic respiratory or gastrointestinal disease. Some are brachycephalic breeds. Rarely, they have a history of fainting after vomiting. Rarely, carotid sinus massage results in reproduction of clinical signs. Exaggerated vagal tone may produce acute vasodilation without a bradyarrhythmia.

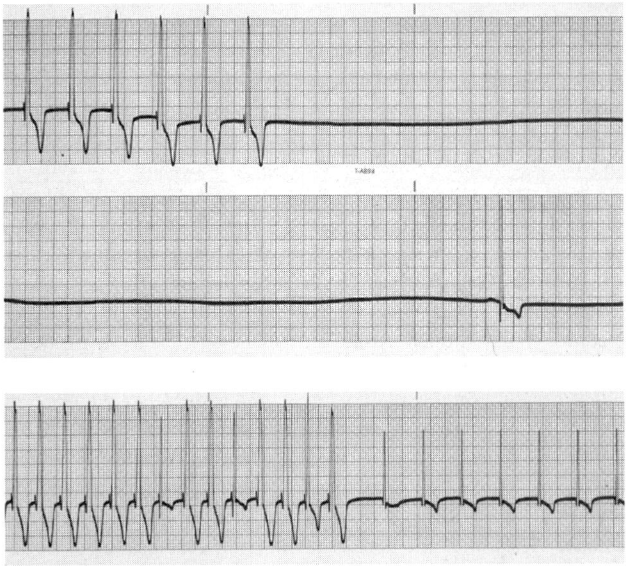

FIGURE 28-2 ECG tracings from a 12-year-old American cocker spaniel. The dog was "fainting" 3 times a week. The dog had periods of sinus arrest that responded to atropine administration. Instead of medical therapy, the owner opted to have a pacemaker implanted. **A,** A temporary pacemaker was placed, and the dog was anesthetized. The rate of the temporary pacemaker was set at approximately 100 beats/min for 1 minute, and then the pacemaker was abruptly turned off. A long period (6.3 seconds) of sinus arrest occurred. **B,** The procedure in **A** was repeated after administration of atropine 0.04 mg/kg IV. The sinus node promptly (less than 0.4 seconds) recovered after pacing was terminated (i.e., the sinus node recovery time was normal). This proved that the bradyarrhythmia in this dog was vagally mediated.

Carotid sinus syncope is a well-described abnormality in humans.[4] Although it may occur in dogs, it is poorly documented. The carotid sinus is a baroreceptor organ that lies at the origin of the internal carotid artery, where it branches from the common carotid artery. Carotid sinus hypersensitivity occurs most commonly in older men who have coronary artery disease and hypertension. Pressure on the carotid sinus by tight collars, shaving, and sudden turning of the head results in a reflex increase in vagal tone. The increase in vagal tone may result in brief periods of asystole, acute vasodilation, or both. These result in syncope. The diagnosis is generally made when pressure over a carotid sinus reproduces the syncopal event. Because the common and internal carotid arteries lie deep beneath the neck musculature, next to the trachea in dogs and cats, it is difficult to produce pressure on this region. One of the authors has reproduced periods of sinus arrest by carotid sinus massage in several dogs presented for syncope. Atropine has abolished this response. Whether these dogs had increased vagal tone for other reasons exacerbated by the carotid sinus massage or they had carotid sinus syncope is unknown. They did not appear to have an inherent sinus node dysfunction, because their heart rates increased into the normal range after atropine administration.

Cough syncope is an ill-defined but well recognized abnormality in both humans and dogs. In humans, cough syncope is seen predominantly in middle-age men who smoke and have chronic lung disease.[12] In dogs, cough syncope is usually seen in geriatric small-breed dogs that have mitral regurgitation and chronic lung or airway disease. These dogs have a paroxysm of coughing that culminates in syncope. Two mechanisms for cough syncope have been proposed. The first is that increased intrathoracic and intraabdominal pressures increase venous pressures, which are transmitted to the spinal and intracranial veins. The brain is encased in the rigid skull and surrounded by noncompressible fluid. Consequently, the increased venous pressure results in an acute and severe increase in the intracranial pressure. Cerebral perfusion pressure is determined by the difference between arterial blood pressure and intracranial pressure. When intracranial pressure is acutely increased to a level greater than arterial blood pressure, cerebral perfusion is acutely decreased. Two other things probably also occur during coughing. First, coughing increases intrathoracic pressure, resulting in decreased venous return and decreased cardiac output. Secondly, prolonged coughing probably also produces hypocapnia, a known stimulus of cerebral vasoconstriction.[13] The acute decrease in cerebral blood flow with coughing has been documented in one study of three humans with cough syncope.[12] Each of these individuals had no major alteration in systemic hemodynamics during coughing and subsequent fainting. Cerebral blood flow was measured with a Doppler technique and actually reversed (went back toward the heart) in these individuals during coughing at the time of their syncopal events. This mechanism is used on occasion by adolescents who make each other pass out through hyperventilation and chest compression. In this "game," the individual hyperventilates to produce hypocapnia and then a friend acutely squeezes the individual's chest while the individual keeps his or her glottis closed (forced Valsalva maneuver). The individual then "passes out." The other theory is that coughing results in vagal afferent neural transmission to the vasomotor center in the medulla, with subsequent stimulation of vagal efferent nerves to the heart and blood vessels.[6] In dogs with pulmonary edema secondary to mitral regurgitation, cough-induced syncope usually can be alleviated by controlling the heart failure. In other cases, treating or suppressing the cough may control clinical signs. Cough syncope, although frightening to the owner, is usually benign. We have never observed an instance of sudden death associated with cough syncope.

Diagnostic Evaluation

HISTORY

Syncope is a frequent owner complaint in a busy cardiology referral practice. Because syncope is episodic and often infrequent, syncopal events are only rarely observed by a veterinarian. Consequently, a detailed query of the owner is required to identify the timing and the appearance of the "episode." Many owners are not good observers, whereas others are not good observers during such an event because they panic. Owners commonly report that they thought their animal was going to die or was dying during a syncopal event. Many attempt resuscitation procedures, including thoracic compression and mouth-to-mouth resuscitation. Owners also commonly exaggerate the time that an event lasted.

The clinician should allow the owners to tell their version of the event(s) initially. Then he or she should specifically ask questions regarding any activity leading up to the event, any observed abnormalities before the event, how the animal acted after the event, what occurred during the event, and how long it lasted. Syncope and seizure activity are often difficult to differentiate based on historical findings. In some cases, even when the event is witnessed by a veterinarian, the distinction is difficult or even impossible. One of our neurologists observed one dog that appeared to him to have a grand mal seizure. The dog was ultimately proved to have syncope. One might think that feeling the pulse, feeling the apex beat of the heart, or ausculting the heart might help distinguish syncope from seizure. However, the initiating arrhythmia occurs before the animal falls over and may last for only a short time during the event. Consequently, by the time an owner or veterinarian tries to find evidence of cardiac activity, the arrhythmia is no longer present, leading to the false conclusion that an arrhythmia is not responsible. Seizures classically have a prodromal period in which the patient "feels" the seizure coming on and a postictal period in which the patient is disoriented after the seizure. During the seizure, a tonic (stiffening) phase is classically seen, followed by a clonic (twitching) phase that can last for seconds to being continuous. Autonomic stimulation usually results in salivation, urination, and defecation. The animal may vocalize. The animal becomes unconscious and breathing stops. Syncopal events, on the other hand, classically do not produce any abnormalities before or after the event. Instead the animal appears normal and then either becomes weak, retaining consciousness, or collapses and loses consciousness. Classically the animal is "limp" while it is unconscious, with no seizure activity. As in all other aspects of medicine, not all cases are classic cases, and there is a tremendous amount of overlap between these two extremes that can make the differentiation of seizure activity from syncopal activity difficult in an individual patient. Patients that faint can experience cerebral hypoxia and start to seize or at least have muscle twitches once they are unconscious. Patients with seizures may not have any evidence of abnormalities before or after a seizure. Dogs that seize may not have the classic tonic-clonic movements of a grand mal seizure. A careful neurologic examination, careful auscultation, resting ECG, and Holter monitor recording may help distinguish a bout of syncope from a seizure. The cause of syncope in humans is never definitively diagnosed in up to 40% of cases. This figure is probably similar in small animal veterinary medicine.

If an accurate history can be obtained, the owner will often relate that the animal was normal and then fell over on its side. The episode may have no precipitating event or may be precipitated by excitement or coughing. Some dogs will not fall over but appear to collapse in the rear legs or collapse into sternal recumbency. These animals do not lose consciousness. Animals that collapse onto their side may or may not be unconscious. Animals that are unconscious may still have their eyes open and may appear to the owner to be conscious. The eyes may rotate upward. During the episode, the animal may appear and feel flaccid to the owner or may have clonic movements (twitches). The animal may appear flaccid during the initial stage of the syncopal episode and then develop muscle twitches toward the end. Opisthotonos may occur. However, generalized tonus followed by clonic seizure movement occurs only rarely. Micturition may occur as the urethral sphincters relax. Most syncopal events last less than 10 seconds, although they can last longer. To an owner witnessing a syncopal episode, especially if it is for the first time, the time seems much longer, and the owner will commonly report that the event lasted for 30 seconds to a minute. Although this can occur, it is probably unlikely. Owners often continue to hold the animal, although the animal has recovered, or will continue resuscitation procedures after the animal has recovered and do not realize that recovery has occurred. Once an event is completed, most animals recover very quickly. There is no postictal disorientation or abnormal behavior in most cases. Instead, the animal appears normal and resumes its normal activity.

PHYSICAL EXAMINATION

The physical examination of an animal presented for syncope may be normal. This is most often the case in dogs with tachyarrhythmias leading to syncope and may be the case in dogs with increased vagal tone. The most common abnormality identified on a physical examination is an arrhythmia. In dogs with third-degree atrioventricular block, the heart rate is too slow. Pauses in the rhythm may occasionally be noted. Most dogs with sick sinus syndrome have a bradyarrhythmia and, usually, evidence of sinus arrest. Supraventricular tachyarrhythmias may also be present. Ventricular tachyarrhythmias in dogs may range from no ECG abnormalities at the time of examination to isolated premature ventricular contractions to sustained ventricular tachycardia. Most dogs with cough syncope have evidence of respiratory disease or mitral regurgitation with or without left heart failure. Vagal maneuvers, such as eyeball pressure and carotid sinus massage, may exacerbate bradyarrhythmias.

RESTING ELECTROCARDIOGRAM

A resting ECG should be obtained in any patient suspected of experiencing a syncopal episode. The rhythm should be evaluated for at least a minute if not longer and may be evaluated when the animal is calm and when it is excited. In dogs with bradyarrhythmias, the ECG must be evaluated before and after the administration of atropine 0.04 mg/kg or more SC or IV. Dogs with sick sinus syndrome either do not respond to atropine or have an increase in heart rate, but the increase is not into the expected range of 140 to 220 beats/min. Dogs with high vagal tone consistently have an increase in heart rate to greater than 160 beats/min. In dogs with third-degree atrioventricular block, the atrial rate may increase, but the escape rhythm is usually not affected.

Most dogs do not faint while the ECG is being recorded. Consequently, an absolute association between the syncopal event and an arrhythmia cannot be made. However, in animals with severe and consistent arrhythmia, the resting ECG provides a high index of suspicion for the diagnosis. Dogs with third-degree atrioventricular block or periods of sinus arrest or the correct breeds of dogs with ventricular arrhythmias associated with cardiomyopathy have syncope resulting from the observed or associated abnormality until proved otherwise. Consequently, they should be treated appropriately. Syncopal events almost always disappear after pacemaker implantation in dogs with third-degree atrioventricular block or sick sinus syndrome. Boxers with syncope as a result of malignant ventricular arrhythmias usually respond to sotalol administration. Many animals have intermittent arrhythmias that cause their syncope. In these animals, the resting ECG may be normal.

PROLONGED ELECTROCARDIOGRAPHIC MONITORING

In patients in which the resting ECG is normal or doubt exists as to the relationship between an arrhythmia and the observed events, Holter monitoring or event monitoring can aid the diagnosis. A Holter monitor consists of electrodes attached by wires (leads) to a tape-recording device that records the ECG continuously, usually for 24 hours (Color Plates 109 and 110). The recorder is carried in a pack by the dog or taped to the dog (Color Plate 111). The leads must be carefully covered to prevent access by the dog, because dogs will readily chew the leads. The recording tape is analyzed by a technician and a computer to detect any rhythm abnormalities that occurred during the recording. The results are generally reported as printouts of the abnormalities noted during the recording and reports of trends in heart rate, premature beats, and so on. This modality is commonly available through commercial laboratories (Roche Laboratories, Nutley, N.J.) and usually costs less than $250. The laboratory supplies the equipment, analyzes the tape, and provides the analysis. Holter monitoring frequently provides clues to the origin of syncopal events. However, syncopal events often occur infrequently. Consequently, a syncopal event may not occur during the time that the recording is taking place. If a syncopal event does occur, an event marker can be depressed by the owner to signify when the event occurred so that an attempt can be made to correlate the ECG recording and the event. If syncope does not occur during the recording, significant arrhythmias may still be present and provide clues as to the origin of the syncopal events.

Some normal findings on Holter recordings can be mistaken for significant arrhythmias. Normal dogs commonly have very slow heart rates when they are asleep. Heart rates less than 40 beats/min are common, and heart rates of 20 to 30 beats/min can occur.[14] One study documented a heart rate as slow as 17 beats/min in one normal dog.[15] Sinus arrest is common. In one study of 16 randomly selected dogs, all dogs had a period of sinus arrest that lasted longer than 2 seconds and the longest pause was 5.7 seconds.[15] The periods of sinus arrest were invariably associated with marked sinus arrhythmia. Second-degree atrioventricular block is normal in puppies.[16] In one study of 90 normal beagles, 9% of the males and 20% of the females had at least one instance of second-degree atrioventricular block.[14] Ventricular arrhythmias, other than infrequent single premature beats, are uncommon in normal dogs or cats. In one study, ventricular ectopy was observed in about 20% of 90 normal beagles.[14] The total number of premature ventricular beats per 24 hours was less than 10 in all but two of these dogs. In these two otherwise normal dogs, there were 751 and 101 ectopic beats per 24 hours. It is most likely that the number observed in these two dogs represented an abnormality. In another study, 3 of 16 dogs had more than 10 premature ventricular beats per 24 hours, numbering 16, 27, and 52 in dogs that were otherwise normal.[15] Supraventricular premature beats are rare in normal dogs. However, it is common for a human laboratory to report frequent atrial or supraventricular premature beats in dogs with marked sinus arrhythmia. Visual inspection of the recording is required in this instance to determine the correct diagnosis. Sinus tachycardia occurs during excitement and exercise. Maximum heart rates varied between 110 and 300 beats/min in one study.[15]

Event recorders or intermittent loop recorders can be used in patients that have infrequent but recurrent syncopal episodes. Event recorders continuously record the ECG but also continuously erase older portions of the recording. These recorders can be placed on a patient for several days to several weeks. When an event is observed by an owner, the owner can activate the device to save the recording of the patient's rhythm for the previous several minutes. We have little experience with these devices, but theoretically they should be useful in patients with recurrent but infrequent episodes that have owners who regularly witness the events.

OTHER DIAGNOSTIC TESTS

Any animal suspected of having a primary neurologic event should have a thorough neurologic examination. Animals with seizures as a result of organic brain disease may have other neurologic abnormalities. Animals with idiopathic epilepsy, however, usually have a normal neurologic examination.

A serum chemistry panel is generally indicated in animals presented for syncope. Evidence of hypoglycemia, electrolyte abnormalities, or other abnormalities may give one clues as to the origin of the clinical signs.

Other tests to identify or exacerbate arrhythmias are generally impractical in veterinary medicine. In human medicine, recording the ECG during a standardized exercise test or electrophysiologic testing may help identify an offending rhythm disturbance.[6] Recording a signal-averaged ECG to detect late potentials in humans is about 80% sensitive at detecting patients with ventricular arrhythmias. Upright tilt testing is used in humans to identify ventricular mechanoreceptor-stimulated bradycardia and vasodilation. These tests are generally impractical in dogs or cats.

Treatment

Treatment of syncope depends on the underlying cause. Vagally mediated bradyarrhythmias can be treated with orally active or parenteral vagolytic agents, orally active β-agonists such as terbutaline, or pacemaker implantation (see Figure 28-2). Weak anticholinergic agents, such as propantheline, can be tried, but they are often too weak to produce the desired effects. Atropine tablets are no longer manufactured but some pharmacies may still have some. We have effectively administered the parenteral form of atropine orally. This compound is extremely bitter and must be diluted (usually 10:1) in corn syrup. The dose is 0.04 mg/kg q8-12h. Alternatively, glycopyrrolate tablets (Robinul, A. H. Robins Company, Richmond, Va.) can be tried. It is supplied as 1- and 2-mg tablets. However, we have no experience administering this drug in this manner and are unaware of an effective dose. Transdermal scopolamine has been used successfully in humans.[6] The dose for an adult human is one patch every 2 to 3 days. This dose must be reduced markedly in most patients with vagally mediated syncope, because most of these dogs are small (less than 15 kg). Any anticholinergic agent has the potential to produce side effects, which include dry mouth, photophobia caused by pupil dilation, and constipation. These effects seem to be mild or nonexistent in most of the dogs we have treated. Terbutaline (Brethine, Geigy Pharmaceuticals, Summit, N.J.; Bricanyl, Marion Merrell Dow, Kansas City, Mo.), a β_2-receptor agonist, can also be used in these dogs to abolish episodes of sinus arrest and increase the sinus rate. This drug probably works because it has some β_1-adrenergic stimulating properties and because the sinus node has β_2-receptors that increase the sinus node rate. The dose is 1.25 to 5 mg/dog q8-12h. The most common side effects are nervousness and tremors. Terbutaline should be used cautiously if at all in dogs with mitral regurgitation caused by myxomatous mitral valve degeneration. We have not noted complications with this drug in this setting but have noted acute pulmonary edema in dogs treated with albuterol, another β_2-agonist. The pulmonary edema in these dogs was most likely due to acute chordal rupture. Some dogs do not respond well to anticholinergic or sympathomimetic treatment. These dogs usually respond to pacemaker implantation. One must be cognizant, however, that syncope secondary to increased vagal tone can be primarily due to vasodilation. If this is the case, syncope could still occur following pacemaker implantation.

Syncope secondary to third-degree atrioventricular block and sick sinus syndrome should be treated with pacemaker implantation. Some dogs with sick sinus syndrome have a partial response to anticholinergic or sympathomimetic agents. Some of these dogs have cessation of their syncopal activity when these agents are administered chronically. Most, however, become refractory to drug administration, many within a short time.

Dogs with syncope secondary to malignant ventricular arrhythmias are at risk for sudden death. Antiarrhythmic therapy is indicated. Many classic antiarrhythmic drugs used in this situation are ineffective at preventing sudden death, in our experience. If the data from human medicine can be extrapolated to veterinary medicine, many of these drugs may actually exacerbate the incidence of sudden death in this population. Consequently, we rarely use drugs such as procainamide and quinidine in dogs with syncope secondary to ventricular arrhythmia. Sotalol (Betapace, Berlex Laboratories, Wayne, N.J.) appears to be very effective in boxers with malignant ventricular arrhythmias and without severe myocardial failure. It is dosed at 40 to 80 mg q12h. Amiodarone (Cordarone, Wyeth-Ayerst, Philadelphia, Pa.) and possibly mexiletine (Mexitil, Boehrenger Ingelheim, Ridgefield, Conn.) may be effective drugs in dogs with ventricular arrhythmias and moderate-to-severe primary myocardial failure (dilated cardiomyopathy).

Cough syncope in dogs should be treated by treating the underlying disease. If pulmonary edema resulting from congestive heart failure is present, the heart failure should be treated appropriately. Chronic pulmonary disease should be treated appropriately. If these measures are ineffective, cough suppressants should be tried.

Dogs with subaortic stenosis and syncope should be closely evaluated for evidence of malignant ventricular arrhythmias. Generally, a Holter monitor should be employed. If ventricular arrhythmias are present, they should be treated appropriately. If syncope is associated with excitement or exercise and no ventricular arrhythmias are present, stimulation of ventricular mechanoreceptors may be the reason for this type of event. Drugs used in humans to alter the reflex pathway in this event include β-adrenergic blocking drugs and anticholinergic agents. β-Adrenergic blockers prevent the initial increase in sympathetic tone to the heart, decreasing the reflex increase in contractility and therefore the marked increase in systolic intraventricular pressure that stimulates the mechanoreceptors. Anticholinergic drugs prevent the reflex increase in vagal tone. However, the increase in heart rate associated with these drugs in dogs with subaortic stenosis would probably have long-term detrimental effects. Theophylline has also been successful in human patients.[6] The mechanism is unknown but it may block the vasodilatory effects of adenosine.

REFERENCES

1. O'Laughlin MP, McNamara DG: Syncope. In Garson AJ, Bricker JT, McNamara DG, eds: *The science and practice of pediatric cardiology,* Philadelphia, 1946, Lea & Febiger.
2. O'Brien DP, Kroll RA: Metabolic encephalopathies. In Kirk RW, Bonagura JD, eds: *Kirk's current veterinary therapy, XI: small animal practice,* Philadelphia, 1992, WB Saunders.

3. Feldman EC, Nelson RW: Hypoglycemia. In Feldman EC, Nelson RW, eds: *Canine and feline endocrinology and reproduction,* Philadelphia, 1987, WB Sanders.
4. Braunwald E: Hypotension and syncope. In Braunwald E, ed: *Heart disease: a textbook of cardiovascular medicine,* ed 4, Philadelphia, 1992, WB Saunders.
5. Schlant RC, Sonnenblick EH: Syncope: pathophysiology, recognition, and treatment. In Hurst JW, Schlant RC, Rackley CE et al, eds: *The heart,* ed 7, New York, 1990, McGraw-Hill.
6. Kapoor WN: Syncope and hypotension. In Braunwald E, ed: *Heart disease: a textbook of cardiovascular medicine,* ed 5, Philadelphia, 1997, WB Saunders.
7. Johnson LR, Boon J, Orton EC: Pulmonary hypertension in dogs, 1992-1996: a Doppler echocardiographic study, *J Vet Intern Med* 11:139, 1997 (abstract).
8. Liu SK, Maron BJ, Tilley LP: Canine hypertrophic cardiomyopathy, *J Am Vet Med Assoc* 174:708, 1979.
9. Bright JM, Toal RL, Blackford LA: Right ventricular outflow obstruction caused by primary cardiac neoplasia: clinical features in two dogs, *J Vet Intern Med* 4:12, 1990.
10. DeLellis LA: Excitement-induced syncope in a dog, personal communication, 1996.
11. Sapire DW, Casta A, Safley W et al: Vasovagal syncope in children requiring pacemaker implantation, *Am Heart J* 106:1406, 1983.
12. Mattle HP, Nirkko AC, Baumgartner RW et al: Transient cerebral circulatory arrest coincides with fainting in cough syncope, *Neurology* 45:498, 1995.
13. Nollert G, Mohnle P, Tassani-Prell P et al: Determinants of cerebral oxygenation during cardiac surgery, *Circulation* 92:II327, 1995.
14. Ulloa HM, Houston BJ, Altrogge DM: Arrhythmia prevalence during ambulatory electrocardiographic monitoring of beagles, *Am J Vet Res* 56:275, 1995.
15. Hall LW, Dunn JK, Delaney M et al: Ambulatory electrocardiography in dogs, *Vet Rec* 129:213, 1991.
16. Branch CE, Robertson BT, Williams JC: Frequency of second-degree atrioventricular heart blocks in dogs, *Am J Vet Res* 36:925, 1975.

CHAPTER 29

Drugs Used in Treatment of Cardiac Arrhythmias

Mechanisms by Which Antiarrhythmic Drugs Abolish Tachyarrhythmias

REENTRANT ARRHYTHMIAS

Reentrant arrhythmias are created by labile electrical circuits. There are many ways to interrupt these circuits; therefore antiarrhythmic therapy is often successful at abolishing them. On the other hand, reentrant circuits are probably responsible for most ventricular arrhythmias that produce sudden death, even when patients are on antiarrhythmic medication. Although antiarrhythmic drugs are effective at suppressing reentrant arrhythmias, they probably are not very good at abolishing them or effectively keeping them suppressed.

Reentrant circuits are initiated and maintained by regions of slowed conduction and conduction block with refractory periods that are normal or shorter than normal in undamaged tissue. Antiarrhythmic drugs can disrupt these circuits in the following ways: (1) creating a bidirectional block (either by slowing conduction to the point that it decrements to no conduction or by increasing the refractory period of the abnormal segment); (2) improving conduction or shortening the refractory period of the abnormal segment to the point that there is no unidirectional block; (3) prolonging the refractory period of the normal tissue to the point that it is still refractory when confronted by the reentrant impulse; (4) speeding conduction in the normal segment; (5) slowing conduction in the circuit to the point that an electrical impulse from another site (usually the sinus node) depolarizes the circuit before it has time to complete its path; and (6) increasing the sinus rate to the point that the normal electrical impulse depolarizes the circuit before it completes its path. Almost all antiarrhythmic drugs can accomplish one or more of these goals. For example, in ventricular myocardium, quinidine can depress conduction in the abnormal segment to the point that a bidirectional block occurs. Quinidine can also prolong the refractory period of either the abnormal segment or normal tissue. The former results in a bidirectional block, and the latter keeps the normal tissue from being restimulated. Because depressed conduction is one feature of both reentrant circuits and antiarrhythmic drugs, it should be noted that not only can antiarrhythmic drugs interrupt reentrant circuits, they may also create them.

ABNORMAL AUTOMATICITY

Arrhythmias resulting from abnormal automaticity can be abolished by antiarrhythmic drugs.[1,2] This can be accomplished by altering membrane currents responsible for spontaneously depolarizing these cells (e.g., the i_f current or the chloride current). It can also be accomplished by decreasing the excitability of these damaged cells or bringing resting membrane potential back toward normal. The exact mechanisms by which these are accomplished are unclear. It appears that lidocaine is one of the most successful drugs at suppressing abnormal automaticity. Other class I agents are less successful.

TRIGGERED ACTIVITY

Arrhythmias resulting from early afterdepolarizations (EADs) can theoretically be abolished by drugs that shorten the action potential duration or speed the heart rate. Action potential duration can be decreased by agents that enhance repolarization by slowing the slow inward calcium current during phase 2 of the action potential or by increasing the potassium current, i_x.[3] Magnesium and catecholamine stimulation are known to reduce the formation of EADs. Increasing the heart rate is another effective means of suppressing EADs.[4]

Delayed afterdepolarizations (DADs) can theoretically be suppressed by drugs that increase potassium flux out of the cell during repolarization.[3] Because DADs are often caused by cellular calcium overload, drugs that decrease intracellular calcium would be expected to be antiarrhythmic as well. Verapamil can suppress ventricular arrhythmias induced by DADs in experimental dogs with digitalis intoxication.[5] However, the dose used in these experimental dogs (0.5 to 1.0 mg/kg IV) is approximately 10 times that used clinically. This dose could produce a profound decrease in contractility and should not be tried clinically. Lidocaine reduces the amplitude of DADs, but the mechanism is unexplained.[6,7] It is the drug of choice for digitalis intoxication–induced DADs. Phenytoin is also used for digitalis intoxication and so is likely able to suppress DADs.

Drugs Used to Treat Tachyarrhythmias

CLASSES OF ANTIARRHYTHMIC AGENTS

The drugs used to treat supraventricular and ventricular tachyarrhythmias can be divided into separate classes based on their generalized mechanisms of action. Antiarrhythmic drugs exert their effects primarily by blocking sodium, potassium, or calcium channels or β-receptors. These drugs are commonly subclassified. This classification scheme is somewhat helpful clinically when deciding to use particular drugs for specific arrhythmias. However, the actions of antiarrhythmic drugs are usually studied in vitro using somewhat arbitrary concentrations of drugs on isolated normal Purkinje fibers.

Because most arrhythmias are not generated in normal Purkinje fibers, any findings in these preparations must be interpreted cautiously. Consequently, clinical experience with these drugs is the more important means of determining efficacy to suppress tachyarrhythmias. A table of the common arrhythmias, the mechanisms responsible for their generation, and the drugs most commonly effective clinically are listed in Table 29-1. The doses of the common antiarrhythmic agents are listed in Table 29-2.

Class I. Class I drugs are the so-called membrane stabilizers. Their common mechanism of action is the blockade of a certain percentage of the fast sodium channels in myocardium. Sodium channel blockade results in a decrease in the upstroke (phase 0) velocity of the action potential in atrial and ventricular myocardium and Purkinje cells. The upstroke velocity is a major determinant of conduction velocity. Consequently, class I drugs slow conduction velocity in normal cardiac tissue, abnormal cardiac tissue, or both. Class I agents have variable effects on repolarization. Some of them prolong repolarization, whereas others shorten it or have no effect. Primarily based on differences in repolarization effects, class I agents are subdivided into classes Ia, Ib, and Ic. Class Ia agents include quinidine, procainamide, and disopyramide. These agents depress conduction in normal and abnormal cardiac tissue and prolong repolarization. Class Ib agents include lidocaine and its derivatives, tocainide, and mexiletine. Phenytoin is also in this class. Class Ib agents do not prolong conduction velocity in normal cardiac tissue nearly as much as class Ia drugs. They do, however, have profound effects on conduction velocity in abnormal cardiac tissue.[8] They also shorten the action potential duration by accelerating repolarization in Purkinje fibers. A greater degree of shortening occurs in fibers that have a longer action potential duration.[9] They have little effect on the effective refractory period of normal atrial and ventricular muscle.[10,11] In contrast, lidocaine may prolong the effective refractory period of damaged myocardium.[12] Class IC antiarrhythmic drugs include encainide and flecainide. These drugs slow conduction and have little effect on action potential duration.

Class II. Class II drugs are the β-adrenergic blocking drugs. Class II drugs are useful for both supraventricular and ventricular tachyarrhythmias. Although few tachyarrhythmias are the direct result of catecholamine stimulation, β-adrenergic receptor stimulation by catecholamines commonly exacerbates abnormal cellular electrophysiology. This can result in initiation or enhancement of a tachyarrhythmia. Drugs that block β-adrenergic receptors do not have direct membrane effects at clinically relevant concentrations. Consequently, their action is indirect and related to blocking catecholamine enhancement of abnormal electrophysiology or related to other effects of the drug. An example of the latter is β-adrenergic receptor blockade resulting in a decrease in myocardial contractility and therefore in myocardial oxygen consumption. The resultant improvement in myocardial oxygenation might improve cellular electrophysiology and reduce arrhythmia formation.

Class II drugs are most commonly used to alter the electrophysiologic properties of the atrioventricular (AV) junction in patients with supraventricular tachyarrhythmias. β-receptor blockade at the AV junction results in an increase in conduction time through the AV junction and an increase in the time that the AV junction is refractory to depolarization. Both changes effectively disrupt reentrant circuits that use the AV node as part of the circuit. An increase in AV junctional refractoriness decreases the number of depolarizations

TABLE 29-1

Arrhythmias: mechanisms for generation and commonly effective drugs for treatment

Arrhythmia	*Mechanism*	*Vulnerable parameter*	*Effective drugs*
Inappropriate sinus tachycardia	Enhanced normal automaticity	Decrease phase 4 depolarization	β-Adrenergic blockers, digitalis
Ectopic atrial tachycardia	Abnormal automaticity	Maximum diastolic potential or phase 4 depolarization	Digitalis, class I (not lidocaine), class IV
Accelerated idioventricular rhythm	Abnormal automaticity	Maximum diastolic potential or phase 4 depolarization	Usually don't treat; lidocaine, other class I agents, possibly class IV
Ventricular tachycardia in German shepherds	Early afterdepolarizations (EADs)	Arrhythmias occur at slow heart rate	β-Agonists or atropine (increase sinus rate)
Digitalis-induced arrhythmias	Delayed afterdepolarizations (DADs)	Suppress DADs or decrease calcium overload	Lidocaine or phenytoin, possibly class IV (verapamil)
Supraventricular tachycardia resulting from pre-excitation	Reentry (long or short excitable gap or calcium channel–dependent)	Prolong the refractory period or depress calcium channel–dependent conduction	Class I except Ib, class III, class IV, digitalis
Primary (slow) atrial fibrillation	Reentry (short excitable gap)	Prolong refractory period of atrial myocardium	Quinidine, class III
Secondary (fast) atrial fibrillation	Reentry with AV block	Prolong refractory period of AV node to slow ventricular rate	Digitalis, β-adrenergic blockers, diltiazem
Sustained monomorphic ventricular tachycardia	Reentry (long excitable gap)	Depress conduction and excitability to suppress; prolong refractory period to prevent ventricular fibrillation	Mexiletine, class III, lidocaine for short-term suppression
Nonsustained polymorphic ventricular tachycardia	Reentry (short excitable gap)	Prolong refractory period to suppress and prevent ventricular fibrillation	Class III, possibly mexiletine, lidocaine for short-term suppression
Ventricular fibrillation	Reentry (short excitable gap)	Prolong refractory period to prevent fibrillation	Class III
AV nodal reentrant (most supraventricular) tachycardias	Reentry (calcium channel dependent)	Depress conduction and excitability	Class IV, class II, digitalis

Modified from: The Sicilian gambit, Taskforce of the Working Group on Arrhythmias of the European Society of Cardiology, *Circulation* 84:1831, 1991.
AV, Atrioventricular.

TABLE 29-2
Common antiarrhythmic agents

Drug (trade name)	*Species*	*Route*	*Dose*
β-Adrenergic blockers			
Atenolol (Tenormin)	Dog	PO	6.25-50 mg q12h (total dose; start low; titrate)
Atenolol (Tenormin)	Cat	PO	6.25-12.5 mg q12-24h (total dose; start low; titrate)
Esmolol (Brevibloc)	Both	IV	0.25-0.5 mg/kg (slow bolus) 10-200 μg/kg/min infusion
Propranolol (Inderal)	Dog	PO	0.1-2.0 mg/kg q8h (start low and titrate to effect in atrial fibrillation; higher doses used for other arrhythmias)
Propranolol (Inderal)	Cat	PO	2.5-10 mg (total dose; start low; titrate)
Propranolol (Inderal)	Both	IV	0.01-0.1 mg/kg (start low; titrate to effect for supraventricular arrhythmias)
Sotalol (Betapace)	Dog	PO	1-3 mg/kg q12h
Calcium channel blockers			
Diltiazem (Cardizem)	Dog	PO	0.5-1.5 mg/kg q8h (start low; titrate to effect for atrial fibrillation)
Diltiazem (Cardizem)	Dog	PO	0.5-3 mg/kg (start low; titrate to effect for supraventricular tachycardia)
Diltiazem (Cardizem)	Dog	IV	0.05-0.25 mg/kg (administer initial 0.05 mg/kg dose over 2-3 min; repeat every 5 min up to cumulative dose of 0.25 mg/kg)
Diltiazem (Cardizem)	Cat	PO	7.5-15 mg q8h (total dose)
Verapamil (many)	Dog	IV	0.05-0.25 mg/kg (administer initial 0.05 mg/kg dose over 2-3 min; repeat every 5 min up to cumulative dose of 0.15 mg/kg)
Positive chronotropes			
Atropine (many)	Both	IV, SC	0.02-0.04 mg/kg
Glycopyrolate (Robinul)	Both	IV, SC	0.005-0.01 mg/kg
Isoproterenol (many)	Both	IV	0.01-0.1 μg/kg/min (constant-rate infusion; alternatively 1 mg diluted into 500 mL of 5% dextrose or lactate Ringer's solution and infuse to effect)
Terbutaline (Brethine, Bricanyl)	Dog	PO	2.5-10 mg (total dose; start low; titrate)
Ventricular antiarrhythmics			
Amiodarone (Cordarone)	Dog	PO	Loading dose: 10-30 mg/kg q24h for 7-10 days; maintenance dose: 5-15 mg/kg q24h
Lidocaine (Xylocaine)	Dog	IV	Loading dose: 2-4 mg/kg slow bolus over 1 to 3 minutes maintenance dose: 40-100 μg/kg/min
Mexiletine (Mexitil)	Dog	PO	5-10 mg/kg q8h
Phenytoin (Dilantin)	Dog	PO	20-35 mg/kg q8h
Procainamide (Pronestyl; Pronestyl-SR)	Dog	PO	10-30 mg/kg q6-8h
Procainamide (Pronestyl)	Dog	IV, IM	5-20 mg/kg (administer slowly; start low; titrate)
Quinidine (many)	Dog	PO, IM	6-16 mg/kg q6-8h
Tocainide	Dog	PO	10-15 mg/kg q8h

reaching the ventricles from the atria in atrial fibrillation and flutter. Class II drugs are also commonly used with other agents to suppress ventricular arrhythmias.

Class III. Class III drugs act primarily by prolonging the action potential duration and refractory period. Therefore they increase the fibrillation threshold and are used primarily to prevent sudden death resulting from ventricular tachyarrhythmias. They may, however, also have the ability to suppress ventricular arrhythmias. Examples of class III drugs are amiodarone, bretylium, and sotalol. Neither we nor others have enough experience using class III drugs in veterinary patients. The use of these drugs is evolving in veterinary medicine.

Class IV. Class IV drugs are the calcium channel blocking drugs. They are also known as *calcium entry blockers, calcium channel antagonists,* and *slow-channel inhibitory blockers.* They act by inhibiting the function of the L-type calcium channels in cardiac cell membranes. Slow calcium channels are responsible for depolarization of sinus node and AV junctional tissues and for initiation of excitation-contraction coupling in myocardial cells. Calcium channel blocking drugs slow the upstroke velocity of sinus node and AV junctional cell action potentials, resulting in slowing of sinoatrial and AV junctional conduction times.[13] They may also slow the depolarization rate of the sinus node. Calcium channel blocking drugs prolong the time for recovery from inactivation of the slow calcium channel and as a result markedly prolong the refractory period of the AV junctional tissue. Calcium channel blocking drugs are also negative inotropic agents because of their effects on L-type slow calcium channels during phase 2 of the action potential in myocardial cells.

Because the primary effects of the calcium channel blocking drugs are on the sinus node and the AV junction, these drugs are most effective for treating supraventricular tachyarrhythmias. Although they have been shown to suppress DADs that occur secondary to digitalis intoxication and to depress automaticity in abnormally automatic cells, clinically they are generally considered not to be efficacious for treating ventricular tachyarrhythmias.[14]

CLASS I ANTIARRHYTHMIC DRUGS

Lidocaine

Actions. Lidocaine is a class Ia antiarrhythmic agent that is also used for local anesthesia. It has little effect on atrial conduction or refractoriness and is not used for atrial tachyarrhythmias. Lidocaine can abolish both automatic and reentrant ventricular arrhythmias.

Lidocaine can abolish ventricular reentrant arrhythmias by either increasing or decreasing conduction velocity within the circuit or prolonging the refractory period. The cellular actions of lidocaine are dependent on the extracellular potassium concentration.[15] When the resting membrane potential is decreased, such as when potassium concentration is high, lidocaine acts by suppressing fast sodium channel activity similarly to quinidine and procainamide. Lidocaine has more marked effects on automaticity, conduction velocity, and refractoriness in damaged cells (where resting membrane potential is also often decreased) than in normal cells.[16-18] Lidocaine can also hyperpolarize partially depolarized cells and so can improve conduction in a region of damaged myocardium.[19] The multitude of potential actions on variables that produce reentrant arrhythmias make lidocaine an especially effective drug for abolishing reentrant arrhythmias. In arrhythmias caused by abnormal automaticity in ventricular myocardium, lidocaine's ability to hyperpolarize these partially depolarized cells gives it the ability to suppress these arrhythmias (e.g., accelerated idioventricular rhythm).[19] Although lidocaine has no direct effect on EADs, it may hyperpolarize or accelerate repolarization in cells with EADs, indirectly terminating the arrhythmia.[20] However, in German shepherds with ventricular arrhythmias caused by EADs lidocaine is not very effective. Lidocaine is effective at suppressing DADs resulting from digitalis intoxication.[7] Because of this ability and because of its ease of use, lidocaine is the preferred drug for the acute termination of digitalis-induced ventricular tachyarrhythmias.

Pharmacokinetics. Lidocaine's half-life in dogs is 90 to 100 minutes. Total body clearance is approximately 60 mL/min/kg.[21] Lidocaine is primarily metabolized by the liver with less than 5% of the clearance occurring through the kidneys. Clearance and half-life are prolonged by liver disease or poor hepatic perfusion (e.g., heart failure, shock, propranolol administration). The volume of distribution is approximately 6 L/kg. Heart failure may also reduce the volume of distribution, resulting in a higher serum concentration. Therapeutic serum concentration is thought to be between 2 and 6 μg/mL.[22]

Clinical use. Lidocaine is used clinically to treat acute life-threatening ventricular arrhythmias in many different clinical settings. Its rapid onset of action, effectiveness, safety, and short half-life make it ideal for acute interventions. Lidocaine's short half-life also allows quick changes in serum concentration, so that its effects can be titrated quickly. It is usually the most effective antiarrhythmic drug for treatment of a ventricular arrhythmia. It does not affect supraventricular tachyarrhythmias.

ECG effects. Lidocaine produces very few electrocardiographic changes except for a possible shortening of the Q-T interval. Unless the sinoatrial node is diseased, lidocaine does not affect its automaticity. It should be avoided in dogs with sick sinus syndrome. It does slow the rate of phase 4 depolarization in Purkinje fibers, resulting in a slowing of the rate of escape beats.[9] For this reason, lidocaine (or for that matter any other antiarrhythmic drug) should never be administered to a patient dependent on an escape focus, such as a patient with a third-degree AV block. Lidocaine has fewer proarrhythmic effects than other antiarrhythmic agents.[23]

Administration and dosage. Lidocaine is administered parenterally because it has a short half-life and is extensively metabolized by the liver to toxic metabolites after oral administration. Although intramuscular lidocaine administration is feasible in the dog, clinical experience is limited at this time.

Lidocaine is generally administered as an initial intravenous loading dose followed by a constant intravenous infusion. If a loading dose is not administered, maximum infusion rates will take 1 to 2 hours to achieve a therapeutic concentration. The initial loading dose in dogs is 2 to 4 mg/kg IV administered over 1 to 3 minutes, followed by an infusion of 25 to 100 μg/kg/min (Figure 29-1). The dose is titrated while observing the ECG. When the arrhythmia is suppressed, drug administration is discontinued. It may be necessary to repeat half the initial loading dose in 20 to 40 minutes if the arrhythmia recurs. In cats the initial dose is 0.25 to 0.75 mg/kg IV, followed by an infusion administered at 10 to 40 μg/kg/min. Cats more commonly develop seizures with lidocaine, and it must be used cautiously.

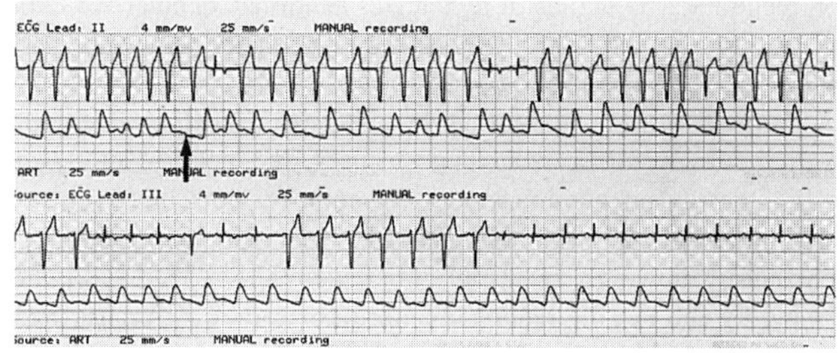

FIGURE 29-1 Simultaneous recordings of an ECG and systemic arterial pressure from a dog that developed a ventricular arrhythmia after being hit by a car. The top tracing shows runs of nonsustained ventricular tachycardia (rate = 150 to 300 beats/min) with pulse deficits (e.g., after the sixth QRS complex *[arrow]*) and alternating pulse pressure. Three 2 mg/kg boluses of lidocaine had been administered over 20 minutes, followed by 50 μg/kg/min with no response. Lidocaine was administered because of the very fast depolarizations. The infusion rate was increased to 100 μg/kg/min for 2.5 hours *(bottom trace)*. The rhythm is now well controlled, with short runs of accelerated idioventricular rhythm. By the following day the arrhythmia had abated. The poor response to the initial lidocaine bolus probably occurred because it was infused too slowly over too long a period.

Toxicity. Lidocaine exerts toxic effects on the central nervous system, producing signs of drowsiness, emesis, nystagmus, muscle twitching, and seizures. Dogs administered infusion rates at the upper end of the dosage range are commonly sedate. Toxic effects can be particularly severe in the cat. Treatment for toxicity is lidocaine withdrawal and, when necessary, intravenous diazepam administration (0.25 to 0.5 mg/kg IV) for seizure control. Lidocaine can depress ventricular function in severe myocardial failure, produce AV block in conduction system disease, and exacerbate sinus bradycardia and arrest in patients with sick sinus syndrome. It must be used with care in dogs with AV or ventricular conduction disorders. Prolonged lidocaine infusions during concurrent propranolol administration prolong lidocaine's half-life.

Supply. Lidocaine is supplied for direct intravenous administration as 10- and 20-mg/mL-concentrations (Lidocaine Hydrochloride Injection For Cardiac Arrhythmias, IMS South El Monte, Calif.; Xylocaine IV Injection for Ventricular Arrhythmias, Astra, Westborough, Mass.; Fujisawa SmithKline Corp., Deerfield, Ill.). It is also supplied at higher concentrations of 40 mg/mL (Xylocaine IV Injection For Ventricular Arrhythmias, Astra, Westborough, Mass.), and 100 and 200 mg/mL (Lidocaine Hydrochloride Injection For Cardiac Arrhythmias, Abbott, North Chicago, Ill.) for preparation of intravenous infusions only. Preparations containing epinephrine used for local anesthesia should never be used intravenously. Lidocaine is absorbed by the polyvinyl chloride in the plastic bags used to store intravenous solutions.

Phenytoin

Actions. Phenytoin, when used as an antiarrhythmic, shares many properties with lidocaine. It reduces normal automaticity in Purkinje fibers, abolishes abnormal automaticity resulting from digitalis intoxication, and has effects identical to those of lidocaine on reentrant arrhythmias. It repolarizes abnormal, depolarized cells, reduces sympathetic nerve effects, and may modify parasympathetic nerve activity in digitalis toxicity.[24]

Indications. Phenytoin may be effective in treating ventricular arrhythmias resulting from many causes, but because of dosing difficulties when administered intravenously, lidocaine is generally preferred for acute termination of ventricular arrhythmias.[25] Phenytoin, however, is useful, when administered at a dose of 50 mg/kg q8h PO, for treating digitalis intoxication.[25] Because it can be administered orally, phenytoin can in theory be administered prophylactically to patients that may be easily intoxicated with digitalis (e.g., severe myocardial failure patients).[25]

Administration and dosage. The oral phenytoin dosage is 30 to 50 mg/kg q8h.[25,26] Phenytoin absorption is erratic, slow, and incomplete from both the gastrointestinal tract and intramuscular injection sites.[26] The half-life is 3 to 4 hours. Serious arrhythmias require intravenous treatment in intermittent doses of 2 mg/kg administered over 3 to 5 minutes to prevent hypotension and cardiac arrest from the propylene glycol vehicle. The total dose should not exceed 10 mg/kg. Because phenytoin in solution has a pH of 11, phlebitis will occur unless a large vein is used and flushed immediately with normal saline. The drug should not be added to intravenous fluids because of lack of solubility and resultant precipitation.

Drug interactions. Phenytoin is metabolized by the liver. Any drugs affecting microsomal enzymes will therefore also affect the phenytoin metabolism. Chloramphenicol administration increases serum phenytoin concentration, and, in one study, it increased the half-life from 3 hours to 15 hours.[27] Phenytoin may also decrease serum quinidine concentration.

Toxicity. Long-term phenytoin administration at 50 mg/kg q8h results in an increase in serum alkaline phosphatase concentration.[28] Histologic changes consist of increased hepatic cell size. This appears to be due to increased glycogen storage.

Supply. Phenytoin (Diphenylan Sodium, Lannett, Philadelphia, Pa.; phenytoin podium, various manufacturers) is supplied as 30- and 100-mg capsules. For parenteral administration, phenytoin sodium (Phenytoin Sodium, Elkins-Sinn, Cherry Hill, N.J.; Dilantin, Parke-Davis, Morris Plains, N.J.) is supplied as injectable solutions of 50 mg/mL in 2- and 5-mL ampules or vials.

Quinidine. Quinidine is an optical isomer of quinine. It was originally prepared by Pasteur to treat malaria in 1853.[8] It was not until 1918 that quinidine was recognized as an effective agent for treating atrial fibrillation in humans.[8]

Actions. Quinidine is a class Ia antiarrhythmic agent that can be effective against automatic and reentrant supraventricular and ventricular tachyarrhythmias in dogs. Its primary action is to decrease the movement of sodium through the fast sodium channel during phase 0.[29] This results in a decrease in the upstroke velocity of the action potential and a consequent decrease in cardiac electrical impulse conduction velocity. This effect is enhanced by increasing extracellular potassium concentration because of the decreased resting membrane potential.[30] Quinidine prolongs the refractory period in atrial, ventricular, and Purkinje cells, which can effectively interrupt reentrant pathways. Quinidine also acts to decrease the slope of phase 4 and increase the threshold potential toward 0 in automatic cells.[31] In so doing it suppresses normal automaticity in Purkinje fibers and suppresses cardiac excitability. Sinus node automaticity is unchanged or may even increase because of decreased vagal tone in normal patients (vagolytic effect). There is a paucity of literature on the effects of quinidine on abnormal automaticity. Quinidine can suppress DADs in the Purkinje system, but it can also increase the amplitude of DADs in atrial myocardium.[8] Quinidine is used experimentally to produce EADs and so is unlikely to have beneficial effects with rhythms generated by this mechanism.[32,33]

Pharmacokinetics. Quinidine is about 85% protein-bound and has a half-life of 5 to 6 hours in the dog. A steady-state serum concentration is achieved approximately 24 hours after initiating therapy, but the serum concentration is commonly within the therapeutic range following the first dose (Figure 29-2). Pharmacokinetics have not been studied in cats. Quinidine is metabolized in the liver to some cardioactive and some inactive metabolites and is also excreted by the kidneys. Renal disease and heart failure may elevate the serum concentration. Microsomal enzyme–inducing drugs, such as anticonvulsants, may shorten the half-life of quinidine. Concomitant administration of the antacids aluminum hydroxide or magnesium oxide with quinidine decreases the maximum plasma quinidine concentration in dogs.[34]

Indications. Quinidine has been used most commonly for the long-term suppression of ventricular premature depolarizations and ventricular tachyarrhythmias. Chronic oral therapy of ventricular arrhythmias is most commonly aimed at preventing sudden death. Because quinidine does not appear, to us, to be very effective at preventing sudden death in dogs and, in humans, may increase the incidence of sudden death, use of this drug as a chronic agent has plummeted in our clinic in the past 5 years.[35,36] Quinidine can also be used acutely to abolish ventricular arrhythmias and is occasionally effective in the control of atrial premature depolarizations and paroxysmal supraventricular tachycardia. However, other drugs (e.g., digitalis, β-blockers, calcium channel blockers) are generally more effective in the dog for supraventricular arrhythmias. Quinidine is ineffective in dogs with atrial fibrillation secondary to cardiac disease. However, it can be quite effective at converting atrial fibrillation to sinus rhythm in dogs without underling cardiac disease (primary atrial fibrillation) (see Chapter 27).[37]

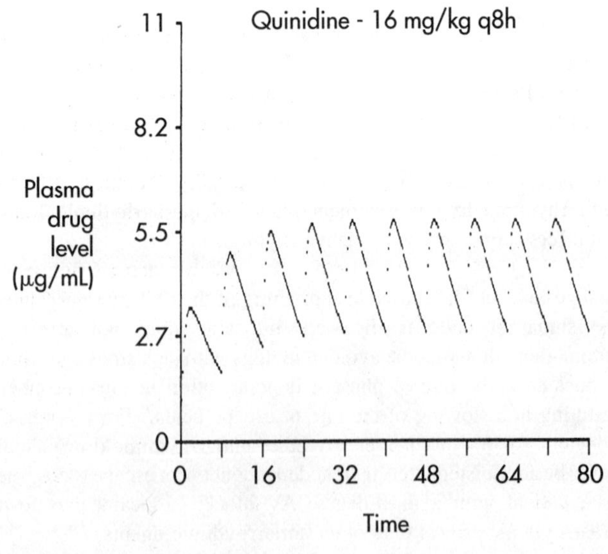

FIGURE 29-2 Computer-generated theoretical graph of plasma quinidine concentration over time following the administration of quinidine 16 mg/kg q8h PO to a dog. The volume of distribution was set at 2.9 L/kg and the elimination half-life at 5.6 hours. The bioavailability was assumed to be 80%. The therapeutic plasma concentration for quinidine is 3 to 5 μg/mL. Steady-state plasma concentration is achieved within 24 hours. The trough concentration is approximately 3 μg/ml, and the peak concentration is slightly above 5 μg/mL.

Administration and dosage. In dogs, the chronic oral dose of quinidine for treatment of ventricular arrhythmias is 6 to 16 mg/kg q8h. Quinidine sulfate is more rapidly absorbed than quinidine gluconate. Quinidine gluconate may also be administered parenterally, but rapid intravenous injections may cause dangerous hypotension. Lidocaine and procainamide are preferred over quinidine for parenteral administration. The parenteral dose is 5 to 10 mg/kg IM or IV.

Drug interactions. Quinidine displaces digoxin from binding sites throughout the body and reduces digoxin renal clearance, resulting in a higher digoxin serum concentration.[38,39] This is an important drug interaction and can lead to clinical signs of digitalis intoxication.[39] Most of the digitalis toxicity in this situation is due to central nervous system stimulation (e.g., vomiting resulting from stimulation of the chemoreceptor trigger zone). Brain concentration of digoxin increases by 50% when quinidine is administered, whereas digoxin concentration decreases in all other tissues.[40] Myocardial digoxin concentration also decreases after quinidine administration, so myocardial toxicity is not expected.[40] However, a decrease in efficacy might be expected because of this fact. Quinidine does not increase serum digitoxin concentration.[41]

Toxicity. Gastrointestinal disturbances are the most common toxic effects observed following quinidine administration. These appear to be direct effects of the drug on the gastrointestinal tract. Gastrointestinal side effects have been reported to occur in approximately 25% of dogs administered quinidine.[42] Cardiovascular toxicity is frequently reported in human medicine. Findings in humans have frequently been extrapolated to the veterinary literature. Quinidine toxicity is manifested as QRS and Q-T interval prolongation. However, we have not noted a clinically significant prolongation in QT interval or QRS complex duration, even in dogs that we have made toxic to the point of producing seizures. We have noted P-R prolongation and seizures at toxic serum concentrations during conversion of atrial fibrillation (see Box 27-1). One dog with aplastic anemia following quinidine administration is described in the literature.[43] The most important clinical problem that we have noted (although rarely) is an exacerbation of heart failure after starting quinidine administration. Presumably this is due to the negative inotropic effects of quinidine. In general, we avoid the use of quinidine in dogs with severe myocardial failure or in dogs that have or have had heart failure.

Supply. Quinidine is available as quinidine gluconate, quinidine sulfate, and quinidine polygalacturonate. Quinidine sulfate (Quinora, Key Pharmaceuticals, Kenilworth, N.J.) is available as 200- and 300-mg tablets. Quinidine polygalacturonate (Cardioquin, Purdue Frederick Co., Norwalk, Conn.) tablets contain 275 mg, which is equivalent to 200 mg of quinidine sulfate. Quinidine gluconate comes as a solution for parenteral use (Quinidine Gluconate Injection, Eli Lilly, Indianapolis, Ind.) containing 80 mg/mL.

Procainamide

Actions. Procainamide is a class Ia antiarrhythmic agent with properties very similar to those of quinidine. Procainamide decreases the upstroke velocity of phase 0 depolarization in normal action potentials and in action potentials produced by abnormal automaticity.[44] This slows conduction in these tissues. Reentrant tachyarrhythmias may be terminated by procainamide either slowing conduction or producing a bidirectional block in the abnormal segment of the reentrant pathway. This effect is enhanced as extracellular potassium concentration is increased.[45] This means that procainamide may be more effective in a patient with hypokalemia if the serum potassium concentration is normalized. Procainamide shifts the threshold potential to more positive values. This reduces the excitability of cardiac tissue.[46] It also increases the duration of repolarization and the effective refractory period.[47] The increase in effective refractory period is greater than the increase in action potential duration. Theoretically, this function should increase fibrillation threshold and make procainamide an effective drug for preventing sudden death as a result of ventricular fibrillation. However, clinically this does not appear to be the case in human or veterinary medicine. Procainamide can suppress digitalis-induced DADs.[48] This should theoretically make it effective for treating digitalis intoxication–induced tachyarrhythmias. Although it does suppress these arrhythmias in dogs, it appears that a very high serum concentration is required.[49] Procainamide was not effective against DADs produced by a means other than digitalis intoxication in one in vitro study.[50] It does not appear to suppress automatic atrial arrhythmias.[51] Procainamide has vagolytic properties.[52] These properties, however, are less than those observed with quinidine and are rarely clinically significant.

Pharmacokinetics. Procainamide has a short half-life of approximately 3 hours in the dog.[53,54] The short half-life is problematic when administering procainamide orally to a dog. To maintain a serum concentration within the therapeutic range generally requires administering the drug at least every 6 hours per os (Figures 29-3 and 29-4). The volume of distribution is approximately 2 L/kg. The vast majority of the drug is metabolized in the liver. Parenteral and oral routes of administration are used, but intravenous injections must be administered slowly to prevent circulatory collapse from peripheral vasodilation and decreased cardiac contractility. Procainamide pharmacokinetics have not been studied in the cat.

A sustained release preparation is available. It has the same half-life as procainamide but has a longer time to peak concentration (longer absorption half-life).[54] This enables q8h administration

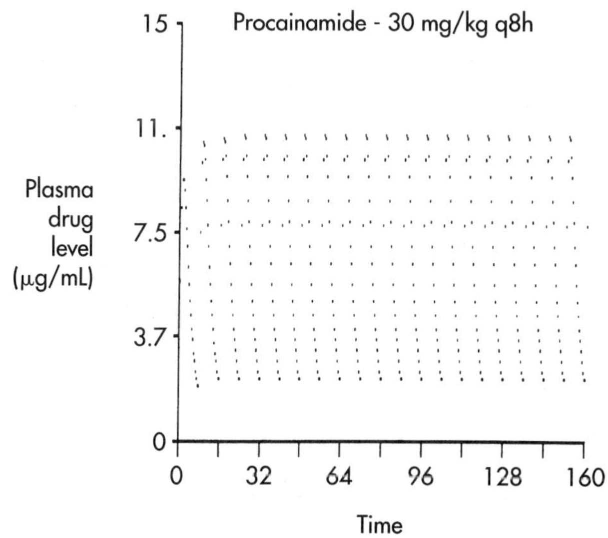

FIGURE 29-3 Similar graph to that shown in Figure 29-1 following the administration of procainamide 30 mg/kg q8h PO. The volume of distribution was set to be 2.1 L/kg and the elimination half-life to be 2.4 hours. It was assumed that the bioavailability was 100%. The therapeutic plasma concentration for procainamide is 4 to 20 μg/mL. This dosage regimen results in a peak serum concentration that is within the therapeutic range but a trough concentration that is subtherapeutic.

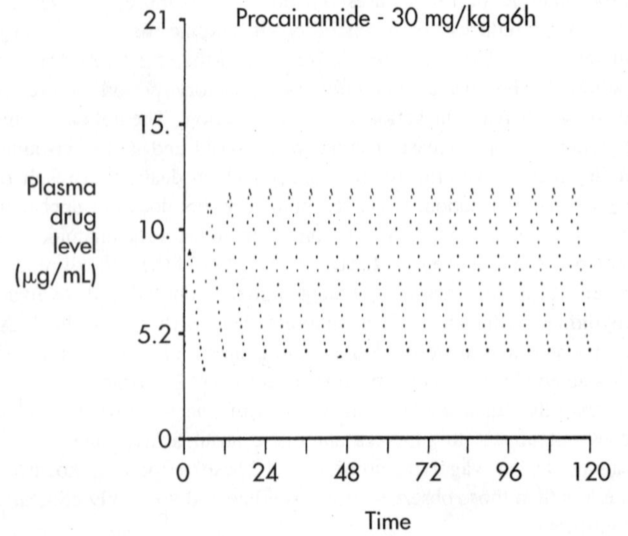

FIGURE 29-4 Graph shown in Figure 29-2 but with the dosing frequency increased to q6h. Peak and trough plasma concentrations are within the therapeutic range.

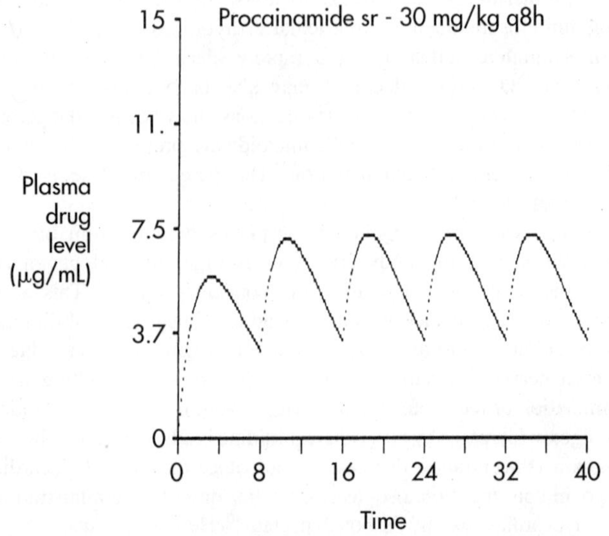

FIGURE 29-5 Similar graph to that shown in Figure 29-2. The absorption half-life has been increased to 2 hours to simulate administering sustained-release procainamide 30 mg/kg q8h PO. The peak plasma concentration is less than in Figure 29-2, but the trough concentration is higher and within therapeutic range.

(Figure 29-5). However, the peak serum concentration achieved with the sustained-release preparation is lower than with the regular preparation when administered at the same dose. Consequently, it has been recommended that the dose of the sustained-release preparation should be higher.[54]

Indications. Procainamide is effective against ventricular tachyarrhythmias and may be effective against some supraventricular tachyarrhythmias in dogs.[55] We have no experience using this drug in cats. Although it is often effective at decreasing the frequency and rate of ventricular tachyarrhythmias, procainamide does not appear to be very effective at preventing sudden death in patients with severe underlying cardiac disease. It may have proarrhythmic effects in certain patients. Consequently, we do not recommend its use in Doberman pinschers and boxers with dilated cardiomyopathy or dogs with subaortic stenosis that are prone to sudden death because of ventricular tachyarrhythmias. Procainamide is more rationally used in dogs in the intensive care unit with malignant ventricular tachycardia that is unresponsive to lidocaine administration or in anesthetized dogs that have a serious ventricular tachyarrhythmia that is unresponsive to lidocaine.

There is one report in the literature in which procainamide has been used successfully to treat one dog with a supraventricular tachycardia resulting from an accessory pathway (preexcitation syndrome).[55] We have had a similar experience in one dog. Procainamide has also been used in human medicine to treat a variety of supraventricular arrhythmias, including atrial fibrillation, and to prevent the recurrence of supraventricular tachyarrhythmias, such as atrial fibrillation, following successful conversion to sinus rhythm.[22]

Administration and dosage. Despite many years of clinical use, the oral dose of procainamide in the dog is still not well established. Previous recommendations of 8 to 20 mg/kg q6-8h PO are almost certainly too low.[56] The fact that we have never observed a case of procainamide cardiotoxicity suggests that even the doses that we use today (20 to 30 mg/kg q6-8h PO) could be too low. Studies of procainamide administration in a dog model of ventricular arrhythmia induced by ouabain administration, suggests that the serum concentration required to suppress this arrhythmia is much higher than the therapeutic serum concentration in humans.[49] In humans, the therapeutic procainamide serum concentration is generally 4 to 8 μg/mL. A serum concentration of 12 to 16 μg/mL is potentially toxic, and a concentration greater than 16 μg/mL is often toxic.[22] In the aforementioned study, a serum concentration between 25 μg/mL and 48.5 μg/mL was required to abolish the ventricular tachyarrhythmia in dogs. These dogs were anesthetized, so toxic effects could have been missed. Consequently, it is unclear whether all dogs with ventricular arrhythmias may require a concentration this high or if ventricular tachycardia resulting from digitalis intoxication is very resistant to the antiarrhythmic effects of procainamide. There is a report of one dog in the veterinary literature that required a serum concentration of approximately 20 μg/mL to control an arrhythmia associated with preexcitation.[55] No untoward effects were reported in this dog. This young adult male Labrador retriever required a dose of procainamide in the 30- to 40-mg/kg q8h PO range. Clinically, we usually use a dose of approximately 30 mg/kg q6h PO for procainamide hydrochloride and q8h for the sustained-release preparation. We rarely observe any clinically significant toxicity at these doses and can usually document efficacy.

One reason that humans may have beneficial effects from procainamide at lower doses and at a lower serum concentration is because they metabolize procainamide to a metabolite, N-acetyl procainamide (NAPA), which has antiarrhythmic properties. Dogs cannot acetylate aromatic and hydrazine amino groups and therefore are incapable of producing NAPA.[49]

When administered intravenously, intermittent boluses of 2 to 4 mg/kg should be administered slowly (over 2 minutes), up to a total dose of 12 to 20 mg/kg until the arrhythmia is controlled. This can be followed by a constant-rate infusion of 10 to 40 μg/kg/min.

Toxicity. Theoretically, procainamide can produce cardiotoxicity manifested as QRS and Q-T interval prolongation. We, however, have never observed this clinically. In humans, procainamide can have a proarrhythmic effect in some patients.[35] This has never been documented in dogs, although it is suspected. A toxic concentration can depress myocardial contractility and produce hypotension. The only means by which we can envisage this happening is with rapid intravenous administration. In humans, procainamide can induce systemic autoimmune reactions. It has been documented that experimental dogs (beagles) administered procainamide at 25 to 50 mg/kg q6h for 1 to 5 months develop antinuclear antibodies (ANA).[57] No one has examined this issue in clinical patients. Within the past 15 years, we have observed two possible immune-mediated abnormalities in dogs. We have observed granulocytopenia in one dog administered procainamide that resolved when procainamide administration was discontinued. We have also documented lymphadenopathy and a positive ANA test in one dog that resolved after procainamide administration was discontinued. Both dogs had been on procainamide for several years.

Supply. Procainamide hydrochloride (Pronestyl, Princeton Pharmaceuticals, Princeton, N.J.; Procainamide, various manufacturers) is available for oral administration in tablets or capsules containing 250, 375, or 500 mg and for parenteral administration in 10-mL vials containing 100 mg/mL and 2-mL vials containing 500 mg/mL. A sustained-release preparation is available in 500-mg tablets (Pronestyl-SR Filmlok, Princeton Pharmaceuticals, Princeton, N.J.) and as 250-, 750-, and 1000-mg tablets (Procan SR, Parke-Davis, Morris Plains, N.J.). The intravenous preparation may become light yellow, but can still be used. If the solution becomes amber, however, the drug has deteriorated and the solution should not be used.

Disopyramide

Actions. Disopyramide is an oral antiarrhythmic agent with properties almost identical to those of quinidine and procainamide.[58] Because procainamide is as effective as disopyramide and is safer, disopyramide is almost never used in canine patients.

Pharmacokinetics. In the dog, disopyramide has a half-life of only approximately 3 hours, which makes effective dosing difficult.[59] It is rapidly absorbed, and its bioavailability is 70%.[59]

Administration and dosage. When used as an antiarrhythmic in dogs, 7 to 30 mg/kg is administered q4h PO.

Toxicity. In experimental dogs, all doses prolong the PR interval.[60] Doses of 15 and 30 mg/kg q8h prolong the Q-T interval, and the 30-mg/kg q8h dose also prolongs the QRS complex duration.[60] Doses of 15 and 30 mg/kg q8h significantly decrease the echocardiographic shortening fraction.[60] Disopyramide is contraindicated in heart failure patients because it decreases myocardial contractility and increases peripheral vascular resistance, a potentially lethal combination.[61] Disopyramide is such a potent negative inotropic agent that it is used in humans with hypertrophic cardiomyopathy to reduce systolic anterior motion of the mitral valve.[62] Disopyramide possesses significant anticholinergic properties that may produce toxic effects.[63] It also decreases the serum glucose concentration in a dose-dependent manner (approximately a 15% decrease at a dose of 30 mg/kg).[64]

Supply. Disopyramide phosphate (Norpace, Searle Laboratories, Chicago, Ill.) is available in 100- and 150-mg capsules.

Mexiletine

Actions. Mexiletine is an analogue of lidocaine that is not extensively metabolized on its first pass through the liver. It was first used as an antiarrhythmic agent in Europe in 1969. Mexiletine can interrupt reentry circuits by slowing conduction and depressing membrane responsiveness, as is true of other class I drugs.[65] Abnormal automaticity is suppressed by mexiletine.[66] It can also suppress digitalis-induced DADs.[66,67] Most important, mexiletine can increase the fibrillation threshold in the dog ventricle. In one study of experimental dogs with myocardial infarction, ventricular fibrillation or a rapid ventricular tachycardia could be induced in six of 10 dogs at baseline by stimulating the heart with two premature beats.[68] These arrhythmias could not be induced after mexiletine administration.

Combination therapy is sometimes more effective than administration of one drug alone. In one study a combination of mexiletine and quinidine was more effective at preventing induced ventricular arrhythmias in experimental dogs with myocardial infarction than was either drug alone.[69]

Pharmacokinetics. Mexiletine is well absorbed from the gastrointestinal tract in dogs and has a bioavailability of approximately 85%.[67] Approximately 80% is excreted in the urine in dogs, and 10% is metabolized by the liver and excreted in the feces.[67] It has a plasma half-life of 3 to 4 hours in the dog.[67] Therapeutic serum concentration is thought to be between 0.5 and 2 μg/mL.

Indications. Mexiletine is indicated for chronically treating ventricular tachyarrhythmias in dogs. One group of investigators has reported limited success at suppressing ventricular arrhythmias with mexiletine in canine patients.[15] Another group has reported good efficacy.[70] However, in the latter report, many dogs had what appeared to be benign and self-limiting ventricular tachyarrhythmias, therefore knowing whether the drug was effective is difficult. Calvert has reported that mexiletine appears to be effective at controlling ventricular tachyarrhythmias and preventing sudden death in Doberman pinschers with dilated cardiomyopathy.[71] Although this has not been tested in any clinical trials, this report is encouraging and is consistent with the reported increase in the fibrillation threshold.[68]

ECG effects. In humans, mexiletine has no effect on sinus rate, PR interval, and QRS duration in patients without preexisting conduction system disease. In human patients with sinus node or conduction system disease, bradycardia and AV block can be produced.[8] In dogs, mexiletine has been studied in normal dogs at doses ranging from 3 mg/kg to 15 mg/kg for 13 weeks.[67] No effects on heart rate, PR interval, QRS complex duration, or QT interval were noted. No clinical signs of toxicity were seen.

Administration and dosage. The dose in dogs is 5 to 10 mg/kg q8h PO. An effective serum concentration may be achieved after three doses.[71]

Toxicity. Toxic effects can include vomiting and disorientation or ataxia but are uncommon at the suggested dosage range.[15,71] A dose of 25 mg/kg per os to dogs can induce seizure activity.[67] A dose of 40 mg/kg per os consistently produces ataxia, tremor, and salivation within 10 minutes after administration.[67] These signs last for up to 2.5 hours. Tonic-clonic spasms often begin within 15 to 40 minutes after administration and last for up to 1 hour. Vomiting and diarrhea can be seen at doses of 15 to 30 mg/kg.[67]

Supply. Mexiletine (Mexitil, Boehrenger Ingelheim, Ridgefield, Conn.) is supplied as 150-, 200-, and 250-mg capsules.

Tocainide

Actions. Tocainide is structurally similar to lidocaine. The major difference is that it is not metabolized extensively on its first pass through the liver after absorption (first pass effect).[72] Its actions on the normal action potential are almost identical to lidocaine.[73] Although its effects on abnormal action potentials have not been well studied, they are most likely also similar to lidocaine's effects. The depression of the sodium current is more pronounced in abnormal than in normal myocardial tissue. Tocainide does increase the fibrillation threshold.[74]

Pharmacokinetics. The half-life of the drug after oral administration is dose dependent.[75] After oral doses of 50 and 100 mg/kg the half-life is 8.5 and 12 hours, respectively. These doses are much higher than those used clinically, so the half-life of the drug at clinical doses is unknown but probably shorter. Tocainide is metabolized by the liver and excreted in the urine.[72] About 30% of an intravenous dose is excreted unchanged in the urine.[72] Therapeutic plasma concentration is thought to range between 4 and 10 μg/mL.[22]

ECG effects. In humans, tocainide produces little effect on the electrocardiogram in patients without conduction system disease. It has been documented to produce asystole when administered concurrently with a β-adrenergic blocking agent in human patients with sinus node dysfunction.[76] It produces no adverse effects in human patients with preexisting conduction abnormalities.[77]

Administration, dosage, and toxicity. Clinical experience with the use of tocainide in small animal veterinary medicine is limited. Doses required to adequately suppress ventricular arrhythmias in Doberman pinschers range between 15 and 25 mg/kg q8h PO.[78] These doses produce a serum tocainide concentration between 6.2 and 19.1 μg/mL 2 hours after dosing and between 2.3 and 11.1, 8 hours after dosing. At these doses, about 25% of dogs acutely develop anorexia. About 10% to 15% develop central nervous signs of ataxia or head tremor. Chronically, these doses produce the intolerable side effects of corneal dystrophy in 10% to 15% of dogs and renal failure in about 25% of dogs within 4 months. Apparently, smaller doses are not effective. We have used doses ranging between 10 and 15 mg/kg q8h PO in our clinic without evidence of toxicity. However, we have not been impressed with the efficacy of this drug at these doses. Consequently, it does not appear that tocainide is a drug that should be used in dogs for the suppression of ventricular arrhythmias and the prevention of sudden death.

Supply. Tocainide (Tonocard, Merck, West Point, Pa.) is supplied as 400- and 600-mg tablets.

CLASS II ANTIARRHYTHMIC DRUGS (β-ADRENERGIC BLOCKERS)

Class II antiarrhythmic drugs competitively bind with β-adrenergic receptors and therefore are termed *β-blockers.* All β-blockers exert their antiarrhythmic effects by inhibiting the effects of the adrenergic system on the heart. Cardiac adrenergic stimulation increases the heart rate, increases the conduction velocity through all regions of the conduction system and myocardium, and decreases the refractoriness of cardiac tissues. In addition, it enhances normal automaticity of subsidiary pacemaker tissue.

Three types of β-receptors, termed β_1-, β_2-, and β_3-receptors are present in the body. The β_1-receptors are primarily located within the heart and adipose tissue. Stimulation of these receptors results in increases in heart rate, myocardial contractility, atrioventricular conduction velocity, and automaticity of subsidiary pacemakers. The β_2-receptors are primarily in bronchial and vascular smooth muscle, where they produce relaxation. However, β_2-receptors are also in the sinus and AV nodes, where they contribute to the increase in heart rate and increased conduction velocity.[79] They are also present in myocardium, where stimulation results in increased contractility.[80] In addition, they are present in kidney and pancreas, where they mediate renin and insulin release. The β_3-receptors were discovered only recently and appear to depress myocardial contractility.[81]

Classes. Numerous β-blockers are marketed for pharmacologic use. They differ in ability to block β-receptor types. Some, in addition to their ability to block β-receptors, also can mildly stimulate β-receptors. Some are said to have membrane stabilizing effects, but these effects occur only at very high doses. Consequently, this is of no clinical significance. Some β-blockers also weakly inhibit α-receptors and so have mild vasodilating properties.[82]

Many β-blockers have been developed to selectively block β_1-adrenergic receptors. This is primarily because bronchospasm develops in humans with asthma that receive a β_2-adrenergic blocking drug. Dogs do not develop asthma. Consequently, no advantage to using a specific β_1-blocking drug exists from this standpoint in this species. This may be a reason to use a specific β_1-blocking drug in cats with asthma. Drugs that block β_2-receptors also limit the ability of patients with diabetes mellitus to respond to hypoglycemia with glycogenolysis. Consequently, drugs that block β_2-receptors should be avoided in diabetic patients. Drugs that block β_2-receptors also have the potential of blocking the peripheral vasodilating response to β-agonists. Consequently, peripheral vascular resistance may increase.[83]

In veterinary medicine, very few individuals have any clinical experience with the vast majority of the β-blockers. The two primary drugs in use today are propranolol and atenolol. Propranolol blocks both β_1- and β_2- receptors, whereas atenolol blocks only β_1-receptors. These drugs are equipotent, but their pharmacokinetics are different. Esmolol, a β-blocker with a very short half-life, is also used on occasion as an intravenous agent for short-term management of arrhythmias.

Veterinary use. In veterinary medicine, β-blockers are used to treat both supraventricular and ventricular tachyarrhythmias and prevent sudden death caused by ventricular tachyarrhythmias. Besides their uses as antiarrhythmic agents, β-blockers are used to treat hypertrophic cardiomyopathy in cats. They are occasionally used to treat systemic arterial hypertension. They may be more effective in cats than in dogs for controlling blood pressure.[84] Amlodipine, however, is more effective than propranolol for this purpose in cats. In our experience, β-blockers are usually ineffective for treating systemic hypertension secondary to renal disease in dogs.

As antiarrhythmic drugs, β-blockers are most commonly used to slow the ventricular rate in patients with atrial fibrillation, abolish supraventricular tachycardia, slow the sinus rate in cats with hyperthyroidism, prevent sudden death in dogs with severe subaortic stenosis (see Chapter 16), chronically treat ventricular tachyarrhythmias, and treat the cardiac effects of pheochromocytoma. They are used as sole agents or in combination with other antiarrhythmic drugs.

Actions. Drugs that block β-adrenergic receptors do not produce many of the specific cellular membrane changes observed with other antiarrhythmic drugs. At doses that induce β-adrenergic blockade, there is no change in resting membrane potential, amplitude of the action potential, or velocity of depolarization.[85] In the dog, however, atenolol does prolong the refractory period.[86] This change, along with the inhibition of sympathetic input, reduces the ability of induced premature beats to produce ventricular tachycardia and fibrillation in experimental dogs 7 to 30 days following induced myocardial infarction, at a time that ventricular arrhythmias are due to reentry.[86]

With all β-blockers, no simple correlation exists between dose or serum concentration and therapeutic effect.[22] The serum concentration required to produce a beneficial effect depends on the prevailing sympathetic tone and on β-adrenergic receptor density and sensitivity. These variables differ widely from patient to patient. In addition, the pharmacokinetics of β-blockers vary widely among patients. In humans, there can be 20-fold differences in plasma concentration in patients receiving the same oral dose.[87] In one study in normal dogs, a fivefold difference between dogs being administered the same dose was reported.[88] Because hepatic blood flow is a major determinant of propranolol clearance and half-life, this variability can be expected to be worse in cardiac patients in which hepatic blood flow is compromised. Consequently, the dose required to produce a therapeutic effect varies widely. Because of this, the dosage must be titrated to an effective endpoint.

Toxicity. In patients subjected to chronic increases in circulating catecholamine concentrations and increased sympathetic nervous system activity (e.g., patients with heart failure), β-adrenergic receptors decrease in number, internalize into the cell membrane, and become less efficient at producing cAMP.[89] These changes are commonly lumped together and termed *receptor down-regulation.* In these patients, fewer receptors are present to which a β-blocker may bind. However, many of these patients are dependent on the stimulated β-receptors to maintain a given degree of myocardial contractility. The acute administration of medium-to-high doses of a β-blocker to patients with compromised myocardial function (e.g., patients with dilated cardiomyopathy) that are dependent on β-receptor stimulation can result in lethal decreases in contractility and heart rate.

Propranolol

Actions. Propranolol is the prototype β-receptor blocking agent. Propranolol has antiarrhythmic effects that depend on its ability to block β-receptor stimulation. It reduces catecholamine-dependent automatic (normal and abnormal) rhythms and slows conduction in abnormal ventricular myocardium. Propranolol also increases the refractory period and slows conduction velocity in AV nodal tissues. This slows the ventricular response to atrial fibrillation and flutter and effectively abolishes supraventricular arrhythmias resulting from AV nodal reentry. By reducing contractility, propranolol reduces myocardial oxygen consumption, which may reduce myocardial hypoxia and arrhythmia formation in patients with subaortic stenosis. Propranolol also abolishes supraventricular and ventricular tachyarrhythmias resulting from pheochromocytoma and thyrotoxicosis.

Pharmacokinetics. Propranolol is lipid-soluble and therefore is almost completely absorbed by the small intestine. It is largely metabolized by the liver.[90] Oral propranolol undergoes a variable but extensive first pass hepatic metabolism. As a result, its bioavailability for the first dose ranges from only 2% to 17% for oral administration in the dog.[88] Serum half-life after the first dose is about 1.5 hours in the dog. Chronic oral dosing increases half-life to about 2 hours and results in serum concentrations 1.25 to 10 times greater than after initial doses because of an increase in bioavailability. This increase is probably due to saturation of the metabolic process involved in metabolizing the drug on its first pass through the liver after absorption.

Propranolol, like any β-blocker, produces dosage-dependent decreases in myocardial contractility. This does not occur after an intravenous dose of 0.02 mg/kg in normal dogs (this would be comparable to an oral dose of 0.2 mg/kg).[83] An intravenous dose of 0.08 mg/kg (comparable oral dose = 0.8 mg/kg) decreases dP/dt, an index of myocardial contractility, by approximately 30%. Propranolol does have a profound effect on peripheral vascular resistance in normal, conscious experimental dogs. At an intravenous dose of 0.02 mg/kg, peripheral vascular resistance increases to almost twice the baseline.[83] There is no further increase with a dose of 0.08 mg/kg. These effects have not been studied in dogs with heart failure, but it is apparent that larger doses of propranolol must be avoided in these patients. Propranolol appears to have a greater effect on the sinus rate in normal dogs than drugs that specifically block β_1-receptors.[83] This is probably because β_2-receptors are also present in the sinus node and help modulate the sinus rate.

Indications. Propranolol administration is indicated in canine and feline patients with ventricular and supraventricular tachyarrhythmias. It is commonly used with digoxin to slow the ventricular rate in patients with atrial fibrillation. It is effective for terminating and preventing the recurrence of supraventricular tachycardia. Propranolol can be effective as the sole agent for terminating ventricular tachyarrhythmias but is generally more effective when used in combination with other antiarrhythmic agents. Propranolol is effective for decreasing the sinus rate in patients with hyperthyroidism, pheochromocytoma, and heart failure. Few antiarrhythmic drugs can be used in cats. Propranolol has been used with moderate success to treat both supraventricular and ventricular tachyarrhythmias in cats.

Administration and dosage. The dosage of propranolol depends on the situation for which it is used. In dogs with atrial fibrillation resulting from severe underlying cardiac disease, the oral dose is from 0.1 to 0.5 mg/kg q8h. At this dosage range, the negative inotropic effects of propranolol appear to be negligible.[83] We have never witnessed exacerbation of heart failure at this dosage range in dogs with dilated cardiomyopathy or severe mitral regurgitation, even when the patient was not being administered a concomitant positive inotropic agent, such as digoxin. In canine patients with supraventricular or ventricular tachyarrhythmias and normal myocardial function, doses as high as 2 mg/kg q8h are well tolerated and often required. Doses in this range are contraindicated in patients with severe myocardial failure. Duration of drug effect is longer than the drug's half-life because of active propranolol metabolites and receptor binding of the drug.[91] Consequently, administering the drug every 8 hours appears to be effective. The feline oral dose is 2.5 to 10 mg q8h for the control of tachyarrhythmias. The intravenous dose in dogs is administered as intermittent boluses to effect. The initial intravenous dose of 0.02 mg/kg is much lower than an oral dose, and the total dose should not exceed 0.1 mg/kg. Intravenous doses of propranolol must be administered cautiously to heart failure patients because a decrease in contractility may acutely worsen hemodynamics. The therapeutic endpoint for propranolol is abolition or improvement of a tachyarrhythmia, slowing of the sinus rate, or slowing of the ventricular response to atrial fibrillation.

Toxicity. Toxicity of propranolol is related to its β-blocking actions. Patients with myocardial failure or heart failure as a result of severe volume overload may have their failure state exacerbated by propranolol, especially if it is administered intravenously. These patients usually receive propranolol for control of heart rate, and only low oral doses generally are needed. If acute heart failure is precipitated, catecholamines cannot reverse the problem, so calcium or digitalis must be used. Digitalis plus propranolol can cause varying degrees of AV block.

Propranolol should not be administered to patients with conduction disturbances or abnormal inherent pacemaker function. Propranolol will exacerbate the sinus node dysfunction in patients with sick sinus syndrome. It will also exacerbate AV nodal dysfunction in patients with first- and second-degree AV block, potentially creating third-degree AV block. In patients with third-degree AV block, it will decrease the rate of the subsidiary pacemaker, a potentially lethal effect.

Propranolol should not be used in patients with asthma or chronic lower airway disease, because increases in lower airway resistance may occur with β-blockade. Propranolol should also be used with caution in diabetic patients receiving insulin, because propranolol reduces sympathetic compensation for hypoglycemia. Acute propranolol withdrawal may exacerbate the original problem for which the drug was being administered, so gradual withdrawal should be performed.[92] As an example, we have witnessed sudden death in a boxer with ventricular arrhythmia following the acute cessation of propranolol administration. β-Blockers should not be administered to patients with hyperkalemia, because the β-blockade reduces the potassium flux from intravascular to extravascular spaces.[93]

Supply. Propranolol hydrochloride (Inderal, Wyeth-Ayerst Laboratories, New York, N.Y.) is available as 10-, 20-, 40-, 60-, 80-, and 90-mg tablets for oral administration and in 1-mL ampules containing 1 mg for intravenous administration. When administered intravenously for therapy of acute arrhythmias, ECG and blood pressure should be monitored and the drug should be administered slowly. The intravenous preparation of the drug rapidly decomposes in alkaline solutions.

Atenolol

Actions and pharmacokinetics. Atenolol is a specific β_1-adrenergic blocking drug. It has the same potency as propranolol but different pharmacokinetics. Atenolol is more water-soluble than propranolol. In the dog, bioavailability appears to be approximately 80%.[94] Atenolol is eliminated unchanged in the urine.[94] There is very little hepatic metabolism. The half-life of atenolol is longer than the half-life of propranolol, being 5 to 6 hours in the dog.[94] This is somewhat shorter than the half-life in humans, which is 6 to 9 hours.[90] In the cat, atenolol has a half-life of 3.5 hours.[95,96] Its bioavailability is high, at 90%, and the pharmacokinetic variability from cat to cat is small. When administered to cats at a dose of 3 mg/kg, atenolol attenuates the increase in heart rate produced by isoproterenol for 12 but not for 24 hours.

Indications. Atenolol is used in both dogs and cats. In dogs, it is most commonly used in conjunction with digoxin to slow the heart rate in patients with atrial fibrillation. It is also used in dogs to treat supraventricular tachycardia and ventricular tachyarrhythmias and is used in an attempt to prevent sudden death in dogs with severe subaortic stenosis. It is used in cats most commonly to decrease systolic anterior motion of the mitral valve in feline hypertrophic cardiomyopathy and to treat ventricular tachyarrhythmias.

Administration and dosage. In humans, once-a-day dosing is adequate to maintain efficacy. This is unknown in the dog. Because of its shorter half-life in the dog, we administer atenolol q12h to our patients. The atenolol dose for dogs is 6.25 to 50 mg/dog q12h PO. In large dogs with atrial fibrillation, we usually start with a dose of 12.5 mg q12h PO and titrate upward until the heart rate is less than 160 beats/min. In small dogs, we start with a dose of 6.25 mg q12h PO. If used to treat ventricular arrhythmias in dogs without underlying myocardial failure or in an attempt to prevent sudden death in dogs with subaortic stenosis, the dose should be on the higher end of the dosage range. In cats with hypertrophic cardiomyopathy, atenolol can be used to decrease the subaortic pressure gradient that occurs secondary to systolic anterior motion of the mitral valve. In these cases, we start with a dose of 6.25 mg q12h PO and titrate upward. We have titrated as high as 25 mg q12h PO in one cat, with no untoward effects.

Supply. Atenolol (Tenormin, Zeneca, Inc., Wilmington, Del.) is supplied as 25-, 50-, and 100-mg tablets. It is also supplied as a solution of 0.5 mg/mL for intravenous injection. The intravenous dosage is not known for dogs and cats.

Esmolol

Actions and pharmacokinetics. Esmolol is an ultra–short-acting (half-life less than 10 minutes) β_1-adrenergic blocking drug used for intravenous administration. It has the basic structure of a β-adrenergic blocking drug but contains an ester on the phenoxypropanolamine nucleus that is rapidly hydrolyzed by red blood cell esterases.[83] The major metabolite of esmolol is ASL-8123. It has a half-life in dogs of 2.1 hours.[83] This metabolite has 1/1500 the β-blocking activity of esmolol, which is clinically insignificant.

Steady-state β-blockade is produced within 10 to 20 minutes after starting intravenous administration of esmolol in dogs.[83] After discontinuation of drug administration, no detectable β-blockade is apparent at 20 minutes postinfusion, regardless of the dose administered. Esmolol decreases the sinus node rate. At an infusion rate of 25 µg/kg/min, approximately 30% of the effect of isoproterenol-induced tachycardia is inhibited. This value increases to approximately 60% with a 50 µg/kg/min dose and to approximately 70% with a 100 µg/kg/min infusion rate. Myocardial contractility is depressed with esmolol.[83] In normal conscious dogs, an infusion rate of 10 µg/kg/min does not change dP/dt. An infusion rate of 40 µg/kg/min decreases dP/dt by approximately 30%, and an infusion rate of 160 µg/kg/min decreases it by 50%. Because esmolol only blocks β_1-adrenergic receptors, it produces no increase in peripheral vascular resistance.

Indications. Esmolol can be used in several clinical situations. It can be used for the acute termination of supraventricular tachycardia. It can also be used, at low doses, acutely to decrease the heart rate in dogs with severe tachycardia (heart rate greater than 250 beats/min) resulting from atrial fibrillation. In cats with hypertrophic cardiomyopathy (HCM), it has been used as an agent to determine if β-blockade will reduce the dynamic left ventricular outflow tract obstruction resulting from systolic anterior motion of the mitral valve.[97]

Administration and dosage. In dogs, esmolol can be administered in two ways. An initial loading dose of 0.25 to 0.5 mg/kg (250 to 500 µg/kg) can be administered intravenously as a slow bolus over 1 to 2 minutes and then followed by a constant-rate infusion of 10 to 200 µg/kg/min.[98] Alternatively, a constant-rate infusion of 10 to 200 µg/kg/min can be started without a loading dose. In this manner, maximal effect should be apparent within 10 to 20 minutes. With the loading dose, an effect should be apparent more quickly. An initial loading dose and the high end of the dosage range should only be used in dogs with normal cardiac function or cats with HCM. In dogs with severe dilated cardiomyopathy or severe mitral regurgitation and atrial fibrillation with a very fast ventricular rate, we recommend that esmolol only (no loading dose) should be infused and that the infusion should start at 10 to 20 µg/kg/min and be titrated upward every 10 minutes to an effective endpoint.

Supply. Esmolol hydrochloride (Brevibloc, Anaquest, Madison, Wis.) is supplied as a solution containing 10 mg/mL for injection and a concentrated solution containing 250 mg/mL for dilution in solution for intravenous infusion.

CLASS III ANTIARRHYTHMIC DRUGS

There is an increasing amount of data in human medicine that class I antiarrhythmic agents are ineffective for preventing sudden death and in some instances may increase the incidence of sudden death in patients with organic heart disease and ventricular arrhythmias.[99] Because of this, the use of these drugs in human medicine has plummeted within the past 5 years. At the same time, other drugs have been examined more vigorously. β-Blockers are effective agents for preventing sudden death in human patients with myocardial infarction.[100] Class III drugs act primarily by prolonging the refractory period. In so doing, they theoretically reduce the ability for microreentrant circuits to develop and therefore make it more difficult for ventricular fibrillation to develop.

Amiodarone

Actions. Amiodarone is a benzofurane derivative. It is structurally related to thyroxine and has a high iodine content. It is metabolized to desethylamiodarone in the dog.[101] Desethylamiodarone has important antiarrhythmic effects because of its ability to block fast sodium channels. It is more effective than amiodarone at suppressing ventricular arrhythmias 24 hours after myocardial infarction in experimental dogs.[102]

Amiodarone was first introduced into human medicine in 1961 as an antianginal agent.[103] Its antiarrhythmic properties were recognized in 1970. Since then, it has been used for this purpose extensively in human medicine in European countries. It is currently being used more frequently in human medicine in the United States to treat patients at risk for sudden death resulting from ventricular arrhythmia. This increased use is due primarily to the reports of proarrhythmia and increased mortality in patients with ventricular tachyarrhythmias receiving class I antiarrhythmic agents and to the recognition that antifibrillatory actions may be more important than antiarrhythmic action in preventing sudden death.[104-106] No one in veterinary medicine has any reasonable amount of clinical experience using this drug in dogs.

Electrophysiologically, amiodarone's primary effect is to prolong the refractory period of atrial and ventricular myocardium and the AV junction without changing resting membrane potential when administered chronically.[107,108] This may result in an increase in the PR interval and the QT interval on the ECG. Because of its effect on refractory period in myocardium, amiodarone has a marked antifibrillatory effect. Consequently, its primary clinical use is to prevent sudden death. In automatic cells, amiodarone reduces the slope of phase 4 of the action potential. This results in a decrease in the sinus rate. Amiodarone also can suppress tachyarrhythmias. Prolongation of the refractory period can interrupt reentrant circuits. In addition, amiodarone has sodium channel blocking properties (class I effects) that can slow conduction and interrupt reentrant circuits.[107] Amiodarone also noncompetitively blocks α- and β-receptors and appears to have some ability to block slow calcium channels.[109,110]

Pharmacokinetics. Amiodarone has bizarre pharmacokinetics. After repeated administration the drug has a long half-life of 3.2 days in the dog.[111] It is very lipophilic and accumulates to up to 300 times the plasma concentration in adipose tissue.[111] Once drug administration is discontinued, amiodarone is cleared rapidly from all tissues except adipose tissue. Myocardial concentration of the drug is approximately 15 times that of plasma.[112] The long half-life of the drug means that it takes a prolonged time to produce a significant effect once administration starts. It also takes a prolonged time for drug effect to dissipate once administration is discontinued. For example, the time to reach one half of the peak value ultimately achieved for the increase in left ventricular refractory period in dogs is 2.5 days.[113] The time to come down to one-half the peak value after drug administration is discontinued is 21 days in dogs. Because of the long time to onset, loading doses of amiodarone are commonly administered in human medicine. In humans it may take 1 to 3 weeks to observe an onset of action, even with loading doses.[22] Antiarrhythmic effects are present for weeks to months after discontinuing the drug in humans.

Indications. In dogs, amiodarone has been suggested as one possible drug to use in dogs with dilated cardiomyopathy that are at risk for sudden death.[71] We have not had enough experience with the drug to make this recommendation. However, the drug is potentially useful and may become more popular in small animal medicine as veterinarians gain more experience with it.

Administration and dosage. The effective dose for amiodarone in the dog is unknown. Because of its bizarre and variable pharmacokinetics, predicting the ultimate serum concentration is difficult and predicting the myocardial concentration is impossible. For years, amiodarone was administered to humans at higher doses than currently used. More recently, lower doses have proved efficacious. This was discovered through clinical use. Because amiodarone has not been used extensively in clinical veterinary medicine, it is unknown whether lower doses than those used in experimental studies are effective. It is known that an oral dose of approximately 10 mg/kg/day to experimental dogs increases the defibrillation threshold after 9 days.[114] No established relationship between plasma concentration and efficacy in humans exists.[22] However, a plasma concentration less than 1 mg/L is often not effective, and a plasma concentration greater than 2.5 mg/L is usually not needed. A plasma concentration greater than 2.5 mg/L is associated with a higher incidence of side effects in humans.[115] It is known that the plasma concentration was 1.9 ± 1.1 mg/L within 3 weeks in experimental dogs administered 40 mg/kg/day PO for 10 days, followed by 30 mg/kg/day PO for 4 days, followed by 20 mg/kg/day PO for 6 weeks.[112] It is also known that this dose was effective at preventing inducible ventricular tachycardia/fibrillation in these dogs with experimentally induced myocardial infarction. From these data, it appears that this dose may be effective in clinical canine patients. However, lower doses were not tested in this study, so it is unknown whether a lower dose might have been equally effective. The dose outlined above resulted in a plasma concentration greater than 2.5 mg/L in some dogs. This may suggest that a lower dose might be safer. However, low-dose (5 mg/kg/day) amiodarone therapy, which is what is used most commonly today in humans, results in a serum concentration of approximately 2.5 mg/L.[116] This may suggest that the pharmacokinetics are quite different in the dog and that a higher dose may be required in dogs compared with humans. One veterinary clinician reported that a dose of 10 to 15 mg/kg q12h (20 to 30 mg/kg/day) PO for 7 days followed by 5 to 7.5 mg/kg q12h (10 to 15 mg/kg/day) PO has produced an improvement in ventricular arrhythmias in a few dogs treated in this manner.[71]

Toxicity. Numerous side effects of amiodarone have been reported in the human literature. Amiodarone's side effect profile in dogs is poorly documented. Gastrointestinal disturbances have been reported in dogs.[71] In humans that receive more than 400 mg/day of amiodarone (400 mg is approximately 6 mg/kg/day), 75% experience adverse reactions, and 7% to 18% discontinue the drug because of side effects. Most of the adverse sequelae occur after 6 months of drug administration.

Adverse reactions in humans consist of neurologic problems (20% to 40%); gastrointestinal disturbances (25%); visual disturbances, including corneal microdeposits (4% to 9%); dermatologic reactions, including photosensitivity and blue discoloration to the skin (5%); cardiovascular reactions, including congestive heart failure and bradycardia (3%); abnormal liver function tests (4% to 9%); pulmonary inflammation and fibrosis (4% to 9%); and hypothyroidism and hyperthyroidism. Pulmonary fibrosis is the most common severe sequela to amiodarone administration. Pulmonary fibrosis, heart failure, and elevation of liver enzymes necessitate discontinuing the drug in humans. We can find no studies of chronic toxicity of amiodarone in dogs. Lung changes comparable to those seen in humans are induced in rats and mice. Pulmonary toxicity appears to be multifaceted, but inhibition of phospholipase A with resultant phospholipidosis is one mechanism responsible for producing pulmonary lesions.[117] Dyslipidic lesions can be produced in dogs in the gastrointestinal tract by amiodarone administration but only at very high doses (greater than 50 mg/kg/day for 30 days).[118] It is also known that amiodarone increases the phospholipid content of feline myocardium.[119] Consequently, it is suspected that chronic amiodarone toxicity could occur in dogs and cats.

Amiodarone can result in either hypothyroidism or hyperthyroidism in humans. Amiodarone inhibits T_4 and T_3 secretion from canine thyroid glands.[120,121] Consequently, thyroid function should be monitored when amiodarone is chronically administered in veterinary patients.

Drug interactions. Amiodarone alters the pharmacokinetics and increases the serum concentrations or the effects of several drugs in humans, including digoxin, quinidine, procainamide, phenytoin, and warfarin.[22,122] Amiodarone administration increases the bioavailability of diltiazem and decreases total body clearance and volume of distribution of the drug in the dog.[123] This results in an increased serum diltiazem concentration and could produce a toxic concentration. This combination should be used cautiously and the dose of diltiazem reduced.

Supply. Amiodarone (Cordarone, Wyeth-Ayerst, Philadelphia, Pa.) is supplied as 200-mg tablets.

Bretylium

Actions. Bretylium was first developed as an antihypertensive agent. In 1966, it was noted that bretylium increased the fibrillation threshold.[124] Since then, it has found limited usefulness as an antiarrhythmic and antifibrillatory agent in human medicine. Bretylium's primary effect is prolongation of the action potential duration and refractory periods in myocardium. It also decreases the disparity in action potential duration between normal and diseased myocardium. Bretylium is taken up by and concentrated in adrenergic nerve terminals. This initially results in norepinephrine release and a brief sympathomimetic effect. This is followed by an inhibition of norepinephrine release. Bretylium's major effect on cardiac tissues is to prolong the action potential duration and refractory period of atrial and ventricular myocardium and Purkinje fibers.[125] In so doing, it increases the fibrillation threshold.[126] Bretylium produces a biphasic effect on impulse initiation and conduction and on hemodynamics. Sinus rate, myocardial contractility, and blood pressure increase transiently for 10 to 15 minutes.[8] These variables then tend to decrease as sympathetic tone decreases. These antiadrenergic effects prolong atrioventricular conduction time in dogs.[8]

Indications. Bretylium is used for the emergency treatment of life-threatening ventricular tachycardia or ventricular fibrillation that recurs despite direct current shock and lidocaine. It is generally ineffective against supraventricular arrhythmias. Bretylium appears to have no use as an agent to produce chemical defibrillation in dogs.[127,128]

Pharmacokinetics. In the dog, bretylium has a biologic half-life of approximately 16 hours.[129] However, plasma concentration declines rapidly after intravenous administration of 15 mg/kg from approximately 20 μg/mL at 6 minutes to less than 2 μg/mL after 1 hour. The drug is cleared from the body through renal elimination.[130] The antifibrillatory action correlates with myocardial concentration, which increases slowly after intravenous administration to reach a peak 1.5 to 6 hours after dosing.[130] Consequently, antifibrillatory actions also peak in 1.5 to 6 hours.

Administration and dosage. Because the oral route of administration results in erratic absorption, the drug is only administered intravenously. The intravenous dose in dogs is 2 to 6 mg/kg. This dose increases fibrillation threshold 5 to 18 times the baseline.[130] Toxicity is rare, although hypotension can occur. In experimental dogs, this dose is effective at preventing ventricular fibrillation and tachycardia when administered every 12 hours chronically.[131,132] This, however, is not a practical means of treating canine patients. When administered to dogs during cardiopulmonary resuscitation, bretylium takes time to produce antifibrillatory effects.[133] Lidocaine produces a more rapid but less pronounced antifibrillatory effect. A combination of lidocaine (2 mg/kg) and bretylium (5 mg/kg) may have a more beneficial effect than either drug alone.[133,134]

Toxicity. Hypotension may occur following administration. Blood pressure should be monitored and dopamine or norepinephrine administered if systolic blood pressure falls below 75 mm Hg. Transient hypertension and arrhythmia exacerbation may occur after the initial dose because of norepinephrine release from nerve terminals.

Supply. Bretylium tosylate (Bretylol, DuPont Pharmaceuticals, Wilmington, Del.; bretylium tosylate injection, various manufacturers) is supplied as a solution containing 50 mg/mL. Bretylium tosylate in dextrose (Bretylium Tosylate in 5% Dextrose Injection, Abbott Laboratories, North Chicago, Ill., and Baxter Healthcare Corp., Deerfield, Ill.) is supplied as 2 mg/mL and 4 mg/mL solutions.

Sotalol

Very few individuals in veterinary medicine have adequate experience with the clinical use of sotalol. The information provided on this drug in this chapter is based on studies reported from its administration to experimental animals, on reports of its use in human medicine, on limited clinical experience, and on anecdotal reports from individuals that have used the drug. Sotalol is potentially a very useful drug in small animal veterinary medicine, but this potential has not yet been fully explored.

Actions. Sotalol is a potent and nonselective β-adrenergic blocking drug that also prolongs the action potential duration and increases the refractory period of both atrial and ventricular myocardium (class III effect).[135] In human medicine it is useful for treating a variety of arrhythmias and for increasing the fibrillation threshold. The drug has been used extensively to treat humans in Europe.[136] It has recently been approved for human use in the United States.

Sotalol is marketed as the racemic mixture of its stereoisomers, *d*- and *l*-sotalol. The *d* isomer has less than 1/50 the β-blocking activity of the *l* isomer. The *l* isomer's potency is similar to propranolol. The *d* and *l* isomers prolong action potential duration and refractoriness.[137] The increase in action potential duration is caused by blockade of potassium channels.[136]

Sotalol, when administered intravenously or at high doses orally, increases the QT interval on the ECG in experimental dogs.[138] As for any β-blocker, the heart rate is decreased with sotalol administration. It also prolongs the AV nodal refractory period and the PR interval because of its β-blocking effect.[139] Sotalol increases the atrial and the ventricular fibrillation threshold in experimental dogs.[140,141] The effect on atrial refractoriness should make it a good drug for preventing atrial fibrillation in dogs, especially those with primary atrial fibrillation after cardioversion. The effect on the ventricular fibrillation threshold should make it an effective agent for preventing sudden death in dogs. Its effects on defibrillation are less well understood. In one study, sotalol decreased the success rate for defibrillation, whereas in another study it decreased the energy required for defibrillation.[135,142]

The hemodynamic effects of sotalol are mixed. Because it is a β-blocker, a decrease in myocardial contractility is expected and has been identified in anesthetized, experimental dogs with normal hearts and in experimental dogs after myocardial infarction.[143,144] However, in isolated cardiac tissues, sotalol does not have any negative inotropic effect and may have a modest (20% to 40% increase) positive inotropic effect in catecholamine-depleted experimental cats.[145] This effect may be due to the prolongation of the action potential allowing more time for calcium influx in systole.[136] In experimental dogs, sotalol has less of a negative inotropic effect than propranolol.[146] In humans with compromised myocardial function, sotalol can induce or exacerbate heart failure, but the incidence is much lower that one might expect. In one study, heart failure was aggravated by sotalol in only 3% of human patients.[136] The potential negative inotropic effects of sotalol could theoretically produce myocardial depression and produce or aggravate heart failure in small animal patients. As in human patients, the dose must be carefully titrated, and canine or feline patients with moderate-to-severe cardiac disease must be monitored carefully.

Indications. In human medicine, sotalol is effective for treating various arrhythmias. It is not as successful as quinidine for converting primary atrial fibrillation to sinus rhythm.[136] It is, however, as effective as quinidine at preventing recurrence of atrial fibrillation after electrical cardioversion. Sotalol is effective at terminating supraventricular tachycardia resulting from AV nodal reentry or preexcitation in humans. In human patients with ventricular tachycardia, sotalol may be one of the more effective agents for terminating or slowing the tachycardia. It also appears to be efficacious for preventing sudden death.[136] These effects, however, are not profound and have required large clinical trials to reach statistical significance.

A major indication in veterinary medicine is boxers with severe ventricular tachyarrhythmias and syncope. Sotalol, in our experience and that of others, has been very effective at suppressing the arrhythmias and stopping the syncopal events in this breed.[147] We have limited experience with sotalol for the treatment of supraventricular arrhythmias.

Pharmacokinetics. In experimental dogs, sotalol is rapidly absorbed and has a bioavailability in the 85% to 90% range.[138,148] Consequently, the intravenous dose and the oral dose should be comparable. Less than 1% of the drug is metabolized. Elimination is via renal clearance and is linearly related to the glomerular filtration rate. Consequently, the drug dose must be reduced in patients with compromised renal function from any cause. Sotalol is not protein-bound in plasma of dogs. The elimination half-life is 4.8 ± 1.0 hours. The apparent volume of distribution is in the 1.5- to 2.5-L/kg range.

Following the oral administration of sotalol at 5 mg/kg q12h for 3 days (when steady state is reached in experimental dogs), the plasma concentration is 1.1 to 1.6 mg/L.[138] In humans administered the same dose, the plasma concentration is 2 to 3 mg/L. This discrepancy probably occurs because the elimination half-life in humans is longer (7 to 18 hours).[149] This suggests that the dose in dogs should be roughly double that used in humans. The human dosage recommendation is to administer 40 to 80 mg q12h as an initial dose. This dose then can be increased as necessary every 3 to 4 days. The maximum dose is 320 mg q12h. Assuming an average weight of 70 kg for humans, the dose starts at approximately 0.5 to 1.0 mg/kg q12h and can achieve a maximum dose of approximately 5 mg/kg q12h.

A plasma concentration of 0.8 mg/L is needed to produce half-maximal β-adrenergic blockade in experimental dogs.[150] This suggests that a dose of 5 mg/kg q12h PO to a dog should result in near maximal blockade. The plasma concentration required to prolong cardiac refractoriness is higher. In humans, a plasma concentration of 2.6 mg/L is necessary to increase the QT interval.[136] Doses between 2 and 5 mg/kg q12h PO in humans prolong the QT interval 40 to 100 ms. In experimental dogs, a dose of 5 mg/kg q12h PO also prolongs the QT interval.[138]

Doses used in experimental dogs. If the above data are accurate, the dose of sotalol in the dog should be somewhere between 1 and 10 mg/kg administered per os q12h. However, we do not recommend that the high end of this dosage be used before more clinical experience is gained. We advise extreme caution in veterinary patients with dilated cardiomyopathy or a severe volume overload. The manufacturer's recommendations for humans include starting therapy in an environment where the patient can be monitored.

In one study in experimental dogs, sotalol successfully converted atrial flutter to sinus rhythm in 14 of 15 dogs at a dose of 2 mg/kg IV administered over 15 minutes.[151] Atrial flutter was produced by intercaval crush and rapid atrial pacing. Quinidine only converted 9 of the 15 dogs at a dose of 10 mg/kg IV over 15 minutes. In a study to examine sotalol's ability to terminate and to prevent atrial fibrillation, sotalol was administered intravenously to dogs with induced atrial fibrillation.[152] At a dose of 2 mg/kg IV, sotalol did not terminate or prevent atrial fibrillation. At a cumulative dose of 8 mg/kg, however, it terminated the arrhythmia in seven of eight dogs and prevented its reinduction in all eight dogs. This effect was due to a prolongation of atrial refractory period.

Similarly, sotalol at relatively high doses suppresses the formation of ventricular arrhythmias in experimental dogs. In one study of conscious experimental dogs 3 to 5 days after myocardial infarction, four doses of 8 mg/kg *d*-sotalol administered intravenously successfully prevented the induction of ventricular tachycardia by programmed electrical stimulation in six of nine dogs and slowed the rate of the tachycardia in two of the three remaining dogs.[141]

Sotalol also effectively increases the ventricular fibrillation threshold in experimental dogs with myocardial infarction. Again, the dose required to produce this beneficial effect appears to be quite high, although the data are conflicting and lower doses were not used in most studies. In one study that examined conscious dogs, four doses of *d*-sotalol 8 mg/kg PO were administered over 24 hours. This dose prevented ventricular fibrillation secondary to ischemia produced distal to a previous myocardial infarction.[141] The use of lower doses was not reported. In another study using conscious dogs subjected to distal myocardial ischemia and infarction, sotalol was administered at 2 mg/kg and at 8 mg/kg IV. Although the two groups were not reported separately, it appears that both doses prevented ventricular fibrillation and sudden death. In the group of dogs that was administered sotalol, 13 of 20 dogs survived, whereas only one of 15 dogs administered a placebo lived.[153]

Clinical experience with sotalol doses. Although some experimental studies might suggest that high doses of sotalol are required to treat ventricular arrhythmias and prevent sudden death, anecdotal evidence from others and our own experience suggests that lower doses are effective and probably produce fewer adverse effects. Anecdotal reports and our experience suggest that boxers with severe ventricular arrhythmias and syncope with or without myocardial failure often respond favorably to the administration of sotalol. Syncopal episodes have ceased, and a marked reduction in ventricular arrhythmias has occurred. Doses used range from 40 mg q12h to 120 mg q12h (approximately 1 to 4 mg/kg q12h) PO.[147] The dose used in boxers is comparable to that used in human pediatric patients of 50 mg/m^2 of body surface area q12h PO.[154] One veterinary cardiologist has used this dose extensively in boxers with category 2 cardiomyopathy (see Chapter 20).[147] Boxers in category 2 have severe ventricular arrhythmias, syncope, and may or may not have myocardial failure. He has used it in boxers with shortening fractions as low as 5% with no apparent untoward effects. His protocol is to hospitalize the patient and place it on a continuous ECG monitor. The sotalol dose is titrated by administering 40 mg q12h PO for at least 1 day while monitoring the ECG. The dose is increased to 80 mg in the morning and 40 mg in the evening and then to 80 mg q12h until the ventricular arrhythmia is markedly suppressed. He occasionally has to increase the dose to as high as 120 mg q12h. During the titration period he carefully monitors the patient for any signs of low cardiac output but rarely experiences any difficulty.

One anecdotal report suggests that sotalol may significantly depress myocardial function in some dogs with depressed myocardial function.[155] In this situation, a Doberman pinscher with mild myocardial failure (shortening fraction = 20%; *E*-point–to–septal separation [EPSS] = 8 to 10 mm) was administered sotalol. Three weeks later the dog's myocardial function had deteriorated (shortening fraction = 15%; EPSS = 14 mm). Sotalol administration was discontinued, and myocardial function returned to the baseline. We have had one dog with a supraventricular tachycardia and a shortening fraction of 20% die within 12 hours after starting sotalol administration. Although the death could have been unrelated, the dog appeared to die of low cardiac output and no other cause of death was apparent. *Consequently, we recommend that patients with myocardial failure be monitored very carefully during the initial stages of sotalol administration, as outlined above.* In our experience, in dogs with myocardial failure, the most common response to a relative overdose is weakness, presumably secondary to a low cardiac output. In patients in heart failure, exacerbation of edema can occur. In most cases, withdrawal of the drug should be the only action required if evidence of low cardiac output or exacerbation of the edema becomes apparent. If this does not suffice or if the clinical abnormalities are severe, the administration of a bipyridine compound, calcium, or glucagon may be beneficial. Administration of a catecholamine, such as dobutamine or dopamine, will not produce the desired response, because β-receptors are blocked by sotalol.

Toxicity. Adverse effects of sotalol in humans are related to the negative inotropic effects of sotalol and its ability to prolong the QT interval. As stated earlier, the negative inotropic effects appear to be minor, and very few human patients experience exacerbation of heart failure. The most dangerous adverse effect of sotalol in humans is aggravation of existing arrhythmias or provocation of new arrhythmias. Excessive QT interval prolongation can provoke torsades de pointes in humans (see Chapter 27). Torsades de pointes has also been produced in experimental dogs.[156] It appears to be more difficult to invoke in dogs. For example, one canine model requires that the dog be bradycardic from experimentally induced third-degree AV block and hypokalemic (serum potassium concentration approximately 2.5 mEq/L) before sotalol can produce this serious arrhythmia.[156-158] The arrhythmia in this model can be terminated with intravenous magnesium administration (1 to 2 mg/kg/min for 20 to 30 min). Sotalol apparently can also induce other forms of ventricular tachyarrhythmia because of the prolongation of the QT interval.[159]

As for any other β-blocker, withdrawal of sotalol should be performed gradually over 1 to 2 weeks because of up-regulation of β-receptors. Sudden cessation of use can produce fatal ventricular arrhythmias. The drug should not be used in patients with conduction system disease, such as sick sinus syndrome, AV block, or bundle branch block.

Supply. Sotalol hydrochloride (Betapace, Berlex Laboratories, Wayne, N.J.) is supplied as 80-, 160-, and 240-mg tablets, which are scored.

CLASS IV ANTIARRHYTHMIC DRUGS

Description and discovery. Class IV antiarrhythmic drugs are the calcium channel blocking drugs. These are also known as *calcium entry blockers, slow channel blockers,* and *calcium antagonists.* Verapamil, the prototype calcium channel blocker, was discovered in 1963.[160] Verapamil was being developed as a coronary vasodilator and was discovered to have negative inotropic properties. The negative inotropism could be neutralized by the addition of calcium, β-adrenergic agonists, and digitalis glycosides—measures that increase calcium flux into myocardial cells. It was subsequently discovered in 1969 that verapamil and other drugs with similar effects selectively suppressed transmembrane calcium flow. Today, at least 29 different calcium channel blockers are used in clinical human medicine worldwide. In veterinary medicine, only verapamil and diltiazem have been used with enough frequency to make recommendations regarding therapy of arrhythmias.

Physiology of calcium channels. Calcium channel blockers interfere with the movement of calcium across the cell membrane through slow calcium channels. Charged ions such as calcium do not move across lipid bilayers (e.g., cell membranes). Consequently, they must move through channels in the cell membrane. Channels are protein complexes that span the cell membrane. Calcium moves from the extracellular space into the intracellular space via calcium channels. The movement of calcium through these channels is slow compared with the movement of sodium through sodium channels. Consequently, the calcium channels may be called *slow calcium channels.*

The calcium ion is fundamental in many physiologic processes, including initiation of further calcium release in cells, initiation of muscle contraction, and cellular growth. Extracellular calcium is an important source for intracellular calcium. Calcium gains entry to cells through calcium channels in the cell membrane. The movement of calcium through these channels is passive and occurs when these channels are open. Channels are opened by various physiologic and pharmacologic stimuli. Voltage-sensitive calcium channels are opened by depolarization of cardiac cells. Receptor-operated channels are activated by membrane receptors, independent of changes in membrane potential.[161]

Voltage-gated calcium channels are present in the cell membranes of all excitable tissues (e.g., muscle and nerve) and in the cell membranes of many secretory cells. Several types of calcium channels exist. They are designated as *T* (transient), *N* (neural), *P* (Purkinje [cerebellum]), and *L* (long-lasting).[162] Each channel type is operated by specific channel receptors, has its own molecular structure, is present in particular cell types, and is responsive to particular agonists and antagonists. The *N* channels are found only in neuronal cell membranes, appear to play an important role in neurotransmitter release, and are insensitive to calcium channel blockers. The *T* channels are in smooth muscle, skeletal muscle, and cardiac muscle cells. They do not appear to be involved in intracellular calcium ion homeostasis. This channel type is sensitive to calcium channel blockers but only at very high doses. The *L* channels are present in vascular smooth and cardiac muscle cells. They are the channels that are primarily responsible for regulating calcium ion influx associated with excitation-contraction coupling in cardiac cells and in contraction in vascular smooth muscle. This calcium channel type is extremely sensitive to the effects of calcium channel blockers and is considered the receptor site for these drugs.[161]

Types and actions. Calcium channel blockers have a variety of chemical structures. They can be classified into three groups: phenylalkylamines (e.g., verapamil), benzothiazepines (e.g., diltiazem), and dihydropyridines.[163] The dihydropyridines include nifedipine and amlodipine.

The primary sites of action for calcium channel blockers in cardiovascular medicine are the L-type calcium channels in cardiac cells and L-type calcium channels in vascular smooth muscle cells.[164] In the heart, calcium channel blockers directly decrease myocardial contractility, slow sinoatrial depolarization, and slow AV conduction. In vascular smooth muscle, calcium channel blockers produce relaxation of systemic arterioles, resulting in a decrease in peripheral vascular resistance. The ability of various calcium channel blockers to affect these sites varies tremendously between calcium channel blockers. Verapamil binds equally well to cardiac and vascular smooth muscle sites. The dihydropyridines have very little effect on cardiac calcium channels but have profound effects on vascular smooth muscle. Diltiazem is somewhere between these two extremes, with an intermediate effect on cardiac functions and a mild effect on vascular smooth muscle. In conscious dogs, nifedipine and verapamil increase the heart rate. This is presumably the result of a reflex increase in sympathetic tone caused by the vasodilation.[163] Diltiazem has little effect. Myocardial contractility is increased reflexly by nifedipine, decreased directly by verapamil, and not changed by diltiazem in the normal cardiovascular system. When the autonomic nervous system is blocked with propranolol and atropine, all three drugs decrease contractility and heart rate. These differences are due to slight differences in L-type channel subunit structure between different sites that results in marked differences in channel pharmacology.[165]

Calcium channel blocking agents that affect myocardial channels block the slow inward calcium current during phase 2 of the cardiac cell action potential. This results in a decrease in myocardial contractility. This may be beneficial in certain circumstances, such as in feline patients with hypertrophic cardiomyopathy and dynamic subaortic stenosis. In human patients with normal myocardial function, the negative inotropic effect is generally offset by the reflex increase in sympathetic tone. In human patients with myocardial dysfunction, however, the negative inotropic and negative chronotropic effects of a drug like verapamil cannot be offset by a sympathetic nervous system that is already maximally stimulated. The resultant decrease in contractility and heart rate following calcium channel blockade can be clinically significant.[166]

Because fast sodium channel (phase 0) activity is absent in the sinus node and in portions of the AV node, slow calcium channel activity is responsible for depolarization in these areas. Calcium channel blockers prolong AV conduction; slow the ventricular response to supraventricular tachyarrhythmias, such as atrial fibrillation; and abolish supraventricular arrhythmias when caused by reentry through the AV node. The depolarizing currents of the sinus node and the AV junction are, at least in part, carried by calcium. Calcium channel blockers have the potential of decreasing the sinus rate in patients with tachycardia, but reflex increases in sympathetic tone as a result of the decrease in vascular resistance commonly overcomes this effect. This effect can be lethal in patients that are dependent on escape rhythms to maintain heart rate (e.g., canine patients with third-degree AV block).

Clinical use. In humans, calcium channel blockers are highly effective for treating paroxysmal supraventricular tachycardia and are useful in slowing ventricular response to atrial flutter and fibrillation.[167] This is also their primary use in dogs.[168,169] Calcium channel blockers are effective for suppressing accelerated idioventricular rhythms in dogs following shock-induced myocardial injury and myocardial infarction.[170,171] They have also been effective at suppressing digitalis-induced ventricular arrhythmias in conscious experimental dogs.[5] To our knowledge, however, no reports exist in the veterinary literature concerning the use of calcium channel blockers to suppress ventricular arrhythmias in canine patients.

Verapamil

Actions. Verapamil is a synthetic papaverine derivative. It was one of the first calcium channel blockers discovered and the first to be used in clinical use in human medicine.[160] In human medicine it is used both parenterally and orally to treat supraventricular tachyarrhythmias, systemic arterial hypertension, angina pectoris, and hypertrophic cardiomyopathy.[172] In veterinary medicine, its use is restricted to intravenous administration for the acute control of supraventricular tachycardia in dogs.[168]

Pharmacokinetics. In dogs, verapamil is absorbed well (more than 90%) but undergoes extensive first pass hepatic metabolism, so bioavailability is only 10% to 23%. Verapamil is metabolized to several active and inactive metabolites.[173] Most of the metabolites are excreted in the bile. The half-life of verapamil is 1.8 to 3.8 hours in anesthetized experimental dogs, and the volume of distribution is 2.6 ± 1.0 L/kg.[174] The effective plasma concentration is probably 50 to 200 ng/mL. A plasma concentration of approximately 100 ng/mL increases the pulse rate interval in normal dogs, and a plasma concentration of approximately 200 ng/mL produces second-degree AV block. Myocardial concentration of the drug is linearly related to plasma concentration and is approximately 9 times the plasma concentration.[174] Left ventricular and AV nodal region concentrations are greater than the atrial concentration.[174,175]

Indications. Verapamil is indicated for the acute termination of supraventricular tachycardia in the dog. Although other indications may exist, we have not used this drug to treat any other arrhythmia and there are no reports of its use for other indications in the veterinary literature. The experimental literature suggests that verapamil may be effective for terminating accelerated idioventricular rhythm in patients in intensive care units and for treating digitalis-induced ventricular tachyarrhythmias.[5,170,171]

Administration and dosage. For the acute termination of supraventricular tachycardia, the intravenous dose ranges from 0.05 to 0.15 mg/kg.[168] The initial dose of 0.05 mg/kg should be administered over 1 to 2 minutes while the ECG is monitored. If this initial dose is not effective, the same dose should be repeated 5 to 10 minutes later. If the arrhythmia still is not terminated, a last dose of 0.05 mg/kg (total dose = 0.15 mg/kg) should be administered 5 to 10 minutes after the second dose. This dosage schedule is effective at terminating supraventricular tachycardia in approximately 85% of dogs.[168] The effect following termination of administration is short-lived, often lasting less than 30 minutes. For longer control, the initial bolus injections can be followed by a constant infusion of verapamil at 2 to 10 μg/kg/min.[176]

The ability of verapamil to terminate supraventricular tachycardia is probably due to its effects on the AV junctional tissue. Most likely, most of the supraventricular tachycardias that respond to verapamil use the AV junction as part or all of a reentrant loop. Verapamil has the ability to slow conduction through the AV junction and to prolong the refractory period of this tissue at clinically relevant doses and plasma concentrations.[177] Prolongation of conduction and refractoriness are classic means of terminating reentrant arrhythmias.

Toxicity. Verapamil can depress cardiac contractility and cause peripheral vasodilation and should not be used in patients with severe myocardial failure or patients in heart failure, unless hemodynamic monitoring can be done and immediate administration of calcium or catecholamines can be performed. In patients with mild-to-moderate myocardial failure, verapamil may increase cardiac output by dilating arterioles. Occasionally, severe hypotension and cardiovascular collapse can be induced, especially if the drug is administered too vigorously.[168] Verapamil should not be used in patients with sick sinus syndrome or AV block because of its ability to depress automaticity in these diseased tissues. Adverse effects can be reversed by calcium or catecholamine administration. Catecholamine administration is more effective than calcium for treating calcium channel blocker–induced AV blocks in experimental conscious dogs.[178]

Drug interactions. Several drug interactions occur between verapamil and other drugs. Verapamil and β-blockers should not be used together for several reasons. Coadministration of verapamil and β-blockers results in additive negative inotropic, chronotropic, and dromotropic (conduction properties) effects on the heart. This produces profound myocardial depression, prolonged AV nodal conduction, and depressed heart rate, resulting in severe cardiovascular depression.[179,180] Verapamil can increase the bioavailability of some β-blockers by decreasing first pass hepatic metabolism.[181] Addition of β-blocker administration to dogs with a stable plasma concentration of verapamil results in an increase in the plasma verapamil concentration.[180] Coadministration of verapamil and lidocaine to experimental dogs anesthetized with isoflurane produces profound cardiovascular depression and severe systemic hypotension.[182] Cimetidine decreases total body clearance of verapamil. This increases the plasma concentration of intravenously and orally administered verapamil.[183] This effect probably occurs because of cimetidine's ability to inhibit hepatic microsomal enzymes. Verapamil increases the serum digoxin concentration in humans and probably does the same in dogs.[184] The increase is thought to be due to reduced renal and extrarenal clearances of digoxin.

Supply. Verapamil hydrochloride (Calan, G.D. Searle, Chicago, Ill.; Isoptin, Knoll Pharmaceuticals, Whippany, N.J.; various manufacturers) is supplied for intravenous use in a 2-mL ampule containing 5.0 mg and in 40-, 80-, and 120-mg tablets for oral administration.

Diltiazem

Actions. Diltiazem was developed in Japan in the early 1970s.[185] Diltiazem slows AV conduction and prolongs the AV refractory period to a degree similar to verapamil. It has minimal effects on myocardial contractility at clinically relevant plasma concentrations in normal dogs.[186] Its effects on myocardial contractility in dogs with cardiac disease are outlined below. Diltiazem's effects on peripheral vascular smooth muscle are mild, although it is a potent coronary vasodilator. In veterinary medicine, diltiazem is a popular drug for slowing the heart rate in dogs with atrial fibrillation, for terminating supraventricular tachycardia, and for treating hypertrophic cardiomyopathy in cats.

Pharmacokinetics. In normal experimental dogs, diltiazem is rapidly absorbed from the gastrointestinal tract, reaching a maximum plasma concentration approximately 30 minutes after oral administration.[187] Bioavailability of the tablets is approximately 24% in dogs.[188] The volume of distribution is 7.6 ± 1.1 L/kg.[188] Approximately 70% of the drug is protein-bound. The elimination half-life has been estimated to be 2.3 and 4.2 hours in two different studies.[187,188] The effective plasma concentration for terminating supraventricular tachycardia is probably in the 50- to 200-ng/mL range. For controlling the ventricular rate in atrial fibrillation, a lower plasma concentration may be efficacious. An oral dose of approximately 4 mg/kg results in a plasma concentration of 162 to 176 ng/mL 1 hour after administration.[188] Administration of a sustained-release diltiazem preparation at approximately 4 mg/kg q8h results in steady plasma concentrations between 60 and 100 ng/mL.[187] Intravenous administration of a dose of 0.2 mg/kg results in an average plasma concentration of 138 ng/mL 1 minute after administration. An infusion rate of 7 μg/kg/min produces a plasma concentration of 140 ± 23 ng/mL.[189,190]

In normal experimental dogs, one study found that diltiazem (0.8 mg/kg IV) did not alter left ventricular myocardial contractility but did decrease the peripheral vascular resistance and increased the heart rate in response to a reflex increase in plasma catecholamine concentrations.[191] These effects resulted in an increase in cardiac output. In the same study in experimental dogs with pacing-induced myocardial failure; however, the effects were quite different. In these dogs, diltiazem decreased myocardial contractility and did not change the heart rate. The net result was a decrease in cardiac output. Another study identified similar findings in dogs with left ventricular volume overload induced by creating an aorta-caval fistula.[192] Consequently, diltiazem must be administered cautiously to dogs with moderate-to-severe myocardial failure or heart failure.

In cats, the pharmacokinetics of diltiazem and two sustained-release forms of diltiazem (Cardizem CD and Dilacor XR) have been studied.[95,193] The bioavailability of diltiazem in cats is 94%. Its half-life is approximately 2 hours, with a volume of distribution of 1.88 L/kg. Peak concentration is achieved 30 minutes after oral administration. A dose of 1 mg/kg q8h PO maintains the serum concentration within therapeutic range for 8 hours. Conversely, Cardizem CD (Marion Merrell Dow, Inc., Kansas City, Mo) has a much lower bioavailability in cats (38%) and a much longer half-life (approximately 6.5 hours). Peak serum concentration is not achieved until 6 hours after an oral dose. A dose of 10 mg/kg q24h PO maintains the serum concentration within therapeutic range for 24 hours. The duration of effect for Dilacor XR (Rhone-Poulenc Rorer, Collegeville, Pa.) is approximately 12 hours.

Indications. In veterinary medicine, diltiazem is popular for decreasing the ventricular rate in dogs with atrial fibrillation. In most canine patients, digoxin is administered first and the heart rate response determined once a therapeutic serum concentration is achieved. If an adequate response is not achieved, diltiazem can be added into the treatment protocol. For this purpose, an initial dose of 0.5 mg/kg q8h PO should be administered. If the heart rate does not decrease adequately, the dose can be increased to 1.0 mg/kg q8h PO and, finally, to 1.5 mg/kg q8h PO. In general, the heart rate should be decreased to less than 160 beats/min. At these doses, diltiazem appears to have no or negligible negative inotropic effects, because exacerbation of heart failure at this dose is rare. β-Blockers are also commonly used to assist in heart rate control in dogs with atrial fibrillation. In general, a β-blocker should not be administered in conjunction with diltiazem because of the possibility of increasing plasma concentrations of both drugs and because of the potential for negative inotropic effects, exacerbation of heart failure, and death. In one report, diltiazem, at a dose of 1.5 mg/kg PO, decreased the ventricular rate by an average of 56% in dogs with atrial fibrillation, whereas the combination of digoxin and propranolol 0.5 mg/kg q8h PO only decreased ventricular rate by an average of 11%.[169] The effect of diltiazem occurred within 2 hours of administration and lasted for at least 6 hours.

Diltiazem can also be used in dogs to treat supraventricular tachycardia. For the acute termination of supraventricular tachycardia, our experience suggests that a dosing schedule similar to that used for verapamil is effective (Figure 29-6). Generally we use a dose of 0.05 mg/kg IV, administered over 1 to 2 minutes. We repeat this dose up to 2 times, with 5 minutes between doses. Other veterinary cardiologists use a dose of 0.25 mg/kg administered over 5 minutes. Diltiazem can also be used for the chronic control of supraventricular tachycardia. In our experience, doses higher than those used for heart rate control in atrial fibrillation are needed for supraventricular tachycardia. We have administered doses as high as 4 mg/kg q8h PO to dogs for this purpose. These dogs have not had significant ventricular dysfunction. In general, we titrate the dose, starting at a dose of 1 mg/kg q8h PO. Diltiazem at doses ranging from 2 to 4 mg/kg q8h should probably not be administered to dogs that have moderate-to-severe myocardial failure or dogs with significant cardiac compromise for any reason.

In cats with hypertrophic cardiomyopathy, diltiazem can be administered at doses between 7.5 and 15 mg/cat q8h PO. Alterna-

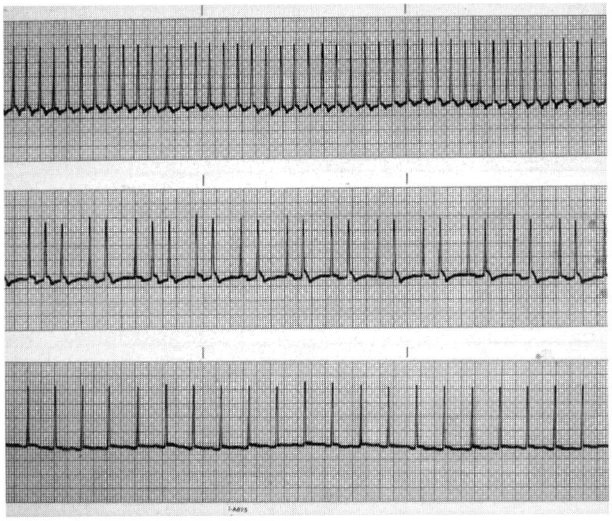

FIGURE 29-6 Electrocardiograms from a 5-year-old golden retriever that had been hit by a car. The top tracing was taken on admission and shows supraventricular tachycardia. The heart rate is 290 beats/min. The middle tracing was taken 20 seconds after a cumulative diltiazem dose of 0.15 mg/kg was administered. The bottom tracing was recorded 1 minute later. The rhythm is sinus. The heart rate is 140 beats/min. (Lead II, paper speed = 25 mm/sec.)

tively, a sustained-release preparation of diltiazem can be administered at a dose of 10 mg/kg q12h PO (Cardizem CD) or 30 mg/cat q24h (Dilacor XR).

Supply. Diltiazem (Cardizem, Marion Merrell Dow, Inc., Kansas City, Mo.) is supplied in 30-, 60-, 90-, and 120-mg sizes. The 30-mg size is not scored but can be quartered for use in cats. Several forms of sustained-release diltiazem are marketed. Cardizem SR is a capsule that contains beads that release the drug over 12 hours in humans. Cardizem SR has not been studied in cats or dogs. Cardizem CD is a dual-release capsule that contains two types of beads of diltiazem hydrochloride. The beads differ in the thickness of the surrounding membranes. The manufacturer states that 40% of the beads release the drug within the first 12 hours after oral administration, and the other 60% (which are surrounded by a thicker membrane) release the drug throughout the next 12 hours. The net effect is a drug that lasts for 24 hours in humans and in cats. Dilacor XR (Rhone-Poulenc Rorer, Collegeville, Pa.) is an extended-release capsule that consists of multiple 60-mg tablets contained in a swellable matrix core that slowly releases the drug over 24 hours in humans and 12 hours in cats.[95] The total capsule contains either 120-, 180-, or 240 mg of diltiazem. The 60-mg tablets can be removed and administered to cats. This dose may be excessive, however. Consequently, most veterinarians cut this tablet in half and administer 30 mg q12h PO.

COMBINATION THERAPY

At times, combinations of two antiarrhythmic drugs may be more effective than one drug alone. For example, the combination of digoxin and a β-blocker or digoxin and diltiazem is often more effective than digoxin alone at controlling the ventricular rate in patients with atrial fibrillation. At times, adding digoxin along with quinidine may be more effective for converting primary atrial fibrillation to sinus rhythm than using quinidine alone. This is an example of a combination in which toxicity can also be produced. Because quinidine decreases renal clearance of digoxin and displaces it from its binding sites, serum digoxin concentration commonly doubles when quinidine is added. This can result in clinical signs of digoxin intoxication.[37] Another example of the combination of two drugs causing clinical problems is the combination of a β-blocker and a calcium channel blocker. Both drug types can produce negative inotropic effects. In combination, this effect is exacerbated and can result in a severe decrease in contractility, worsening of heart failure, and even death.

Combination therapy may be more effective for treating ventricular arrhythmias. Many veterinary cardiologists have had the clinical impression for years that the combination of a class I antiarrhythmic agent and a β-blocker is more effective at controlling ventricular arrhythmias than is the use of either agent alone. In one experimental study using dogs, the combination of quinidine and propranolol was more effective than either drug alone at preventing ventricular fibrillation.[194] Many veterinary cardiologists prefer to use a combination of procainamide and propranolol. In experimental studies, the combination of two class I agents may be more effective at controlling ventricular arrhythmias in dogs than either drug alone.[69] An example is the combination of mexiletine and quinidine. In one study of experimental dogs with myocardial infarction, mexiletine controlled the ventricular arrhythmia in only one of 13 dogs and quinidine successfully suppressed the arrhythmia in only three of 13 dogs. The combination, however, was efficacious in eight of the 13 dogs.[69]

Another example is the combination of mexiletine and sotalol. Mexiletine decreases the QT interval in experimental dogs that have a prolonged QT interval as a result of sotalol administration.[195] One might think that this would counteract the antiarrhythmic efficacy of sotalol. However, in one study, the combination of these two drugs in experimental dogs was more effective at preventing ventricular tachycardia and more effective at slowing the rate of the ventricular tachycardia than was either drug alone.[196] Sotalol was more effective than mexiletine at preventing ventricular fibrillation in this study either alone or in combination with mexiletine.

Drugs Used to Treat Bradyarrhythmias

ANTICHOLINERGIC DRUGS

Anticholinergic agents, such as atropine and glycopyrrolate, can be used diagnostically and therapeutically in veterinary patients with bradyarrhythmias. Increased vagal tone can cause sinus bradycardia, periods of sinus arrest, and second-degree AV block. Whenever a patient presents with one of these abnormalities, an assessment of the response to the administration of an anticholinergic agent is indicated, especially if clinical signs are caused by the bradyarrhythmia. Generally, we administer atropine either subcutaneously or intravenously to determine if a bradyarrhythmia is vagally induced. When administered subcutaneously, we administer 0.04 mg/kg and then place the dog in a cage for 30 minutes before reassessing the cardiac rhythm. For intravenous administration, we also inject 0.04 mg/kg but wait only 5 to 10 minutes. Dogs with vagally mediated sinus node depression (either sinus bradycardia or arrest) respond by increasing their sinus rate to greater than 150 beats/min. Dogs with intrinsic sinus node disease (sick sinus syndrome) may have no response to atropine administration or may have a partial response (e.g., the heart rate may increase to 110 beats/min). Second-degree AV block disappears following atropine administration to dogs with vagally mediated second-degree AV block. Although we commonly administer atropine to dogs with third-degree AV block to assess their response, we have never identified a dog that had a significant response.

Vagal tone can be increased by numerous factors. Anesthesia, central nervous system lesions, abnormal carotid sinus function (hypersensitive carotid sinus syndrome in humans), and respiratory disease are common. Often the cause is unknown (idiopathic). Parenteral anticholinergic therapy can be used to control bradyarrhythmias in situations in which vagal tone is increased for only a short period (e.g., during anesthesia). In patients with chronically increased vagal tone that are symptomatic because of their bradyarrhythmia, one alternative is to administer the anticholinergic agent parenterally. This is no more involved than teaching a client to administer insulin to a pet with diabetes mellitus. Oral administration of anticholinergic agents can also be tried in these patients. Some patients do very well on oral anticholinergic therapy. However, oral anticholinergic therapy is not always successful, and parenteral administration, administration of a sympathomimetic, or pacemaker implantation may be required. The oral anticholinergic drugs can be ranked in order of effect. Drugs with weak anticholinergic effects are commonly used as antidiarrheal drugs in veterinary medicine. They include isopropamide iodide (Darbid, Smith, Kline, French Laboratories, Philadelphia, Pa.) and propantheline bromide (Pro-banthine, Schiapparelli Searle, Chicago, Ill.). These drugs are only rarely effective for chronically treating vagally induced bradyarrhythmias. Atropine and glycopyrrolate are more potent vagolytics and much more effective agents. Atropine tablets used to be available and, in our experience, were often effective. They are no longer manufactured but occasionally can be found. The parenteral atropine solution can also be administered per os, but is extremely bitter. To administer it per os, it must be diluted in a sweet substance, such as corn syrup, to disguise the taste. We have found that a dose of 0.04 mg/kg q8h can be effective. Glycopyrrolate (Robinul, A.H. Robins, Richmond, Va.) is available as 1- and 2-mg tablets. Although this product should be effective, we have little experience with its use.

Vagolytic substances can produce side effects. These include mydriasis, constipation, dry mouth, and keratoconjunctivitis sicca. In our experience, however, these side effects are often remarkably inapparent.

SYMPATHOMIMETIC DRUGS

Sympathomimetics can also be used to treat bradyarrhythmias. Isoproterenol is a pure β-agonist that stimulates both β_1- and β_2-adrenergic receptors. In so doing, it increases the sinus node rate, increases the rate of subsidiary pacemakers in the heart and increases conduction velocity in the AV node. Isoproterenol can be used temporarily to increase the heart rate in dogs with sick sinus syndrome or third-degree AV block. This is done only in dogs that are severely bradycardic or are symptomatic. Isoproterenol is infrequently used in our clinic to increase the heart rate in dogs that are waiting to have a pacemaker implanted. It is more frequently used in dogs that become severely bradycardic under anesthesia before pacemaker implantation. Isoproterenol is administered intravenously as a constant-rate infusion at a dose of 0.05 to 0.2 μg/kg/min. Isoproterenol also stimulates β-receptors in systemic arterioles, producing vasodilation. This can cause hypotension. Isoproterenol can also stimulate tachyarrhythmias. The dose must be titrated, and the lowest effective dose should be used. Oral administration of isoproterenol is not effective because it is almost completely metabolized by the liver before it reaches the systemic circulation.

Numerous drugs that stimulate β_2-receptors are available. These drugs are used as bronchodilators and are effective after oral administration. They are generally formulated not to produce many cardiac effects. However, this is impossible because β_2-receptors are present in the heart and play an important role in modulating the sinus rate. Consequently, these drugs can also be used to treat bradyarrhythmias. Most of our experience is with the use of terbutaline (Brethine, Geigy Pharmaceuticals, Summit, N.J.; Bricanyl, Marion Merrell Dow, Kansas City, Mo.) in dogs with vagally mediated sinus bradycardia and sinus arrest. In these dogs, terbutaline can be effective at increasing the sinus rate and eradicating the sinus pauses. The dose must be titrated, usually starting with 2.5 mg/dog q8h PO and increasing as needed. Side effects include hyperactivity and gastrointestinal disturbances. Brethine and Bricanyl are supplied as 2.5- and 5-mg tablets. Terbutaline should be used cautiously if at all in dogs with mitral regurgitation resulting from myxomatous mitral valve degeneration. We have not noted complications with this drug in this setting but have noted acute pulmonary edema, possibly secondary to ruptured chordae tendineae, in dogs treated with albuterol, another β_2-agonist.

REFERENCES

1. Fazekas T, Vos MA, Leunissen JD et al: Effects of magnesium and ethmozin on ventricular tachycardia induced by ouabain and ventricular pacing in conscious dogs with complete atrioventricular block, *Acta Physiol Hung* 81:59, 1993.
2. Hashimoto H, Katoh H, Nakashima M: Effects of flecainide on ventricular arrhythmias, abnormal automaticity and activation in a canine model of myocardial infarction, *J Pharmacobiodyn* 15:191, 1992.
3. Carlsson L, Abrahamsson C, Drews L et al: Antiarrhythmic effects of potassium channel openers in rhythm abnormalities related to delayed repolarization, *Circulation* 85:1491, 1992 (comments).
4. Levy MN, Wiseman MN: Electrophysiologic mechanisms for ventricular arrhythmias in left ventricular dysfunction: electrolytes, catecholamines and drugs, *J Clin Pharmacol* 31:1053, 1991.
5. Vos MA, Fazekas T, Gorgels AP et al: Action of MgSO4 differs from moricizine and verapamil on ouabain-induced ventricular tachycardia in normomagnesemic conscious dogs, *J Cardiovasc Pharmacol* 23:252, 1994.
6. Kane KA, Berdeja Garcia GY, Sanchez-Perez S et al: Electrophysiological effects of lidocaine, l-chlorpheniramine, and bepridil on normal and ouabain-intoxicated canine Purkinje fibers, *J Cardiovasc Pharmacol* 5:109, 1983.
7. Rosen MR, Danilo PJ: Effects of tetrodotoxin, lidocaine, verapamil, and AHR-2666 on ouabain-induced delayed afterdepolarizations in canine Purkinje fibers, *Circ Res* 46:117, 1980.
8. Danilo P, Rosen MR: Pharmacodynamics of antiarrhythmic drugs. In Chatterjee K, Cheitlin MD, Karliner J et al, eds: *Cardiology: an illustrated text reference,* Philadelphia, 1991, JB Lippincott Company.
9. Wittig J, Harrison LA, Wallace AG: Electrophysiological effects of lidocaine on distal Purkinje fibers of canine heart, *Am Heart J* 86:69, 1973.
10. Davis LD, Temte JV: Electrophysiological actions of lidocaine on canine ventricular muscle and Purkinje fibers, *Circ Res* 24:639, 1969.
11. Mandel WJ, Bigger JT: Electrophysiologic effects of lidocaine on isolated canine and rabbit atrial tissue, *J Pharmacol Exp Ther* 178:81, 1971.
12. Gettes LS, Reuter H: Slow recovery from inactivation of inward currents in mammalian myocardial fibres, *J Physiol (Lond)* 240:703, 1974.
13. Wit AL, Cranefield PF: Effect of verapamil on the sinoatrial and atrioventricular nodes of the rabbit and the mechanism by which it arrests reentrant atrioventricular nodal tachycardia, *Circ Res* 35:413, 1974.
14. Cranefield PF, Aronson RS, Wit AL: Effect of verapamil on the normal action potential and on a calcium-dependent slow response of canine cardiac Purkinje fibers, *Circ Res* 34:204, 1974.

15. Muir WW, Sams RA: Pharmacology and pharmacokinetics of antiarrhythmic drugs. In Fox PR, ed: *0* New York, 1988, Churchill Livingstone.
16. Hondeghem LM, Grant AO, Jensen RA: Antiarrhythmic drug action: selective depression of hypoxic cardiac cells, *Am Heart J* 87:602, 1974.
17. Lazzara R, Hope RR, el-Sherif N et al: Effects of lidocaine on hypoxic and ischemic cardiac cells, *Am J Cardiol* 41:872, 1978.
18. el-Sherif N, Scherlag BJ, Lazzara R et al: Re-entrant ventricular arrhythmias in the late myocardial infarction period. IV. Mechanism of action of lidocaine, *Circulation* 56:395, 1977.
19. Gadsby DC, Cranefield PF: Two levels of resting potential in cardiac Purkinje fibers, *J Gen Physiol* 70:725, 1977.
20. Moe GK: Evidence for reentry as a mechanism for cardiac arrhythmias, *Rev Physiol Biochem Pharmacol* 72:56, 1975.
21. Muir WW, Sams R: Pharmacodynamics of cardiac drugs. Columbus, Ohio 1979 Ohio State University.
22. In: Amsterdam EA, ed: *Cardiology drug facts,* New York, 1989, JB Lippincott.
23. Anderson KP, Freedman RA, Mason JW: Use of antiarrhythmic drugs: general principles. In Chatterjee K, Cheitlin MD, Karliner J et al, eds: *Cardiology: an illustrated reference,* Philadelphia, 1991, JB Lippincott.
24. Rosen MR, Danilo PJ, Alonso MB et al: Effects of therapeutic concentrations of diphenylhydantoin on transmembrane potentials of normal and depressed Purkinje fibers, *J Pharmacol Exp Ther* 197:594, 1976.
25. Keene BW, Hamlin RL: Prophylaxis and treatment of digitalis-enhanced dysrhythmias with phenytoin in the dog, *Proc ACVIM,* 1980, p 118 (abstract).
26. Sanders JE, Yeary RA: Serum concentrations of orally administered diphenylhydantoin in dogs, *J Am Vet Med Assoc* 172:153, 1978.
27. Sanders JE, Yeary RA, Fenner WR et al: Interaction of phenytoin with chloramphenicol or pentobarbital in the dog, *J Am Vet Med Assoc* 175:177, 1979.
28. Keene BW, Hamlin RL, Rogers WA: Safety of orally administered phenytoin for one month in the dog, *Proc ACVIM,* 1980, p 119 (abstract).
29. Grant AO, Starmer CF: Antiarrhythmic drug action: blockade of the inward sodium current, *Circ Res* 55:427, 1984.
30. Singh BN, Hauswirth O: Comparative mechanisms of action of antiarrhythmic drugs, *Am Heart J* 87:367, 1974.
31. Hoffman BF, Rosen MR, Wit AL: Electrophysiology and pharmacology of cardiac arrhythmias. VII. Cardiac effects of quinidine and procaine amide, *B Am Heart J* 90:117, 1975.
32. Sicouri S, Antzelevitch C: Drug-induced afterdepolarizations and triggered activity occur in a discrete subpopulation of ventricular muscle cells (M cells) in the canine heart: quinidine and digitalis, *J Cardiovasc Electrophysiol* 4:48, 1993.
33. Roden DM, Hoffman BF: Action potential prolongation and induction of abnormal automaticity by low quinidine concentrations in canine Purkinje fibers: relationship to potassium and cycle length, *Circ Res* 56:857, 1985.
34. Remon JP, Belpaire F, Van Severen R et al: Interaction of antacids with antiarrhythmics. V. Effect of aluminium hydroxide and magnesium oxide on the bioavailability of quinidine, procainamide and propranolol in dogs, *Arzneimittelforschung* 33:117, 1993.
35. Velebit V, Podrid P, Lown B et al: Aggravation and provocation of ventricular arrhythmias by antiarrhythmic drugs, *Circulation* 65:886, 1982.
36. Morganroth J, Goin JE: Quinidine-related mortality in the short-to-medium-term treatment of ventricular arrhythmias: a meta-analysis, *Circulation* 84:1977, 1991 (comments).
37. Pyle RL: Conversion of atrial fibrillation with quinidine sulfate in a dog, *J Am Vet Med Assoc* 151:582, 1967.
38. Warner NJ, Leahey EB, Hougen TJ et al: Tissue digoxin concentrations during the quinidine-digoxin interaction, *Am J Cardiol* 51:1717, 1983.
39. De Rick A, Belpaire F: Digoxin-quinidine interaction in the dog, *J Vet Pharmacol Ther* 4:215, 1981.
40. Doherty JE, Straub KD, Murphy ML et al: Digoxin-quinidine interaction: changes in canine tissue concentration from steady state with quinidine, *Am J Cardiol* 45:1196, 1980.
41. Peters DN, Hamlin RL, Powers JD: Absence of pharmacokinetic interaction between digitoxin and quinidine in the dog, *J Vet Pharmacol Ther* 4:271, 1981.
42. Sisson DD: The clinical management of cardiac arrhythmias in the dog and cat. In Fox PR, ed: *Canine and feline cardiology,* New York, 1988, Churchill Livingstone.
43. Weiss DJ, Klausner JS: Drug-associated aplastic anemia in dogs: eight cases (1984-1988), *J Am Vet Med Assoc* 196:472, 1990.
44. Ehring GR, Hondeghem LM: Antiarrhythmic structure activity relationships in a series of lidocaine procainamide derivatives, *Proc West Pharmacol Soc* 24:221, 1981.
45. Rosen MR, Gelband H, Hoffman BF: Canine electrocardiographic and cardiac electrophysiologic changes induced by procainamide, *Circulation* 46:528, 1972.
46. Arnsdorf MF, Bigger JT: The effect of procaine amide on components of excitability in long mammalian cardiac Purkinje fibers, *Circ Res* 38:115, 1976.
47. Sada H, Kojima M, Ban T: Effect of procainamide on transmembrane action potentials in guinea-pig papillary muscles as affected by external potassium concentration, *Naunyn Schmiedebergs Arch Pharmacol* 309:179, 1979.
48. Hewett K, Gessman L, Rosen MR: Effects of procaine amide, quinidine and ethmozin on delayed afterdepolarizations, *Eur J Pharmacol* 96:21, 1983.
49. Papich MG, Davis LE, Davis CA: Procainamide in the dog: antiarrhythmic plasma concentrations after intravenous administration, *J Vet Pharmacol Ther* 9:359, 1986.
50. Dangman KH: Effects of procainamide on automatic and triggered impulse initiation in isolated preparations of canine cardiac Purkinje fibers, *J Cardiovasc Pharmacol* 12:78, 1988.
51. Hordof A, Edie R, Malm J et al: Effects of procainamide, quinidine, and ethmozin on delayed afterdepolarizations, *Pediatr Res* 9:267, 1975
52. Pearle DL, Souza JD, Gillis RA: Comparative vagolytic effects of procainamide and N-acetylprocainamide in the dog, *J Cardiovasc Pharmacol* 5:450, 1983.
53. Papich MG, Davis LE, Davis CA et al: Pharmacokinetics of procainamide hydrochloride in dogs, *Am J Vet Res* 47:2351, 1986.
54. Kaufman GM, Weirich WE, Mayer PR: The pharmacokinetics of regular and sustained release procainamide in the dog, *Proc ACVIM,* 1983, p 42 (abstract).
55. Atkins CE, Kanter R, Wright K et al: Orthodromic reciprocating tachycardia and heart failure in a dog with a concealed posteroseptal accessory pathway, *J Vet Intern Med* 9:43, 1995.
56. Kittleson MD: Drugs used in the therapy of cardiac arrhythmias. In Kirk RW, ed: *Kirk's current veterinary therapy, VIII: small animal practice,* Philadelphia, 1983, WB Saunders.
57. Balazs T, Robinson CJ: Procainamide-induced antinuclear antibodies in beagle dogs, *Toxicol Appl Pharmacol* 71:299, 1983.
58. Arnsdorf MF, Mehlman DJ: Observations on the effects of selected antiarrhythmic drugs on mammalian cardiac Purkinje fibers with two levels of steady-state potential: influences of lidocaine, phenytoin, propranolol, disopyramide and procainamide on repolarization, action potential shape and conduction, *J Pharmacol Exp Ther* 207:983, 1978.
59. Karim A, Kook C, Novotney RL et al: Pharmacokinetics and steady-state myocardial uptake of disopyramide in the dog, *Drug Metab Dispos* 6:338, 1978.
60. Crosby HH, Hamlin RL, Strauch SM: Effects of disopyramide on the electrocardiogram and ventricular function in the unanesthetized dog, *J Vet Pharmacol Ther* 7:167, 1984.
61. Walsh RA, Horwitz LD: Adverse hemodynamic effects of intravenous disopyramide compared with quinidine in conscious dogs, *Circulation* 60:1053, 1979.
62. Sherrid M, Delia E, Dwyer E: Oral disopyramide therapy for obstructive hypertrophic cardiomyopathy, *Am J Cardiol* 62:1085, 1988.

63. Konishi T, Kadoya M, Ikeguchi S et al: Combined effect of disopyramide and bethanechol: use of bethanechol to prevent anticholinergic side effects of disopyramide without reduction of antiarrhythmic efficacy, *J Cardiovasc Pharmacol* 14:341, 1989.
64. Means JR, Hjelle JJ, Kotsonis FN: The effects of disopyramide phosphate on serum glucose and glucose counterregulation in the dog, *Fundam Appl Toxicol* 5:539, 1985.
65. Yamaguchi I, Singh BN, Mandel WJ: Electrophysiological actions of mexiletine on isolated rabbit atria and canine ventricular muscle and Purkinje fibres, *Cardiovasc Res* 13:288, 1979.
66. Weld FM, Bigger JT, Swistel D et al: Electrophysiological effects of mexiletine (Ko1173) on ovine cardiac Purkinje fibers, *J Pharmacol Exp Ther* 210:222, 1979.
67. Mexiletine: clinical investigator's brochure, 1989, (abstract).
68. Yoon MS, Han J: Electrophysiologic effects of mexiletine on normal and ischemic ventricles, *J Electrocardiol* 15:109, 1982.
69. Duff HJ: Mexiletine-quinidine combination: enhanced antiarrhythmic and electrophysiologic activity in the dog, *J Pharmacol Exp Ther* 249:617, 1989.
70. Lunney J, Ettinger SJ: Mexiletine administration for management of ventricular arrhythmia in 22 dogs, *J Am Anim Hosp Assoc* 27:597, 1991.
71. Calvert CA: Diagnosis and management of ventricular arrhythmias in Doberman pinschers with cardiomyopathy. In Bonagura JD, ed: *Kirk's current veterinary therapy, XII: small animal practice,* Philadelphia, 1995, WB Saunders.
72. Berlin-Wahlen A, Barcus JC, Keenhagen JB: Elimination of N-(2-aminoacyl)-2,6-xylidines after intravenous infusion in dogs, *Acta Pharm Suec* 14:417, 1977.
73. Man RY, Bril A: Effects of class I anti-arrhythmic drugs in infarcted tissue, *Clin Invest Med* 14:466, 1991.
74. Steinberg JS, Sahar DI, Rosenbaum M et al: Proarrhythmic effects of procainamide and tocainide in a canine infarction model, *J Cardiovasc Pharmacol* 19:52, 1992.
75. Coltart DJ, Berndt TB, Kernoff R et al: Antiarrhythmic and circulatory effects of Astra W36095, a new lidocaine-like agent, *Am J Cardiol* 34:35, 1974.
76. Ikram H: Hemodynamic and electrophysiologic interactions between antiarrhythmic drugs and beta blockers, with special reference to tocainide, *Am Heart J* 100:1076, 1980.
77. Anderson JL, Mason JW, Winkle RA et al: Clinical electrophysiologic effects of tocainide, *Circulation* 57:685, 1978.
78. Calvert CA, Jacobs GJ: Use of tocainide for ventricular tachyarrhythmias in Doberman pinscher dogs with cardiomyopathy, *J Vet Intern Med* 9:199, 1995 (abstract).
79. Takei M, Furukawa Y, Narita M et al: Sympathetic nerve stimulation activates both $beta_1$- and $beta_2$-adrenoceptors of SA and AV nodes in anesthetized dog hearts, *Jpn J Pharmacol* 59:23, 1992.
80. Altschuld RA, Starling RC, Hamlin RL et al: Response of failing canine and human heart cells to $beta_2$-adrenergic stimulation, *Circulation* 92:1612, 1995.
81. Gauthier C, Tavernier G, Charpentier F et al: Functional $beta_3$-adrenoreceptors in the human heart, *J Clin Invest* 98:556, 1996.
82. Eichhorn EJ, Bristow MR: Practical guidelines for initiation of beta-adrenergic blockade in patients with chronic heart failure, *Am J Cardiol* 79:794, 1997.
83. Reynolds RD, Gorczynski RJ, Quon CY: Pharmacology and pharmacokinetics of esmolol, *J Clin Pharmacol* 26(suppl A):A3, 1986.
84. Ross LA, Labato MA: Use of drugs to control hypertension in renal failure. In Kirk RW, ed: *Kirk's current veterinary therapy, X: small animal practice,* Philadelphia, 1989, WB Saunders.
85. Davis LD, Temte JV: Effects of propranolol on the transmembrane potentials of ventricular muscle and Purkinje fibers of the dog, *Circ Res* 22:661, 1968.
86. Uprichard AC, Harron DW: Atenolol, but not mexiletine, protects against stimulus-induced ventricular tachycardia in a chronic canine model, *Br J Pharmacol* 96:220, 1989.
87. Nies AS, Shand DG: Clinical pharmacology of propranolol, *Circulation* 52:6, 1975.
88. Kates RE, Keene BW, Hamlin RL: Pharmacokinetics of propranolol in the dog, *J Vet Pharmacol Therap* 2:21, 1979.
89. Wisler PL, Green FJ, Watanabe AM: Cardiovascular adrenergic and muscarinic cholinergic receptors. In Chatterjee K, Cheitlin MD, Karliner J et al, eds: *Cardiology, an illustrated text/reference,* Philadelphia, 1991, JB Lippincott.
90. Frishman WH: Clinical differences between beta-adrenergic blocking agents: implications for therapeutic substitution, *Am Heart J* 113:1190, 1987.
91. McDevitt DG, Shand DG: Plasma concentrations and the time-course of beta blockade due to propranolol, *Clin Pharmacol Ther* 18:708, 1975.
92. Shand DG: Editorial: Propranolol withdrawal, *N Engl J Med* 293:449, 1975.
93. Hiatt N, Chapman LW, Davidson MB et al: Insulin and beta receptor modulation of K homeostasis in nephrectomized dogs with hyperkalemia, *Horm Metab Res* 14:299, 1982.
94. McAinsh J, Holmes BF: Pharmacokinetic studies with atenolol in the dog, *Biopharm Drug Dispos* 4:249, 1983.
95. Keene BW: Feline cardiovascular drugs: which drug/which dose? *Proc Annu Vet Med Forum,* 1997, p 155.
96. Quinones M, Dyer DC, Ware WA et al: Pharmacokinetics of atenolol in clinically normal cats, *Am J Vet Res* 57:1050, 1996.
97. Bonagura JD, Stepien RL, Lehmkuhl LB: Acute effects of esmolol on left ventricular outflow obstruction in cats with hypertrophic cardiomyopathy, *J Vet Intern Med* 5:123, 1991 (abstract).
98. The International Small Animal Cardiac Health Council: *Recommendations for the diagnosis of heart disease and the treatment of heart failure in small animals,* The Council, 1994, (abstract).
99. Singh BN: Controlling cardiac arrhythmias by lengthening repolarization: historical overview, *Am J Cardiol* 72:18F, 1993.
100. Kendall MJ, Lynch KP, Hjalmarson A et al: Beta-blockers and sudden cardiac death, *Ann Intern Med* 123:358, 1995.
101. Latini R, Reginato R, Burlingame AL et al: High-performance liquid chromatographic isolation and fast atom bombardment mass spectrometric identification of Di-N-desethylamiodarone, a new metabolite of amiodarone in the dog, *Biomed Mass Spectrom* 11:466, 1984.
102. Nattel S, Davies M, Quantz M: The antiarrhythmic efficacy of amiodarone and desethylamiodarone, alone and in combination, in dogs with acute myocardial infarction, *Circulation* 77:200, 1988.
103. Podrid PJ: Amiodarone: reevaluation of an old drug, *Ann Intern Med* 122:689, 1995.
104. Nicklas JM, McKenna WJ, Stewart RA et al: Prospective, double-blind, placebo-controlled trial of low-dose amiodarone in patients with severe heart failure and asymptomatic frequent ventricular ectopy, *Am Heart J* 122:1016, 1991.
105. Anderson JL: Symposium on the management of ventricular dysrhythmias: antifibrillatory versus antiectopic therapy, *Am J Cardiol* 54:7A, 1984.
106. Morganroth J: Early and late proarrhythmia from antiarrhythmic drug therapy, *Cardiovasc Drugs Ther* 6:11, 1992.
107. Gallagher JD, Bianchi J, Gessman LJ: A comparison of the electrophysiologic effects of acute and chronic amiodarone administration on canine Purkinje fibers, *J Cardiovasc Pharmacol* 13:723, 1989.
108. Varro A, Nakaya Y, Elharrar V et al: The effects of amiodarone on repolarization and refractoriness of cardiac fibers, *Eur J Pharmacol* 154:11, 1988.
109. Bauthier J, Broekhuysen J, Charlier R et al: Nature of the inhibition by amiodarone of isoproterenol-induced tachycardia in the dog, *Arch Int Pharmacodyn Ther* 219:45, 1976.
110. Takanaka C, Singh BN: Barium-induced nondriven action potentials as a model of triggered potentials from early afterdepolarizations: significance of slow channel activity and differing effects of quinidine and amiodarone, *J Am Coll Cardiol* 15:213, 1990.
111. Brien JF, Jimmo S, Brennan FJ et al: Disposition of amiodarone and its proximate metabolite, desethylamiodarone, in the dog for oral administration of single-dose and short-term drug regimens, *Drug Metab Dispos* 18:846, 1990.

112. Abdollah H, Brien JF, Brennan FJ: Antiarrhythmic effect of chronic oral amiodarone treatment in dogs with myocardial infarction and reproducibly inducible sustained ventricular arrhythmias, *J Cardiovasc Pharmacol* 15:799, 1990.
113. Tuna IC, Qi AC, Gornick C et al: Kinetics of electrophysiologic changes during oral loading of amiodarone and after withdrawal of amiodarone in the unsedated dog, *Circulation* 72:1380, 1985.
114. Frame LH: The effect of chronic oral and acute intravenous amiodarone administration on ventricular defibrillation threshold using implanted electrodes in dogs, *PACE Pacing Clin Electrophysiol* 12:339, 1989.
115. Rotmensch HH, Belhassen B, Swanson BN et al: Steady-state serum amiodarone concentrations: relationships with antiarrhythmic efficacy and toxicity, *Ann Intern Med* 101:462, 1984.
116. Staubli M, Bircher J, Galeazzi RL et al: Serum concentrations of amiodarone during long term therapy: relation to dose, efficacy and toxicity, *Eur J Clin Pharmacol* 24:485, 1983.
117. Hostetler KY, Reasor MJ, Walker ER et al: Role of phospholipase A inhibition in amiodarone pulmonary toxicity in rats, *Biochim Biophys Acta* 875:400, 1986.
118. Vic P, Gouy D, Lacheretz F et al: Intestinal pathology in the dog induced by sublethal doses of amiodarone, *Arch Toxicol Suppl* 8:104, 1985.
119. Shaikh NA, Downar E: Effects of chronic amiodarone treatment on cat myocardial phospholipid content and on in vitro phospholipid catabolism, *Mol Cell Biochem* 78:17, 1987.
120. Pasquali D, Tseng FY, Rani CS et al: Inhibition of intermediary metabolism by amiodarone in dog thyroid slices, *Am J Physiol* 259:E529, 1990.
121. Laurberg P: Amiodarone inhibits T4 and T3 secretion but does not affect T4 deiodination to T3 in perfused dog thyroid lobes, *Thyroidol Clin Exp,* 1988, p 1.
122. Lesko LJ: Pharmacokinetic drug interactions with amiodarone, *Clin Pharmacokinet* 17:130, 1989.
123. Ben David J, Bialer M: Pharmacokinetic interaction between diltiazem and amiodarone in the dog, *Biopharm Drug Dispos* 10:423, 1989.
124. Bacaner M: Bretylium tosylate for suppression of induced ventricular fibrillation, *Am J Cardiol* 17:528, 1966.
125. Bigger JT, Jaffe CC: The effect of bretylium tosylate on the electrophysiologic properties of ventricular muscle and Purkinje fibers, *Am J Cardiol* 27:82, 1971.
126. Sanna G, Arcidiacono R: Chemical ventricular defibrillation of the human heart with bretylium tosylate, *Am J Cardiol* 32:982, 1973.
127. Elenbaas RM, Mattson K, Cole H et al: Bretylium in hypothermia-induced ventricular fibrillation in dogs, *Ann Emerg Med* 13:994, 1984.
128. Breznock EM, Kagan K, Hibser NK: Effects of bretylium tosylate on the in vivo fibrillating canine ventricle, *Am J Vet Res* 38:89, 1977.
129. Kamath BL, Gibson TP, Look ZM et al: Pharmacokinetics of bretylium in dogs and the effect of hemoperfusion on elimination, *J Pharm Sci* 71:1294, 1982.
130. Anderson JL, Patterson E, Conlon M et al: Kinetics of antifibrillatory effects of bretylium: correlation with myocardial drug concentrations, *Am J Cardiol* 46:583, 1980.
131. Holland K, Patterson E, Lucchesi BR: Prevention of ventricular fibrillation by bretylium in a conscious canine model of sudden coronary death, *Am Heart J* 105:711, 1983.
132. Patterson E, Gibson JK: Prevention of chronic canine ventricular tachyarrhythmias with bretylium tosylate, *Circulation* 64:1045, 1981.
133. Hanyok JJ, Chow MS, Kluger J et al: Antifibrillatory effects of high dose bretylium and a lidocaine bretylium combination during cardiopulmonary resuscitation, *Crit Care Med* 16:691, 1988.
134. Vachiery JL, Reuse C, Blecic S et al: Bretylium tosylate versus lidocaine in experimental cardiac arrest, *Am J Emerg Med* 8:492, 1990 (comments).
135. Antonaccio MJ, Gomoll A: Pharmacologic basis of the antiarrhythmic and hemodynamic effects of sotalol, *Am J Cardiol* 72:27A, 1993.
136. Hohnloser SH, Woosley RL: Sotalol, *N Engl J Med* 331:31, 1994.
137. Brachmann J, Beyer T, Schmitt C et al: Electrophysiologic and antiarrhythmic effects of D-sotalol, *J Cardiovasc Pharmacol* 20(suppl 2): S91, 1992.
138. Gomoll AW, Lekich RF, Bartek MJ et al: Comparability of the electrophysiologic responses and plasma and myocardial tissue concentrations of sotalol and its d stereoisomer in the dog, *J Cardiovasc Pharmacol* 16:204, 1990.
139. Giudicelli JF, Lhoste F: Beta-adrenoceptor blockade and atrioventricular conduction in dogs: role of intrinsic sympathomimetic activity, *Br J Clin Pharmacol* 13:167S, 1982.
140. Bertrix L, Timour-Chah Q, Lang J et al: Protection against ventricular and atrial fibrillation by sotalol, *Cardiovasc Res* 20:358, 1986.
141. Lynch JJ, Coskey LA, Montgomery DG et al: Prevention of ventricular fibrillation by dextrorotatory sotalol in a conscious canine model of sudden coronary death, *Am Heart J* 109:949, 1985.
142. Wang M, Dorian P: DL and D sotalol decrease defibrillation energy requirements, *PACE Pacing Clin Electrophysiol* 12:1522, 1989.
143. Duker G, Almgren O, Carlsson L: Electrophysiologic and hemodynamic effects of H 234/09 (almokalant), quinidine, and (+)-sotalol in the anesthetized dog, *J Cardiovasc Pharmacol* 20:458, 1992 (erratum 20[6]:1014, 1992).
144. Buchanan LV, Kabell G, Turcotte UM et al: Effects of ibutilide on spontaneous and induced ventricular arrhythmias in 24-hour canine myocardial infarction: a comparative study with sotalol and encainide, *J Cardiovasc Pharmacol* 19:256, 1992.
145. Parmley WW, Rabinowitz B, Chuck L et al: Comparative effects of sotalol and propranolol on contractility of papillary muscles and adenyl cyclase activity of myocardial extracts of cat, *J Clin Pharmacol New Drugs* 12:127, 1972.
146. Hoffmann RP, Grupp G: The effects of sotalol and propranolol on contractile force and atrioventricular conduction time of the dog heart in situ, *Dis Chest* 55:229, 1969.
147. Brown WA, DeLellis LA: Sotalol administration in boxer dogs with dilated cardiomyopathy and syncope, personal communication, 1996.
148. Schnelle K, Garrett ER: Pharmacokinetics of the β-adrenergic blocker sotalol in dogs, *J Pharm Sci* 62:362, 1973.
149. Antonaccio MJ, Gomoll A: Pharmacology, pharmacodynamics and pharmacokinetics of sotalol, *Am J Cardiol* 65:12A, discussion p 35A, 1990.
150. Nattel S, Feder-Elituv R, Matthews C et al: Concentration dependence of class III and beta-adrenergic blocking effects of sotalol in anesthetized dogs, *J Am Coll Cardiol* 13:1190, 1989.
151. Feld GK, Venkatesh N, Singh BN: Pharmacologic conversion and suppression of experimental canine atrial flutter: differing effects of d-sotalol, quinidine, and lidocaine and significance of changes in refractoriness and conduction, *Circulation* 74:197, 1986
152. Wang J, Feng J, Nattel S: Class III antiarrhythmic drug action in experimental atrial fibrillation: differences in reverse use dependence and effectiveness between d-sotalol and the new antiarrhythmic drug ambasilide, *Circulation* 90:2032, 1994.
153. Patterson E, Lynch JJ, Lucchesi BR: Antiarrhythmic and antifibrillatory actions of the beta adrenergic receptor antagonist, dl-sotalol, *J Pharmacol Exp Ther* 230:519, 1984.
154. Parks J: The dose of sotalol in pediatric patients, personal communication, 1997.
155. Calvert CA: Use of sotalol in a Doberman pinscher with mild to moderate myocardial failure, personal communication, 1997.
156. Weissenburger J, Davy JM, Chezalviel F: Experimental models of torsades de pointes, *Fundam Clin Pharmacol* 7:29, 1993.
157. Davy JM, Weissenburger J, Ertzbischoff O et al: [Sotalol-induced torsades de pointe in the conscious dog with atrioventricular block: role of hypokalemia] Torsades de pointe experimentales avec le sotalol chez le chien vigile en bloc auriculo-ventriculaire: role de l'hypokaliemie, *Arch Mal Coeur Vaiss* 81:1117, 1988.
158. Weissenburger J, Davy JM, Chezalviel F et al: Arrhythmogenic activities of antiarrhythmic drugs in conscious hypokalemic dogs with atrioventricular block: comparison between quinidine, lidocaine, flecainide, propranolol and sotalol, *J Pharmacol Exp Ther* 259:871, 1991.

159. Lynch JJ, Wilber DJ, Montgomery DG et al: Antiarrhythmic and antifibrillatory actions of the levo- and dextrorotatory isomers of sotalol, *J Cardiovasc Pharmacol* 6:1132, 1984.
160. Fleckenstein A: History of calcium antagonists, *Circ Res* 52:I3, 1983.
161. Triggle DJ, Swamy VC: Calcium antagonists: some chemical-pharmacologic aspects, *Circ Res* 52:I17, 1983.
162. Sperelakis N, Josephson I: Slow action potential and properties of the myocardial slow Ca channels. In Sperelakis N, ed: *Physiology and pathophysiology of the heart,* ed 3, Boston, 1995, Kluwer.
163. Millard RW, Grupp G, Grupp IL et al: Chronotropic, inotropic, and vasodilator actions of diltiazem, nifedipine, and verapamil: a comparative study of physiological responses and membrane receptor activity, *Circ Res* 52:I29, 1983.
164. Liu SK, Hsu FS, Lee RCT: *An atlas of cardiovascular pathology,* Tainan, Taiwan, 1989, Pig Research Institute of Taiwan.
165. Welling A, Kwan YW, Bosse E et al: Subunit-dependent modulation of recombinant L-type calcium channels: molecular basis for dihydropyridine tissue selectivity, *Circ Res* 73:974, 1993.
166. van Zwieten PA, Pfaffendorf M: Similarities and differences between calcium antagonists: pharmacological aspects, *J Hypertens Suppl* 11:S3, 1993.
167. Myerburg RJ, Kessler KM: Clinical assessment and management of arrhythmias and conduction disturbances. In Hurst JW, Schlant RC, eds: *The heart,* ed 7, New York, 1995, McGraw-Hill.
168. Kittleson M, Keene B, Pion P et al: Verapamil administration for acute termination of supraventricular tachycardia in dogs, *J Am Vet Med Assoc* 193:1525, 1988.
169. Hamlin RL: Clinical use of diltiazem for dogs in atrial fibrillation, *Proc Annu Vet Med Forum,* 1988, p 759 (abstract).
170. Ishibashi H, Fu L, Namiki T et al: Induction and the possible mechanism of ventricular tachycardia after catheter ablation with direct current shocks in dogs, *Eur Heart J* 14:1132, 1993.
171. Vos MA, Gorgels AP, Leunissen JD et al: Programmed electrical stimulation and drugs identify two subgroups of ventricular tachycardias occurring 16-24 hours after occlusion of the left anterior descending artery, *Circulation* 85:747, 1992.
172. Rosing DR, Kent KM, Borer JS et al: Verapamil therapy: a new approach to the pharmacologic treatment of hypertrophic cardiomyopathy. I. Hemodynamic effects, *Circulation* 60:1201, 1979.
173. Neugebauer G: Comparative cardiovascular actions of verapamil and its major metabolites in the anaesthetised dog, *Cardiovasc Res* 12:247, 1978.
174. Keefe DL, Kates RE: Myocardial disposition and cardiac pharmacodynamics of verapamil in the dog, *J Pharmacol Exp Ther* 220:91, 1982.
175. Schwartz JB, Todd E, Abernethy DR et al: Steady state verapamil tissue distribution in the dog: differing tissue accumulation, *Pharmacology* 32:307, 1986.
176. McAllister RG, Bourne DW, Dittert LW: The pharmacology of verapamil. I. Elimination kinetics in dogs and correlation of plasma levels with effect on the electrocardiogram, *J Pharmacol Exp Ther* 202:38, 1977.
177. Traunecker W: His bundle electrography in the dog: normal values and findings with verapamil, *Arzneimittelforschung* 38:509, 1988.
178. Sabatier J, Pouyet T, Shelvey G et al: Antagonistic effects of epinephrine, glucagon and methylatropine but not calcium chloride against atrio-ventricular conduction disturbances produced by high doses of diltiazem, in conscious dogs, *Fundam Clin Pharmacol* 5:93, 1991.
179. Kapur PA, Matarazzo DA, Fung DM et al: The cardiovascular and adrenergic actions of verapamil or diltiazem in combination with propranolol during halothane anesthesia in the dog, *Anesthesiology* 66:122, 1987.
180. Hamann SR, Kaltenborn KE, McAllister RG: Hemodynamic and pharmacokinetic aspects of the interactions between verapamil and pindolol, *Pharmacology* 34:326, 1987.
181. Murthy SS, Nelson WL, Shen DD et al: Pharmacokinetic interaction between verapamil and metoprolol in the dog: stereochemical aspects, *Drug Metab Dispos* 19:1093, 1991.
182. Kapur PA, Grogan DL, Fournier DJ: Cardiovascular interactions of lidocaine with verapamil or diltiazem in the dog, *Anesthesiology* 68:79, 1988.
183. Johnson LM, Lankford SM, Bai SA: The influence of cimetidine on the pharmacokinetics of the enantiomers of verapamil in the dog during multiple oral dosing, *J Vet Pharmacol Ther* 18:117, 1995.
184. Klein HO, Lang R, Weiss E et al: The influence of verapamil on serum digoxin concentration, *Circulation* 65:998, 1982.
185. Sato M, Nagao T, Yamaguchi I et al: Pharmacological studies on a new 1,5-benzothiazepine derivative (CRD-401), *Arzneimittelforschung* 21: 1338, 1971.
186. Millard RW, Lathrop DA, Grupp G et al: Differential cardiovascular effects of calcium channel blocking agents: potential mechanisms, *Am J Cardiol* 49:499, 1982.
187. Kohno K, Takeuchi Y, Etoh A et al: Pharmacokinetics and bioavailability of diltiazem (CRD-401) in dog, *Arzneimittelforschung* 27:1424, 1977.
188. Piepho RW, Bloedow DC, Lacz JP et al: Pharmacokinetics of diltiazem in selected animal species and human beings, *Am J Cardiol* 49:525, 1982.
189. Skarvan K, Priebe HJ: Cardiovascular effects of diltiazem in the dog, *Br J Anaesth* 60:660, 1988.
190. Nakamura S, Suzuki T, Sugawara Y et al: Metabolic fate of diltiazem: distribution, excretion and protein binding in rat and dog, *Arzneimittelforschung* 37:1244, 1987.
191. Su J, Renaud N, Carayon A et al: Effects of the calcium channel blockers, diltiazem and Ro 40-5967, on systemic haemodynamics and plasma noradrenaline levels in conscious dogs with pacing-induced heart failure, *Br J Pharmacol* 113:395, 1994.
192. Porter CB, Walsh RA, Badke FR et al: Differential effects of diltiazem and nitroprusside on left ventricular function in experimental chronic volume overload, *Circulation* 68:685, 1983.
193. Atkins C, Johnson L, Keene B et al: Diltiazem pharmacokinetics and pharmacodynamics in cats, *J Vet Intern Med* 8:144, 1994 (abstract).
194. Lawson JW, Wojciechowski NJ: Comparative antiarrhythmic activity of quinidine combined with propranolol and with sotalol, *Arch Int Pharmacodyn Ther* 249:72, 1981.
195. Chezalviel-Guilbert F, Davy JM, Poirier JM et al: Mexiletine antagonizes effects of sotalol on QT interval duration and its proarrhythmic effects in a canine model of torsade de pointes, *J Am Coll Cardiol* 26:787, 1995.
196. Chezalviel F, Weissenburger J, Guhennec C et al: Antiarrhythmic effect of a sotalol-mexiletine combination on induced ventricular tachycardia in dogs, *J Cardiovasc Pharmacol* 21:212, 1993.

CHAPTER 30

Interventional Antiarrhythmic Therapy

Interventional techniques for the treatment of arrhythmias were introduced in human medicine in the 1930s, and the first self-contained artificial pacemaker was implanted in 1957.[1] The first reported pacemaker to be placed in a dog with naturally occurring disease was nearly 11 years later, in 1968, and was originally reported in cats in 1985.[2,3] Today more than 1 million human patients rely on implanted pacemakers, and such devices have become the definitive therapy for treatment of symptomatic bradyarrhythmias in both dogs and cats. Although pacemaker technology continues to advance, recent interest has also focused on the use of implantable cardioverter-defibrillators and interventional catheter techniques for the diagnosis and treatment of a variety of arrhythmias.[4-6]

Cardiac Pacemaker Therapy

A pacemaker is a device that delivers battery-supplied electrical stimuli through electrodes in contact with the myocardium to produce an artificially triggered depolarization. Since the first implantable pacemakers were developed, the equipment and techniques available have improved dramatically.[1,4] Recent advances in pacemaker technology include new lead designs, microprocessor-based circuitry, long-life batteries, telemetric manipulation, and newer pacing routines that allow rate-responsive adaptations and dual-chamber pacing. Cardiac pacemakers are now much smaller and more durable than before, and newer batteries can provide up to 12 years of continuous function.[7] Probably the most important technologic advance has been the refinement of percutaneous transvenous pacing leads that can be introduced into the heart through a peripheral vein.[8] Before this development, reliable pacemaker implantation required thoracotomy and surgical application of the lead directly to the epicardium.

INDICATIONS

The primary indications for artificial pacing in both humans and animals are symptomatic bradyarrhythmias and conduction disturbances that are unresponsive to medical control.[4,9] In veterinary patients the most common arrhythmias treated with artificial pacing include sinus bradycardia/sinus arrest (usually resulting from sick sinus syndrome or high vagal tone), high-grade second-degree and complete atrioventricular blocks, and persistent atrial standstill.[10]

The indications for cardiac pacing are outlined in Box 30-1. This material presented in Box 30-1 has been modified from the paper published in 1991 by the Joint Committee in the American College of Cardiology and the American Heart Association (ACC/AHA) outlining the indications for permanent pacing in humans.[11] Although indications are not always clear-cut, we have modified the indications in humans to provide a classification system for use in dogs. The information in Box 30-1 is based on the reference cited and on our clinical experience. In class I are the conditions for which there is general agreement that a permanent pacemaker should be placed. Class II includes conditions for which pacemakers are used frequently but opinion diverges as to their necessity. Class III includes those conditions for which there is general agreement that a pacemaker is not necessary. Both arrhythmia definition and symptom correlation may be confusing, and differences of opinion exist regarding which patients should receive artificial pacemakers.[11-13] In most patients, the decision is based on the assessment of the resting ECG or a Holter monitor recording, clinical signs, the predicted response to artificial pacing, and the general health of the patient. It is important for the clinician to understand that the recognition of an abnormal electrocardiographic (ECG) rhythm alone is not an indication for artificial pacing.[11,12] Clearly, in animals with documented ECG abnormalities and associated clinical signs (episodic weakness, syncope, etc.), artificial pacing is the preferred method of therapy when medical therapy is unrewarding. In patients with documented ECG abnormalities and clinical signs in which a definite correlation cannot be made, artificial pacing should be considered, but ultimately may not be pursued.[11] However, because of the cost, potential complications, and life-long special care inherent to permanent artificial pacing, it is not always rational therapy in asymptomatic animals, even when documented ECG abnormalities exist.[12]

CONTRAINDICATIONS

There are no absolute contraindications for pacemaker implantation; however, clinical and personal factors may preclude the decision to implant a pacemaker. Relative contraindications include debilitating generalized diseases and poor cardiac function secondary to a preexisting cardiac disorder.[4,10] Other serious medical problems may place the patient at an increased anesthetic risk or may significantly alter the patient's prognosis even if pacemaker implantation is successful. Some patients have congestive heart failure or other cardiac manifestations of their underlying cardiac disorder that may not be controlled by artificial pacing (e.g., persistent atrial standstill). The cost of new pacemaker hardware is prohibitive in veterinary medicine. The use of previously used generators and donation of outdated components by pacemaker manufacturing companies provides free generators.[14] Lead donations are more difficult to identify and may cost between $700.00 and $800.00.

BOX 30-1

Indications for permanent pacing in dogs

Class I

1. AV block
   - Permanent third degree (complete) AV block with clinical signs
   - Permanent or intermittent second degree AV block with clinical signs
2. Sick sinus syndrome
   - Sinus node dysfunction with documented bradycardia and clinical signs
3. Malignant vagal syndromes
   - Recurrent syncope and periods of asystole of >3 seconds in duration with or without carotid sinus stimulation (unusual in dogs)

Class II

1. AV block
   - Permanent complete AV block without clinical signs with a heart rate <40 beats/minute.
   - Permanent or intermittent type II second degree AV block without clinical signs (unusual in dogs).
   - Bundle branch block or bifascicular block with syncope when other causes for the syncope are not identified (unusual in dogs).
2. Sick sinus syndrome
   - Sinus node dysfunction associated with bradycardia but where a clear association between clinical signs and the bradycardia have not been established.
3. Malignant vagal syndromes
   - Recurrent syncope associated with bradycardia that is atropine-responsive but that is not controlled with medical therapy or medical therapy produces adverse clinical signs.
4. Persistent atrial standstill
   - Recurrent syncope or persistent weakness or fatigue associated with a slow heart rate. The owner must be made aware that the disease often progresses so that pacemaker therapy is only a temporary means of controlling clinical signs.

Class III

1. AV block
   - Type I second degree AV block.
2. Sick sinus syndrome
   - Sinus node dysfunction where clinical signs are clearly documented to not be associated with a slow heart rate.
   - Sinus node dysfunction due to drug therapy.
3. Malignant vagal syndromes
   - Recurrent syncope associated with bradycardia that is atropine-responsive and that is controlled with anticholinergic therapy.
   - Vagally-mediated bradycardia that produces no clinical signs.

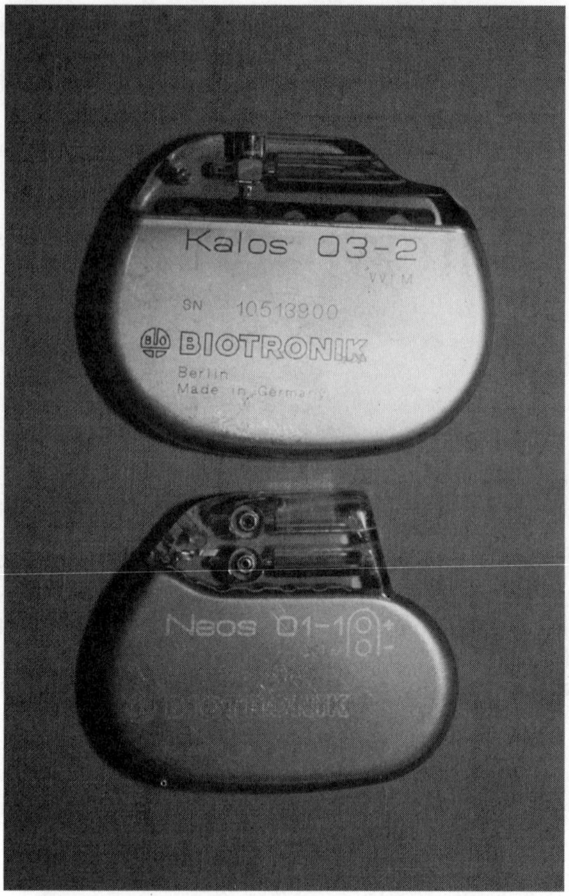

FIGURE 30-1 Implantable pulse generators. The upper pulse generator is unipolar, and the lower pulse generator is bipolar (notice the two connection ports). Many newer bipolar pulse generators are coaxial, with only one connection port.

Dogs with hyperadrenocorticism (iatrogenic or naturally-occurring) have more complications than dogs without hyperadrenocorticism, in our experience. Dogs with hyperadrenocorticism have compromised immune function that makes the patient more susceptible to infection. They also often have very thin skin that predisposes the patient to having problems with wound healing of the area where the generator is implanted.

CASE SELECTION

The primary clinical goal for patients with symptomatic bradyarrhythmias is to prevent clinical signs related to bradycardia or episodic cessation of cardiac activity. Complete resolution of episodic weakness and syncope is a reasonable goal in properly selected candidates. A secondary goal may be to increase the heart rate such that a normal cardiac output can be maintained at rest or over a wide range of activity levels. In human patients, some asymptomatic patients with cardiac arrhythmias are predisposed to sudden death and receive pacemakers to prevent this occurrence.

All patients should receive a complete medical screening and a complete cardiovascular evaluation before implantation of a pacemaker. At minimum, a biochemical panel, a complete blood count, an ECG before and after atropine administration, and thoracic radiographs should be performed. Patients with preexisting cardiac abnormalities or abnormal findings on thoracic radiographs should be evaluated echocardiographically. The main rationale behind a complete patient evaluation is to identify problems that may affect anesthesia or significantly alter the long-term prognosis of the patient. If other significant medical problems exist, artificial pacing may not be pursued.

PACEMAKER EQUIPMENT

The basic pacing system consists of an implantable pulse generator (IPG) that houses the circuitry and power supply and a pacing lead or electrode that transmits the electrical information between the IPG and the myocardium. Other ancillary equipment is necessary for proper implantation and maintenance of the pacing system.

Pulse generator. The IPG is a sophisticated power pack that carries all the necessary electronics for pacing, hermetically sealed in a titanium or stainless steel casing (Figure 30-1). Modern pulse generators are compact, reliable, and long-lived. The lithium anode

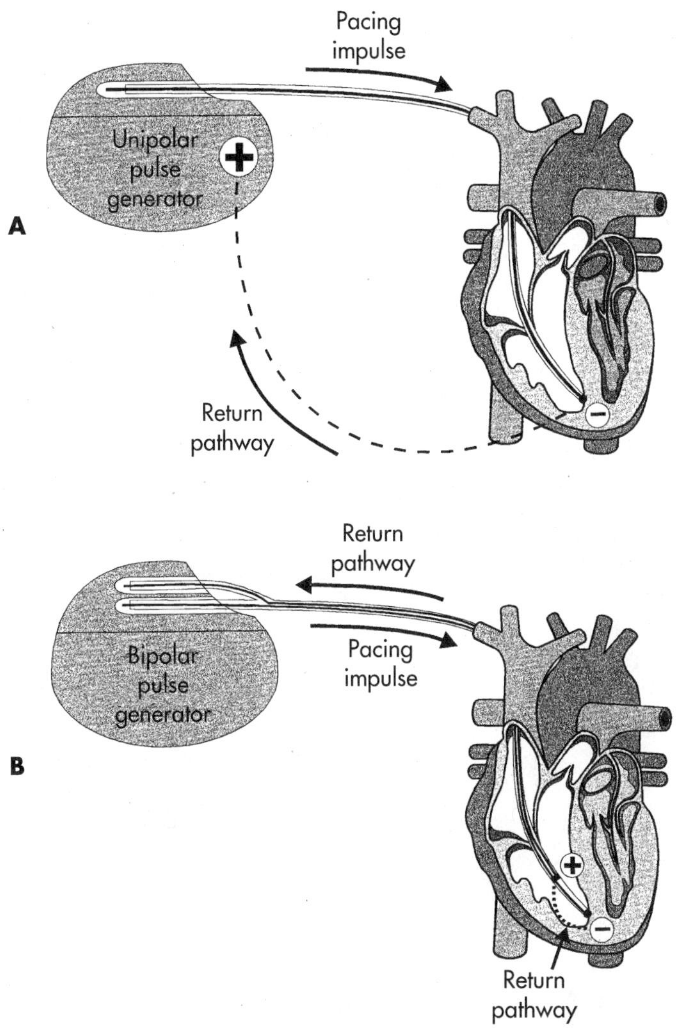

FIGURE 30-2 Schematic representation of unipolar and bipolar pacing systems. **A,** Unipolar leads provide one electrode (cathode) within the heart. Impulses travel through the lead to the myocardium and return to the IPG casing (anode) to complete the circuit. **B,** Bipolar leads provide two closely spaced electrodes, both of which lie within the heart. The distal electrode is usually the cathode and the proximal electrode is a ring anode.

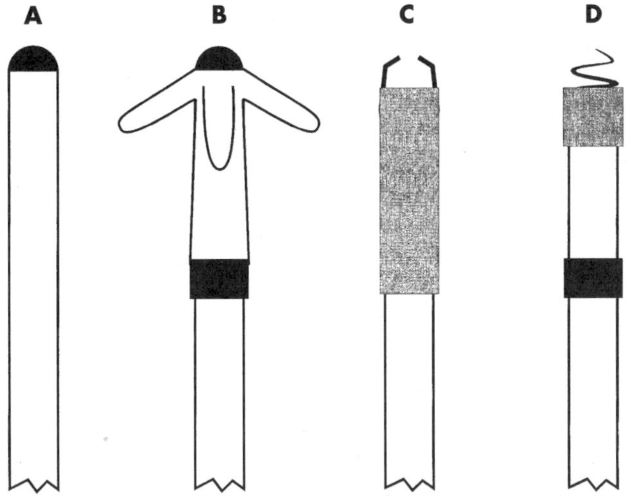

FIGURE 30-3 Representative transvenous ventricular leads. **A,** Unipolar lead with no fixation device (passive fixation). **B,** Bipolar lead with silastic tines (passive fixation). **C,** Unipolar lead with retractable metallic barbs (active fixation). **D,** Bipolar lead with screw-in tip (active fixation).

battery (usually lithium iodide) has become the industry standard power supply.[4,7] The major advantages are small size, long life, reliability, and a satisfactory voltage output for up to 90% of the battery's life.

Three basic electronic circuits are housed within the IPG. The timing circuit controls the pacing interval, the output circuit controls the charging and discharging of the electrical impulse, and the sensing circuit is responsible for the recognition of spontaneous intracardiac signals.[4] Most modern pacing circuits are further modified by a variety of other electrical accessories, including filters, protective devices, and the complex circuitry required for programmability, telemetry, memory, and rate-adaptive functions. Pacemaker pulse generators also contain a special electromagnetic switch that allows pacemaker function to be temporarily converted to asynchronous mode by placing it in a strong magnetic field.

Pacing lead. The pacing lead is an insulated wire or set of wires that delivers the pulse stimuli from the generator to the myocardium and conducts intracardiac potentials to the sensing circuit. Originally, epicardial or epimyocardial leads were surgically affixed to the external surface of the heart. To eliminate the need for thoracotomy, transvenous leads are now preferred. There are two major types of lead systems. Unipolar leads provide one electrode (cathode) within the heart. Impulses travel through the lead to the myocardium and return to the IPG casing (anode) to complete the circuit (Figure 30-2, *A*). The potential advantages of unipolar leads are smaller design and theoretical sensing superiority. Because of the larger distance between the electrodes, the unipolar system uses a large sensing area. The major disadvantage of unipolar systems is the proximity of skeletal muscle to the circuit. Skeletal muscle may twitch as it is stimulated by the IPG discharge. This can be diminished by insulating a portion of the IPG and in many situations is only a temporary inconvenience that resolves when the IPG is walled off by fibrosis.[4] Bipolar leads provide two closely spaced electrodes, both of which lie within the heart. The distal electrode is usually the cathode, and the proximal electrode is a ring anode (Figure 30-2, *B*). Although many bipolar pacemakers require two connections at the generator, causing slightly larger generator size, coaxial bipolar leads (one connection at the generator) on newer systems have overcome this problem. Bipolar leads are generally preferred because of a greater signal-to-noise ratio, less sensitivity to extraneous interference, and avoidance of skeletal muscle stimulation.[7]

Lead fixation to the myocardium may be active (invading the myocardium) or passive (promote fixation by indirect means) (Figure 30-3). Active leads provide myocardial penetration by grasping screws or small retractable prongs and are used for both transthoracic and transvenous implantation. Passive leads use tines or fins to enhance entanglement within the trabeculae of the right ventricle during transvenous placement.[7] The choice of fixation is largely personal, because equally good performance is obtained with both active and passive fixation when the leads are implanted properly.[15] Several enhancements in lead design, including smaller surface-area tips, porous electrodes, and steroid-eluding leads, have been developed to reduce stimulation threshold and increase pacemaker efficiency.[4,7]

Ancillary equipment. The use of appropriate testing and programming techniques and other ancillary equipment can improve the chances of a successful pacemaker implantation (Figure 30-4). A temporary pacemaker is helpful, especially in patients with an increased anesthetic risk. Temporary pacing can usually be achieved in a lightly sedated patient and can be used to support the patient until the permanent system can be implanted, including anesthetic induction. A pacing magnet is helpful for troubleshooting in malfunctioning pacemakers because it forces the pulse generator to function in asynchronous mode (VOO).

Lead electrical studies at the time of placement allow selection of the optimal electrode stimulation and sensing site. Using a pacing systems analyzer (PSA), such testing is simple. A PSA is a special type of temporary pacemaker that allows the electrical characteristics of the pacing circuit (lead and lead placement position) to be analyzed. Guidelines regarding optimal values for threshold voltage and current, *R* wave sensitivity, system impedance, and IPG integrity have been reported for both humans and dogs.[4,16]

The use of multiprogrammable pacing generators allows greater battery efficiency and the use of rate-adaptive functions that are more physiologic than fixed-rate systems. For optimal use of these newer pacemakers, a telemetric pacing system programmer, with modules for the appropriate model(s) of IPG, is necessary unless only the default settings are to be employed. Telemetry (reading

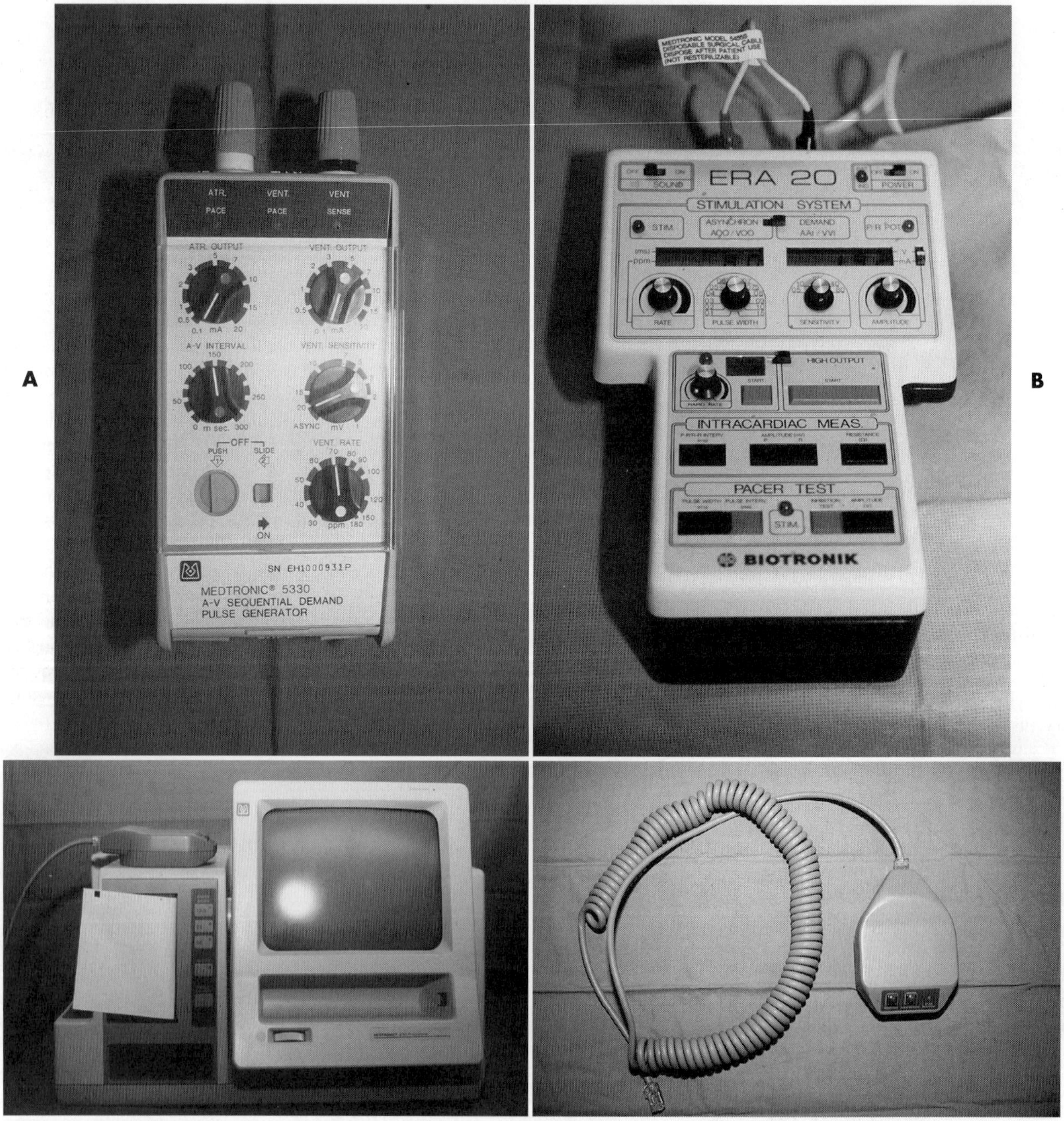

FIGURE 30-4 **A,** Temporary pacemaker. **B,** Pacing system analyzer. **C,** Pacing system programmer. **D,** Pacing system programming magnetic head.

the values programmed into the generator) is virtually indispensable because it provides information on all programmed values, as well as real-time and previously recorded data on how the pacemaker is operating. Programming provides the capability of changing pacemaker settings noninvasively. This is important because settings incorporated into the pacemaker during implantation are not always optimal for the duration of the life of the patient. Data that can be retrieved telemetrically include information on the output circuit (current, voltage, resistance), battery parameters, sensor activity (for rate-adaptive units), diagnostic information regarding interaction between the pacemaker and the patient over an extended period, event markers, and direct recording of electrograms. Event markers depicting pacing and sensing can be displayed simultaneously with the ECG and allow real-time troubleshooting of the pacing system.

Pacing system programmers consist of a magnetic scanner (usually hand-held), a microprocessor with stored parameters and information regarding the specific model of pacemaker, a cathode ray tube (CRT) or liquid crystal display (LCD) screen for display of parameters, and a keyboard for interaction with the programmer. Almost every pacing parameter can be manipulated within a range of accepted settings, although each model has individual differences in programming capability. The three most important parameters for single-chamber pacemakers are rate, output (voltage and pulse width), and sensitivity. It may be necessary to increase the rate if the initial rate selection results in inability to exercise appropriately. It may be necessary to increase the voltage and pulse width if the pacing threshold changes over time in a patient. The threshold commonly increases as fibrous tissue forms around the tip of the lead. Conversely, output can often be decreased 2 to 3 months after implanting a pacemaker. Reducing output increases battery life and the longevity of the pacemaker. Chronic skeletal muscle stimulation ("twitch") may also be reduced or eliminated by reducing the output of unipolar generators. The sensing function of the pacemaker should normally be set to half the sensing threshold. Oversensing of the *T* wave or other electrical events can be remedied by decreasing the sensitivity (increasing the number toward the threshold value).

MODES OF CARDIAC PACING

The early pacemakers employed a single lead implanted in the ventricle, which was paced at a fixed rate without ventricular sensing.[4,17] With the development of more complex pacing systems, the broad array of pacing modes available can be used to optimize pacemaker therapy for a wide range of clinical problems. However, this flexibility also makes device selection more complex. To relieve difficulties with terminology, a classification system was developed in which pacemakers are categorized according to the site and mode of pacing and sensing.[18] Originally a three- letter code, later modified to a five-letter code with the advent of programmability and antitachycardia pacing, was used to discriminate between different types of pacing systems (Table 30-1).[19] The first three positions of the code describe the chamber paced, the chamber sensed, and the mode of response to sensing, respectively. The fourth position describes programmable functions, and the fifth position relates tachyarrhythmia devices. The latter two positions are usually omitted when irrelevant.

Asynchronous ventricular pacing (VOO) was the original mode. In this mode the ventricle is paced at a fixed rate, with no relationship to the underlying spontaneous rhythm. The pacemaker does not sense spontaneous ventricular activity and therefore fires completely independent of any other modification. Most programmable pacemakers can be forced to function in asynchronous mode by placing the pacemaker within a strong magnetic field. This is often done for diagnostic purposes.[7]

Fixed-rate, single-chamber ventricular-inhibited pacing (VVI) is used most commonly in veterinary patients.[10] In this mode, also called *ventricular demand pacing,* the ventricle is paced at a fixed rate but continuously senses for spontaneous ventricular electrical activity (electrical activity generated in the ventricle that travels back through the lead to the generator). When the spontaneous underlying rate is below the set rate of the pacemaker, the pacemaker controls the heart rate. When the spontaneous ventricular rate exceeds the generator rate, the generator is temporarily suppressed and does not fire. The initial portion of the pacing cycle consists of a refractory period (usually 200 to 350 ms) during which the pacing generator is insensitive to any sensed signals.[7] This prevents the pacemaker from sensing its own stimulus or the paced or spontaneous discharge. Beyond the refractory period, a sensed QRS potential will inhibit the pacemaker. When this occurs, the pacing output circuit is reset to the baseline and pacing stimuli resume at the fixed rate and fixed interval following cessation of spontaneous QRS potentials. The VVI system allows conservation of battery power when underlying spontaneous rhythms are adequate and prevents competitive rhythms that may have fatal consequences.[4,7] Newer ventricular demand systems are programmable (VVIP or VVIM) and allow the fixed rate and output settings to be reprogrammed for longer battery life and optimal function. The principal advantages of VVI systems include straightforward device operation and simple follow-up procedures. Additionally, only a single pacing lead is required, and its placement is easily learned. The disadvantages of the VVI mode are its inability to provide chronotropic responsiveness or a normal atrioventricular

TABLE 30-1

International generic pacemaker code (modified in 1987)[19]

Code Positions				
I Chamber paced	*II* Chamber sensed	*III* Response to sensing	*IV** Programmable functions	*V*** Antitachycardia functions
O = None	O = None	O = None	O = None	O = None
A = Atrium	A = Atrium	T = Triggers pacing	P = Rate or output	P = Pacing
V = Ventricle	V = Ventricle	I = Inhibits pacing	M = Multiprogrammable	S = Shock
D = Dual (A + V)	D = Dual (A + V)	D = Dual (T + I)	C = Communicating (telemetric control)	D = Dual (P + S)
			R = Rate-adaptive	

*Under common usage position 4 is only indicated if the device is rate-adaptive because almost all modern pacemakers have P/M/C.
**Position 5 is rarely used because this mode of pacing is uncommon.

relationship.[17] For these reasons, the functional capacity of patients with VVI pacemakers may be limited. This, however, is rarely a problem in veterinary patients.

Rate-responsive, multiprogrammable pacemakers (VVIR) were introduced in the mid-1980s and have received substantial worldwide acceptance in human medicine.[17] Rate-adaptive pacemakers have been used in dogs, and, with more units becoming available for veterinary use, will likely become more popular.[20,21] However, the benefits of these systems over traditional modes and the optimal settings for these systems have not been evaluated in clinical animals. Rate-adaptive functions allow the rate of the pacing stimulus to be dynamically modified by some external factor. Many sensor systems have been evaluated and developed, but few have gained widespread acceptance. Early rate-adaptive systems employed an atrial electrode that sensed the atrial activity and adjusted the ventricular rate in accordance with physiologic changes in the sinus node (VDDR mode). Obviously, this type of sensing is not applicable to patients with sinus node dysfunction or patients with atrial arrhythmias, which severely limited the use of the early rate-adaptive systems.[4,17] The most common type of rate-responsive pacing system used in humans is called *activity pacing*.[4] These systems employ a piezoelectric crystal within the pacing generator that senses patient movement. Detection of movement results in an increase in the rate of the pacing stimulus, with a resultant increase in cardiac output. Although considered by some to be nonphysiologic, the simplicity and reliability of the activity pacing systems have led to them becoming well accepted. Other sensors incorporated into rate-adaptive pacemakers include respiratory sensors (respiration rate or minute volume), temperature sensors, ventricular repolarization (QT interval) sensors, sensors of myocardial contractility (e.g., stroke volume, dV/dt, dP/dt, preejection period), sensors of venous oxygen saturation, and pH sensors.[4,7] Most of these systems require special sensing leads to be incorporated into the pacing system, and many are not approved for clinical use.[7]

Dual-chamber (right atrium and right ventricle) pacing (DDI[R] and DDD[R] modes) offers the most physiologic form of pacing currently available, especially when rate-adaptive functions are also available.[17] These modes provide maintenance of atrioventricular synchrony at rest and during exercise, resulting in preservation of the atrial contribution to ventricular stroke volume. Maintenance of atrioventricular synchrony is also advantageous in humans to reduce the incidence of atrial arrhythmias and thromboembolism associated with pacemaker therapy.[17] The principal disadvantages to dual-chamber pacing are the need for two pacing leads and the reduced generator longevity. Programming and follow-up are complex for these types of units. The use of dual-chamber pacing has been reported in one dog.[22]

TEMPORARY PACING

Temporary pacing can be achieved percutaneously, epicardially, or via the esophagus. Although the components of the system are the same (i.e., a pulse generator and lead), temporary generators are bulky, not implantable, and tend to have less versatility than implantable devices (see Figure 30-4, *A*). Temporary pacing is indicated in patients that require hemodynamic stabilization of acute clinical signs before implantation of the permanent pacemaker, in patients with a high risk of developing severe complications (e.g., asystole) during anesthetic induction, and in patients suspected of having a transient arrhythmia producing the clinical signs.[7,23]

Transvenous temporary pacing is done through percutaneous puncture of a jugular or lateral saphenous vein using a balloon-tipped bipolar electrode. Percutaneous placement of a temporary lead via the jugular vein may be difficult in uncooperative patients.[24] The lateral saphenous vein is preferable in patients in which the jugular vein(s) will later be used for placement of the permanent pacing lead. Accessing and threading the catheter in a lateral saphenous vein can be problematic in small patients. We prefer to place the temporary pacing lead via the lateral saphenous vein. This usually can be accomplished in most patients using a 14-gauge, over-the-needle catheter. Whatever the site of access, the lead tip is placed into the right ventricular apex using fluoroscopic guidance.[25] In patients with normal atrioventricular conduction, the lead tip may be positioned in the right auricle. Temporary pacing systems are usually set to VVI with a ventricular rate between 100 to 120 beats/min. During placement of a permanent pacemaker, the rate of the temporary pacemaker should be set to a rate below that of the IPG to prevent competing rhythms.[7] Temporary pacing can be continued for several days; however, the lead should be replaced and repositioned in accordance with standards of indwelling catheter care to prevent the development of infections and phlebitis.

TRANSVENOUS (ENDOCARDIAL) IMPLANTATION

Transvenous implantation of permanent pacemakers is the preferred method in both human and veterinary medicine (Color Plate 112).[10,26,27] Most patients requiring artificial pacing are old and are poor surgical and anesthetic candidates because of their arrhythmia, coexisting cardiac disease, and other unrelated medical problems.[10,23] The primary advantage of transvenous application is that it is less invasive (in reality only a minor surgical procedure), with reduced anesthesia and recovery times compared with thoracotomy and direct epicardial lead placement. In appropriate patients, transvenous pacing systems can be implanted using only light sedation and local anesthesia.[28] However, general anesthesia is preferred to minimize breaks in aseptic technique. There is less morbidity associated with transvenous pacing, leading to shorter periods of hospitalization. Shortened surgery and anesthesia times and the need for fewer surgical supplies reduce the cost compared with other methods of pacemaker implantation. However, there is a higher potential for improper lead placement or lead dislodgment because of the inability to directly attach the lead to the myocardium. These limitations can be minimized by strict adherence to proper technique and proper lead placement at the time of implantation. Transvenous pacemaker implantation requires fluoroscopic equipment, which is often unavailable. Fluoroscopy also carries the risk of exposure to radiation.

Patient preparation. Many patients are a high anesthetic risk, and temporary pacing should be considered.[10,23] The majority of our patients have a temporary lead placed before anesthetic induction. In those that do not, an infusion setup of isoproterenol is prepared to increase the heart rate if required, because an exacerbation of a bradyarrhythmia is common during induction and the subsequent anesthetic period. Provisions for emergency transvenous pacing should be made for those patients not receiving a temporary pacemaker, although placement during a crisis is difficult. Preanesthetic medications and the choice of an anesthetic induction regimen should be based on the patient's general condition, the patient's underlying problems, and the familiarity of the anesthetist with the agents to be used.[29-32] The external jugular vein is almost always used for placing the permanent lead. The patient should be positioned in right or left lateral recumbency, depending on which jugular vein is to be used. The right jugular vein is preferred because of the occasional patient that has a persistent left cranial vena cava. The lateral cervical region and lateral thorax (if this site is to be used to bury the IPG) should be clipped thoroughly from the crest to the ventral midline and the skin prepared for aseptic surgery. Electrocautery should not be used during pacemaker implantation, because it can cause ventricular fibrillation and damage the generator if used when the generator or lead are in place.

Lead placement. A small (3- to 5-cm) incision is made in the skin over the right or left jugular vein, which is exposed and prepared as described in Chapter 7 (Color Plate 32). The jugular vein is ligated cranially, and a small venotomy is made caudal to the ligature. An endocardial lead, stiffened by a wire stylet, is introduced through the venotomy and advanced under fluoroscopic guidance until the tip is positioned in the right ventricular apex, close to the diaphragm (see Figure 30-5, Color Plate 112, *A*). If the lead is difficult to advance across the tricuspid valve, a subtle, sweeping bend can be made in the wire stylet or the lead may be advanced without the stylet. When tined-tipped leads are used, the electrode tip should wedge within the trabecular muscles by gently rotating and advancing the lead with the stylet in place. If the tined lead is positioned and wedged properly, gentle traction on the lead should be met with subtle resistance.[10] There are various procedures for attaching active-fixation leads to the endocardium. Once the lead is positioned properly, sensitivity and threshold measurements can be made using a PSA, if available. Alternatively, adequate lead placement may be judged by identifying its placement using fluoroscopy and observing for evidence of pacing activity (observing regular cardiac contractions on fluoroscopy, observing an arterial pulse rate equal to the preprogrammed pacing rate, or identifying normal pacing and sensing functions on a simultaneously recorded surface ECG).[10] The most common mistake is to place the lead too far forward in the body of the right ventricle or in the right ventricular outflow tract. Lead dislodgement into the pulmonary artery is a common sequela to improper placement.

Lead analysis. Using a pacing system analyzer, the threshold voltage and current, *R* wave sensitivity and amplitude, system impedance, and integrity of the pulse generator can be quickly and easily determined. This gives measurements of the electrical nature of the pacing system at the time of placement. The major problem with relying on this type of device is that these characteristics change, often dramatically, as the tissue around the lead tip becomes inflamed and scar tissue forms.

The endocardial *R* wave size should be measured first, before pacing, because pacemaker dependence may occur immediately, making it difficult to reestablish a satisfactory spontaneous rhythm after measuring pacing thresholds.[33] An *R* wave amplitude greater than 10 mV is ideal, but anything over 4 mV is adequate for proper sensing. In dogs, positioning the lead tip in the right ventricular outflow tract is associated with significantly smaller *R* wave amplitudes than the right ventricular caudal wall or right ventricular apex. In some cases this may be inadequate for proper sensing function.[16]

To measure the lead threshold, the PSA is set at a discharge amplitude of 5 V and a pulse duration of 0.5 ms. The pacing rate is set at a level at which steady, regular pacing is achieved (usually around 100 beats/min). The voltage output is slowly reduced until loss of capture occurs. The voltage at this point is the *stimulation threshold*. The voltage and current are recorded. The voltage output is then increased until consistent pacing is reestablished; this is the *pacing threshold*. There is almost always a slight difference between the two measurements, with the pacing threshold being slightly higher. There is no standard convention for deciding which of the two thresholds is better suited for optimal lead characteristics. An acute voltage threshold between 0.3 and 1.0 V is acceptable.[33] Next the voltage is returned to 5 V, and a similar current threshold is recorded by varying the current. An acceptable acute *current threshold* is between 0.3 and 2.0 mA.[33] All endocardial positions in the canine right ventricle commonly provide acceptable voltage and current thresholds, based on the above ranges reported in humans.[16]

To measure the impedance (resistance) of the system, the voltage is set to 5 V. Newer analyzers simply have a button that provides a digital display of the resistance when pushed. If a direct measurement is not available, the current and voltage are recorded and the impedance is calculated using Ohm's law. The normal range for impedance is 250 to 1000 Ω.[33]

If the measured parameters are unsatisfactory, the lead should be repositioned and reanalyzed until a satisfactory location is found. Once satisfactory lead positioning is obtained, the lead is examined under fluoroscopy and advanced slightly to place a small bend in the lead in the right atrium to allow for neck movement that might otherwise exert traction on the lead. The lead is secured in position by placing several encircling nonabsorbable ligatures around the lead and jugular vein. The neck incision should remain open until after placement of the IPG. The lead is then secured to the vein and surrounding tissues using nonabsorbable ligatures.

Generator placement. The IPG is placed into a subcutaneous pocket either in the neck or lateral thorax. For placement in the neck, a separate incision is made in the dorsolateral aspect of the neck, cranial to the lead insertion in the jugular vein.[9,34] For placement on the lateral thorax, an incision through the skin and cutaneous trunci muscle is made in the dorsal one third of the thorax at the sixth or seventh intercostal space. A pocket is created beneath the cutaneous trunci muscle by blunt dissection (note that this position is not immediately beneath the skin). The pacing lead is passed through a tunnel connecting the two incisions and connected to the IPG. For tunneling between the neck and lateral thorax, special instrumentation is usually helpful. Any type of large, long, strong forceps can be used to create the tunnel, from the thoracic end. These forceps can then be used to grasp the lead tip and pull it back through the tunnel. The lead should not be grasped nor retracted forcefully because separation of the lead coils and lead dysfunction may result. We prefer to use a large trocar type of chest tube to create the tunnel (Color Plate 112, *B*). The trocar is removed, and the lead is fed through the chest tube without excessive tension (Color Plate 112, *C*). If a bipolar generator is being used, the lead can be attached to the generator and the temporary pacemaker can be inactivated at this time (Color Plate 112, *D*). When using a unipolar pacemaker, temporary pacing should be maintained until the generator has been permanently placed in the subcutaneous pocket, because contact of the IPG casing with the patient is required to complete the pacing circuit. The IPG is placed into the pocket and sutured to the deep musculature using the provided anchor hole and large nonabsorbable suture. Although not used routinely, synthetic Dacron pouches may be used to cover the IPG for placement.[28] The excess lead is coiled and placed beneath the generator, and both incisions are closed routinely, taking special care to minimize dead space around the IPG to minimize seroma formation.

Postoperative care. Postoperative care is minimal. Systemic antibiotics, usually a cephalosporin or potentiated penicillin, may be prophylactically administered for 7 to 10 days to prevent infection at the surgery sites. The incisions should be kept clean and dry until the sutures are removed.[35] Patients are usually discharged from the hospital within 24 to 48 hours after surgery. Patient activity should be restricted, to minimize the chance of lead dislodgement before permanent fibrosis is achieved (Color Plate 113). In extreme cases, heavy sedation or cage confinement may be necessary, but are preferable to replacement of the pacemaker lead. Patients should be restrained from disturbing the incisions before complete healing, which may require bandages or Elizabethan collars.

EPICARDIAL (EPIMYOCARDIAL) IMPLANTATION

Epicardial implantation is an established technique that requires surgical exposure of the heart and direct implantation of the lead into the epimyocardium. Epicardial pacing leads were used almost exclusively in dogs before the widespread availability and acceptance of transvenous endocardial pacing leads. Epicardial leads are now usually only used at our institution when a patient is also undergoing thoracotomy for another reason or in patients with repeated dislodgement of transvenous endocardial leads.[24] Epicardial lead placement offers the advantage of secure, active myocardial fixation and, other than a standard surgery pack, no need for fluoroscopy. However, the need for general anesthesia and thoracotomy with inherently extended anesthetic and recovery times are unfavorable, and transvenous pacing is still preferred and is generally less costly. Depending on the site of IPG placement, inaccessibility for reprogramming or replacement is another potential limitation of epicardial implantation.[23]

Surgical approach and pulse generator placement. The following three approaches for epicardial pacemaker implantation have been described in dogs: (1) lateral thoracotomy[9,36-38]; (2) midline celiotomy/sternotomy[9,23,36]; and (3) the ventral abdominal transdiaphragmatic approach.[9,39,40] Each approach has inherent strengths and weaknesses, but the transdiaphragmatic approach is more commonly used because of its simplicity, reduced tissue trauma, and shorter anesthesia time.[40]

The lateral thoracotomy approach may be performed from either the right or left fifth intercostal space. An incision is made in the skin, and the thorax is accessed in a standard fashion. The heart is isolated, and a small pericardiotomy is made at the cardiac apex to expose the relatively avascular left ventricular apical epicardial surface. The heart is elevated and cradled in the operator's hand. Alternatively, two partial-thickness stay sutures may be placed in the left ventricular apex. The stay sutures can then be used to raise the heart slightly and will allow the heart to rest normally when not being manipulated. After the lead is affixed to the myocardium, separate incisions are made behind the last rib and caudodorsally on the lateral thoracic wall. A subcutaneous pocket is created by blunt dissection, and the lead is tunneled between the two incisions. The IPG is connected to the lead and sutured within the subcutaneous pocket.

For the midline celiotomy with caudal third sternotomy, a midline incision is made from the cranial third of the abdomen to the caudal third of the sternum, extending through the xiphoid cartilage and xiphoid process to the level of the sixth sternebra. If the generator is to be placed in an abdominal location, the incision is extended to the umbilicus. A retractor is used to spread the sternum, allowing direct visualization of the cardiac apex. A small pericardiotomy is performed, and the lead is implanted, as detailed later in this section. The lead is passed through the diaphragm into the peritoneum and is connected to the IPG. The IPG may be inserted in a subcutaneous pocket in the flank or may be left free in the abdomen. Subcutaneous placement is preferable because it allows easier programming or replacement of the IPG. However, in some small dogs, abdominal placement is unavoidable if a larger generator must be used.[23]

The ventral abdominal transdiaphragmatic approach was developed to reduce surgery time, reduce the postoperative infection rate, and reduce tissue trauma.[39,40] It is a simpler technique than those previously described. A ventral midline incision is made from the umbilicus to the xiphoid. A 3- to 5-cm longitudinal incision is made in the muscular portion of the diaphragm, extending from the ventral midline to the central tendon and allowing exposure of the cardiac apex. A pericardiotomy is performed, and the edges are stabilized with Allis forceps or stay sutures. The epicardial lead is implanted in the myocardium, and the lead is passed into the abdominal cavity. A small length of redundant lead is left in the thorax to reduce traction, and a double purse-string suture is placed through the diaphragm and around the lead to stabilize it. The IPG is left to float free in the abdomen, and the diaphragmatic and abdominal incisions are closed in routine fashion.

Lead attachment. The site of epicardial lead attachment is variable; it can be placed anywhere on the right or left ventricle, preferably near, but not on, the apex. A site in a region of thick myocardium and away from the coronary arteries should be identified and if possible should not lie directly under the sternum. The apex should be avoided to prevent undue stress on the electrode tip and to reduce the possibility of rupture of the thin myocardium in this region.[41] Two general types of epicardial leads are used—those requiring sutures and those not requiring sutures.[42] The coiled spring leads are the most commonly used sutured leads. These leads have a spring electrode tip emanating from a synthetic disc containing holes for stay sutures. With this type of lead, a small partial-thickness stab incision is made in the myocardium to allow insertion of the electrode, and the disc is affixed to the myocardium with three or four fine nonabsorbable sutures.[42] The sutureless screw-in design is the epicardial lead used most commonly. These leads have a corkscrew tip surrounded by a Dacron ring that promotes fibrosis.[42] Screw-in epicardial leads are implanted using an insertion tool preloaded with the lead by the manufacturer. The tip of the lead is placed against the myocardium at the predetermined site and is inserted by turning it clockwise 2½ turns, with gentle pressure against the myocardium. The lead is dislodged from the tool and the tip inspected for proper placement. The Dacron pad should rest firmly against myocardium. If not, the insertion tool can be reapplied and an extra turn can be placed. Once the lead is positioned properly, sensitivity and threshold measurements can be made using a PSA, if available.

Postoperative care. The principles of postoperative care for patients receiving an epicardial implant are similar to those described for transvenous implantation. There is much less of a concern of lead dislodgement, and strict measures to restrict activity are usually unnecessary. The postoperative hospital stay is usually 3 to 5 days to allow full recovery from surgery. The use of prophylactic antibiotics and measures to facilitate proper wound healing are identical to those described above.

PACEMAKER FOLLOW-UP

The IPG is usually set at fairly high settings at the time of implantation. We recommend turning off rate-adaptive functions and leaving the output settings at the factory defaults (usually pulse amplitude = 5.0 V, pulse width = 0.5 ms), at least until the time of suture removal. This approach helps to ensure the pacemaker will capture the ventricle properly while healing occurs. The pacing threshold usually increases shortly after implantation, because inflammation and edema separate the tip from the myocardium.[7] Chronically, most of the increase in the threshold is due to the formation of nonexcitable fibrous tissue around the electrode. The threshold reaches a maximum value 10 to 20 days after implantation.[7] The fixed rate also allows the owners to track the heart rate at home without confusion from the variability of rate-adaptive functions. Thoracic radiographs should be taken on the first postoperative day to confirm lead position and provide a baseline for follow-up studies (Figure 30-5). An ECG should be recorded and evaluated for the proper pacing interval (pacing rate), capture (should

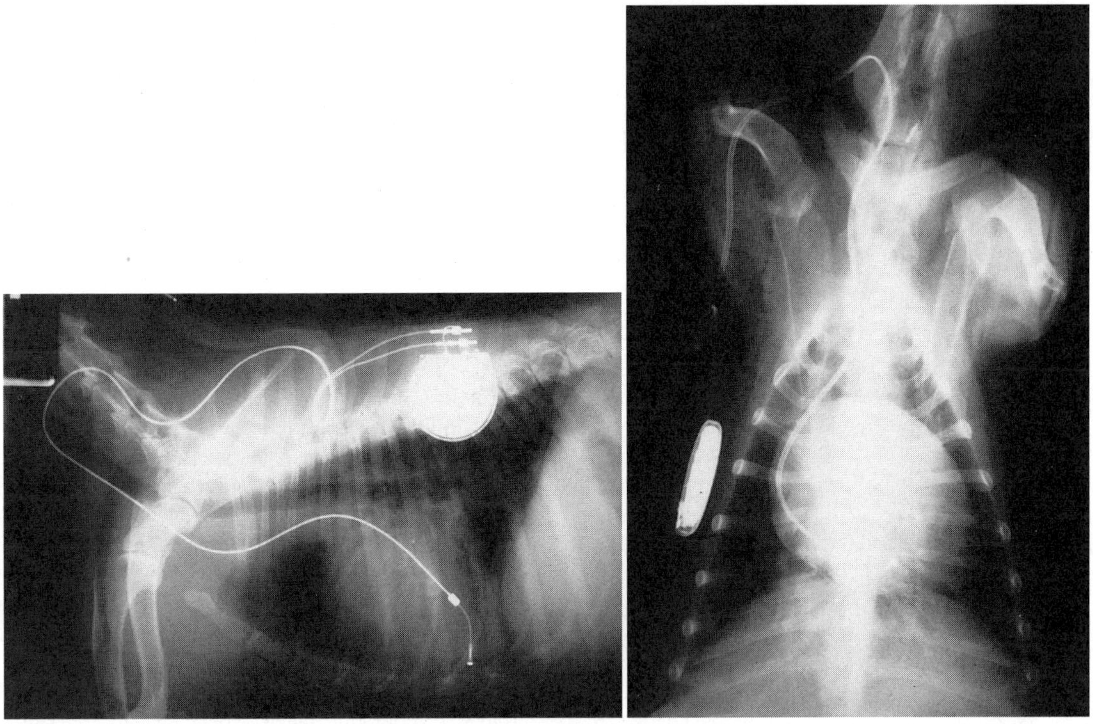

FIGURE 30-5 Thoracic radiographs from a dog with a transvenous pacemaker. **A,** Lateral thoracic radiograph showing placement of the IPG on the right lateral thorax. The lead courses in the subcutaneous tissues of the lateral thorax and neck and enters the cardiovascular system through the right jugular vein. The lead tip is fixed in position in the right ventricular apex. **B,** Dorsoventral thoracic radiograph from the dog shown in **A.**

be 100%), and sensing functions. The morphology of the pacing-induced QRS complex should be noted for comparison with follow-up studies.

Sutures should be removed 10 to 14 days postoperatively, at which time thoracic radiographs and an ECG should be repeated and compared with the initial postoperative studies. Dislodgement of endocardial leads usually occurs within the first few weeks following implantation.[10] If the lead is still in the proper position, it is very unlikely that dislodgement will occur. At this time, we turn on the rate-adaptive functions, if available, and inform the owners of the rate limits, so that casual heart rate monitoring can be done at home. However, the output settings should be left at factory defaults, because stabilization of the pacing threshold does not occur until 1 to 2 months after implantation.[7,41] Typically, thoracic radiographs and electrocardiography are repeated in 3 months, and output settings are set to the lowest reliable settings based on telemetric threshold measurements to extend battery life. The patient is then rechecked biannually with thoracic radiography and electrocardiography, and programmable functions are evaluated. If a programmable pacemaker is not used, if a programmer is not available, or if long-term survival of the patient is not expected, biannual rechecks may commence after the 2-week recheck and reprogramming the output settings can be overlooked.

PACEMAKER ELECTROCARDIOGRAPHY

Electrocardiographic recordings represent the single most valuable means of analyzing pacemaker function. The ECG patterns encountered in patients with pacemakers are different from normal patterns. Of primary importance is the critical distinction between ECG patterns of pacemaker dysfunction and variations of normal patterns.

QRS patterns associated with ventricular pacing. An ECG wave form with three distinct components is produced by a ventricular-generated pacing stimulus, a stimulus artifact followed by a depolarization wave (QRS complex) and a repolarization wave (*T* wave). The stimulus artifact is the initial deflection preceding the QRS complex. It represents between 2.5 and 5 V delivered to the heart for approximately 0.5 ms. With a unipolar lead system, the ECG records a perpendicular deflection of about 2 to 3 mV followed by a voltage decay curve that represents the exponential dissipation of energy through the body's tissues (Figure 30-6, *A*).[4] In some cases this decay curve may dramatically distort the QRS-T morphology, making it difficult if not impossible to determine the mean electrical axis.[43] With a bipolar lead system, however, the stimulus artifact is much smaller and may not be recorded in all leads (Figure 30-6, *B*).

The morphology of the QRS complex varies depending on the site of lead placement. Endocardial or epicardial placement of the lead into the right ventricular apex generally leads to a left bundle branch block configuration to the QRS complex in the frontal leads and a frontal plane vector that is normal or shifted to the left. If the pacing lead dislodges toward the right ventricular outflow tract, the QRS maintains a left bundle branch block pattern, but the frontal plane axis may shift to the right.[4,43] A right bundle branch pattern associated with a right ventricular endocardial lead suggests dislodgement of the lead into the coronary sinus and direct stimulation of the left ventricular myocardium.[43] Epicardial placement of the lead onto the left ventricle results in a right bundle branch configuration and a shift in the frontal plane vector to the right.

A pacing fusion beat results from simultaneous stimulation of the myocardium by a spontaneous impulse and a paced impulse. This

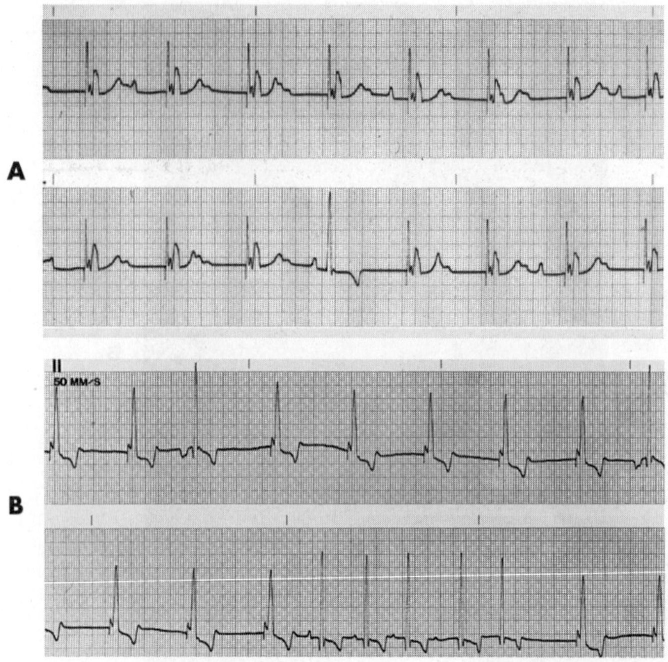

FIGURE 30-6 **A,** Electrocardiogram from a dog with third-degree atrioventricular block after placement of a transvenous unipolar pacemaker set in VVI mode with a rate of 100 beats/min (lead II; 50 mm/sec; 1 cm = 1 mV). Notice that the interval between pacing spikes (automatic interval) is exactly 30 mm. Notice that the unipolar pacemaker produces a large pacing spike preceding each QRS complex. Spontaneous *P* waves that occur independent of the pacing system can be seen in the baseline. The fourth beat from the left on the bottom tracing is a spontaneous sinus beat. Notice that the pacemaker was inhibited and regained capture at the predetermined escape interval of 600 ms (30 mm) after the spontaneous beat. See text for details. **B,** Electrocardiogram from a dog with sick sinus syndrome after placement of a transvenous bipolar pacemaker set in VVI mode with a rate of 100 beats/min (lead II; 50 mm/sec; 1 cm = 1 mV). Notice that the interval between pacing spikes (automatic interval) is exactly 30 mm. Notice that the bipolar pacemaker produces a small pacing spike preceding each QRS complex. Although this tracing appears rather erratic, the pacemaker is functioning normally. In dogs with sick sinus syndrome there is a lot of spontaneous activity that can inhibit the pacemaker. The third complex from the left and the last beat in the top tracing are junctional escape beats. Notice that the escape interval (interval between the *Q* wave of the spontaneous beat and the next pacing spike) is exactly 30 mm, indicating that the pacemaker sensed the beat and reset. The pacemaker is inhibited for a longer period in the bottom tracing by a short run of atrial tachycardia. See text for details.

may occur in normally functioning pacemakers when the spontaneous beat occurs at a similar time as the paced impulse, with insufficient time for sensing.[43] Pseudofusion beats occur when the stimulus artifact is superimposed on a QRS complex generated from a nonpaced focus. The stimulus artifact does not contribute to the depolarization. This may or may not represent an abnormal sensing ability of the system.

Ventricular asynchronous pacing. When a ventricular pacemaker is in asynchronous mode, pacing stimuli appear at a constant, predetermined rate regardless of the spontaneous rhythm. The pacemaker stimuli will capture the ventricles (cause ventricular depolarization and a resultant QRS-T on the ECG) if they fall outside the ventricular refractory period of the spontaneous beats. Stimuli that occur during the refractory period of spontaneous beats are ineffective and do not cause ventricular depolarization. Potentially serious arrhythmias may result from competing rhythms, as when a pacing-induced ventricular depolarization occurs on the end of the *T* wave.[43]

Ventricular demand pacing. When a VVI pacemaker senses a spontaneous beat, the output of the pacemaker is inhibited and recycled to discharge after a set interval. A pacing spike will only be delivered on demand after a set interval during which no spontaneous ventricular depolarization is sensed. As a result, three characteristic pacing intervals can be measured in patients with VVI pacing systems (see Figure 30-6).[43] The *automatic,* or *pacing,* interval is the time between two consecutive pacing discharges and is equal to the preset heart rate of the system. The pacemaker *escape* interval is measured from the instant a spontaneous discharge is sensed to the subsequent pacing spike. In most VVI systems, the escape interval is equal to the automatic interval. However, on the surface ECG the escape interval is measured from the onset of the spontaneous discharge and may therefore actually be slightly longer than the measured automatic interval (up to 120 ms). This occurs because the precise moment within the QRS that the sensing mechanism was activated cannot be determined on the surface ECG.[4] Pacemakers programmed to operate with hysteresis may have an escape interval that is longer than the automatic interval (positive-rate hysteresis). The rationale behind this programming, which is rarely used because of sensing complications, is to give the heart a slightly longer opportunity to maintain a spontaneous cardiac rhythm. The third is the *fixed-rate* pacing interval. The fixed-rate interval is the automatic interval that results from activation of the magnetic reed switch by an external magnetic source (i.e., asynchronous mode). The fixed-rate interval is the most stable and reliable of the three and is the recommended rate to follow to assess battery function.[43] In some VVI systems the automatic interval and the fixed-rate interval are equal; in other systems the fixed-rate interval may be as much as 30 ms shorter or longer than the automatic interval.[43] Because of competitive rhythms when using a magnet, most manufacturers use a magnet rate (fixed-rate) faster than the automatic rate to override spontaneous rhythms.[33] The ECG features of the rate-adaptive modes in dogs (VVIR) are similar to those described above, with the exception that the automatic rate is variable between a preset minimum and a preset maximum. It is highly recommended that rate-adaptive pacemakers be evaluated with telemetric programming systems so that pacing trends can be accurately determined.

COMPLICATIONS

Complications related to permanent cardiac pacemakers fall into the following three general categories: (1) complications of venous access, (2) complications of lead placement and pocket formation, and (3) a mechanical or an electrical malfunction of the device. Complications in the third category are largely unavoidable but may be minimized by careful inspection of all components before implantation. Complications in the former two categories can be prevented by strict adherence to proper surgical technique and maintaining a regular schedule of follow-up maintenance and evaluation after implantation.

The proper determination of pacemaker dysfunction must initially rest with the proper and accurate evaluation of the ECG features, both in synchronous (demand) and asynchronous (magnet or test) modes. Three principles must be fulfilled to establish that a pacing system is functioning normally: (1) A normal stimulus artifact must be regularly produced at the preset rate in asynchronous mode. (2) Each stimulus artifact must be followed by a QRS-T complex in synchronous mode (100% capture). (3) The pacemaker must sense normally based on measurements of the escape interval.[4] If ECG and electronic testing are normal, then the clinical features may suggest the problem is not related to pacemaker dysfunction. Once abnormal pacemaker function has been established by ECG, thoracic radio-

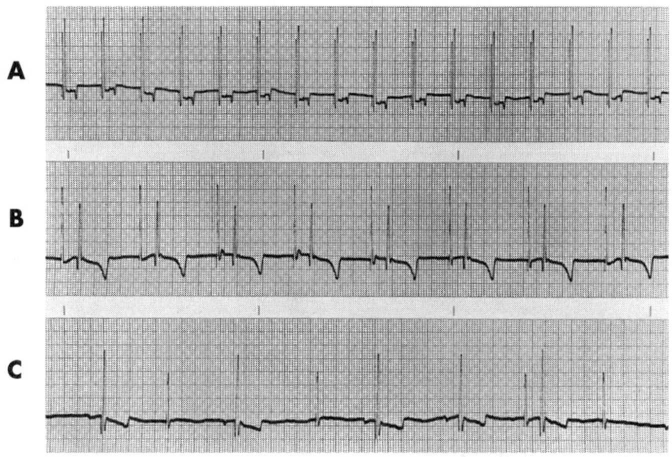

FIGURE 30-7 **A,** Electrocardiogram from a dog with a unipolar pacemaker set in VVI mode at a rate of 100 beats/min (lead II; 25 mm/sec; 1 cm = 1 mV). The pacemaker is functioning normally, with 100% capture at a rate of 100 beats/min. **B,** Electrocardiogram from the dog shown in **A,** with the lead tip dislodged into the right atrium (lead II; 50 mm/sec; 1 cm = 1 mV). The pacemaker is still functioning properly with 100% capture; however, the pacing impulses are stimulating the right atrium, as evidenced by negative *P* waves and a short delay before a normal-appearing QRS complex. **C,** In this tracing, the lead is still in the right atrium but is floating free within the chamber. There is loss of capture, with most pacing spikes occurring without activation of the heart. See text for details.

graphs and IPG assessment using a programmer are used to further characterize the malfunction.

The most common complications reported in dogs include lead dislodgement, infection, hematoma formation, skeletal muscle stimulation, ventricular arrhythmia, migration of the IPG, and skin erosion, all of which are related to improper implantation.[10,36] Although reports of only four cats exist, similar complications include lead displacement, seroma formation, and migration of the IPG.[3]

Complications of lead placement and pocket formation. Major complications associated with lead placement include displacement, myocardial perforation, and venous thrombosis.[7] With percutaneously implanted pacing systems the most common complication is lead dislodgement.[10] Predisposing factors include the use of passive fixation leads, operator inexperience, and inadequate stabilization of the IPG, resulting in the pacemaker twiddle syndrome (see below).[10] If the lead dislodges from the right ventricular apex it may either remain free in the chamber, resulting in intermittent or complete failure to capture, or it may migrate and lodge elsewhere, usually the right atrium or pulmonary artery, where it will not capture properly (Figure 30-7).[10] In dogs, lead dislodgement usually occurs within the first few weeks following the initial implantation, most frequently within the first 48 hours.[10,36] Electrocardiographic evidence of lead displacement includes intermittent or complete loss of pacing and sensing functions and may include ventricular arrhythmias resulting from myocardial irritation by the free lead tip. Lead dislodgement or migration can usually be confirmed by comparing thoracic radiographs with those taken at the time of implantation. Correction requires an operation to reposition the endocardial lead. In dogs with repeated dislodgment, it may be necessary to place an epicardial lead. The likelihood of lead displacement can be minimized by using active-fixation or tined-tip leads, leaving appropriate slack in the cervical portion of the lead, and by strictly minimizing patient activity for the first few weeks after implantation.

Myocardial perforation is rare. It may produce no demonstrable clinical signs or may cause intermittent or complete failure to pace and sense and may even produce diaphragmatic pacing.[7,43] Although cardiac tamponade is a rare occurrence, if it occurs, it is usually at the time of insertion or within the first 24 hours. If myocardial perforation is documented during the initial insertion, the lead should be carefully withdrawn and safely repositioned. In most cases, the perforation will self-correct and no other intervention is necessary. Occasionally, pericardiocentesis or thoracotomy and surgical correction are necessary.

Contraction of the diaphragm can occur with or without lead perforation, and skeletal muscle stimulation is frequently observed in dogs receiving unipolar pacemakers.[7,10] Diaphragmatic stimulation is usually easily controlled by reprogramming the pulse generator to a lower output value. Skeletal muscle stimulation is usually self-limiting and resolves once the subcutaneous pocket insulates the generator with fibrous tissue. However, it may be necessary to reset the pacemaker to a lower output in some cases.[4,10]

Complications related to the IPG pocket include infection, seroma/hematoma formation, skin erosion, IPG migration, and pacemaker twiddle.[7,10,37] Infections developing at the site of pacemaker implantation are usually related to improper surgical technique or concomitant immune system suppression (Color Plate 114).[44] Management of infected pacemaker sites includes removal of the IPG and lead and appropriate antibiotic therapy and drainage.[10,45] After stabilization of the patient, a new IPG and lead can be implanted using the other jugular vein. The risk of postimplant infections can be greatly minimized by using standard aseptic and atraumatic tissue handling techniques.[10,35]

Hematomas and seromas may form at either surgical site, but especially at the site of IPG placement. If a seroma or a hematoma develop, care should be taken not to contaminate the IPG pocket by introducing a needle for fluid sampling or drainage. Hematomas and seromas should be managed conservatively using compresses and prophylactic antibiotics to prevent infection. Most seromas and hematomas can be prevented by properly closing the dead space around the IPG during implantation. Skin erosion, IPG migration, and pacemaker twiddle may also result from a relatively large subcutaneous pocket or from improper stabilization of the IPG in the subcutaneous pocket (Color Plate 115).[7,10,44] In our experience, skin erosion and pacemaker migration have occurred most commonly when we placed the generator in the neck. Skin erosion occurs because of pressure necrosis of the skin. Pacemaker twiddle syndrome is a unique complication described in humans, in which continuous rotation of the IPG by the patient leads to a spiral twisting and shortening of the lead.[44] Dogs may mimic this situation by scratching the region where the generator is placed. Eventually the lead-tip may dislodge or the lead may fail secondary to lead fracture or disruption of the insulation (Figure 30-8). Corrective measures require either transection and splicing of the lead or lead replacement and reimplantation of the IPG in a stable pocket.

Lead extraction. Occasionally, infection or malfunction requires that a pacemaker system be removed. Lead extraction can be problematic. When this is required in our clinic, we usually remove the generator and extrude the lead from the neck incision. Most of the lead is cut and removed. Moderate traction is then placed on the lead and a C clamp placed at the junction of the lead and the neck to maintain traction. On subsequent days the lead is pulled out further and the C clamp replaced to maintain traction. Within several days, the lead will dislodge with further moderate traction.

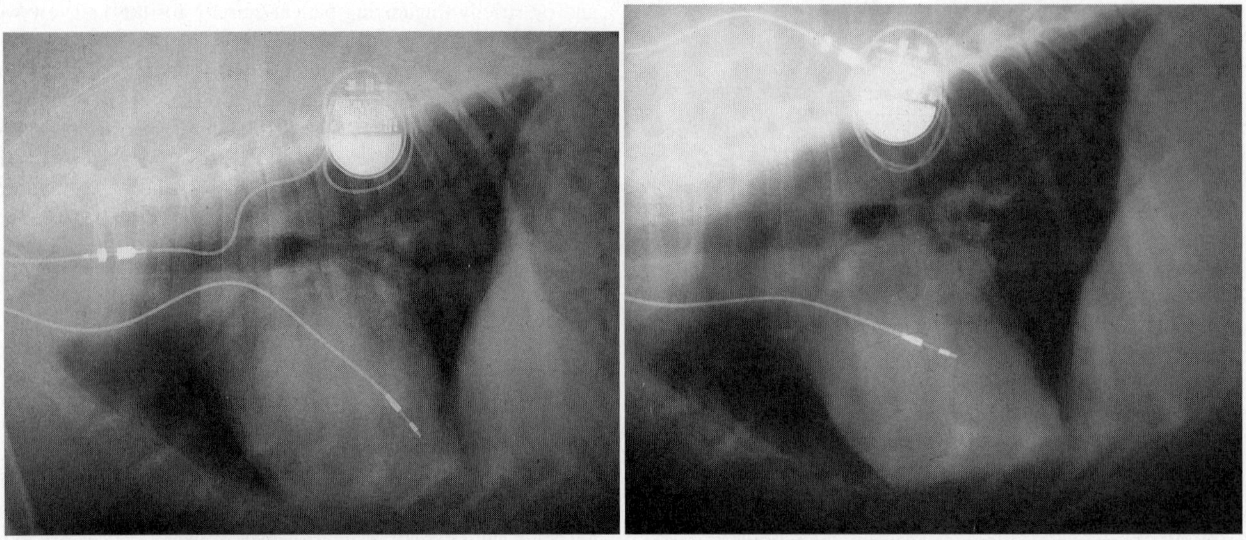

FIGURE 30-8 **A,** Lateral thoracic radiograph from a dog with a transvenous pacemaker. The lead tip and generator are in proper position. **B,** Lateral thoracic radiograph from the dog shown in **A**, taken several months later. Notice that the lead tip has been dislodged from the right ventricular apex and that there is no longer slack in the cervical portion of the lead compared with **A.** Also, there are more coils of the lead around the pacing generator on the lateral thorax. It was suspected that the pacemaker was turning within the subcutaneous pocket and "winding" up the lead, eventually leading to dislodgement of the lead tip. This is similar to the pacemaker twiddle syndrome described in humans.

If the lead is not infected, it may not require extraction. The lead can be cut and the end "capped" with plastic. There are two potential problems with this practice. Usually another lead is placed in the opposite jugular vein once the first has failed. With the original lead in place, the new lead may become entangled in the original lead. Alternatively, the original lead can become dislodged from its moorings in the neck and migrate into the heart. We have observed one dog that required surgery to remove such an aberrant lead because it was creating tricuspid regurgitation.

Pacemaker malfunction

Abnormal pacing rate. Although current pacing systems are quite complex, few device failures occur with any frequency. A change in the pacing rate or an erratic pacing rate is usually the result of normal function (e.g., low programmed rate, rate-adaptive function, application of a magnet, special functions, etc.). Pacemaker malfunctions (e.g., battery failure, component failure, change in mode because of external interference, phantom reprogramming, etc.) are detected by exclusion.[7] The most common device failure leading to an abnormal pacing rate is battery depletion.[37] Most dogs, because of old age and concurrent medical problems, only live a few years after pacemaker implantation, and battery failure is usually of little or no concern. However, when older, used pacemakers are implanted or when pacemakers are implanted in relatively young and otherwise healthy patients, battery failure may occur. Fortunately, modern pacing systems have built in warnings (an end-of-life indicator) that alert the clinician of impending battery failure. The key to identifying the warning stages of battery failure is to follow a regular schedule of rechecks and to have the owner count the heart rate periodically if the patient has a VVI pacemaker. The universal indicator of power source depletion (end-of-life [EOL] indicator or elective replacement indicator [ERI]) is an increase in the automatic or fixed-rate intervals (i.e., decreased rate). Using the test mode and measuring the fixed-rate interval is more reliable than measuring the automatic interval during synchronous pacing because of the higher potential for mild, but normal, variance in the automatic interval under normal operating conditions.[33,43] Although the decline is variable among manufacturers, the most common is a 6% to 10% decrease from the programmed automatic rate (VVI mode) or reversion to demand pacing at a preset fixed-rate (VVIR mode) (Figure 30-9). For example, if a particular generator experiences a 10% decrease in its rate when the battery life is low and the pacing rate is set at 100 beats/min, the heart rate will decrease to 90 beats/min when the generator must be changed.

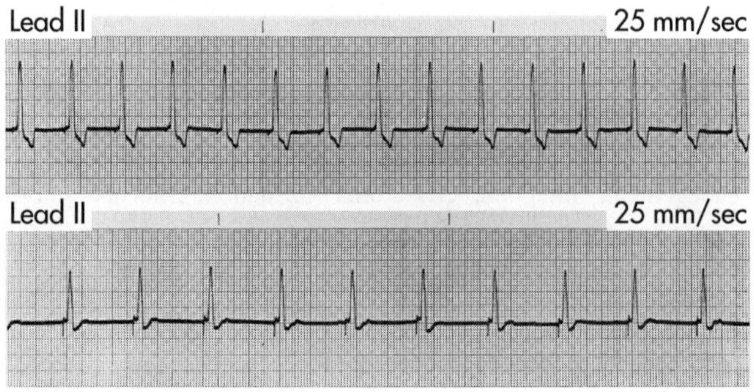

FIGURE 30-9 Electrocardiograms from a dog with a transvenous bipolar pacemaker set in VVI mode at a rate of 90 beats/min (lead II; 25 mm/sec, 1 cm = 1 mV). The top tracing was taken just after implantation of the pacing system. Notice that there is 100% capture with fixed rate of 90 beats/min. The bottom tracing was taken 3 ½ years later during a routine recheck evaluation. Although there is still 100%. capture, the fixed rate has decreased to 65 beats/min, which was the elective replacement indicator for this model of pacemaker.

Loss of capture. Loss of capture is simply an inability for the pacing system to produce a ventricular depolarization. This may occur with a visible pacing spike on the ECG without an associated QRS complex or may occur without a visible pacing spike on the

ECG (see Figure 30-7).[7] Many abnormalities that occur with visible pacing spikes are related to changes in the electrode-tissue interface that increases the resistance to current flow to the point of producing a block in electrical current flow (exit block). Exit block usually occurs because of excessive myocardial fibrosis at the lead tip (Figure 30-10).[36,43,46] Most pacemakers discharge currents that exceed the ventricular threshold; however, excessive fibrosis may be severe enough to increase the threshold above the discharge threshold, resulting in complete exit block and failure to capture. Although excessive myocardial fibrosis can be neither predicted nor prevented, it can sometimes be treated successfully with corticosteroids. Increasing the output voltage from the generator or increasing the pulse width often takes care of the problem. In some cases of chronic elevation of the pacing threshold, lead replacement may be required.[7,46] Other causes of failure to capture are lead displacement, unstable lead position, and myocardial perforation. Correction of these requires reoperation and repositioning of the lead.

Absence of pacing stimuli is usually due to interruption of the circuit, with no current flow, secondary to lead fracture with intact insulation.[7,37] Lead fractures may be detected on radiographs and can be confirmed by surgical exploration or interrogation with a programmer (i.e., increased resistance). Corrective measures require either splicing or replacing the lead. Apparent loss of capture may be misjudged if the intrinsic heart rate is faster than the programmed rate of the pacing system (VVI), resulting in total inhibition of the IPG output (normal operation). Occasionally a bipolar pacing spike is small enough to be overlooked on the ECG (pseudomalfunction).[7] Loss of capture without pacing stimuli may also result from loose or improper connections between the IPG and lead, complete battery depletion, component failure within the IPG, poor anodal contact (unipolar pacemakers), extreme electromagnetic interference (external), and oversensing.[7,46]

Abnormalities of sensing. When the pacing system fails to respond to an intrinsic depolarization in the appropriate fashion (i.e., inhibition or triggering of the IPG output) it is referred to as *undersensing.*[7] Failure of a VVI pacemaker to sense an intrinsic QRS complex results from either the delivery of an inadequate ventricular depolarization to a normally functioning pacemaker or from delivery of an adequate QRS signal to a malfunctioning pacemaker. Most modern pacing systems require only a 2- to 3-mV signal for proper sensing. Low-amplitude electrograms recorded from the site of lead insertion are the most common cause. Other causes include lead displacement and low-amplitude signals from premature ventricular complexes. These situations can usually be remedied by reprogramming the IPG to a lower sensitivity value. Undersensing may also be a result of component failure, electrolyte imbalances, antiarrhythmic drug effects, lead or insulation fracture, or inappropriate programming of the IPG, which may require reprogramming or replacement of damaged components.

One major cause of intermittent pauses in pacemaker function is oversensing. This is a failure of the system to deliver a stimulus at the anticipated time according to the programmed automatic interval resulting from inappropriate inhibition. Oversensing should always be suspected in the presence of irregular lengthening of the automatic interval.[43] It is confirmed electrocardiographically by normal magnet-induced conversion to the asynchronous mode.[7] The unwanted signals responsible for inhibition can arise from several sources, either intrinsic or extrinsic, including atrial depolarizations sensed by a lead displaced into the right ventricular outflow tract, *T* wave sensing, polarization voltage or afterpotential at the electrode-tissue interface, or abrupt changes in resistance caused by loose connections or partial lead fractures.[7,43] Erratic pacing behavior with pauses of varying length and pauses in asynchronous mode that are exact multiples of the magnet-induced interval is virtually diagnostic of an intermittent lead fracture or electrode problem. Loose lead connections may be aggravated or otherwise influenced by wriggling the IPG in its pocket. Corrective measures, including reprogramming of the IPG or replacement of malfunctioning components must be tailored to the individual.

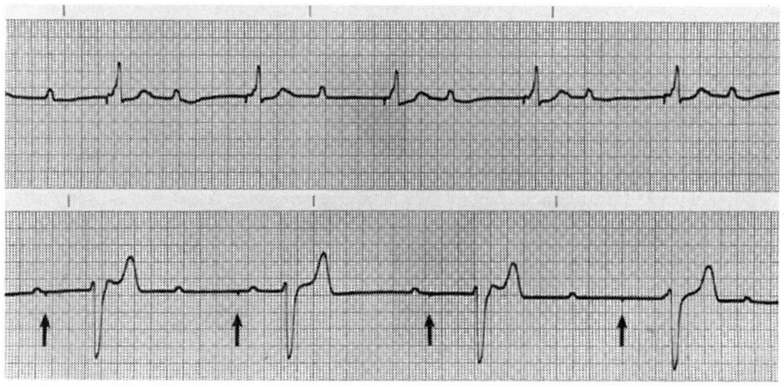

FIGURE 30-10 Electrocardiograms from a dog with a transvenous bipolar pacemaker set in VVI mode at 65 beats/min (lead II; 50 mm/sec; 1 cm = 1 mV). In the top tracing pacemaker function is normal. Notice the small bipolar pacing spike preceding each QRS complex. Spontaneous *P* waves can be seen following each *T* wave. In the bottom tracing the underlying rhythm is third-degree atrioventricular block with ventricular escape beats. This tracing was taken 2 weeks later. Upon close inspection, bipolar pacing spikes can be seen in the baseline *(arrows).* However, they do not capture the ventricle. It is apparent that the lead is still in contact with the ventricle because the escape interval is normal (45 mm). This is an example of exit block. It was later determined that the lead tip had developed an abscess.

External interference. Electromagnetic or other signals from the environment can be sensed by the pacemaker and may lead to a transient or permanent pacemaker malfunction. Common sources of external interference include transthoracic cardioversion or defibrillation, surgical electrocautery, radiation therapy, and magnetic resonance imaging.[7] Cardioversion or defibrillation in patients with permanent pacemakers may damage pacing circuits, with partial or complete destruction of the pulse generator, induction of the end-of-life state, reversible or irreversible alteration of microprocessor programming, or acute, temporary increases in the pacing threshold. Electrocautery may produce permanent loss of the stimulus output, random failures, phantom reprogramming, or reset of the pacemaker to VOO mode as a normal response to high-intensity interference. It can also cause electrical and thermal burns at the electrode-myocardial interface, which can cause ventricular fibrillation or a chronic increase in pacing threshold. Because rapid pacing, inhibition, and transient reed switch malfunction may produce no output or extremely rapid pacing, the use of MRI is contraindicated in patients with permanent pacemakers.[7]

Antitachycardia Devices

Implantable electrical devices may also be used to treat medically refractory tachycardias by either preventing the onset of the arrhythmia or terminating the tachycardia after it has developed.[7] The former type of control is only applicable to those tachyarrhythmias that can be suppressed by pacing the heart at normal or mildly increased rates. These so-called bradycardia-dependent tachyarrhythmias (e.g., torsades de pointes) are quite uncommon in veterinary patients. Chronic control of other refractory tachycardias by this method is rarely successful. Dual-chamber pacing with short atrioventricular conduction can be used to prevent some arrhythmias that rely on the atrioventricular node to maintain the arrhythmia. Some slow atrial tachycardias can be controlled by pacing the atria at rates that are rapid enough to produce a functional atrioventricular nodal block and so limit the ventricular response.[7] However, in most cases, ablative or surgical procedures are preferable for treating supraventricular tachycardias. Rapid pacing techniques and premature stimulation can also be used to terminate many atrioventricular tachycardias, atrial flutter and fibrillation, and many ventricular tachycardias.[7] Early devices of this type required manual activation; however, newer units now incorporate automatic detection and control. In human medicine, roughly half the patients treated with antitachycardia pacemakers have a favorable response. These types of devices have not been critically evaluated in clinical veterinary patients.

Implantable Cardiac Defibrillators

Termination of ventricular fibrillation and hemodynamically unstable ventricular tachycardia requires application of an electrical countershock to the myocardium. The effectiveness of this therapy depends on the immediate availability of equipment and personnel, conditions that are rarely satisfied outside hospital settings. Because of the high numbers of sudden cardiac deaths outside of hospitals in humans, the Automatic Implantable Cardioverter-Defibrillator (AICD) was developed.[5]

An AICD is a self-contained diagnostic-therapeutic system that identifies malignant ventricular arrhythmias and then delivers corrective discharges (shocks) to restore normal sinus rhythm. The automatic nature of the device eliminates the need for trained personnel, and its implantable nature allows out-of-hospital resuscitation. In addition, the growing reports of adverse effects of pharmacologic therapy from several studies have further supported the need for such devices.[47] The clinical utility of such devices has been further enhanced by multifunctional design. These devices are capable of antitachycardia pacing, bradycardia pacing, cardioversion, and defibrillation.[7,47] Early units were large and bulky and required thoracotomy for implantation, but improved lead design and newer circuitry have fostered the growth of several transvenous devices.[7,47]

Several studies, although not randomized, have shown these devices effectively reduce the incidence of sudden death in humans.[7] In patients with AICD, the 1-year mortality rate is approximately 2% compared with the 27% to 66% 1-year mortality in historical controls. The 5-year rate of sudden death is 5% compared with 20% for similar drug refractory human patients.[5,7,47] The use of AICD devices is feasible and effective in research dogs predisposed to sudden cardiac death.[48] To date, design and expense have limited the use of these devices in clinical patients. As these devices become smaller and as transvenous systems become available, either from human sources or manufacturers, implantation is almost inevitable in certain canine patients at risk for sudden death.

Interventional Electrophysiology

During the first half of this century, clinical electrocardiography gained widespread acceptance and allowed a better understanding of many important concepts of cardiac impulse conduction and modern electrophysiology. More recently, the focus has shifted to gaining a better understanding of the mechanisms of various arrhythmias with the use of invasive electrophysiologic diagnostic techniques, and interventional therapy (surgical or catheter ablation) has become the gold standard by which other methods are compared.[6]

A variety of catheter techniques have been recently introduced for the management of drug-resistant arrhythmias in humans, including the use of electrode catheters to both localize arrhythmia foci and deliver electrical energy to ablate these areas.[49] Before catheter techniques, control of refractory arrhythmias was limited to surgical intervention, which was associated with high morbidity and variable results.[50] The principal advantage of catheter ablative techniques is that control of refractory arrhythmias may be achieved without exposure to the risk and expense of open heart surgery.

Interest in electrophysiologic testing is growing in veterinary medicine, and catheter ablative techniques have been used clinically for the treatment of refractory supraventricular tachyarrhythmias in dogs.[51-53] Future directions in these areas should allow further understanding of the mechanisms and treatment of arrhythmias in veterinary patients.

REFERENCES

1. Schechter DC: Background of clinical electrostimulation. VII. Modern era of artificial cardiac pacemakers, *N Y State J Med* 72:1166, 1972.
2. Buchanan JW, Dear MG, Pyle RL et al: Medical and pacemaker therapy of complete heart block and congestive heart failure in a dog, *J Am Vet Med Assoc* 152:1099, 1968.
3. Fox PR, Moise NS, Woodfield JA et al: Techniques and complications of pacemaker implantation in four cats, *J Am Vet Med Assoc* 199:1742, 1991 (erratum 200(5):701, 1992).
4. Mond HG, Sloman JG: The indications for and types of artificial cardiac pacemakers. In Hurst JW, Schlant RC, Rackley CE et al, eds: *The heart, arteries and veins,* ed 7, New York, 1990, McGraw Hill.
5. Mirowski M: The implantable cardioverter-defibrillator. In Hurst JW, Schlant RC, Rackley CE et al, eds: *The heart, arteries and veins,* ed 7, New York, 1990, McGraw Hill.
6. Josephson ME: Historical perspectives. In Josephson ME, ed: *Clinical cardiac electrophysiology: techniques and interpretations,* ed 2, Philadelphia, 1993, Lea & Febiger.
7. Barold SS, Zipes DP: Cardiac pacemakers and antiarrhythmic devices. In Braunwald E, ed: *Heart disease: a textbook of cardiovascular medicine,* ed 4, Philadelphia, 1992, WB Saunders.
8. Parsonnet V, Bernstein AD: Transvenous pacing: a seminal transition from the research laboratory, *Ann Thorac Surg* 48:738, 1989.
9. Schollmeyer M: Pacemaker therapy. In Fox PR, ed: *Canine and feline cardiology,* New York, 1988, Churchill Livingstone.
10. Sisson DD, Thomas WP, Woodfield J et al: Permanent transvenous pacemaker therapy in forty dogs, *J Vet Intern Med* 5:322, 1991.
11. Dreifus LS, Fisch C, Griffin JC et al: Guidelines for implantation of cardiac pacemakers and antiarrhythmia devices: a report of the American College of Cardiology/American Heart Association Task Force on Assessment of Diagnostic and Therapeutic Cardiovascular Procedures (Committee on Pacemaker Implantation), *J Am Coll Cardiol* 18:1, 1991.
12. Roberts WC: Guidelines for cardiac pacing, *J Electrophysiol* 1:35, 1987.
13. Frye RL, Collins JJ, DeSanctis RW et al: Guidelines for permanent cardiac pacemaker implantation: a report of the Joint American College of Cardiology/American Heart Association Task Force on Assessment of Cardiovascular Procedures (Subcommittee on Pacemaker Implantation), *Circulation* 70:331A, 1984.
14. Mond HG, Tartaglia S, Cole A et al: The refurbished pulse generator, *PACE Pacing Clin Electrophysiol* 3:311, 1980.
15. Masterson MM, Maloney JD, Tuzcu EM et al: Atrial pacemaker leads compared, *Cleve Clin J Med* 57:433, 1990.
16. Tobias AH, Pion PD: Pacing system analysis for transvenous pacemaker implantation in the dog, *Proceedings of the Thirteenth Annual House Officer Seminar Day,* 1991, p 21 (abstract).

17. Bendit DG: Current pacing modes: a brief review of their features and indications. In Bendit DG, ed: *Rate-adaptive pacing,* Cambridge, Mass, 1993, Blackwell Scientific.
18. Parsonnet V, Furman S, Smyth NP: Report of the Inter-Society Commission for Heart Disease Resources: Implantable cardiac pacemakers—status report and resource guideline, *Am J Cardiol* 34:487, 1974.
19. Bernstein AD, Camm AJ, Fletcher RD, et al: The NASPE/BPEG generic pacemaker code for antibradyarrhythmia and adaptive-rate pacing and antitachyarrhythmia devices, *PACE Pacing Clin Electrophysiol* 10:794, 1987.
20. Roberts DH, Tennant B, Brockman D et al: Successful use of a QT-sensing rate-adaptive pacemaker in a dog, *Vet Rec* 130:471, 1992.
21. Cobb MA, Nolan J, Brownlie SE et al: Use of a programmable, activity-sensing, rate regulating pacemaker in a dog, *J Small Anim Pract* 31:398, 1990.
22. Darke PG, Been M, Marks A: Use of a programmable, 'physiological' pacemaker in a dog with total atrioventricular block, *J Small Anim Pract* 26:295, 1985.
23. Tilley LP: Special methods for treating arrhythmias: cardiopulmonary arrest and resuscitation, pacemaker therapy. In Tilley LP, ed: *Essentials of canine and feline electrocardiography: interpretation and treatment,* ed 3, Philadelphia, 1992, Lea & Febiger.
24. Sisson DD: Permanent transvenous pacemaker implantation in the dog, *Proc Annu Vet Med Forum,* 1986, p 13.
25. Falk RH, Zoll PM, Zoll RH: Safety and efficacy of noninvasive cardiac pacing: a preliminary report, *N Engl J Med* 309:1166, 1983.
26. Parsonnet V, Bernstein AD, Galasso D: Cardiac pacing practices in the United States in 1985, *Am J Cardiol* 62:71, 1988.
27. Darke PG, McAreavey D, Been M: Transvenous cardiac pacing in 19 dogs and one cat, *J Small Anim Pract* 30:491, 1989.
28. Darke PG: Update: transvenous cardiac pacing. In: Kirk RW, Bonagura JD, eds: *Kirk's current veterinary therapy, XI: small animal practice,* Philadelphia, 1992, WB Saunders.
29. Bednarski RM: Anesthetic concerns for patients with cardiomyopathy, *Vet Clin North Am Small Anim Pract* 22:460, 1992.
30. Evans AT: Anesthesia for severe mitral and tricuspid regurgitation, *Vet Clin North Am Small Anim Pract* 22:465, 1992.
31. Haskins SC, Klide AM: Anesthesia for very old patients, *Vet Clin North Am Small Anim Pract* 22:467, 1992.
32. Wilson DV: Anesthesia for patients with severe systemic debilitation, *Vet Clin North Am Small Anim Pract* 22:491, 1992.
33. Mond HG, Strathmore NF: The technique of using cardiac pacemakers: implantation, testing, and surveillance. In Hurst JW, Schlant RC, Rackley CE et al, eds: *The heart, arteries and veins,* ed 7, New York, 1990, McGraw Hill.
34. Haskins SC: Opinions in small animal anesthesia, *Vet Clin North Am Small Anim Pract* 22:245, 1992.
35. Muers MF, Arnold AG, Sleight P: Prophylactic antibiotics for cardiac pacemaker implantation: a prospective trial, *Br Heart J* 46:539, 1981.
36. Bonagura JD, Helphrey ML, Muir WW: Complications associated with permanent pacemaker implantation in the dog, *J Am Vet Med Assoc* 182:149, 1983.
37. Lombard CW, Tilley LP, Yoshioka MM: Pacemaker implantation in the dog: survey and literature review, *J Am Anim Hosp Assoc* 17:751, 1981.
38. Yoshioka MM, Tilley LP, Harvey HJ, et al: Permanent pacemaker implantation in the dog, *J Am Anim Hosp Assoc* 17:746, 1981.
39. Fox PR, Matthiesen DT, Purse D, et al: Ventral abdominal, transdiaphragmatic approach for implantation of cardiac pacemakers in the dog, *J Am Vet Med Assoc* 189:1303, 1986.
40. Fingeroth JM, Birchard SJ: Transdiaphragmatic approach for permanent cardiac pacemaker implantation in the dog, *Vet Surg* 15:329, 1986.
41. Keller W, Duehren WH: Engineering aspects of cardiac pacing. In Samet P, El-Sherif N, ed: *Cardiac pacing,* ed 2, New York, 1980, Grune and Stratton.
42. Stokes K, Stephenson NL: The implantable cardiac pacing lead: just a simple wire? In Barold SS, Mugica J, eds: *The third decade of cardiac pacing: advances in technology and clinical applications,* Mount Kisco, 1982, Futura.
43. El-Sherif N, Javier RP, Gann D et al: Pacemaker electrocardiography. In Samet P, El-Sherif N, eds: *Cardiac pacing,* ed 2, New York, 1980, Grune and Stratton.
44. Hill RC, Buchanan JW: Infection and twiddler syndrome in a dog with Addison's disease, complete heart block and wandering artificial pacemakers, *J Am Anim Hosp Assoc* 26:25, 1990.
45. Wade JS, Cobbs CG: Infections in cardiac pacemakers, *Curr Clin Top Infect Dis* 9:44, 1988.
46. Snyder PS, Atkins CE, Sato T: Syncope in three dogs with cardiac pacemakers, *J Am Anim Hosp Assoc* 27:611, 1991.
47. Klein LS, Miles WM, Zipes DP: Antitachycardia devices: realities and promises, *J Am Coll Cardiol* 18:1349, 1991.
48. Moise NS, Fain ES, Flanders JA, et al: Automatic implantable cardioverter defibrillators in German shepherds with inherited sudden cardiac death, *Proc 10th ACVIM Forum,* 1992, p 797 (abstract).
49. Scheinman MM: Treatment of cardiac arrhythmias with catheter ablative techniques. In Hurst JW, Schlant RC, Rackley CE et al, eds: *The heart, arteries and veins,* ed 7, New York, 1990, McGraw Hill.
50. Walter PF, Jones EL: Surgical treatment of cardiac arrhythmias. In Hurst JW, Schlant RC, Rackley CE et al, eds: *The heart, arteries and veins,* ed 7, New York, 1990, McGraw Hill.
51. Wright KN: Cardiac electrophysiology and catheter ablation techniques, 1995, p 289-291.
52. Scherlag BJ, Wang X, Nakagawa H, et al: Radiofrequency ablation of a concealed accessory pathway as treatment for incessant supraventricular tachycardia in a dog, *J Am Vet Med Assoc* 203:1147, 1993.
53. Atkins CE, Kanter R, Wright K, et al: Orthodromic reciprocating tachycardia and heart failure in a dog with a concealed posteroseptal accessory pathway, *J Vet Intern Med* 9:43, 1995.

CHAPTER 31

Thromboembolic Disease

Systemic Arterial Thromboembolism

Systemic arterial thromboembolism (STE) is a relatively common and usually very serious sequela to feline cardiac disease. Although systemic thromboembolism can occur in dogs and can also occur in cats that do not have cardiac disease, more than 90% of cases seen in veterinary small animal practice are in cats with cardiac disease.[1] The vast majority of these cats have left atrial enlargement when examined using echocardiography.[1] The left atrium is usually the site of thrombus formation. Systemic thromboembolism used to be a common complication of dilated cardiomyopathy in cats. Because the incidence of this disease has decreased dramatically, the incidence of STE has decreased. However, STE is still a common complication of hypertrophic cardiomyopathy and the unclassified or restrictive forms of feline cardiac disease. It occasionally occurs in cats with hyperthyroidism.[1,2]

Most cats (approximately 90%) presented with STE have the thromboembolus lodged at the terminal abdominal aorta (the aortic trifurcation) (Color Plates 116 and 117). This type of thromboembolus commonly extends down the external iliac arteries, giving it the appearance of a saddle. Consequently, these are commonly called *saddle thromboemboli.* Thromboembolism of the terminal aorta produces acute caudal limb paresis/paralysis and pain, with a loss of the femoral pulses and pale or cyanotic pads (pain, paralysis, pulselessness, and pallor). Some cats, however, have smaller thromboemboli that lodge in one femoral artery, a brachial artery, or another smaller artery. Occasionally a large thromboembolus lodges more proximally in the aorta, above the renal arteries, resulting in acute renal failure. In other cats, a very large thromboembolus lodges in the mitral valve orifice, the left ventricle, or the proximal aorta at the region of the brachiocephalic trunk, causing sudden death.[3]

Systemic thromboembolism and systemic thrombosis are rare events in dogs. Whereas the vast majority of cats that present with STE have an acute onset of clinical signs, only about 50% of dogs present acutely.[4] The others present with a history of lameness that usually progresses to paralysis. Dogs with STE may also have underlying cardiac disease as the predisposing factor, but most have other causes. Infective endocarditis is one of the most common cardiac reasons for STE in dogs. It is an unusual cause in cats. Protein-losing glomerulonephropathy, atherosclerosis, neoplasia, chronic exogenous corticosteroid administration, and hyperadrenocorticism are other primary causes of STE in dogs. Further detail about predisposing causes to thromboembolism in dogs is presented below in the discussion of pulmonary thromboembolism.

Because the vast majority of veterinary patients examined with STE are cats, the remainder of this section is dedicated to the feline patient. Usually, the pathophysiology, diagnosis, and treatment are very similar in cats and dogs.

PATHOPHYSIOLOGY

A thrombus is an aggregation of platelets and fibrin with entrapped blood cells. STE occurs when a thrombus forms in some region of the left heart or systemic circulation and then breaks loose to become an embolus and travel to a distal region of the systemic circulation. It lodges in the systemic circulation and partially or completely occludes blood flow distal to the thromboembolus. Intravascular thrombus formation is an unusual event and requires predisposing factors to allow it to occur. Thrombus formation in cats usually occurs in the left atrium, most commonly in the left auricle.

Intravascular thrombus formation. Reasons for intravascular thrombus formation include sluggish blood flow, endothelial damage, and increased blood coagulability. One study documented increased platelet aggregability in some cats with cardiomyopathy.[5] A specific reason for this finding has not been elucidated. When observed at a postmortem examination, atria from cats with cardiac disease and thromboembolism are very large and may be somewhat fibrotic. Usually no evidence of endothelial damage or other factors that might stimulate thrombus formation are present. The left atrium is usually enlarged in cats with STE. In one study it was severely enlarged in 57%, moderately enlarged in 14%, and mildly enlarged in 22% of cats with STE.[1] Only 5% had a normal left atrial size.

The most plausible explanation for thrombus formation in cats is sluggish blood flow in the left atrium. The amount of blood that flows through the left atrium in cats with cardiomyopathy is normal to low. Normal-to-low blood flow through an enlarged chamber results in a lower-than-normal blood flow velocity. An analogy to explain why blood flow velocity is low in an enlarged left atrium is a canoe floating down a river that is a fixed width and a fixed depth, with a water flow velocity of 1 foot per second. As you float down the river in your canoe, it will also move at 1 foot per second. If the Army Corps of Engineers comes in and widens one section of the river, you will notice that the velocity (speed) at which your canoe travels will decrease in the area where the river is wider because the same amount of water is coming into a larger area. The same is true for the left atrium. This is especially true in regions such as the left auricle. An analogy for flow in the left auricle is a cove along one bank of a river. Here flow is slower than in the rest of the river because of its semi-isolation. Only small eddy currents with very low flow velocities would exist.

When blood flow slows to a certain velocity, red cells and other blood factors clump together. This can be easily demonstrated by performing an ultrasound examination of the heart of an animal

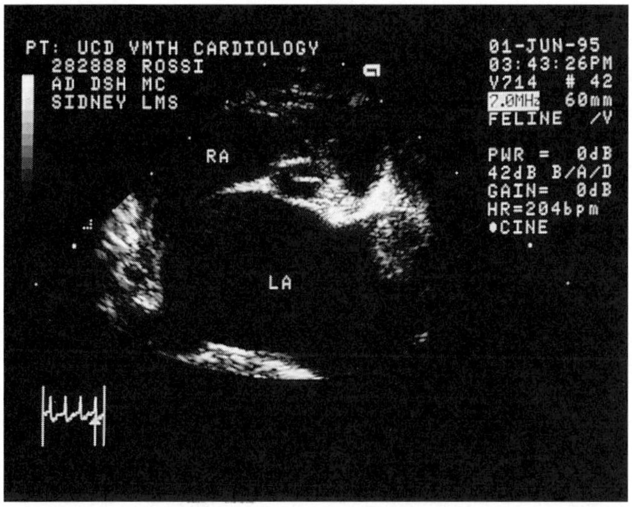

FIGURE 31-1 Two-dimensional echocardiogram from a cat with hypertrophic cardiomyopathy, left atrial *(LA)* enlargement, and a thrombus in the left auricle. The thrombus is on the right side of the image. The cat also had hypertrophic cardiomyopathy. *RA,* Right atrium.

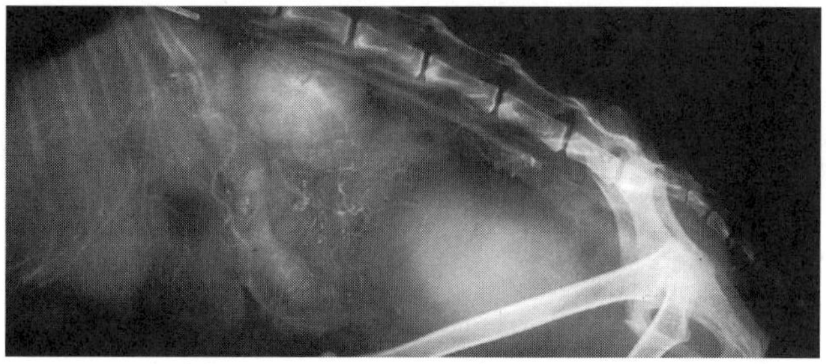

FIGURE 31-2 Angiogram from a cat with a thromboembolus lodged at the terminal aorta. The contrast material has been injected through a catheter in the proximal portion of the abdominal aorta. No contrast material flows through the aorta past the region of the sixth lumbar vertebra. Contrast material can be seen in the third through the sixth lumbar arteries. A small amount of contrast material can be seen in sacral arteries, dorsal to the pelvis. There is contrast material in the renal pelvis and numerous abdominal arteries.

during euthanasia. When the heart stops beating, the cardiac chambers fill with a hazy, amorphous density as blood cells clump. A similar density is often observed in an enlarged left atrium in cats with severe cardiac disease. This abnormality is also recognized in humans with cardiomyopathies, atrial fibrillation, or mitral stenosis and is termed *spontaneous echocardiographic contrast* (also known euphemistically as "smoke"). In the living animal or human, this contrast swirls in the left atrium. In humans, spontaneous echo contrast is associated with increased left atrial size and with reduced left atrial blood flow velocity.[6] It is the factor most strongly associated with left auricular thrombus formation and systemic embolic events. No studies have been performed in veterinary medicine. However, in our experience, finding a thrombus in the left atrium or left auricle in a cat with spontaneous echo contrast on an echocardiogram is common. Sometimes they are obvious. At other times one must search for them, especially when they are confined to the left auricle (Figure 31-1). The stasis of blood also allows activated coagulation factors to accumulate, and intermittent movement of viscous blood may induce platelet activation. If low blood flow velocity is such an important factor, one might also expect dogs with dilated cardiomyopathy to be prone to left atrial thrombus formation. Systemic thromboembolism is rare in dogs with dilated cardiomyopathy. The reason for this discrepancy may be species differences in erythrocyte aggregability. One study documented that normal cat red cells are more aggregable than those of dogs, rats, rabbits, humans, and gerbils.[7] Feline platelets are also more reactive than those of other species. Feline platelets undergo spontaneous aggregation in vitro and are more responsive to serotonin-induced aggregation than are platelets from other species.[8,9] Cats also have a greater volume of platelets per body weight than other species.[8]

Thromboembolism. Once a left atrial thrombus has formed, it can do one of the following three things: (1) it can remain static and cause no problem, (2) it can dislodge and become an embolus, or (3) it can grow very large and occlude intracardiac blood flow. The incidence of the first and third outcomes is unknown. If a thrombus causes no clinical abnormalities, the thrombus usually goes undetected. If it occludes intracardiac flow, it causes death; if a postmortem examination is not done, the cause of death is never known. Only the second scenario results in clinical signs for which owners commonly seek medical attention for their pets.

The clinical signs produced depend primarily on the site occluded by the thromboembolus, whether the occlusion is total or partial, and the amount of collateral circulation. Bilateral renal embolization can cause renal failure. Embolization of the cerebral arteries causes central nervous system signs. Embolization of a brachial artery causes forelimb pain and paresis. Most left atrial thrombi apparently become quite large before they dislodge. These thromboemboli are larger than any artery exiting off the aorta. Consequently, blood flow pushes them the length of the aorta. They lodge at the aortic trifurcation, where the aorta divides into the two external iliac arteries and the common origin of the internal iliac arteries. Here they obstruct blood flow to the hind limbs.

Constriction of collateral vessels. Physical obstruction is only a part of the pathophysiology. Experimentally, the terminal aorta has been ligated in an attempt to reproduce the disease.[10,11] Surprisingly, cats with aortic ligation exhibit no pain and walk following surgery, although the femoral pulses are absent and caudal limb blood flow is only 30% of the baseline.[12] Slight weakness and hyporeflexia are present, but even these resolve within 72 hours, when caudal limb blood flow is 90% of the baseline. Aortograms in these cats confirm the presence of collateral blood flow through the lumbar vertebral arteries and the cranial and caudal epigastric arteries. The disease can be reproduced, however, if a thrombus is created within the terminal aorta.[11,12] Aortograms from these experimental cats are identical to those from spontaneous clinical cases. Both demonstrate very poor collateral flow beyond the region of the thromboembolus (Figure 31-2). Pretreatment with an antiserotoninergic agent or with indomethacin prevents the loss of collateral circulation, and serotonin or thromboxane A_2 injection reproduces the clinical situation when injected into a caudal aortic segment.[10,13-15] It is hypothesized that thromboemboli release serotonin and thromboxane A_2, agents present in platelets and known to produce intense vasoconstriction, and disrupt collateral flow.[16] Antiserotonin agents (e.g., cyproheptadine) and indomethacin prevent vasoconstriction distal to the thromboembolus when administered before producing an experimental thrombus.[14,17] Administering such agents after a thromboembolus is present apparently has no effect.

CLINICAL PRESENTATION

Signalment. The majority of cats seen with STE are domestic varieties.[1] Because more hypertrophic cardiomyopathy is seen in males, more male cats are seen with STE.

History. Most cats with STE have heart disease, but up to 90% have no evidence of this disease before developing acute pain and hind limb paresis/paralysis.[1] Owners often think that their cat has experienced an acute traumatic event. At the onset of STE, the cat may fall off a structure on which it was lying, which reinforces this belief. At other times, the cat is found unable to walk and in pain. Cats vocalize because of the pain during the initial stages of the event.

Physical examination. Auscultation often reveals a heart murmur or gallop sound at presentation.[1] Many cats are in heart failure and therefore are tachypneic and dyspneic. Some cats are also hypothermic.

In cats with a large thromboembolus at the aortic trifurcation, the femoral artery pulses are absent to very weak, the muscles are painful and firm, and there is loss of motor function to the hind limbs (paresis/paralysis). Sensation in the hind limbs is lost over time and reflexes are also lost. The legs are cool, and the nail beds are pale or very dark. Femoral artery pulses in most cats with STE (78% in one study) are absent upon presentation.[1] In some cats, however, a smaller thromboembolus may lodge in one external iliac artery, resulting in cessation of blood flow to only one leg and loss of the femoral pulse on that side only. In other cats, especially ones in which the thromboembolus lodged days before presentation, the femoral artery pulses may be present but very weak because of recanalization of the aorta. In some cats it is difficult to determine whether a pulse is present, and a false diagnosis of thromboembolism in a cat with neurologic disease is common.[18] A Doppler blood flow detection device is helpful in this situation to identify the presence or absence of blood flow. In cats that have no sensation in their distal limbs, a nail can be cut back to the "quick" to determine whether bleeding occurs. Once a thromboembolus lodges in the terminal aorta, ischemic damage to the skeletal muscles and peripheral nerves occurs. Initially, the ischemic damage to the muscles of the caudal legs results in intense pain. The cranial tibial and gastrocnemius muscles are most severely affected and are commonly swollen, turgid, and painful when palpated. The pain usually subsides as sensory nervous input is lost.

Most aortic thromboemboli lodge terminally in the aorta, where they disrupt blood flow to the spinal canal beyond L_5. This means that blood supply to the spinal cord is not disrupted. Instead, perfusion is lost to the cauda equina and the peripheral nerves that originate from this area. Loss of motor function is due to lower motor neuron disease. Motor function loss to the caudal body is variable. Many cats retain the ability to move their tail. Some cats lose the ability to move their caudal legs starting at the hip, whereas others only lose the ability to move the limbs distal to the stifles or distal to the hock (Color Plate 118). These latter cats can extend and flex their hips and so "walk" on their stifles. Loss of cutaneous sensation occurs relatively early and follows the pattern of motor loss. Some cats only lose cutaneous sensation in their limbs distal to the stifle, whereas others lose all sensation. The patellar reflex is lost in many cats, but remains intact in others. Anal tone and the anal reflex are usually normal. Bladder function is often normal. Some cats may have urine retention, but the bladder can usually be easily emptied by external manual compression. In cats with experimental thrombosis of the terminal aorta, neurologic function (patellar reflex, withdrawal reflex, thigh adduction, digit extension, caudal limb weight bearing, locomotive ability, and cutaneous sensation) to the caudal limbs is completely lost in 80% of cases.[12] The remaining cats have very little neurologic function remaining. Presumably, the cats seen clinically with some remaining neurologic function must have some collateral flow to explain their neurologic findings. Acute ligation of the aorta in experimental cats, before collateral circulation becoming fully developed, produces cessation of blood flow to the distal portion of the caudal limbs, whereas proximal flow remains apparently normal.[12] This mimics the situation observed in some feline patients that have function remaining in the proximal portion of their caudal limbs.

After the acute embolic event, thrombolysis occurs. In some cats with small thromboemboli, thrombolysis is rapid and complete such that function returns within hours. In other cats, the thromboembolus is large, and the thrombolytic activity of the cat is low, resulting in permanent loss of perfusion to the caudal limbs. These cats remain paralyzed. Regions of necrotic skin and muscle often develop, and muscle contracture takes place over time. Between these two extremes are cats that recover function over time with no untoward events and cats that partially recover function but develop skin and muscle necrosis (Color Plate 119). The latter cats may require surgery to debride open wounds or amputate toes or parts of limbs. Cats that have complete and lasting occlusion of blood supply to only one limb do very well with limb amputation.

Coagulopathies can occur in cats with STE, although they are usually not severe enough to produce clinical signs.[19] Platelet counts are generally within the normal range, and there is no evidence of fibrin degradation products. Individual clotting factors, however, may be low in certain cases.

Cats with thromboemboli commonly have severe underlying cardiac disease. Acute terminal aortic blockade by the thromboembolus increases afterload to the left ventricle. This can increase left heart filling pressures and resultant pulmonary edema. Consequently, it is common for cats with acute aortic thromboembolism to also present in respiratory distress. The heart failure must be treated appropriately. If pulmonary edema is severe, it worsens the short-term prognosis.

DIAGNOSIS

Definitive diagnosis of thromboembolism. The diagnosis of STE in cats is usually based on the presence of typical clinical signs. These include an acute onset of pain associated with lack of femoral pulses, cold legs, pale or cyanotic pads, and neurologic deficits (Color Plate 120). When we were studying t-PA therapy in cats with STE, we actively sought cases from referring veterinarians and noted that 20% to 30% of cases referred for STE had primary neurologic disease instead. From this experience it does not appear that a diagnosis based only on clinical signs is accurate. Consequently, some effort should be placed into doing more definitive diagnostic tests in these cats. In most cases, simply cutting a nail back to the "quick" is adequate. Cats without blood flow to the caudal limbs will not have any bleeding from a cut nail. Cats with severely compromised flow will have a small amount of black-colored blood ooze from their cut nail. A Doppler device that is usually used to measure systolic blood pressure (Parks Electronics, Aloha, Ore.) can also be used to determine the presence of blood flow to affected limbs. The Doppler crystal is placed over a distal artery, and the operator then listens for a typical flow pattern. Cats with complete aortic obstruction have no evidence of flow. This device can also be used to document that flow is returning to a limb. Imaging of the affected regional vessels by intravenous or intraarterial angiography or nuclear tracers is the definitive diagnostic procedure for thromboembolic disease. Risks to the patient must be considered when contemplating angiography. Stabilizing the patient is the primary consideration before attempting invasive diagnostic procedures. An experienced ultrasonographer may be able to see the thromboembolus in the terminal aorta. Color flow Doppler imaging of the area may demonstrate lack of flow or severely compromised flow.

Ancillary tests. Radiographs reveal cardiomegaly in almost 90% of cats with STE and evidence of heart failure in about 70%.[1]

A

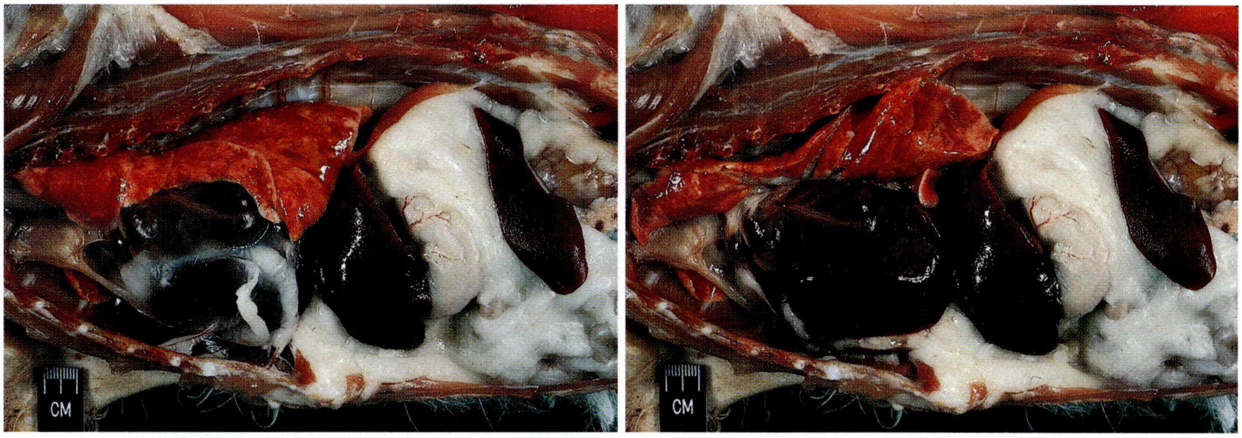

B

COLOR PLATE 99 Necropsy specimens from a kitten with a pericardioperitoneal diaphragmatic hernia. The body is in right lateral recumbency, and the left thoracic and abdominal walls have been dissected. **A,** The lungs are displaced dorsally, and the pericardial sac appears to be enlarged. There is an open communication through the diaphragm and an apparently small liver in the abdomen. **B,** The pericardium has been incised and it is now apparent that several liver lobes have herniated through the diaphragm into the pericardial sac. The heart is displaced dorsally. (Courtesy Dr. Brad Gavashan.)

A

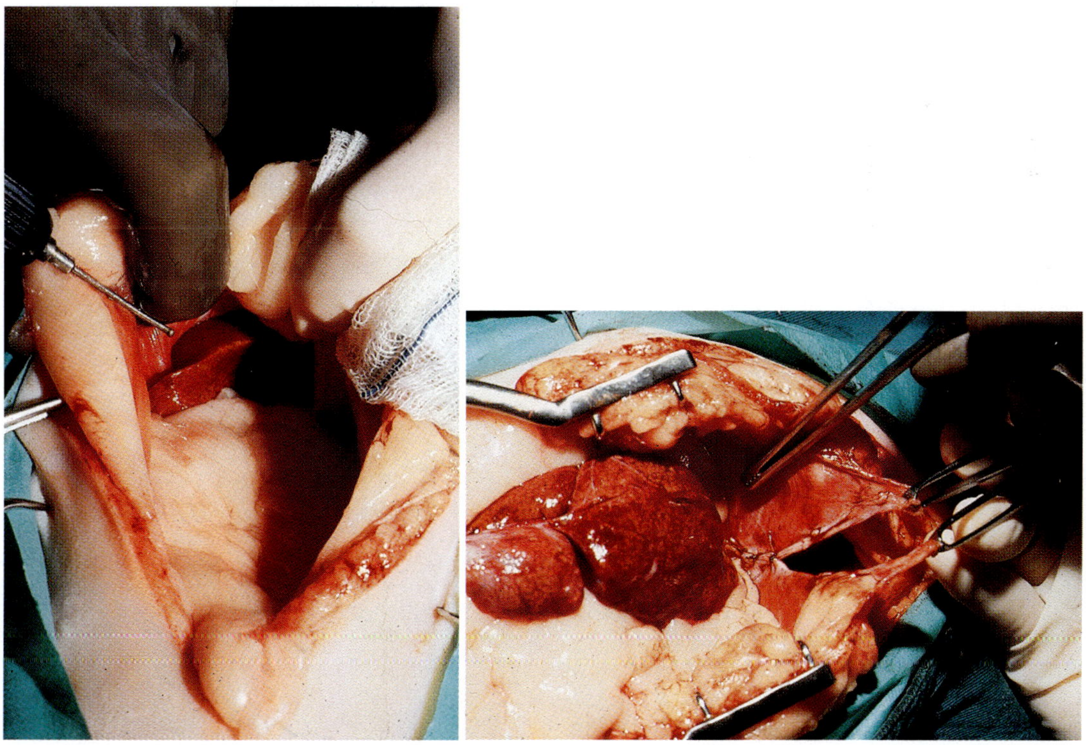

B

COLOR PLATE 100 Surgical correction of a pericardioperitoneal diaphragmatic hernia. **A,** A midline celiotomy has been performed. A defect in the diaphragm with herniated liver can be seen. **B,** The liver has been returned to the abdominal cavity, and the defect is being sutured. (Courtesy Dr. Brad Gavashan.)

A

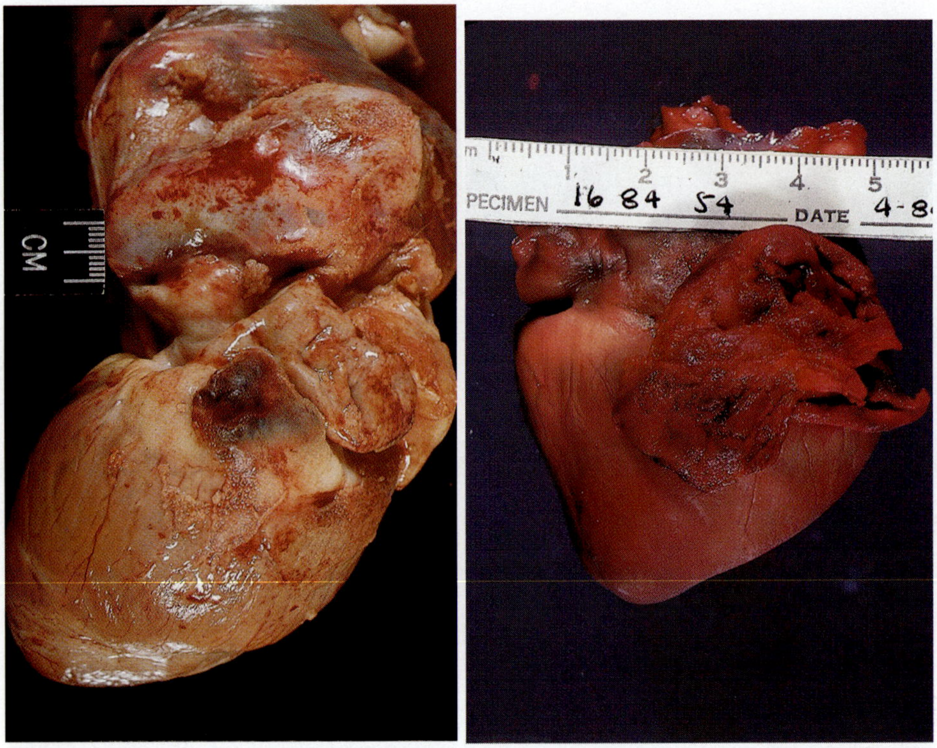

B

COLOR PLATE 101 Gross pathologic specimens from dogs with necropsy-confirmed hemangiosarcomas. **A,** View of the heart from the right side, with the pericardium reflected dorsally. A roughly 1-cm raised hemorrhagic nodule can be seen at the right atrioventricular junction just caudal and ventral to the right auricle. **B,** View of the heart from the right side with the pericardium removed. A large hemorrhagic mass extends from the right auricle.

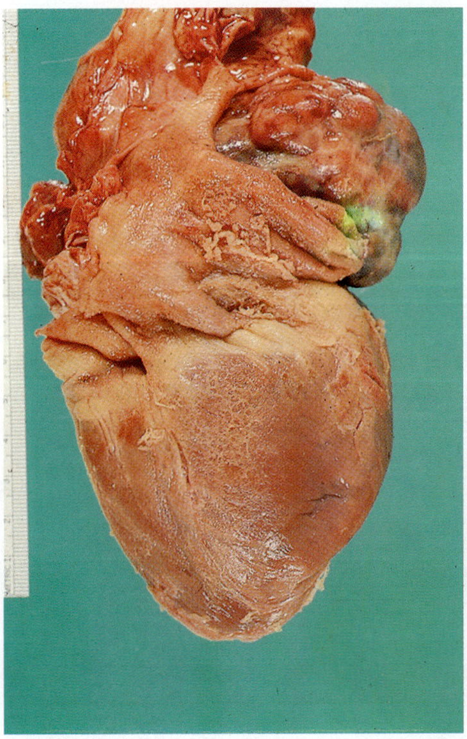

COLOR PLATE 102 Gross pathologic specimen from a dog with a heart base tumor. The heart is viewed from the left side, with the pericardium removed. A large soft tissue mass is seen extending from the base of the heart caudal to the aortic arch and dorsal to the left atrium.

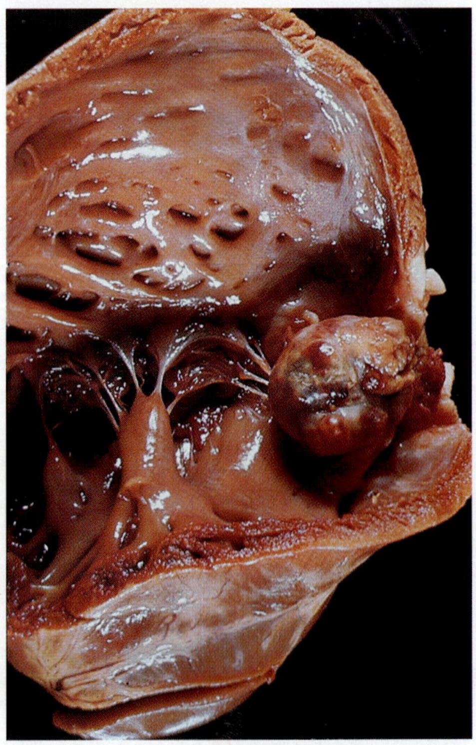

COLOR PLATE 103 Pathologic specimen from the dog shown in Figure 25-8. The right ventricular free wall has been reflected dorsally. A large soft tissue mass is seen within the right ventricular outflow tract just below the pulmonic valve.

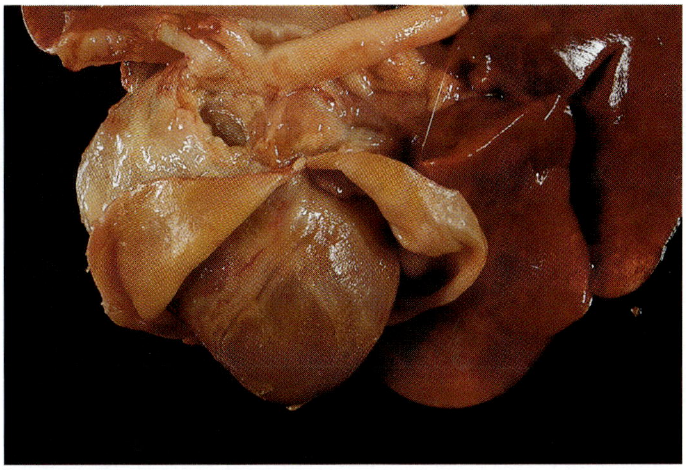

COLOR PLATE 104 Gross pathologic specimen from a dog with constrictive-effusive pericarditis. The pericardium has been bisected and reflected dorsally. Note the thickening and discoloration of the pericardium, suggesting an extreme inflammatory response. The epicardial surface of the heart is also thickened and irregular.

A

B

C

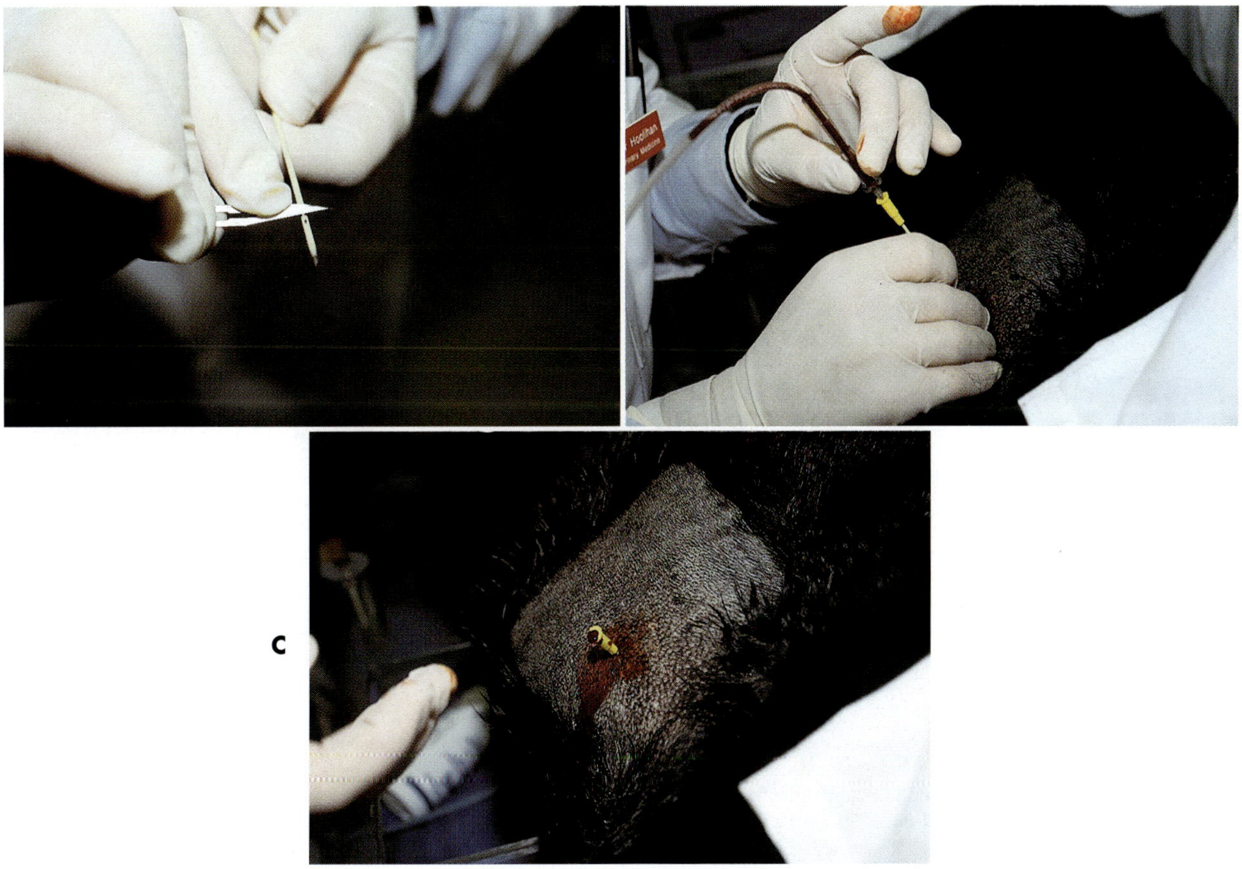

COLOR PLATE 105 Technique for pericardiocentesis in the dog. **A.** Extra side-holes are cut in the catheter using a no. 11 scalpel blade, taking care not to leave burrs on the edges of the cut holes. **B,** The catheter is inserted through a small stab incision and is slowly advanced while applying a mild suction to the syringe. **C,** When fluid is obtained, the catheter is fully advanced over the needle into the pericardial space, the needle is removed, and the stopcock is connected directly to the catheter.

A 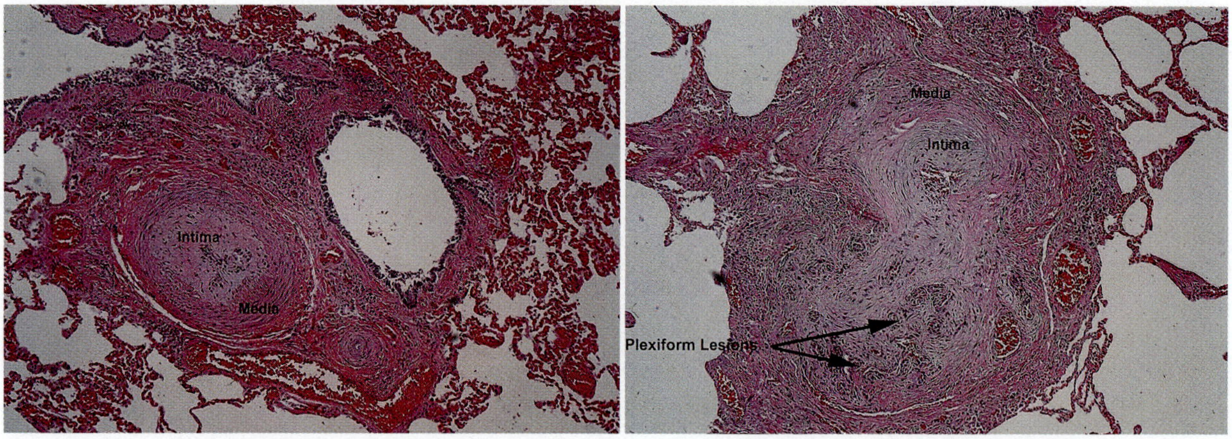 B

COLOR PLATE 106 Photomicrographs of pulmonary arteriolar lesions from a dog with a right-to-left patent ductus arteriosus. **A,** Cross-sections of a pulmonary arteriole and venule. Note the medial hypertrophy and cellular intimal proliferation in the arteriole. **B,** Plexiform lesions are identified within this arteriole.

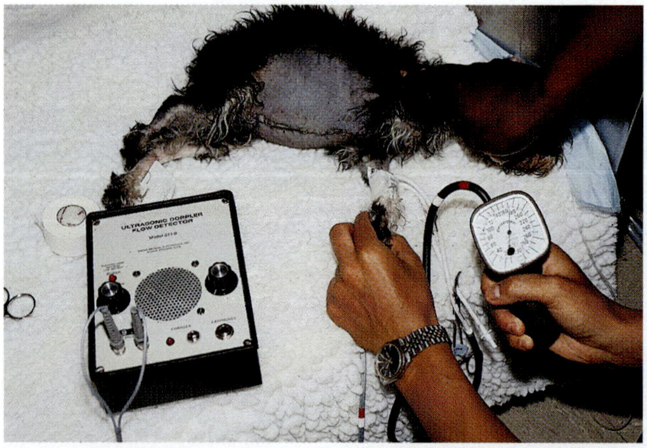

COLOR PLATE 107 Technique of measuring systolic blood pressure using a Doppler device to detect blood flow and an inflatable cuff. The Doppler crystal is being held in place by digital pressure. The cuff is placed above the artery. It has been inflated to a suprasystemic pressure of approximately 170 mm Hg. This occludes flow. The cuff is then gradually deflated. The systolic pressure is read when flow can again be detected by the Doppler device.

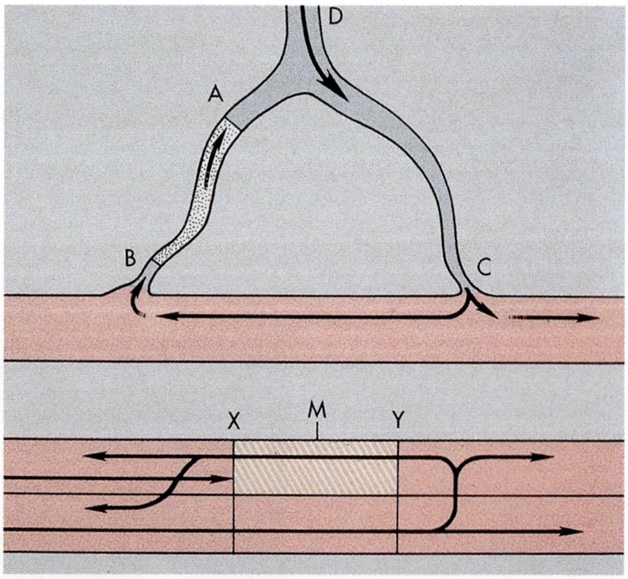

COLOR PLATE 108 Schematic drawing of reentry. The top panel depicts reentry in a branched Purkinje fiber. Normally, depolarization *(arrows)* should conduct from *D* to *B* and *C* uniformly. In this example, a region of tissue is damaged between *A* and *B,* causing antegrade conduction through this region to be blocked. By the time depolarization has proceeded from *D* to *C* to *B,* the diseased tissue has repolarized to the point that it can conduct slowly from *B* to *A.* By the time conduction reaches *A,* the normal tissue has fully repolarized and so can be depolarized again as the depolarization wave 'reenters' this area to produce a premature depolarization. Similarly, in the lower panel, parallel circuits in which one circuit is damaged results in reentry. (From Chatterjee K, Cheitlin MD, Karliner J et al: *Cardiology: an illustrated text/reference,* Philadelphia, 1991, JB Lippincott.)

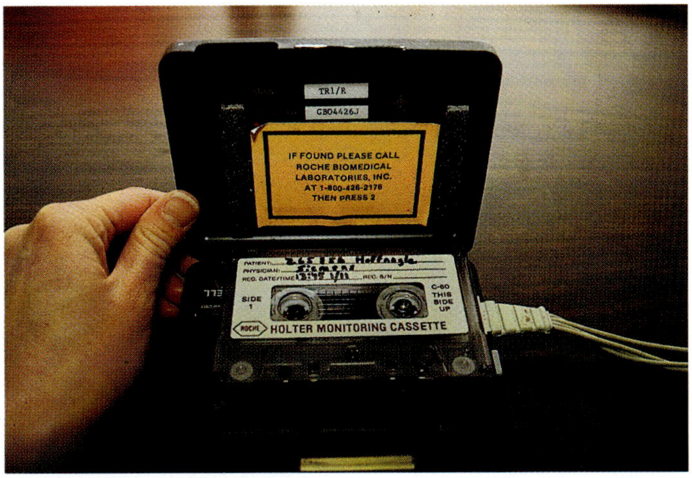

COLOR PLATE 109 A Holter recorder is a small tape-recording device that records electrical signals (e.g., an ECG) instead of sound. The tape will hold at least 24 hours of recording.

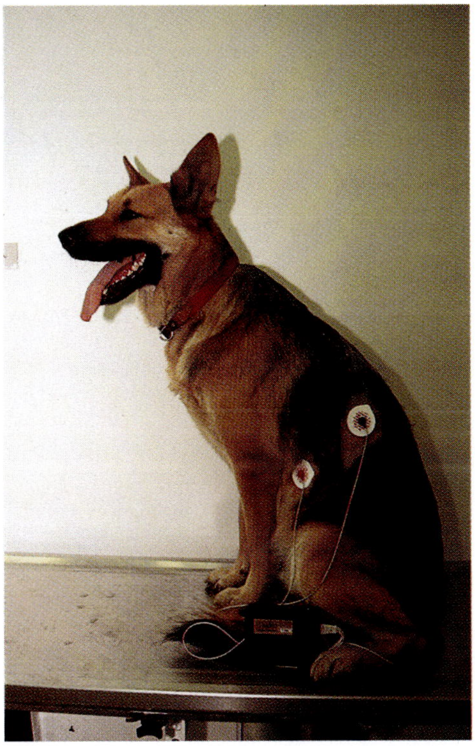

COLOR PLATE 110 Adhesive electrodes are attached to shaved areas of the dog's skin. The electrodes are attached by insulated wires to the recorder.

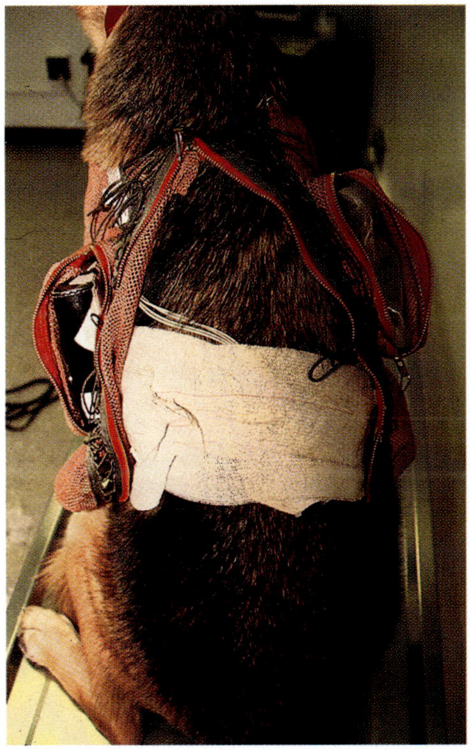

COLOR PLATE 111 Electrodes and wires are placed under elastic tape to prevent damage. The recorder is placed in a pocket (left) in a mesh vest, and the wires are fed through the mesh and attached to the recorder. A bag of fluid is placed on the contralateral side (right) for balance.

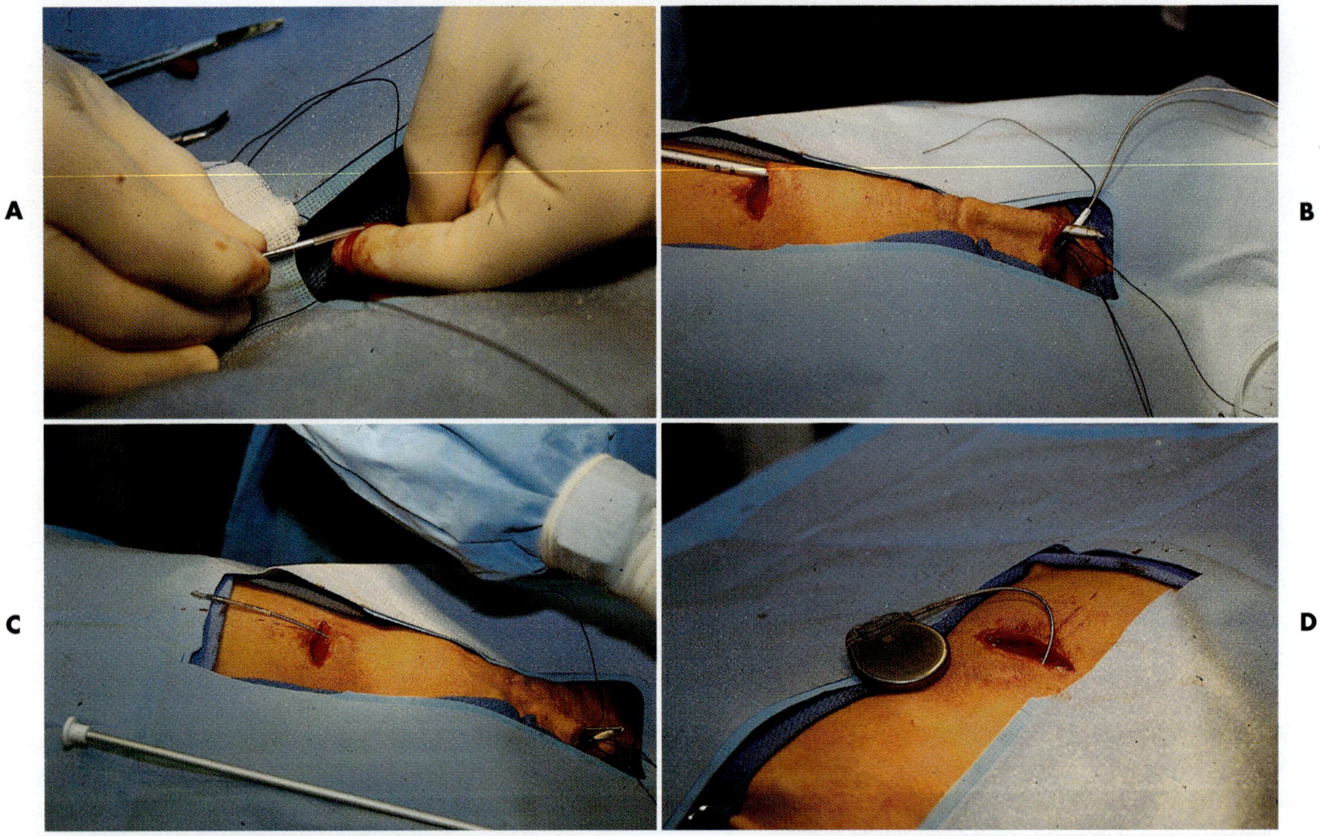

COLOR PLATE 112 Transvenous pacemaker implantation. **A,** The jugular vein is exposed and ligated, and a small venotomy is made. An endocardial lead, stiffened by a wire stylet, is introduced through the venotomy and advanced. **B,** A tunnel is made between the cervical and thoracic incisions using a trochar chest tube. **C,** The lead is extended to the thoracic incision through the chest tube, and the chest tube is removed. **D,** The lead is attached to the generator, which will be placed in a subcutaneous pocket on the laterl thorax.

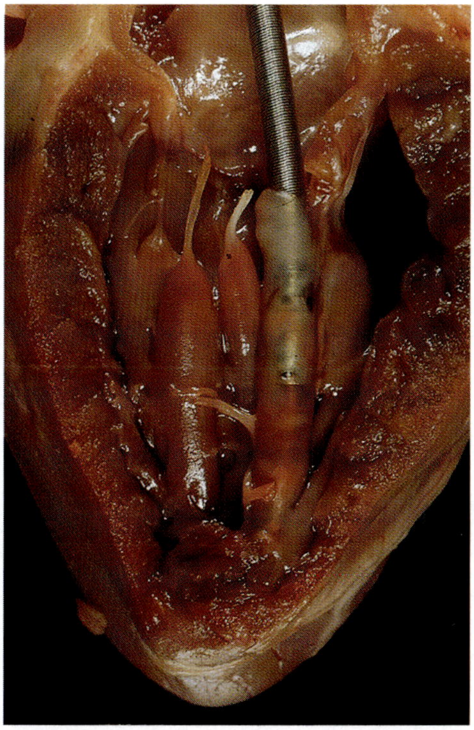

COLOR PLATE 113 Postmortem specimen from a dog with a transvenous pacemaker. The right ventricle and atrium have been opened. The lead in the right atrium crosses the tricuspid valve and is held in place at the right ventriuclar apex by a layer of fibrous tissue.

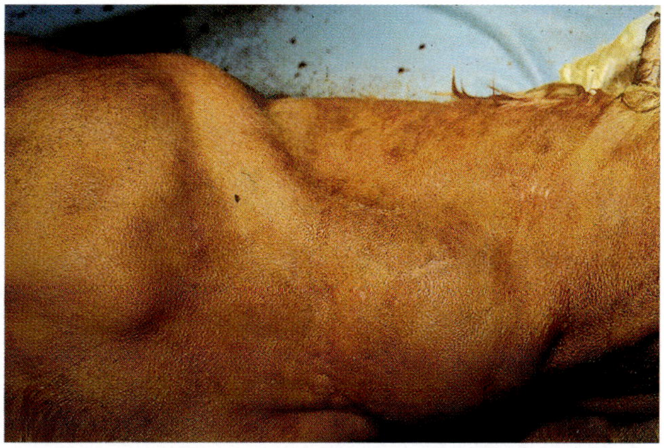

COLOR PLATE 114 Infection along the external portion of the pacing lead and pulse generator.

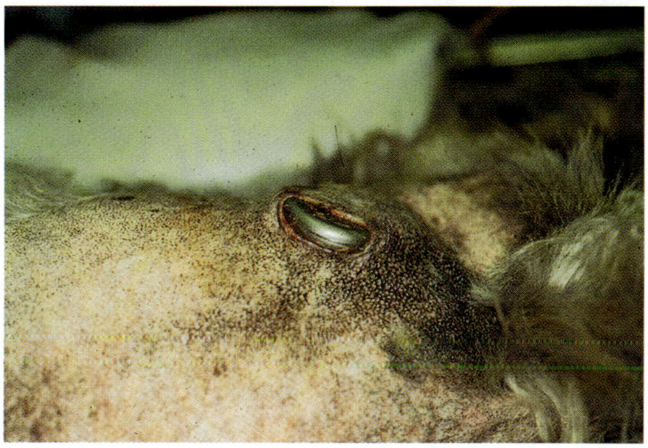

COLOR PLATE 115 Skin erosion in a dog with a pacemaker generator implanted in the subcutaneous tissues of the neck. The generator can be seen extruding through the eroded area of skin.

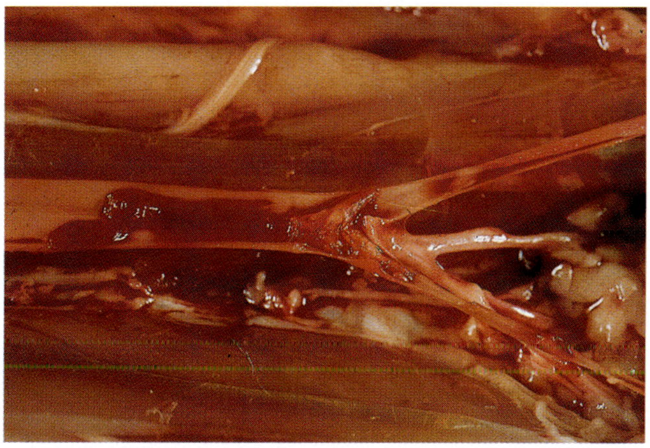

COLOR PLATE 116 Postmortem specimen of a terminal aorta with a thromboembolus from a cat with hypertrophic cardiomyopathy and an acute onset of caudal limb pain and paresis. The thromboembolus is lodged at the terminal aorta ("saddle" thromboembolus), with portions extending into the external iliac arteries. (Courtesy Dr. Mark Rishniw.)

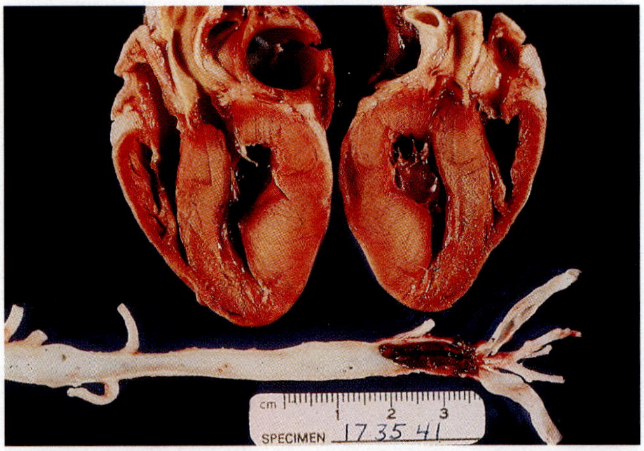

COLOR PLATE 117 Postmortem specimens of the heart and aorta from a cat with hypertrophic cardiomyopathy and an aortic thromboembolus. There is a large thrombus in the left ventricular cavity. (Courtesy Dr. Richard A. LeCouteur.)

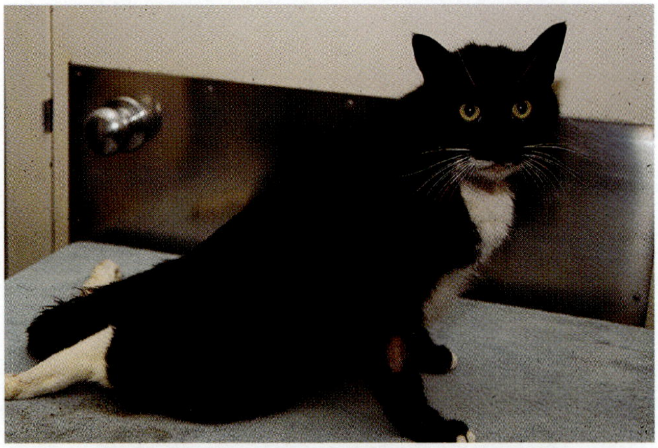

COLOR PLATE 118 Cat with a terminal aortic thromboembolus, approximately 8 hours after the initial event. The cat had no pain sensation and no motor activity beyond the stifles at this stage. It was able to move its proximal caudal limbs and its tail. The cat had hypertrophic cardiomyopathy and an enlarged left atrium.

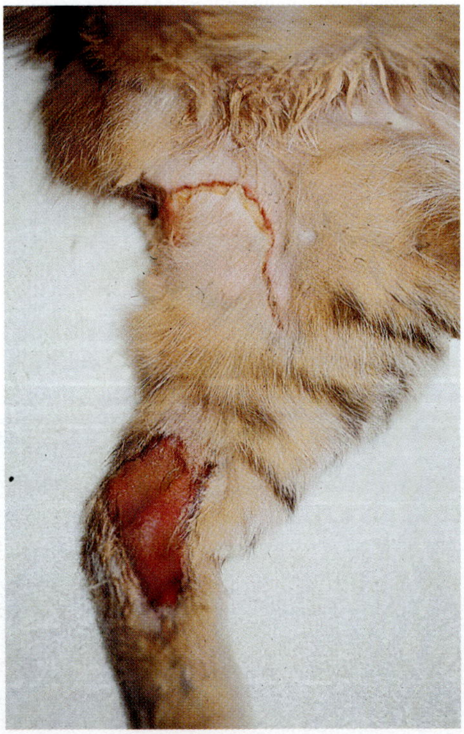

COLOR PLATE 119 Dry gangrene of the skin in a cat 2 weeks following systemic thromboembolism of the caudal limbs.

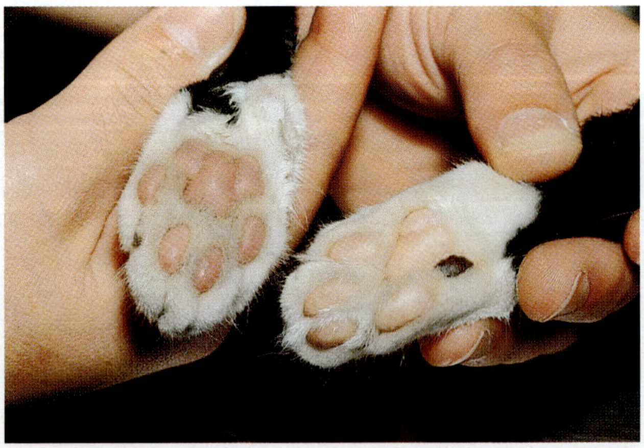

COLOR PLATE 120 Pads from a cat with a smaller thromboembolus that lodged in the right external iliac artery, obstructing flow to the right caudal leg. The pads on this foot are pale compared with the normally perfused left foot. (Courtesy Dr. George Eyster.)

Most cats (85% in one study) have ECG abnormalities.[1] The most common are evidence of left ventricular enlargement and conduction system abnormalities. The most common cardiac rhythms at presentation are sinus rhythm and sinus tachycardia.

Echocardiography is used to identify the underlying cardiac disease. In one study, about 60% of cats had hypertrophic cardiomyopathy and 25% had an unclassified form of cardiomyopathy.[1] The remaining cats had either restrictive cardiomyopathy, dilated cardiomyopathy, or hyperthyroidism.

Laboratory abnormalities are common in cats with STE.[1] Most have increases in serum aspartate aminotransferase and alanine aminotransferase concentrations and serum glucose concentration. The former is due to muscle necrosis, and the latter is due to stress. Increased serum urea nitrogen and creatinine concentrations are often increased, presumably as a result of reduced renal perfusion, although they may be increased in some cats because of the thromboembolus lodging in the aorta in the region of the renal arteries. Numerous other abnormalities can be identified occasionally in some cats.

TREATMENT

Palliative therapy. Most cats with STE receive only palliative therapy for their thromboembolus. The outcome of arterial occlusion depends on the extent of occlusion and the time to spontaneous reperfusion, either via the primary vessel or collateral circulation. Cats may lose an affected leg because of ischemic necrosis, die of toxemia, remain paralyzed from peripheral nerve damage, or regain full or partial function of their legs. About 50% of cats that are not treated definitively will regain all or most caudal limb motor function within 1 to 6 weeks.[20] The return of function in this situation is due to the cat's own fibrinolytic system disrupting the thromboembolus. The degree and rapidity of the dissolution depend on the activity of a particular cat's fibrinolytic system and the size of the thromboembolus. Usually, cats that present with some evidence of caudal limb flow recover more rapidly than do cats with no evidence of flow. Presumably this is because the size of the thromboembolus in cats with some flow is smaller than in those cats in which total occlusion is present. With total occlusion, some cats recanalize within days, whereas others never recanalize. This extreme variability makes it very difficult to render a prognosis for a particular patient at the time of presentation.

Palliative therapy can consist of only cage rest or can include administering drugs such as heparin, aspirin, or arteriolar dilators, along with cage rest. No drugs administered for palliation have any proven benefit over cage rest alone. Heparin is commonly administered in the hope of preventing new thrombus formation on top of the thromboembolus. Heparin does not aid in thrombolysis. There is no evidence in cats that heparin does or does not provide benefit. New thrombus formation may or may not occur in feline STE. One experimental study noted that the thrombi produced at surgery were not significantly larger 3 days later at postmortem examination, which makes the theory of clot extension questionable in this situation.[12] On the other hand, when thromboemboli are examined at a postmortem examination, they often have a shape that conforms to the shape of the aorta and proximal iliac arteries. This is more typical of a thrombus and might suggest that additional thrombus has formed at the site. If new thrombus formation does occur, it is known that approximately 20 times more heparin is required to inactivate fibrin-bound thrombin than to inactivate free thrombin. Consequently, more heparin is required to prevent extension of a venous thrombus than to prevent the formation of a new thrombus.[21] Heparin can be administered at an initial dose of 220 U/kg IV, followed by a maintenance dose of 70 to 200 U/kg SC q6h. The dose should be tailored to each individual cat to increase the activated partial thromboplastin time (aPTT) to at least 1.5 times baseline.

Indomethacin is effective at preventing vasoconstriction distal to the thromboembolus when administered to experimental cats before creating an aortic thrombus. Theoretically aspirin could do the same thing. There is no evidence that it does or does not improve collateral blood flow once the thromboembolus is in place. Presumably this has been attempted in experimental cats but the negative results never reported. The administration of drugs that dilate systemic arterioles (e.g., hydralazine, acepromazine) has been advocated to open collateral blood vessels in cats with STE. Again there is no proven benefit, only conjecture that it might help. These drugs act by relaxing the smooth muscle in systemic arterioles. The exact anatomy of collateral vessels is not well described, but they are probably larger vessels than arterioles. However, they must contain smooth muscle because they can open and close. The ability of arteriolar dilators to counteract serotonin and thromboxane A_2-induced vasoconstriction is unknown.

Definitive therapy

Surgery. Definitive treatments for STE in cats include administration of exogenous fibrinolytic agents, balloon embolectomy, and surgery. Surgical removal of systemic thromboemboli is associated with high mortality. Cats with STE commonly have underlying cardiac disease exacerbated by the increase in afterload produced by blocking the aorta. Consequently, they are commonly in heart failure and are poor anesthetic risks.

More important, when a thromboembolus is removed acutely, the caudal legs are suddenly reperfused. The muscles of the legs before removal are undergoing necrosis. The cellular breakdown releases potassium and hydrogen ions from the cells into the interstitial spaces, where they accumulate. Sudden reperfusion carries these ions into the systemic circulation. The same thing can occur with fibrinolytic therapy. Following the administration of tissue plasminogen activator (t-PA) we have observed the serum potassium concentration to increase from the normal range into the 9- to 11-mEq/L range within 5 minutes. We have also noted the blood pH to decrease into the 6.9- to 7.1-mEq/L range within the same time span. Unless treated immediately and aggressively, these perturbations are often lethal. Before studying t-PA administration in cats with STE, the presence of this "reperfusion" syndrome was not appreciated in cats with thromboembolic disease. Now that it is known that this occurs, surgical intervention may be a viable option in a patient that is not in severe heart failure. This could be done if the legs could be "flushed" with sterile saline before allowing reperfusion (saline infused into the arterial tree and the blood/saline wash removed via cannulas in the femoral veins) or if treatment with insulin/glucose or calcium could be initiated immediately upon reperfusion, with careful monitoring. We have not tried these approaches, so caution is advised.

Balloon embolectomy. The procedure of choice in human medicine is balloon embolectomy.[22] We have had limited experience with balloon embolectomy. In this procedure, the femoral arteries are isolated and a small balloon embolectomy catheter is passed from one femoral artery into the aorta. Contrary to what one might think, the femoral arteries are not extremely difficult to isolate if one has had experience isolating them previously. The catheter is pushed past the thromboembolus, and the balloon is then inflated and the catheter withdrawn, along with thromboembolic material. The catheter is passed sequentially, first in one artery and then in the other. Usually this sequence must be repeated several times. Reperfusion syndrome may occur with balloon embolectomy, and therefore appropriate precautions apply.

Thrombolytic therapy. Thrombolytic therapy is possible in cats with STE using fibrinolytic agents. Thromboemboli are composed of red cells, platelets, and strands of fibrin. Fibrinolytic agents cleave plasminogen to plasmin. Plasmin hydrolyzes fibrin and fibrinogen. The hydrolysis of fibrin results in thrombolysis. Different agents vary in ability to bind specifically to fibrin-bound plasminogen and in half-life. Clinically, however, efficacy and complication rates appear to be very similar in humans.[23] Complications consist primarily of hemorrhage and rethrombosis. Fibrinolytic agents can be very effective at lysing systemic thromboemboli. However, we currently treat very few cats with STE with thrombolytic agents, because reperfusion syndrome and rethrombosis are common.

The common thrombolytic agents used in veterinary medicine include tissue plasminogen activator (t-PA) and streptokinase. Tissue plasminogen activator is an intrinsic protein present in all mammals. Recently, because of recombinant DNA techniques, it has become possible to manufacture large quantities of t-PA, making its use as a therapeutic thrombolytic agent possible. There are numerous reports of the use of t-PA for the lysis of thrombi as therapy for acute myocardial infarction, pulmonary thromboembolism, and peripheral vascular obstruction in humans and experimental animals.[23] The activity of genetically engineered t-PA in feline plasma is 90% to 100% of that seen in human plasma. The half-life of t-PA is quite short. Consequently, heparin must be administered concomitantly to prevent acute rethrombosis. Heparin need not be administered with streptokinase because it has a longer half-life, allowing it to be active for a longer time. Our clinical trials at the University of California, Davis, with t-PA in cats with aortic thromboemboli have shown acute thrombolytic efficacy (shortened time to reperfusion and ambulation) associated with the administration of t-PA at a rate of 0.25 mg to 1 mg/kg/hr for a total dose of 1 to 10 mg/kg IV.[24] Forty-three percent of cats treated survived therapy and were walking within 48 hours of presentation. Angiograms performed after t-PA administration demonstrated resolution of the primary vascular occlusion. Thus, acutely, t-PA effectively decreased the time to reperfusion and return to function in cats with aortic thromboemboli. However 50% of the cats died during therapy, which raises extreme concerns regarding acute thrombolysis (Box 31-1). Fatalities resulted from reperfusion syndrome (hyperkalemia, metabolic acidosis [70%]), congestive heart failure (15%), and sudden arrhythmic death, presumed to result from embolization of an echocardiographically identifiable left atrial thrombus to a coronary artery (15%). Two cats that died of reperfusion syndrome also had renal arterial occlusion by the original thromboembolus followed by severe hemorrhage into and around the kidney after renal blood flow was reestablished. These cats died of hyperkalemia complicated by severe anemia that could not be controlled with repeated transfusions. The cats that successfully completed t-PA therapy exhibited signs of increasing neuromuscular function and ambulatory ability within 2 days of presentation. This contrasts with 1 to 6 weeks before seeing similar signs of improvement in most cats exhibiting spontaneous resolution.

Mortality resulting from reperfusion syndrome can probably be reduced if the patient can be observed continuously by an individual trained to identify clinical and electrocardiographic evidence of hyperkalemia, if intensive monitoring of electrolytes can be performed, and if aggressive medical therapy for hyperkalemia and metabolic acidosis can be initiated promptly. In our experience, this means having a cardiologist, a cardiology resident, or other trained individual dedicated to treating a particular patient observe the animal 24 hours a day until the thrombolus is lysed. Complete thrombolysis may take only 3 hours or as long as 48 hours.

BOX 31-1

Reperfusion syndrome: a case study

A 4-year-old male domestic shorthaired cat presented with a history of 24 hours of posterior paresis and 12 hours of paresis and tonic flexion of the right forelimb. The cat was dyspneic and hypothermic. Affected limbs were cool, and the toe pads were cyanotic. The gastrocnemius muscles felt firm, and the cat exhibited pain when affected limbs were manipulated. No femoral pulses were palpable. An electrocardiogram revealed a heart rate of 210 beats/min, wide QRS complexes (0.06 seconds), and atrioventricular dissociation resulting from an accelerated junctional rhythm. An echocardiogram demonstrated severe dilated cardiomyopathy. Thoracic radiographs revealed marked generalized cardiomegaly and a mixed interstitial-alveolar pattern in the right dorsocaudal lung, compatible with pulmonary edema. An injection of 0.5 mCi of technetium-99m into the left cephalic vein while the patient was lying on a gamma camera demonstrated complete occlusion of the abdominal aorta just distal to the left renal artery. There was also complete occlusion of the right axillary artery. Heparin (100 U/kg SC) was administered, and an infusion of tissue plasminogen activator (t-PA) was administered at a rate of 1 mg/kg over 1.5 hours, followed by 0.5 mg/kg over the next 3 hours. At that time, the patient's condition deteriorated rapidly. The heart rate decreased to 130 beats/min, and the following laboratory values were obtained:

Values	*Patient*	*Reference range*
Serum potassium	8.33 mEq/L	(3.5-4.5)
Packed cell volume	42%	(24-45)
Total protein	6.2 mg/dL	(5.4-7.8)
Venous blood pH	7.11	(7.31-7.42)
Venous PCO_2	37.6 mm Hg	(35-45)
Venous PO_2	20.7 mm Hg	(30-45)
Calculated base deficit	16.5 mEq/L	(–4-+4)

These data were interpreted as hyperkalemia with metabolic acidosis along with venous hypoxemia resulting from poor cardiac output. The hyperkalemia and metabolic acidosis probably originated from the release of intracellular potassium and hydrogen ions secondary to ischemic skeletal muscle in avascular tissue followed by reperfusion (reperfusion syndrome). The acidemia may also have contributed to the hyperkalemia because of mass action movement of cations across cell membranes. Treatment for the hyperkalemia and metabolic acidosis was difficult because of the cat's compromised cardiac function creating a limitation on the amount of intravenous fluids and sodium load that could be administered safely. Therapy included sodium bicarbonate (0.5 mEq/kg IV), dextrose (1 g IV), and furosemide (1 mg/kg IV). One hour later the acid-base analysis was unchanged but the serum potassium concentration had decreased to 6.1 mEq/L. The patient's attitude was greatly improved, and the heart rate was 250 beats/min. Two hours into the t-PA infusion, the cat's heart rate began to decrease rapidly from greater than 225 to 125 beats/min. Hyperkalemia secondary to reperfusion of the affected limbs was suspected. Therapy consisted of 20 mg of calcium chloride, 1 g of dextrose, and 0.2 mg of atropine intravenously. The heart rate increased to 150 beats/min but soon decreased to 60 beats/min, followed by cardiac arrest and death. Serum potassium concentration at the time of arrest was 8 mEq/L.

If reperfusion syndrome was the only major complicating factor in cats treated with thrombolytic agents, continued use in selected patients might be warranted. However, 90% of the cats that we have successfully treated with t-PA have rethrombosed within 1 to 3 months. Rethrombosis has occurred despite aspirin, warfarin, or heparin administration. Consequently, we have not been recommending thrombolytic therapy for STE in cats.

Our, and others, impression has been that the incidence of STE in cats with hypertrophic cardiomyopathy has decreased since the advent of using diltiazem. This may or may not be true. However, calcium channel blockers do have antiplatelet activity in humans, cats, and cattle.[25-27] In addition, diltiazem could have beneficial effects on left atrial hemodynamics. However, subacute oral diltiazem administration did not prevent platelet aggregation in normal cats in one study, whereas aspirin administration did.[28] We believe that diltiazem could still be efficacious in cats with cardiac disease. Consequently, we have considered using thrombolytic agents again, but not with t-PA because it is very expensive.

Streptokinase has efficacy very similar to t-PA in human patients with coronary artery thrombosis.[23] Streptokinase is a less expensive product and so may be a feasible agent to use in veterinary medicine. There are no reports of streptokinase use for STE in veterinary patients. However, one experimental study produced promising results.[29] In this study, a thrombus was created at the terminal aorta by temporarily ligating the aorta at two sites, immediately proximal to the aortic trifurcation and at the branching of the caudal mesenteric artery. Thrombin was injected between the two ligatures to create a thrombus, and the ligatures were removed. Streptokinase was administered as a loading dose at 90,000 IU followed by 45,000 IU/hr for 3 hours. This dose produced evidence of systemic fibrinolysis in a separate group of normal cats without evidence of severe fibrinolysis or bleeding. Efficacy was judged by examining angiograms and skin temperature before and after streptokinase administration. In most cats there was no change in the angiogram and no improvement in limb temperature. There was a tendency for the thrombus weight to be lower in the treated cats compared with control cats at postmortem examination in this small study. From our experience with t-PA, we do not believe that streptokinase was administered long enough to result in complete lysis of the thrombi in these cats. Consequently, we believe that this drug may still be effective when administered at this dose.

Another possible approach to thrombolytic therapy is to administer a dose of a thrombolytic agent that only partially dissolves the clot. Following this, palliative therapy is administered while the cat's inherent fibrinolytic system breaks down the remaining thrombus more slowly. We and others have administered a loading dose of streptokinase (90,000 IU) followed by 45,000 IU/hr for 3 hours and then stopped. Although it is difficult to judge efficacy, we have seen several cases that appeared to benefit from this approach.

Adjunctive therapy. At presentation, many cats are in intense pain. The pain commonly subsides as sensory nervous function is lost. Treatment of pain is mandatory during the initial stages of the disease. Choices include oxymorphone (0.05 to 0.15 mg/kg q6h IM or IV) and butorphanol tartrate (0.1 mg/kg IV or 0.02 to 0.4 mg/kg q4h IM or SC). Oxymorphone may produce excitement in some cats. The analgesic properties of butorphanol are 5 times that of morphine It has recently been reclassified as a scheduled drug by the Food and Drug Administration. Its respiratory depressant effects equal that of morphine. Consequently, one must be careful with administering this drug to a patient with severe pulmonary edema or pleural effusion. Acepromazine (0.05 to 0.1 mg/kg IV) may be administered in addition to an analgesic as an anxiolytic agent to cats that still appear distressed following the administration of the analgesic.

Cats with STE are commonly in heart failure at the time of presentation. Medical therapy with furosemide and an angiotensin converting enzyme inhibitor is often indicated. Cats with hypertrophic cardiomyopathy may benefit from diltiazem or β-blocker administration. Cats that are in pain usually do not eat or drink. Fluid therapy is warranted in this situation, but care must be taken not to aggravate or produce heart failure with overzealous fluid administration.

Cats that take a long time to recover caudal limb function or that only attain partial function may develop regions of skin and muscle necrosis, especially on the distal limbs. These regions may require surgical debriding. Cats that lose the function of only one leg or that do not regain function of one leg benefit from amputation of that leg. Cats that have permanently lost muscle function distal to the hock may benefit from arthrodesis.

Prognosis. The short-term prognosis for life is good in cats without heart failure. The prognosis for continued life in cats with STE and heart failure is guarded and depends on the ability to control the heart failure. One of the most common causes of death within the first 24 hours is euthanasia. Faced with the guarded-to-poor prognosis and the immediate pain that the cat is feeling, many owners opt for euthanasia as a rational means of dealing with the problem. In one study, about 30% of cats with acute STE died during the initial hospitalization and about 35% were euthanized. The long-term prognosis for survival is highly variable with cats living from 3 to 30 months after the initial episode in one report.[1] The average survival time was about 10 to 12 months in this report. The long-term prognosis for limb function depends on the ability of the cat to lyse its own clot or on the success of intervention. Many biologic variables determine whether reperfusion will spontaneously occur. Of the 50% of the cats that regain adequate caudal limb function following STE, some will go on to do well, whereas others will develop complications such as open skin lesions, gangrene, and muscle contractures. Some cats will develop a new thromboembolus days to months after recovery.

Prophylaxis. Feline patients with myocardial disease, especially those with enlarged left atria, should be considered at risk for developing intracardiac thrombi and signs of peripheral arterial thromboembolism. Preventing peripheral thrombosis is one of the most important therapeutic objectives for the veterinarian managing cats with myocardial disease. The ideal means of preventing thrombosis would be resolution of the underlying myocardial disease. This is usually not possible except in a cat with dilated cardiomyopathy secondary to taurine deficiency.

At present, the only option available is to manipulate the patient's coagulation system in an attempt to alter the delicate balance between the pathways that promote clotting and those that inhibit thrombus formation to reduce the patient's thrombogenic potential. At this time, antiplatelet and anticoagulant therapy are the only means of preventing thrombus formation in cats with myocardial disease. Unfortunately, they are often ineffective and, in the case of warfarin, can produce serious side effects.[30] Experience is similar in human medicine.[31]

Antiplatelet therapy: aspirin. Prostaglandins enhance platelet aggregation via activation of cAMP. Aspirin (acetylsalicylic acid) acetylates platelet cyclooxygenase, preventing the formation of thromboxane A_2, a potent prostaglandin-like platelet aggregating substance.[21] Aspirin also inhibits cyclooxygenase in vascular endothelium and prevents the formation of prostacyclin, a potent prostaglandin-like compound that inhibits platelet aggregation. Thus, aspirin's action upon platelets inhibits thrombotic tendencies and prolongs bleeding time, whereas its action upon vascular endothelium inhibits prostacyclin-induced platelet inhibition, favoring local thrombosis. This paradox can be used therapeutically because of the different kinetics of the two systems. The inhibition of platelet cyclooxygenase is irreversible, and bleeding time is restored to normal only after the production of new platelets. The inhibition of endothelial cyclooxygenase is reversible. The practice of administering aspirin every second or third day may in theory allow the patient to have maximal platelet inactivation (a beneficial effect) while minimizing endothelial cyclooxygenase inhibition and thrombotic tendencies (a detrimental effect). The dose of aspirin recommended in cats is 25 mg/kg every third day. Whether this dose allows

BOX 31-2

Failure of aspirin to prevent rethrombosis: a case study

A 2-year-old intact female domestic shorthaired cat without previous medical problems was presented with a 12-hour history of tachypnea and posterior paresis progressing to severe dyspnea and posterior paralysis over the next 6 hours. The cat was vocalizing, and the caudal limbs were painful and cool to the touch. A femoral pulse was not palpable in either caudal leg, the gastrocnemius muscles felt firm, and the toe pads were cyanotic. When the claws of two digits were cut back to the ungual processes, they did not bleed. Thoracic auscultation revealed a 3/6 systolic murmur heard best just to the left of the sternum. The respiratory rate was 64 breaths/min. Crackles were auscultable in the caudal lung fields. Thoracic radiography revealed moderate cardiomegaly with an enlarged left atrium and pulmonary infiltrates compatible with pulmonary edema. Echocardiography confirmed a diagnosis of hypertrophic cardiomyopathy. A thrombus was not visualized in the left atrium. Furosemide (3 mg/kg) was administered intravenously, and the patient was placed in an oxygen cage. Three hours later the respiratory rate had decreased to 48 breaths/min. The patient was tranquilized with intravenous ketamine and diazepam, and digital angiography of the distal aorta and femoral arteries was diagnostic for a thrombus at the aortic trifurcation, partially obstructing perfusion to both caudal limbs. Heparin was administered (5 U/kg IV followed by 100 U/kg IM every 6 hours) and an infusion of t-PA was administered at a rate of 1 mg/kg/hr IV for 1.5 hours, followed by 0.5 mg/kg/hr for 3.5 hours. A femoral pulse was palpable in both legs 3 hours after beginning the t-PA infusion. The cat could ambulate 6 hours after admission. A digital angiogram performed 12 hours after admission revealed resolution of the aortic thromboembolus with partial obstruction of the right femoral artery. The cat was released 48 hours after admission with a mild conscious proprioceptive deficit in the right caudal limb. Medication consisted of furosemide (1.0 mg/kg q8h), captopril (0.5 mg/kg q8h), and aspirin (25 mg/kg q72h). The serum potassium concentration remained normal during the entire course of therapy. Eighteen days later the cat had another episode of posterior paresis and was euthanized by the referring veterinarian.

endothelial cyclooxygenase to recover in cats is undetermined. At this dose, aspirin has a half-life of 45 hours in the cat. In humans, doses as low as 20 to 100 mg/day inhibit platelet cyclooxygenase, but there is no evidence that this low dose has any more benefit than conventional daily doses of 625 to 1250 mg. In fact, after examining more than 18,000 patients in human medicine there is still controversy about whether aspirin is effective at preventing coronary thrombosis.[32] There is no evidence that any dose of aspirin is effective at preventing intracardiac or peripheral arterial thrombosis in cats with myocardial disease. However, compared with the human doses commonly used for this purpose, the cat dose may be quite high, especially for a species that has such a long aspirin half-life. Clinical impression of aspirin's efficacy varies between clinicians. In our experience, aspirin, at the dose cited above, does not prevent recurrence of peripheral thromboembolism in cats with a history of aortic thromboembolism associated with myocardial disease (Box 31-2).

Anticoagulant therapy. Available anticoagulants include heparin and the coumarins. Heparin's anticoagulant properties are indirect, resulting from augmentation of antithrombin III activity. Heparin forms a 1:1 stoichiometry complex with antithrombin III. Factor Xa bound to platelets and thrombin bound to fibrin are protected from activation by the heparin-antithrombin III complex.[21] Heparin is destroyed in the gastrointestinal tract and is therefore not effective for long-term oral therapy. Heparin may be administered intravenously or subcutaneously. Repeated intramuscular injection is discouraged because local hemorrhage may result. Some owners can administer heparin subcutaneously at home, but the method is not ideal. We have noted rethrombosis with heparin therapy in some cats with cardiac disease. The dose of heparin for preventing thrombosis in cats is unknown.

Warfarin sodium (Coumadin, DuPont Pharmaceuticals, Wilmington, Del.) is an oral anticoagulant that inhibits the synthesis of vitamin K–dependent clotting factors (II, VII, IX, X).[21] It does this by inhibiting vitamin K-2,3 synthesis in the liver.[21] Warfarin exerts no anticoagulant effect in vitro. In vivo, inhibitory effects on synthesis of clotting factors begin immediately. However, clotting is unaffected until already existing clotting factors decline. Therefore there is a delay between initial administration and effect on the prothrombin time. The coumarins are highly bound to plasma albumin (95% to 99% in humans). Historically, oral anticoagulant therapy has been monitored with the prothrombin time. This test measures the activity of factors II, VII, and X. The factor depressed most quickly and profoundly (usually factor VII) determines the prothrombin time during the initial days of therapy. Prothrombin time or partial thromboplastin time may be used to determine the adequacy of a chronic oral anticoagulant dose. The PIVKA (proteins induced by vitamin K antagonists) test is a more sensitive and specific test.[18] The PIVKA test detects the presence of inactive precursors of factors II, VII, IX, and X. If available, this is the assay of choice for monitoring oral anticoagulant therapy. The anticoagulant action of warfarin types of compounds is consistent with the view that they compete with the fat-soluble vitamin K for a receptor in the liver that controls synthesis of factors II, VII, IX, and X. When the anticoagulant effect is excessive, it can be counteracted by administering vitamin K_1. However, once synthesis of factors II, VII, IX, and X is reinstituted, time must elapse before factors achieve concentrations in the plasma that will adequately reverse the bleeding tendency. If serious bleeding occurs during therapy with coumarins, it may be stopped immediately by administering fresh blood or plasma that contain the missing clotting factors. Other drugs can modify the anticoagulant actions of coumarins by altering the bioavailability of vitamin K; by altering the absorption, distribution, or elimination of the coumarins; by affecting synthesis or degradation of clotting factors; or by altering protein binding of the coumarins. Therefore, the maintenance dose should be evaluated daily during the initial titration (3 days), then every other day (twice), and then weekly, until a safe and stable dosage regimen is determined. The therapeutic effect should be reevaluated periodically (at least once per month). Evaluation should be based upon the APTT or PT (or PIVKA, if available). The recommended initial dose is 0.5 mg q24h to a 3- to 5-kg cat. It can take up to 1 week for new steady-state conditions to be achieved. In humans, overregulation of the administered dose can lead to wide fluctuations in clotting test parameters.[21]

Besides its well-known effect on coagulation factors, warfarin reduces the concentration of protein C, a naturally occurring antithrombotic protein. Protein C has a short plasma half-life similar to factor VII. Therefore, in the early stages of warfarin therapy, a potential exists for a transient hypercoagulable state before other vitamin K-dependent factors (II, IX, and X) are affected. During this potential hypercoagulable period, in which protein C is diminished and the intrinsic clotting pathway factors are relatively unaffected, heparin should be used concurrently.

The efficacy of warfarin at preventing recurrent thrombosis in cats with cardiac disease has been reported.[1,2] Both reports have come from the Angell Memorial Animal Hospital in Boston. In one report, out of 23 cats examined retrospectively, 10 experienced new thromboembolic episodes while being administered warfarin. Two of these cats had at least two new episodes. In the other report, 8 of 18 cats on warfarin experienced a new thromboembolic episode. This may be some improvement over the 75% recurrence rate reported for aspirin alone following t-PA therapy, but these results are still disappointing.[18] In the first report, besides the cats that experienced rethrombosis, four cases died suddenly (which can be caused by thromboembolism). Three of these cats did not have postmortem examinations. The one cat that did have a postmortem examination had a thrombus present in its left atrium. One cat died of a renal infarct that produced renal failure. Four cats appeared to have bleeding complications. In the second report, one cat died of a hemoabdomen and one was suspected to have an acute intracranial hemorrhage resulting in death. As evidenced by these cases, warfarin therapy can produce fatal complications, something that is rare with aspirin.

Pulmonary Thromboembolism

Pulmonary thromboembolism (PTE) is caused by the formation of a thrombus in the systemic venous system or right heart that breaks loose to be carried by blood flow to the pulmonary arteries. It lodges in the pulmonary arteries, producing a decrease in or cessation of blood flow to a variable amount of lung. Pulmonary embolism can be caused by foreign bodies (e.g., intravenous catheters), air, or fat. This chapter is devoted to the embolism of pulmonary arteries by thrombi not caused by heartworm disease. Of the diseases diagnosed in human and veterinary medicine, PTE is one of the most difficult to diagnose correctly. In human patients, studies have shown that only 30% of anatomically important pulmonary thromboemboli are diagnosed correctly.[33] Pulmonary thromboembolism is a diagnostic challenge because clinical signs are often ambiguous, mimicked by other diseases, or masked by those of other cardiopulmonary diseases. Dogs lyse pulmonary thromboemboli rapidly, and by the time diagnostic tests are performed, the disease may have resolved. Thromboemboli lyse after death and therefore may not be present at postmortem examination. The clinical signs produced by PTE are nonspecific, and PTE may often be confused with other respiratory diseases. In one series of cases of confirmed or suspected PTE, out of 47 cases, 16 had no clinical signs referable to PTE and were only diagnosed at postmortem examination.[24] Twenty-two of these cases were suspected of having PTE, but the diagnosis could not be confirmed.

PATHOPHYSIOLOGY AND CLINICAL PRESENTATION

Diseases most commonly associated with PTE in dogs are cardiac disease, neoplasia, pancreatitis, disseminated intravascular coagulopathy, autoimmune hemolytic anemia, sepsis, glomerular disease, diabetes mellitus, and hyperadrenocorticism.[24,34,35] Most likely, in all these diseases, a thrombus develops within the systemic venous system. Potential reasons for thrombus formation are multiple and include venous stasis, injury to vascular endothelial lining, and systemic hypercoagulability. Dogs with glomerular disease may have a decreased antithrombin III concentration because of urinary loss.[36,37] The cause of thrombosis in immune-mediated hemolytic anemia is unknown, but it has been suggested in humans that endothelial damage by antierythrocyte antibodies triggers thrombosis.[21] Concentrations of clotting factors V and X and of fibrinogen are increased in dogs with hyperadrenocorticism.[38] Proteolytic enzymes may gain access to the vascular space in pancreatitis. They are normally bound by α-macroglobulins and removed by the reticuloendothelial system. If this system fails, these enzymes can lead to activation of the coagulation cascade.[35] Serum antithrombin III and plasminogen concentrations and platelet counts are decreased in experimental pancreatitis.[39] Neoplasia can cause local endothelial damage or venous stasis.

Once a thrombus lodges in a pulmonary artery, it releases serotonin and thromboxane A_2, causing vasoconstriction distal to the thrombus. If only one thromboembolus lodges in a distal artery, there may be no clinical sequelae. However, if multiple thromboemboli lodge in several pulmonary arteries or a large thromboembolus lodges in a major branch or in the main pulmonary artery, clinical sequelae can be severe. Major clinical sequelae include pulmonary hypertension and ventilation/perfusion mismatching. The degree of pulmonary hypertension produced depends on the number of thromboemboli and their location. More than half the pulmonary circulation must be obstructed by an embolus before pulmonary artery pressure will increase at rest.[40] Pulmonary hypertension can be severe, however, and can cause right heart failure. Ventilation/perfusion mismatching produces arterial hypoxemia in dogs with experimentally induced PTE.[41] In human medicine, hypoxemia is usually but not always seen in patients with PTE. Arterial Pco_2 is usually normal or low because of hyperventilation. It has been suggested that the difference in Pco_2 between arterial blood and end-tidal gas might be a useful test for detecting PTE. However, this has not worked well in practice.[40]

Clinical signs of PTE are nonspecific. Acute, unexplained dyspnea is one of the more common presentations in patients presented for examination and hospitalized patients. Dyspnea in a canine patient that has no or little radiographic pulmonary changes should always make one suspicious of PTE, once airway obstruction has been ruled out. Other possible clinical signs include tachypnea, tachycardia, coughing, fever, weakness, and restlessness, presumably as a result of chest pain. Evidence of right heart failure can occur but is rare. A right-sided heart murmur may suddenly appear. Dogs with massive embolism may be hypotensive or cyanotic and can die suddenly.

It has been known for more than 30 years that pulmonary thromboemboli are broken down in dogs much more rapidly than they are in humans.[42] This fact makes the dog a poor experimental model of acute PTE. In humans, resolution of massive pulmonary embolism is usually incomplete after 1 year, whereas in the dog it is complete within 6 weeks.[42] Single experimentally produced pulmonary thromboemboli are completely degraded within 5 days.[43] The ability to rapidly lyse thrombi is due to several factors.[42] The net activity of plasminogen activators (PA), especially u-PA, is much higher in canine blood fractions than in human blood fractions. In addition, canine platelets have 50 times more lytic activity than human platelets. Human platelets primarily inhibit plasminogen activator activity. Along with this, canine pulmonary endothelial cells secrete u-PA. The canine carotid artery and aorta secrete very little u-PA. One must be aware that pulmonary thromboemboli can be rapidly lysed in dogs, because this knowledge can change therapeutic plans and prognoses.

Acute right heart failure can occur secondary to massive PTE and acute, severe pulmonary hypertension. Acute severe pulmonary and right ventricular hypertension in experimental dogs results in inadequate right ventricular myocardial blood flow creating right ventricular myocardial hypoxia and ischemia.[44] The resultant myocardial failure combined with the marked increase in afterload results in right heart failure.

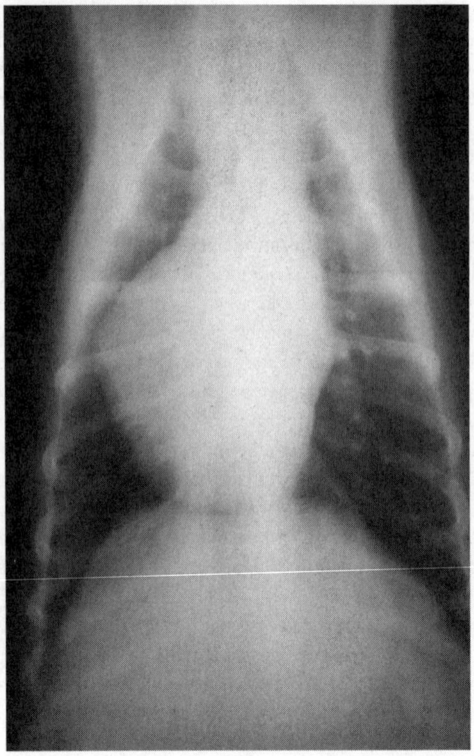

FIGURE 31-3 Dorsoventral thoracic radiograph from a 10-year-old golden retriever presented because it had been coughing for the previous 2 months. The radiograph taken the day of admission revealed right heart enlargement and lack of pulmonary blood vessels on the right side of the thorax. The tentative diagnosis was pulmonary thromboembolism. (Courtesy Dr. Bill Hornof.)

DIAGNOSIS

The antemortem diagnosis of PTE is difficult and often requires specialized diagnostic tests. Thoracic radiographs are variable. They are often normal.[35] Any dog with tachypnea, dyspnea, or hypoxemia that has a normal chest radiograph or only mild changes should be suspected of having PTE, once airway obstruction is ruled out. Thoracic radiographs may, on the other hand, show more specific evidence of PTE. The more common findings include abrupt loss of pulmonary vasculature in a region of lung, increased proximal pulmonary artery size, blunting (pruning) of a pulmonary artery, and lobar pulmonary infiltrates resulting from hemorrhage or edema (infarction) (Figure 31-3).[45] Occasionally, mild pleural effusion, main pulmonary artery enlargement, or right heart enlargement are present.

Arterial blood gas analysis is a sensitive test for PTE but is nonspecific, because one would expect most dyspneic dogs to be hypoxemic regardless of the etiology. Consequently, it is little value except to document the degree of hypoxemia.

Other laboratory tests are of little value in making the diagnosis of PTE but are valuable for detecting predisposing diseases and for detecting sequelae. Blood testing should be performed at the discretion of the clinician and should be guided by clinical signs and physical examination. Evaluation of a clotting profile may be indicated in certain cases.

Large thromboemboli are occasionally identified on two-dimensional echocardiography if they are in the main pulmonary artery or proximal major branches (Figure 31-4; Box 31-3). A Doppler examination can identify pulmonary hypertension if there is tricuspid or pulmonary regurgitation. Pulmonary hypertension does

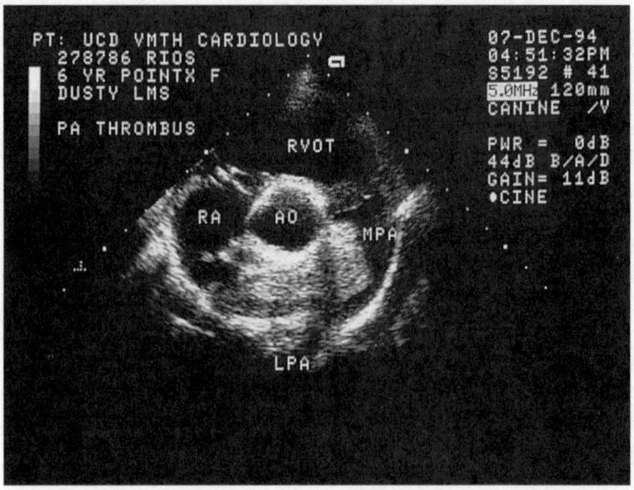

FIGURE 31-4 Two-dimensional echocardiogram from a 6-year-old German shorthaired pointer dog with a large pulmonary thromboembolus or thrombus lodged in the main pulmonary artery *(MPA)*. The echocardiogram is a right parasternal, cross-sectional, basilar view. The entire case is presented in Box 31-3. *RA*, Right atrium; *RVOT*, right ventricular outflow tract; *AO*, aorta.

BOX 31-3

Severe pulmonary embolism: a case study

A six-year-old female German shorthaired pointer cross was presented to the referring veterinarian for dyspnea that the owners noted on returning from vacation. At presentation the dog was dyspneic and respiratory rate was 64 breaths/min. The dog was also depressed and hypothermic (rectal temperature = 95° F). Thoracic radiographs showed an enlarged heart with no pulmonary pathology. She was referred to the University of California, Davis, Veterinary Medical Teaching Hospital Cardiology Service for an echocardiogram. At presentation she was active and alert, with a normal rectal temperature and mild dehydration. She was mildly dyspneic, with increased bronchovesicular sounds. She had jugular pulses that went one third of the way up the neck. However, the jugular veins filled and emptied normally when occluded at the thoracic inlet and released. The patient had a sinus tachycardia (HR = 180 beats/min). Heart sounds were normal. The echocardiogram revealed an enlarged right ventricle that was moderately concentrically and eccentrically hypertrophied. The interventricular septum was flattened in diastole. The region of the foramen ovale was aneurysmal, and color flow Doppler suggested laminar left-to-right shunting between the atria. A contrast echocardiogram using air bubbles injected intravenously demonstrated very mild right-to-left shunting. Moderate tricuspid regurgitation was present on color flow Doppler examination of the right heart. The velocity of the tricuspid regurgitation jet was 4.2 m/sec, which translated into a pressure gradient across the tricuspid valve in systole of 70 mm Hg. We assumed that the right atrial pressure was mildly increased and therefore between 5 and 10 mm Hg. This meant that the right ventricular systolic pressure was approximately 75 to 80 mm Hg (70 mm Hg difference in pressure between the right ventricle and right atrium plus 5 to 10 mm Hg right atrial pressure). There was no evidence of pulmonic stenosis. This meant the dog had pulmonary hypertension with a pulmonary artery systolic pressure of 75 to 80 mm Hg (normal = 15 to 30 mm Hg). Echocardiography of the main pulmonary artery and main branches revealed a large thrombus or thromboembolus that occluded a large part of the main pulmonary artery and almost completely occluded the right pulmonary artery branch (see Figure 31-4). The urine protein:creatinine ratio was markedly increased at 28, indicating a protein-losing glomerulonephropathy as the underlying cause of the PTE. The owner opted not to pursue any definitive treatment for the PTE or the glomerulonephropathy. Two days later, the dog seemed to be doing fine but suddenly collapsed and died. Postmortem examination was not allowed.

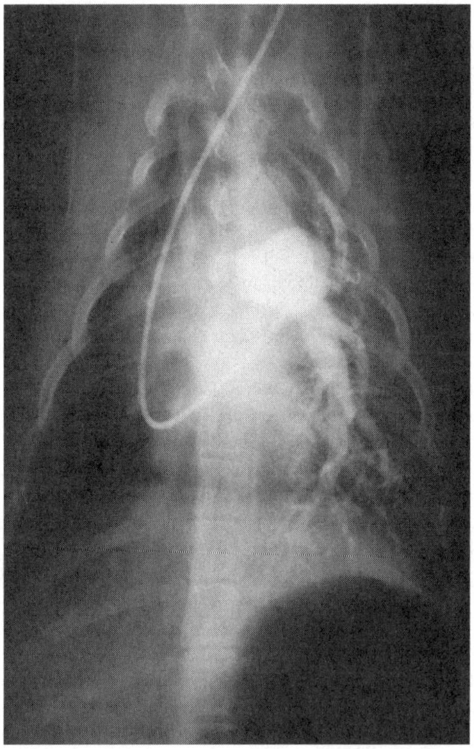

FIGURE 31-5 Dorsoventral view of a pulmonary angiogram from the dog shown in Figure 31-3. A radiopaque contrast agent has been injected into the main pulmonary artery through a catheter that was introduced via a jugular vein. The main pulmonary artery and left branches are outlined normally with the contrast medium because blood flow through them is normal. There is no apparent flow in the vessels on the right side. The diagnosis was a large pulmonary thromboembolus occluding the right main branch of the pulmonary artery. (Courtesy Dr. Bill Hornof.)

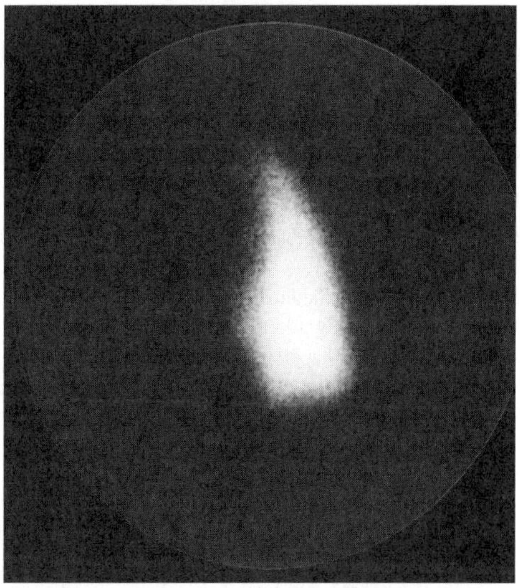

FIGURE 31-6 Dorsoventral view of a pulmonary perfusion scan from the dog shown in Color Plate 120 and Figure 31-4. Radiolabeled albumin was injected into a peripheral vein while the dog was lying on a gamma camera. There is no apparent blood flow to the lungs on the right side of the thorax. Blood flow to the lung on the left side of the thorax appears normal. (Courtesy Dr. Bill Hornof.)

not always exist in dogs with PTE. If severe pulmonary hypertension is present, the right ventricular chamber is usually enlarged on a two-dimensional echocardiogram. The main pulmonary artery or pulmonary artery branches may also be enlarged. The interventricular septum may be flattened, especially in systole, on a two-dimensional echocardiogram. Paradoxical septal motion may be identified on an M-mode echocardiogram.

The definitive diagnosis of PTE can be made with pulmonary angiography, ventilation and perfusion scans, or postmortem examination. Pulmonary angiography is best performed selectively, with the tip of the catheter placed in the pulmonary artery before the injection of contrast media (Figure 31-5). The pulmonary artery pressure should be measured before the injection. Dogs with severe pulmonary hypertension can die acutely following the injection of contrast media into the pulmonary circulation. Consequently, if severe pulmonary hypertension is present, the risk of injecting contrast media must be weighed carefully against the benefit of making a definitive diagnosis. Nonselective angiography can also be used to make a diagnosis, but results are often less than satisfactory. In a dog with PTE, angiography reveals a filling defect or defects if the thromboembolus completely occludes a vessel. Because pulmonary thromboemboli dissolve so rapidly in dogs, angiography should be performed as soon as possible if it is to be used.

Ventilation and perfusion scanning with radioisotopes can also be used to diagnose PTE, but the access to this type of testing is very limited (Figure 31-6; Box 31-4). This type of testing is noninvasive and is associated with very little morbidity or mortality. Perfusion scanning is performed by injecting radiolabeled albumin intravenously. These particles are trapped proximal to the pulmonary capillaries in a distribution pattern identical to blood flow distribution. If the perfusion scan is normal, significant PTE at the time of the scan can be ruled out. Previous PTE cannot be excluded. If the perfusion scan is abnormal, a ventilation scan should be done. Any pulmonary disease that results in regional hypoventilation can produce a region of hypoperfusion by creating regional vasoconstriction. To diagnose PTE one must identify a region of hypoperfusion that is not hypoventilated. Unfortunately, even in university centers, ventilation scanning may not be available. If it is unavailable, making sure that there is no radiographic evidence of pulmonary disease in the region of hypoperfusion may be used in an attempt to rule out regional hypoventilation as the cause of hypoperfusion.

TREATMENT

The primary therapy of canine PTE is supportive and palliative. This is probably appropriate because of the ability of dogs to lyse their own thromboemboli rapidly. In some cases, if life can be supported for several days, resolution of clinical signs may occur. This is especially true if predisposing factors can be controlled. Dogs with massive PTE or dogs with serious underlying disease will not fare as well.

Supportive care for canine patients with PTE includes strict cage rest to reduce tissue oxygen consumption, oxygen therapy to treat the hypoxemia, and treatment of any underlying disease. Fluid therapy is indicated to maintain hydration.

Patients with PTE are at risk for developing more thrombi. Consequently, anticoagulant therapy is usually indicated. Anticoagulants have no thrombolytic activity. Heparin is most commonly used. Doses of 100 to 300 U/kg q 6-8h SC can be used to maintain the partial thromboplastin time at 1.5 to 2.5 times normal or activated clotting time at 1.2 to 1.4 times normal. Clotting times should be measured at baseline and 4 hours after subcutaneous administration.

BOX 31-4

Bleeding complications following anticoagulant therapy: a case study

A 10-year-old golden retriever that weighed 25 kg was presented because of a 2-month history of gradually worsening coughing. The dog had run away for 5 days before the onset of the cough. The pulmonary blood vessels to the right lung lobes on a dorsoventral thoracic radiograph were extremely small to nonexistent (see Figure 31-3). Pulmonary thromboembolism was suspected. To confirm the diagnosis, technetium-labeled albumin was injected into a peripheral vein while the dog was lying on a gamma camera, and the passage of the radiolabeled albumin to the capillaries of patent pulmonary vasculature was observed. The radionuclide angiogram revealed no apparent blood flow to the lung lobes on the right side of the thorax (see Figure 31-6). This was confirmed by anesthetizing the dog and performing a pulmonary angiogram using a iodinated contrast agent (see Figure 31-5). There was no apparent blood flow in the right pulmonary circulation. Consequently, the diagnosis was thromboembolism of the right branch of the pulmonary artery. Hyperadrenocorticism and a protein-losing glomerulonephropathy were ruled out. A baseline coagulation study was performed and the dog was administered coumadin 5 mg (0.2 mg/kg) q24h. Three days later the prothrombin time was 3 times the baseline value. Four days later the prothrombin time was 2.5 times the baseline value. Two weeks later she was presented because of an acute onset of depression and dyspnea. The prothrombin time was 4 times the baseline value, although the owners had not administered the coumadin for the past 2 days. Thoracic radiographs were unchanged. The dog was started on aspirin (25 mg/kg q24h) and dipyridamole (1 mg/kg q8h), an antiplatelet agent. The dog died 2 days later. At necropsy, there was approximately 2 L of blood in the thoracic cavity and hemorrhage in the mesentery, retroperitoneal space, and subcutaneous tissue of the trunk and neck. The intestinal tract contained bloody fecal material. The right branch of the pulmonary artery was occluded by a green-brown thrombus that started 4 cm distal to the pulmonic valve and extended to the origins of the arteries supplying the right lung lobes. The right heart was enlarged, presumably secondary to the pulmonary hypertension. Histopathologic examination of the kidneys revealed a moderate amount of amyloid deposition in the glomeruli. Whether this was severe enough to result in renal loss of antithrombin III was unknown. The dog apparently died of hemorrhagic complications of its anticoagulant therapy.

Bleeding time is usually not affected. Heparin may be less effective in patients with decreased plasma antithrombin III concentration. Administration of fresh or fresh frozen plasma may be helpful in these cases. Heparin should be used only when PTE is confirmed or highly suspected. A heparin overdose can cause bleeding complications, and dogs with serious systemic disease may be at greater risk of developing these complications. Bleeding complications are treated by discontinuing heparin therapy and administering protamine sulfate. Protamine sulfate has an anticoagulant effect when administered alone. When administered with heparin, a stable salt forms, resulting in loss of anticoagulant activity. Protamine's effects are almost immediate and last for about 2 hours. Overdosage results in anticoagulation. Protamine sulfate 1 mg neutralizes about 100 USP units of heparin.

Although warfarin has been recommended for PTE patients in the veterinary literature, we are not aware of anyone that is currently using this drug in dogs with PTE often enough to make recommendations. Recommendations appear to be made on a theoretical basis only.

Thrombolytic agents are used to lyse pulmonary thromboemboli in human medicine.[23] Experience in veterinary medicine is extremely limited and should only be tried as investigational therapy.

REFERENCES

1. Laste NJ, Harpster NK: A retrospective study of 100 cases of feline distal aortic thromboembolism: 1977-1993, *J Am Anim Hosp Assoc* 31:492, 1995.
2. Harpster NK, Baty CJ: Warfarin therapy of the cat at risk of thromboembolism. In Bonagura JD, ed: *Kirk's current veterinary therapy, XII: small animal practice,* Philadelphia, 1995, WB Saunders.
3. Griffiths IR, Duncan ID: Ischaemic neuromyopathy in cats, *Vet Rec* 104:518, 1979.
4. van Winkle TJ, Hackner SG, Liu SM: Clinical and pathological features of aortic thromboembolism in 36 dogs, *Vet Emerg Crit Care* 3:13, 1993.
5. Helenski CA, Ross JN: Platelet aggregation in feline cardiomyopathy, *J Vet Intern Med* 1:24, 1987.
6. Fatkin D, Kelly RP, Feneley MP: Relations between left atrial appendage blood flow velocity, spontaneous echocardiographic contrast and thromboembolic risk in vivo, *J Am Coll Cardiol* 23:961, 1994.
7. Ohta K, Gotoh F, Tomita M et al: Animal species differences in erythrocyte aggregability, *Am J Physiol* 262:H1009, 1992.
8. Weiser MG, Kociba GJ: Platelet concentration and platelet volume distribution in healthy cats, *Am J Vet Res* 45:518, 1984.
9. Tschopp TB: Aggregation of cat platelets in vitro, *Thromb Diath Haemorrh* 23:601, 1970.
10. Butler HC: An investigation into the relationship of an aortic embolus to posterior paralysis in the cat, *J Small Anim Pract* 12:141, 1971.
11. Imhoff RK: Production of aortic occlusion resembling acute aortic embolism syndrome in cats, *Nature* 192:979, 1961.
12. Schaub RG, Meyers KM, Sande RD et al: Inhibition of feline collateral vessel development following experimental thrombolic occlusion, *Circ Res* 39:736, 1976.
13. Schaub RG, Gates KA, Roberts RE: Effect of aspirin on collateral blood flow after experimental thrombosis of the feline aorta, *Am J Vet Res* 43:1647, 1982.
14. Olmstead ML, Butler HC: Five-hydroxytryptamine antagonists and feline aortic embolism, *J Small Anim Pract* 18:247, 1977.
15. Schaub RG, Meyers KM, Sande RD: Serotonin as a factor in depression of collateral blood flow following experimental arterial thrombosis, *J Lab Clin Med* 90:645, 1977.
16. Dodds WJ: Platelet function in animals: species specificities. In deGaetano G, Garattini S, eds: *Platelets: a multidisciplinary approach,* New York, 1978, Raven.
17. Helenski C, Schaub RG, Roberts R: Improvement of collateral circulation after arterial thrombosis with indomethacin therapy, *Thromb Haemost* 44:69, 1980.
18. Pion PD, Kittleson MD: Therapy for feline aortic thromboembolism. In Kirk RW, ed: *Kirk's current veterinary therapy, X: small animal practice,* Philadelphia, 1989, WB Saunders.
19. Fox PR, Dodds WJ: Coagulopathies observed with spontaneous aortic thromboembolism in cardiomyopathic cats, *Proc ACVIM,* 1982, p 83 (abstract).
20. Fox PR: Feline thromboembolism associated with cardiomyopathy, *Proc Annu Vet Med Forum,* 1987, p 714.
21. Fuster V, Verstraete M: Hemostasis, thrombosis, fibrinolysis. and cardiovascular disease. In Braunwald E, ed: *Heart disease: a textbook of cardiovascular medicine,* ed 5, Philadelphia, 1997, WB Saunders.
22. Lindsay Jr J, Beall AC, DeBakey ME: Disease of the aorta. In Hurst JW, Schlant RC, Rackley CE et al, eds: *The heart, arteries, and veins,* ed 7, New York, 1990, McGraw Hill.
23. Marder VJ, Sherry S: Thrombolytic therapy: current status, *N Engl J Med* 318:1512, 1988.
24. LaRue MJ, Murtaugh RJ: Pulmonary thromboembolism in dogs: 47 cases (1986-1987), *J Am Vet Med Assoc* 197:1368, 1990.
25. Lippton HL, Horwitz PM, McNamara DB et al: Influence of verapamil and diltiazem on aggregatory responses in cat and rabbit platelet rich plasma, *Prostaglandins Leukot Med* 16:121, 1984.
26. Utoh J, Zajkowski-Brown JE, Harasaki H: Effect of oral and intravenous diltiazem on whole blood platelet aggregability, *J Invest Surg* 7:533, 1994.

27. Zucker ML, Budd SE, Dollar LE et al: Effect of diltiazem and low-dose aspirin on platelet aggregation and ATP release induced by paired agonists, *Thromb Haemost* 70:332, 1993.
28. Behrend EN, Grauer GF, Greco DS et al: Comparison of the effect of diltiazem and aspirin on platelet aggregation in cats, *J Vet Intern Med* 9:203, 1995 (abstract).
29. Killingsworth CR, Eyster GE, Adams T et al: Streptokinase treatment of cats with experimentally induced aortic thrombosis, *Am J Vet Res* 47:1351, 1986.
30. Pion PD: Feline aortic thromboemboli: t-PA thrombolysis followed by aspirin therapy and rethrombosis, *Vet Clin North Am Small Anim Pract* 18:262, 1988.
31. Jivegard L, Holm J, Schersten T: Arterial thromboembolectomy: should anticoagulants be administered? *Acta Chir Scand* 152:493, 1986.
32. Handin RI, Loscalzo J: Hemostasis, thrombosis, fibrinolysis, and cardiovascular disease. In Braunwald E, ed: *Heart disease: a textbook of cardiovascular medicine,* ed 4, Philadelphia, 1992, WB Saunders.
33. Goldhaber SZ, Hennekens CH, Evans DA et al: Factors associated with correct antemortem diagnosis of major pulmonary embolism, *Am J Med* 73:822, 1982.
34. Hargis AM, Stephens LC, Benjamin SA et al: Relationship of hypothyroidism to diabetes mellitus, renal amyloidosis, and thrombosis in purebred beagles, *Am J Vet Res* 42:1077, 1981.
35. Keyes ML, Rush JE, Knowles KE: Pulmonary thromboembolism in dogs, *Vet Emerg Crit Care* 3:23, 1993.
36. Greco DS, Green RA: Coagulation abnormalities associated with thrombosis in a dog with nephrotic syndrome, *Compend Cont Educ Pract Vet* 9:653, 1987.
37. Rasedee A, Feldman BF, Washabau R: Naturally occurring canine nephrotic syndrome is a potentially hypercoagulable state, *Acta Vet Scand* 27:369, 1986.
38. Feldman BF, Feldman EC, Cowgill LD: Thrombotic disease in canine Cushing's and nephrotic syndromes, *Proc ACVIM,* 1982, p 84 (abstract).
39. Feldman BF, Attix EA, Strombeck DR et al: Biochemical and coagulation changes in a canine model of acute necrotizing pancreatitis, *Am J Vet Res* 42:805, 1981.
40. West JB: *Pulmonary pathophysiology: the essentials,* Baltimore, 1978, Williams & Wilkins.
41. Dantzker DR, Wagner PD, Tornabene VW et al: Gas exchange after pulmonary thromboembolization in dogs, *Circ Res* 42:92, 1978.
42. Lang IM, Marsh JJ, Konopka RG et al: Factors contributing to increased vascular fibrinolytic activity in mongrel dogs, *Circulation* 87:1990, 1993.
43. Dalen JE, Mathur VS, Evans H et al: Pulmonary angiography in experimental pulmonary embolism, *Am Heart J* 72:509, 1966.
44. Vlahakes GJ, Turley K, Hoffman JI: The pathophysiology of failure in acute right ventricular hypertension: hemodynamic and biochemical correlations, *Circulation* 63:87, 1981.
45. Fluckiger MA, Gomez JA: Radiographic findings in dogs with spontaneous pulmonary thromboembolism or embolism, *Vet Radiol* 25:124, 1984.

CHAPTER 32

The Effects of Systemic Disease on the Cardiovascular System

The effects of certain systemic, metabolic, and endocrine abnormalities on cardiac performance and function are well chronicled in the human literature. Although many of the same disorders are recognized in dogs and cats, the effects on the cardiovascular system are not well described, either because they are less clinically apparent in animals or they do not occur. This chapter discusses the effects of noncardiovascular disorders that are *frequently* recognized in the dog and cat on cardiovascular performance. This chapter is not intended to be exhaustive but includes only clinically important and well-recognized disorders. Further, this material is not intended to be a comprehensive review of each of these disorders.

Vascular Disease

The effect of most vascular diseases is to create either a pressure or volume overload on the heart, thereby invoking the mechanisms for either eccentric or concentric hypertrophy and, if severe enough, leading to secondary changes and effects. Most of the peripheral or pulmonary vascular disorders that are recognized with any frequency in dogs and cats have been discussed in previous chapters. These include cor pulmonale, pulmonary hypertension, pulmonary thromboembolism, and systemic hypertension (see Chapter 26) and heartworm disease and caval syndrome (see Chapter 23).

ARTERIOVENOUS SHUNTS (FISTULAS)

An arteriovenous shunt (fistula) is an abnormal vascular communication that allows blood to flow from an artery to a vein without traversing a capillary bed. Extracardiac arteriovenous shunts may be congenital, which occur as single or multiple communications, or acquired, which are typically single communications.[1] The most common form of a congenital arteriovenous fistula in dogs and cats is a patent ductus arteriosus (see Chapter 12). Acquired arteriovenous shunts are usually the result of blunt or penetrating trauma or neovascularization associated with neoplastic growths.[2] Although they typically involve the extremities, arteriovenous shunts can occur anywhere in the body.[1]

The local and systemic effects of arteriovenous shunts result from the shunting of blood from the high-resistance systemic arterial system into the low-resistance systemic venous system. Regionally, venous blood is hyperoxygenated and may cause proliferation in the affected vessels and therefore increase the number of arteriovenous communications.[1] The effected region may feel warmer than surrounding areas, may be edematous and swollen, and may be painful. Dermatologic abnormalities such as necrosis, ulceration, and abnormal pigmentation in the skin overlying the region have also been reported.[1,2] Turbulence within the communication results in a continuous bruit (murmur) and fremitus (palpable thrill).

Systemically, the continuous shunting of blood, if of significant volume, may lead to a generalized volume overload with increased blood volume and eccentric hypertrophy of all cardiac chambers. Typically systolic function is maintained and is often hyperdynamic. With very large shunts, the increase in end-diastolic pressure may be enough to produce signs of congestive heart failure. Cardiac output is typically elevated, such that the clinical syndrome may be called *high-output cardiac failure.*[3] Ultimately, systolic myocardial failure may develop further, exacerbating the signs of congestive heart failure. When the arteriovenous shunt is in the systemic circulation, signs of right heart failure may predominate, although pulmonary edema is also usually present.

The ideal therapy is to surgically ligate the communicating vessels. However, surgical correction is often limited by multiple microscopic connections and the physical location of the shunt. In patients with congestive heart failure the use of diuretics may be palliative.

Thyroid Dysfunction

Thyroid hormone has profound effects on metabolic processes in many tissues. The myocardium is particularly sensitive to the effects of thyroid hormone, and increased or decreased concentrations of circulating thyroid hormone can produce clinically significant changes in the cardiovascular system.

The thyroid gland secretes two biologically active hormones: triiodothyronine (T_3) and thyroxine (T_4). Triiodothyronine is the major mediator of thyroid actions. Thyroxine is less active than T_3 and serves primarily as a circulating reservoir for conversion into T_3. Most evidence suggests that one of the major sites of action of thyroid hormone is within the cell nucleus, where it binds to a chromatin-bound nonhistone nucleoprotein, creating alterations in protein synthesis.[4,5] In many tissues, the biologic response includes changes in the activity of membrane-bound Na^+,K^+- ATPases and Ca^+-ATPases and altered responsiveness to the sympathetic nervous system.[6]

EFFECTS OF THYROID HORMONE ON THE HEART

Several studies have identified direct effects of thyroid hormone on the myocardium.[7-11] The results of these and other studies suggest that the major physiologic actions of thyroid hormone on the myocardium are (1) a direct positive inotropic effect, (2) stimulation of myocardial hypertrophy, and (3) increased responsiveness to adrenergic stimulation.

Thyroid hormone increases the activity of sarcolemmal Na^+,K^+-ATPase by more than 50% when administered to hypothyroid rats.[12] Some authors suggest this is due to an increase in functional enzyme complexes related to the increased rate of protein synthesis. Increased synthesis of ventricular myosin and alterations in myosin structure result in a predominance of a myosin isoenzyme with fast ATPase activity that in part explains the changes in the myocardial contractile properties.[6] Increased myocardial oxygen consumption is thought to result from an increase in protein synthesis and increased glucose and calcium transport rather than a direct effect of thyroid hormone on the mitochondria, as previously believed.[6]

The effect of thyroid hormone on myocardial contractility is also mediated through changes in cellular calcium handling as a result of increases in the number of L-type calcium channels in the sarcolemma and an enhanced efficiency of sarcoplasmic reticulum calcium uptake and release.[6]

Overall, the clinically recognizable effects of excess thyroid hormone include increased heart rate, increased inotropic state of the myocardium, and increased ventricular size and mass.[6,7] These opposite influences are evident when thyroid hormone is deficient.

RELATIONSHIPS BETWEEN THYROID HORMONE, THE SYMPATHETIC NERVOUS SYSTEM, AND THE HEART

Although there are many documented direct effects of thyroid hormone on the heart, it has been postulated that some effects are secondary, mediated through changes in the interaction of the thyroid hormone with the sympathetic nervous system. Such theories stem from the fact that many of the effects of hyperthyroidism can be abolished or reduced by β-adrenergic blockade.[6]

Several reports have shown that administration of thyroid hormone can cause the number or affinity of β-adrenergic receptors to increase. These effects vary across species and tissues.[6,13,14] The changes in receptor number and affinity in the myocardium correlate with changes in the sensitivity of the myocardium of hyperthyroid animals to β-adrenergic receptor agonists.[13] It remains unclear whether thyroid hormone also exerts additional effects that could alter sensitivity to adrenergic stimuli. It has also been proposed that thyroid hormone may increase the activity of the sympathoadrenal system.[14]

HYPOTHYROIDISM

The "myxedema" heart in humans was first described in 1918 by a physician who noted a dilated cardiac silhouette, slow indolent heart action, and low electrocardiographic voltage, which were all corrected by thyroid hormone replacement therapy. Although invasive and noninvasive studies have confirmed that thyroid hormone deficiency is associated with a reversible decrease in myocardial contractility, it remains controversial whether hypothyroidism alone can cause myocardial failure (dilated cardiomyopathy) and congestive heart failure in dogs.[15,16]

Three ventricular myosin isoenzymes are known to exist (see Chapter 2), and their expression is dictated not only by stage of development (fetal vs. adult) but also by thyroid hormone status. The regulation of the isoenzymes is accomplished through control of the genes coding for the α and β myosin heavy chains (MHC).[15] In rats with induced hypothyroidism, MHC β mRNA is the predominant message, with only slightly detectable expression of MHC α mRNA. This leads to a change in the predominant form of MHC expressed from V_1 to V_3. Administration of T_3 to hypothyroid animals leads to significant increases in MHC α mRNA within only a few hours of administration and return to normal values within 24 hours.[17] Myosin isoenzymes in adult dogs and humans are different from those in rodents and, although not as extensively studied as in the rat, thyroid hormone is thought to alter myosin isoenzyme gene expression in a manner analogous to rodents.[15,18]

In recent years the availability of highly specific radioligands has permitted the identification and direct quantitation of α- and β-adrenergic receptors in hypothyroidism. It is also possible to examine biochemical and physiologic outcomes of receptor occupancy and to assess the influence of thyroid hormone deficiency on the receptor-adenylate cyclase complex. The adrenergic effects of hyperthyroidism are well known, and many of the effects seen with hypothyroidism are opposite in direction and related to decreased responsiveness to catecholamines. The number of β-receptors in the hypothyroid rat myocardium is reduced 30% to 40%. No change in receptor affinity has been reported in mammals.[13] The maximal response to isoproterenol has also been shown to be reduced.[19,20] Similarly, it has been reported that the chronotropic and inotropic responses of hypothyroid rat atria to isoproterenol are significantly reduced and that normal responses can be restored by the administration of thyroid hormone.[20] Thus deficiency of thyroid hormone reduces both cardiac β-receptor number and physiologic responsiveness, with the reduction in effect being almost entirely the result of decreased receptor number. The decreases in cardiac β-receptor number parallels decreases observed in the genes coding for the receptor, as well as the level of β-receptor mRNA.[6,15]

Clinical manifestations. Hypothyroidism is a commonly recognized endocrinopathy in the dog. Idiopathic atrophy and immune-mediated thyroiditis are the most common causes in the dog.[21] Clinical signs usually develop in middle-age and are variable. In adult dogs, signs of decreased cellular metabolism (e.g., mental dullness, exercise intolerance, and lethargy) predominate. Signs involving the skin, reproductive system, and neuromuscular system are also frequently recognized. Ocular, cardiovascular, gastrointestinal, and clotting abnormalities are uncommon manifestations of canine hypothyroidism.[21] The most commonly reported cardiovascular signs include bradycardia, a weak cardiac apex beat, and cardiac arrhythmias.[22,23] Human patients with thyroid deficiency have a threefold increased incidence of systemic hypertension, but this association has not been reported in canine hypothyroidism to our knowledge.[24]

Changes in the electrocardiogram (ECG) are usually only evident with severe hypothyroidism. In humans, electrocardiographic changes associated with hypothyroidism include sinus bradycardia, conduction disturbances, low QRS complex voltage, deviations of the mean electrical axis, prolongation of the QRS complex interval, and flattened or inverted *T* waves.[25] In dogs with spontaneous primary hypothyroidism, the most frequently observed ECG abnormalities are low QRS voltage, inverted *T* waves, and sinus bradycardia.[26] In dogs with experimentally induced hypothyroidism, prolongation of the PR interval suggests there may be abnormalities of atrioventricular nodal conduction associated with thyroid hormone deficiency.[27] However, this has not been documented in dogs with spontaneous disease. Uncommonly, atrial fibrillation or other arrhythmias may develop. Many of these abnormalities reverse with thyroid hormone supplementation, and there appears to be a correlation between ECG changes and the severity of thyroid deficiency.[26]

Myocardial changes induced by hypothyroidism are measurable in vivo and in vitro as reductions in the velocity of contraction, the force developed during contraction, and the rate of relaxation. In humans with hypothyroidism, reversible reductions in ventricular pump function have been documented; however, congestive heart failure is rare in the absence of underlying heart disease.[28] Similarly, reduced left ventricular pump function has been demonstrated in dogs with experimentally induced hypothyroidism.[16,29] Abnormal echocardiographic findings in dogs include thinning of the left ventricular posterior wall and septum, reduced shortening fraction, decreased left ventricular posterior wall excursion, and alterations in systolic and diastolic time intervals.[16] In a study of echocardiographic variables in eleven dogs with spontaneous hypothyroidism, end-systolic left ventricular dimension was mildly increased and left ventricular shortening fraction was mildly decreased, with values returning to normal after thyroid replacement in all but one dog.[30] Administration of thyroid hormone to normal dogs did not result in significant alteration in echocardiographic measures.[31]

In dogs, atherosclerosis of the coronary vessels resulting from derangements in serum lipid and cholesterol profiles may be an inciting factor leading to the development of arrhythmias[32] and reductions in left ventricular pump function.[33,34] Despite the above abnormalities, there have been no reports of echocardiographic, hemodynamic, or pathologic abnormalities suggestive of congestive heart failure in dogs with spontaneous hypothyroidism. Hypothyroidism is rare in the cat.

Role of hypothyroidism in dilated cardiomyopathy. Patients with dilated cardiomyopathy have a poor long-term prognosis. As demonstrated with taurine deficiency in cats and American cocker spaniels and carnitine deficiency in a small population of humans and dogs, identification of a specific and treatable underlying metabolic abnormality can lead to reversal of the hemodynamic and morphologic abnormalities.[35-37] It has been suggested that hypothyroidism may play a role in the development of canine idiopathic dilated cardiomyopathy. Currently, the relationship between hypothyroidism and canine dilated cardiomyopathy has not been documented convincingly, and no relationship has yet been drawn between hypothyroidism and overt congestive heart failure. In a study of 13 dogs with dilated cardiomyopathy, only five were found to have subnormal serum thyroid hormone concentration.[33] Only one of these dogs had an abnormally low response to a thyroid-stimulating hormone test.

Until a relationship between hypothyroidism and canine dilated cardiomyopathy is proved, care must be taken when evaluating the results of thyroid hormone screening in dogs with congestive heart failure, because any severe illness can falsely lower the basal thyroid hormone concentration when thyroid function is actually normal (euthyroid sick syndrome).[38]

HYPERTHYROIDISM

Unlike hypothyroidism, hyperthyroidism is commonly associated with significant cardiovascular manifestations that must be considered in the management of individual patients. These may include but are not limited to increased susceptibility to dysrhythmias during anesthetic procedures, ventricular hypertrophy (concentric or eccentric), systemic hypertension, and congestive heart failure.[39]

The cardiac changes associated with hyperthyroidism are mediated by both direct and indirect effects on the heart and vasculature. The sums of these effects are a heart that operates at a faster rate (tachycardia), is larger (hypertrophied), can contract faster and more powerfully (enhanced contractility), and has a propensity to develop abnormal electrical depolarizations (tachyarrhythmias). Although many of these might, at first glance, sound like beneficial changes (larger, faster, stronger, more excitable), the thyrotoxic state strains the energy economy of the heart and increases the overall work of the heart. Additionally, the thyrotoxic heart, although hyperkinetic when the patient is at rest has less "reserve capacity" available when increased cardiac work is necessary (e.g., exercise).[40] This situation, especially when placed on top of preexisting cardiac disease, results in many significant clinical cardiac manifestations in hyperthyroid patients.[40]

Many direct actions of thyroid hormone on the heart are amplified during hyperthyroidism.[6,24] These include increased myocardial protein synthesis (mitochondrial, ion pump, and contractile proteins), alteration of myosin subtype ("slow" to "fast" types of myosin; V_3 to V_1), less efficient energy conversion from chemical (ATP) energy to mechanical (force) energy by the myocardium, increased rate of calcium cycling by the sarcoplasmic reticulum, up-regulation of cardiac β-receptors, enhanced rate of spontaneous depolarization by sinoatrial node cells, and a shortened action potential duration.

Myocardial hypertrophy is a prominent feature of feline hyperthyroidism and is attributed to the combined effects of chronic volume overload, high sympathetic tone, systemic hypertension, and direct stimulation of contractile protein synthesis by thyroid hormone.[6,24,40,41] There is evidence that hyperthyroidism increases the synthesis of myosin and alters its structure. The alteration of its structure leads primarily to an increase in its contractile properties, particularly by increasing the faster myosin isoenzyme V_1. In hypothyroid rats, the mRNA for α MHC is substantially reduced, whereas the β MHC, which primarily forms the slower V_3 myosin isoform, is substantially increased.[42]

Thyrotoxicosis greatly increases the number of sarcolemmal slow calcium channels that augment transarcolemmal calcium influx in cultured ventricular cells.[6] In ferret ventricles, hyperthyroidism increases peak tension and prolongs the duration of contraction in association with changes in cytosolic calcium that are increased and prolonged in relation to euthyroid animals.[6]

Thus the heart responds to thyrotoxicosis by increasing synthesis of the fast myosin isoform, with enhanced ATPase activity and enhanced cycling and recycling of calcium. The augmented myosin ATPase activity and alterations in intracellular calcium handling appear to directly contribute to the thyroid-induced changes in myocardial contractile function.

As previously stated, it has been proposed that thyroid hormone may alter the relationship between the sympathetic nervous system and the cardiovascular system, either by increasing sympathetic activity or by enhancing the response of the cardiac tissue to adrenergic stimuli. It has also been suggested that adrenergic stimuli merely exert a direct additive effect to that produced by thyroid hormone itself.[6] Furthermore, there is evidence that chronic hyperthyroidism may actually reduce the sensitivity of cardiac tissue to sympathetic stimuli.[6]

In humans, plasma and urine concentrations of catecholamines and β-hydroxylase are either low or normal in patients with hyperthyroidism, suggesting that the sympathomimetic features of the disease are not simply the result of increased adrenergic activity.[43] This suggests that the increased sympathetic activity associated with hyperthyroidism may stem from increased β-adrenergic receptor number or affinity or postreceptor events.

Tissues derived from hyperthyroid human patients demonstrate enhanced adenylate cyclase activity (membrane homogenates) and force of contraction (muscle strips) in response to isoproterenol.[6] Enhanced β-adrenergic activity has also been demonstrated in vivo in hyperthyroid dogs, which had greater reductions in heart rate and myocardial contractility in response to propranolol compared with euthyroid dogs.[11]

Enhanced metabolic activity in other tissues results in a "high cardiac output state" in which the heart must increase its throughput to meet the increased demands of the peripheral tissues resulting from excess circulating thyroid hormone.[6,24] Thus reduced systemic vascular resistance plays an important role in the overall cardiac status of patients with hyperthyroidism. Resistance is reduced, and intravascular volume is increased. Reduced systemic vascular resistance in the presence of an increased intravascular volume (not documented in cats to our knowledge) leads to significant increases in cardiac output. This high cardiac output state can (especially in the presence of underlying primary cardiac pathology) progress to result in clinically apparent signs of congestive heart failure in human hyperthyroid patients.

Atrial natriuretic factor is elevated in hyperthyroid humans.[44] Atrial natriuretic factor was found to be elevated in some hyperthyroid cats with left ventricular concentric hypertrophy, suggesting concurrent systemic hypertension.[45] Atrial natriuretic factor in hyperthyroid cats decreased significantly after treatment. The significance of changes in atrial natriuretic factor concentration in hyperthyroid patients is unknown but may influence the clinical status both before (hypertension) and after (reduced glomerular filtration rate and azotemia) treatment.

Clinical manifestations. Hyperthyroidism is one of the most common feline endocrine disorders, with a reported incidence from one source of 1 out of 300 cats.[22] Functional thyroid adenoma (adenomatous hyperplasia) involving one or both thyroid lobes is the primary abnormality found in hyperthyroid cats. In contrast, most canine thyroid tumors are malignant (adenocarcinoma), and nonfunctional and clinical hyperthyroidism in dogs is quite rare.

Abnormalities of the cardiovascular system are detected in most hyperthyroid cats, and some develop signs of congestive heart failure.[39-41,46] In early studies, congestive heart failure was detected in as many as 20% of affected cats. The prevalence of this complication appears to have declined with increased awareness and earlier diagnosis.[47] A variety of clinical signs may be observed in cats with hyperthyroidism, many of which are relatively mild and are manifestations of the increased cardiac output rather than overt or impending heart failure.[24,39-41,48-50] Increased resting heart rate is one of the most consistent clinical findings in hyperthyroid cats. The intensity of the heart sounds and the force of the precordial impulse are often accentuated. Some affected cats exhibit open-mouth breathing (dyspnea) when stressed, even in the absence of congestive heart failure. Other common findings include strong-to-bounding arterial pulses, mildly distended jugular veins, a jugular venous pulse, an apical systolic murmur, cardiac dysrhythmias, and gallop sounds.[24,39-41,48,49]

Despite the statement of reduced systemic vascular resistance in hyperthyroid patients, hypertension, rather than hypotension, is observed in many hyperthyroid cats.[51,52] Increased systolic blood pressure in hyperthyroidism results primarily from an increased peak rate of left ventricular ejection and increased stroke volume. Because most hyperthyroid cats are old, aortic vascular compliance may also be diminished, contributing to the increased peak systolic pressure. Pronounced elevation in both systolic and diastolic pressures is observed in some hyperthyroid cats.[24,51] Hypertension resolves in most treated cases once a euthyroid state is reached. Increased systemic vascular resistance may develop in some affected cats as a result of the combined influences of age, renal disease, high sympathetic outflow, and vascular remodeling.

Numerous ECG abnormalities have been reported in cats with hyperthyroidism (in one study 80% of cats had at least one abnormal finding).[46,48,50,53] The most frequently reported abnormalities include sinus tachycardia and increased QRS complex voltage. Supraventricular and ventricular arrhythmias, probably the result of increased β-adrenergic sensitivity, and conduction abnormalities (left axis deviation, increased QRS complex duration, etc.) are occasionally observed.[46,50,53]

Recently, it has been reported that there was a reduced prevalence of sinus tachycardia and increased *R* wave voltage in a group of 95 cats with hyperthyroidism evaluated in 1992 versus cats evaluated between 1979 and 1982.[47] It was suggested that these changes were due to either earlier diagnosis or the diagnosis of a population of previously untested, mildly affected cats.

Both the direct actions of thyroid hormone and the influence of the sympathetic nervous system probably account for the ECG changes associated with elevated thyroid hormone levels. The ability of β-adrenergic antagonists to restore normal resting heart rates in hyperthyroid cats provides indirect evidence for the contribution of the sympathetic nervous system.[54-56] Many of the arrhythmias resolve after successful restoration of the euthyroid state.

Thoracic radiographs in cats with hyperthyroidism often reveal generalized cardiomegaly. Pleural effusion or pulmonary edema, resulting from congestive heart failure, may also be observed in some patients.[50]

Echocardiographic changes reported in hyperthyroid cats include biatrial enlargement, increased dimensions of the aortic root, thickening of the interventricular septum and left ventricular posterior wall, increased diastolic dimension of the left ventricle, increased or decreased systolic dimension of the left ventricle, and an increased or decreased fractional shortening.[57,58] The echocardiographic changes that, in our experience, most typify hyperthyroidism are hyperkinetic left ventricular free wall and septal motion with left ventricular dilation (eccentric hypertrophy) and varying degrees of left atrial enlargement. In general the left ventricular wall and septal thicknesses are not excessive in relation to the chamber dimensions and do not resemble the typical changes associated with hypertrophic cardiomyopathy.

In our experience, many cats with hyperthyroidism and marked left ventricular concentric hypertrophy are also hypertensive. However, there are occasional nonhypertensive hyperthyroid cats with marked left ventricular concentric hypertrophy. Whether the hypertrophy in these cases is a result of the hyperthyroidism or coincident primary hypertrophic cardiomyopathy in a hyperthyroid cat is unknown.

There are reports of hyperthyroid cats with myocardial failure, demonstrating marked increases in left ventricular end-diastolic and end-systolic dimensions, moderate-to-severe left atrial enlargement and a reduction in shortening fraction.[39] The relationship of this presentation to a deficiency of the amino acid taurine is unknown. However, this presentation, albeit rare, has persisted since cat food manufacturers rectified dietary deficiencies of taurine in cats.

Canine thyrotoxicosis is clinically variable with abrupt or insidious onset. Signs range in severity, with polyuria and polydipsia predominating.[21] Cardiovascular manifestations are subtle and include hyperkinetic femoral pulses and apical precordial beats.[59] Overt congestive heart failure is rare in dogs with hyperthyroidism. Heart rates seldom exceed the normal range, and, although ECG evidence of left ventricular enlargement may be observed, the ECG is usually normal in dogs with hyperthyroidism.[60] Although there have been no reports of radiographic or echocardiographic findings in dogs with hyperthyroidism, it is expected they are similar to those reported in cats.

Many of the clinical manifestations of hyperthyroidism are reversible with restoration of a euthyroid state.[51,57] Even some cats with severe congestive heart failure may, after successful treatment of their hyperthyroidism, no longer require cardiac medications. However, we have seen at least one cat with severe myocardial failure worsen following successful treatment of the hyperthyroidism.

Adrenal Dysfunction

HYPOADRENOCORTICISM (ADDISON'S DISEASE)

Addison's disease is produced by a deficiency of either cortisol or mineralocorticoid secretion from the adrenal gland. Cortisol is gluconeogenic, catabolic, has antiinsulin activity, stimulates erythropoiesis, and reduces calcium absorption from the gastrointestinal tract by interfering with vitamin D activity.[6] Cortisol also plays a role in vascular tone by maintaining vascular integrity and responsiveness to circulating vasoconstrictors. Aldosterone controls extracellular fluid volume by its modulation of sodium excretion and potassium absorption in the renal collecting ducts.[6] Adrenal insufficiency has been associated with decreased cardiac wall motion, cardiac output, heart rate, and peak left ventricular work.[22] These cardiac manifestations are primarily related to the volume depletion associated with aldosterone deficiency and the bradycardia and electrocardiographic abnormalities associated with hyperkalemia.[6,22] Electrocardiographic changes include tall, peaked *T* waves, reduced amplitude or absent *P* waves (sinoventricular conduction), increased PR and QT intervals, increased QRS duration, and low-amplitude complexes (see Chapter 5).[22] Although stress in patients with Addison's disease has been known to cause cardiovascular collapse and death, congestive heart failure is only rarely identified in humans.[61] Musselman[62] reported heart failure in dogs with Addison's disease and identified reversible echocardiographic myocardial failure in cats with suspect hypocortisolism. In our experience, these findings are extremely rare.

HYPERADRENOCORTICISM (CUSHING'S DISEASE OR SYNDROME)

Canine hyperadrenocorticism is most often secondary to functional pituitary tumors but may also be primary, associated with benign or malignant functional adrenal tumors.[24] Heart failure secondary to severe hypertension has been reported in humans with hyperadrenocorticism.[63] The hypertension is felt to reflect increased sodium and water retention, increased vascular sensitivity to vasopressors, and cortisol-induced activation of the renin-angiotensin system.[6] Reportedly, 50% of dogs with hyperadrenocorticism are hypertensive at the time of diagnosis.[62,64]

Dogs with hyperadrenocorticism have also been reported to have radiographic and echocardiographic evidence of cardiomegaly and a coincident occurrence of congestive heart failure.[22] However, hyperadrenocorticism tends to occur in aged dogs and in breeds that are prone to acquired myxomatous valvular disease. In our experience, cardiomegaly and congestive heart failure are uncommon in dogs with Cushing's syndrome without concomitant valvular disease. However, in those patients with concomitant valvular disease, hypertension, if present, certainly may worsen the mitral regurgitation.

Probably the most common and serious cardiac complication of hyperadrenocorticism is pulmonary thromboembolism (see Chapter 31). Although the incidence of pulmonary thromboembolism in dogs with Cushing's syndrome is relatively low, the majority of dogs with confirmed pulmonary thromboembolism that have a cause identified have hyperadrenocorticism.

PRIMARY ALDOSTERONISM

Primary aldosteronism (Conn's disease) has been reported in one dog and two cats.[24,65,66] In humans, excessive aldosterone secretion produces hypernatremia, hypokalemia, and systemic hypertension.[6,63] Cardiovascular manifestations include left ventricular concentric hypertrophy secondary to the systemic hypertension and electrocardiographic changes associated with the electrolyte abnormalities, including various arrhythmias. The one affected dog had borderline systemic hypertension, hypernatremia and mild hypokalemia. Sinus tachycardia and ST segment depression with a mildly increased *P* wave amplitude were noted on ECG.[65] The reported cats exhibited severe hypokalemia, atrioventricular conduction abnormalities, and increased QRS and QT interval durations. One cat also had hypertensive retinopathy, a cardiac murmur, and prominent *U* waves. The other cat had hypernatremia, paroxysmal ventricular tachycardia, and diminished *T* wave amplitude.[24,66]

PHEOCHROMOCYTOMA

Functional adrenal medullary tumors are extremely rare in both humans and animals.[6,67] However, when present, they can have profound and serious cardiac manifestations and carry a relatively poor prognosis unless surgical removal is possible. Cardiac manifestations may be related to local invasion, usually of the caudal vena cava, or the effects of excessive catecholamine release. Local invasion of the caudal vena cava is common, reported in five of 13 cases in one report.[67] In this same study, two of these five dogs also had ascites associated with caudal vena caval obstruction. In humans, renal, hepatic, and adrenal vessels are also commonly invaded by the tumor. Multiple cardiovascular manifestations are reported in humans, including systemic hypertension with left ventricular concentric hypertrophy, orthostatic hypotension, and various electrocardiographic abnormalities. Dogs usually present with nonspecific signs involving multiple organ systems. In the report cited above, two dogs died suddenly and two manifested signs of congestive heart failure. Systemic hypertension is identified in approximately 50% of dogs in which systemic blood pressure is measured, and left ventricular enlargement and atrial and ventricular ectopic arrhythmias appear common.[67,68] Sinus tachycardia is the most common electrocardiographic finding in dogs, occurring in 15% to 54% of reported cases.[67,68]

Acromegaly

Growth hormone excess is recognized in both dogs and cats.[69,70] Although rare in both species, it is more commonly recognized in cats. In cats the most common etiology is a functional pituitary adenoma, whereas in dogs it is more commonly associated with prolonged progesterone use.[69,70] Many biologic effects are influenced by growth hormone and the somatomedins it simulates. Most are mitigated through an increase in protein synthesis and a reduction in protein catabolism or modulations in glucose utilization and storage. Growth hormone is also a potent diabetogenic hormone, and therefore diabetes mellitus is the most commonly recognized clinical syndrome in affected animals.

In a study of 14 cats with acromegaly, Peterson et al[70] identified thirteen as having "cardiomyopathy." Systolic murmurs and/or gallop sounds were detected in nine, radiographic cardiomegaly was identified in 12, and echocardiographic ventricular concentric hypertrophy was identified in seven of eight cats examined. Signs referable to congestive heart failure were reported in six cats. A postmortem diagnosis of dilated cardiomyopathy was made in one cat from this study. At our institution, we have noted that cardiac changes are only rarely noted in cats with pituitary tumors and signs consistent with acromegaly.

One report describes a cat with hypersomatotropism without clinical evidence of acromegaly or diabetes mellitus that had hypertrophic cardiomyopathy, hyperinsulinemia, glucose intolerance, and signs of congestive heart failure.[71] A more recent study examined the relationship between hypertrophic cardiomyopathy and hypersomatotropism in 31 cats.[72] Mean serum growth hormone concentration was significantly elevated in cats with hypertrophic cardiomyopathy (HCM) compared with normal cats and cats with other cardiac disorders. However, only half of the cats with HCM in this study had growth hormone levels outside the normal reference range. None of these cats had signs referable to acromegaly or diabetes mellitus, and of the eight cats that were necropsied, none had pituitary adenomas. Although there may be a relationship between HCM and hypersomatotropism in some cats, these findings suggest that the cardiac hypertrophy seen in cats with acromegaly is different from idiopathic HCM, and that the increase in serum growth hormone concentration in some cats with HCM is more likely an effect, rather than a cause, of the heart disease.

Little is known about hypersomatatropism in dogs because of its rare occurrence and milder clinical presentation than in cats. Cardiomegaly, but not heart failure, has been reported in dogs with hypersomatotropism.[22]

Diabetes Mellitus

A multitude of significant cardiovascular abnormalities are recognized in humans with diabetes mellitus. Most notably, humans with type I and type II diabetes have an increased incidence of systemic hypertension, cardiac arrhythmias, and coronary atherosclerosis.[6] Further, myocardial infarctions are more severe in diabetic patients, resulting in increased morbidity and mortality compared with nondiabetic patients.[73] It is felt that a combination of coronary microvascular and macrovascular disease, systemic hypertension, autonomic neuropathy, and a greater incidence of stroke and peripheral vascular thrombosis are responsible for more severe cardiac disease in diabetic patients. Also, the existence of a unique cardiomyopathy, diabetic cardiomyopathy, is now well accepted.[73] This form of cardiomyopathy is associated with coronary microvascular disease in a prolonged diabetic state with histologic changes characterized by myocyte hypertrophy, fibrosis, glycoprotein accumulation, and coronary microvascular endothelial and subendothelial proliferation. The pathogenesis of the syndrome is still largely unresolved. However, more recently it has been shown that diabetic cardiomyopathy is milder in patients without coronary macrovascular disease or systemic hypertension. Further, a large multicenter study determined that diabetic cardiomyopathy in its isolated form is mild, uncommon, and significantly related only to age and duration of disease.[74]

Dogs with diabetes mellitus are at increased risk of developing systemic hypertension and pulmonary thromboembolism. An increased risk of coronary artery disease has not been demonstrated in diabetic dogs or cats.[75] Mild reductions in left ventricular systolic function in experimentally induced diabetes has been shown in the dog.[24] Further, an inverse correlation was identified between glycosylated hemoglobin and left ventricular fractional shortening in these dogs.[24] Congestive cardiac failure has not been reported secondary to diabetes mellitus in domestic dogs or cats.

Electrolyte Abnormalities

Virtually any electrolyte that influences ion movements across the sarcolemma may induce electrocardiographic abnormalities when present in either excessive or diminished concentrations. However, the severity and clinical significance of the abnormalities vary considerably. The most important electrolyte imbalances that have cardiovascular manifestations are imbalances in calcium, potassium, and magnesium. The electrocardiographic changes associated with hyperkalemia are discussed in Chapter 27. Calcium is also important in excitation-contraction coupling and vascular smooth muscle tone. Consequently, calcium imbalances can have profound influence on cardiovascular function (see Chapter 2).

Synchronous contraction of the diaphragm with the heart beat (synchronous diaphragmatic flutter) has been reported in humans and animals.[76-79] It is believed that the syndrome results from excitation of the pericardial segment of the phrenic nerve(s) by the electrical activity of the heart. It is noted as forceful rhythmic abdominal contractions that occur with the heart beat and is typically confirmed by auscultation and fluoroscopy. Although rare in dogs, it most commonly occurs in association with persistent vomiting.[77] It is theorized that alkalosis or hypocalcemia associated with prolonged vomiting may lead to hyperirritability in the phrenic nerve. We have seen several cases in our hospital, most commonly associated with hypocalcemia.

Renal Disease

Humans with end-stage renal disease often exhibit cardiac dysfunction or signs of congestive heart failure associated with several cardiac complications, such as coronary atherosclerosis, systemic hypertension, lipid abnormalities, and complications associated with chronic hemodialysis.[80] It has been suggested that uremic toxins may possess direct cardiotoxic effects, producing a so-called uremic cardiomyopathy.[80] Uremic cardiomyopathy is not universally accepted as a specific disease entity because it is difficult to document in view of the many other possible causes of cardiac dysfunction in such patients.[80] Although many dogs and cats with renal disease may develop systemic hypertension and some animals have complications associated with pulmonary thromboembolism, overt congestive heart failure secondary to isolated renal disease and its complications has not been documented in animals. In one report, two of 150 dogs with renal failure were described as having "uremic endocarditis," suggesting that some animals may have direct cardiac complications associated with renal failure.[81]

Acute and chronic uremia have long been associated with pericardial inflammation.[80] The exact mechanisms of uremic pericarditis are not well understood, but likely are related to pericardial serositis secondary to the accumulations of uremic toxins. In most humans the pericardial effusion is hemorrhagic and small compared with the occurrence in other pericardial disorders.[80] In some patients the amount of pericardial fluid is severe, leading to signs of cardiac tamponade, and a small number of patients develop chronic constrictive pericarditis. A pericardial friction rub is present in almost all human patients that develop uremic pericarditis.[80]

Uremic pericarditis occurs in animals, but is very uncommon and is rarely a significant complication. In our experience, pericardial friction rubs are common, and the amount of effusion is typically trivial. In one report in cats, seven of 66 cats with chronic renal failure had pericardial effusion.[82] Dogs were reported to have pericardial effusion in one of 42 cases in one report and 11 of 150 in another.[81,83] To our knowledge, cardiac tamponade secondary to uremic pericarditis has not been reported in animals.

Gastrointestinal Disease

PANCREATITIS

It has been postulated that the pancreas releases a myocardial depressant factor (MDF) with acute pancreatitis. This substance is thought to have a negative inotropic effect and therefore produce a reduction in cardiac output in patients with pancreatitis. Significant cardiac complications have not been reported in animals with pancreatitis.

GASTRIC DILATATION-VOLVULUS

Cardiac complications associated with arrhythmias and reduced ventricular function in patients with gastric dilatation-volvulus (GDV) are commonly reported.[24] Cardiac arrhythmias are reported to occur in 42% of patients with GDV, most of which develop after surgical decompression.[84] Reported arrhythmias include atrial and ventricular premature depolarizations, sinus tachycardia, atrial fibrillation, and, uncommonly, bradyarrhythmias. Suggested mechanisms that induce these arrhythmias include myocardial ischemia associated with hypotension and caudal caval compression; autonomic imbalance; fluid, electrolyte, and acid-base imbalances; and the release of MDF from the pancreas.[24] Myocardial lesions, including myocardial degeneration, fibrosis, and necrosis, are frequently observed on histologic examinations.[85] Most of these dogs were also reported to have arrhythmias before death. In experimental dogs, six of eight developed subendocardial necrosis, four of which had ventricular arrhythmias.[85]

Two comprehensive studies on the hemodynamic alterations in dogs with GDV suggest that there are both cardiostimulatory and cardioinhibitory humoral factors involved, that they are released after decompression, and that the net effect in most dogs is an overall reduction in cardiac performance.[86,87] Experimentally, GDV has been shown to reduce cardiac output, myocardial contractility, mean arterial pressure, total peripheral resistance, coronary perfusion, and myocardial oxygen consumption.[86,88] Most of these variables normalize after surgical decompression; however, cardiac output and mean arterial pressure tend to remain reduced, and the indices of cardiac contractility tend to rise to levels above that of baseline. It is postulated that the increased contractility is mediated by the sympathetic nervous system but is counteracted by alterations in heart rate and rhythm, reduced preload, and increased afterload such that the net effect is a reduction in cardiac output. Plasma taken from dogs with GDV has been shown to produce inconsistent depression of isolated papillary muscle when harvested after decompression but not if harvested during GDV.[87] This suggests that the cause of reduced cardiac performance is humoral and that the substances are either not produced initially or are sequestered before decompression.

Recent evidence from humans suggests that tumor necrosis factor and interleukin-1 are the factors responsible for myocardial depression in humans with septic shock. Similar to the situation in GDV, serum from human patients with septic shock depresses myocardial performance in vitro. Immunoabsorption of these substances from the serum removes all myocardial depressant activity from the serum. Further evidence suggests that these inflammatory cytokines mediate their myocardial depression through the induction of nitric oxide synthesis and resultant nitric oxide formation in the myocardium.[89]

There is little controversy that ventricular arrhythmias occur in the majority of patients with GDV. However, the clinical significance of these arrhythmias and the frequency of other cardiac complications and heart failure in dogs with GDV and no preexisting cardiac disease deserves further scrutiny. Although the mortality rate in patients with GDV has been reported to be 43%, most of these animals succumb to complications associated with hypovolemia, shock, endotoxemia, and disseminated vascular coagulation. Documented death directly attributable to direct cardiac complications is relatively rare and usually occurs in breeds of dogs that are also predisposed to dilated cardiomyopathy.[24] In general, we do not recommend therapy for ventricular arrhythmias in dogs recovering from surgery for GDV unless preexisting dilated cardiomyopathy is present or unless the ventricular arrhythmias appear malignant. In most patients the arrhythmias consist of accelerated idioventricular rhythms (i.e., ventricular tachycardia with rates between 100 and 180 beats/min) that resolve within 72 hours after surgery, as do the hemodynamic alterations.

Hematologic Disease

ANEMIA

Anemia is the most common cause of high cardiac output state in humans and may lead to high-output failure in patients with underlying heart disease.[3] The mechanisms responsible for the development of heart failure in patients whose cardiac output is initially elevated is complex and largely depends on the specifics of the underlying condition. In anemic patients, the reduced red cell mass and hemoglobin concentration lead to a reduced oxygen delivery to the tissues. The heart is stimulated to pump an abnormally large volume of blood to provide metabolizing tissues with adequate amounts of oxygen. This increased volume load exerts an effect on the myocardium similar to the volume overload of regurgitant lesions or congenital left-to-right shunts, leading to eccentric hypertrophy (typically of all cardiac chambers), hyperdynamic ventricular function, and sinus tachycardia. In animals, clinically significant complications only occur with chronic severe anemia (packed cell volume less than 20%). In these patients, cardiac enlargement can be documented but heart failure is rare (see Figure 4-23). Animals with moderate-to-severe anemia commonly have a soft cardiac murmur, and a few have a gallop sound. The precordial impulse may be increased.

HYPERVISCOSITY

In humans, both polycythemia and hyperglobulinemias, the two alterations that are most commonly associated with hyperviscosity, are known to increase ventricular afterload and may lead to high-output cardiac failure.[24] Polycythemia from any cause is known to increase blood oxygen content, cardiac output, and blood volume in humans.[90] Several cases of hyperviscosity syndrome have been reported in the veterinary literature.[24] Of these, only one had congestive heart failure and, although not clear, likely had acquired valvular disease as well. Although there is little evidence of significant cardiac complications of hyperviscosity in animals without underlying cardiac disease, polycythemia and hyperviscosity most likely contribute to the cardiac dysfunction and clinical signs seen in cyanotic congenital heart disease.

REFERENCES

1. Suter PF: Peripheral vascular disease. In Ettinger SJ, ed: *Veterinary internal medicine,* ed 3, Philadelphia, 1989, WB Saunders.
2. Grossman W, Braunwald E: Clinical aspects of heart failure. In Braunwald E, ed: *Heart disease,* ed 4, Philadelphia, 1990, WB Saunders.
3. Katz AM: Cardiomyopathy of overload, *N Engl J Med* 322:100, 1990.
4. Apriletti JW, Davidlouye Y, Baxter JD: Physiochemical characterization of intranuclear receptors. In Oppenheimer JH, Sammuels HH, eds: *Molecular basis of thyroid hormone action,* New York, 1983, Academic Press.
5. Jump DB, Oppenheimer JH: Association of thyroid hormone with chromatin, *Mol Cell Biochem* 55:159, 1983.
6. Williams GH, Braunwald E: Endocrine and nutritional disorders and heart disease. In Braunwald E, ed: *Heart disease: a textbook of cardiovascular medicine,* Philadelphia, 1992, WB Saunders.
7. Buccino RA, Spann JF, Pool PE et al: Influence of the thyroid state on the intrinsic contractile properties and the energy stores of the myocardium, *J Clin Invest* 46:1669, 1967.
8. Josephson RA, Spurgeon HA, Lakatta EG: The hyperthyroid heart: an analysis of systolic and diastolic properties in single rat ventricular myocytes, *Circ Res* 66:773, 1990.
9. Markowits C, Yater WM: Response of explanted cardiac muscle to thyroxine, *Am J Physiol* 100:162, 1932.
10. Murayama M, Goodkind MJ: Effect of thyroid hormone on the frequency-force relationship of atrial myocardium from the guinea pig, *Circ Res* 23:743, 1968.
11. Rutherford JP, Vatner SF, Braunwald E: Adrenergic control of myocardial contractility in conscious dogs, *Am J Physiol* 237:H590, 1979.
12. Philipson KD, Edelman IS: Thyroid hormone control of NA^{+},K^{+}-ATPase and K+-dependant phosphatase in the rat heart, *Am J Physiol* 232:C196, 1977.
13. Bilezikian JP, Loeb JN: Increased myocardial beta receptors and adrenergic responsiveness, *Endocr Rev* 4:378, 1983.
14. Hammond HK, White FC, Buxton ILO et al. Increased myocardial beta receptors and adrenergic responses in hyperthyroid pigs, *Am J Physiol* 252:H283, 1987.
15. Ladenson PW, Sherman SI, Baughman KL et al. Reversible alterations in myocardial gene expression in a young man with dilated cardiomyopathy and hypothyroidism, *Proc Natl Acad Sci U S A,* 89:5321, 1992.
16. Miller CW, Boon JA, Soderberg SA et al: Echocardiographic assessment of cardiac function in beagles with experimentally produced hypothyroidism, *J Ultrasound Med* 3(suppl):157, 1984.
17. Everett AW, Sinha AM, Umeda PK, et al: Regulation of myosin synthesis by thyroid hormone: relative changes in alpha- and beta-myosin heavy chain mRNA levels in rabbit heart, *Biochemistry* 23:1596, 1984.
18. Tsika RW, Bahl JJ, Leinwand LA et al: Thyroid hormone regulates expression of a transfected human alpha-myosin heavy-chain fusion gene in fetal rat heart cells, *Proc Natl Acad Sci U S A,* 87:379, 1990.
19. Macleod KM, McNeill JH: The influence of altered thyroid hormone levels on guinea pig cardiac adrenoreceptors and histamine receptors, *Can J Physiol Pharmacol* 59:1039, 1981.
20. Simpson WW, Rodgers RL, McNeill JH: Cardiac responsiveness to alpha and beta adrenergic amines: effects of carbochol and hypothyroidism, *J Exp Pharm Ther* 219:231, 1981.
21. Nelson RW: Disorders of the thyroid gland. In Nelson RW, Couto CG, ed: *Essentials of small animal internal medicine,* St Louis, 1992, Mosby.
22. Fox PR, Nichols CER: Cardiac involvement in systemic disease. In Fox PR, ed: *Canine and feline cardiology,* New York, 1988, Churchill Livingstone.
23. Manning PJ: Thyroid gland and arterial lesions in beagles with familial hypothyroidism and hyperlipoproteinemia, *Am J Vet Res* 40:820, 1979.
24. Atkins CE: The role of noncardiac disease in the development and precipitation of heart failure, *Vet Clin North Am Sm Anim Pract* 21:1035, 1991.
25. Braunwald E, Sonnenblick EH, Spann JF et al: Effects of heart failure, ventricular hypertrophy and alterations in thyroid state on contractility of isolated cardiac muscle, *Ann NY Acad Sci* 156:379, 1969.
26. Nijhuis AH, Stokhuf AA, Huisman GH et al: ECG Changes in dogs with hypothyroidism, *Tijdschr Diergeneesk* 103:736, 1985.
27. Goel BG, Hanson CS, Han BS: Atrioventricular conduction in hypothyroid dogs, *Am Heart J* 83:504, 1972.
28. Santos AD, Miller RP, Mathew PK: Echocardiographic characterization of the reversible cardiomyopathy of hypothyroidism, *Am J Med* 68:675, 1980.
29. Taylor RR, Covell JW, Ross J: Influence of the thyroid state on left ventricular tension-velocity relations in the intact, sedated dog, *J Clin Invest* 48:775, 1969.
30. Panciera DL: M-Mode echocardiographic and electrocardiographic findings before and after levothyroxine treatment in hypothyroid dogs, *J Vet Intern Med* 7:115, 1993 (abstract).
31. Panciera DL: Administration of levothyroxine to euthyroid dogs does not affect echocardiographic and electrocardiographic measurements, *Res Vet Sci* 58:130, 1992.
32. Liu SK, Tilley LP, Tapp JP et al: Clinical and pathologic findings in dogs with atherosclerosis: 21 cases, *J Am Vet Med Assoc* 189:227, 1986.
33. Calvert CA, Chapman WL, Toal RL: Congestive cardiomyopathy in Doberman pinscher dogs, *J Am Vet Med Assoc* 181:598, 1982.
34. Patterson JS, Rusley MS, Zachary JF: Neurologic manifestations of cerebrovascular atherosclerosis associated with primary hypothyroidism in a dog, *J Am Vet Med Assoc* 186:499, 1985.
35. Pion PD, Kittleson MD, Rodgers QR et al: Myocardial failure in cats associated with low plasma taurine: a reversible cardiomyopathy, *Science* 237:764, 1987.
36. Campos Y, Huertas R, Lorenzo G et al: Plasma carnitine insufficiency and effectiveness of L-carnitine therapy in patients with mitochondrial myopathy, *Muscle Nerve* 16:150, 1993.
37. Keene BW, Panciera DL, Atkins CE et al: Myocardial L-carnitine deficiency in a family of dogs with dilated cardiomyopathy, *J Am Vet Med Assoc* 198:647, 1991.
38. Peterson ME, Ferguson DC: Thyroid diseases. In Ettinger SJ, ed: *Textbook of veterinary internal medicine,* Philadelphia, 1989, WB Saunders.
39. Jacobs G, Hutson C, Dougherty J et al: Congestive heart failure associated with hyperthyroidism in cats, *J Am Vet Med Assoc* 188:52, 1986.
40. Bond BR: Hyperthyroidism and other high output states. In Fox PR, ed: *Canine and feline cardiology,* New York, 1988, Churchill Livingstone.
41. Jacobs G, Panciera DL: Cardiovascular complications of feline hyperthyroidism. In Kirk RW, Bonagura JD, eds: *Kirk's current veterinary therapy, XI: small animal practice,* Philadelphia, 1992, WB Saunders.
42. Gustafson TA, Markham BE, Morkin E: Effects of thyroid hormone on alpha-actin and myosin heavy chain gene expression in cardiac and skeletal muscles of the rat: measurement of mRNA content using synthetic oligonuleotide probes, *Circ Res* 59:194, 1986.
43. Nishizawa Y, Hamada N, Fujii S, et al: Serum dopamine-beta-hydroxylase activity in thyroid dysfunction, *J Clin Endocrinol Metab* 39:599, 1974.
44. Shigematsu S, Iwasaki T, Aizawa T et al: Plasma atrial natriuretic peptide, plasma renin activity and aldosterone during treatment of hyperthyroidism due to Graves' disease, *Hormone Met Res* 9:514, 1989.
45. Hodges RD, Lothrop CD: Atrial natriuretic factor concentration in the cat, *J Vet Intern Med* 5:129, (abstract).
46. Peterson ME, Keene BW, Ferguson DC, et al: Electrocardiographic findings in 45 cats with hyperthyroidism, *J Am Vet Med Assoc* 180:934, 1982.
47. Fox PR, Broussard JD, Peterson ME: Electrocardiographic and radiographic changes in cats with hyperthyroidism: comparison of populations evaluated during 1979-1982 vs 1992, *J Vet Intern Med* 7:118, 1993, (abstract).
48. Harpster HK: The cardiovascular system. In Holzworth J, ed: *Diseases of the cat,* Philadelphia, 1986, WB Saunders.
49. Harpster HK: Feline myocardial diseases. In Kirk RW, ed: *Current veterinary therapy,* Philadelphia, 1986, WB Saunders.

50. Peterson ME, Kintzer PP, Cavanaugh PG et al: Feline hyperthyroidism: pretreatment clinical and laboratory evaluation of 131 cases, *J Am Vet Med Assoc* 183:103, 1983.
51. Kobayashi DL, Peterson ME, Graves TK et al: Hypertension in cats with chronic renal failure or hyperthyroidism, *J Vet Intern Med* 4:58, 1990.
52. Lesser M, Fox PR, Bond BR: Assessment of hypertension in 40 cats with left ventricular hypertrophy by Doppler-shift sphygmomanometry, *J Small Anim Pract* 33:55, 1992.
53. Moise N, Dietze AE, Mezza LE et al: Echocardiography, electrocardiography, and radiography of cats with dilation cardiomyopathy, hypertrophic cardiomyopathy, and hyperthyroidism, *Am J Vet Res* 47:1476, 1986.
54. Dillman WH: Thyroid hormones and the heart, *Thyroid Today* 6:1, 1983.
55. Forfar JC, Caldwell GC: Hyperthyroid heart disease, *Clin Endocrinol Metab* 14:491, 1985.
56. Klein, I, Levey GS: New perspectives on thyroid hormone, catecholamines, and the heart, *Am J Med* 76:167, 1985.
57. Bond BR, Fox PR, Peterson ME et al: Echocardiographic findings in 103 cats with hyperthyroidism, *J Am Vet Med Assoc* 192:1546, 1988.
58. Moise NS, Dietze AE: Echocardiographic, electrocardiographic, and radiographic detection of cardiomegaly in hyperthyroid cats, *Am J Vet Res* 47:1487, 1986.
59. Fox PR: Canine myocardial diseases. In Fox PR, ed: *Canine and feline cardiology,* New York, 1988, Churchill Livingstone.
60. Rijnberk A, Leav I: Thyroid tumors. In Kirk RW, ed: *Kirk's current veterinary therapy, VI: small animal practice,* Philadelphia, 1977, WB Saunders.
61. Knowlton AI, Baer L: Cardiac failure in Addison's disease, *Am J Med* 74:829, 1984.
62. Musselman EE: Endocrine cardiomyopathies, *Proc Acad Vet Cardiol,* 1990, p 18.
63. Snyder DW: Cardiac manifestations of noncardiac disease in the elderly. In Messerli FH, ed: *Cardiovascular disease in the elderly,* Boston, 1988, Martinus Nijhoff.
64. Kallet A, Cowgill LD: Hypertensive states in the dog, *Proc ACVIM,* 1982, p 79. 65.
65. Breitschwerdt EB, Meuten DJ, Greenfield CL et al: idiopathic hyperaldosteronism in a dog, *J Am Vet Med Assoc* 187:841, 1985.
66. Eger CE, Robinson WF, Huxtable CR: Primary aldosteronism (Conn's syndrome) in a cat: a case report and review of comparative aspects, *J Small Anim Pract* 24:293, 1983.
67. Bouyard H, Feeny DA, Caywood DD: Pheochromocytoma in dogs: 13 cases (1980-1985), *J Am Vet Med Assoc* 191:1614, 1987.
68. Twedt DC, Wheeler SL: Pheochromocytoma in the dog, *Vet Clin North Am* 14:767, 1984.
69. Feldman EC, Nelson RW: Growth hormone. In Feldman EC, Nelson RW, eds: *Canine and feline endocrinology and reproduction,* Philadelphia, 1987, WB Saunders.
70. Peterson ME, Taylor RS, Gieco DS et al: Acromegaly in 14 cats, *J Vet Intern Med* 4:192, 1990.
71. Kittleson MD, Pion PD, Lathrop CD, et al: Hypersomatotropism in a cat presenting with hypertrophic cardiomyopathy (HCM) and insulin resistance but without diabetes mellitus (DM), *Proc ACVIM,* 1989, p 1038 (abstract).
72. Kittleson MD, Pion PD, DeLellis LA et al: Increased serum growth hormone concentration in feline hypertrophic cardiomyopathy, *J Vet Intern Med* 6:320, 1992.
73. Fein FS, Sonnenblick EH: Diabetic cardiomyopathy, *Prog Cardiovasc Dis* 27:255, 1985.
74. Follansbee WP, Curtiss EL, Schulman DS et al: Diabetic cardiomyopathy: final results of diabetes complications study, *Circulation* 80:206, 1989, (abstract).
75. Atkins CE, Engerman RL, Kern TS: Diabetic cardiomyopathy, Proc ACVIM, 2:9, 1988.
76. Bohn FK, Patterson DF: Long-standing unilateral contraction of the diaphragm synchronous with the heart beat, *J Am Vet Med Assoc* 156:1411, 1970.
77. Detweiler DK: Contraction of the diaphragm synchronous with the heart beat in dogs, *J Am Vet Med Assoc* 126:445, 1955.
78. Smith LK: Contraction of the diaphragm synchronous with the heartbeat in a dog, *J Am Vet Med Assoc* 146:611, 1965.
79. Ettinger SJ, Suter PF, Gould L: Synchronous myocardial and diaphragmatic contractions in a dog, *J Am Vet Med Assoc* 208:2475, 1969 (letter).
80. Pastan SO, Braunwald E: Renal disorders and heart disease. In Braunwald E, ed: *Heart disease: a textbook of cardiovascular medicine,* ed 4, Philadelphia, 1992, WB Saunders.
81. Madewell BR, Norrdin RW: Renal failure associated with pericardial effusion in the dog, *J Am Vet Med Assoc* 167:1091, 1975.
82. Rush JE, Keene BW, Fox PR: Pericardial disease in the cat: a retrospective evaluation of 66 cases, *J Am Anim Hosp Assoc* 26:39, 1990.
83. Berg RJ, Wingfield WE: Pericardial effusion in the dog: a review of 42 cases, *J Am Anim Hosp Assoc* 20:721, 1984.
84. Muir WW: Gastric-dilatation-volvulus in the dog, with emphasis on cardiac arrhythmias, *J Am Vet Med Assoc* 180:739, 1983.
85. Muir WW, Weisbrode SE: Myocardial ischemia in dogs with gastric dilatation-volvulus, *J Am Vet Med Assoc* 181:363, 1987.
86. Orton EC, Muir WW: Hemodynamics during gastric dilatation-volvulus in dogs, *Am J Vet Res* 44:1512, 1983.
87. Orton EC, Muir WW: Isovolumetric indices and humoral cardioactive substance assay during clinical and experimental induced gastric dilatation-volvulus in dogs, *Am J Vet Res* 44:1516, 1983.
88. Horne WA, Gilmore DR, Dietze AE et al: Effects of gastric dilatation-volvulus on coronary blood flow and myocardial oxygen consumption in the dog, *Am J Vet Res* 46:98, 1985.
89. Parrillo JE: The Asmund S. Laerdal Memorial Lecture: myocardial depression in sepsis—a journey with answers, *Proceedings of the 27th Educational and Scientific Symposium of the Society of Critical Care Medicine,* 1998, p 7.
90. Rosenthal DS, Braunwald E:. Hematological-oncological disorders and heart disease. In Braunwald E, ed: *Heart disease: a textbook of cardiovascular medicine,* ed 4, Philadelphia, 1992, WB Saunders.

Index

Italics indicate illustration, t indicates table.

B

C

E

G

I

J

K

L

M

Q

R

T